CONTENTS

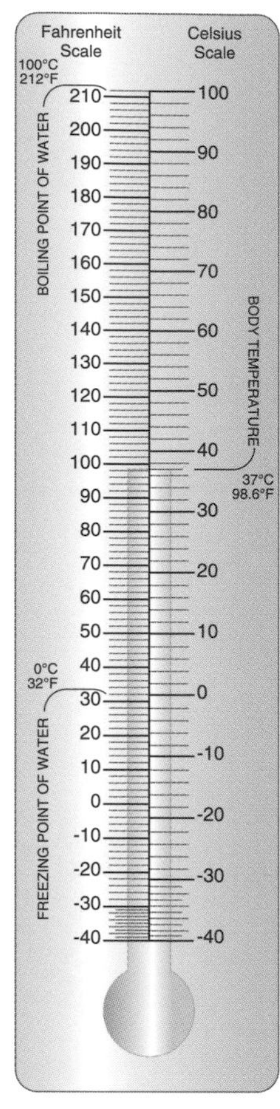

Temperature Measurement: Celsius-Fahrenheit Scales
You can use this diagram to convert from one temperature scale to the other. For instance, locate 32° on the Fahrenheit scale. Read the equivalent number on the Celsius scale (0° C). Another example: locate 100° on the Celsius scale. Read the equivalent number on the Fahrenheit scale (212° F). Body temperature is therefore 98.6° F or 37° C.

Units of Measurement

Unit	Metric Equivalent	US Equivalent
Units of Length		
1 meter (m)	100 cm, 1000 mm	39.4 inches
1 centimeter (cm)	10 mm	0.39 inches
1 inch (in)	2.54 cm	0.08 foot
Units of Weight		
1 kilogram (kg)	1000 g	2.2 lb
1 pound (lb)	454 g, 0.454 kg	16 ounces (oz)
1 gram (g)	1000 mg	0.002 lb
Units of Volume		
1 liter (L)	1000 ml	1.06 quarts (qt)
1 deciliter (dL)	100 ml	3.33 oz
1 quart (qt)	0.946 L	32 oz
1 ounce (oz)	29.6 ml	0.03 qt

cm, Centimeter; *dL*, deciliter; *g*, gram; *in*, inch; *kg*, kilogram; *L*, liter; *lb*, pound; *m*, meter; *mg*, milligram; *ml*, milliliter; *mm*, millimeter; *oz*, ounce; *qt*, quart.

The Human Body in Health and Illness

Third Edition

The Human Body in Health and Illness

Third Edition

Barbara Herlihy, PhD, RN
Professor
University of the Incarnate Word
School of Nursing and Health Professions
San Antonio, Texas

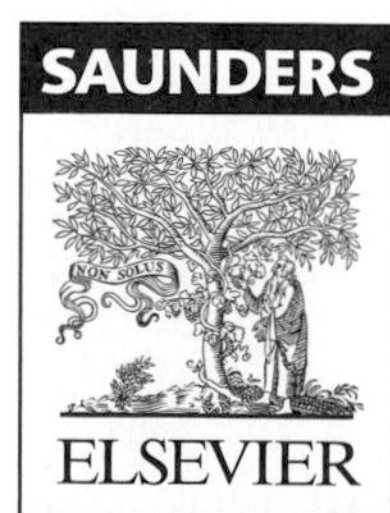

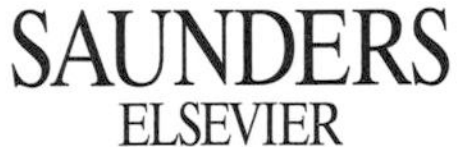

11830 Westline Industrial Drive
St. Louis, Missouri 63146

THE HUMAN BODY IN HEALTH AND ILLNESS, THIRD EDITION ISBN-13: 978-1-4160-2886-4
ISBN-10: 1-4160-2886-2

Notice

Knowledge and best practice in this field are constantly changing. As new research and experience broaden our knowledge, changes in practice, treatment and drug therapy may become necessary or appropriate. Readers are advised to check the most current information provided (i) on procedures featured or (ii) by the manufacturer of each product to be administered, to verify the recommended dose or formula, the method and duration of administration, and contraindications. It is the responsibility of the practitioner, relying on their own experience and knowledge of the patient, to make diagnoses, to determine dosages and the best treatment for each individual patient, and to take all appropriate safety precautions. To the fullest extent of the law, neither the Publisher nor the Author assumes any liability for any injury and/or damage to persons or property arising out or related to any use of the material contained in this book.

The Publisher

ISBN-13: 978-1-4160-2886-4

ISBN-10: 1-4160-2886-2

Executive Editor: Thomas J. Wilhelm
Managing Editor: Jeff Downing
Developmental Editor: Allison Brock
Publishing Services Manager: Deborah L. Vogel
Project Manager: Katherine Hinkebein
Design Direction: Paula Ruckenbrod
Cover Designer: Mark Oberkrom
Text Designer: Paula Ruckenbrod

Printed in Canada

Last digit is the print number: 9 8 7 6 5 4 3 2 1

To my family and closest friends:

Husband, Jerry

Children, Joseph (Earthmover) and Kellie (NICU nurse and overall princess)

Grandsons, Grey (4-year-old, AKA "Jabber Jaw") and Case (new on the block, AKA "Doodle Bug")

Daughter-in-law, Kristan (a great mother to Jabber and Doodle)

Furry friends: cats, Minky (very sweet) and Julia (alpha animal); dogs, Annie, Lucy (Boston terriers), Kenner (mutt), and Doofus (Blue heeler)

Barbara

Acknowledgments

The publishing and republishing of an anatomy and physiology text requires the combined efforts of persons with diverse talents. I have been blessed to work with many generous and talented individuals at Elsevier and offer my grateful thanks, especially to

- Jeff Downing for his direction, trust, and encouragement. His ability to create a relaxed and friendly environment made the writing experience a joy.
- Allison Brock for her day-to-day pleasant, "get-it-done" approach ... a coordinating genius! I especially appreciate her willingness to accommodate my quirky sense of humor; she let me do my thing.
- Katherine Hinkebein for her meticulous editing and gentle suggestions. The editing process was smoooooth!
- Caitlin Duckwall of Duckwall Productions, for the beautiful illustrations. We acknowledge with gratitude that the telling of the story of the human body is told as much through the art as through the written word.
- Paula Ruckenbrod, Designer.

Many thanks to my students and friends at the University of the Incarnate Word. They have listened to me whine my way through three editions and, for the most part, still love me. Thanks to my husband, Jerry, for living with an author ... and all the fallout. He graciously adjusted to books and papers littered throughout the house. He also constructed tables, proofread, and offered many helpful tips—he, too, is a physiologist. Thanks to my children and grandchildren for their insistence on leisure and play; they are in charge of my mental health. I highly recommend "granny-hood"; it is beyond joy! Last, but not least, thanks to my furry friends Annie, Lucy, Kenner, and Doofus (woof) and Minky and Julia (meow) for the hours they hovered around me and my laptop. Two Jack Russell terriers (Keike and Mollie) were frequent visitors and contributed to the overall chaos. A special acknowledgment to my beloved dachshund, Pretzyl, who labored so hard on the first two editions. Pretzyl died last summer and is missed so much.

Also, many thanks to those who used previous editions and were kind enough to forward comments and suggestions. Your assistance is so appreciated. Keep the comments coming!

To the Instructor

She's getting older and better (with the help of your comments and suggestions)! After minor surgery and a speedy recovery, the second edition of *The Human Body in Health and Illness* has given way to the third edition ... and she hasn't lost her sense of humor.

The Human Body in Health and Illness tells the story of the human body with all its parts and the way these parts work together. It is a story that we have told many times in our classes. It is also a story that gets better with each telling as the body continues to reveal its mysteries and how marvelously it has been created. I hope that you enjoy telling the story as much as I do.

The Human Body in Health and Illness is a basic anatomy and physiology text that is addressed to the student who is preparing for a career in the health professions. The text is written for students with minimal preparation in the sciences; no prior knowledge of biology, chemistry, or physics is required. The text provides all the background science information needed for an understanding of anatomy and physiology. The basic principles of chemistry and biochemistry are presented in Chapters 2 and 4, and they set the stage for an understanding of cellular function, fluid and electrolyte balance, endocrine function, and digestion. Chapter 5, Microbiology Basics, presents clinically relevant microbiological topics. Check out the stories "Rick, Nick, and the Sick Tick" and "Dr. Semmelweis Screams: 'Wash Those Mitts!'" "Wash Those Mitts" is an amusing presentation of a sad tale in the history of medicine; it corresponds to the current problem of handwashing and nosocomial infection.

The anatomy and physiology content is presented in a traditional order, from simple to complex. The text begins with a description of a single cell and progresses through the various organ systems. There are two key themes that run throughout the text. The first theme is the relationship between structure and function—the student must understand that an organ is anatomically designed to perform a specific physiological task. The second major theme is homeostasis—the role that each organ system plays in sustaining life, and what happens when that delicate balance is disturbed.

The text addresses two concerns about the selection of content. The first concern has to do with the amount of content. The field of anatomy and physiology is huge. Therefore, there must be a selection of context that can be mastered in the short period of time that a semester (or two) allows. This text focuses on the physiology that is basic and most clinically relevant. Pathophysiology is introduced primarily to clarify physiologic function. For instance, the different types of anemias illustrate the various steps in the making of the red blood cell. A second concern has to do with the recognition that you are not preparing physiologists; instead, you want the student to be able to use the physiology to understand more clinically relevant content such as pathophysiology, physical assessment, diagnostics, and pharmacology. An understanding of physiology is crucial for advancement in the medically related sciences.

TEXTBOOK STRENGTHS

I believe that this text has many strengths:

- The anatomy and physiology are clearly and simply explained. A beautiful set of illustrations, complete with cartoons, supports the text. In fact, the story of the body is told as much through the art as through the written word.
- The text truly integrates pathophysiology; it is not merely boxed in or tacked on at the end. The integrated pathophysiology is used primarily to amplify the normal anatomy and physiology.
- In addition to the pathophysiology, other topics are liberally integrated throughout the text. These include common diagnostic procedures such as blood count, lumbar puncture, urinalysis, and electrocardiography. Pharmacological topics are also introduced and, like the pathophysiology, are used to amplify the normal anatomy and physiology. For instance, the discussion of the neuromuscular junction is enhanced by a description of the effects of the neuromuscular-blocking agents. Because of the effort of the text to make clinical correlations, it sets the stage for the more advanced health science courses, including pharmacology and medical-surgical nursing.
- Medical terminology is introduced, defined, and used throughout the text. Common clinical terms such as *hyperkalemia, vasodilation, hypertension*, and *diagnosis* are defined and reused so that the student gradually builds up a substantial medical vocabulary.

- The text incorporates many amusing anecdotes from the history of medicine. Although the human body is perfectly logical and predictable, we humans think, do, and say some strange things. Tales from the medical crypt provide some good laughs and much humility.

FEATURES

OBJECTIVES

The objectives identify the goals of the chapter.

KEY TERMS

The key terms are identified and thoroughly explained in the chapter and defined in the Glossary.

Do You Know...

Most of these boxed vignettes refer to clinical situations; others relate to interesting and amusing historical events.

As You Age

These numbered statements identify the major physiological changes that occur with aging.

SUMMARY OUTLINE

A detailed summary outline at the end of each chapter serves as an excellent review and helps the student pull together the content of the chapter.

Review Your Knowledge

The matching and multiple-choice questions review the major points of the chapter and ask the student to integrate key concepts.

Sum It Up!

Sum-it-up paragraphs appear regularly throughout the chapters and help the student pull together key concepts.

Disorders of the Skeletal System

These tables describe specific disorders related to individual body systems.

Appendixes. The three appendixes provide information about medical terminology, common laboratory values, and answers to the Review Your Knowledge questions.

- **Appendix A** includes an introduction to medical terminology and a listing of eponymous terms. A table of prefixes, suffixes, and word roots provides ample information for a beginning course in medical terminology.
- **Appendix B** lists common laboratory values for blood and urine. Laboratory values for common blood tests include hemoglobin, hematocrit, and a white blood cell differential count. Also included are the values for a routine urinalysis.
- **Appendix C** contains answers to all Review Your Knowledge questions found in the textbook.

Glossary. The glossary includes a pronunciation guide and a brief definition of all key terms and many other words in the text.

ANCILLARY PACKAGE

Study Guide. The Study Guide for *The Human Body in Health and Illness* offers something for students at all levels of learning. Each chapter includes three parts: Part I, Mastering the Basics, with matching, labeling, and coloring exercises; Part II, Putting It All Together, containing multiple-choice practice quizzes, completion exercises, and case studies; and Part III, Challenge Yourself!, which has grouping exercises and word puzzles. Textbook page references are included with the questions, and the answer key is located in the Instructor's Electronic Resource CD-ROM.

Instructor's Electronic Resource (IER) CD-ROM. The Instructor's Electronic Resource CD-ROM includes the following:

- Instructor's Manual
- Computerized Test Bank of over 1300 questions
- PowerPoint presentations with over 200 text and image slides
- Electronic Image Collection, featuring full-color illustrations from the book
- Answers to the Study Guide questions

The Instructor's Manual consists of Lecture Notes and Self-Paced Learning Modules. Lecture Notes outline the chapter and reference specific images within the PowerPoint slides and text. Scattered and highlighted throughout the Lecture Notes are clinical correlates that the lecturer might want to introduce. Self-Paced Learning Modules focus on reinforcement and remediation and are broken up by chapter. These contain:

1. A series of short-answer questions; the student should be able to work through these questions independently.
2. A practice unit exam for each chapter
3. An objective unit exam for each chapter

The Instructor's Electronic Resource CD-ROM is free to adopters of the textbook. Contact your Elsevier sales representative for information.

Materials from both the Study Guide and Instructor's Electronic Resource CD-ROM can be used to:

1. Remediate students who are having difficulty in grasping the content
2. Remediate students who have missed classes
3. Review students who are engaged in pathophysiology and pharmacology and need to refresh the physiology

TEACH. Instructors who adopt the textbook will also be eligible to receive the TEACH Lesson Plan Manual, which links all parts of the Herlihy educational package by providing customizable lesson plans and lecture outlines based on learning objectives drawn from the text.

The TEACH lesson plans are keyed to the chapter-by-chapter organization of *The Human Body in Health and Illness* and can be modified or combined to meet your school's scheduling and teaching needs. Each lesson plan features:

- Teaching Focus summaries that identify essential lesson goals
- Lesson preparation checklists that make planning your class quick and easy
- Pretests and background assessment questions that gauge student readiness
- Critical-thinking questions to focus and motivate students
- Teaching resources that cross-reference all of Elsevier's curriculum solutions
- Class activities designed to engage students in the learning process

In addition to the lesson plans, you'll discover unique lecture outlines to complete your TEACH experience. Whether you're a seasoned veteran or a new instructor, you'll certainly benefit from having these PowerPoint outlines at your fingertips. Each lecture outline features:

- Practical, concise talking points that complement the slides
- Thought-provoking questions to stimulate classroom discussions
- Unique ideas for moving beyond traditional lectures and getting students involved

To the Student

This book will take you on an amazing journey through the human body. You will learn many body parts, and more importantly, how they work in an integrated manner to keep you going. Hopefully you will use this information in your clinical practice when human beings become ill with disorders of those structures. To help make learning this enjoyable and fun, we've spotlighted the following special features for you:

> **KEY TERMS**
>
> **Abdominopelvic cavity,** p. 10
> **Anatomical position,** p. 7
> **Anatomy,** p. 2

- A list of **Key Terms** opens each chapter. Terms are in bold type in the book and are defined in the Glossary.

> **OBJECTIVES**
>
> 1. Define the terms *anatomy* and *physiology.*
> 2. List the levels of organization of the human body.

- **Objectives** for learning at the beginning of each chapter give you goals to keep in mind while you read.

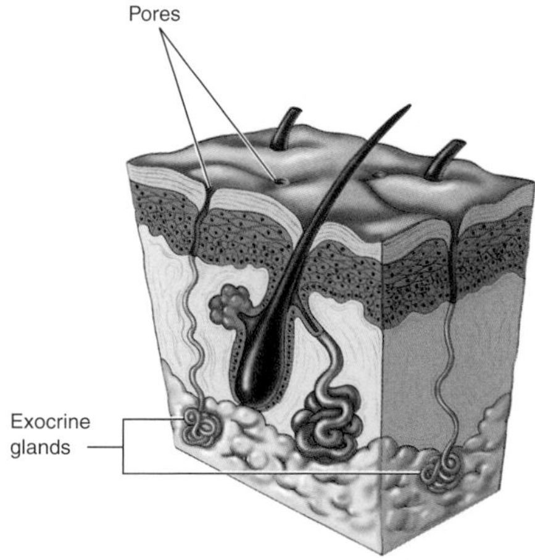

- **Original, full-color illustrations** help you make sense of anatomy and physiology structure, function, and concepts.

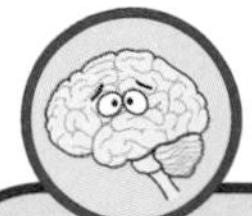

Do You Know...

Why this toe needs this leech?

This toe was accidentally severed from its owner. In reattaching the toe to the foot, the surgeon recognized that the toe graft would be successful only if the blood supply to the toe was good.

- **Do You Know...** boxes, often illustrated, pique your interest with novel background information related to anatomy and physiology.

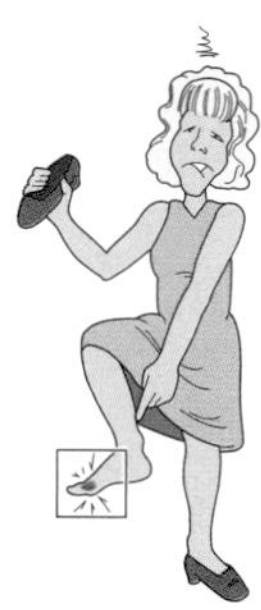

- **Full-color cartoons** bring anatomy and physiology closer to you with humor, clarity, and insight.

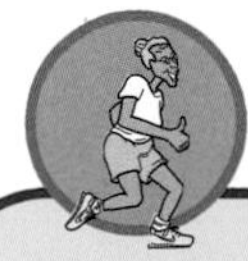

As You Age

1. Beginning at the age of 30, the number of neurons decreases. The number lost, however, is only a small percentage of the total number of brain cells.

- **As You Age** sections contain numbered lists describing how human anatomy and physiology is affected by the aging process.

Disorders of Cellular Growth

Atrophy	Atrophy is a decrease in the size of the cells.
Hyperplasia	Overgrowth in the numbers of cells.

- **Disorders of the ...** are pathophysiology tables that describe disorders related to specific body systems.

Sum It Up!

The purpose of the heart valves is to keep blood flowing forward. There are four heart valves: two atrioventricular valves and two semilunar valves. The heart sounds are due to the closure of the valves.

- **Sum It Up!** paragraphs throughout each chapter help you to quickly scan and review the key concepts.

SUMMARY OUTLINE

- The **Summary Outline** at the end of each chapter serves as a study tool. Use it to review your reading and prepare for exams.

Review Your Knowledge

- **Review Your Knowledge** questions are at the end of each chapter so you can test your comprehension.

GLOSSARY

Abdominopelvic cavity (ăb-Dŏm-ĭ-nō-PĔL-vĭk KĂ-vĭ-tē) - Part of the ventral cavity that lies inferior to the diaphragm; includes upper abdominal cavity and lower pelvic cavity.

Zygote (ZĪ-gōt) - Fertilized ovum.

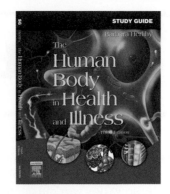

Enhance your learning of the textbook content with the accompanying **Study Guide to *The Human Body in Health and Illness.*** The Study Guide has something to offer students at all levels of learning, from labeling and coloring exercises to multiple-choice practice tests and case studies.

Contents

CHAPTER 1

Introduction to the Human Body

KEY TERMS

Abdominopelvic cavity, p. 10
Anatomical position, p. 7
Anatomy, p. 2
Cranial cavity, p. 9
Dorsal cavity, p. 9
Frontal plane, p. 8
Homeostasis, p. 4
Morphology, p. 2
Organ, p. 3
Physiology, p. 2
Sagittal plane, p. 8
Spinal (vertebral) cavity, p. 9
Thoracic cavity, p. 10
Transverse plane, p. 8
Ventral cavity, p. 10
Viscera, p. 9

OBJECTIVES

1. Define the terms *anatomy* and *physiology.*
2. List the levels of organization of the human body.
3. Describe the 11 major organ systems.
4. Define *homeostasis.*
5. Describe the anatomical position.
6. List common terms used for relative positions of the body.
7. Describe the three major planes of the body.
8. List anatomical terms for regions of the body.
9. Describe the major cavities of the body.

The human body is a wonderful creation. Millions of microscopic parts work together in a coordinated fashion to keep you going, day in and day out, for about 75 years. Most of us are curious about our bodies—how they work, why they do not work, what makes us tick, and what makes us sick. As you learn more about the body, you will sometimes feel like this cartoon character: "What is this? Why do I need it? How does it work? Why don't I have one?" As you study anatomy and physiology, you will learn the answers to these questions.

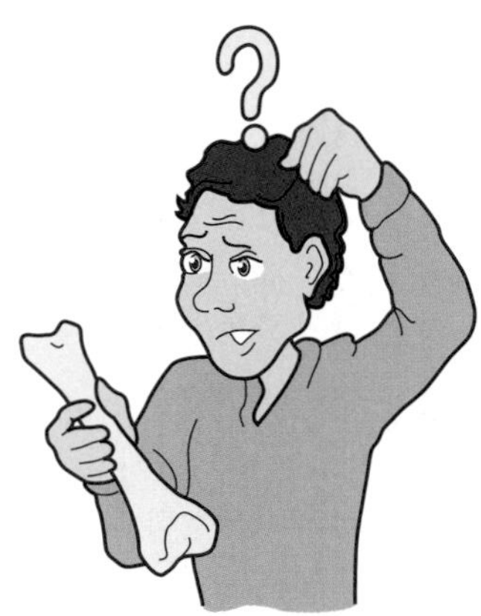

ANATOMY AND PHYSIOLOGY: WHAT THEY ARE

WHAT'S IT MEAN?

Anatomy (ă-NĂT-ă-mē) is the branch of science that studies the structure, or **morphology,** (mōr-FŎL-e-jē) of the body. For example, anatomy describes what the heart looks like, how big it is, what it is made of, how it is organized, and where it is located. The word *anatomy* comes from the Greek word meaning to dissect. The science of anatomy arose from observations made by scientists as they dissected the body.

Physiology (fĭz-ē ŎL-ĕ-jē) is the branch of science that describes how the body works, or functions. For instance, physiology describes how the heart pumps blood and why the pumping of blood is essential for life. **Pathophysiology** is the branch of science that describes the consequences of the improper functioning of the body parts—that is, how a body part functions when a person has a disease. Pathophysiology would describe what happens during a heart attack, when the heart functions poorly, or not at all.

WHY DO I NEED TO KNOW THIS?

Why study anatomy and physiology as part of your professional curriculum? Unless you gain a good understanding of normal anatomy and physiology, you cannot understand the diseases and disorders experienced by your patients, nor can you understand the basis for the various forms of treatment such as drug therapy and surgical procedures. You want to give your patients the best possible care, so you must have a sound understanding of the human body.

Anatomy and physiology are closely related. Structure and function go together. When you examine the anatomy of a body part, ask yourself how its structure relates to its function. The structure of the hand is related to its function: its ability to grasp an object (Figure 1-1). The heart pumps blood, and the long, strong, flexible tail of the monkey allows it to hang from the tree. Structure and function go together.

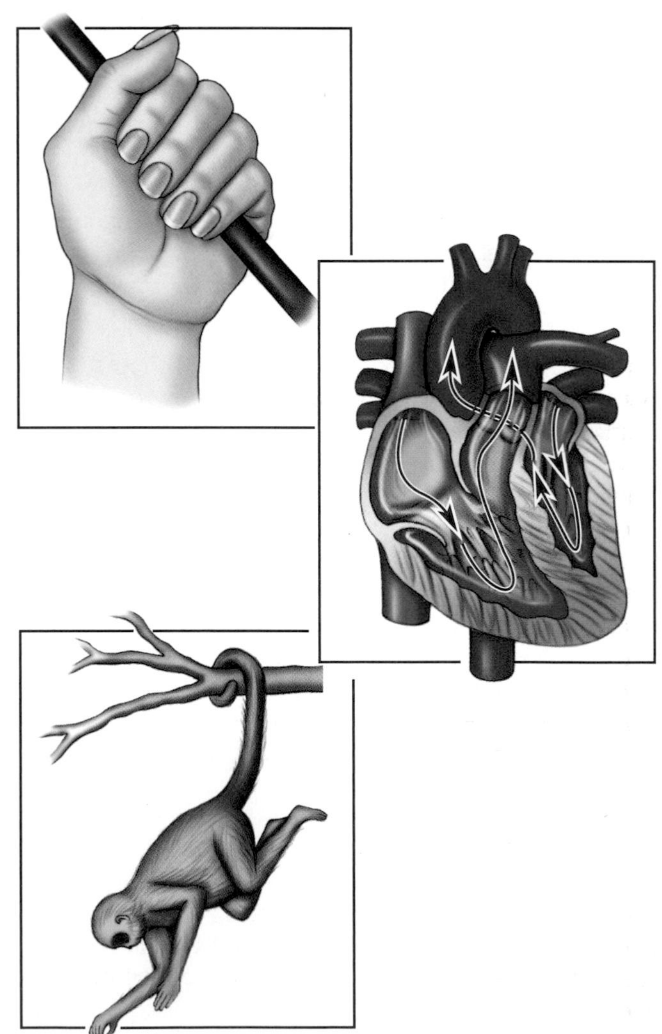

FIGURE 1-1 Structure and function are closely related.

Do You Know...

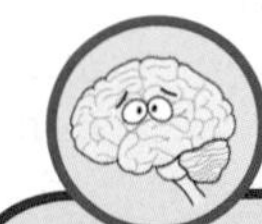

Why this grave is being robbed, and why the grave robber is in big, big trouble?

Dissection of the human body during medieval times was not allowed. Thus, the only way that the early anatomists had of obtaining human bodies for dissection was to rob graves. Medieval scientists hired people to rob graves. Punishment for robbing graves was swift and severe. This lad will be in big, big trouble if he is caught, and it looks as if he will be.

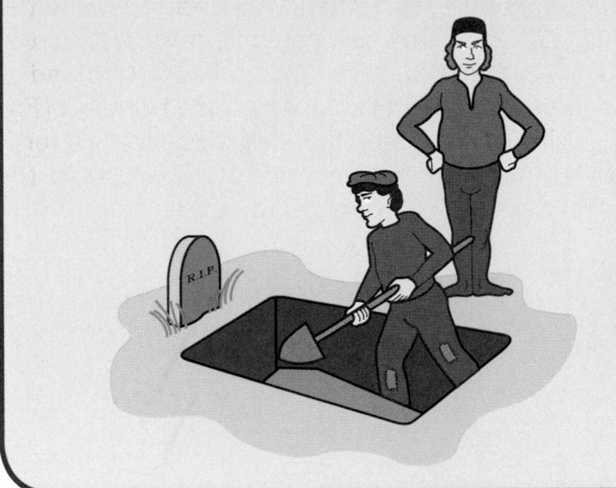

THE BODY'S LEVELS OF ORGANIZATION

ORGAN TO ORGAN SYSTEM

The body is organized from the very simple to the complex, from the microscopic atom to the complex human organism. Note the progression from simple to complex in Figure 1-2. Tiny atoms form molecules. These in turn form larger molecules. The larger molecules are eventually organized into **cells,** the basic unit of life. Specialized groups of cells form **tissues.** Tissues are then arranged into **organs** such as the heart, stomach, and kidney. Each organ has a function, such as digestion, excretion, or reproduction. Groups of organs, in turn, create **organ systems.** All of the organ systems together form the human organism. From simple to complex, the body is built from the tiny atom to the human being.

MAJOR ORGAN SYSTEMS

Eleven major organ systems make up the human body. Each has a specific function. Refer to Figure 1-3 and identify the location and distribution of the organs of each system.

- The **integumentary system** consists of the skin and related structures such as hair and nails. The integumentary system forms a covering for the body, helps regulate body temperature, and contains some of the structures necessary for sensation.
- The **skeletal system** forms the basic framework of the body. It consists primarily of bones, joints, and cartilage. The skeleton protects and supports body organs.
- The **muscular system** consists of three types of muscles. Skeletal muscles attach to the bones and are responsible for movement of the skeleton and the maintenance of body posture.
- The **nervous system** consists of the brain, spinal cord, nerves, and sense organs. Sensory nerves receive information from the environment and bring it to the spinal cord and brain, where it is interpreted. Decisions made by the brain and spinal cord are transmitted along other nerves to various body structures.
- The **endocrine system** consists of numerous glands that secrete hormones and chemical substances that regulate body activities such as growth, reproduction, metabolism, and water balance.
- The **circulatory system** consists of the heart and blood vessels. This system pumps and transports blood throughout the body. Blood carries nutrients and oxygen to all the body's cells and also carries the waste away from the cells to the organs of excretion.

Do You Know...

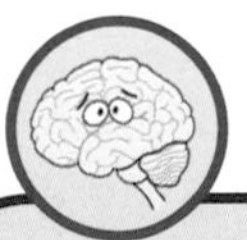

Why this famous anatomy laboratory was built over a small river in Italy?

Because dissection of the human body was illegal during the Middle Ages, the anatomy laboratories were routinely raided by the police. In the event of a raid, the partially dissected body was lowered through a hole in the floor of the laboratory onto a barge on the river. The body (and incriminating evidence) then floated away.

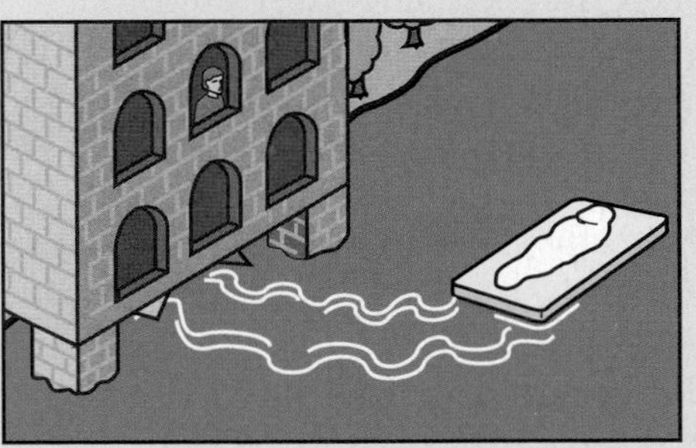

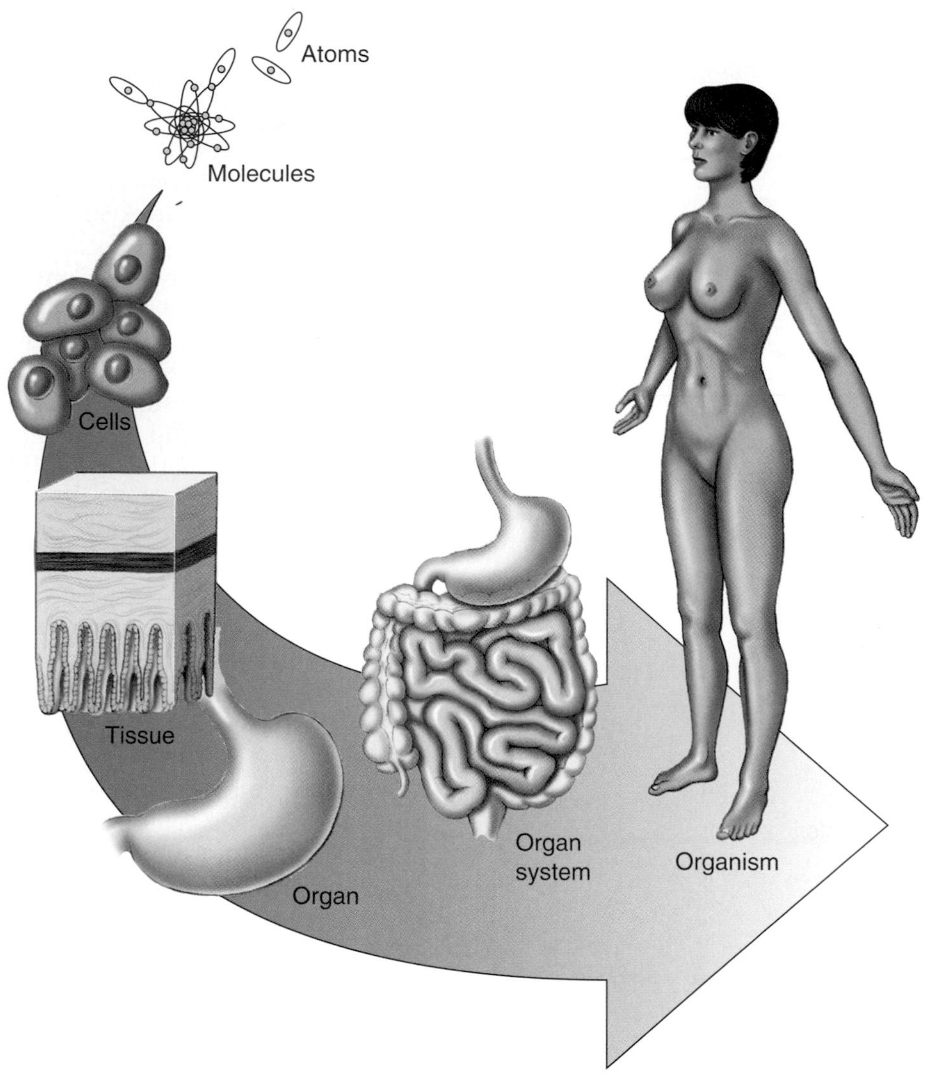

FIGURE 1-2 Levels of organization: from atom to human organism.

- The **lymphatic system** consists of the lymph nodes, lymphatic vessels, lymph, and other lymphoid organs. Lymph and lymphoid structures play an important role in fluid balance and in the defense of the body against pathogens and other foreign material.
- The **respiratory system** consists of the lungs and other structures that conduct air to and from the lungs. Oxygen-rich air moves into the lungs and carbon dioxide-rich air (waste) moves out of the lungs.
- The **digestive system** consists of organs designed to eat food, break it down into substances that can be absorbed by the body, and eliminate the waste.
- The **urinary system** consists of the kidneys and other structures that help excrete waste products from the body through the urine. The urinary system helps control the amount and composition of water and other substances in the body.
- The **reproductive system** consists of organs and structures that enable humans to reproduce.

HOMEOSTASIS: STAYING THE SAME

Homeostasis (hō-mē-ō-STĀ-sĭs) literally means staying (stasis) the same (homeo). The term refers to the body's ability to maintain a stable internal environment in response to a changing external environment. When your body achieves homeostasis, the conditions in your body remain the same, despite the many changes outside. For instance, in a healthy person, body temperature stays around 98.6° F (37° C) even when room temperature increases to 100° F or decreases to 60° F. The amount of water in your cells stays the same whether you drink 2, 3, or 4 liters (L) of water per day. Your blood sugar remains within normal limits whether you have just eaten a turkey dinner or have fasted for 6 hours.

Mechanisms that help maintain homeostasis are called **homeostatic mechanisms.** The body has hundreds of homeostatic mechanisms, including those for temperature control, blood sugar control, water balance, blood pressure regulation, and regulation of plasma sodium levels. When homeostatic mechanisms

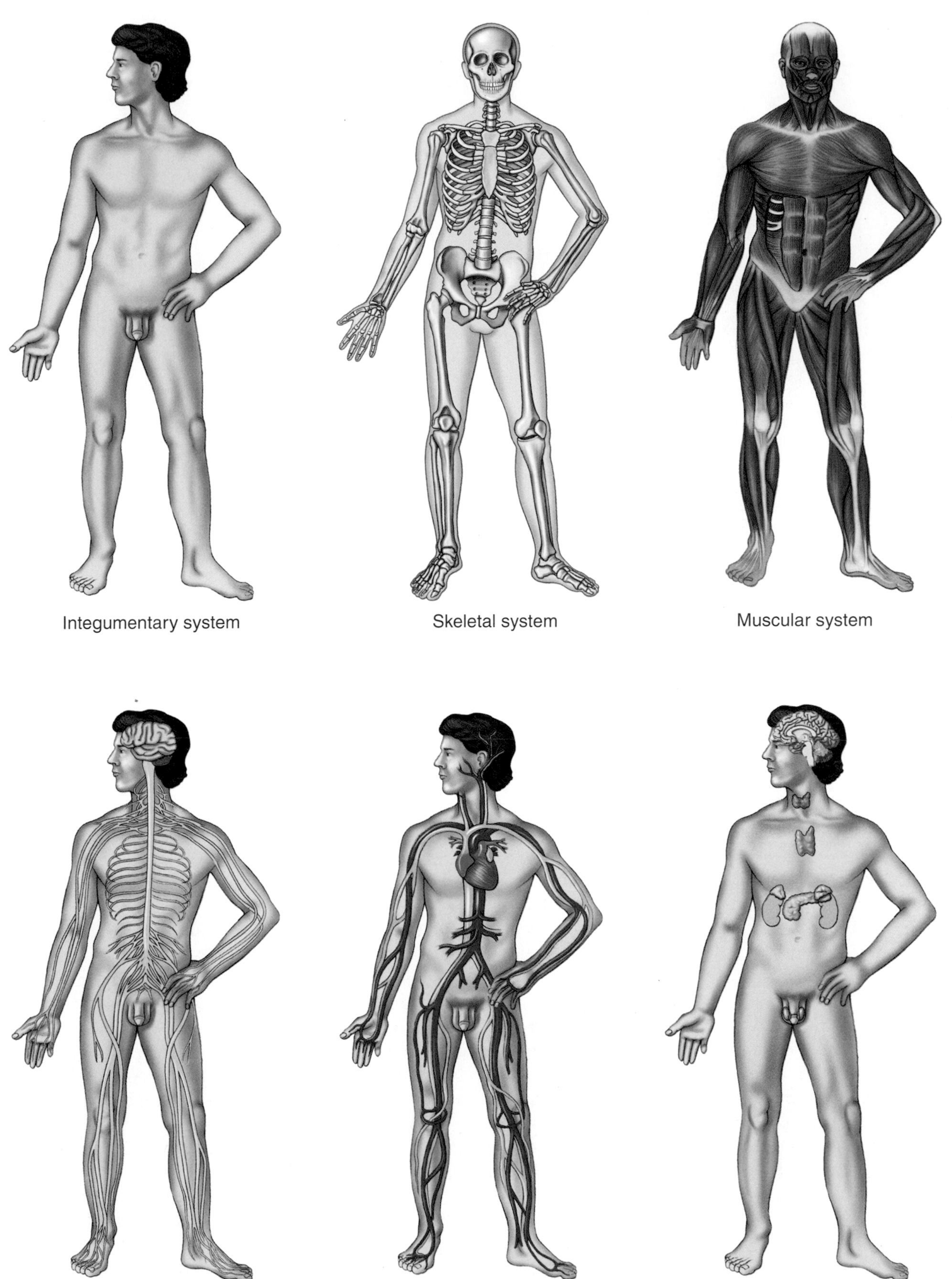

FIGURE 1-3 Major organ systems of the body.

Continued

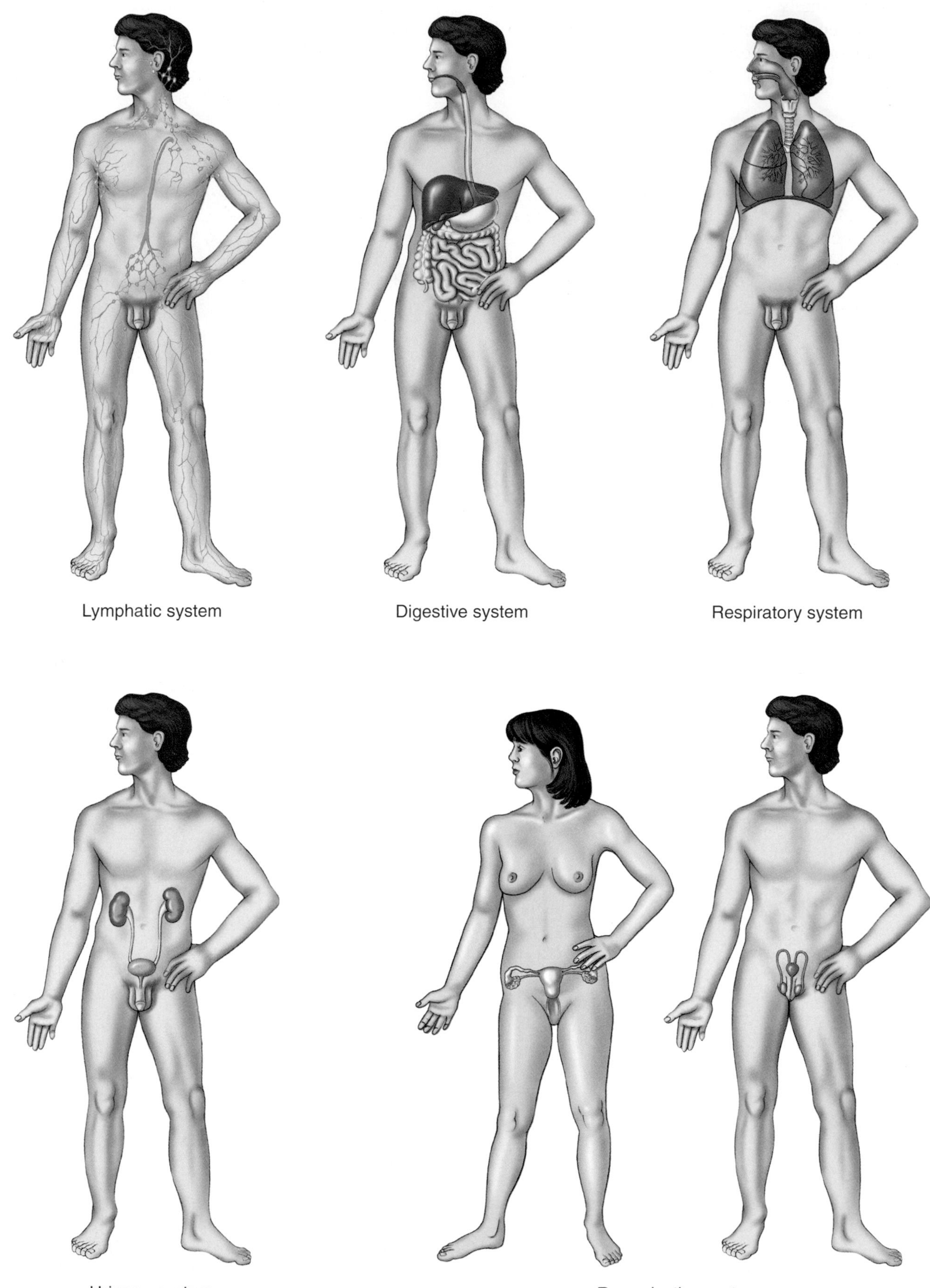

FIGURE 1-3, cont'd Major organ systems of the body.

do not work normally, the result can be disease or dysfunction. **Homeostatic imbalance** is therefore associated with various disorders.

ANATOMICAL TERMS: TALKING ABOUT THE BODY

Special terms describe the location, position, and regions of body parts. Because these terms are used frequently, you should become familiar with them now. People in the medical field are often accused of speaking their own language. Indeed, we do! We always use these terms as if the body were standing in its anatomical position.

ANATOMICAL POSITION

In its **anatomical position** the body is standing erect, with the face forward, the arms at the sides, and the toes and palms of the hands directed forward (Figure 1-4).

RELATIVE POSITIONS

Specific terms describe the position of one body part in relation to another body part. These are directional terms. They are like the more familiar directions of north, south, east, and west; however, while you can correctly describe Canada as located north of the United States, you would sound strange if you described the head as north of the chest. Therefore, in locating body parts, we use other terminology. The terms come in pairs. Note that the two terms in each pair are generally opposites.

- *Superior and inferior.* **Superior** means that a part is above another part or is closer to the head. For example, the head is superior to the chest. **Inferior** means that a part is located below another part or is closer to the feet. The chest, for example, is inferior to the head.
- *Anterior and posterior.* **Anterior** means toward the front surface (the belly surface). **Posterior** means toward the back surface. For example, the heart is anterior to the spinal cord. The heart is posterior to the breastbone. Another word for anterior is **ventral.** Another word for posterior is **dorsal.** Consider the dorsal fin of a fish. It is the dorsal part of the shark that can be seen moving effortlessly and very quickly toward your surfboard!
- *Medial and lateral.* Imagine a line drawn through the middle of your body, dividing it into right and left halves. This is the midline point. **Medial** means toward the midline of the body. The nose, for example is medial to the ears. **Lateral** means away from the midline of the body. For example, the ears are lateral to the nose.
- *Proximal and distal.* **Proximal** means that the structure is nearer the point of attachment, often the trunk of the body. Because the elbow is closer to the point of attachment than is the wrist, it is described as proximal to the wrist. The wrist is proximal to the fingers, meaning that the wrist is closer to the point of attachment than are the fingers. **Distal** means that a part is farther away from the point of attachment than is another part. For example, the wrist is distal to the elbow, and the fingers are distal to the wrist.
- *Superficial and deep.* **Superficial** means that a part is located on or near the surface of the body. The skin is superficial to the muscles. **Deep** means that the body part is away from the surface of the body. The bones, for example, are deep to the skin.
- *Central and peripheral.* **Central** means that the part is located in the center. **Peripheral** means away from the center. The heart, for example, is located centrally, while the blood vessels are located peripherally (away from the center and extending toward the limbs).

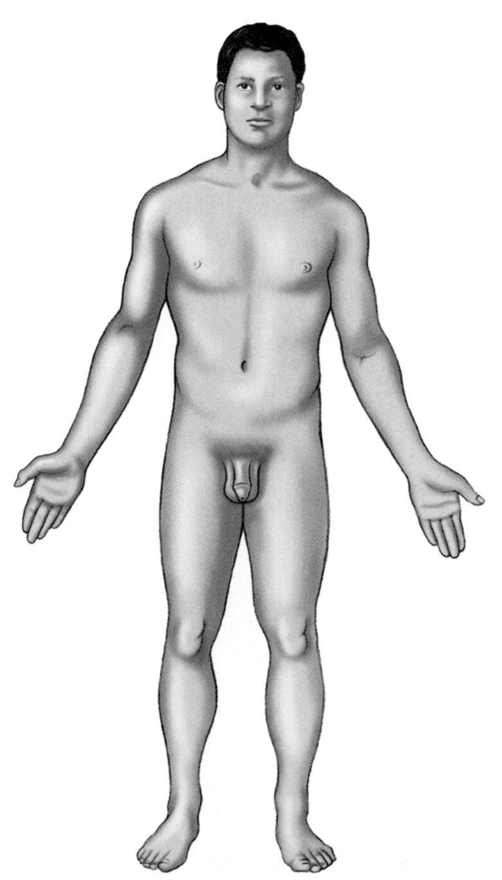

FIGURE 1-4 Anatomical position.

Sum It Up!

Specific terms describe the relative positions of one body part to the other. The terms are paired as opposites and include superior and inferior, anterior (ventral) and posterior (dorsal), medial and lateral, proximal and distal, superficial and deep, and central and peripheral.

PLANES AND SECTIONS OF THE BODY

When we refer to the left side of the body, the top half of the body, or the front of the body, we are referring to the planes, or sections, of the body. Each plane divides the body with an imaginary line in one direction. Figure 1-5 shows the following three important planes:

1. Sagittal plane (see Figure 1-5, *A*). The **sagittal** (SĂJ-ĭ-tl) **plane** divides the body lengthwise into right and left portions. If the cut is made exactly down the midline of the body, the right and left halves of the body are equal. This division is a midsagittal section.
2. Frontal plane (see Figure 1-5, *B*). The **frontal plane** divides the body into anterior (ventral) and posterior (dorsal) portions. This plane creates the front part of the body and the back part of the body. The frontal plane is also called the coronal plane. Why? Coronal means crown. The imaginary line for the coronal plane is made across the part of the head where a crown sits and then downward through the body.
3. Transverse plane (see Figure 1-5, *C*). The **transverse plane** divides the body horizontally, creating an upper (superior) and a lower (inferior) body. When the body or an organ is cut horizontally or transversely, it is called a cross section.

REGIONAL TERMS

Specific terms describe the different regions or areas of the body. Figure 1-6 illustrates the terms used to identify the regions on the anterior and posterior surfaces of the body.

On the anterior surface, identify the following regions:

Abdominal: anterior trunk just below the ribs
Antecubital: area in front of the elbow
Axillary: armpit
Brachial: arm
Buccal: cheek area, specifically between the gum and cheek
Cephalic: head
Cervical: neck region
Cranial: nearer to the head
Digital: fingers, toes
Femoral: thigh area
Flank: fleshy area along each side between the lower ribs and the top of the hip bones
Inguinal: area where the thigh meets the trunk of the body
Oral: mouth
Orbital: area around the eye
Patellar: front of the knee
Pedal: foot

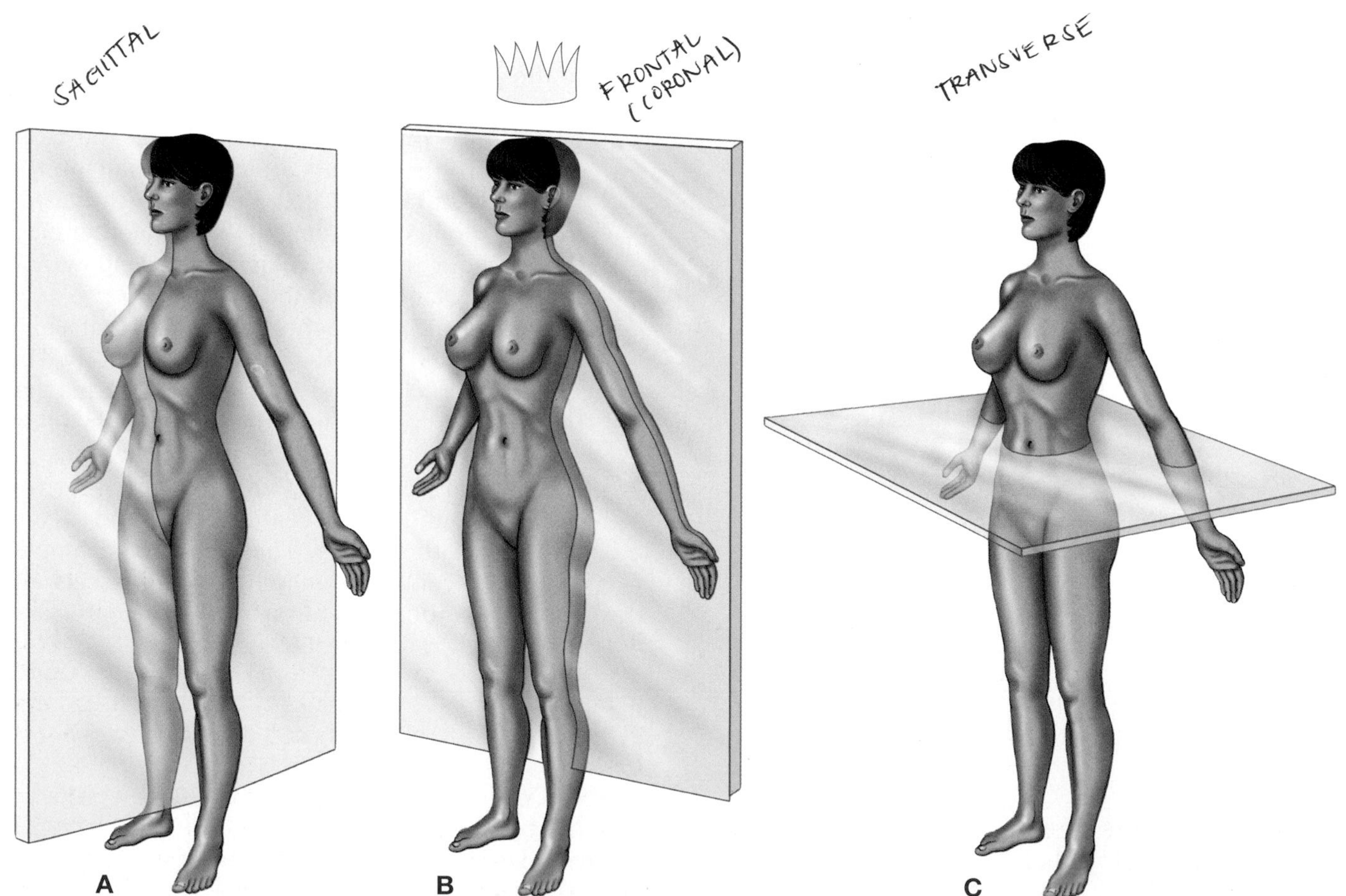

FIGURE 1-5 Planes of the body. **A,** Sagittal. **B,** Frontal (coronal). **C,** Transverse.

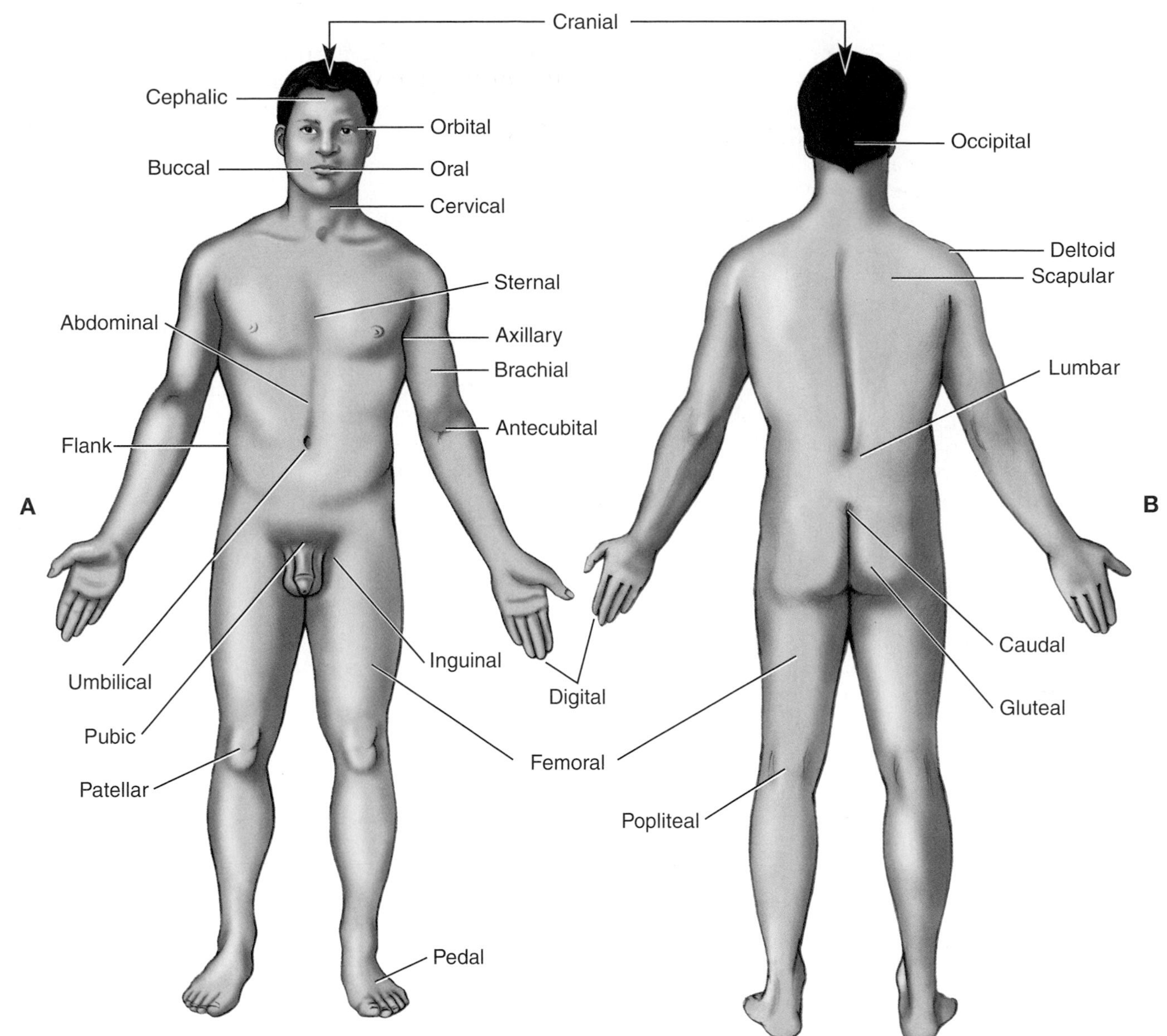

FIGURE 1-6 Regional terms. **A,** Anterior view. **B,** Posterior view.

Pubic: genital area
Sternal: middle of the chest (over the breastbone area)
Umbilical: navel

On the posterior surface, identify the following regions:

Caudal: nearer to the lower region of the spinal column (near your tailbone)
Deltoid: rounded area of the shoulder closest to the upper arm
Gluteal: buttocks
Lumbar: area of the back between the ribs and the hips
Occipital: back of the head
Popliteal: behind, or back of, the knee area
Scapular: shoulder blade area

CAVITIES OF THE BODY

DORSAL CAVITY

The organs, called **viscera,** are located within the cavities of the body. Cavities are large, internal spaces. The body contains two major cavities: the dorsal cavity and the ventral cavity (Figure 1-7). The **dorsal cavity** is located toward the back of the body and has two divisions, the **cranial cavity** and the **spinal (vertebral) cavity.**

The cranial cavity is located within the skull and contains the brain. The spinal, or vertebral, cavity extends downward from the cranial cavity and is surrounded by bony vertebrae; it contains the spinal cord. These two areas form one continuous space.

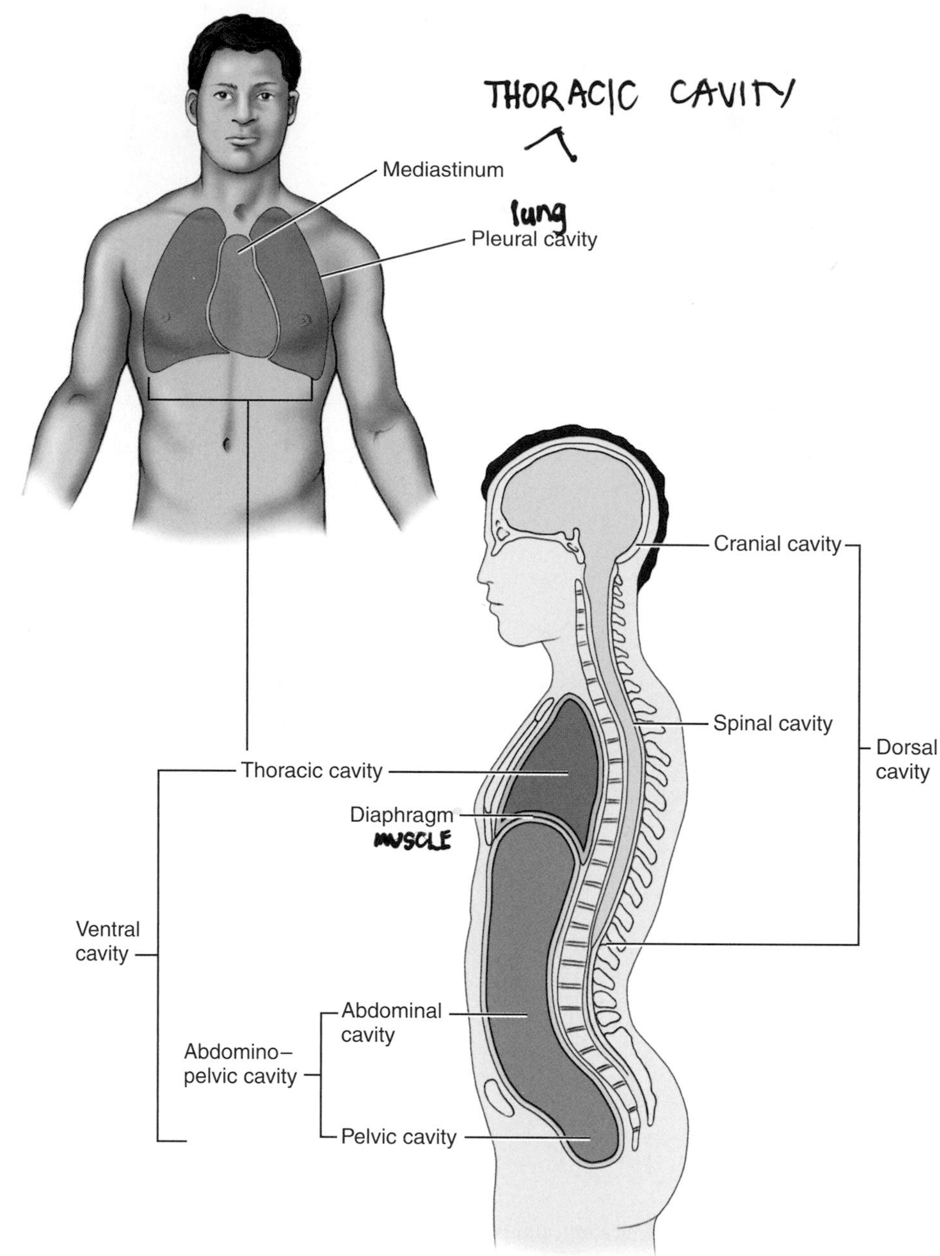

FIGURE 1-7 Major body cavities.

VENTRAL CAVITY

The larger **ventral cavity** is located toward the front of the body and has two divisions, the **thoracic** (thō-RĂS-ĭk) **cavity** and the **abdominopelvic** (ăb-Dŏm-ĭ-nō-PĔL-vĭk) **cavity.**

Thoracic Cavity

The thoracic cavity is located above the diaphragm and is surrounded by the rib cage. The thoracic cavity is divided into two compartments by the **mediastinum,** a space that contains the heart, esophagus, trachea, thymus gland, and large blood vessels attached to the heart. The right and left lungs are located on either side of the mediastinum in the **pleural cavities.** The lungs occupy most of the space within the thoracic cavity.

Abdominopelvic Cavity

The abdominopelvic cavity is located below the diaphragm. The upper portion of this cavity is the **abdominal cavity.** It contains the stomach, most of the intestine, liver, gallbladder, pancreas, spleen, and kidneys. The lower portion of the abdominopelvic cavity is called the **pelvic cavity.** It extends downward from

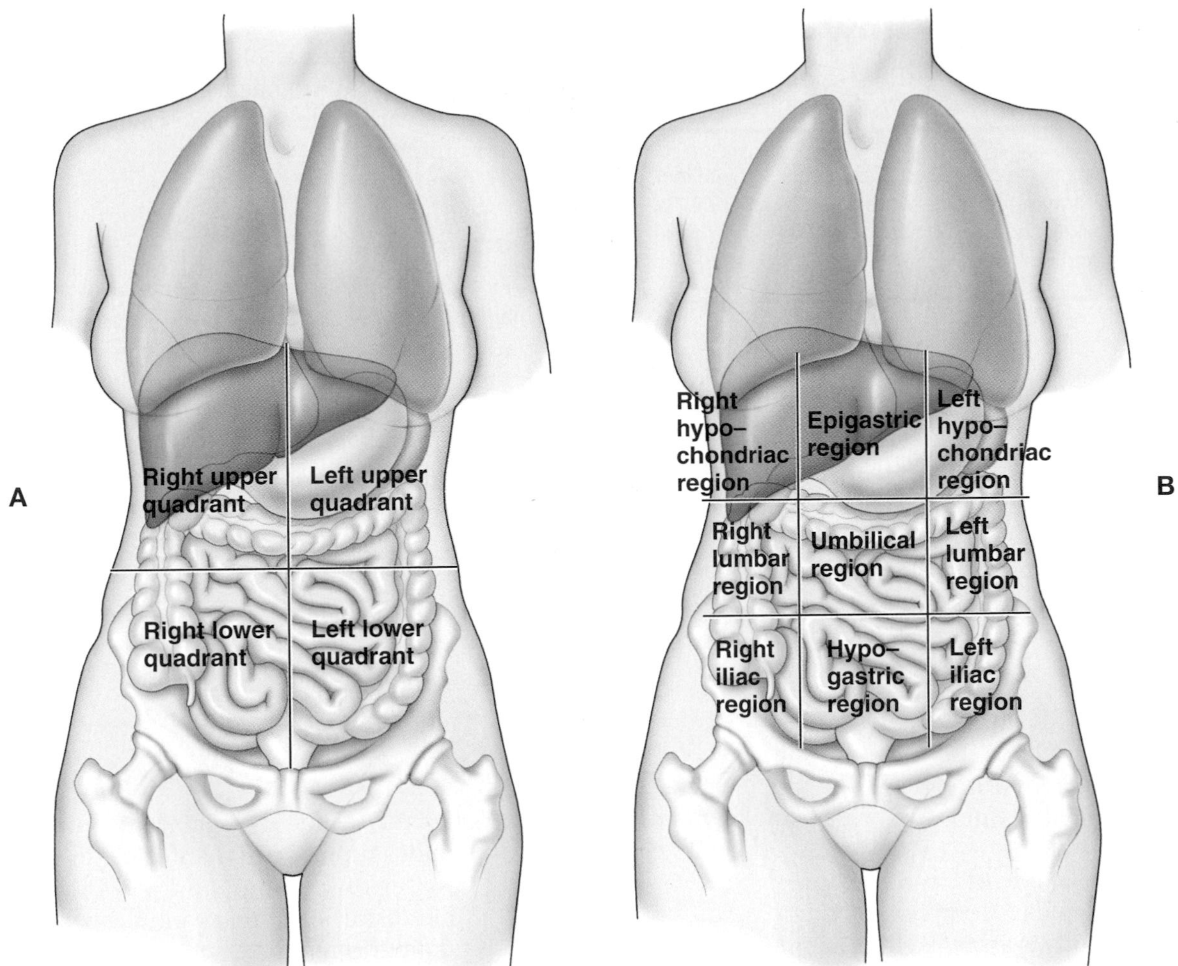

FIGURE 1-8 Areas of the abdomen. **A,** Four quadrants. **B,** Nine regions.

the level of the hips and includes the remainder of the intestines, the rectum, urinary bladder, and internal parts of the reproductive system.

Because the abdominopelvic cavity is so large, it is subdivided into smaller areas for study. Quadrants and regions divide the abdominopelvic cavity. Note the organs located in each quadrant or region, as shown in Figure 1-8.

Division into Quadrants. The abdominopelvic cavity can be divided into four **quadrants** (see Figure 1-8, *A*). The quadrants are named for their positions: right upper quadrant (RUQ), left upper quadrant (LUQ), right lower quadrant (RLQ), and left lower quadrant (LLQ).

Quadrant terms are used frequently in the clinical setting. For instance, a patient who presents in the emergency room with acute pain in the RLQ may be diagnosed with appendicitis. Note that the RLQ appears to be on your left. This is similar to looking in a mirror. Keep this in mind when you are studying the diagrams in the text.

Division into Regions. A second system divides the abdominopelvic cavity into nine separate regions that resemble the squares for tic-tac-toe (see Figure 1-8, *B*). The three central regions (from top to bottom) include the epigastric, umbilical, and hypogastric regions. The epigastric region is located below the breastbone. Epigastric literally means upon (epi) the stomach (gastric). The umbilical region is the centermost region and surrounds the umbilicus, or navel. The hypogastric region is located just below the umbilical region. Hypogastric literally means below (hypo) the stomach (gastric).

Six regions are located on either side of the central regions. They include the hypochondriac, lumbar, and iliac regions. The right and left hypochondriac regions are located on either side of the epigastric region and overlie the lower ribs. The word hypochondriac literally means below (hypo) the cartilage (chondro) and refers to the composition of the ribs (cartilage). The right and left lumbar regions are located on either side of the umbilical region and are inferior to the hypochondriac regions. The right and left iliac regions are also called

Do You Know...

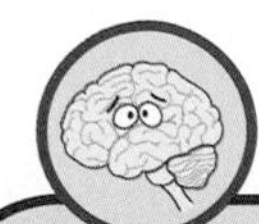

What your postsurgical patient has done if he eviscerated?

His internal organs have protruded through his surgical incision. This word comes from the word viscera (organs). The organs must be kept moist and sterile until they can be returned to their home cavity.

the right and left inguinal regions. They are located on either side of the hypogastric region and inferior to the lumbar regions. A knowledge of these regions helps you understand terms such as epigastric pain and umbilical hernia.

Other Cavities

Four smaller cavities are located in the head. They include the oral cavity, nasal cavities, orbital cavities, and middle ear cavities. (These cavities are described in later chapters.)

Sum It Up!

The organs are located within body cavities. The two major cavities are the dorsal cavity, located toward the back of the body, and the larger ventral cavity, located in the front of the body. The dorsal cavity is subdivided into the cranial cavity and the spinal cavity. The ventral cavity is divided by the diaphragm into the thoracic cavity and the abdominopelvic cavity.

SUMMARY OUTLINE

Anatomy is the study of structure; physiology is the study of function.

I. The Body's Levels of Organization

- A. From Simple to Complex
  1. The body is arranged from simple to complex.
  2. Structure and function are related.
- B. Major Organ Systems
  1. An organ system is a group of organs that help each other to perform a particular function.
  2. There are 11 major organ systems.
     - a. The integumentary system
     - b. The skeletal system
     - c. The muscular system
     - d. The nervous system
     - e. The endocrine system
     - f. The heart and circulatory systems
     - g. The lymphatic system
     - h. The respiratory system
     - i. The digestive system
     - j. The urinary system
     - k. The reproductive system
  3. Homeostasis refers to the body's ability to maintain a stable internal environment in response to a changing external environment.

II. Anatomical Terms: Talking About the Body

- A. Anatomical Position
  1. The anatomical position is the body standing erect, arms by the side, with palms facing forward.
  2. Paired terms that describe direction include superior and inferior, anterior and posterior, medial and lateral, proximal and distal, superficial and deep, and central and peripheral.
  3. The three planes are the sagittal plane, frontal (coronal) plane, and transverse plane.
  4. Regional terms are listed in Figure 1-6.
- B. Cavities of the Body
  1. Dorsal cavity
     - a. The cranial cavity contains the brain.
     - b. The spinal cavity, or vertebral cavity, contains the spinal cord.
  2. Ventral Cavity
     - a. The thoracic cavity is above the diaphragm and contains the lungs; it also contains the mediastinum.
     - b. The abdominopelvic cavity is located below the diaphragm.
     - c. The abdominal cavity is the upper part that contains the stomach, most of the intestines, liver, spleen, and kidneys.
     - d. The pelvic cavity is the lower part that contains the reproductive organs, urinary bladder, and lower part of the intestines.
     - e. For reference, the abdominopelvic cavity is divided into four quadrants and nine regions.

Review Your Knowledge

Matching: Directions of the Body

Directions: Match the following words with their descriptions below. Some words may be used more than once.

a. posterior
b. distal
c. medial
d. anterior
e. proximal
f. superior
g. deep

1. ____ Toward the midline of the body; opposite of lateral
2. ____ A structure is nearer to the trunk than is another part; opposite of distal
3. ____ The part of the radius (arm bone) that is closer to the wrist than to the elbow
4. ____ The lung is above the diaphragm; above is described as
5. ____ Toward the front (the belly surface); another word is ventral

Matching: Regional Terms

Directions: Match the following words with their descriptions below.

a. inguinal
b. oral
c. lumbar
d. axillary
e. buccal
f. patellar
g. flank
h. antecubital
i. sternal
j. scapular

1. ____ Armpit
2. ____ Kneecap area
3. ____ Breastbone area
4. ____ Front part of the elbow area
5. ____ Fleshy area along the side between the ribs and the hip bone
6. ____ Pertaining to the mouth
7. ____ Lower back area extending from the chest to the hips
8. ____ Pertains to the space between the cheek and the gum
9. ____ Groin region
10. ____ Shoulder blade area

Multiple Choice

1. This part of the humerus (upper arm bone) is closer to the elbow than to the axillary region.
   a. Anterior
   b. Superior
   c. Distal
   d. Proximal
2. The lung is located in the thoracic cavity. Describe the relationship of the lung to the diaphragm.
   a. Distal
   b. Deep
   c. Anterior
   d. Superior
3. The umbilical area is located
   a. inferior to the inguinal region.
   b. superior to the RUQ.
   c. inferior to the diaphragm.
   d. within the midepigastric region.
4. The sternal area is
   a. superior to the diaphragm.
   b. the breastbone area.
   c. superficial to the mediastinum.
   d. all of the above are true.
5. Which of the following is not descriptive of the mediastinum?
   a. Thoracic cavity
   b. Dorsal cavity
   c. Ventral cavity
   d. Superior to the diaphragm

CHAPTER 2

Basic Chemistry

KEY TERMS

Acid, p. 22
Adenosine triphosphate (ATP), p. 24
Atom, p. 15
Base, p. 22
Catalyst, p. 22
Compound, p. 20
Covalent bond, p. 17
Electrolyte, p. 19
Element, p. 15
Energy, p. 24
Enzyme, p. 22
Hydrogen bond, p. 19
Ionic bond, p. 17
Isotope, p. 17
Matter, p. 15
Molecule, p. 20
pH, p. 22
Solution, p. 25
Suspension, p. 26

OBJECTIVES

1. Define the terms *matter* and *element*.
2. List the four elements that compose 96% of body weight.
3. Describe the three components of an atom.
4. Describe the role of electrons in the formation of chemical bonds.
5. Differentiate among ionic, covalent, and hydrogen bonds.
6. Explain the differences among electrolytes, ions, cations, and anions.
7. Explain the difference between a molecule and a compound.
8. List five reasons why water is essential to life.
9. Define *energy* and describe the role of adenosine triphosphate (ATP) in energy transfer.
10. Explain the role of catalysts and enzymes.
11. Differentiate between an acid and a base.
12. Define *pH.*
13. Differentiate between a mixture, solution, suspension, and colloidal suspension.

Why a chapter on chemistry? Because our bodies are made of different chemicals. The food we eat, the water we drink, and the air we breathe are all chemical substances. We digest our food, move our bodies, experience emotions, and think great thoughts because of chemical reactions. To understand the body, we must understand some general chemical principles.

MATTER, ELEMENTS, AND ATOMS

MATTER

Chemistry is the study of matter. **Matter** is anything that occupies space and has weight. Anything that you see as you look around is matter.

Matter exists in three states: solid, liquid, and gas. Solid matter has a definite shape and volume. Skin, bones, and teeth are examples of solid matter. Liquid matter takes the shape of the container it is in. Liquid matter includes blood, saliva, and digestive juices. A gas, or gaseous matter, has neither shape nor volume. The air we breathe is matter that exists as gas.

Matter can undergo both physical and chemical changes. The logs in a fireplace illustrate the difference between a physical and a chemical change (Figure 2-1). The logs can undergo a **physical change** by being chopped into smaller chips of wood with a hatchet. The wood chips are smaller than the log, but they are still wood. The matter (wood) has not essentially changed. Only the physical appearance has changed. A **chemical change** occurs when the wood is burned. When burned, the wood ceases to be wood. The chemical composition of the ashes is essentially different from that of wood.

The body contains many examples of physical and chemical changes. For example, digestion involves both physical and chemical changes. Chewing breaks the food into smaller pieces; this is a physical change. Potent chemicals digest or change the food into simpler substances; this is a chemical change.

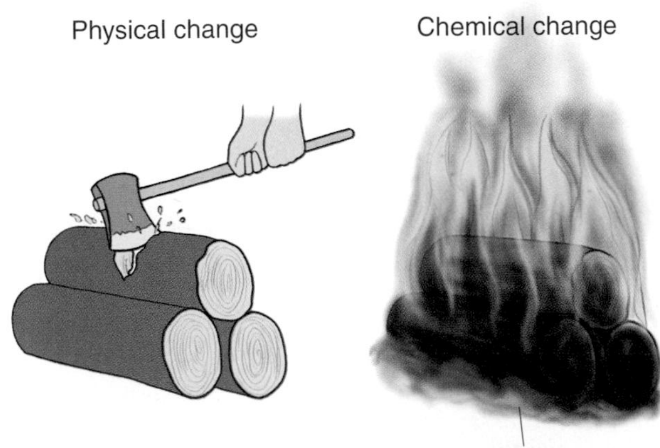

FIGURE 2-1 Changes in matter.

ELEMENTS

All matter, living or dead, is composed of elements. An **element** is a fundamental substance that cannot be broken down into a simpler form by ordinary chemical reactions. Even a very small amount of an element contains millions and millions of identical atoms, and the same name is used for the element and the atom. For example, all atoms of the element sodium are identical, and sodium is used for both the element and the atom. Although more than 100 elements exist, only about 25 elements are required by living organisms.

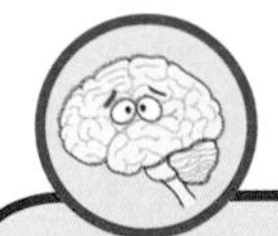

Do You Know...

Why children should not be allowed to play in traffic and chew on old paint?

Aside from the obvious safety issues, old paint and emissions from motor vehicles contain high amounts of lead. Exposure to high levels of lead causes lead poisoning, a serious condition that causes degeneration of major organs, including the brain, liver, kidney, and bone marrow. The old name for chronic lead poisoning is **plumbism,** from the Latin word for lead *(plumbum).* The chemical symbol for lead is **Pb.** Why does plumbism have such a great history? Lead was used to make pipes that carried water and to make pottery, particularly drinking vessels. This practice killed many famous names, including King Tut, and those wealthy enough to afford leaded wine goblets. Because of the toxic nature of lead, pipes and pottery are no longer made of lead, and gasoline and paint are now legally lead free. By the way, a plumber is called a plumber because the ancient water pipes were made of lead!

The most abundant elements found in the body are listed in Table 2-1. Four elements—carbon, hydrogen, oxygen, and nitrogen—make up 96% of the body weight. The **trace elements** are present in tiny amounts. Despite the small amounts required, the trace elements are essential for life. (Not all of the trace elements appear in the table.)

Each of the elements included in Table 2-1 is represented by a symbol. For example, the symbol O is for oxygen, N is for nitrogen, Na is for sodium, K is for potassium, and C is for carbon. The first letter of the symbol is always capitalized. These symbols are used frequently. You should memorize the symbols of the major elements. You will need to use them.

ATOMS

Atomic Structure

Elements are composed of atoms. An **atom** is the smallest unit of an element with that element's chemical characteristics. It is the basic unit of matter. An atom is composed of three subatomic particles: protons, neutrons, and electrons.

Table 2-1 Common Elements in the Human Body

Element	Symbol	Percentage of Body Weight (%)
Oxygen	O	65.0
Carbon	C	18.5
Hydrogen	H	9.5
Nitrogen	N	3.2
Calcium	Ca	
Phosphorus	P	
Potassium	K	
Sulfur	S	
Sodium	Na	
Chlorine	Cl	
Magnesium	Mg	
Iron	Fe	
Iodine*	I	
Chromium*	Cr	
Cobalt*	Co	
Copper*	Cu	
Fluorine*	F	
Selenium*	Se	
Zinc*	Zn	

*Trace elements.

The arrangement of the subatomic particles resembles the sun and planets (Figure 2-2, *A*). The sun is the center. The planets constantly move around the sun in orbits, or circular paths. The atom is composed of a nucleus (the sun) and shells, or orbits, that surround the nucleus (see Figure 2-2, *B*).

Where are the subatomic particles located? The protons and the neutrons are located in the nucleus (see Figure 2-2, *C*). **Protons** carry a positive (+) electrical charge; **neutrons** carry no electrical charge. The electrons are located in the shells, or orbits, surrounding the nucleus like planets. **Electrons** carry a negative (−) electrical charge. In each atom, the number of protons (+) is equal to the number of electrons (−). The atom is therefore electrically neutral; it carries no net electrical charge.

All protons are alike; all neutrons are alike; and all electrons are alike. So what makes one atom different from another atom? The difference is primarily due to the numbers of protons and electrons in each atom. For instance, hydrogen is the simplest and smallest atom. It has one proton and one electron. Helium has two protons and two electrons. Lithium has three protons and three electrons. Hydrogen, helium, and lithium are different atoms because of the different numbers of protons and electrons.

Other Characteristics of Atoms

Two terms describe individual atoms. The **atomic number** is the number of protons in the nucleus. Thus

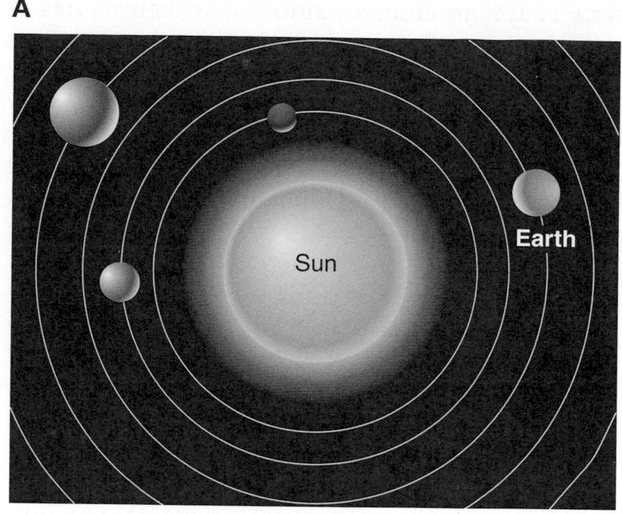

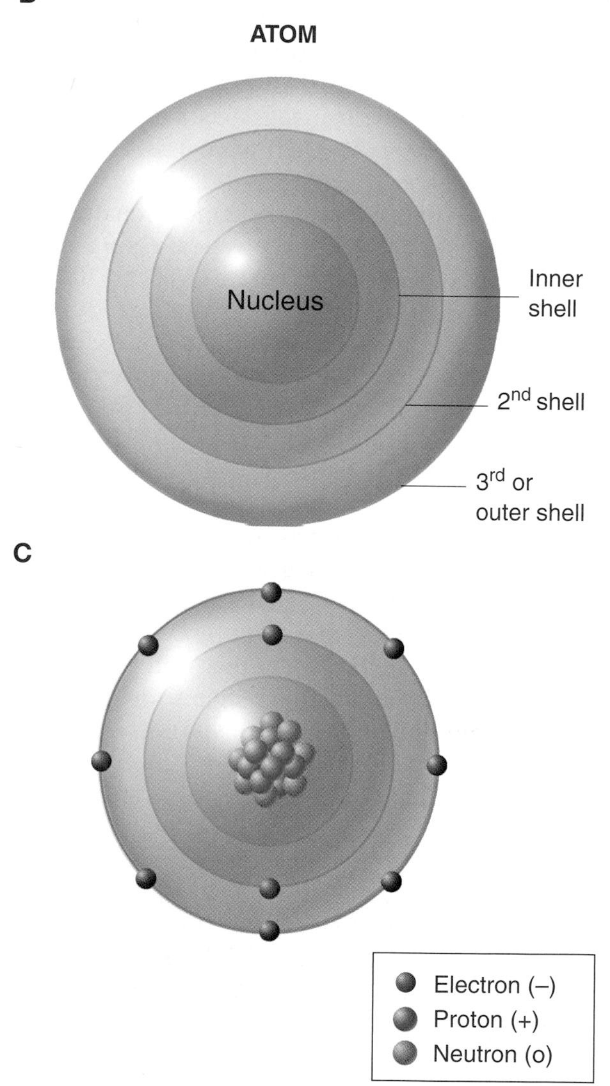

FIGURE 2-2 Structure of the atom. **A,** Subatomic particles arranged like the sun and the planets. **B,** Nucleus and electron shells. **C,** Protons and neutrons located in the nucleus and electrons encircling the nucleus in orbits.

hydrogen has an atomic number of 1; helium has an atomic number of 2, and lithium has an atomic number of 3. The **atomic weight** of an atom is determined by adding the numbers of protons and neutrons in the nucleus. Thus the atomic weight of hydrogen is also 1 because the hydrogen nucleus contains one proton and no neutrons. The atomic weight of helium is 4 because the nucleus contains two protons and two neutrons.

What is an isotope? An **isotope** (Ī-sŏ-tōp) is a different form of the same atom. For example, hydrogen has different forms. Hydrogen has an atomic number of 1 and an atomic weight of 1; it has one proton and no neutrons in the nucleus. A second and less common form of hydrogen is called heavy hydrogen. It has one proton and one neutron in its nucleus; thus its atomic number is 1, but its atomic weight is 2. Because its atomic number is 1, it is still a hydrogen atom. The additional neutron in the nucleus, however, makes it heavy and changes its atomic weight. Heavy hydrogen is an isotope of hydrogen. Remember that an isotope has the same atomic number as an atom but a different atomic weight. An isotope of an atom varies only in the number of neutrons.

Isotopes are often unstable and their nuclei break down, or decay, giving off particles or energy waves. By emitting particles or energy waves, the unstable nuclei become more stable. Unstable isotopes are called **radioisotopes.** The process of spontaneous breakdown (decay) is called **radioactivity.** Radioisotopes are damaging to tissue and are used clinically to destroy cells. For instance, radioactive iodine is used to destroy excess thyroid tissue. Other radioisotopes are used to destroy cancer cells.

Electron Shells

Electrons surround the nucleus in orbits called energy levels or electron shells (see Figure 2-2, *C*). The number of shells varies from one atom to the next. Some atoms, like hydrogen, have only one shell; other atoms, like sodium, have three shells. Each shell can hold a specific number of electrons. The inner shell closest to the nucleus can hold only two electrons. The second and third shells each hold eight electrons.

The only electrons that are important for chemical bonding are the electrons in the outermost shell. If it is not filled with its proper number of electrons, the outer shell becomes unstable. It then seeks either to give up electrons so as to empty the shell or to acquire electrons so as to fill the shell. The tendency of the outer shell to want to become stable forms the basis of chemical bonding.

CHEMICAL BONDS

Atoms are attracted to each other because they want to achieve a stable outer electron shell. In other words, they want either to fill or empty the outer electron shell. The force of attraction between the atoms is similar to the force of two magnets. When you try to separate the magnets, you can feel the pull. The electrical attraction between atoms is a **chemical bond.** The three types of chemical bonds are ionic bonds, covalent bonds, and hydrogen bonds.

IONIC BONDS

The **ionic** (ī-ŎN-ĭk) **bond** is caused by a transfer of electrons between atoms. The interaction of the sodium and the chlorine atoms illustrates an ionic bond (Figure 2-3, *A*). The sodium atom has 11 protons in the nucleus and 11 electrons in the shells. Two electrons are in the inner shell, eight in the second shell, and only one in the outer shell. The single electron makes the outer shell unstable. To become more stable the sodium atom would like to donate the single electron. Donating an electron forms a bond between the two atoms. Sodium often bonds with chlorine.

The chlorine (Cl) atom has 17 protons in the nucleus and 17 electrons orbiting in its shells. The electrons are positioned as follows: two electrons in the inner shell, eight in the second shell, and seven in the outer shell. The seven electrons make the outer shell unstable. The chlorine atom would like to add a single electron. The electrical attraction occurs between the outer shells of the sodium and chlorine atoms.

The single electron in the outer shell of the sodium (Na) atom is attracted to the seven electrons in the outer shell of the chlorine atom. Thus the sodium atom and the chlorine atom bond ionically to form sodium chloride (NaCl), or table salt.

COVALENT BONDS

A second type of chemical bond is the **covalent** (Kō-VĀ-lĕnt) **bond.** Covalent bonding involves a sharing of electrons by the outer shells of the atoms. Covalent bonding is like joining hands (see Figure 2-3, *B*). The formation of water from hydrogen and oxygen atoms illustrates covalent bonding. Oxygen has eight electrons, two in the inner shell and only six in the outer shell. An oxygen atom needs two electrons to complete the outer shell. Hydrogen has only one electron and requires one electron to complete its inner shell.

Water is formed when two hydrogen atoms, each with one electron, share those electrons with one oxygen atom. By sharing the electrons of the oxygen, each of the two hydrogen atoms has completed the inner shells (capacity is two electrons). By sharing the electrons of two hydrogen atoms, the outer shell of the oxygen is completed with eight electrons. Water is represented as H_2O (two hydrogen and one oxygen).

Carbon atoms always form covalent bonds. A carbon atom has four electrons in the outer shell. Carbon

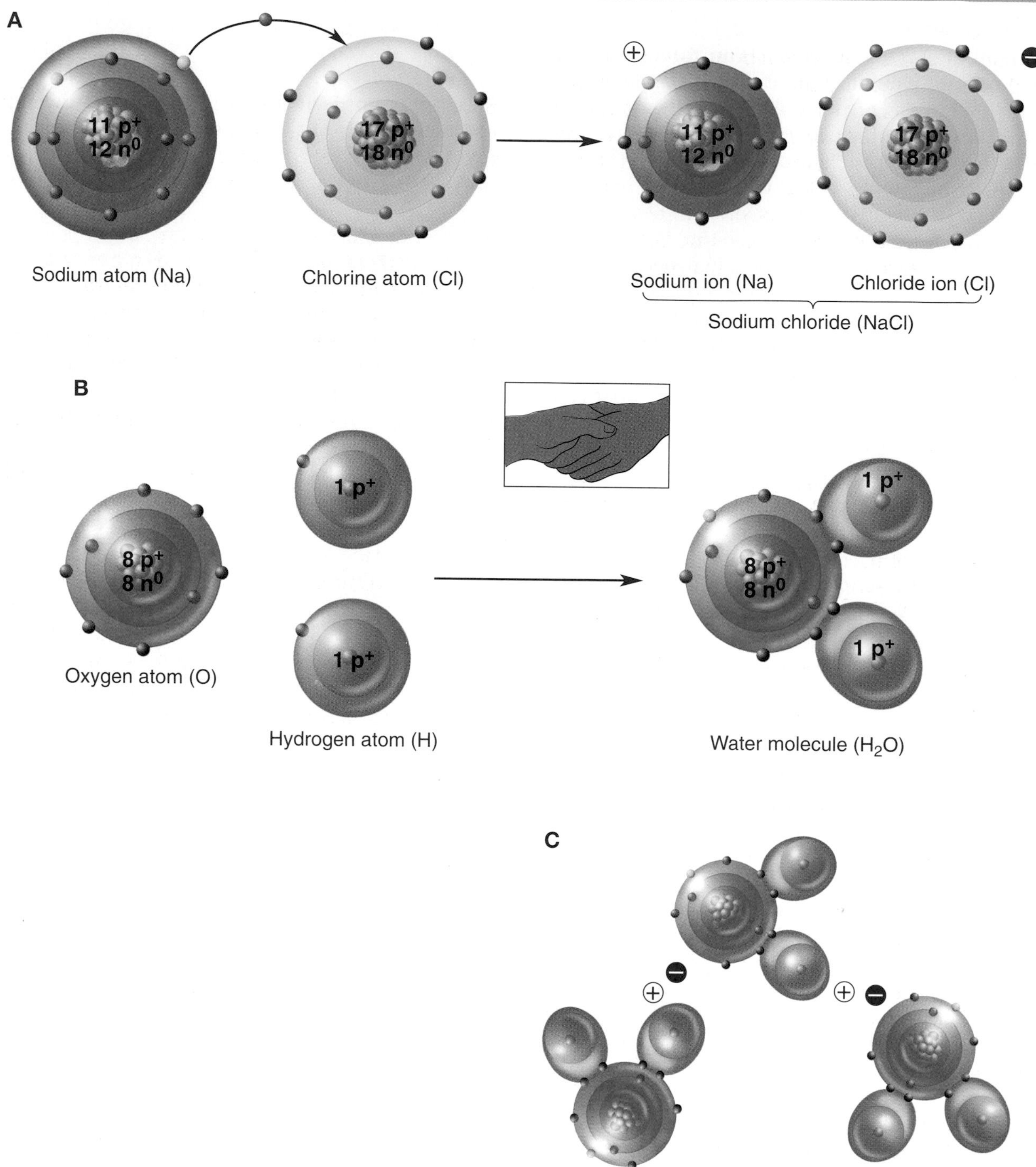

FIGURE 2-3 Chemical bonds. **A,** Ionic bond. **B,** Covalent bond. **C,** Hydrogen bond.

most commonly bonds with hydrogen (H), oxygen (O), nitrogen (N), and other carbon (C) atoms. Carbon is one of the major elements in the body. Covalent bonding of carbon with hydrogen, oxygen, and nitrogen forms complex molecules such as proteins and carbohydrates. Covalent bonds are strong and do not break apart in an aqueous (water) solution. The strength of these bonds is important because the protein produced by the body must not "fall apart" when exposed to water.

Many proteins, such as hormones, are transported around the body by blood, which is mostly water. If the covalent bonds of the protein broke apart in water, the hormones would be unable to accomplish their tasks. So many chemical reactions in the body involve carbon that a separate branch of chemistry studies only carbon-containing substances. The study of carbon-containing substances is called **organic chemistry.** In contrast, **inorganic chemistry** studies non–carbon-containing substances.

HYDROGEN BONDS

A third type of bond is a **hydrogen bond** (see Figure 2-3, *C*). It differs from the ionic and covalent bonds in that the hydrogen bond is not caused by either the transfer or the sharing of electrons of the outer shells of atoms. A hydrogen bond is best illustrated by the weak attraction between water molecules. Water is composed of hydrogen and oxygen. The weak positive charge around the hydrogen of one water molecule is attracted to the weak negative charge of the oxygen in a second water molecule.

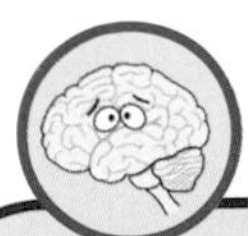

Do You Know...

What the patient's "lytes" are?

This is medical talk for electrolytes. One of the most important clinical tools is the assessment of the patient's electrolytes. Actually, the "lytes" are really ions such as Na^+ (sodium), K^+ (potassium), Cl^- (chloride), Mg^{2+} (magnesium), HCO_3^- (bicarbonate), etc. The terms electrolytes and ions are used interchangeably in the clinical setting. (Sloppy terminology, but acceptable!)

Water engages in hydrogen bonding because it is a polar molecule. What makes water a polar molecule? Because of the uneven sharing of electrons within a water molecule, there is a slight positive (+) charge around the hydrogen end of the water and a slight negative (−) charge around the oxygen end. Note in Figure 2-3, *C*, how lopsided the water molecule appears; more importantly, the charges are lopsided. A **polar molecule** is defined as a molecule that has a lopsided charge: a (+) end and a (−) end. The lopsided charge means the positive (+) end—hydrogen—of one water molecule is attracted to the negative (−) end—oxygen—of a second water molecule.

IONS

CATIONS, ANIONS, AND ELECTROLYTES

Several other terms are related to the activity of the electrons in the outer shells of the atoms. If the negatively charged electrons are lost from or gained by the outer shell of an atom, the electrical charge of the atom changes. In other words, the electrical charge of the atom or element changes from a neutral charge (i.e., no charge) to either a positive (+) charge or a negative (−) charge. Elements that carry an electrical charge are called **ions.** If the ion is positively charged, it is a **cation.** If the ion is negatively (−) charged, it is an **anion.**

An **electrolyte** is a substance that forms ions when it is dissolved in water. Electrolytes, as the name implies, are capable of conducting an electrical current. For instance, the electrocardiogram (ECG) and the electroencephalogram (EEG) record electrical events in the heart and brain.

ION FORMATION

Ions are formed when electrons in the outer shell are either lost or gained. For instance, the sodium atom has 11 protons (positive charge) and 11 electrons (negative charge). If a single electron is donated, the sodium is left with 11 positive (+) charges and only 10 negative (−) charges. Sodium is said to carry a net charge of +1. The sodium ion is therefore a cation. It is represented as Na^+.

The chlorine atom has 17 protons (positive charge) and 17 electrons (negative charge). If an electron is gained, the chlorine then contains 17 (+) charges and 18 (−) charges. Chlorine is said to carry a net charge of −1 and is called an anion. The chlorine anion is called chloride and is represented as Cl^-. Some atoms may give up more than one electron and have a stronger positive charge. Calcium, for instance, gives up two electrons. It is represented as Ca^{2+}. Table 2-2 presents other important ions. Note that combinations of atoms, such as bicarbonate (HCO_3^-) carry an electrical charge and are therefore ions.

Table 2-2 Common Ions

Name	Symbol	Function
Cations		
Sodium	Na^+	Fluid balance (principal extracellular cation); nerve-muscle function
Calcium	Ca^{2+}	Component of bones and teeth; blood clotting; muscle contraction
Iron	Fe^{2+}	Component of hemoglobin (oxygen transport)
Hydrogen	H^+	Important in acid-base balance
Potassium	K^+	Nerve and muscle function; chief intracellular cation
Ammonium	NH_4^+	Important in acid-base regulation
Anions		
Chloride	Cl^-	Primary extracellular anion
Bicarbonate	HCO_3^-	Important in acid-base regulation
Phosphate	PO_4^{3-}	Component of bones and teeth; component of ATP (energy)

ATP, Adenosine triphosphate.

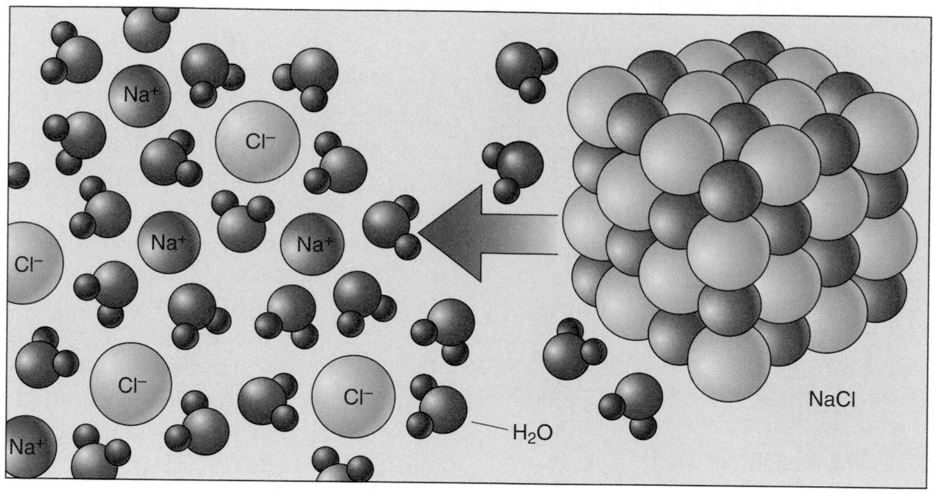

FIGURE 2-4 Ionization.

IONIZATION

When an electrolyte splits, or breaks apart in solution, the electrolyte is said to dissociate (Figure 2-4). For example, NaCl is an electrolyte. In the solid state, it appears as tiny white granules. When dissolved in water, however, the table salt dissociates. What is happening?

$$\underset{\text{salt}}{NaCl} \rightarrow \underset{\substack{\text{sodium ion}\\ \text{(cation)}}}{Na^+} + \underset{\substack{\text{chloride ion}\\ \text{(anion)}}}{Cl^-}$$

When the salt is placed in water, the ionic bonds holding the sodium and chlorine together weaken. The solid NaCl then splits into Na^+ (sodium ion) and Cl^- (chloride ion). In other words, the NaCl dissociates. Because the products of this dissociation are ions, this dissociation process is referred to as ionization. Only electrolytes ionize.

MOLECULES AND COMPOUNDS

MOLECULES

When two or more atoms bond together, they form a **molecule.** Two identical atoms may bond. For instance, one atom of oxygen may bond with another atom of oxygen to form a molecule of oxygen, which is designated O_2. The same bonding is true for nitrogen (N_2) and hydrogen (H_2) (Figure 2-5). A molecule can also be formed when atoms of different elements combine. For example, when two atoms of hydrogen combine with one atom of oxygen, a molecule of water (H_2O) is formed.

COMPOUNDS

A substance that contains molecules formed by two or more different atoms is called a **compound.** For example, if two atoms of hydrogen combine with one atom of oxygen, water is formed. Water is considered both a molecule and a compound.

SOME IMPORTANT COMPOUNDS AND MOLECULES

Water

Water is the most abundant compound in the body. It constitutes approximately two thirds of an adult's body weight and even more of a child's body weight. Water is essential for life. Although we can last for many weeks without food, we can last only a few days without water. What makes water so special?

- **Water as the universal solvent.** Water is called the universal solvent because most substances dissolve in water. Its use as a solvent is one of the most important characteristics of water. The ability to dissolve substances is due largely to the polar structure of water (positive charge on one end, negative charge on the other end). For instance, the plasma protein albumin carries a negative (−) charge. It is attracted to the positive (+) end of the water molecule. The attraction of the electrical charges allows albumin to dissolve in water. Many molecules dissolve in water for transport throughout the body.
- **Water as temperature regulator.** Water has the ability to absorb large amounts of heat without the temperature of the water itself increasing dramatically. This ability means that heat can be removed from heat-producing tissue, like exercising muscle, while the body maintains a normal temperature. Water, therefore, plays an important role in the body's temperature regulation.
- **Water as an ideal lubricant.** Water is a major component of mucus and other lubricating fluids. Lubricating fluids decrease friction as two structures slide past each other.
- **Water in chemical reactions.** Water often plays a crucial role in chemical reactions. For instance, water is necessary to break down carbohydrates during digestion.

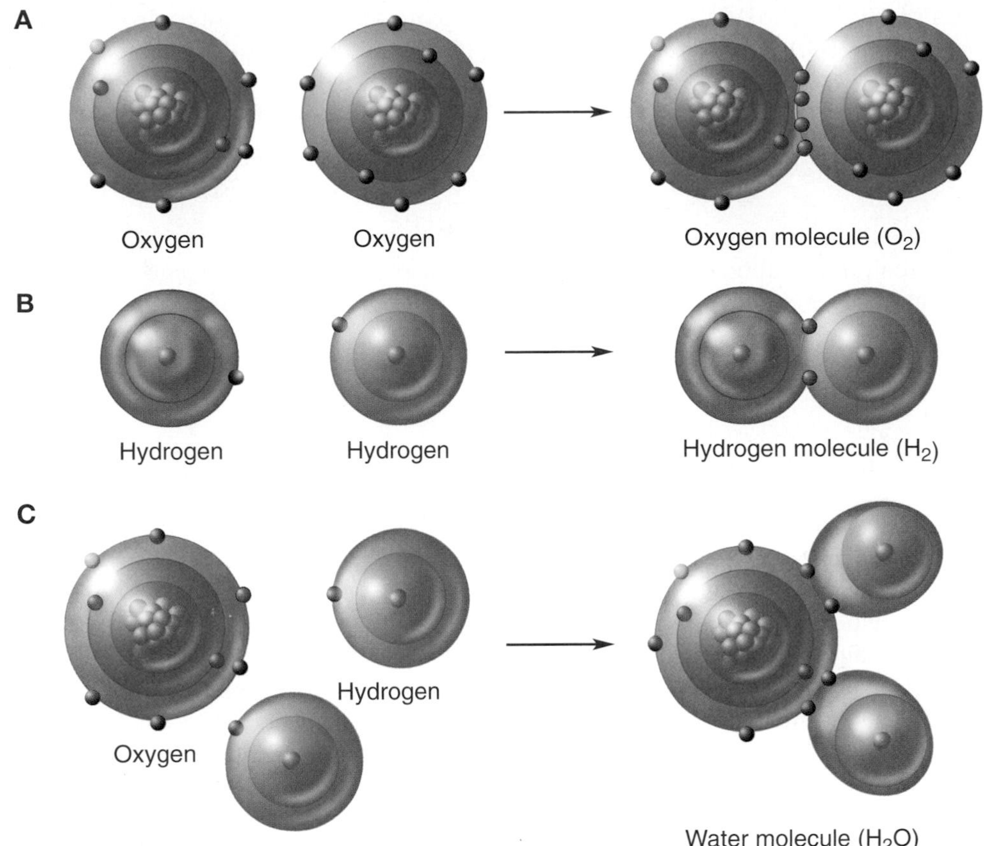

FIGURE 2-5 Molecules and compounds. **A,** Oxygen (O_2). **B,** Hydrogen (H_2). **C,** Water (H_2O).

- **Water as a protective device.** Water may also be used to protect an important structure. For instance, the cerebrospinal fluid surrounds and cushions the delicate brain and spinal cord. Likewise, the amniotic fluid surrounds and cushions the developing infant in the mother's womb.

Oxygen

Oxygen (O_2), a molecule composed of two oxygen atoms, exists in nature as a gas. The air we breathe contains 21% oxygen. Oxygen is essential for life; without a continuous supply, we would quickly die. The oxygen we breathe in is used by the cells to liberate the energy from the food we eat. This energy powers the body. Like an engine, if the body has no energy, it stops running. The importance of oxygen accounts for the urgency associated with cardiopulmonary resuscitation (CPR). If the heart stops beating, the delivery of oxygen to the tissue ceases and the brain dies.

Carbon Dioxide

Carbon dioxide (CO_2) is a compound that consists of one carbon atom and two oxygen atoms, hence the name carbon dioxide (*di-* means "two"). CO_2 is a waste product, so it must be eliminated from the body. It is made when food is chemically broken down for energy.

Sum It Up!

Chemistry is the study of matter. Matter is composed of elements such as hydrogen, oxygen, carbon, and nitrogen. Each element is composed of millions of identical atoms. Atoms are composed of subatomic particles called protons, neutrons, and electrons. Chemical bonds are formed through the interaction of one atom with another, particularly with electrons. The three chemical bonds are ionic, covalent, and hydrogen bonds. The transfer of electrons is also responsible for the formation of ions (cations and anions). Molecules and compounds are formed when atoms interact in a particular fashion.

CHEMICAL REACTIONS

A **chemical reaction** is a process whereby the atoms of molecules or compounds interact to form new chemical combinations. For instance, glucose interacts with oxygen to form carbon dioxide, water, and energy. This chemical interaction is characterized by the breaking of the chemical bonds of glucose and oxygen and the making of new bonds as carbon dioxide and water are formed. The reaction is represented as follows:

$C_6H_{12}O_6$ +	O_2	→	CO_2	+ H_2O	+ energy
glucose	oxygen		carbon dioxide	water	

The rates of chemical reactions (how fast they occur) are important. Chemical substances called **catalysts** (KĂT-ă-lĭsts) speed up the rate of a chemical reaction. When proteins perform the role of catalysts, they are called **enzymes.** Most chemical reactions require a catalyst.

ACIDS AND BASES

A normally functioning body requires a balance between substances classified as acids and as bases. Acid–base balance is important because the chemical reactions in the body occur only when these substances are in balance. Imbalances of acids and bases cause life-threatening clinical problems. An understanding of the chemistry of acids and bases is crucial to understanding acid–base balance.

ACIDS

We all recognize the sour taste of an acid. Grapefruit juice, lemon juice, and vinegar are acids. In addition to a sour taste, very strong acids, such as hydrochloric acid (HCl), can cause severe burns. Acid splashed in your eye, for instance, can damage the eye tissue to the point of blindness.

An **acid** is an electrolyte that dissociates into a hydrogen ion (H^+) and an anion. Its dissociation is represented as follows:

HCl	→	H^+	+	Cl^-
hydrochloric acid		hydrogen ion		chloride ion

In this reaction, HCl dissociates into H^+ and the chloride ion (Cl^-). For our purposes, the most important component is the H^+. The amount of H^+ in a solution determines its acidity.

A **strong acid** dissociates completely into H^+ and an anion. HCl, found within the stomach, is a strong acid; it yields many hydrogen ions. A **weak acid** does not dissociate completely. Vinegar, or acetic acid, is a weak acid. Vinegar dissociates slightly into H^+. Most of the vinegar remains in its undissociated form. Its dissociation is represented as follows:

$$\text{Vinegar} \rightleftharpoons H^+ + \text{acetate}^-$$

The heavy arrow pointing to the left indicates that the vinegar remains as vinegar, forming very little H^+. Because the number of hydrogen ions (H^+) determines the acidity of a solution, vinegar is classified as a weak acid. This weakness is the reason that vinegar does not burn your hand. HCl is so strong that it can actually burn a hole through your hand.

BASES

A **base** has a bitter taste and is slippery like soap. Bases are substances that combine with H^+. Bases usually contain the hydroxyl ion (OH^-), such as sodium hydroxide (NaOH). NaOH dissociates into sodium ion (Na^+) and the hydroxyl ion (OH^-) as follows:

$$NaOH \rightarrow Na^+ + OH^-$$

OH^- is a hydrogen ion eliminator. In other words, the OH^- soaks up a hydrogen ion. The addition of a base makes a solution less acidic.

NEUTRALIZATION OF ACIDS AND BASES

When an acid is mixed with a base, as in the following example, the H^+ of the acid combines with the OH^- of the base to form water. In addition, the Na^+ and the Cl^- combine to form a salt, NaCl. The reaction is important because the H^+ is converted to water. In other words, the acid has been neutralized. This chemical reaction is represented as follows:

HCl	+ NaOH	→	H_2O	+ NaCl
acid	base		water	salt

MEASUREMENT: THE pH SCALE

pH is a unit of measurement that indicates how many H^+ are in a solution. The **pH scale** ranges from 0 to 14 (Figure 2-6). At the midpoint of the scale, pH 7, the number of H^+ in pure water is equal to the number of OH^-. Therefore the solution is neutral. A pH that measures less than 7 on the scale indicates that the solution has more H^+ than OH^-. The solution is then said to be acidic.

Note the pH of lemon juice and vinegar on the scale. They are both less than 7. A pH measuring more than 7 indicates fewer H^+ than OH^-. These substances are bases, and the solution is said to be **basic,** or **alkaline.** The pH scale measures the degree of acidity or alkalinity.

Reading the pH Scale

Each pH unit represents a 10-fold change in H^+ concentration. For instance, a change in 1 pH unit (from 7 to 6) represents a 10-fold increase in H^+, whereas a change in 2 pH units (from 7 to 5) represents a 100-fold increase in H^+ concentration. The important point is this: very small changes in the pH reading indicate very large changes in the H^+ concentration.

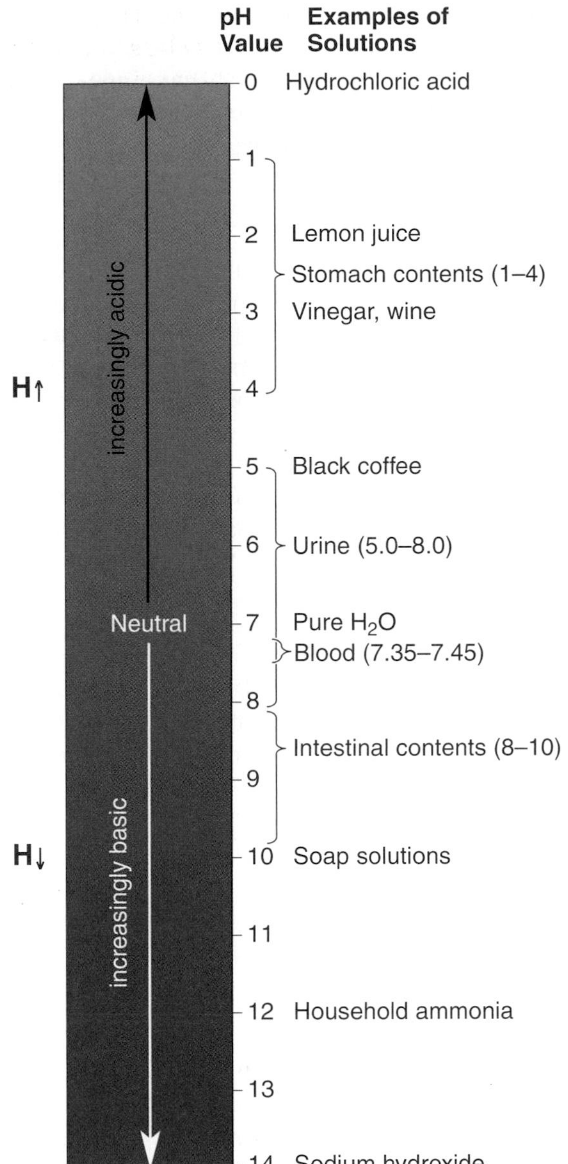

FIGURE 2-6 pH scale. The scale indicates the H^+ concentration. A pH of 0 is most acidic, whereas a pH of 14 is most alkaline. The *pink coloring* indicates the acidic range. The *blue coloring* indicates the basic, or alkaline, range. Note the pH of various substances.

pH of Body Fluids

Note the pH of some of the body fluids (see Figure 2-6). The stomach contents are very acidic, with a pH of 1 to 4. The pH of urine is normally acidic, with a pH range of 5 to 8, although a number of conditions, including diet, can change urinary pH. The intestinal secretions are alkaline, with a pH range of 8 to 10.

Blood pH is maintained within a narrow range of 7.35 to 7.45, a slightly alkaline pH. Because the blood pH is normally slightly alkaline, a blood pH of less than 7.35 is more acidic than normal, and the patient is said to be acidotic. If the patient's blood pH is greater than 7.45, the patient is said to be alkalotic. Because all of the body enzymes work best at a normal blood pH, both **acidosis** and **alkalosis** cause serious clinical problems and must be corrected. The need to maintain the body's normal alkaline state is the reason for monitoring blood pH closely during the course of a patient's illness.

The blood pH is regulated on a minute-by-minute basis by three means: a buffer system, the lungs, and the kidneys. (These processes of regulation are described in Chapters 24 and 25.)

Do You Know...

Why antacids are used?

Patients with ulcers often have excess stomach acid. The stomach acid (HCl) can be neutralized with a drug that contains a base. Because these drugs oppose acids, they are called antacids. One of the most commonly used antacids contains aluminum hydroxide. The hydroxyl ion of the drug combines with the H^+ of the stomach acid, thereby neutralizing the acid.

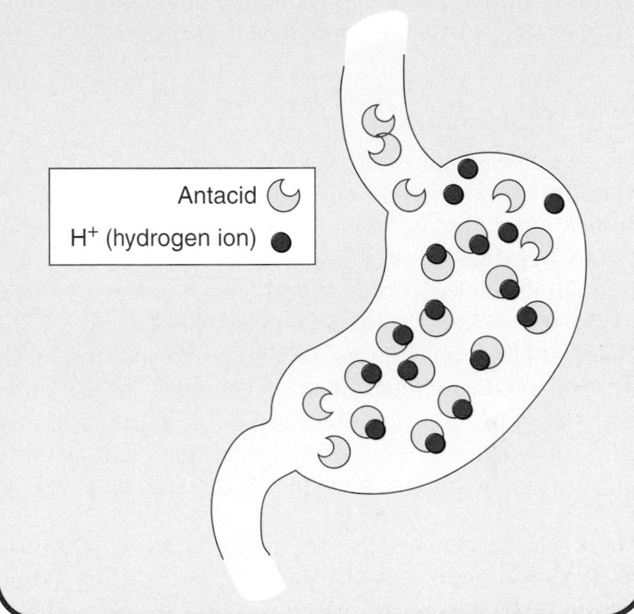

Sum It Up!

Chemical reactions are processes whereby one chemical substance is converted into a different chemical substance. The rate of a chemical reaction can be increased by a catalyst, or enzyme. A normally functioning body requires a balance between acids and bases. Hydrogen ion concentration is measured by pH. Normal blood pH is 7.35 to 7.45 and is therefore slightly alkaline. When pH falls below 7.35, the person is said to be acidotic; when pH rises above 7.45, the person is said to be alkalotic. Blood pH is regulated within normal limits by three mechanisms: buffers, lungs, and kidneys.

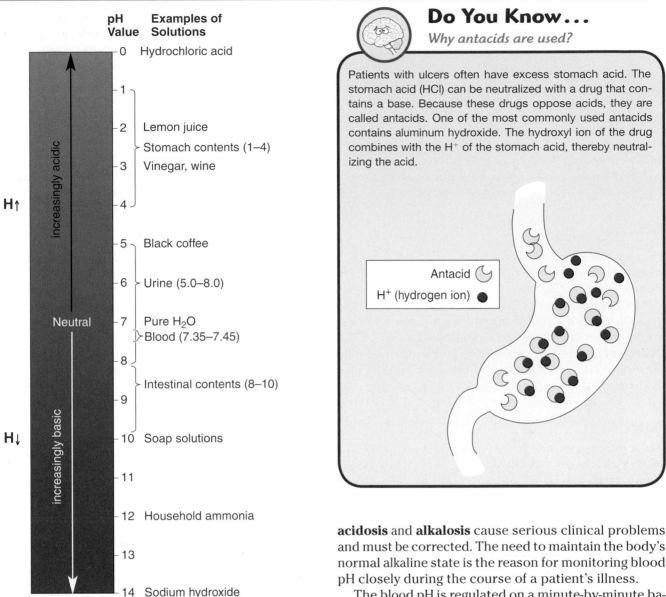

ENERGY

Energy is the ability to perform work. The body depends on a continuous supply of energy. Even at rest, the body is continuously working and using up energy. Heart muscle, for instance, is contracting and forcing blood throughout a large network of blood vessels. Nerve and muscle cells are continuously pumping sodium out of the cells. This effort sets the stage for the formation of nerve impulses. The cells of the pancreas are continuously making enzymes so that we can digest our food. Without energy, the body ceases to function.

FORMS OF ENERGY

There are six forms of energy, summarized in Table 2-3. **Mechanical energy** is expressed as movement. For instance, when the leg muscles contract, you are able to walk. **Chemical energy** is stored within the chemical bonds holding the atoms together. When the chemical bonds are broken, chemical energy is released. The released energy can then be used to perform other kinds of work, such as digesting food. This process is similar to the running of a car's engine. The energy released from the burning, or breakdown, of the gas is used to turn the engine; the running engine then moves your car.

CONVERSION OF ENERGY

Energy is easily converted from one form to another. For instance, when a log burns, the chemical energy stored in it is converted to heat **(thermal energy)** and light **(radiant energy).** In a similar way, the chemical energy stored in the muscle is converted into mechanical energy when the muscle contracts and moves your leg.

The conversion of energy in the body is generally accompanied by the release of heat. For instance, when muscles contract during strenuous exercise, chemical energy is converted into both mechanical energy (running) and heat. Recall how hot you get while exercising. (Body temperature is further described in Chapter 7.)

ENERGY TRANSFER: THE ROLE OF ADENOSINE TRIPHOSPHATE

The energy used to power the body comes from the food we eat (Figure 2-7, *A*). As the food is broken down, energy is released. This energy, however, cannot be used directly by the cells of the body. The energy must first be transferred to another substance called **adenosine triphosphate** (ă-DĔN-ō-sēn trī-FŎS-fāt) (ATP). ATP is an energy transfer molecule.

ATP is composed of three parts: a base, a sugar, and three phosphate groups (see Figure 2-7, *B*). The phosphate groups are the most important part of the ATP molecule. The phosphate groups have unique chemical bonds. The "squiggly" lines connecting the second and third phosphate groups indicate that these bonds are high-energy bonds. When these bonds are broken, a large amount of energy is released. More importantly, the energy released from ATP can be used directly by the cell to perform its tasks.

The energy stored within the high-energy bonds is similar to the energy stored in a loaded mousetrap (see Figure 2-7, *C*). Energy is stored in the trap when you set the metal bar in its loaded position. When the trap is set off by the mouse, the metal bar snaps back into its original position, thereby releasing the stored energy. Similarly, when energy is needed by the body, ATP is split. The energy that was stored in ATP is released. In other words, the bond that holds the end phosphate group is broken, and energy is released. With the release of energy, the splitting of ATP also yields adenosine diphosphate (ADP) and phosphate (P). This process is indicated as follows:

$$\text{ATP} \rightarrow \text{Energy} + \text{ADP} + \text{P}$$

ADP is almost identical to ATP, but the molecule now has one less phosphate group. ATP is replenished when energy, obtained from burning food, reattaches the end phosphate to ADP as follows:

$$\text{ADP} + \text{P} + \text{Energy} \rightarrow \text{ATP}$$

Table 2-3 Forms of Energy

Form of Energy	Description	Example
Mechanical	Energy that causes movement	Movement of legs in running, walking; contraction of heart muscle, causing movement of blood
Chemical	Energy stored in chemical bonds	Fuel to do work, like running
Electrical	Energy released from the movement of charged particles	Electrical signal involved in the transmission of information along nerves
Radiant	Energy that travels in waves	Light: stimulates the eyes for vision; ultraviolet radiation from the sun for tanning
Thermal	Energy transferred because of a temperature difference	Responsible for body temperature
Nuclear	Energy released during the decay of radioactive substances such as isotopes	Not useful physiologically

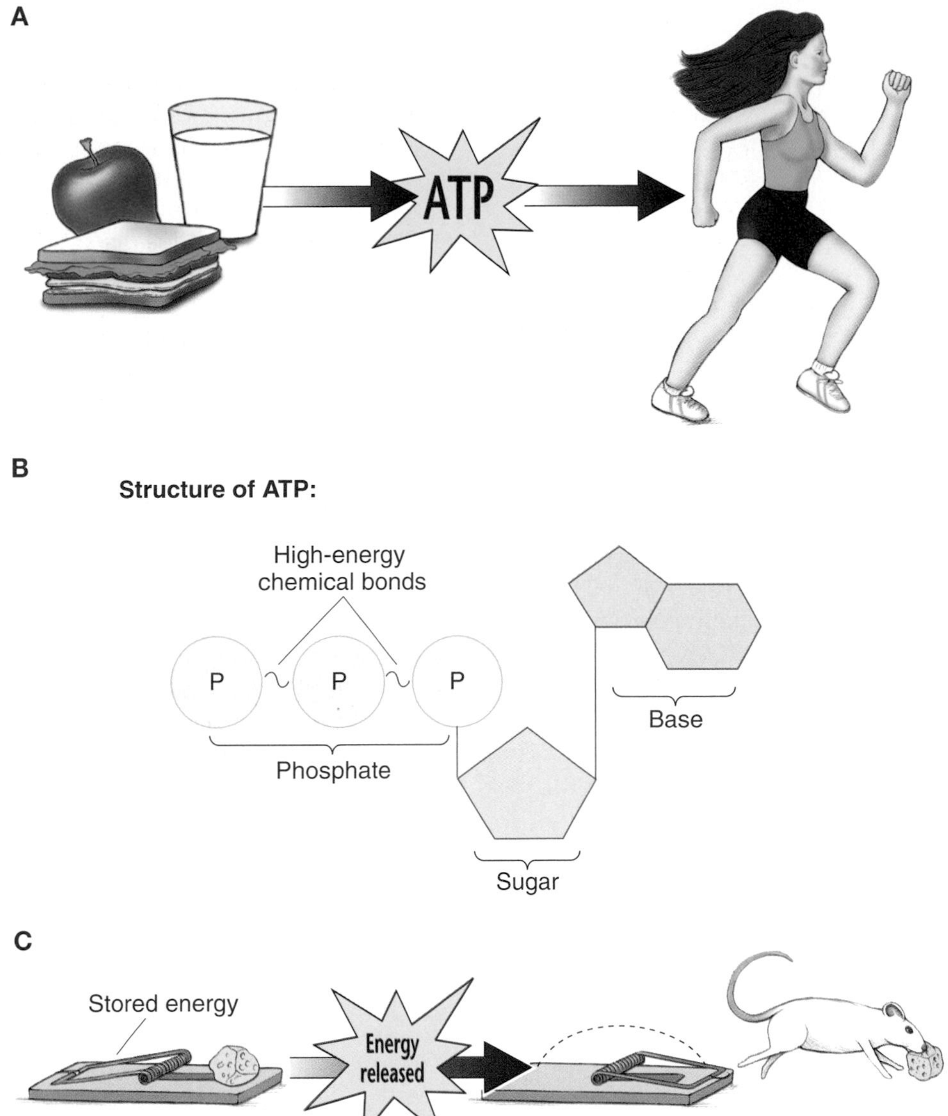

FIGURE 2-7 Energy. **A,** Source of energy. **B,** Storage of energy within the high-energy bonds of ATP. **C,** Release of energy.

MIXTURES, SOLUTIONS, AND SUSPENSIONS

You will encounter several other chemical terms in clinical situations.

MIXTURES

Mixtures are combinations of two or more substances that can be separated by ordinary physical means. When separated, the substances retain their original properties. For instance, imagine that you have a mixture of sugar and little bits of iron. A magnet is then moved close to this sugar-iron mixture. The magnet pulls all of the iron away from the sugar, thereby separating the two substances. Note that the two substances have retained their original properties. The sugar is still sugar, and the iron is still iron.

SOLUTIONS

Solutions are mixtures. In a solution, the particles that are mixed together remain evenly distributed. Salt water is an example of a solution. A solution has two parts, a solvent and a solute. The **solute** is the substance present in the smaller amount; it is the substance being dissolved. The salt in the salt water is the solute. The solute can be solid, liquid, or gas.

The **solvent** is the part of the solution present in the greater amount. It does the dissolving. Water is the solvent in salt water. The solvent is usually liquid or gas. If water is the solvent, the solution is referred to as an **aqueous solution.** If alcohol is the solvent, the solution is referred to as a **tincture.** A solution is always clear, and the solute does not settle to the bottom.

SUSPENSIONS

Suspensions are mixtures. In a suspension the particles are relatively large and tend to settle to the bottom unless the mixture is shaken continuously. For instance, if sand and water are shaken together and then allowed to sit undisturbed, the sand gradually settles to the bottom.

In a **colloidal suspension,** the particles do not dissolve, but they are so small that they remain suspended within the liquid, even when not being shaken. A **colloid** is a gel-like substance that resembles egg whites. The body contains many colloidal suspensions. Blood plasma is a colloidal suspension because the proteins remain suspended within the plasma. Other examples of colloidal suspensions include mayonnaise and jelly.

Sum It Up!

Energy is the ability to do work. Without an adequate supply of energy, the body cannot work, and it dies. Energy is derived from food and transferred to high-energy bonds in ATP. When needed, the energy is released from ATP and used to power the body. Chemical combinations include mixtures, solutions, and suspensions.

SUMMARY OUTLINE

Our bodies are made of different chemicals. To understand the body, you need to understand some general chemical principles.

I. Matter, Elements, and Atoms
- A. Matter
  1. Matter is anything that occupies space and has weight.
  2. Matter exists in three states: solid, liquid, and gas.
  3. Matter can undergo physical and chemical changes.
- B. Elements
  1. An element is a fundamental substance that cannot be broken down into a simpler form by ordinary chemical means.
  2. Four elements (carbon, hydrogen, oxygen, and nitrogen) make up 96% of the body weight.
- C. Atoms
  1. An atom is the basic unit of matter.
  2. An atom is composed of three subatomic particles: neutrons, protons, and electrons.
  3. The atomic number: the number of protons. The atomic weight: the number of the neutrons and protons.
  4. An isotope is an atom with the same atomic number but a different atomic weight. A radioisotope is an unstable isotope.

II. Chemical Bonds
- A. Electron Shells and Bonding
  1. Each electron shell holds a specific number of electrons.
  2. Ionic bonds are formed as electrons are transferred to stabilize the shells of the atoms.
  3. Covalent bonds are formed as the electrons of the outer shells are shared by the interacting atoms.
  4. Hydrogen bonds are intermolecular bonds.

III. Ions
- A. An ion is an atom that carries an electrical charge. A cation is a positively charged ion. An anion is a negatively charged ion.
- B. An electrolyte is a substance that forms ions when dissolved in water.

IV. Molecules and Compounds
- A. A molecule is a substance formed by two or more atoms (O_2, H_2O).
- B. A compound is a substance that forms when two or more different atoms bond (H_2O).
- C. Important molecules and compounds include water, oxygen, and carbon dioxide.

V. Acids and Bases
- A. An acid is an electrolyte that dissociates into hydrogen ion (H^+).
- B. A base is a substance that combines with H^+ and eliminates H^+; a base neutralizes an acid by producing a salt and water.
- C. The pH scale measures acidity and alkalinity. A pH of 7 is neutral. A pH less than 7 is acidic, and a pH greater than 7 is basic, or alkaline.
- D. The normal pH of the blood is 7.35 to 7.45. A person with a pH less than 7.35 is acidotic, and a person with a pH greater than 7.45 is alkalotic.
- E. Blood pH is regulated by buffers, the respiratory system, and the kidneys.

VI. Energy
- A. Definition: The Ability to Do Work
- B. Forms of Energy
  1. The six forms of energy: see Table 2-3.
  2. Most energy is released as heat.
- C. Role of Adenosine Triphosphate (ATP)
  1. ATP is an energy-transfer molecule.
  2. The energy is stored in high-energy phosphate bonds.

VII. **Mixtures, Solutions, and Suspensions**
   A. A mixture is a blend of two or more substances that can be separated by ordinary physical means.
   B. Solutions, suspensions, and colloidal suspensions are types of mixtures.

Review Your Knowledge

Matching: Atoms and Elements

Directions: Match the following words with their descriptions below.

a. atom
b. K
c. matter
d. Na
e. ion

1. ____ Composed of three particles: protons, neutrons, and electrons
2. ____ The symbol for potassium
3. ____ The symbol for sodium
4. ____ Exists in three states: liquid, solid, and gas
5. ____ Formed when sodium loses an electron

Matching: Structure of the Atom

Directions: Match the following words with their descriptions below. Some words may be used more than once, others not at all.

a. atomic weight
b. isotope
c. protons
d. electrons
e. neutrons
f. atomic number

1. ____ The number of protons in the nucleus
2. ____ The sum of the protons and neutrons
3. ____ A different form of the same element: same atomic number but a different atomic weight
4. ____ In each atom the number of these is equal to the number of protons
5. ____ Circulate in orbits around the nucleus

Matching: Ions and Electrolytes

Directions: Match the following words with their descriptions below.

a. cation
b. ions
c. electrolyte
d. anion
e. ionization

1. ____ Classification of KCl
2. ____ Classification of K^+ and Cl^-
3. ____ K^+ is an ion that is classified as a (an)
4. ____ Cl^- is an ion that is classified as a (an)
5. ____ The dissociation of $KCl \rightarrow K^+ + Cl^-$

Matching: Acids and Bases

Directions: Match the following words with their descriptions below. Some words may be used more than once, others not at all.

a. alkalosis
b. pH
c. H^+
d. base
e. acid
f. acidosis

1. ____ An electrolyte that dissociates into H^+ and an anion
2. ____ The ion that makes a solution more acidic
3. ____ A measurement of hydrogen ion concentration $[H^+]$
4. ____ The condition characterized by a pH less than 7.35
5. ____ The condition caused by excess H^+

Multiple Choice

1. The ionization of salt (NaCl)
   a. is called a neutralization reaction.
   b. lowers pH.
   c. produces a cation (Na^+) and an anion (Cl^-).
   d. causes acidosis.
2. Which of the following is true of iodine and radioactive iodine?
   a. Both have the same atomic numbers.
   b. Both have the same atomic weights.
   c. Neither have electrons in their orbitals.
   d. Both create radiation hazards.
3. Which of the following is not true of Na^+?
   a. It's called the sodium ion.
   b. It has more protons than electrons.
   c. It's called a cation.
   d. It is measured by pH.
4. Which of the following is true of water?
   a. It is a molecule.
   b. It is an aqueous solvent.
   c. It is a compound.
   d. All of the above.
5. Which of the following best describes ATP?
   a. It is a buffer, removing H^+ from solution.
   b. It is an energy-transfer molecule.
   c. It is a radioactive isotope of phosphate.
   d. It ionizes to H^+, thereby lowering pH.

6. Which of the following has donated an electron?
   a. H_2O
   b. Cl^-
   c. Na^+
   d. HCO_3^-
7. Which of the following is least descriptive of the nucleus of the atom?
   a. Contents determine the atomic number.
   b. Contents determine the atomic weight.
   c. It is "home" of the electrons.
   d. It is "home" of the protons.
8. Which of the following is descriptive of the patient with a blood pH of 7.28?
   a. He has a deficiency of H^+.
   b. pH is within normal limits.
   c. He is acidotic.
   d. He is dehydrated.

CHAPTER 3

Cells

KEY TERMS

Active transport, p. 35
Cell cycle, p. 41
Cell membrane, p. 30
Cells, p. 30
Cytoplasm, p. 33
Differentiate, p. 42
Diffusion, p. 36
Endocytosis, p. 40
Endoplasmic reticulum, p. 33
Equilibrium, p. 36
Exocytosis, p. 40
Facilitated diffusion, p. 36
Filtration, p. 39
Golgi apparatus, p. 34
Lysosomes, p. 34
Mitochondria, p. 33
Mitosis, p. 41
Nucleus, p. 33
Organelle, p. 33
Osmosis, p. 36
Passive transport, p. 35
Ribosomes, p. 33

OBJECTIVES

1. Label a diagram of the main parts of a typical cell.
2. Describe the functions of the main organelles of the cell.
3. Explain the role of the nucleus.
4. Identify the structure of the cell membrane.
5. Describe the active and passive movement of substances across a cell membrane.
6. Define *tonicity* and compare isotonic, hypotonic, and hypertonic solutions.
7. Describe the phases of the cell cycle, including mitosis.
8. Explain what is meant by cell differentiation.

What do this monk and a cell have in common? While looking at a piece of cork under a microscope in the 1600s, Robert Hooke observed cube-like structures that resembled the rooms, or cells, occupied by monks in a monastery. Hooke therefore called his structures **cells.**

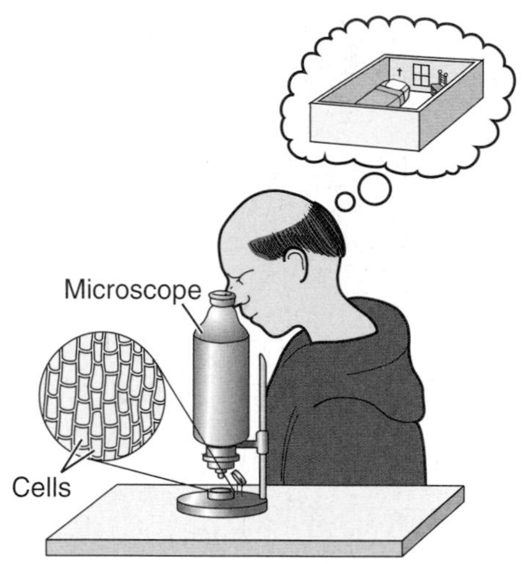

The cell is the structural and functional unit of all living matter. Cells vary considerably in size, shape, and function. A red blood cell, for instance, is tiny, whereas a single nerve cell may measure 4 feet in length (Figure 3-1). The shapes and structures of the cells are also very different. The red blood cell is shaped like a Frisbee and is able to bend. The shape allows it to squeeze through tiny blood vessels and deliver oxygen throughout the body. Some nerve cells are very long and many resemble bushes or trees. Their shapes enable them to conduct electrical signals quickly over long distances. Cell structure and function are closely related.

A TYPICAL CELL

Despite the differences, cells have many similarities. Figure 3-2 is a typical cell with all known cellular components. Each specialized cell, such as a nerve cell, possesses some or all of the properties of the typical cell.

The cell is encased in a membrane. Many smaller structures are inside the cell. Table 3-1 summarizes the functions of these cellular components.

CELL MEMBRANE

The cell is encased by a **cell membrane,** also called the plasma membrane. The cell membrane separates intracellular (inside the cell) material from extracellular

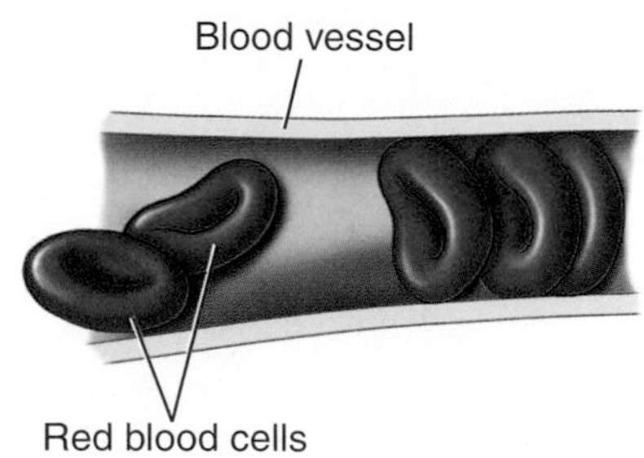

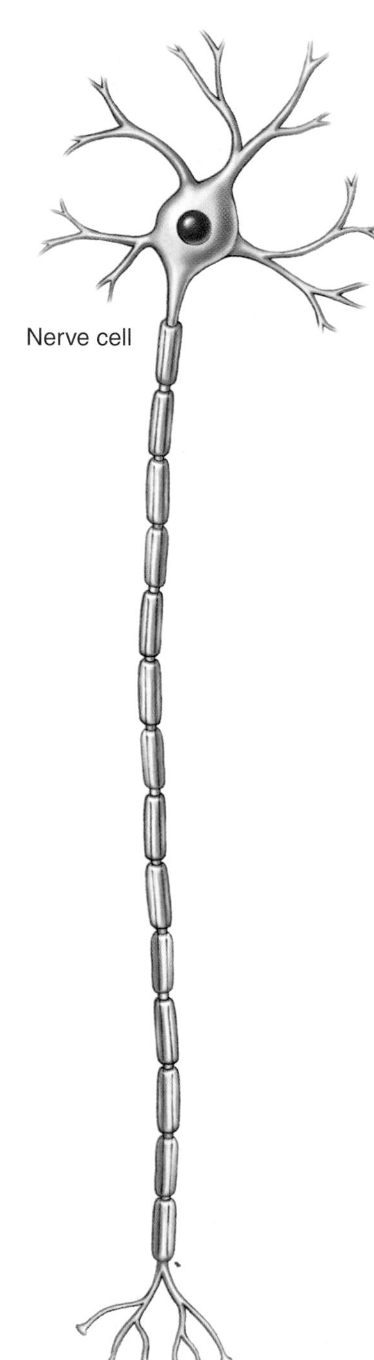

FIGURE 3-1 Cells come in all shapes and sizes.

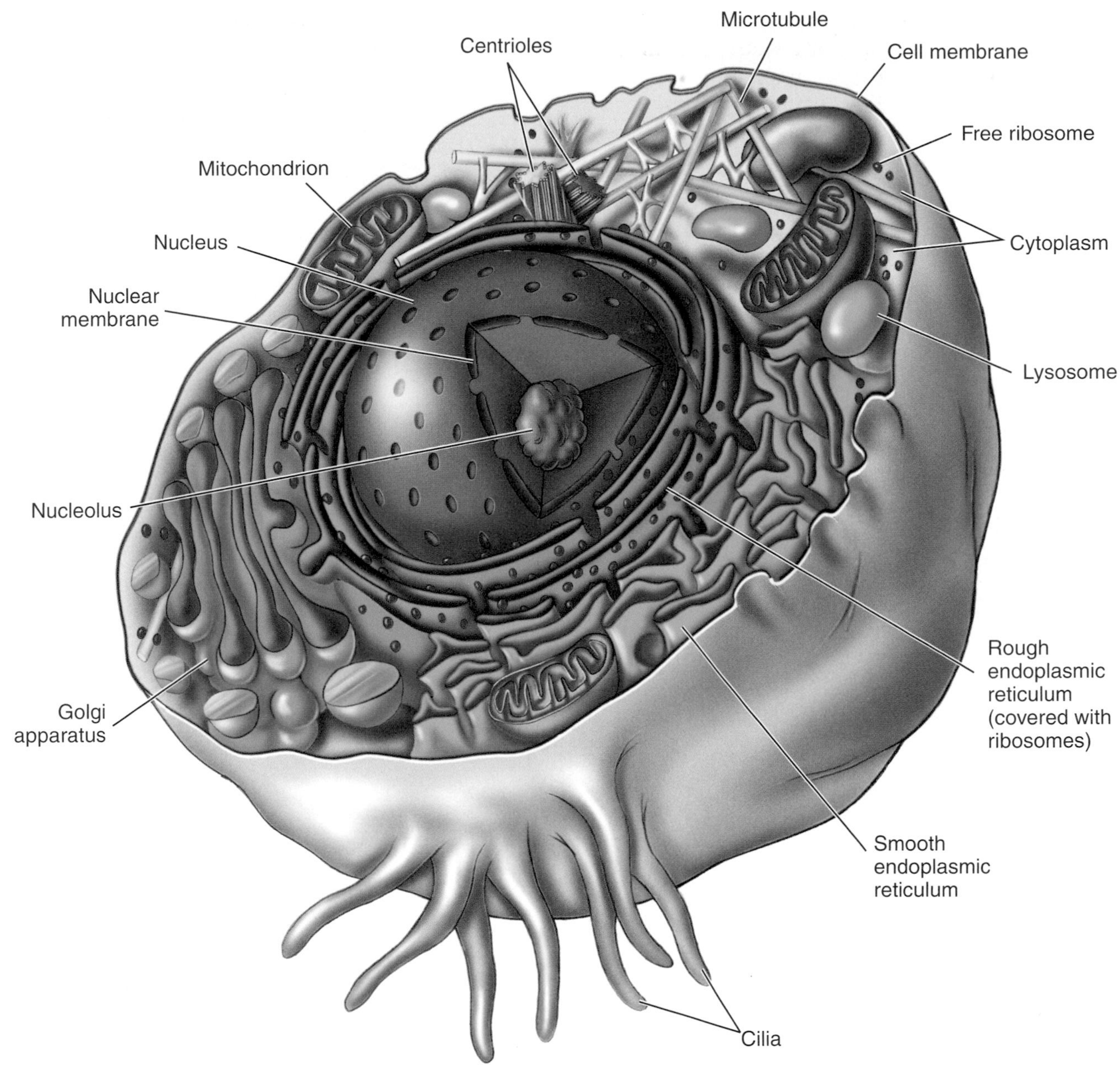

FIGURE 3-2 A typical cell.

(outside the cell) material. In addition to physically holding the cell together, the cell membrane performs other important functions. One of its chief functions is the selection of substances allowed to enter or leave the cell. Because the membrane chooses the substances allowed to cross it, the membrane is said to be selectively permeable, or **semipermeable.**

What is a cell membrane made of? The cell membrane is composed primarily of phospholipids and protein (Figure 3-3). The phospholipids are arranged in two layers. The protein molecules in the membrane perform several important functions: they provide structural support for the membrane, act as binding sites for hormones, and poke holes, or pores, through the lipid membrane. These pores form channels through which water and dissolved substances can flow.

Substances move across the selectively permeable membrane either by dissolving in the lipid portion of the membrane, as oxygen and carbon dioxide do, or by flowing through the pores. Electrically charged substances such as sodium and chloride cannot penetrate the lipid membrane and must use the pores. The size of the pores also helps select which substances cross the membrane. Substances larger than the pores cannot cross the membrane, whereas smaller substances such as sodium and chloride flow through easily.

Table 3-1 Cell Structure and Function

Cell Structure	Function
Cell membrane	Contains cellular contents: regulates what enters and leaves the cell
Cytoplasm	Surrounds and supports organelles; medium through which nutrients and waste move
Nucleus	Contains genetic information; control center of the cell
Endoplasmic reticulum (ER)	Transports material through the cytoplasm
• Rough	Contains the ribosomes where protein is synthesized
• Smooth	Site of steroid synthesis
Mitochondria	Convert energy in nutrients to ATP (power plants of the cell)
Golgi apparatus	Packages protein in membrane; puts the finishing touches on protein
Ribosomes	Sites of protein synthesis
Lysosomes	"Housekeeping" within the cell; phagocytosis through powerful enzymes
Cytoskeleton	Provides for intracellular shape and support
Centrioles	Help separate the chromosomes during mitosis
Cilia	Create movement over the cell surface
Flagella	Create movement of cell (e.g., allow the sperm to swim)

ATP, Adenosine triphosphate.

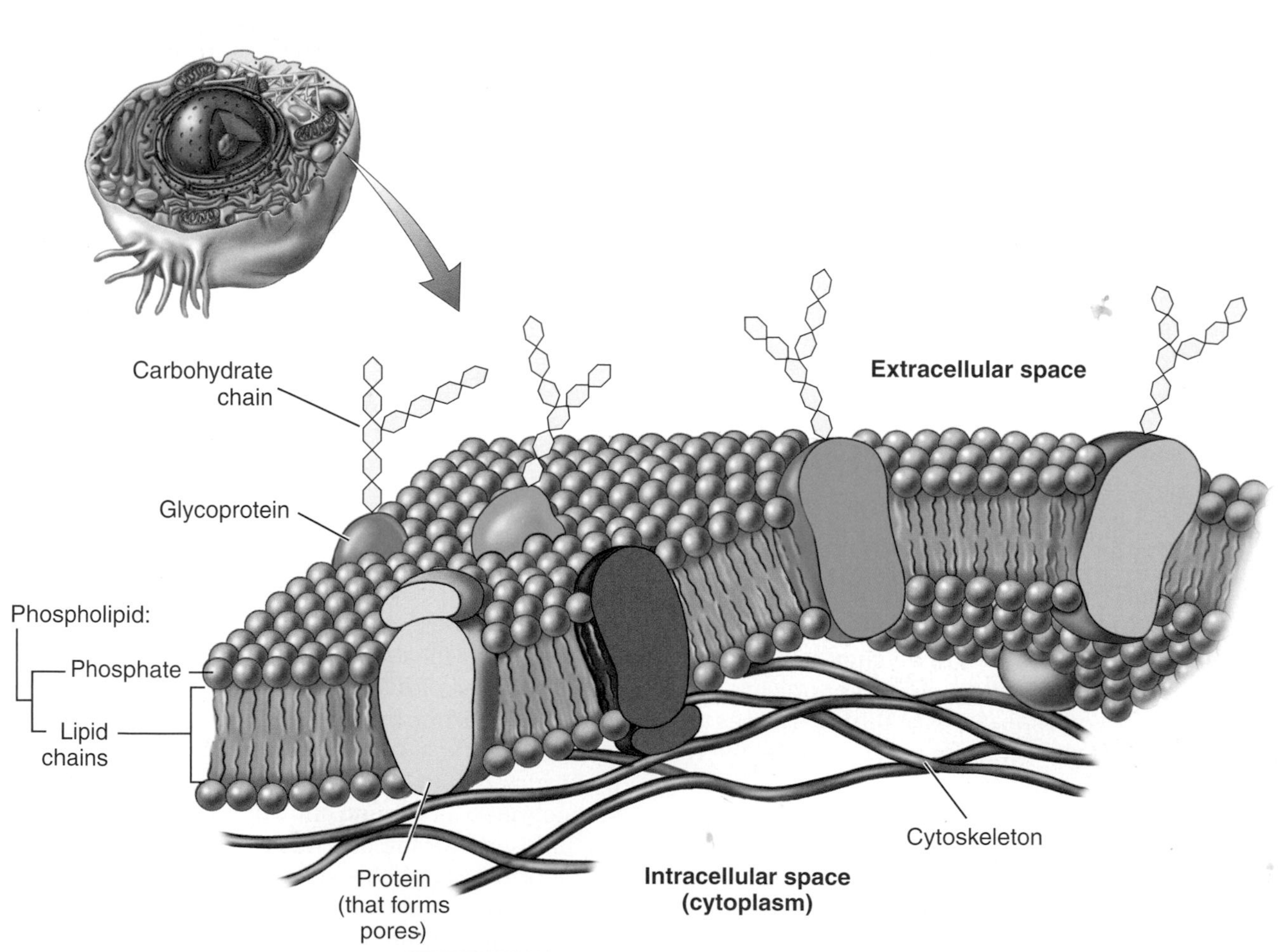

FIGURE 3-3 Structure of the cell membrane.

INSIDE THE CELL

The inside of the cell is divided into two compartments: the nucleus and the cytoplasm. The inside of the cell resembles the inside of a raw egg. The yellow yolk is like the nucleus, and the white is like the cytoplasm.

Nucleus

The **nucleus** is the control center; it controls the workings of the entire cell (see Figure 3-2). In particular, the nucleus contains the genetic information and controls all protein synthesis. Most adult cells have one nucleus. Only mature red blood cells have no nucleus. Surrounding the nucleus is a double-layered **nuclear membrane.** The nuclear membrane contains large pores that allow the free movement of certain substances between the nucleus and the cytoplasm.

The nucleus is filled with a substance called **nucleoplasm.** It also contains two other structures: (1) the nucleolus, or little nucleus, and (2) chromatin, which are threadlike structures that contain genes.

Cytoplasm

Cytoplasmic Gel. The **cytoplasm** (CĪ-tŏ-plăzm) is a gel-like substance found inside the cell but outside the nucleus (it's like the white of a raw egg). The "gel in the cell" is composed primarily of water, electrolytes, and nutrients. The cytoplasm contains numerous organelles and inclusion bodies. The **organelles** (ŏr-gă-NĔLZ), or little organs, each have a specific role. The inclusion bodies are temporary structures that appear and disappear. These include water vacuoles, secretory vesicles, and various granules. Locate the organelles in Figure 3-2.

Cytoplasmic Organelles

Mitochondria. The **mitochondria** (mī-tō-KŎN-drē-ă) are tiny, slipper-shaped organelles. The number of mitochondria per cell varies, depending on the metabolic activity of the cell (how hard the cell works). The more metabolically active the cell, the greater the number of mitochondria. The liver, for instance, is very active and therefore has many mitochondria per cell. Bone cells are less active metabolically and have fewer mitochondria.

The mitochondrial membrane has two layers (Figure 3-4). The outer layer is smooth, whereas the inner layer has many folds, referred to as **cristae.** The enzymes associated with ATP production are located along the cristae. Because the mitochondria produce most of the energy (ATP) in the body, they are referred to as the "power plants" of the cell. (See Chapter 2 for an explanation of ATP.)

Ribosomes. Ribosomes (RĪ-bō-sōmz) are cytoplasmic organelles concerned with protein synthesis, which is explained in Chapter 4. Some ribosomes are attached to the endoplasmic reticulum. Others float freely within the cytoplasm.

Endoplasmic Reticulum. The **endoplasmic reticulum** (ĕn-dō-PLĂS-mĭk rĕ-TĬK-ū-lŭm) **(ER)** is a network of membranes within the cytoplasm (see Figure 3-2). These long, folded membranes form channels through which substances move. The two types of ER include the kind containing ribosomes along its surface; it is called **rough endoplasmic reticulum (RER)** because of its rough, sandpaper-like appearance. The RER is primarily concerned with protein synthesis. Protein synthesized along the RER is transported through the

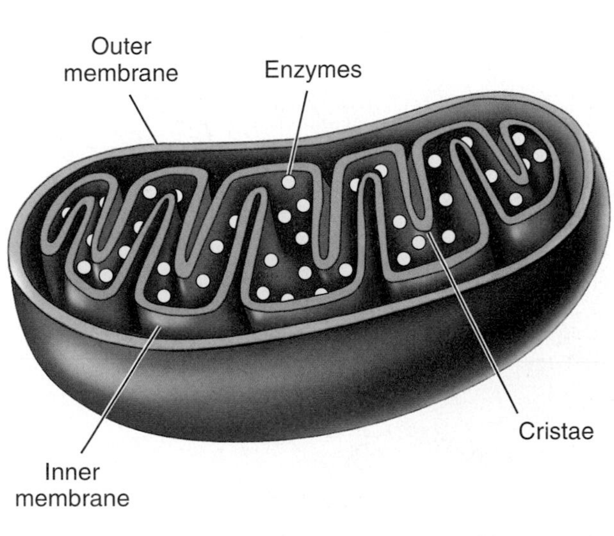

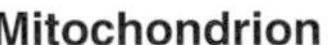

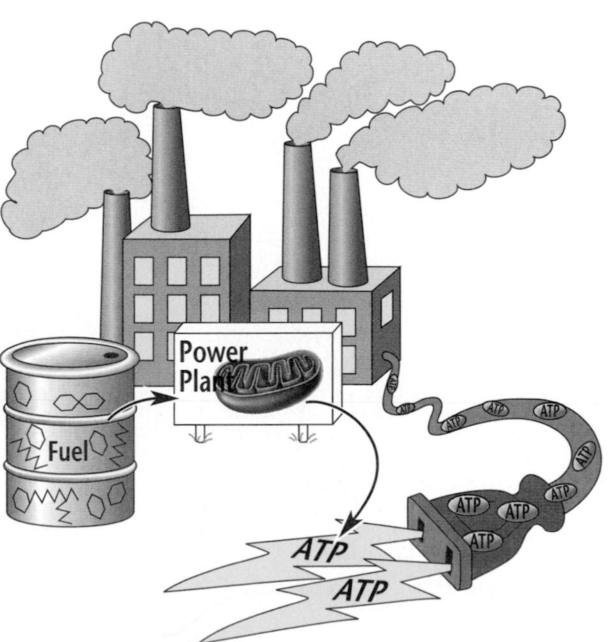

FIGURE 3-4 Mitochondria are the power plants of the cells.

channels to the Golgi apparatus for further processing. The ER that does not contain ribosomes on its surface appears smooth; it is therefore called **smooth endoplasmic reticulum (SER).** SER is primarily concerned with the synthesis of lipids and steroids.

Golgi Apparatus. The **Golgi** (GŌL-jē) **apparatus** is a series of flattened membranous sacs (Figure 3-5). Proteins synthesized along the RER are transported to the Golgi through channels formed by the ER. The Golgi put the finishing touches on the protein. For example, a glucose molecule may be attached to a protein within the Golgi apparatus. A segment of the Golgi membrane then wraps itself around the protein and pinches itself off to form a secretory vesicle. In this way the Golgi apparatus packages the protein for secretion.

Lysosomes. Lysosomes (LĪ-sō-sōmz) are membranous sacs containing powerful enzymes. Lysosomes are digestive organelles. Lysosomal enzymes break down intracellular waste and debris and thus help to "clean house." Lysosomal enzymes perform several other functions. For instance, they participate in the destruction of bacteria, a process called phagocytosis.

Cytoskeleton. The **cytoskeleton** is composed of threadlike structures called microfilaments and microtubules (tiny tubelike structures). The cytoskeleton helps to maintain the shape of the cell and assists the cell in various forms of cellular movement. Cellular movement is particularly evident in muscle cells, which contain large numbers of microfilaments.

Centrioles. Centrioles are paired, rod-shaped microtubular structures that play a key role in cellular reproduction.

ON THE CELL MEMBRANE

Cilia

Cilia are short, hairlike projections on the outer surface of the cell. Cilia use wavelike motions to move substances across the surface of the cell. For instance, cilia are abundant on the cells that line the respiratory

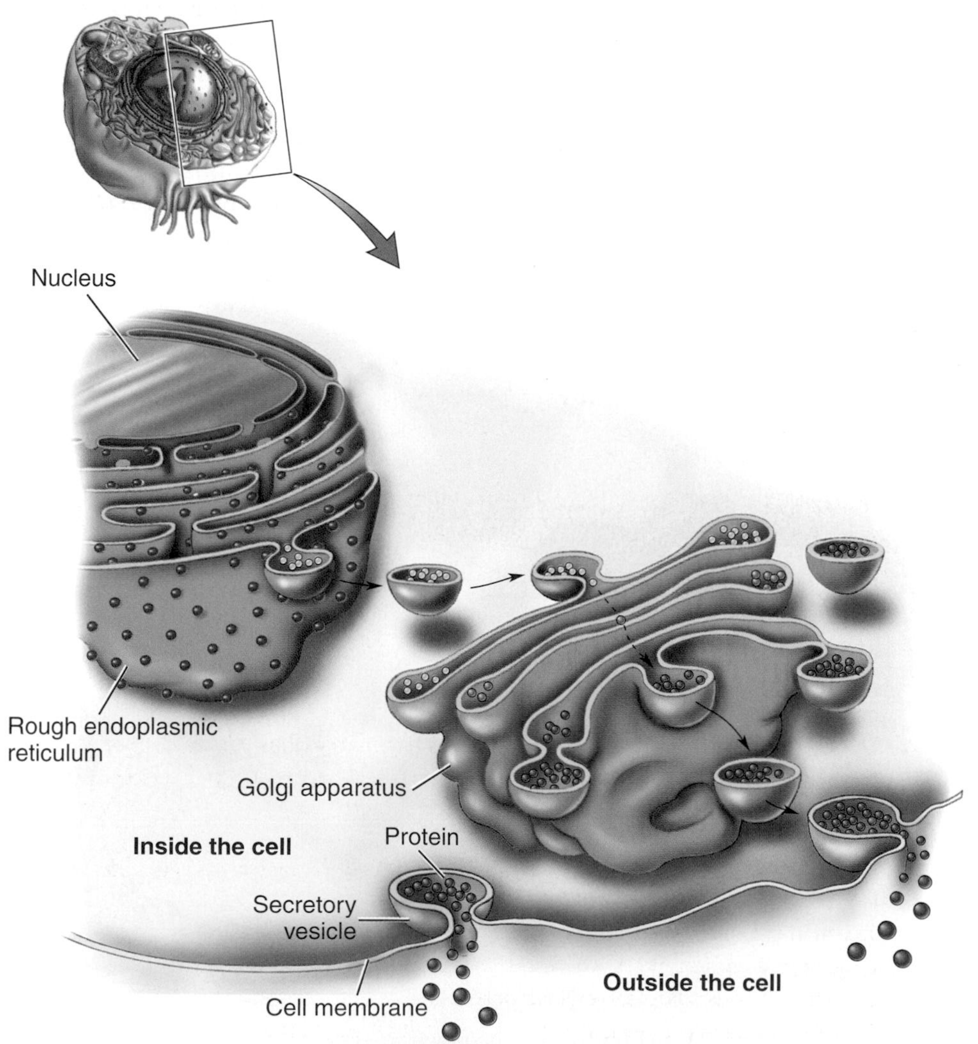

FIGURE 3-5 The Golgi apparatus.

passages. The cilia help move mucus and trapped dust and dirt toward the throat, away from the lungs. Once in the throat, the mucus can be removed by coughing. The cilia therefore help to keep the respiratory passages clean and clear. Cigarette smoking damages the cilia and thus deprives the smoker of this benefit.

Flagella

Flagella (meaning whiplike) are similar to cilia in that both are hairlike projections. Flagella, however, are thicker, longer, and fewer in number; they help move the cell. The tail of the sperm is an example of a flagellum; the tail enables the sperm to swim.

> **Sum It Up!**
>
> The cell is the structural and functional unit of all living matter. Although cells differ considerably, they also share many similarities. The cell is surrounded by a cell membrane. The inside of the cell is divided into the nucleus and the cytoplasm. The nucleus is the control center of the cell. The cytoplasm contains many little organs, or organelles, each of which has a special task to perform.

MOVEMENT ACROSS THE CELL MEMBRANE

Cells are bathed in an extracellular fluid that is rich in nutrients such as oxygen, glucose, and amino acids. These nutrients are needed within the cell and must therefore be able to cross the cell membrane. The cell's waste, which accumulates within the cell, must also be able to cross the cell membrane. Wastes are eventually eliminated from the body.

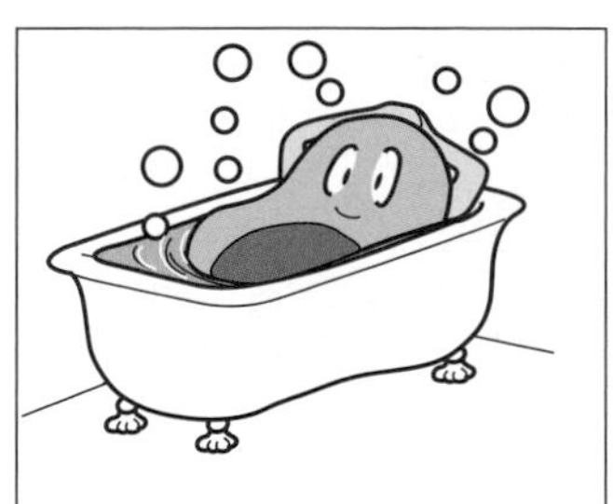

A number of mechanisms assist in the movement of water and dissolved substances across the cell membrane. The transport mechanisms can be divided into two groups: **passive transport** and **active transport** mechanisms. Table 3-2 summarizes both kinds of transport.

The passive transport mechanisms require no additional energy in the form of ATP. Passive transport is something like the downward movement of a ball (Figure 3-6, *A*). The ball is at the top of the hill. Once released, the ball rolls downhill. The ball does not need to be pushed; it moves passively, without any input of energy. Passive transport mechanisms cause water and dissolved substances to move without additional energy, like a ball rolling downhill.

Active transport mechanisms require an input of energy in the form of ATP. Active transport is like the upward movement of a ball (see Figure 3-6, *B*). For the ball to move uphill, it must be pushed, therefore requiring an input of energy.

PASSIVE TRANSPORT MECHANISMS

The passive mechanisms that move substances across the membrane include diffusion, facilitated diffusion, osmosis, and filtration.

Table 3-2 Transport Mechanisms

Mechanism	Description
Passive	
Diffusion	Movement of a substance from an area of high concentration to an area of low concentration
Facilitated diffusion	A helper molecule within the membrane assists the movement of substances from an area of high concentration to an area of low concentration
Osmosis	Movement of water (solvent) from an area with more water to an area with less
Filtration	Movement of water and dissolved substances from an area of high pressure to an area of low pressure; the water and dissolved substances are pushed
Active	
Active transport pumps	Movement of a substance uphill (from an area of low concentration to an area of high concentration). Requires an input of energy (ATP)
Endocytosis	Taking in or ingestion of substances by the cell membrane
Phagocytosis	Engulfing of solid particles by the cell membrane (cellular eating)
Pinocytosis	Engulfing of liquid droplets (cellular drinking)
Exocytosis	Secretion of cellular products (e.g., protein, debris) out of the cell

ATP, Adenosine triphosphate.

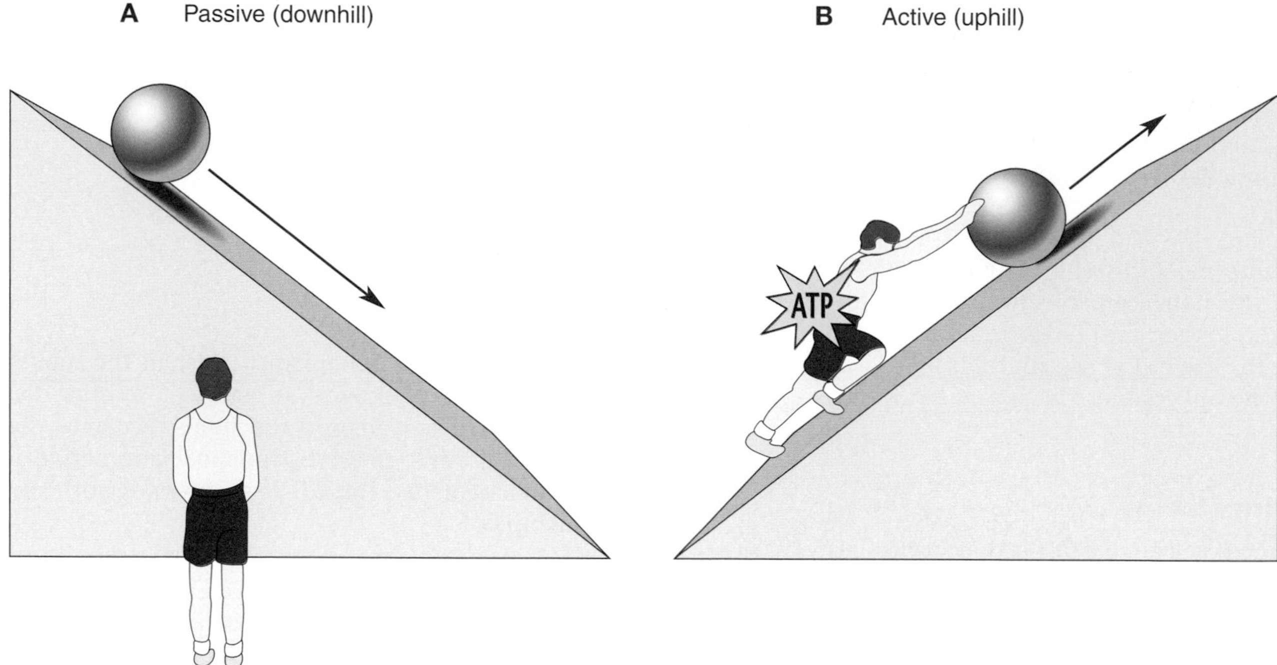

FIGURE 3-6 Transport mechanisms. **A,** Passive transport mechanisms: the ball rolls downhill on its own. **B,** Active transport mechanisms: the ball must be pushed uphill.

Diffusion

Diffusion (dĭ-FŪ-zhŭn) is the most common transport mechanism. Diffusion is the movement of a substance from an area of higher concentration to an area of lower concentration. For instance, a tablet of red dye is placed in a glass of water (Figure 3-7, *A*). The tablet dissolves, and the dye moves from an area where it is most concentrated (glass number 1) to an area where it is less concentrated (glasses number 2 and 3). Diffusion continues until the dye is evenly distributed throughout the glass. The point at which no further net diffusion occurs (glass number 3) is called **equilibrium.**

The scent of our pet skunk, Perfume, also illustrates diffusion (see Figure 3-7, *B*). Perfume's scent does not take long to permeate the area! Diffusion is involved in many physiological events. For instance, diffusion causes oxygen to move across the membrane of an alveolus of the lung into the blood (see Figure 3-7, *C*). Oxygen diffuses from the alveolus because the concentration of oxygen is greater within the alveolus than within the blood. Conversely, carbon dioxide, a waste product that accumulates within the blood, diffuses in the opposite direction (carbon dioxide moves from the blood into the alveolus). The lungs then exhale the carbon dioxide, thereby eliminating waste from the body. Thus the process of diffusion moves oxygen into the blood and carbon dioxide out of the blood.

Facilitated Diffusion

Facilitated diffusion is a form of diffusion and is responsible for the transport of many substances. As in diffusion, substances move from a higher concentration toward a lower concentration (Figure 3-8). In facilitated diffusion, however, the substance is helped across the membrane by a molecule within the membrane. (Facilitate means to help.) The helper molecule increases the rate of diffusion. The transport of glucose by facilitated diffusion is illustrated by a boy carrying the glucose. Note that he is moving downhill, indicating that facilitated diffusion is a passive transport process.

Osmosis

Osmosis (ŏz-MŌ-sĭs) is a special case of diffusion. Osmosis is the diffusion of water through a selectively permeable membrane. A selectively permeable—or semipermeable—membrane allows the passage of some substances while restricting the passage of others. During osmosis, the water diffuses from an area with more water to one with less. The dissolved substances, however, do not move.

Two different solutions in the glass illustrate osmosis. The glass is divided into two compartments (A and B) by a semipermeable membrane (Figure 3-9). Compartment A contains a dilute glucose solution, whereas compartment B contains a more concentrated glucose solution. The membrane is permeable only to water. The glucose cannot cross the membrane and is therefore confined to its compartment.

During osmosis, the water moves from compartment A to compartment B (from the area where there is more water to the area with less). The following two effects occur: (1) the amount, or volume, of water in compartment B becomes greater than the volume in compartment A, and (2) the concentrations of the

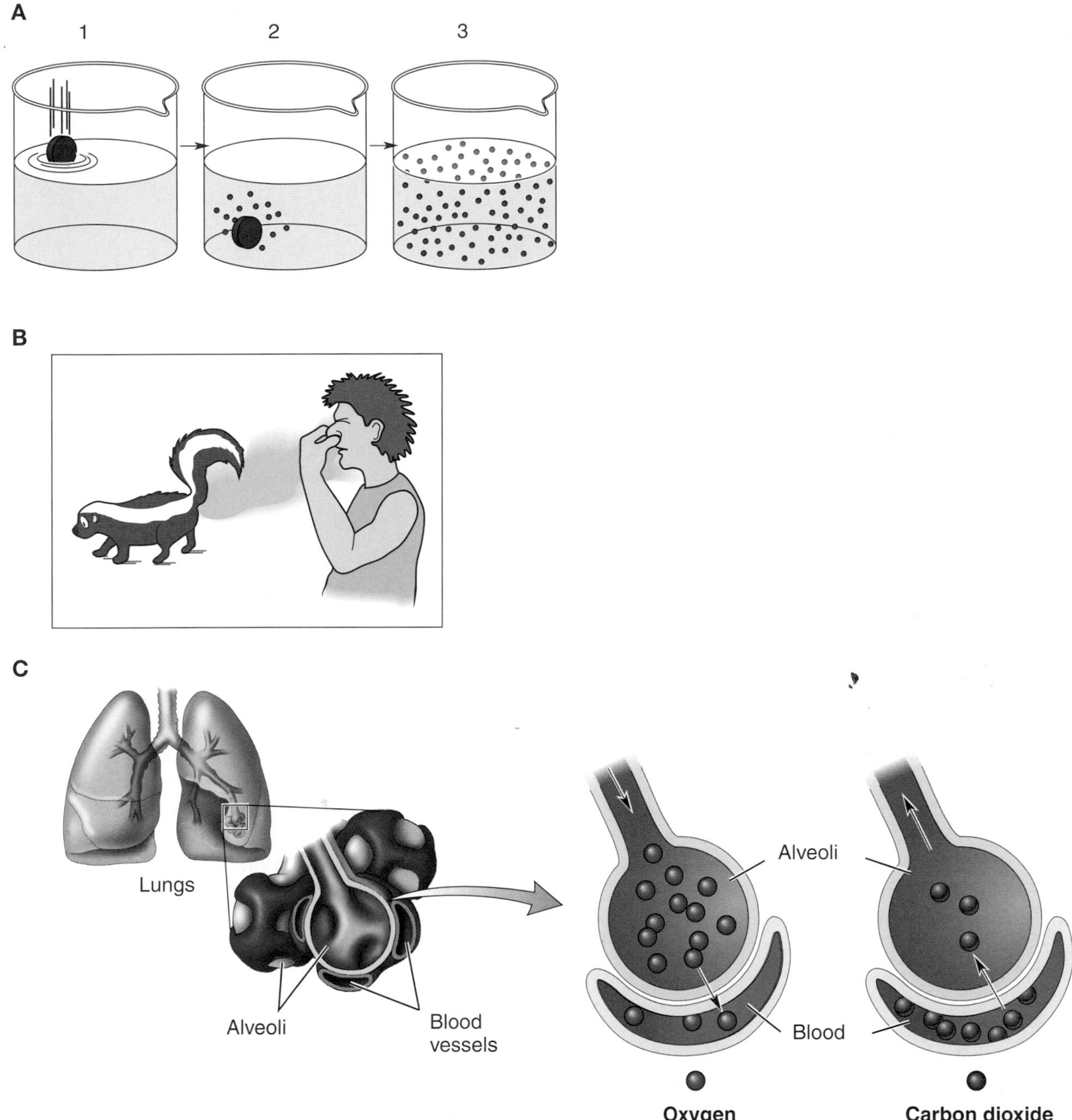

FIGURE 3-7 Diffusion. **A,** A red tablet is placed in glass 1. Given enough time, the red dye diffuses until it is evenly distributed throughout glass 3. **B,** Diffusion of Perfume's "perfume." **C,** Diffusion of oxygen and carbon dioxide in the lung.

solutions in both compartments change. The solution in compartment A becomes more concentrated, whereas the solution in compartment B becomes more dilute.

Whenever dissolved substances such as glucose or protein are confined in a space by a selectively permeable membrane, they can pull water into the compartment by osmosis.The strength of the osmotic pull is related directly to the concentration of the solution. The greater the concentration, the greater the pulling, or osmotic pressure. In other words, the more concentrated solution has more osmotically active particles.

Because osmotic pressure pulls water into a compartment, it can cause swelling. For example, tissue injury causes leakage and accumulation of proteins within the tissue spaces. The confined proteins act osmotically, pulling water toward them. This process causes an accumulation of water in the tissue spaces. The accumulation of water is referred to as edema.

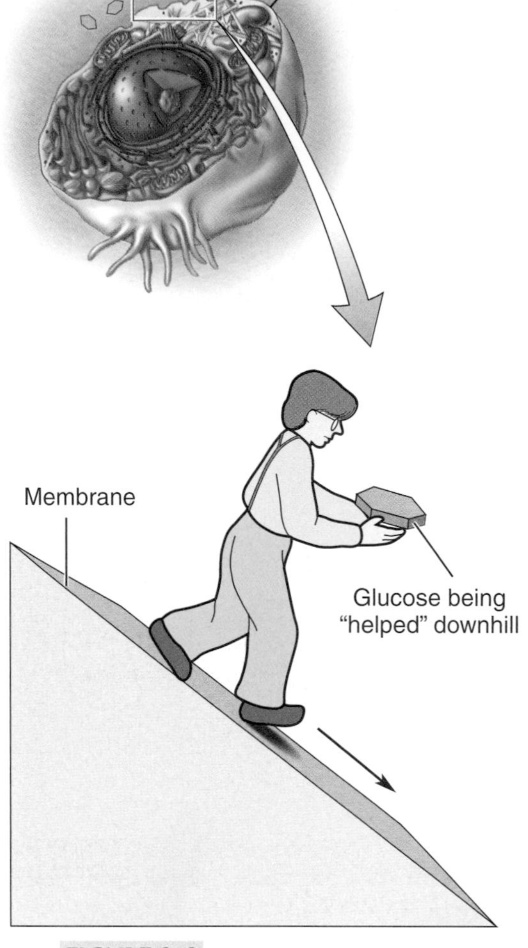

FIGURE 3-8 Facilitated diffusion.

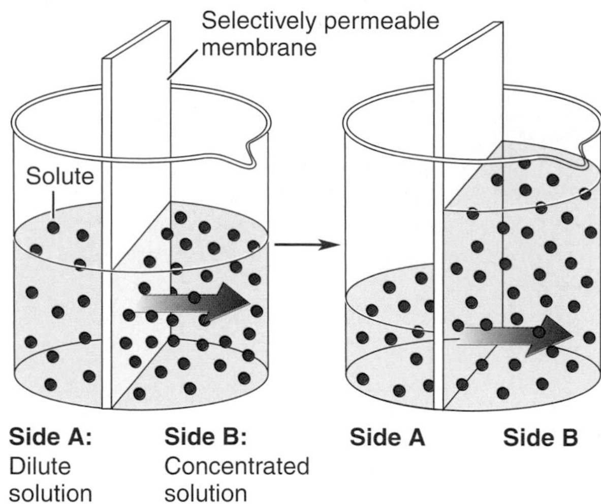

FIGURE 3-9 Osmosis. The glass is sectioned into side **A** and **B** by a membrane that is permeable only to water. The water moves from side **A** to side **B**, thereby creating unequal volumes.

Tonicity

Tonicity is the ability of a solution to affect the volume and pressure within a cell. Note what happens when a cell is placed in solutions of different concentrations (Figure 3-10). The following three terms are used to illustrate tonicity: isotonic, hypotonic, and hypertonic.

Isotonic Solution. An **isotonic solution** has the same concentration as intracellular fluid. (*Iso* means "same.") Consider an RBC placed in an isotonic solution. Because the solution is isotonic, no net movement of water occurs; the cell neither gains nor loses water.

Hypotonic Solution. If an RBC is placed in pure water (a solution containing no solute), water moves into the cell by osmosis (from where there is more water to where there is less). The pure water, being more dilute

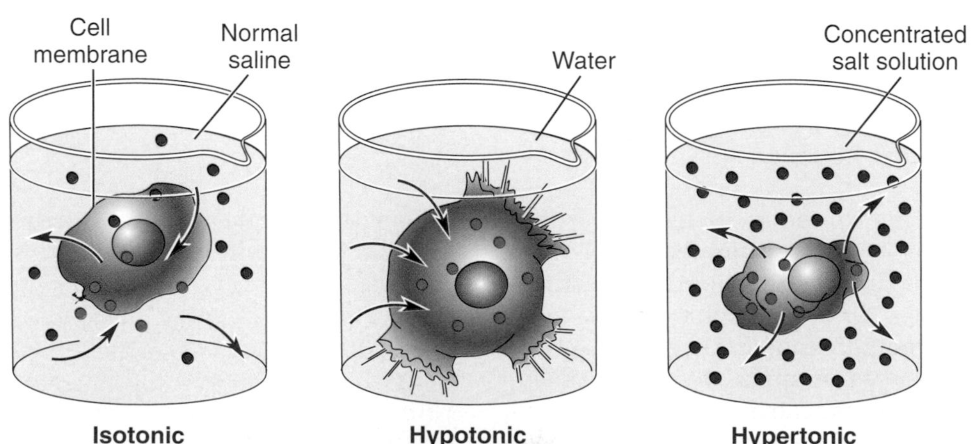

FIGURE 3-10 Effects of osmosis: isotonic, hypotonic, and hypertonic solutions.

Do You Know...

Why a blood clot may continue to "grow" even when the bleeding stops?

The components of the blood clot are osmotically active substances. The blood clot pulls water into itself, thereby expanding. If the expanding blood clot is located within the brain, it presses on the brain tissue, causing a variety of neurologic deficits.

than the inside of the cell, is said to be hypotonic. **Hypotonic solutions** cause RBCs to burst, or lyse. This process is referred to as hemolysis. Because of hemolysis, pure water is not administered intravenously.

A boiled hot dog may also illustrate this bursting effect. The hot dog, which contains a lot of salt, is boiled in plain water. Because the plain water is hypotonic relative to the hot dog, water diffuses into the hot dog and it bursts.

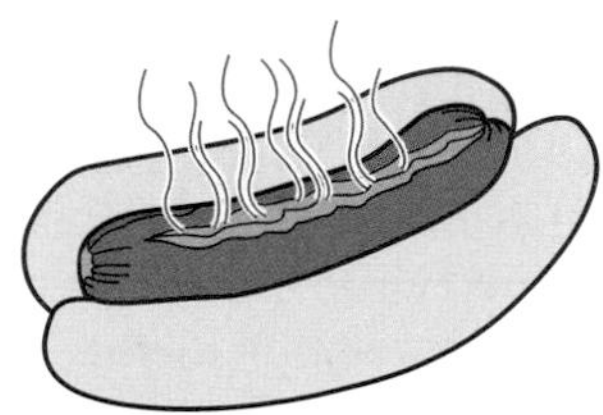

Hypertonic Solutions. If an RBC is placed within a very concentrated salt solution, water diffuses out of the RBC into the bathing solution, causing the RBC to shrink, or crenate. The salt solution is referred to as a **hypertonic solution.**

Why is the tonicity of a solution important? If the cell gains water, the RBC membrane bursts, or lyses. If the RBC loses water, the cell shrinks. In both cases, RBC function is severely impaired. Isotonic solutions do not cause cells to swell or shrink. Isotonic solutions are frequently administered intravenously. Commonly used isotonic solutions include normal saline (0.9% NaCl), 5% D/W (dextrose or glucose in water, or D_5W), and Ringer's solution. Under special conditions, hypotonic or hypertonic solutions may be administered intravenously. Most IV solutions, however, are isotonic.

Filtration

With diffusion and osmosis, water and dissolved substances move across the membrane in response to a difference in concentrations. With **filtration,** water and dissolved substances cross the membrane in response to differences in pressures. In other words, pressure pushes substances across the membrane.

A syringe can illustrate filtration (Figure 3-11). Syringe number 1 is filled with water. If a force is applied to

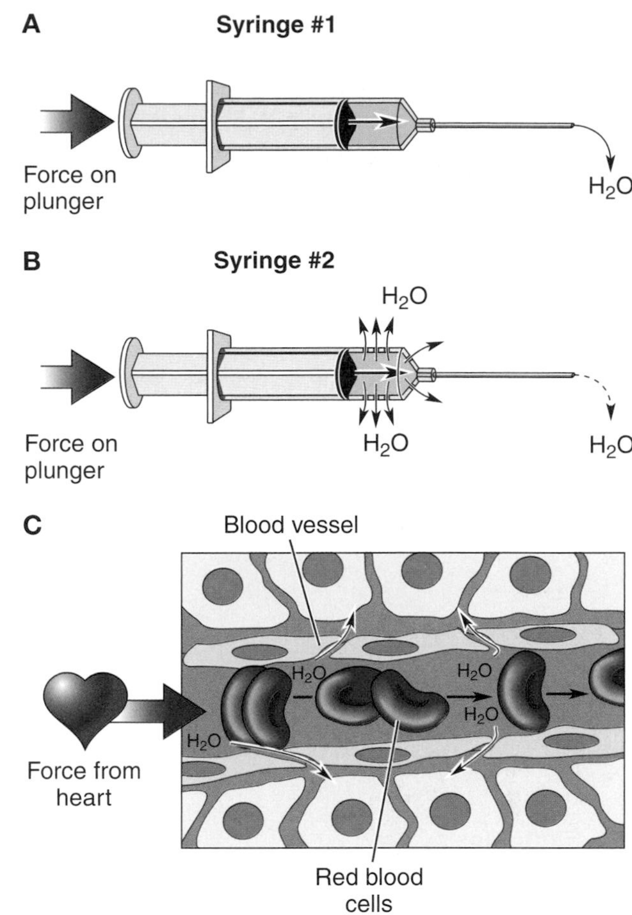

FIGURE 3-11 Filtration. **A,** Water is forced through the needle. **B,** Water is forced through the holes in the barrel of the syringe. **C,** H_2O is forced out of capillary.

the plunger, the water is pushed out through the needle. The water moves in response to a pressure difference, with greater pressure at the plunger than at the tip of the needle. In the second syringe, tiny holes are made in the sides of the barrel. When force is applied to the plunger, water squirts out the sides of the syringe and out the tip of the needle.

Where does filtration occur in the body? The movement of fluid across the capillary wall can be compared with the movement of water in the syringe with holes on

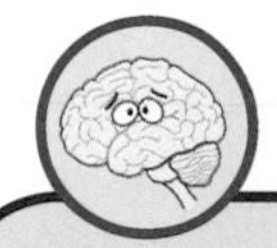

Do You Know...

How to shrink a swollen brain?

By administering a hypertonic solution (e.g., mannitol) intravenously. Because a hypertonic solution contains more solute than is present in the interstitial or tissue fluid of the brain, water leaves the brain tissue in response to osmosis and moves into the blood. As the blood is carried away from the brain, brain swelling (cerebral edema) decreases.

the side (syringe number 2). A capillary is a tiny vessel that contains blood. The capillary wall is composed of a thin layer of cells with many little pores. The pressure in the capillary pushes water and dissolved substances out of the blood and through the pores in the capillary wall into the tissue spaces. This process is filtration; it is movement caused by pushing. (Capillary filtration is further explained in Chapter 19.)

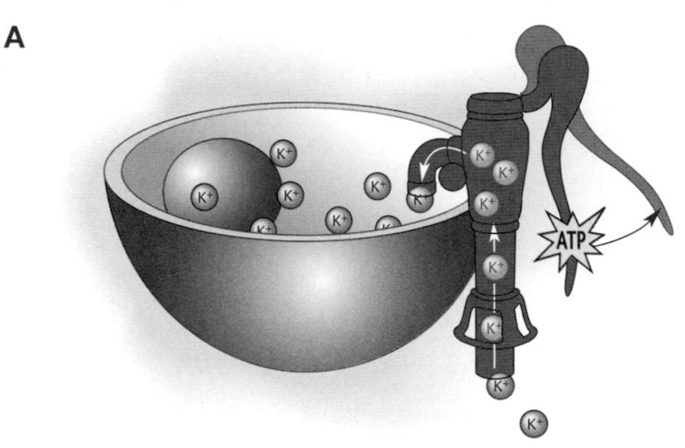

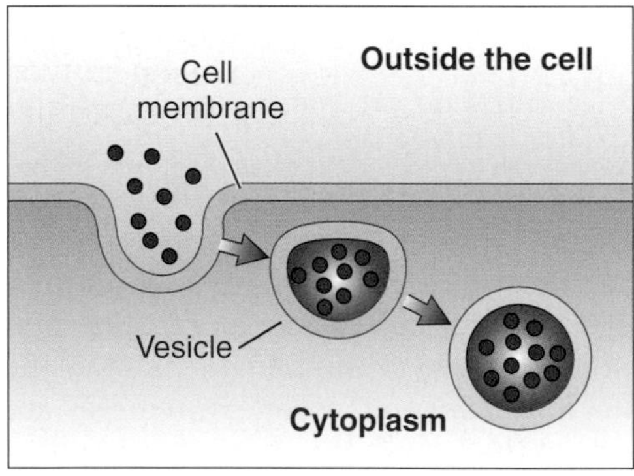

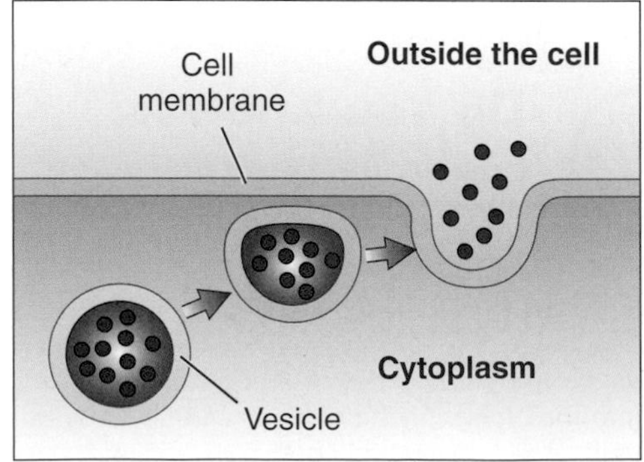

FIGURE 3-12 Active transport. **A,** The active pumping of K^+ into the cell. **B,** Endocytosis. **C,** Exocytosis.

ACTIVE TRANSPORT MECHANISMS

The active transport mechanisms include active transport pumps, endocytosis, and exocytosis.

Active Transport Pumps

Active transport refers to a transport mechanism that requires an input of energy (ATP) to achieve its goal. Why is it necessary to pump certain substances? Because the amount of some substances in the cell is already so great that the only way to move additional substances into the cell is to pump them in. For instance, the cell normally contains a large amount of potassium (K^+). The only way to move additional K^+ into the cell is to pump it in. To move the K^+ from an area of low concentration to an area of high concentration (uphill), energy is invested (Figure 3-12, *A*).

Endocytosis

Endocytosis (ĔN-dō-cī-TŌ-sĭs) is a transport mechanism that involves the intake of food or liquid by the cell membrane (see Figure 3-12, *B*). In endocytosis the particle is too large to move across the membrane by diffusion. Instead, the particle is surrounded by the cell membrane, which engulfs it and takes it into the cell. There are two forms of endocytosis. If the endocytosis involves a solid particle, it is called **phagocytosis** (phago means eating). For instance, white blood cells eat, or phagocytose, bacteria, thereby helping the body to defend itself against infection. If the cell ingests a water droplet, the endocytosis is called **pinocytosis,** or "cellular drinking."

Exocytosis

Whereas endocytosis brings substances into the cells, **exocytosis** (ĕx-ō-cī-TŌ-sĭs) moves substances out of the cells (see Figure 3-12, *C*). For instance, the cells of the pancreas make proteins for use outside the pancreas. The pancreatic cells synthesize the protein and wrap it in a membrane. This membrane-bound vesicle moves toward and fuses with the cell membrane. The protein is then expelled from the vesicle into the surrounding space. This process is exocytosis.

Sum It Up!

Water and dissolved substances must be able to move from one body compartment to another. This movement usually involves passage across cell membranes. Movement of water and dissolved substances is achieved through both passive and active transport mechanisms. Passive transport mechanisms require no investment of energy (ATP) and include diffusion, facilitated diffusion, osmosis, and filtration. The active transport mechanisms require an input of ATP and include the active transport pumps, endocytosis, and exocytosis.

CELL DIVISION

Cell division, or cell reproduction, is necessary for bodily growth and repair. The frequency of cell division varies considerably from one tissue to the next. Some cells reproduce very frequently, whereas other cells reproduce very slowly or not at all. For instance, the cells that line the digestive tract are replaced every few days, and more than 2 million red blood cells are replaced every second. Certain nerve cells in the brain and spinal cord, however, do not reproduce at all.

Two types of cell division are mitosis and meiosis. Meiosis occurs only in sex cells and will be discussed in Chapter 26. **Mitosis** (mī-TŌ-sĭs) is involved in bodily growth and repair. Mitosis is the splitting of one mother cell into two identical "daughter cells." The key word is *identical.* In other words, an exact copy of genetic information, stored within the chromosomes, must be passed from the mother cell to the two daughter cells (Figure 3-13). Mitosis is further described under Cell Cycle.

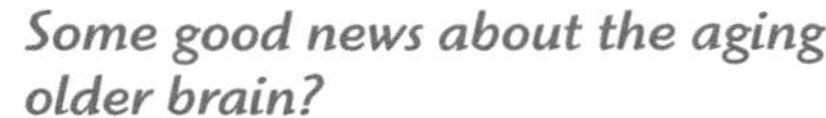

Do You Know...

Some good news about the aging older brain?

Neurons in the brain do not undergo mitosis and therefore don't replicate. Therefore, we have always assumed that there are no "new" brain neurons. Recently, however, "new" neurons in the brain have been identified, even in older brains. The neurons arise from newly discovered stem cells located in the brain. Brain cell replacement is now a possibility.

CELL CYCLE

The cell cycle is the sequence of events that the cell goes through from one mitotic division to the next. The **cell cycle** is divided into two major phases: interphase and mitosis (Figure 3-14).

Interphase

During interphase the cell carries on with its normal functions and gets ready for mitosis through growth and DNA replication. Interphase is divided into three phases: first gap phase (G_1), phase (S), and second gap phase (G_2).

- First gap phase (G_1). During this phase the cell carries on its normal activities and begins to make the DNA and other substances necessary for cell division.
- Phase (S). During the S phase the cell duplicates its chromosomes, thereby making enough DNA for two cells.
- Second gap phase (G_2). This phase is the final preparatory phase for cell division (mitosis); it includes the synthesis of enzymes and other protein needed for mitosis. At the end of G_2 the cell enters the mitotic (M) phase.

Mitosis

During the mitotic (M) phase the cell divides into two cells in such a way that the nuclei of both cells have identical genetic information. Mitosis consists of four phases: prophase, metaphase, anaphase, and telophase. During mitosis the pairs of identical chromosomes (which carry genetic information) line up in the middle of the cell. Threadlike spindles then attach to the chromosomes. As the spindles pull on the chromosomes, each pair of chromosomes splits and is pulled to the left or the right. The result is the separation of

A

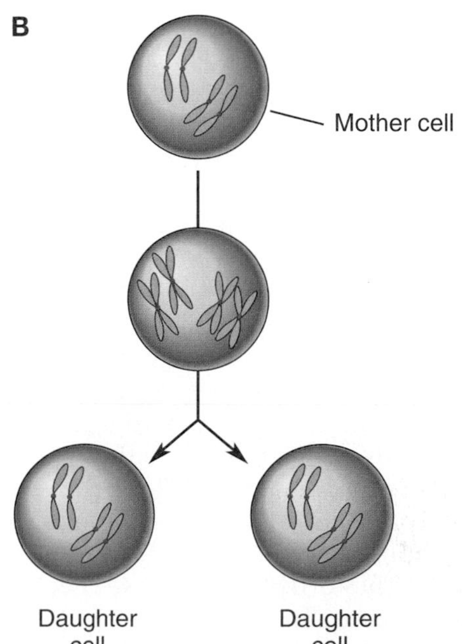

FIGURE 3-13 Mitosis. **A,** Mother and two identical daughters. **B,** The arrangement of chromosomes during mitosis.

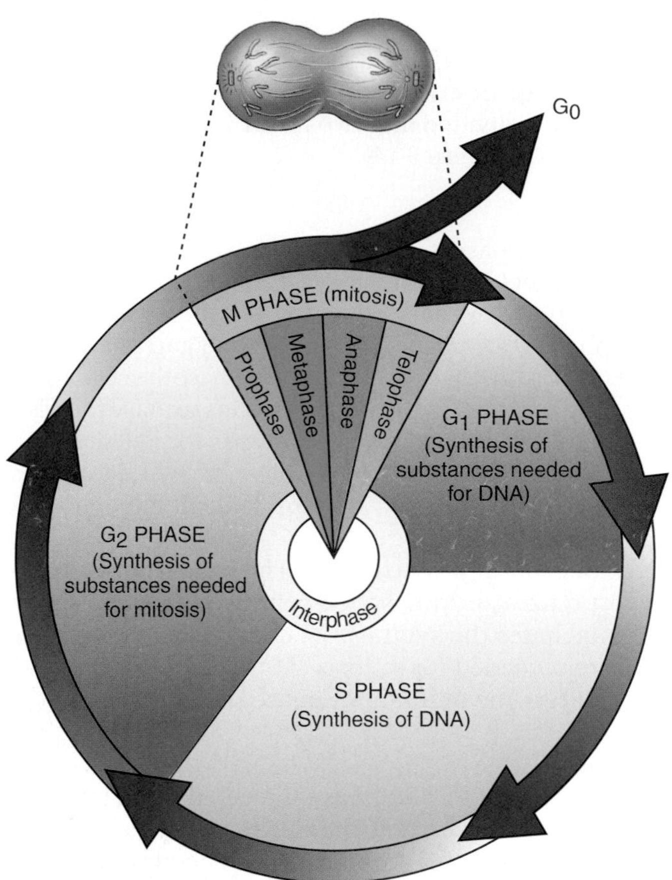

FIGURE 3-14 Cell cycle.

chromosomes into two identical sets, one set at one end of the dividing cell and a second identical set at the other end. Each end of the cell therefore contains the same genetic information. Mitosis ends with cytokinesis, the pinching of the cell membrane to split the cytoplasm into two distinct cells.

At the end of mitosis the daughter cells have two choices. They can enter G_1 and repeat the cycle (and divide again) or they can enter another phase called G-zero (G_0). Cells in G_0 "drop out" of the cell cycle and rest; they do not undergo mitosis. Cells may reenter the cell cycle after days, weeks, or years. The inability to stop cycling and enter G_0 is characteristic of cancer cells. Cancer cells constantly divide and proliferate. Anticancer drugs are more active against cells that are cycling than against cells resting in G_0. Thus, tumors that contain many cycling cells respond best to chemotherapy.

Anticancer drugs are classified according to the cell-cycle phases that they affect. Some anticancer drugs are called cell cycle–phase specific. These drugs affect the cell when it is in a particular phase. Using this terminology, the anticancer drug methotrexate is called S-phase specific. Other drugs are M-phase specific and G_2-phase specific. Some anticancer drugs can act at any phase of the cell cycle and are called cell cycle–phase nonspecific. By knowing the cell-cycle terminology you can better understand anticancer drugs.

CELL DIFFERENTIATION

Mitosis assures us that the division of one cell produces two identical cells. How do we account for the differences in cells like muscle cells, RBCs, and bone cells? In other words, how do cells differentiate or develop different characteristics?

An embryo begins life as a single cell, the fertilized ovum. Through mitosis, the single cell divides many times into identical cells. Then, sometime during their development, the cells start to specialize, or **differentiate** (Figure 3-15). One cell, for instance, may switch on enzymes that produce red blood cells. Other enzymes are switched on and produce bone cells. Whatever the mechanism, you started life as a single, adorable cell and ended up as billions of specialized cells!

What does it mean when a tissue biopsy (surgical removal of tissue for examination) shows many poorly differentiated cells? It means that the tissue cells have failed to differentiate or specialize. In other words, the poorly differentiated cells of a liver tumor do not resemble normal liver cells. Failure to differentiate is characteristic of cancer cells.

STEM CELLS

Stem cells are relatively undifferentiated or unspecialized cells whose only function is the production of additional unspecialized cells. Each time a stem cell divides, one of its daughter cells differentiates, while the other daughter cell prepares for further stem cell division. The rate of stem cell division varies with the tissue type. The stem cells within the bone marrow and skin are capable of dividing more than once a day, while the stem cells in adult cartilage may remain inactive for years. Stem cell research is of particular interest because of the possibility of replacing damaged tissue and growing new organs. How amazing it would be if newly discovered stem cells could be used to repair a damaged spinal cord or restore the dopamine-secreting cells in the brains of persons with Parkinson's disease. Recently an individual, paralyzed after a spinal cord injury, donated her own stem cells taken from deep within her nose. The stem cells were surgically placed within her spinal cord. The stem cells then differentiated into nerve cells. Although it is too early to claim success, some return of spinal cord function has been reported.

ORDER, DISORDER, AND DEATH

Most cell growth is orderly. Cells normally reproduce at the proper rate and align themselves in the correct positions. At times, however, cell growth becomes uncontrolled and disorganized. Too many cells are produced. This process is experienced by the patient as a lump or tumor (tumor means swelling).

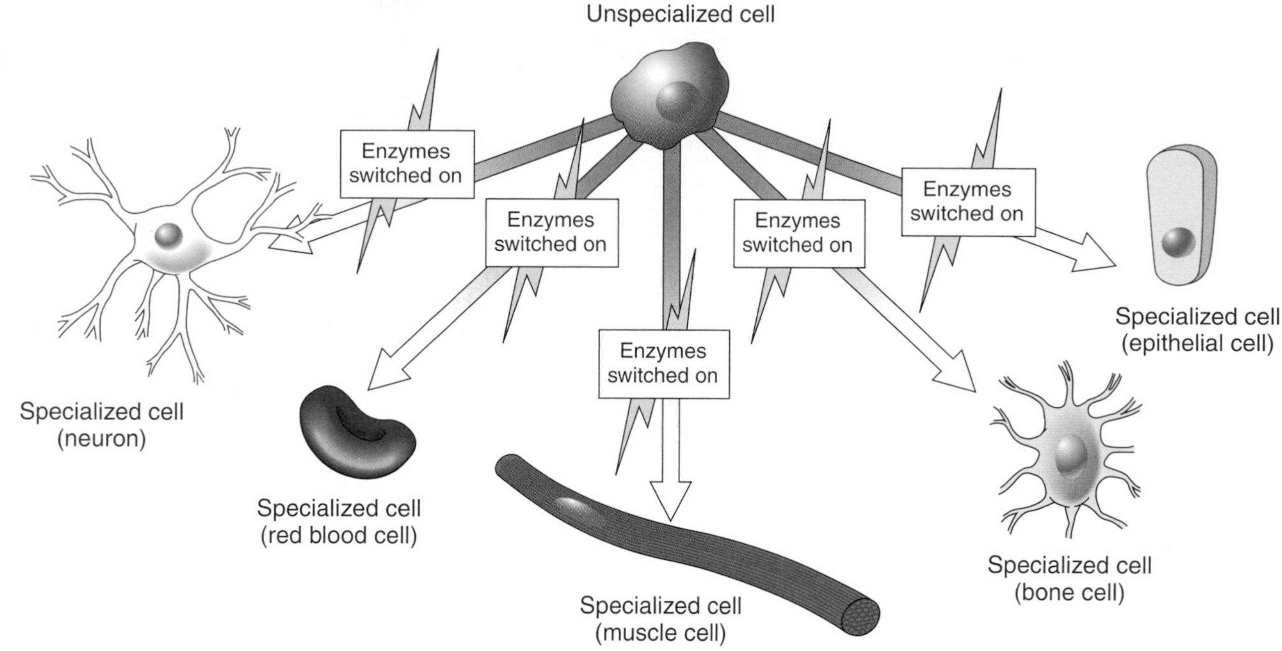

FIGURE 3-15 Cell differentiation.

Tumors may be classified as **benign** (noncancerous) or **malignant** (cancerous). Cancer cells are appropriately named. *Cancer* means "crab"; cancer cells, like a crab, send out clawlike extensions that invade surrounding tissue. Cancer cells also detach from the original tumor (primary site) and spread throughout the body (secondary sites). Widespread invasion of the body by cancer cells often causes death. The spreading of cancer cells is referred to as **metastasis.**

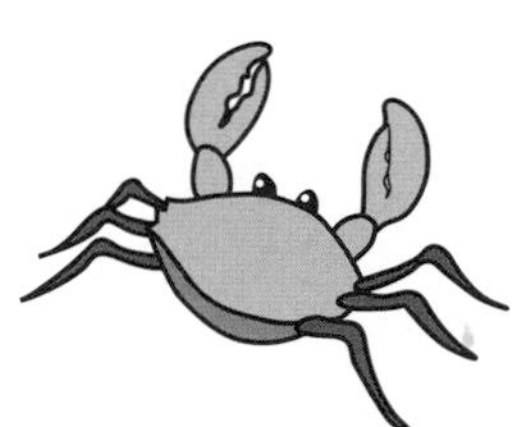

A Pap smear is one of the diagnostic procedures used to detect cancer. A sample of cells (a smear) is obtained, usually from around the cervix in the female. The smear is then examined under a microscope for changes that could indicate cancer. A positive Pap smear can detect cancer in its early stages. Early detection is associated with a very high cure rate.

Sometimes the cells are injured so severely that they die, or necrose (from the Greek word *necros,* meaning death). For instance, the cells may be deprived of oxygen for too long a period, be poisoned, be damaged by bacterial toxins, or suffer the damaging effects of radiation.

Sum It Up!

The union of the sperm and egg forms a single cell that divides by mitosis into billions of identical cells. The cell cycle is the sequence of events that the cell goes through from one mitotic division to the next. The cell cycle is divided into two phases: interphase and the mitotic phase. Mitosis splits a cell into two genetically identical cells. The cells then specialize, or differentiate, into many different types of cells, all of which are needed to perform a wide variety of functions. Most cells grow in an orderly way. Cells can, however, grow abnormally. The result is sometimes a tumor, which may be benign or malignant (cancerous).

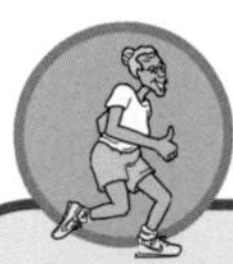

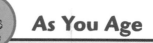

As You Age

1. All cells show changes as they age. The cells become larger, and their capacity to divide and reproduce tends to decrease.
2. Normal cells have built-in mechanisms to repair minor damage; this ability to repair declines in aging cells.
3. When DNA is damaged, changes in membranes and enzymes occur in the cell. Changes in the transport of ions and nutrients occur at the cell membrane. The chromosomes in the nucleus undergo such changes as clumping, shrinkage, and fragmentation.
4. Certain genetic disorders such as Down syndrome are more common in children born to older women.
5. Organelles such as mitochondria and lysosomes are present in reduced numbers as a person ages. In addition, cells function less efficiently.

Disorders of Cellular Growth

Atrophy	Atrophy is a decrease in the size of the cells, leading to a wasting away of tissues and organs.
Dysplasia	Abnormal growth. Dysplasia is an alteration in cell size, shape, and organization. The concern is that these alterations can result in cancer.
Hyperplasia	Overgrowth or increase in the numbers of cells, resulting in an increase in the size of tissues and organs.
Metaplasia	Transformation of one cell type into another (e.g., the change of columnar cells in the breathing passages of a smoker into a different cell type).
Necrosis	Death of cells or groups of cells.
Neoplasm	Abnormal new growth, also called a tumor. A malignant neoplasm is a cancerous tumor, and a benign neoplasm is a noncancerous tumor. Malignant neoplasms are invasive and tend to metastasize from an original (primary) site to another (secondary) site.

SUMMARY OUTLINE

I. A Typical Cell

The cell is the structural and functional unit of all living matter.

A. Cell Membrane (Plasma Membrane)
1. The cell membrane is composed of a two-layer phospholipid and protein.
2. The cell membrane is selectively permeable.

B. Structures Inside the Cell
1. The nucleus is the control center of the cell; it stores the genetic information.
2. The cytoplasm is a gel-like substance inside the cell membrane but outside of the nucleus.
3. Many different organelles are in the cytoplasm.
4. The mitochondria are the power plants of the cell.
5. Ribosomes are concerned with protein synthesis.
6. The endoplasmic reticulum has two types: the rough endoplasmic reticulum (RER) and the smooth endoplasmic reticulum (SER).
7. The Golgi apparatus packages and puts the finishing touches on the newly synthesized protein.
8. Lysosomes act as intracellular housekeepers.
9. The cytoskeleton provides shape and support to the cell.
10. Centrioles play a role in cell reproduction.

C. Structures on the Cell Membrane
1. Cilia are hairlike projections.
2. Flagella are long hairlike projections; the sperm has a flagellum that allows it to swim.

II. Movement Across the Cell Membrane

A. Passive Transport Mechanisms
1. Passive transport mechanisms require no input of energy (ATP).
2. Diffusion causes a substance to move from an area of greater concentration to an area of lesser concentration.
3. Facilitated diffusion is the same as diffusion but uses a helper molecule to increase the rate of diffusion.
4. Osmosis is a special case of diffusion using a semipermeable membrane. Osmosis involves the diffusion of water from an area with more water to an area of less water. The concentrations of a solution are expressed as tonicity. Solutions are isotonic, hypotonic, or hypertonic.
5. Filtration is the movement of water and dissolved substances from an area of high pressure to an area of low pressure.

B. Active Transport Mechanisms
1. Active transport requires an input of energy (ATP).
2. Active transport pumps move substances from an area of low concentration to an area of high concentration.
3. Endocytosis moves substances into a cell; pinocytosis is cellular "drinking" and phagocytosis is cellular "eating."
4. Exocytosis moves substances out of a cell.

III. Cell Division

A. Mitosis: Produces Two Identical Cells

B. Meiosis: Occurs Only in Sex Cells

IV. Cell Cycle
- A. Interphase (G_1, S, and G_2 phases)
- B. Mitosis (M phase)
  1. The splitting of one mother cell into two identical daughter cells.
  2. Four phases of mitosis: prophase, metaphase, anaphase, and telophase.
- C. Cell Cycle–Phase Specific Drugs
  1. Some drugs are aimed at a specific phase of the cell cycle.
  2. Some are cell cycle–phase nonspecific.

V. Cell Differentiation

VI. Stem Cells

VII. Order, Disorder, and Death

Review Your Knowledge

Matching: Cell Structure

Directions: Match the following words with their descriptions below.

a. mitochondria
b. endoplasmic reticulum
c. ribosomes
d. cilia
e. lysosomes
f. nucleus
g. cytoplasm

1. ____ The control center of the cell; contains the DNA
2. ____ Short, hairlike projections on the outer surface of the cell
3. ____ The power plants of the cell; most of the ATP is made here
4. ____ Classified as rough and smooth
5. ____ These organelles are attached to the endoplasmic reticulum and are concerned with protein synthesis
6. ____ Digestive organelles that engage in phagocytosis; intracellular housecleaning
7. ____ The gel in the cell (outside the nucleus)

Matching: Transport and Tonicity

Directions: Match the following words with their descriptions below. Some words may be used more than once.

a. hypotonic
b. diffusion
c. pinocytosis
d. isotonic
e. hypertonic
f. osmosis
g. filtration
h. facilitated diffusion
i. exocytosis

1. ____ A pressure gradient is the driving force for this type of passive transport
2. ____ A passive transport mechanism by which glucose is "helped" across the membrane by a helper molecule within the membrane
3. ____ A protein-containing vesicle within a cell fuses with the cell membrane and ejects the protein
4. ____ Called "cellular drinking"
5. ____ An example of this transport mechanism is the swelling of a blood clot as water is pulled into the clot
6. ____ Describes a solution that is more concentrated than the inside of a cell
7. ____ Solution that causes a red blood cell to swell with water and burst
8. ____ Solution that has the same concentration as the inside of a red blood cell
9. ____ A drop of red dye is added to a beaker of water; in 2 hours the beaker of water is uniformly colored red
10. ____ Because of its salt concentration, normal saline is

Multiple Choice

1. The selectively permeable membrane
   a. permits filtration but not diffusion or osmosis.
   b. determines what substances enter and leave the cell.
   c. allows for the unrestricted movement of water and electrolytes across the cell membrane.
   d. permits diffusion but not osmosis.
2. Which of the following is not true of the mitochondria?
   a. Numbers of mitochondria reflect the metabolic activity of the cell.
   b. Mitochondria are the organelles that make most of the body's ATP.
   c. Mitochondria contain enzymes that work aerobically.
   d. Mitochondria are the sites of protein synthesis.
3. Which of the following is an incorrect statement regarding the cellular organelles?
   a. Most ATP is produced in the mitochondria.
   b. Lysosomes contain potent enzymes that digest cellular waste and debris.
   c. Most DNA is located within the Golgi apparatus.
   d. The RER is concerned with protein synthesis.

4. A beaker contains two compartments. Compartment A contains a 20% salt (NaCl) solution while compartment B contains a 5% salt solution. The membrane is permeable to the salt and water. Which statement is true initially?
   a. The volume in A is greater than the volume in B.
   b. The volume in A is less than the volume in B.
   c. Na^+ diffuses from A to B.
   d. Water diffuses from A to B.
5. With regard to the cell cycle
   a. the M phase is the same as interphase.
   b. cells cannot enter phase G_0 when they complete the cycle.
   c. cell division occurs during the M phase.
   d. prophase, metaphase, anaphase, and telophase occur during phase G_1.

CHAPTER 4

Cell Metabolism

KEY TERMS

OBJECTIVES

1. Define *metabolism, anabolism,* and *catabolism.*
2. Explain the use of carbohydrates, proteins, and fats in the body.
3. Differentiate between the anaerobic and aerobic metabolism of carbohydrates.
4. Describe the structure of a nucleotide.
5. Describe the roles of DNA and RNA in protein synthesis.
6. Describe protein synthesis.

To carry on its function, the cell, like a factory, must bring in and use raw material. The raw material comes from the food we eat and includes carbohydrates, protein, and fat.

METABOLISM

Once inside the cell, the raw materials undergo thousands of chemical reactions. The series of chemical reactions necessary for the use of the raw material is called **metabolism.** Metabolism can be divided into two parts: anabolism and catabolism (Figure 4-1).

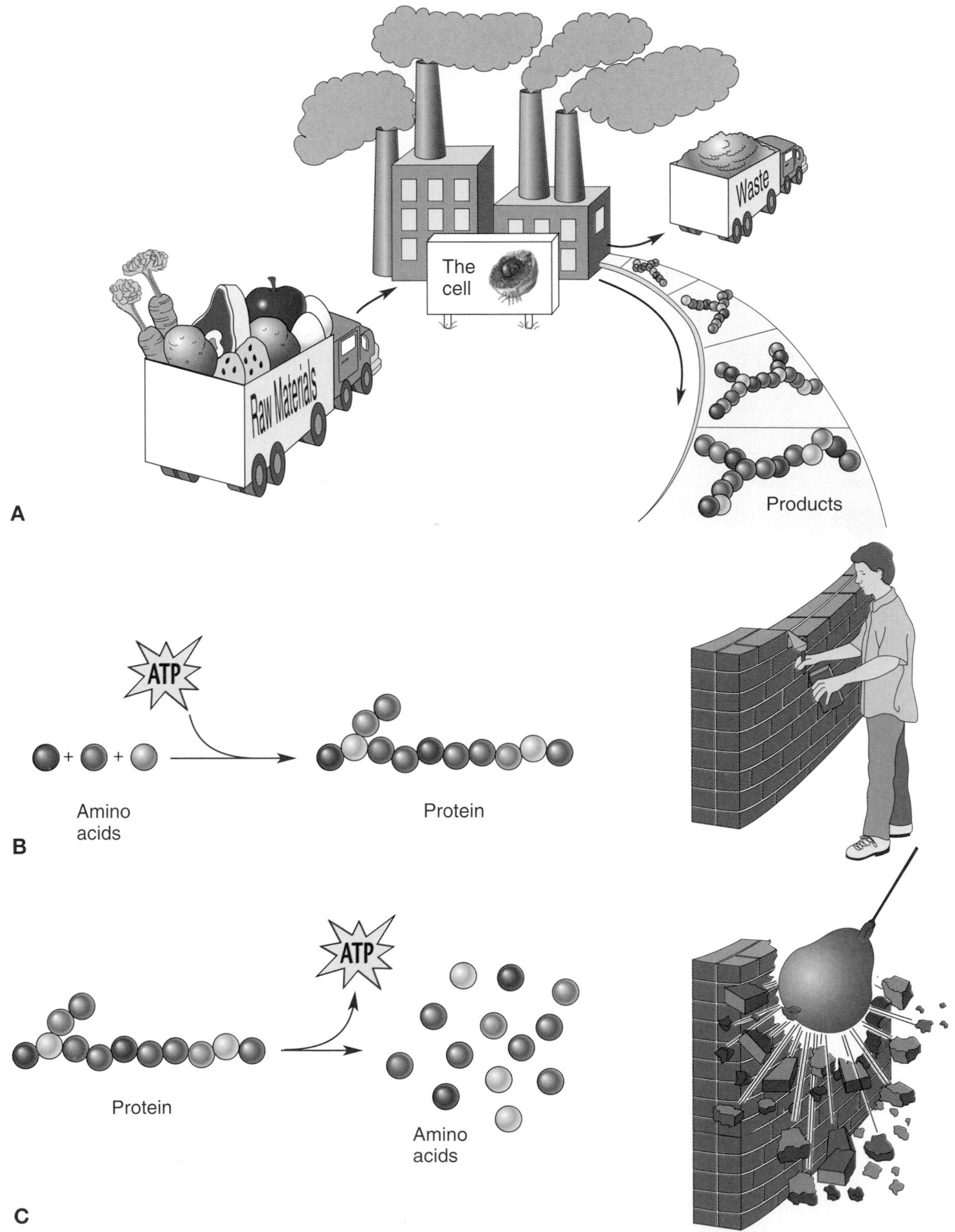

FIGURE 4-1 Metabolism. **A,** Raw materials to run the factory. **B,** Anabolism. **C,** Catabolism.

Anabolism (ă-NĂB-ŏ-lĭzm) includes reactions that build larger, more complex substances from simpler substances. The building of a large protein from individual amino acids is an example of anabolism. The process is similar to the building of a brick wall from individual bricks. Anabolic reactions generally require an input of energy in the form of adenosine triphosphate (ATP).

Catabolism (kă-TĂB-ō-lĭzm) includes reactions that break down larger, more complex substances into simpler substances. The breakdown of a large protein into individual amino acids is an example of catabolism. This process is similar to the knocking down of a brick wall. Catabolism releases energy that is eventually converted into ATP.

CARBOHYDRATES

We have all eaten sugars and starchy food. Bread, potatoes, rice, pasta, and jelly beans are some of our favorite foods. These are all carbohydrates. **Carbohydrates** are organic compounds composed of carbon (C), hydrogen (H), and oxygen (O). Carbohydrates are classified according to size (Figure 4-2). **Monosaccharides** (mŏn-ō-SĂK-ă-rīdz) are single (mono) sugar (saccharide) compounds. **Disaccharides** are double (di) sugars, and **polysaccharides** are many (poly) sugar compounds. The shorter monosaccharides and disaccharides are called sugars, and the longer chain polysaccharides are called starches. The carbohydrates are listed in Table 4-1.

MONOSACCHARIDES

Monosaccharides are sugars containing three to six carbons. The six-carbon simple sugars include glucose, fructose, and galactose. **Glucose** is the most important of the three and is used by the cells as an immediate source of energy.

There are also five-carbon monosaccharides. They include ribose and deoxyribose. These sugars are used in the synthesis of ribonucleic acids (RNA) and deoxyribonucleic acids (DNA).

DISACCHARIDES

Disaccharides are double sugars. They are made when two monosaccharides are linked together (see Figure 4-2, *B*). The disaccharides include sucrose (table sugar), maltose, and lactose. Disaccharides are present in the food we eat. They must be digested, or broken down, into monosaccharides before they can be absorbed across the walls of the digestive tract and used by the cells.

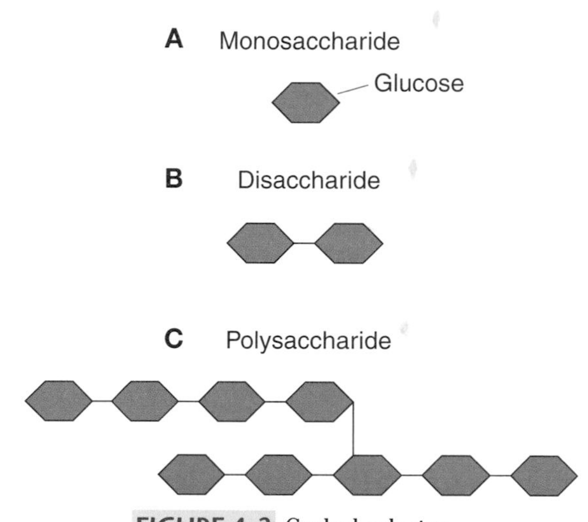

FIGURE 4-2 Carbohydrates.

Table 4-1 Carbohydrates

Name	Function
Monosaccharides (simple sugars)	
Glucose	Most important energy source
Fructose	Converted to glucose
Galactose	Converted to glucose
Deoxyribose	Sugar in DNA
Ribose	Sugar in RNA
Disaccharides (double sugars)	
Sucrose	Split into monosaccharides
Maltose	Split into monosaccharides
Lactose	Split into monosaccharides
Polysaccharides (many sugars)	
Starches	Found in plant foods; digested to monosaccharides
Glycogen	Animal starch; excess glucose stored in liver and skeletal muscle
Cellulose	Nondigestible by humans; forms dietary fiber or roughage

DNA, Deoxyribonucleic acid; *RNA,* ribonucleic acid.

POLYSACCHARIDES

Polysaccharides are made of many glucose molecules linked together. Some are linked together in straight chains, others in branched chains (see Figure 4-2, *C*). The three polysaccharides of interest to us are plant starch, animal starch, and cellulose. Starch is the storage polysaccharide in plants. It is a series of glucose molecules linked together in a branched pattern. Starchy foods such as potatoes, peas, grains, and pasta contain this type of starch.

Do You Know...

Why this termite can digest wood and you can't?

Unlike humans, termites have the enzymes that digest cellulose. The ability to make this enzyme enables the mighty termite to eat your house plank by plank.

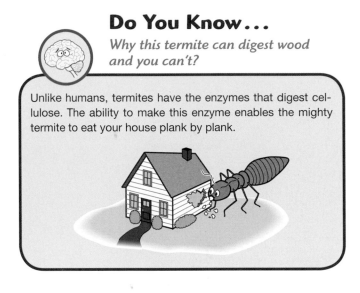

Glycogen (GLĪ-kō-jĕn) is also called animal starch and is a highly branched polysaccharide similar to plant starch. Glycogen is the form in which humans store glucose. Glycogen is stored primarily in the liver and skeletal muscle. When blood sugar levels become low, the glycogen is converted to glucose and released into the blood, where it restores normal blood sugar levels.

Cellulose is a straight-chained polysaccharide found in plants. Although we do not have the enzymes to digest cellulose as a source of nutrients, this polysaccharide plays an important role in our digestive process. The cellulose provides the fiber in our diet and improves digestive function in many ways.

USES OF GLUCOSE

What about that mound of jelly beans, those colored, oval globs of sugar that you just ate? The jelly beans are eaten, digested, and absorbed. Then what? Glucose is used by the body in three ways: (1) it can be burned immediately as fuel for energy, (2) it can be stored as glycogen and burned as fuel at a later time, and (3) it can be stored as fat and burned as fuel at a later time. The "stored as fat" phrase is the most distressing!

The Breakdown of Glucose

Glucose is broken down under the following two conditions: (1) in the absence of oxygen (the process is called **anaerobic catabolism**) and (2) in the presence of oxygen (this process is called **aerobic catabolism**). In the absence of oxygen, glucose is broken down through a series of chemical reactions, first into pyruvic acid and then into lactic acid. This anaerobic process occurs in the cytoplasm and is called **glycolysis** (glī-kōl-Ĭ-sĭs). Because most of the energy is still locked up in the lactic acid molecule, glycolysis produces only a small amount of ATP (Figure 4-3, *A*).

If oxygen is available, glucose is completely broken down to form carbon dioxide, water, and ATP (Figure 4-3, *B*). The glucose is first broken down to pyruvic acid in the cytoplasm. The pyruvic acid molecules then move into the mitochondria, the power plants of the cell. In the presence of oxygen and special enzymes in the mitochondria, the pyruvic acid fragments are completely broken down to carbon dioxide and water. This process is accompanied by the release of a large amount of energy (ATP). There are two sets of enzymes in the mitochondria: the enzymes of the Krebs cycle and the enzymes of the electron transport chain. Both sets of enzymes work to produce ATP aerobically.

Three important points about aerobic catabolism should be remembered. First, the chemical reactions occurring in the mitochondria require oxygen. If the cells are deprived of oxygen, they soon become low in energy and cannot carry out their functions. This need for oxygen is the reason we need to breathe continuously—to ensure a continuous supply of oxygen to the cells. Second, when glucose is broken down completely to carbon dioxide and water, all of the stored energy is released. Thus the aerobic breakdown of glucose produces much more ATP than does the anaerobic breakdown of glucose. Third, if oxygen is not available to the cell, the pyruvic acid cannot enter the mitochondria. Instead, the pyruvic acid is converted to lactic acid in the cytoplasm. The buildup of lactic acid is the reason that a lack of oxygen in a critically ill patient causes lactic acidosis.

THE MAKING OF GLUCOSE

As we have seen, carbohydrates can be broken down in the cells as a source of energy. Cells can also make, or synthesize, glucose from noncarbohydrate substances. Protein, for instance, can be broken down and the breakdown products used to make glucose. The making of glucose from nonglucose sources, especially protein, is called **gluconeogenesis.** Gluconeogenesis is an important mechanism in the regulation of blood sugar. For example, if blood sugar declines, protein is converted to glucose in the liver and released into the blood, thereby restoring blood sugar to normal.

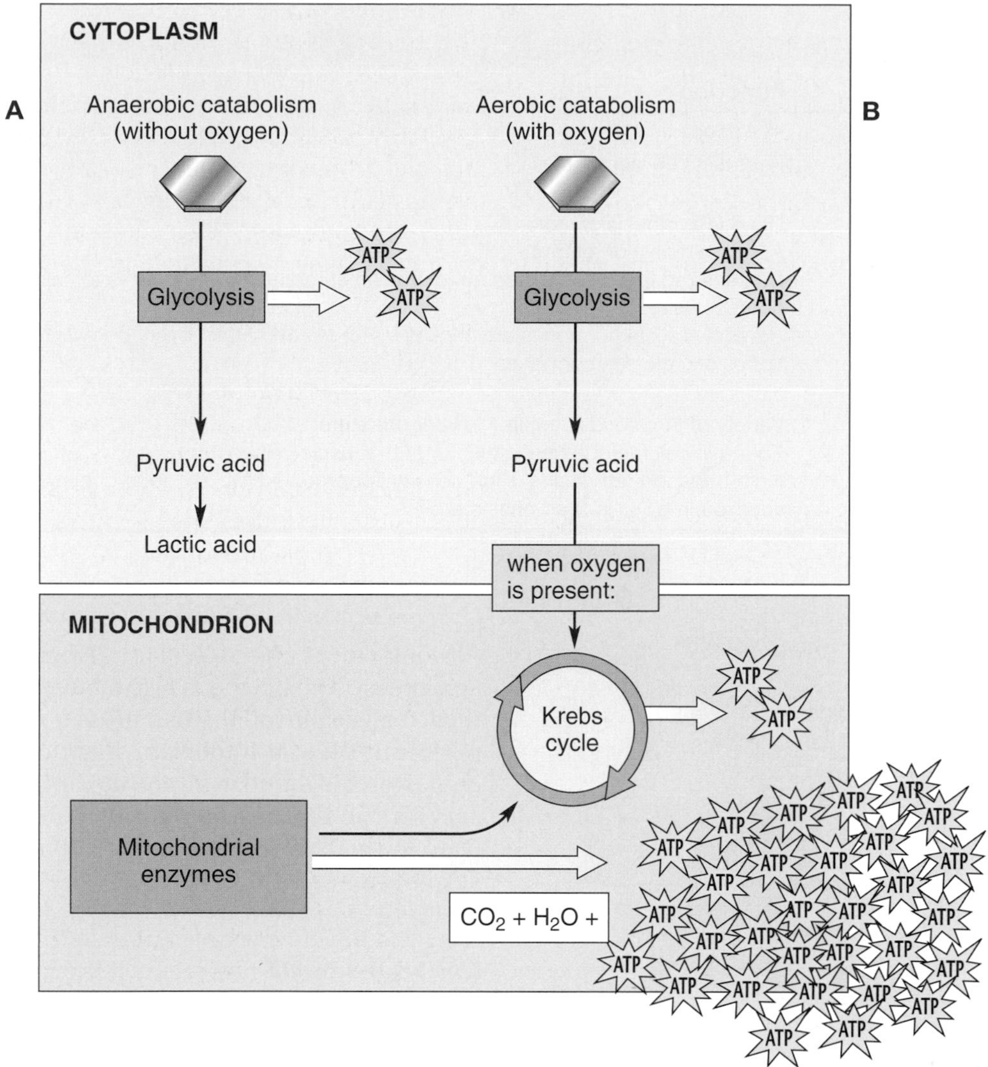

FIGURE 4-3 Breakdown of glucose. **A,** Anaerobic: to lactic acid. **B,** Aerobic: to carbon dioxide, water, and ATP.

Clinical conditions involving glucose breakdown and synthesis are common. In the person with diabetes, the lack of the insulin hormone affects glucose metabolism in two ways. First, because insulin is needed for the transport of glucose into the cell, a lack of insulin deprives the cells of glucose and thus the energy that glucose provides. Second, the lack of insulin causes body protein to be broken down and then converted into glucose (gluconeogenesis). However, because the diabetic cells cannot utilize the glucose, it accumulates in the blood, making the person hyperglycemic (having excess glucose in the blood). Thus the person with diabetes ends up with most of the glucose in the blood and not in the cells, where it is needed for energy. Drugs used to treat diabetes do two things: they increase the uptake of glucose by the cells and they suppress gluconeogenesis by the liver. Both effects lower blood glucose.

LIPIDS (FATS)

Lipids are organic compounds that are commonly called fats and oils. Fats are solid at room temperature while oils are liquid. Most of the lipids are eaten as fatty meats, egg yolk, dairy products, and oils. The lipids found most commonly in the body include triglycerides, phospholipids, and steroids. Other relatives of lipids, called lipoid substances, are listed in Table 4-2.

The building blocks of lipids are fatty acids and glycerol. The lipid illustrated in Figure 4-4, *A,* is a triglyceride. It has three (tri) long chains of fatty acids attached to one small glycerol molecule. A phospholipid is formed when a phosphorus-containing group attaches to one of the glycerol sites (Figure 4-4, *B*). Phospholipids are important components of the cell membrane.

The steroid is a third type of lipid. The most important steroid in the body is cholesterol (Figure 4-4, *C*).

Table 4-2 Lipids

Lipid Type	Function
Triglycerides	In adipose tissue: protect and insulate body organs; major source of stored energy
Phospholipids	Found in cell membranes
Steroids	
Cholesterol	Used in synthesis of steroids
Bile salts	Assist in digestion of fats
Vitamin D	Synthesized in skin on exposure to ultraviolet radiation; contributes to calcium and phosphate homeostasis
Hormones from adrenal cortex, ovaries, and testes	Adrenal cortical hormones are necessary for life and affect every body system; ovaries and testes secrete sex hormones
Lipoid substances	
Fat-soluble vitamins (A, D, E, K)	Variety of functions (identified in later chapters)
Prostaglandins	Found in cell membranes; affect smooth muscle contraction
Lipoproteins	Help transport fatty acids. High density lipoprotein (HDL) is "good cholesterol"; Low density lipoprotein (LDL) is "bad cholesterol"

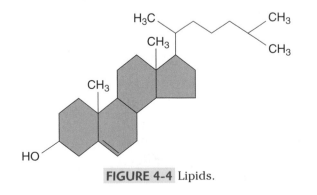

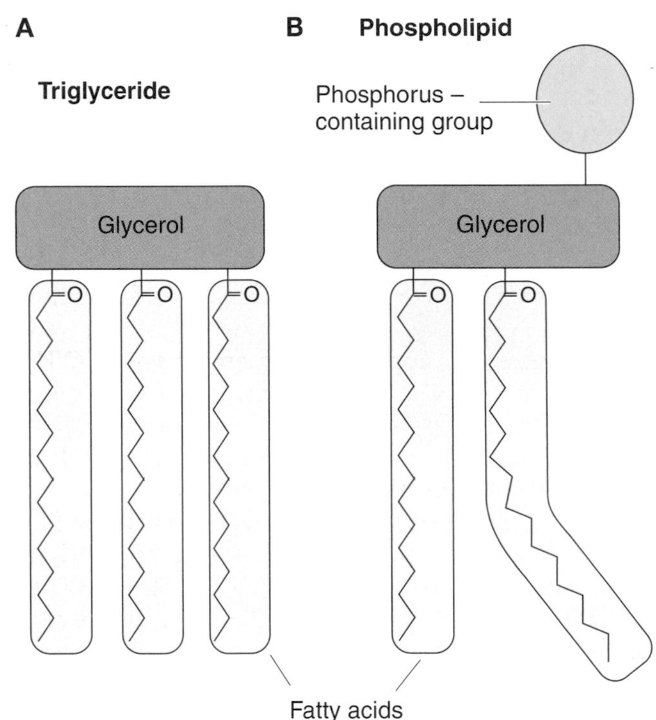

FIGURE 4-4 Lipids.

Although most cholesterol is consumed as meat, eggs, and cheese, the body can also synthesize cholesterol in the liver. Despite all the bad press about it, cholesterol performs several important functions. For instance, cholesterol is found in all cell membranes and is necessary for the synthesis of vitamin D in the skin. It is also used in the ovaries and testes in the synthesis of the sex hormones.

USES OF LIPIDS

What about the bacon you ate for breakfast? There is good news and bad news. The good news is that lipids are needed by the body (1) as a source of energy, (2) as a component of cell membranes and myelin sheath (coverings of nerve cells), and (3) in the synthesis of steroids. The bad news is that fat can be put into long-term storage. Fat can make you fat! It can also be deposited in areas where it is not wanted, such as inside your blood vessels.

METABOLISM OF LIPIDS

Like glucose, fatty acids and glycerol can be broken down so as to release the stored energy. Because the fatty acids are long structures, however, they must be chopped into tiny units before entering the mitochondria and becoming part of the citric acid cycle (Krebs cycle). The aerobic burning of the fatty acid units in the mitochondria releases a huge amount of energy that is captured as ATP. Because the fatty acids are much longer than the glucose molecules, the amount of energy released in the burning of fatty acids is much greater than the amount released in the burning of glucose.

Knowing her lipid metabolism, Mother Nature encourages Griz to overeat and gain weight. By doing so, the grizzly is able to hibernate during the winter

Do You Know...

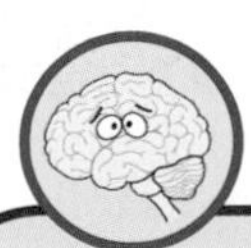

That Griz does not urinate during his hibernating months?

What then about the waste produced by his metabolizing body? The bear has apparently developed the metabolic ability to convert his waste (urea) into a substance that can be used by the body. He literally recycles his urine. An understanding of this recycling process would certainly benefit the many persons who require dialysis because of kidney failure.

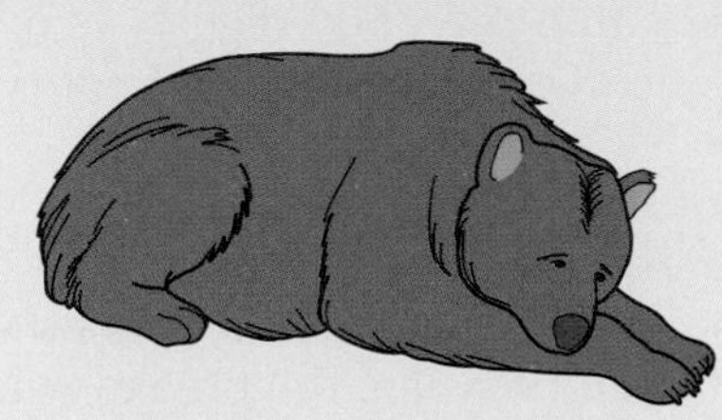

months because he can live off the fat stored during the summer feeding frenzy. While hibernating, the bear's fat is gradually broken down, and the energy that is released is sufficient to keep him alive.

Making Fat

As we all know, fat can also be made. The extra donut eaten today is worn on your hip tomorrow! When excess calories (energy) are consumed, the enzymes that synthesize fat are stimulated. The fat is deposited in adipose tissue throughout the body.

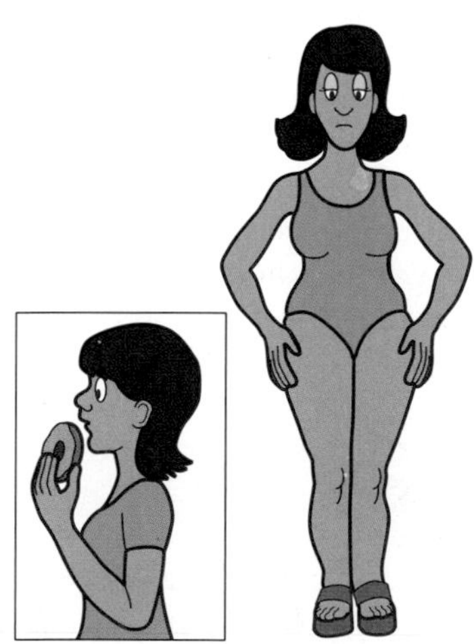

PROTEINS

Protein is the most abundant organic matter in the body. Because proteins are present in so many physiologically important compounds, it is safe to say that they participate in every body function. For instance, almost every chemical reaction in the body is regulated by an enzyme, which is a protein substance. Most hormones are proteins; they exert important widespread effects throughout the body. Hemoglobin, which delivers oxygen to every cell in the body, is a protein. Finally, muscles contract because of their contractile proteins. As you can see, proteins are essential to life.

AMINO ACIDS

The building blocks of protein are **amino acids.** About 20 amino acids are used to build body protein. Most amino acids come from protein foods. Foods such as lean meat, milk, and eggs are excellent sources of protein. More than half of the amino acids can be synthesized by the body. If the diet lacks the amino acid alanine, for instance, alanine can be synthesized within the liver.

Some amino acids, however, cannot be synthesized by the body and must be obtained from dietary sources. Because dietary intake of these amino acids is essential, these amino acids are called **essential amino acids.** The amino acids that can be synthesized by the liver are called **nonessential amino acids,** meaning that these amino acids are not absolutely necessary in the diet. See Table 4-3 for a list of common amino acids. (NOTE: the word *nonessential* does not mean that these amino acids are not essential to the body. The term refers to the ability of the body to synthesize these amino acids when they are not included in the diet.)

Like carbohydrates and lipids, amino acids are composed of carbon, hydrogen, and oxygen. In addition to these three elements, amino acids also contain nitrogen. The nitrogen appears as an amine group (NH_2). At the other end of the amino acid is the acid group (COOH): hence the name amino acid. Note the amine group and the acid group in Figure 4-5, *A,* which includes the amino acid alanine.

Amino acids are joined together by peptide bonds. A **peptide bond** is formed when the amine group (NH_2) of one amino acid joins with the acid (COOH) group of a second amino acid. A **peptide** is formed when several amino acids are joined together by peptide bonds (see Figure 4-5, B). A **polypeptide** is formed when many amino acids are joined together. **Proteins** are very large

Table 4-3 Common Amino Acids

Alanine	Leucine*
Arginine	Lysine*
Asparagine	Methionine*
Aspartic acid	Phenylalanine*
Cysteine	Proline
Glutamic acid	Serine
Glutamine	Threonine*
Glycine	Tryptophan*
Histidine*	Tyrosine
Isoleucine*	Valine*

*Essential amino acids.

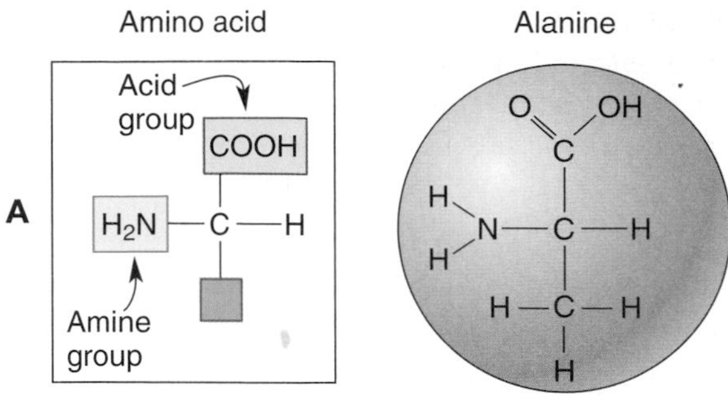

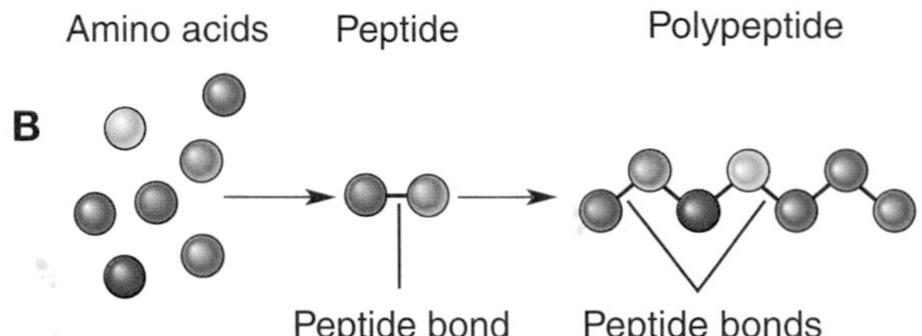

FIGURE 4-5 Amino acids and proteins. **A,** The amino acid, alanine. **B,** The assembly of amino acids to form a polypeptide. Note the peptide bonds.

polypeptides. Most proteins are composed of more than one polypeptide chain. Proteins can bond with other organic compounds. For instance, the combination of a sugar and a protein forms a **glycoprotein,** while the combination of a lipid and protein creates a **lipoprotein.**

USES OF PROTEINS

Proteins are used in three ways. The most important use is in the synthesis of hormones, enzymes, antibodies, plasma and muscle proteins, hemoglobin, and most cell membranes. In one way or another, proteins play a key role in every physiological function. The various types of proteins and their functions are listed in Table 4-4. With such a large demand for protein, most of the amino acids are carefully conserved by the body and used in the synthesis of protein.

The two less common uses of protein are as follows. First, protein can be broken down and used as fuel, as a source of energy for ATP production. This process, however, is not desirable. The preferred energy sources are carbohydrate and fat. Second, protein can be broken down and converted to glucose (gluconeogenesis). This mechanism is used by the body to ensure that the blood glucose level does not become too low to sustain life. In severe starvation the body digests is own protein, including the heart muscle, in order to survive!

Breakdown of Protein and the Problem with Ammonia

Because amino acids contain nitrogen, as well as carbon, hydrogen, and oxygen, the breakdown of protein poses a special problem. Carbon, hydrogen, and oxygen can be broken down into carbon dioxide and water and eliminated from the body. The nitrogen part of the amino acid, however, must be handled in a special way, primarily by the liver. Nitrogen is either recycled and used to synthesize different amino acids or converted to urea and excreted.

Formation of Urea

Some of the nitrogen released by the breakdown of amino acids is converted to urea by the liver (as illustrated in Figure 4-6). Blood then carries the urea, a nitrogenous waste, from the liver to the kidneys, where it is eliminated in the urine. It should be noted that most nitrogen is recycled and not excreted as waste.

Worrying About Ammonia. Why does the liver "worry" about ammonia? Under normal conditions, the liver extracts ammonia (NH_3) from the blood and converts it to urea. Why? Ammonia is toxic to brain cells and causes disorientation (Who am I? Where am I? What time is it?) and a diminished level of consciousness. In liver failure, the extraction of ammonia from the blood

Table 4-4 Proteins

Type	Function
Structural proteins	
Components of cell membranes	Perform many functions: determine pore size; allow hormones to "recognize" cell
Collagen	Structural component of muscle and tendons
Keratin	Part of skin and hair
Peptide hormones (e.g., insulin, growth hormone)	Many hormones are proteins and have widespread effects on many organ systems
Hemoglobin	Transport of oxygen
Antibodies	Protect body from disease-causing microorganisms
Plasma proteins	Blood clotting; fluid balance
Muscle proteins	Enable muscle to contract
Enzymes	Regulate the rates of chemical reactions

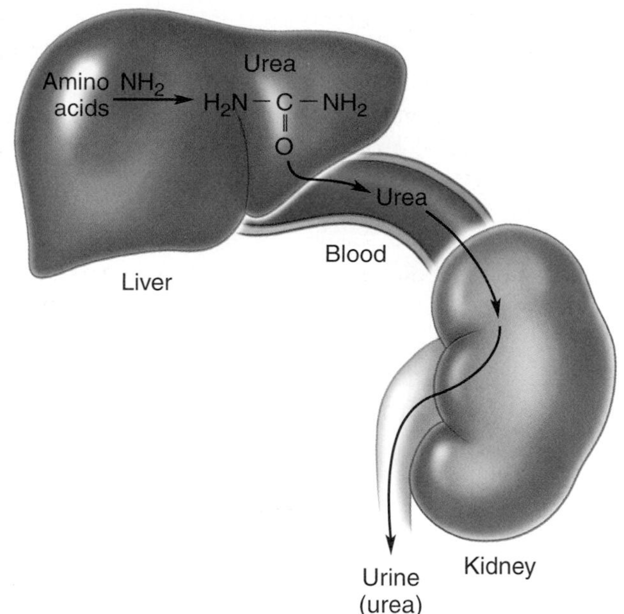

FIGURE 4-6 Urea. Formation in the liver and excretion by the kidney.

is diminished, so blood levels of ammonia rise. The toxic effect of ammonia on the brain has a fancy name: hepatic encephalopathy. A laboratory test called the blood urea nitrogen (BUN) measures the amount of urea in the blood. Because urea is eliminated in the urine, poor kidney function results in elevated BUN.

Sum It Up!

The body, like a factory, requires raw material for growth, repair, and operation. The raw materials for the body come in the form of food—carbohydrates, proteins, and fats. Carbohydrates and fats are the body's primary fuel. The proteins are used primarily in the synthesis of many vital substances, such as hormones, enzymes, antibodies, plasma proteins, and structural components of cells. Metabolism refers to the millions of chemical reactions that make the body run. The anabolic reactions are involved in the buildup, or synthesis, of complex substances from simpler substances. Catabolic reactions break down complex substances into simpler substances, generally in an effort to liberate energy stored within the food substances.

PROTEIN SYNTHESIS AND DNA

Proteins play a crucial role in every body function. You are what your proteins are! Protein synthesis involves the precise arrangement of amino acids in a specific sequence. Because the arrangement of amino acids is so precise, there is an elaborate protein-synthesizing mechanism in each cell. How does the cell know the exact pattern of amino acid assembly? The pattern of amino acid assembly is coded and stored within the **deoxyribonucleic** (dē-ŎK-sē-rī-bō-nū-KLĒ-ĭk) **acid (DNA)** in the nucleus. In fact, the essential role of DNA is to serve as a code for the structure of a protein.

DNA STRUCTURE

DNA is a nucleic acid. Nucleic acids are composed of smaller units called nucleotides (Figure 4-7, *A*). A nucleotide has three parts: a sugar, a phosphate group, and a base. Nucleotides are joined together to form long strands. Two strands of nucleotides are arranged in a twisted ladder formation (the double helix) to form DNA (see Figure 4-7, *B*). The two sides of the DNA ladder are composed of sugar-phosphate molecules. The rungs, or steps, of the ladder are composed of bases, one base from each side. The names of the bases in DNA are adenine (A), cytosine (C), guanine (G), and thymine (T). Note the different shapes of the bases in the rungs of the ladder. Note also that the bases have a particular arrangement. Adenine can pair only with thymine, and cytosine can pair only with guanine. Adenine and thymine are base-pairs, and cytosine and guanine are base-pairs. This system is called **base-pairing.**

The Genetic Code

The protein-synthesizing code is stored within DNA. More specifically, the information is stored, or encoded, within the sequence of bases along one strand (one side of the ladder) of DNA (Figure 4-8). Since the DNA is arranged in hereditary units called genes, the code is called the genetic code. (Genes and heredity are discussed further in Chapter 27.)

Reading the Code. A single strand of DNA reads vertically (according to the bases in the rungs); for example, GACGCCCAA. GAC (a sequence of three bases) codes for a particular amino acid. GCC codes for another amino acid, and CAA codes for a third amino acid. The list of bases in triplicate is called **base-sequencing.** In this way, DNA codes for the proper sequence of amino acids and therefore the synthesis of protein.

NOTE: Do not confuse base-pairing with base-sequencing. Base-pairing describes the way in which two strands of DNA are linked together by the bases. Base-sequencing describes the sequence, or order, of the bases along a single strand of DNA. The code is stored within the sequence of bases.

Copying the Code: mRNA. The code for protein synthesis is stored in the nucleus in the DNA. DNA does not leave the nucleus. Protein synthesis, however, occurs along the ribosomes in the cytoplasm. How does the code get out of the nucleus and into the cytoplasm? The copying and delivery of the code is done by a second nucleic acid called **ribonucleic** (rī-bō-nū-KLĒ-ĭK) **acid (RNA).**

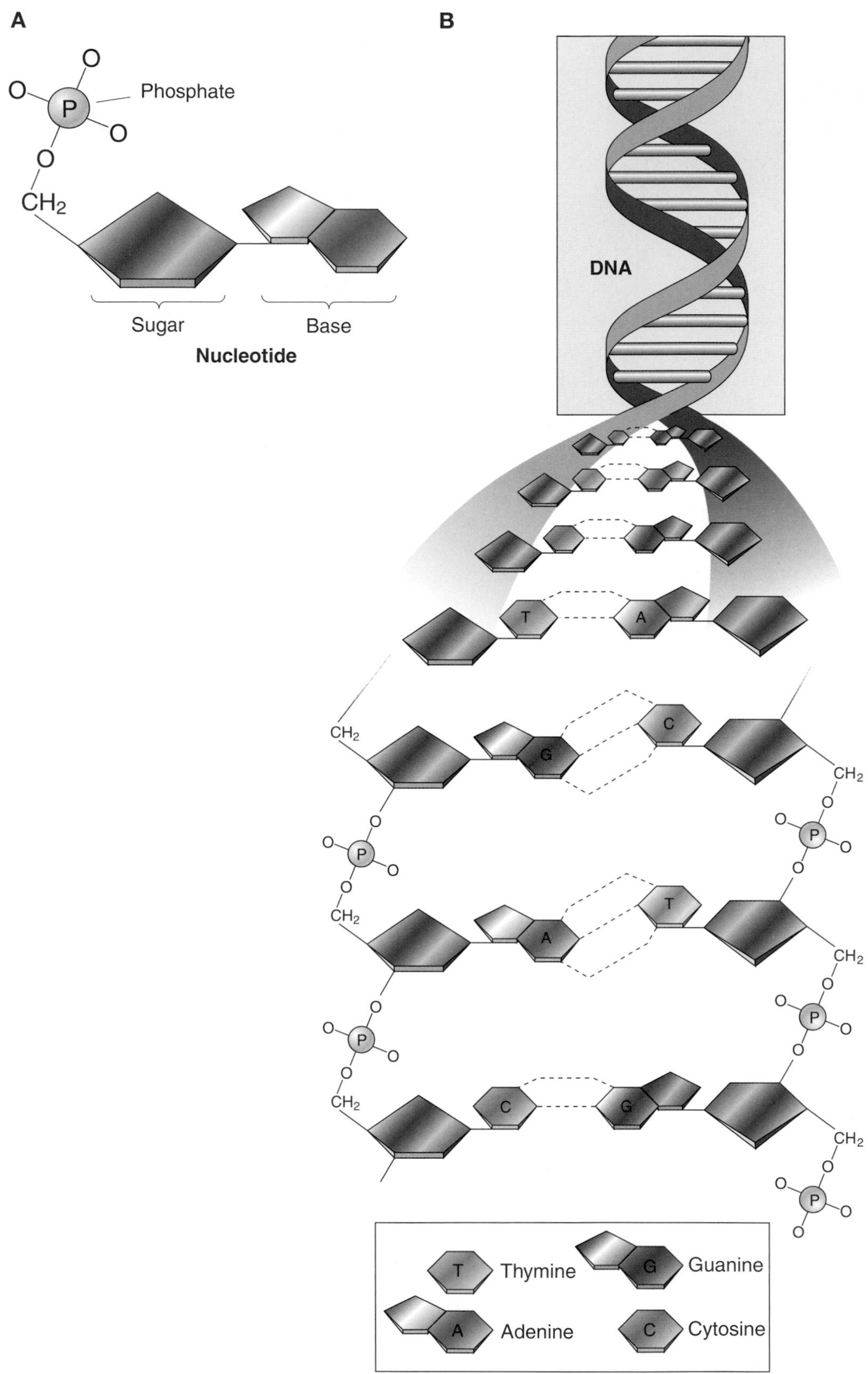

FIGURE 4-7 **A,** Nucleotide. **B,** The ladder structure of DNA. Note the base-pairing of the DNA strands.

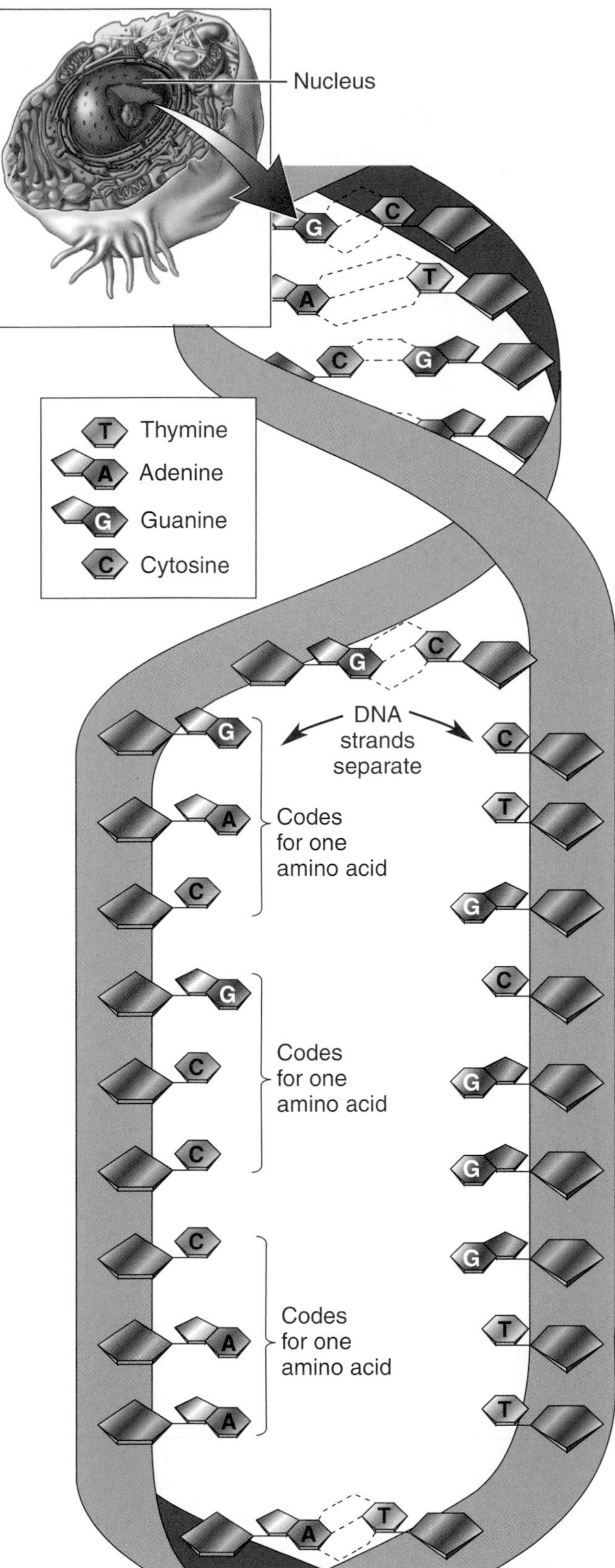

FIGURE 4-8 DNA: genetic code and base sequencing.

RNA is a nucleic acid composed of nucleotides and resembling the structure of DNA. RNA differs from DNA in three ways:

1. The sugars are different. The sugar in DNA is deoxyribose, whereas the sugar in RNA is ribose.
2. DNA has two strands, whereas RNA has only one strand.
3. There is a difference in one of the bases. Both DNA and RNA contain cytosine (C), guanine (G), and adenine (A). The fourth base differs. DNA contains thymine (T), whereas RNA contains uracil (U). The uracil in RNA base-pairs with adenine. The differences between DNA and RNA are summarized in Table 4-5.

There are three types of RNA, but we are concerned with only messenger RNA (mRNA) and transfer RNA (tRNA). Messenger RNA copies the code from DNA in the nucleus and then carries the code, or message, to the ribosomes in the cytoplasm. Because this type of RNA acts as a messenger, it is called mRNA.

Transfer RNA is found attached to individual amino acids within the cytoplasm and can "read" the code on the mRNA sitting on the ribosome. Each individual amino acid is carried by tRNA to its proper site on the mRNA. The amino acids are assembled in the proper sequence as the polypeptide (protein) is formed.

mRNA as Copycat. Refer to Figure 4-8 as we see how mRNA copies the code. DNA separates and exposes the base sequences, GACGCCCAA. A strand of mRNA "reads" the base sequence by forming base pairs. The strand of mRNA has this code: CUGCGGGUU. (The mRNA is not shown.) The copying of the code by mRNA is called **transcription.** Following transcription, the mRNA takes the code to the ribosomes in the cytoplasm, where the amino acids will be assembled.

Purines and Pyrimidines

The bases in the nucleotides that make up DNA and RNA are classified as either purines or pyrimidines. Adenine and guanine are purines, and cytosine, thymine, and uracil are pyrimidines. This terminology is important for you to know because some anticancer drugs are called purine analogs and others pyrimidine analogs. This means that the drugs resemble purines

Table 4-5 Comparison of DNA and RNA Structures

	DNA	RNA
Sugar	Deoxyribose	Ribose
Base	Adenine	Adenine
	Guanine	Guanine
	Cytosine	Cytosine
	Thymine	Uracil
Strands	Double (2)	Single (1)

and pyrimidines. When incorporated in the DNA molecule, the drugs distort the genetic code, impair protein synthesis, and kill the cancer cell. Unfortunately, the drugs are also incorporated into normal cells, thereby causing their death and many of the toxic effects of cancer therapy. No wonder these anticancer drugs are classified as cytotoxic agents.

STEPS IN PROTEIN SYNTHESIS

How do DNA and RNA control protein synthesis? The following five steps are involved in protein synthesis (Figure 4-9):

1. When a particular protein is to be synthesized, the strands of DNA in the nucleus separate. The exposed sequence of bases on the separated DNA strand is copied onto a strand of mRNA (transcription).
2. The mRNA leaves the nucleus and travels to the ribosomes in the cytoplasm.
3. The code on the mRNA (now sitting on a ribosome) determines what amino acids can attach to it. For instance, the code may specify that only the amino acid alanine can bind to site number 1 and only the amino acid cysteine can bind to site number 2.

How does alanine (located in the cytoplasm) know that it should move to the ribosome for protein assembly? Alanine is attached to tRNA. The tRNA contains bases that can recognize and pair with the bases on

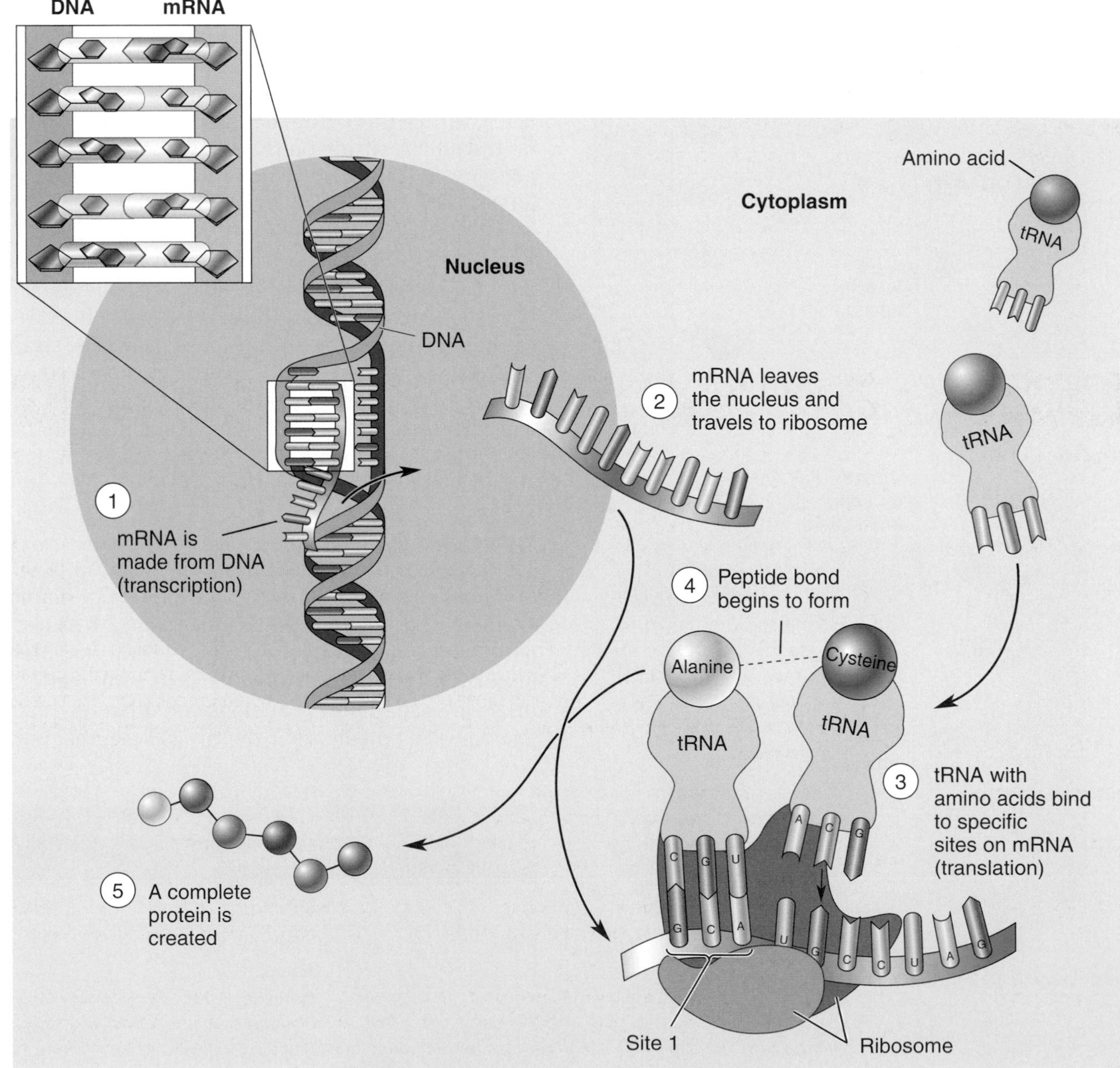

FIGURE 4-9 Steps in protein synthesis (5).

mRNA. For example, if mRNA contains the base sequence GCA, then only a tRNA with the base sequence of CGU can attach to that site. The reading of the mRNA code by tRNA is called **translation.**

NOTE: Transcription refers to the copying of the code of DNA in the nucleus by mRNA. Translation refers to the recognition of the mRNA code by tRNA. This process occurs along the ribosomes in the cytoplasm.

4. The amino acids are lined up in proper sequence along the ribosome. A peptide bond forms between each amino acid, creating a growing peptide chain.
5. When all of the amino acids have been assembled in the exact sequence dictated by the code, the protein chain is terminated. A complete protein has been created. The protein is now ready for use in the cell or for export to another site outside the cell.

Sum It Up!

Body structure and function are largely determined by the specific proteins synthesized by the cells. Because of the crucial roles played by proteins, an elaborate cellular mechanism guides the assembly of the various amino acids into proteins. Your protein blueprint, or genetic code, is stored in the DNA in the nucleus. When there is need for protein synthesis, the code must be transported to the ribosome, where amino acid assembly takes place. Protein synthesis occurs in five steps (see Figure 4-9).

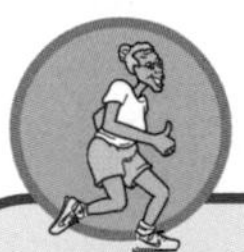

As You Age

1. Age brings a decrease in the number and function of organelles such as mitochondria. Because mitochondria play a key role in metabolism, a decrease in mitochondrial function affects metabolism.
2. In general, metabolism slows with aging. This effect is secondary to a decrease in hormonal secretion, particularly the thyroid hormones. A decreased metabolism has several effects: less tolerance to cold, a tendency to gain weight, and metabolic effects such as a decreased efficiency in using glucose.
3. The rate of protein synthesis decreases. Tissue growth and repair slow down, as does the synthesis of other proteins such as digestive enzymes.

Disorders of Metabolism

Cyanide poisoning	Cyanide is a poison that works by inactivating some of the enzymes in the mitochondria. As a result, oxygen cannot be used, production of ATP stops, and the person dies. A commonly used cardiac drug produces cyanide as a side effect.
Enzyme deficiency diseases	Many diseases are caused by the lack of an enzyme or a defective enzyme. Phenylketonuria is caused by a deficiency of an enzyme that metabolizes the amino acid phenylalanine. Phenylalanine is excreted in the urine, producing phenylketonuria (PKU), a condition that causes severe mental retardation. Cystic fibrosis is caused by defective transporter membrane proteins. This deficiency causes the production of a thick and salty mucus, sweat, and decreased secretion of pancreatic enzymes. The thick mucus in the lungs causes difficulty in breathing. The thick mucus in the pancreas plugs the pancreatic ducts, thereby decreasing the flow of digestive enzymes. Glycogen storage disease is due to an enzyme deficiency that causes excess glycogen to be deposited in the liver and skeletal muscle.
Hormonal disorders	All hormonal disorders are characterized by metabolic changes. In diabetes mellitus, the lack of insulin affects carbohydrate, protein, and fat metabolism; the body burns fat and wastes protein and carbohydrates. Hyperthyroidism increases the metabolic rate; the body speeds up its metabolism, sometimes to the point of causing the heart to fail.
Hypermetabolic state	The hypermetabolic states can develop in patients who have sustained severe burns, in patients with life-threatening infections, and in cachexic patients (patients with advanced cancer who appear wasted).
Lactic acidosis	The amount of oxygen severely decreases in the tissues of a patient in shock. This decrease in oxygen causes the metabolism to shift from an aerobic (with oxygen) to an anaerobic (without oxygen) metabolism. The anaerobic burning of glucose produces lactic acid. An accumulation of lactic acid causes a severe disturbance in blood pH called lactic acidosis.

Matching: Biochemistry Terms

Directions: Match the following words with their descriptions below. Some words may be used more than once.

a. glycolysis
b. Krebs cycle
c. gluconeogenesis
d. enzyme
e. ketone bodies

1. ____ Series of aerobic reactions that occur within the mitochondria
2. ____ Series of anaerobic reactions that occur within the cytoplasm
3. ____ Process of converting protein to glucose
4. ____ Catalyst
5. ____ Series of reactions that converts glucose to lactic acid
6. ____ Metabolic consequence of rapid and incomplete breakdown of fatty acids

Matching: Genetic Code and Protein Synthesis

Directions: Match the following words with their descriptions below.

a. mRNA
b. ribose
c. base-pairing
d. DNA
e. base-sequencing

1. ____ Double-stranded nucleotide that stores the genetic code
2. ____ The manner in which the genetic code is stored
3. ____ The manner by which one strand of a nucleotide interacts with another
4. ____ Single-stranded nucleotide that brings the code from the nucleus to the ribosomes
5. ____ A sugar used in the formation of a nucleotide

Multiple Choice

1. Which of the following is true of the Krebs cycle and electron transport chain enzymes?
   a. Are located within the mitochondria
   b. Function anaerobically
   c. Result in lactic acid production
   d. Are responsible for glycolysis
2. Which of the following is not characteristic of glycolysis?
   a. Occurs within the cytoplasm
   b. Operates anaerobically
   c. Forms lactic acid
   d. Completely metabolizes glucose to CO_2, H_2O, and energy
3. Which of the following is not characteristic of urea?
   a. Formed in the liver
   b. Is nitrogen-containing
   c. Characterized as an essential amino acid
   d. Excreted by the kidneys
4. Which of the following is not true of amino acids?
   a. Joined together by peptide bonds
   b. The building blocks of protein
   c. Classified as monosaccharides, disaccharides, and polysaccharides
   d. Classified as essential and nonessential
5. Monosaccharides
   a. include glucose, fructose, and galactose.
   b. include sucrose, lactose, and maltose.
   c. are classified as saturated and unsaturated.
   d. are the building blocks of protein.
6. Which of the following is descriptive of glycogen?
   a. Can be degraded to glucose thereby elevating blood glucose
   b. Combines with three fatty acids to form a lipid
   c. Is nitrogen-containing
   d. Is a disaccharide

CHAPTER 5

Microbiology Basics

KEY TERMS

Bacteria, p. 64
Carrier, p. 70
Disease, p. 63
Fungus, p. 66
Helminth, p. 66
Infection, p. 63
Normal flora, p. 64
Nosocomial infection, p. 69
Parasite, p. 65
Pathogen, p. 63
Protozoa, p. 66
Rickettsia, p. 65
Spores, p. 65
Sporozoa, p. 66
Vector, p. 66
Virus, p. 65

OBJECTIVES

1. Define *disease* and *infection.*
2. Describe the types of bacteria by shape and staining characteristics.
3. List the characteristics of the different types of pathogens.
4. Define portals of exit and portals of entry.
5. List common ways in which infections are spread.
6. Identify the microbiological principles described in six germ-laden stories.

For as long as humans have roamed the earth, we have been plagued by disease, especially infectious disease. A long and colorful history of medicine relates many tales of how we learned to dose, purge, lance, and incant. Sometimes we managed to arrest and cure the disease, but many times we killed the patient long before we killed the germs. The battle against disease is far from over. The microbial warriors are tough; they mount a great offensive and are very persistent! Although we may not tremble at the thought of the black death that terrorized Europe in the 1300s, we tremble at the thought of other plagues around today, as well as those that can erupt tomorrow. We are living through the terror of acquired immunodeficiency syndrome (AIDS), and we dread an outbreak of avian flu, the contamination of a minor abrasion with flesh-eating streptococcus, and the possibility of contracting mad cow disease, of all things! What about the new generation of life-threatening "super bugs" that are resistant to all antibiotics? This chapter provides background information about microbiology—the world of microorganisms, those tiny critters that keep scientists glued to their microscopes. Chapter 21 describes the body's response to this microbial challenge.

WHAT IS DISEASE?

Disease is a failure of the body to function normally. There are many types of diseases, not all caused by germs. These include inherited diseases, diseases caused by birth defects, age-related degenerative diseases, diseases caused by nutritional deficiencies, tumors, and diseases related to trauma and environmental toxins. This chapter focuses on infectious disease. Although most microorganisms are harmless or even beneficial to the body, some are harmful, causing disease and sometimes death. A leading cause of disease in humans is the invasion of the body by **pathogens,** or disease-producing microorganisms. The invasion of the body by a pathogen and the symptoms that develop in response to this invasion are called an **infection.** A **localized infection** is restricted to a small area, whereas a **systemic infection** is more widespread. A systemic infection is usually spread by the blood; it affects the entire body and generally makes you feel sick. Table 5-1 describes several key terms used in discussing microbiology.

Table 5-1 Key Microbiological Terms

Term	Definition
Antibiotics	Chemicals that are used to treat bacterial infections. A broad-spectrum antibiotic destroys many different types of bacteria, whereas a narrow-spectrum antibiotic destroys only a few types.
Communicable disease	Any disease that can be spread from one host to another. A noncommunicable disease is an infectious disease that cannot be transmitted directly or indirectly from host to host. For instance, a bladder infection due to *E. coli* cannot be spread from the infected person to another person. A contagious disease is a communicable disease that is easily spread from one person to another. Measles and chickenpox are contagious diseases because they are easily spread.
Epidemic disease	A disease acquired by many people in a given area over a short period of time. An endemic disease is always present in a population. A pandemic is a worldwide epidemic.
Epidemiology	The study of the occurrence and distribution of a disease in a population.
Incubation period	The lapsed period of time from the exposure of a person to a pathogen to the development of the symptoms of the disease.
Normal flora	A group of microorganisms that colonize a host without causing disease. Normal flora colonize the mouth, intestinal tract, vagina, nasal cavities, and other areas of the body. Microorganisms that are not pathogenic in one area may become pathogenic when transferred to another area. For instance, when the *E. coli* bacterium that is part of the normal flora of the large intestine is unintentionally transferred to the urinary bladder, it causes a bladder infection. Some body fluids such as blood, urine, and cerebrospinal fluid are sterile and do not have a normal flora.
Nosocomial infection	A hospital-acquired infection.
Reservoir of infection	A continual source of infection. A reservoir of infection can be living organisms such as humans and other animals and nonliving objects or substances that are contaminated with the pathogen. A contaminated nonliving object is called a fomite, such as a dirty glass and used needles. Contaminated soil and water also serve as inanimate reservoirs of infection.
Resistance	The ability to ward off disease. A lack of resistance is called susceptibility.
Sterilization	A process that destroys all living organisms.
Vector	A carrier of pathogens from host to host. The mosquito is the animal vector carrying the plasmodium (malaria) to humans. A contaminated syringe is a nonliving vector (fomite).

TYPES OF PATHOGENS

The groups of microorganisms (some of which are pathogens) are bacteria, viruses, fungi, and protozoa. Other larger, disease-causing organisms include worms and arthropods (Figure 5-1).

MICROORGANISMS (MICROBES)

Bacteria (singular: bacterium) are single-cell organisms found everywhere. They were first observed under the microscope by van Leeuwenhoek, who called them "little beasties." Most bacteria consider living conditions within the human body to be ideal, so they move right in. The good news is that many bacteria perform useful roles. For instance, **normal flora** (organisms that normally and harmoniously live in or on the human body without causing disease) prevents the overgrowth of other organisms, keeping them under control. Some bacteria synthesize needed substances such as vitamin K. The bad news is that bacteria can also cause disease. In fact, bacteria make up the largest group of pathogens. When bacteria successfully invade the human body they cause damage in two ways: (1) by entering and growing in the human cell, and (2) secreting toxins that damage the cells.

Bacteria are classified into three groups based on shape: (1) coccus (round); (2) bacillus (rod-shaped); and (3) curved rod. Rickettsiae and chlamydiae are also classified as bacteria, although they differ in several important ways from cocci, bacilli, and curved rods.

The **cocci** are round cells and are arranged in patterns. Cocci that are arranged in pairs are called **diplococci.** **Streptococci** are arranged in chains, like a chain of beads. **Staphylococci** look like bunches of grapes and are arranged in clusters. The cocci cause many diseases including gonorrhea, meningitis, and pneumonia. The **bacilli** are long and slender and are shaped like a cigar. Diseases caused by bacilli include tetanus, diphtheria, and tuberculosis. The curved rods include the **vibrio,** the **spirillum,** and the **spirochete.** The **vibrios** have a slight curve and resemble a comma. Cholera is caused by a vibrio (*Vibrio cholerae*). The **spirillum** is a long cell that coils like a corkscrew. Tightly coiled spirilla that are capable of waving and twisting motions are called **spirochetes.** The most famous spirochete, *Treponema pallidum,* causes syphilis. Syphilis has been bouncing around for centuries. Its origin, if nothing else, is colorful. The French called syphilis the Italian disease and, of course, the Italians reciprocated, calling it the French disease. The Polish referred to it as the German disease and, you guessed it, the Germans called it the Polish disease! Regardless of its origin, syphilis is well traveled.

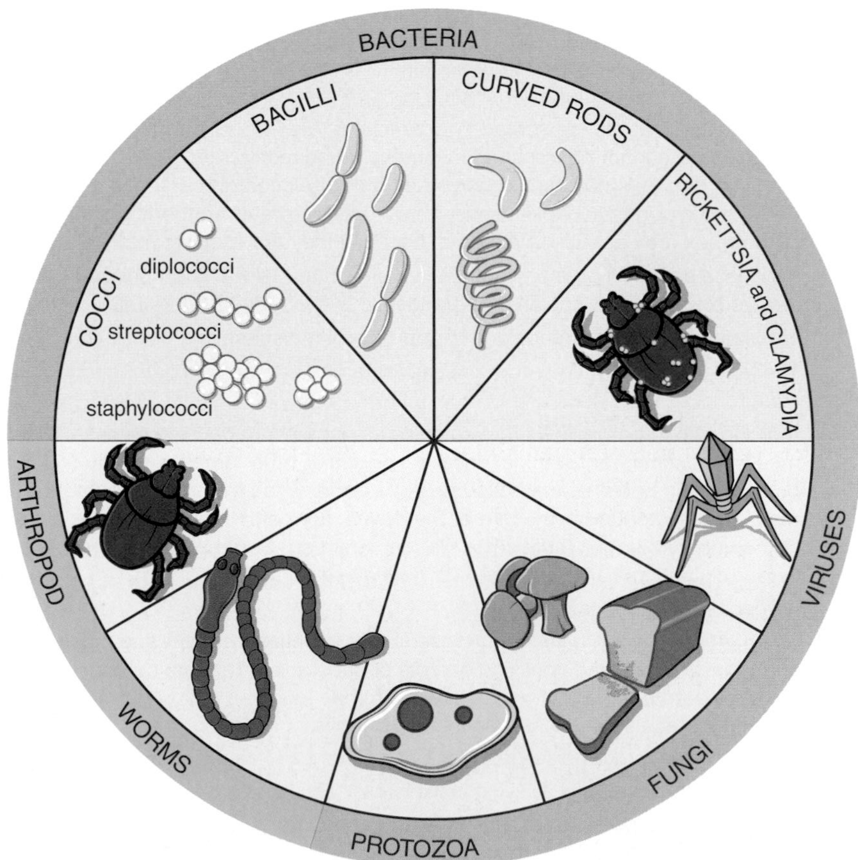

FIGURE 5-1 Pathogens: microorganisms and larger disease-causing organisms.

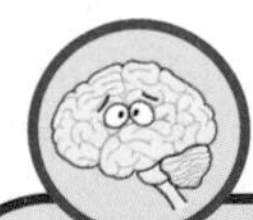

Do You Know...

What Maria, Sophia, and Leah have in common?

"Hey! Maria, Sophia, and Leah . . . y'all got gonorrhea," shouts their main squeeze. Mr. Busy has just been informed that he has gonorrhea, a sexually transmitted infection caused by *N. gonorrhoeae.* As the girls now know, gonorrhea is highly contagious. Today has been hectic for our carrier, Mr. B. He began treatment with the antibiotic ciprofloxacin and is currently burning up the phone lines informing his sexual partners (called contacts in public health jargon) of probable and almost certain infection. It is crucial that all four be treated for gonorrhea to prevent the "Ping-Pong" effect: treatment and cure—reexposure and reinfection. By this time next week, Maria, Sophia, and Leah should also be taking ciprofloxacin and sitting at home in front of the TV contemplating the definition of "safe sex."

No one is "clapping," as in days of old, when the infected were welcomed home by the clapping sounds of their shipmates. (Hence, the nickname "clap" for gonorrhea.)

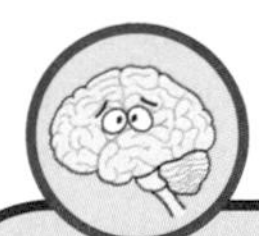

Do You Know...

That Lues, Lues is not a hit tune?

Lues, Lues sounds like an "oldie but goody" hit tune. In fact, it is an oldie, but it is definitely not a goody. Lues refers to syphilis. Lesions associated with syphilis are referred to as luetic lesions. Got lues? Singin' nothing but the blues.

There are two clinically important characteristics of bacteria: (1) the presence of a cell wall and (2) the ability to form spores. Although the human cell is surrounded by the cell membrane, the bacterial cell is surrounded by two structures, a cell membrane and an outer cell wall. The bacterial cell wall is a rigid wall that protects the underlying cell membrane from bursting. If the cell wall is damaged, the cell membrane of the bacterium bursts, killing the bacterium. Enter penicillin! Penicillin prevents cell wall synthesis in the bacterium, causing the cell membrane to burst and the bacterium to die. Since human cells do not have a cell wall, they are not damaged by penicillin; penicillin is therefore relatively safe when administered to humans. Because a virus does not have an outer cell wall, it is not affected by penicillin. So, do not take penicillin for a viral infection—it does not work.

Many bacteria form **spores** that allow them to survive harsh environmental conditions such as drying, heating, and exposure to certain disinfectants. Spores enable the bacteria to exist in a "sleepy," or dormant, state until conditions improve. Then the bacteria wake up, grow, and resume their usual activities. For instance, *Clostridium botulinum,* the organism that causes a deadly form of food poisoning (botulism), is a spore former and can withstand several hours of exposure to boiling water. Obviously, spore-forming microorganisms have great survival skills and present a challenge in infection control procedures.

Rickettsia (rĭ-KĔT-sē-ă) and **chlamydia** are classified as bacteria. However, they are smaller than most bacteria and must reproduce within the living cells of a host. Because they require a living host, they are called **parasites.** The rickettsiae are often carried by fleas, ticks, and body lice. For instance, the rickettsia that causes Rocky Mountain spotted fever is carried by the tick. Body lice carry the rickettsia responsible for epidemic typhus. The chlamydiae are smaller than rickettsiae and cause several important human diseases. One of the most prevalent sexually transmitted diseases in the United States today is caused by *Chlamydia trachomatis.* Chlamydial infection is also responsible for trachoma, a serious eye infection that is a leading cause of blindness in the world. Like other bacterial infections, rickettsial and chlamydial infections are treated with antibiotics.

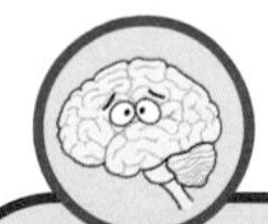

Do You Know...

Who Russ T. Nale is?

Russ T. Nale stepped on one. By stepping on a rusty nail, he accomplished two things. First, he allowed a potentially lethal pathogen, *Clostridium tetani,* to enter his body. Second, he had a deep puncture wound that encouraged the growth of the pathogen. Because little bleeding is associated with a puncture wound, the pathogen was not washed out of the wound. More importantly, however, a deep puncture wound prevents air (oxygen) from entering the wound. Because this pathogen grows anaerobically (without oxygen), the conditions associated with a puncture wound are ideal. Sure hope Russ is up-to-date on his tetanus shots!

Viruses (from the Latin meaning poison) are the smallest of the infectious agents. They are not cells and consist of either ribonucleic acid (RNA) or deoxyribonucleic acid (DNA) surrounded by a protein shell. Since viruses can only reproduce within the living cells of a host, they are parasites. Examples of viral diseases are measles, mumps, influenza, poliomyelitis, and AIDS. Because of the intimacy of the virus-host relationship, the development of nontoxic antiviral agents has been slow and difficult. This point is well illustrated by the drug zidovudine (AZT), used in the treatment of AIDS. While exerting antiviral effects, the drug also causes widespread damage to the host cells. Most upper respiratory infections are viral and are not responsive to antibiotic therapy.

Fungus is a plantlike organism, such as a mushroom, which grows best in dark, damp places. Yeasts and molds (such as bread mold) are types of fungi. Pathogenic fungi cause **mycotic infections** (myco means fungus). Mycotic infections are usually localized and include athlete's foot, ringworm, thrush (in the mouth), and vaginitis. *Candida albicans* is a yeastlike fungus that normally inhabits the mouth, digestive tract, and vagina. When Candida overgrows, it can cause an infection in the mouth (thrush), intestinal symptoms, or vaginitis. Systemic fungal infections are rare, but when they do occur, they are life threatening and difficult to cure.

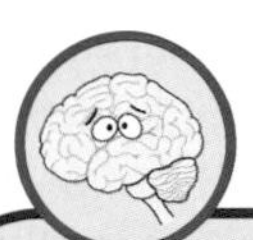

Do You Know...

About the ring of ringworm?

Ringworm is an infection of the skin caused not by worms but a fungus. Why the circular or ring shape? The fungus grows outwards from the center. The fungi in the center of the lesion die before the outer circle of fungi die. This type of fungal growth pattern leaves a clear or healed center surrounded by living fungi.

NOTE: There is a ringworm bush (*Cassia alata*) whose leaves produce a juice that is used as a cure for ringworm and poisonous bites. The two explanations for the name ringworm are as follows: (1) An ancient and mistaken belief existed that worms caused the infection. (2) It was named after the ring-like or circular appearance of the lesion. Both theories have a "ring" of truth.

Protozoa (prō-tō-ZŌ-ă) are single-cell, animal-like microbes. The four main types of protozoa are **amebas, ciliates, flagellates,** and **sporozoa** (spŏr-ō-ZŌ-ă). Protozoa are found in the soil and in most bodies of water. Amebic dysentery and giardiasis are caused by protozoan parasites. The parasites are ingested in contaminated water and food and cause severe diarrhea. Malaria is caused by a sporozoan called a plasmodium. *Plasmodium malariae* is carried by a mosquito. The mosquito is capable of spreading malaria over a wide region. Indeed, malaria still causes more than three million deaths per year in the more tropical regions of the world. Two other members of the sporozoa group pose a serious health threat to those persons with impaired immune systems. *Pneumocystis carinii* and *Cryptosporidium* cause infections in persons with AIDS and other immunocompromised persons. *Pneumocystis carinii* causes pneumonia, and *Cryptosporidium* causes severe diarrhea.

OTHER (MULTICELLULAR) DISEASE-CAUSING ORGANISMS

Other disease-causing organisms that are larger than microorganisms include multicellular organisms such as parasitic worms and arthropods.

Parasitic worms, called **helminths** (HĔL-mĭnths) are multicellular animals that are parasitic and pathogenic to humans. In other words, worms can be germs. The identification of most worm infestations requires microscopic examination of body samples (usually stool) and reveals the presence of either the adult worms or the larval forms. The worms are classified as roundworms or flatworms. Roundworms include ascarides, pinworms, hookworms, trichinae, and the tiny worms that cause filariasis (elephantiasis). Infestation by pinworms is common in children and is very hard to control. The pinworms live in the intestinal tract but lay their eggs on the outer perianal area. The deposition of the eggs causes itching (pruritus). A child may then scratch the anal area and transfer the eggs to his or her mouth and on to others. The eggs are swallowed and the newly hatched pinworms grow into adulthood in the intestine. Most worm infestations are transmitted by the **fecal-oral route.** (Hands contaminated by feces introduce the worms, eggs, or larvae into the mouth.) Trichinosis is transmitted by ingestion of undercooked contaminated pork, and filariasis is transmitted by biting insects.

The flatworms include the tapeworms and the flukes. Tapeworms that live in the intestines may grow from 5 to 50 feet in length. Imagine hosting a 50-foot tapeworm! Flukes are flat, leaf-shaped worms that invade the blood and organs such as the liver, lungs, and intestines. Because these large flatworms feed on the human host, infestation causes weight loss, anemia, and generalized debilitation. Infestation by worms is treated with drugs called anthelmintics (which means against worms).

Arthropods are animals with jointed legs and include insects and ticks. They are of concern for two reasons. Arthropods such as mites and lice are **ectoparasites,** meaning that they live on the surface of the body, the skin, and mucous membranes. Ectoparasites cause itching and discomfort but are not life threatening. More seriously, arthropods such as mosquitoes, biting flies, fleas, and ticks act as vectors of disease. (A **vector** is an object, living or nonliving, that transfers a pathogen from one organism to another.) The bite of the arthropod vector introduces pathogens into the **host** (the person or organism that is infected by a pathogen), causing infection. For instance, the mosquito (arthropod vector) can carry the pathogens for malaria and encephalitis. The tick can carry the pathogens that cause Lyme disease and Rocky Mountain spotted fever.

LABORATORY IDENTIFICATION OF PATHOGENS

Many laboratory procedures and techniques are used to identify pathogens. One of these techniques is called staining and involves the use of dyes. A second technique is a culture.

Many bacteria are classified according to staining characteristics using the **Gram stain** (a dye). A gram-positive bacterium is one that stains purple or blue. Streptococcus is an example of a gram-positive bacterium. A gram-negative bacterium such as *Escherichia coli,* does not absorb the purple Gram stain. Instead, a gram-negative bacterium picks up a pink or red stain. Since most bacteria are either gram-positive or gram-negative, Gram staining is an important first step in the identification of the causative organism of an infection.

Another stain is called the **acid-fast stain.** The bacterium is first stained with a red dye and then washed with an acid. Most bacteria lose the red stain when washed with acid. However, several bacteria retain the red stain and are therefore called acid-fast. The most famous of the acid-fast bacteria is the *Mycobacterium tuberculosis,* the causative organism of tuberculosis (TB). This organism is commonly called the acid-fast bacillus. Some bacteria do not stain with any of the commonly used dyes. Thus spirochetes and rickettsiae must be stained with special dyes and techniques.

Sometimes the physician wants to identify the specific pathogen growing in an infected wound and orders a wound culture to be done. A sample of the wound exudate (pus) is placed on culture medium (food that supports the growth of the pathogens). The pathogens are incubated and allowed to grow and multiply. The pathogens can then be stained and identified. The growth of pathogens in a culture medium is called a **culture.** The cultured pathogens can also be tested for their susceptibility to various antibiotics **(culture and sensitivity test).** For instance, if an antibiotic is placed in the same culture and stops the growth of the pathogen, the pathogen is assumed to be responsive or sensitive to the effects of the antibiotic. The antibiotic is given to the patient to treat the infection. Other antibiotics may have no effect on the growth of the pathogens in the culture and therefore would not be used in the treatment of the infection.

You will often be asked to collect samples for laboratory analysis. Specific rules must be followed for each specimen. For instance, in collecting a urine specimen that will be analyzed for the presence of pathogens, you must be careful not to contaminate the urine with microorganisms from your hands or unsterile containers. The proper identification of the pathogen depends on correct technique.

THE SPREAD OF INFECTION

To understand how infection is spread, we must know how germs move—in, out, and about (Figure 5-2).

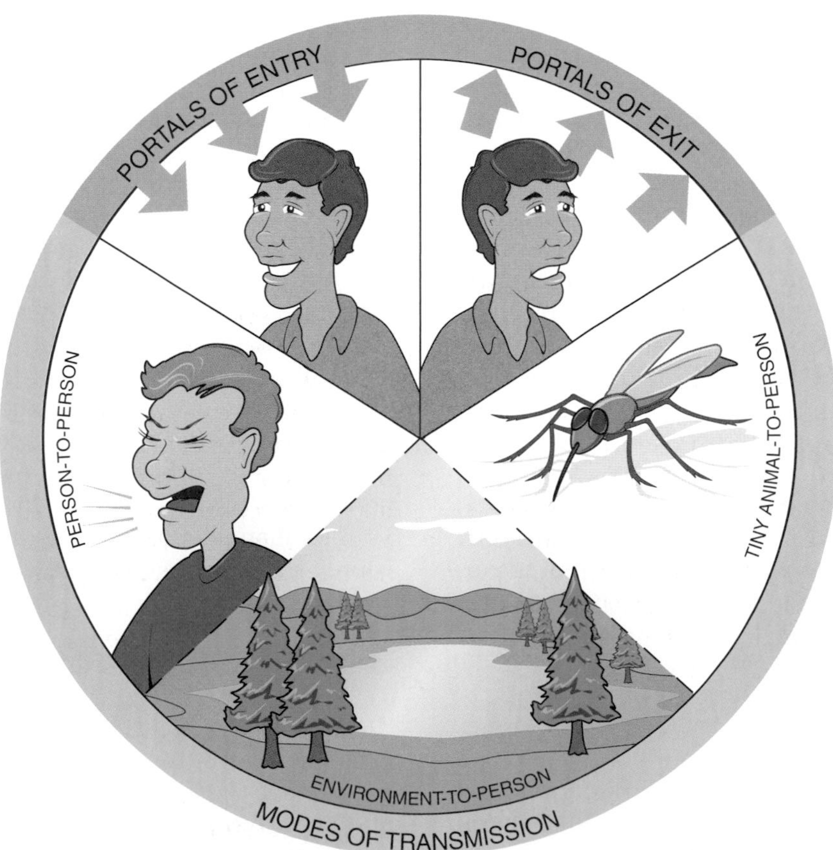

FIGURE 5-2 Spread of infection: portals of entry, portals of exit, and modes of transmission.

PORTALS OF ENTRY AND EXIT

How do pathogens enter the body? Pathogens enter the body by **portals of entry.** The portals of entry include the respiratory, gastrointestinal, and genitourinary tracts; eye (conjunctiva); skin; and parenteral route. The parenteral route includes those injuries that penetrate the skin or mucous membrane, such as bites, cuts, and surgery. A break in the skin is an excellent way for pathogens to enter the body. This is the reason that health-care workers wear gloves when handling blood or other body fluids. In the event that the body fluids are contaminated (with, say, the AIDS or hepatitis viruses) the gloves prevent the entrance of the virus through tiny cuts or abrasions. Most pathogens enter the body through the respiratory tract (inhaled droplets of water and dust) and the gastrointestinal tract (by eating spoiled food or placing contaminated hands in the mouth).

How do pathogens leave the body of an infected person? Pathogens leave an infected body by **portals of exit.** The portals of exit include the respiratory, gastrointestinal, or genitourinary tracts; the skin (intact and broken); eyes (tears); and breasts (milk). The most common portals of exit are the respiratory and gastrointestinal tracts. For example, the common cold virus is often sneezed or coughed into room air from the respiratory passages of the infected person, whereas the salmonella organism in a person with typhoid fever exits the body in the stool. Discharge from the urogenital tract is also an important means of spreading infection (sexually transmitted diseases). By knowing the portal of exit of each pathogen, one can set up procedures for preventing the spread of the infection. For instance, by knowing that *Salmonella typhi* is excreted in the stools, we know that the patient's underwear and bed linens are contaminated with the pathogens. We can then take measures to properly clean the soiled clothing and linens, thereby preventing the spread of the disease. By far, the most important procedure in preventing the spread of infection is **HANDWASHING!**

HOW PATHOGENS SPREAD

We know how pathogens enter and leave the body... but how do they move about or "spread"? Pathogens are spread from person to person, environment to person, and from "tiny animals" (insects) to persons (see Figure 5-2).

Person-to-Person Contact

Suppose you have a cold and go to work. Within a week, everyone in the office has your cold. What happened? First, whenever you sneezed, the cold virus was sprayed into the room air in little droplets of nasal discharge. These droplets were then inhaled by your co-workers. The virus was spread by droplet contact. Second, your hands were contaminated with the virus, and you touched many objects in the office (doorknobs; desktops; and other people's hands, as in handshaking), thereby contaminating these objects. Others touched the contaminated objects and eventually introduced the virus into their own body. The spread of infection from person to person is effective. One of the best ways to prevent respiratory infections is to avoid crowds during cold and flu season. (The doorknob is considered to be both a vector and a fomite. A **vector** is an object, living or nonliving, that transfers a pathogen from one organism to another. A **fomite** is a nonliving vector. Other fomites include soiled handkerchiefs and eating utensils.)

Environment-to-Person Contact

This mode of transmission includes contact with contaminated water, air, food, or soil. For instance, you can develop typhoid fever if you drink a glass of water contaminated by *Salmonella typhi.* Similarly you can develop food poisoning if you eat food contaminated with *Escherichia coli.*

"Tiny Animal"-to-Person Contact

This mode of transmission includes the use of insects (and other "creepy crawlies") in the spread of disease; these tiny animals are living vectors. Example: A mosquito bites a person with malaria. The malaria-causing plasmodium matures in the stomach of the mosquito. The plasmodium-loaded mosquito then bites another person and voila!—malaria. You can understand why the eradication of mosquitoes is key in malaria control. A final stomach-churning example is flies hopping from dog feces to food on a picnic table. The pathogens from the dog feces are transferred by the fly feet to the food, which is then eaten by you.

Note that the mosquito and fly both spread disease. The mosquito, however, plays a more complicated and biological role. The plasmodium (causative organism of malaria) requires the mosquito as part of its life cycle; it matures in the stomach of the mosquito. Because of this role the mosquito is called a **biological vector.** The lowly fly does not participate in the life cycle of the pathogen; it merely walks on the dog feces and the germs stick to the feet of the fly. The fly then flies onto your food and deposits the germs on your food. The fly is only a **mechanical vector.**

SIX GERM-LADEN STORIES

These six stories illustrate important microbiological principles and introduce you to the language of microbiology. Wash those Mitts is a tragic story of handwashing and nosocomial infection. Flora and Her Vaginal Itch addresses the normal flora and superinfection. Rick, Nick, and the Sick Tick describes disease transmission by an arthropod vector and differentiates between a communicable and contagious disease. Why Typhoid Mary Needed to Lose her Gallbladder describes the carrier state and the efficiency of the fecal-oral route in disease transmission. A Pox News Alert focuses on the pox throughout history and some of the current concerns. Finally, The Chief of Staph Reports indicates the clinical challenge of the staphylococcus. As you read the stories, refer to Table 5-1 for the definitions of unfamiliar terms; the table defines and expands the microbiological principles illustrated in the stories.

DR. SEMMELWEIS SCREAMS, "WASH THOSE MITTS!"

Dr. Ignaz Semmelweis was an assistant at the First Obstetrical Clinic in Vienna (circa 1850). At that time, an alarmingly high mortality rate was associated with puerperal fever or childbirth fever. Puerperal fever begins as an infection of the uterus after childbirth and is commonly caused by a strain of beta-hemolytic streptococcus. Puerperal fever progresses from an infection of the uterus to peritonitis and to generalized septicemia, ending in an agonizing death.

Semmelweis made the following two keen observations while caring for his patients:

1. A woman became ill immediately after being examined by a medical student who had previously examined a woman dying of puerperal fever.
2. If a medical student cut himself while attending a woman with puerperal fever, his wound became infected, and he subsequently died of puerperal sepsis.

Dr. Semmelweis concluded that puerperal fever is caused by conveyance to the pregnant woman of "putrid particles derived from living organisms through the agency of the examining fingers." This conclusion was impressive because he linked the disease to the putrid particles—tiny disease-producing critters that would not officially be discovered and linked to disease for another 25 years.

As a result of his observations, Semmelweis demanded that his medical students wash their hands with a disinfectant before examining each patient. "Wash those mitts!" he screamed, and wash they did. What happened? Mortality rates in his clinic decreased from 18% to 1%. You might conclude that Semmelweis eliminated puerperal fever and was honored by his colleagues. Not so! They ridiculed him for his insistence on handwashing. He eventually became so distraught that he deliberately cut his finger and contaminated his injury with the vaginal discharge of a woman with puerperal fever. Ranting and raving, he was committed to the Budapest Insane Asylum where he quickly died of the disease that he had worked so hard to eradicate.

With the passing of Semmelweis, the practice of handwashing was discontinued and the mortality rate from puerperal fever again soared. Puerperal fever, although rarely seen today, is a great example of a nosocomial infection. A **nosocomial** (nō-sō-KŌ-mē-ăl) **infection** is a hospital-acquired infection and is most often transmitted from patient to patient by direct contact (through the agency of the examining finger, according to Semmelweis). Today a nosocomial infection is transmitted by health professionals like us who DO NOT WASH THEIR HANDS. We go from patient to patient carrying germs from one to another. Historically, nosocomial infections have been a tremendous problem. Today, 15% of hospitalized patients develop a nosocomial infection. "Wash those mitts!" echoes through the centuries but generally falls on deaf ears.

FLORA AND HER VAGINAL ITCH

Stuffed up and miserable, Flora went to her physician. She was given an antibiotic for a sinus infection. Within a week the sinus infection was cured; the misery, however, had predictably headed south. Flora now had an antibiotic-induced vaginal discharge.

The vagina is normally inhabited by a population of diverse microbes. These microbes are permanent residents, and when present in normal amounts, they do not produce disease. This population of microbes within the vagina is called the **normal flora.** Other body cavities or areas such as the skin, large intestine, mouth, and respiratory tract contain their own diverse populations of microbes and therefore have their own normal flora.

The presence of a normal flora within the vagina prevents the overgrowth of yeast called *Candida albicans* that is present in small numbers within the vagina. If the normal flora is destroyed by an antibiotic, the yeast grows uncontrollably and causes candidiasis, a vaginal yeast infection, characterized by discharge, odor, and itching. Candidiasis is an example of a **superinfection.** Organisms that do not cause disease in their normal habitat become pathogenic when allowed to overpopulate the area. What was the cause of Flora's itch? Flora's normal flora had become abnormal. Watch those antibiotics!

RICK, NICK, AND THE SICK TICK

One week after returning from a camping trip with his friend Nick, Rick went to his physician feeling awful. He had chills; a high fever; headache; muscle pain; and a red, measleslike spotted rash that was prominent on the palms of his hands and the soles of his feet. On examination the physician removed a tick from Rick's back. He was diagnosed with Rocky Mountain spotted fever (RMSF) and treated with the antibiotic tetracycline. Microbiologically speaking, Rick had become the perfect **host** (an organism who had become infected with a pathogen).

Enough about Rick! What's with the tick? The tick that bit Rick was sick; it was infected with the pathogen called *Rickettsia rickettsii,* the causative organism of RMSF. When the tick bit Rick the infected saliva was injected into the bite site. The rickettsia then feasted on Rick's blood, growing, multiplying, and eventually causing the signs and symptoms that sent Rick to the doctor.

The tick acts as an arthropod vector for RMSF. An **animal vector** is an organism that transmits a pathogen such as rickettsia. An **arthropod** is a class of tiny animals that have jointed legs. In this case the arthropod is the sick tick. The rickettsia is transmitted by saliva (the bite of the tick) or the feces of the tick that are rubbed into the bite.

The tick also serves as a reservoir of infection. A **reservoir of infection** harbors pathogens; in this case the tick is the reservoir.

The tick is not killed by the rickettsia. Mama tick coexists with the rickettsia and passes the rickettsia through her eggs (transovarian passage) to her baby ticks, thereby perpetuating and expanding generations of sick ticks. It should be noted that the tick can live with or without the rickettsia; the rickettsia, however, must get inside the tick to grow and reproduce. Because of this dependency, rickettsiae are said to be obligate intracellular parasites—that is, they require the tick.

Why didn't Nick catch Rick's infection? RMSF is considered a **communicable disease** in as much as the infection can be spread (through the bite of a tick). RMSF, however, is not considered a **contagious disease**—that is, one easily spread from host to host like a common cold or impetigo. Thus Nick remained well, despite his close association with Rick.

One last thing about RMSF: it is an example of **zoonosis,** an animal disease that is transmissible to humans. Other zoonotic diseases include malaria and endemic typhus.

WHY TYPHOID MARY NEEDED TO LOSE HER GALLBLADDER

Mary Mallon (Typhoid Mary) lived in New York in the early 1900s. While employed as a cook, she unintentionally infected many persons with typhoid fever. Hearing several rumors of Mary's unfortunate associations with this disease, her wealthy employer hired a sanitary engineer, George Soper, to investigate the sudden outbreak of typhoid fever within his home. Soper soon informed Mary that she was a **carrier** of the germ that caused typhoid fever. Mary vehemently denied that she was the infecting culprit, since she herself did not feel ill. Understandably, she chased Soper from her kitchen with a carving fork. But Soper was correct. Mary was indeed a carrier of typhoid fever.

The *Salmonella typhi* bacterium, the causative organism of typhoid fever, is transmitted by the fecal-oral route through contaminated food or water. Mary's vocation as a cook was a perfect way to spread the salmonella organism via her contaminated hands touching food. Carriers of typhoid fever never rid their systems of the salmonella. Instead, they harbor the organisms in the bile stored within the gallbladder. Salmonella-laden bile then enters the intestine and contaminates the feces. Removal of the gallbladder rids the body of the salmonella, thereby eliminating the carrier state. Surgical removal of the gallbladder would have made an enormous difference in Mary's life. Unfortunately, Mary was forced into isolation on a coastal island where she lived unhappily for 26 years.

A POX NEWS ALERT!

Pox News, responding to an ancient medieval curse "A pox be upon you," has issued an update on the pox. Here it is, fair and balanced!

- There has been much confusion about the pox throughout history. The ancients referred to any infectious disease as a "dose of the pox." (Since pox infection was so ugly and visible the ancients commonly invoked pox-curses on their enemies.) Later the term pox was restricted to any disease characterized by a vesicular skin lesion. The term pox focuses only on the skin lesion and does not address its cause or treatment. Today the medical focus is placed on the type of virus that causes a pox.
- Pox diseases are not limited geographically, nor are they restricted to humans. There is pox everywhere; there are flocks of pox. There's monkey pox, parrot pox, camel pox, squirrel pox, goat pox, ox pox—even plants have pox (plum pox). Of course, jocks have pox. For sure, Fox have pox.
- Chickenpox, you say. Chickenpox is caused by the Varicella-Zoster virus, a member of the Herpes virus group. It is characterized by a vesicular pox, accompanied by severe pruritis, and capable of causing pock marks. Why the name chickenpox? Explanations abound. In England children were often called chicken. Since chickenpox is primarily a disease of children the pox was dubbed childrenpox. Others suggest that the name derived from the appearance of the pock mark; it looks like the skin has been pecked by a chicken. Others observe the pox as resembling chick peas. No telling what it means.
- Think that's strange? Pox News has just learned that some parents are throwing "pox parties" in which they are deliberately exposing their unvaccinated children to those who currently have chickenpox. What's THAT about? Some parents are convinced that the chickenpox vaccine is unsafe and that the only safe way to build up immunity is to "get" a real case of chickenpox. This is where the "pox party" comes in. When a child contracts chickenpox their friends are invited to a party. Get this! The infected child is told to blow a whistle and to then pass the whistle to his friends. The whistle, acting as a vector, then spreads the virus from child to child. The practice is effective

but dangerous. While most children recover uneventfully from chickenpox some develop serious complications. In particular, children who are immunocompromised may develop a lethal multiple organ infection by the virus; this carries a 17% mortality. Pox parties are probably not the best approach to infectious disease control.

- Poxes come in different sizes. There is the dreaded, lethal smallpox and the infamous Great Pox. Pox News, however, has just learned that the Great Pox is no pox at all; its pocky lesion is a chancre and is caused by a spirochete called the *Treponema pallidum.* Yikes, the Great Pox is syphilis, the source of untold misery. Just ask Beethoven, Hitler and his lovely bunker mate Eva B, Henry VIII and his tower ladies, and Pope Alexander VI, to mention a few. As for the Chief of Grief (syphilis), its etiology was accurately described by the ancients: "It is taken when one pocky person doth synne (sin) in lechery with one another." Prevention is obvious: Sin thou not with a pocky person.
- As for the curse "A pox be upon you," that prompted this news release? Pox News has officially nixed nasty pox curses: "No, no, no," says Mr. O.

THE CHIEF OF STAPH REPORTS . . .

For those of you who have never witnessed a staph meeting, here it is. The committee is meeting in the nostril of Petey Mrsa, a 2-year-old patient in the pediatric unit of a large hospital. Petey was admitted with a severe case of staphylococcus-induced impetigo. The impetigo sprawls from his nostrils to his upper lip. The infection is also apparent on his hands and arms, the natural handkerchief of a 2 year old.

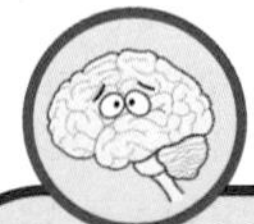

Do You Know . . .

That Dr. Herbie Zoster hung out his shingle?

Meet Dr. Herbie Zoster, a herpes specialist according to his newly hung shingle. Today he is seeing his first patient, Ms. Vera Cella. Ms. Cella is *trés* miserable; she has a string of painful skin lesions around her waist. Dr. Zoster makes an immediate diagnosis: it is shingles, medically known as herpes zoster. Shingles is an acute infection of the peripheral nervous system caused by the varicella-zoster virus, the same virus that causes chickenpox. After a person recovers from chickenpox, the virus hides in a posterior root ganglion. Later in life, often in response to stress or immunosuppressive therapies, the virus leaves the ganglion and travels along the sensory neurons to the skin. This results in a line of skin blisters along the infected nerve and severe pain. As a complication, some persons develop a postherpetic neuralgia (pain that lingers long after the skin lesions have cleared). Yes! Shingles can be triggered by exposure to a child with chickenpox.

The rotund staph members are huddled together in grape-like clusters in Petey's little nose. They appear happy, oozing a honey-colored exudate, and reproducing every 20 minutes. Moreover, they seem indifferent to the antibiotics administered to Petey.

The Chief of Staph is Dr. Aureus, who has an infectious personality and answers to the name Golden Boy (a reference to his ooze). He is eloquently orating on the characteristics of staphylococcal exudates and the expanding numbers of drug-resistant strains of the Gram (+) medical menace. Soon the swelling and oozing staph members begin chanting "MRSA, MRSA, MRSA." The MRSA chant is indeed appropriate; **m**ethicillin-**r**esistant **s**taph **a**ureus is a major cause of resistant nosocomial infection. This is what really hurts! Aureus is acknowledging the cooperation of the hospital staff for its indiscriminate use of antibiotics and for its reluctance to "wash those mitts" (to again quote Dr. Semmelweis).

The Chief of Staph has called for reports from his ad hoc committees.

The Committee on Pimples and Boils is listing its accomplishments, attributing its success to "where they (staph) hang out" on the skin or up noses. It too offers an appreciative nod to shoddy hygienic practices.

The Committee on Resistant Strains is ecstatic. Its greatest achievement? "We've almost got vancomycin out of the picture," spews the Chair. This is a reference to the development of resistance to the most powerful antistaphylococcal drug. Today, we are almost defenseless against staph infections, and lethal staph infections are on the rise.

The Committee on Food Poisoning is bragging about a wedding reception that was forced to reconvene in the emergency room of the local hospital.

One cockeyed coccus who looks particularly mean is reporting on Scalded Skin Syndrome. He is jubilantly describing the peeling away of the layers of skin of a person with a generalized staphylococcal infection.

Whoops! The meeting is adjourned folks. Petey sneezed . . . dispersing the committee far and wide.

Sum It Up!

Infectious disease has plagued us forever. Today the battle continues against the tiny but tough disease-producing organisms called pathogens. Pathogens include bacteria, viruses, fungi, protozoa, parasitic worms, and arthropods. To understand the transmission of an infection one should know the portals of entry (how the pathogen enters the body); the portal of exit (how the pathogen leaves the body); and how the pathogen is spread (person to person, environment to person, or tiny animal to person). Important microbiological principles are illustrated in the six germ-laden stories.

Disorders Caused by Pathogens

Cocci	
Neisseria	*N. gonorrhoeae* causes gonorrhea and inflammation of the mucous membranes of the reproductive and urinary tracts. May cause sterility and pelvic inflammatory disease (PID). Infants of infected mothers may develop ophthalmia neonatorum. *N. meningitidis* causes meningitis, inflammation of the membranes covering the brain and the spinal cord.
Staphylococcus	*S. aureus* causes skin infections such as boils and impetigo, pneumonia, kidney and bladder infections, osteomyelitis, septicemia, and food poisoning. *S. aureus* is a leading cause of nosocomial (hospital-acquired) infections.
Streptococcus	*S. pneumoniae* causes pneumonia, middle ear infection, and meningitis. *S. pyogenes* causes septicemia, strep throat, middle ear infection, scarlet fever, pneumonia, and endocarditis. Immunological response can cause rheumatic fever with permanent damage to the heart valves, and glomerulonephritis.
Bacilli	
Bordetella pertussis	Bordetella causes pertussis (whooping cough), a severe infection of the trachea and bronchi characterized by episodes of violent coughing. The "whoop" is an effort to inhale after the coughing bouts.
Clostridium	*C. botulinum* causes botulism, a potentially fatal form of food poisoning due to improper processing of foods. *C. perfringens* causes gas gangrene, in which death of the tissue is accompanied by the production of a gas. *C. tetani* causes tetanus, or "lockjaw."
Escherichia coli	*E. coli* is part of the normal flora of the intestines. *E. coli* causes local and systemic infections, food poisoning, diarrhea, septicemia, and septic shock; a leading cause of nosocomial infection.
Hemophilus	*H. aegyptius* causes conjunctivitis, a highly contagious infection that occurs in areas where there are many young children. *H. influenzae* causes meningitis in children and upper respiratory infection in older adults.
Helicobacter pylori	*H. pylori* causes gastritis and ulceration of the stomach and duodenum.
Legionella pneumophila	*L. pneumophila* is responsible for legionnaires' disease, a type of pneumonia. The organism contaminates water supplies, as in air-conditioning units.
Mycobacterium tuberculosis	*M. tuberculosis* causes tuberculosis (TB). The organism, also called the tubercle bacillus, causes primary lesions called tubercles. The bacillus most commonly affects the lungs. The incidence of TB is high in the homeless population, persons with AIDS, and closed populations such as in prisons.
Pseudomonas aeruginosa	*P. aeruginosa* is the common cause of wound and urinary infections in debilitated patients such as patients with severe burns, cancer, and other chronic conditions.
Salmonella	*S. enteritidis* causes salmonellosis, food poisoning characterized by severe diarrhea. *S. typhi* causes typhoid fever, an intestinal infection. Typhoid fever is rare in the United States because of the chlorination of the water supply, but the incidence increases during flooding.
Shigella dysenteriae	*S. dysenteriae* causes dysentery.
Curved Rods	
Borrelia burgdorferi	*B. burgdorferi* causes Lyme disease and is characterized by a rash, palsy, and joint inflammation. It is transmitted by a small deer tick.
Treponema pallidum	*T. pallidum* causes syphilis.
Vibrio cholerae	*V. cholerae* causes cholera.
Rickettsia and Chlamydia	
Rickettsia	*R. prowazekii* causes epidemic typhus, which is transmitted to humans by lice. *R. rickettsii* causes Rocky Mountain spotted fever, which is transmitted to humans by ticks. *R. typhi* causes endemic or murine typhus, which is transmitted to humans by fleas.
Chlamydia	*C. trachomatis* causes trachoma, the leading cause of blindness in the world. Another form causes nongonococcal urethritis, the most common sexually transmitted disease in the United States.

Disorders Caused by Pathogens—cont'd

Viruses	
Encephalitis viruses	Encephalitis is the inflammation of the brain.
Hepatitis viruses	Several forms of hepatitis exist causing inflammation of the liver; they are as follows: Hepatitis A is spread by fecal-oral route. Hepatitis B is spread by sexual activity or contact with contaminated blood and body fluids. Hepatitis C is caused by contaminated blood transmitted via transfusions, through needles in drug abuse, and to health-care workers on the job. Hepatitis can become chronic, develop into a carrier state, or deteriorate to hepatic failure.
Herpes simplex viruses	*Type 1*: Cold sores or fever blisters appear on the lip, in the oral cavity, or in the nose. The virus lies dormant in the nerves between attacks. *Type 2*: Genital herpes is a common sexually transmitted disease characterized by painful lesions in the genitalia.
Herpes varicella-zoster	Chickenpox (varicella) is a mild infection characterized by generalized skin lesions. On remission of the infection, the virus becomes dormant and may reactivate in later years as shingles (herpes zoster).
Human papillomavirus (HPV)	HPV causes genital warts, which are transmitted sexually.
Influenza viruses	Influenza or "flu" is caused by different strains of the influenza viruses.
Measles virus	Measles (rubeola) is an acute respiratory inflammation characterized by fever, sore throat, skin rash, and Koplik's spots (white spots in the mouth).
Mumps virus	Mumps are epidemic parotitis.
Polio virus	Poliomyelitis (infantile paralysis) is an acute infection that may destroy nerve cells in the spinal cord, causing paralysis.
Rhabdovirus	Rabies is a fatal disease characterized by headache, fever, seizures, and spasm of the throat muscles while swallowing (hydrophobia). Spread by the saliva of infected animals such as dogs and other wild animals (e.g., bats, raccoons).
Rhinoviruses	Rhinoviruses are responsible for the common cold (coryza).
Rubella virus	German measles; the virus causes severe teratogenic birth defects that occur during the first trimester, such as blindness, deafness, brain damage, and heart defects.
Fungi	
Tinea	Tinea causes ringworm, a highly contagious fungal infection of the skin. One form of ringworm (tinea pedis) is found on the foot and is called athlete's foot. Other forms of ringworm are found on the scalp (tinea capitis) and on the bearded areas of the face and neck (tinea barbae). (Ringworm is not caused by a worm nor is the lesion always ring-shaped.)
Protozoa	
Entamoeba histolytica	*E. histolytica* causes amebic dysentery.
Giardia lamblia	Giardiasis is characterized by gastrointestinal discomfort and diarrhea.
Trichomonas vaginalis	Trichomoniasis is a sexually transmitted disease.
Worms	
Ascaris	Twelve-inch worms that live in the small intestine.
Hookworm (Necator)	Larval worms burrow their way through the skin of a bare foot, migrate to the intestine, and hook onto the intestinal wall. The worms feed on the blood of the host, causing anemia, fatigue, and wasting.
Pinworm (Enterobius)	Pinworm is the most common worm infestation in the United States.
Tapeworms (Taenia, others)	Tapeworms are acquired by eating poorly cooked contaminated food such as beef, fish, and pork.

SUMMARY OUTLINE

The human body is often invaded by disease-producing organisms; these pathogens disrupt normal structure and function and are a common cause of disability and death.

I. Disease and Pathogens
- A. Disease is a failure of the body to function normally.
- B. Infections are diseases caused by pathogens.

II. Types of Pathogens
- A. Microorganisms
  1. Bacteria (Cocci, bacilli, curved rods, chlamydia, rickettsia)
  2. Viruses
  3. Fungi
  4. Protozoa (amebas, ciliates, flagellates, sporozoa)
- B. Other Larger Pathogens
  1. Worms
  2. Arthropods

III. Laboratory Identification
- A. Staining (Gram stain, acid-fast stain)
- B. Culture

IV. Spread of Infection
- A. Portals of Entry (Most pathogens enter the body through the respiratory tract and the gastrointestinal tract).
- B. Portals of Exit (The most common portals of exit are the respiratory and gastrointestinal tracts).
- C. Modes of Transmission
  1. Person to person
  2. Environment to person
  3. Tiny animals to person

V. Six Germ-Laden Stories
- A. Wash Those Mitts
- B. Flora and Her Vaginal Itch
- C. Rick, Nick, and the Sick Tick
- D. Why Typhoid Mary Needed to Lose Her Gallbladder
- E. Pox News Alert!
- F. The Chief of Staph Reports

Review Your Knowledge

Matching: Microorganisms and Other Pathogens

Directions: Match the following words with their descriptions below. Some words are used more than once.

a. virus
b. bacteria
c. arthropods
d. worms
e. fungi
f. protozoa

1. ____ Coccus, bacillus, curved rods
2. ____ RNA or DNA surrounded by a protein shell; parasitic
3. ____ Yeasts and molds
4. ____ Ascarides, trichinae, flukes
5. ____ Helminths
6. ____ Ectoparasites
7. ____ Mycotic infections
8. ____ Chlamydia and rickettsia
9. ____ Animals with jointed legs
10. ____ Arranged in pairs, chains, and bunches of grapes
11. ____ Amebas, ciliates, flagellates, and sporozoa

Multiple Choice

1. A vaginal yeast infection (*Candida albicans*) is most apt to develop
   a. as a consequence to antibiotic therapy.
   b. in response to eating contaminated food.
   c. as an allergic response to penicillin.
   d. in response to being bitten by a "sick tick."
2. The plasmodium
   a. is pathogenic to mosquitoes.
   b. causes malaria.
   c. is an arthropod.
   d. is a biological vector.
3. Cocci, bacilli, and curved rods
   a. are eradicated by anthelmintics.
   b. cause mycotic infections.
   c. are types of bacteria.
   d. always act as pathogens.
4. Which of the following is most descriptive of staphylococcus?
   a. Viral
   b. Parasitic
   c. Gram (+)
   d. Chainlike arrangement
5. Spores
   a. allow the bacterium to stain blue (Gram +).
   b. only develop in parasites.
   c. are characteristic of arthropods.
   d. make a bacterium heat-resistant and hard to kill.

CHAPTER 6

Tissues and Membranes

KEY TERMS

Adipose tissue, p. 81
Areolar tissue, p. 81
Chondrocytes, p. 83
Columnar epithelium, p. 77
Connective tissue, p. 79
Cuboidal epithelium, p. 77
Endocrine gland, p. 79
Epithelial tissue, p. 76
Exocrine gland, p. 79
Ligament, p. 82
Mucous membrane, p. 86
Muscle tissue, p. 83
Nervous tissue, p. 83
Osseous tissue, p. 83
Parietal layer, p. 86
Serous membrane, p. 86
Squamous epithelium, p. 77
Tendon, p. 82
Visceral layer, p. 86

OBJECTIVES

1. List the four basic types of tissues.
2. Describe the functions of epithelial, connective, muscle, and nervous tissue.
3. Explain how epithelial tissue is classified.
4. Differentiate between endocrine and exocrine glands.
5. List the types of epithelial and connective tissue membranes.
6. Differentiate between mucous and serous membranes.

In Chapter 3, we studied a typical cell. We explained how it divides into millions of identical cells and how they differentiate into cells with unique shapes, sizes, and functions. In this chapter, we see how these cells are arranged to perform specific functions.

Tissues are groups of cells that are similar to each other in structure and function. Like the individual tiles arranged as a beautiful floor, cells are placed in various patterns to make different tissues. Four major types of tissues are epithelial, connective, nervous, and muscular. The study of tissues is called **histology.**

EPITHELIAL TISSUE

WHERE IS IT FOUND?

Epithelial (ĕp-ĭ-THĒL-ē-ăl) **tissue,** also called epithelium, forms large, continuous sheets. Epithelial tissue helps form the skin and covers the entire outer surface of the body. Sheets of epithelium also line most of the inner cavities such as the mouth, respiratory tract, and reproductive tract. Types of epithelial tissue are listed in Table 6-1.

WHAT DOES IT DO?

Epithelial tissue is primarily concerned with protection, absorption, filtration, and secretion. The skin, for instance, protects the body from sunlight and from invasion by disease-producing bacteria. The epithelial tissue lining the respiratory passages helps clean inhaled air. The epithelium of the respiratory tract secretes mucus and is lined with cilia. The mucus traps the dust inhaled in the air, and the constantly waving cilia move the dust and mucus toward the throat. The dust and mucus are then either coughed up or swallowed and eliminated in the stools.

Epithelial tissue also functions in the transport of substances across membranes. Epithelium is abundant in organs like those in the digestive tract, which must absorb large amounts of water and digested food. Lastly, epithelial tissue forms glands that secrete a variety of hormones and enzymes.

WHAT IS IT LIKE?

Epithelial tissue has a number of characteristics:

- Epithelial tissue forms continuous sheets (Figure 6-1). The cells fit together snugly like tiles.
- Epithelial tissue has two surfaces. One surface is always unattached, like the surface of the outer

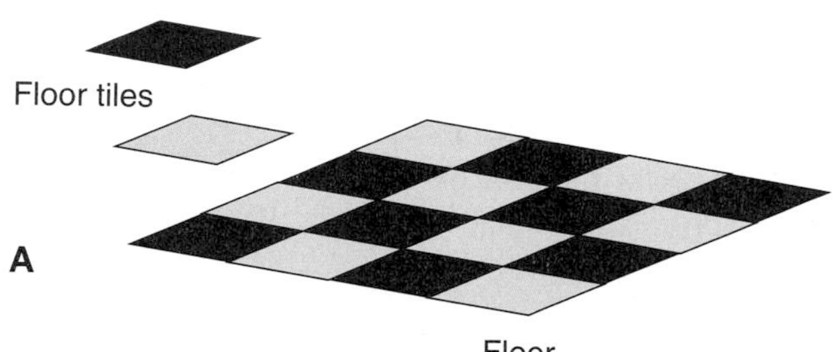

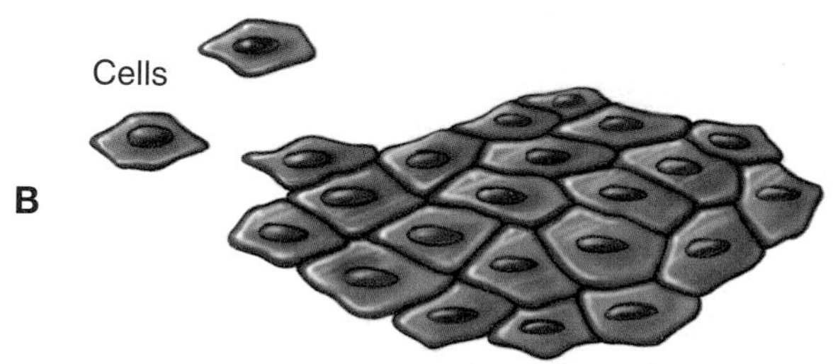

FIGURE 6-1 **A,** A tile floor. **B,** Tight-fitting cells of epithelial tissue.

Table 6-1 Types of Epithelial Tissue

Type	Location	Function
Simple		
Simple squamous	Walls of blood vessels (capillaries)	Permits the exchange of nutrients and wastes
	Alveoli (air sacs in lungs)	Allows diffusion of oxygen and carbon dioxide
	Kidneys	Filtration of water and electrolytes
Simple cuboidal	Lining of kidney tubules	Absorption of water and electrolytes
	Various glands (thyroid, pancreas, salivary glands)	Secretion of enzymes and hormones
Simple columnar	Digestive tract	Protection, absorption, and secretion of digestive juice; often contains goblet cells (mucus)
Pseudostratified columnar	Lining of respiratory tract Lining of reproductive tubes (fallopian tubes)	Protection and secretion; cleans respiratory passages; sweeps egg toward uterus
Stratified		
Stratified squamous	Outer layer of skin Lining of mouth, esophagus, anus, and vagina	Protects body from invading microorganisms; withstands friction
Transitional	Urinary bladder	Permits expansion of an organ

skin or the inner lining of the mouth. The undersurface of the epithelium is attached to a basement membrane. The **basement membrane** is a very thin material that anchors the epithelium to the underlying structure.

- Epithelial tissue has no blood supply of its own; it is avascular. For its nourishment, it depends on the blood supply of underlying connective tissue.
- Because epithelial tissue is so well nourished from the underlying connective tissue, it is able to regenerate, or repair itself, quickly if injured.

CLASSIFICATION

Epithelial tissue is classified according to its shape and the numbers of layers. It has three shapes: squamous, cuboidal, and columnar (Figure 6-2). The **squamous** (SKWĀ-mŭs) **epithelium** cells are thin and flat, like fish scales. (The word squamous comes from squam, meaning scale.) The **cuboidal** (kyū-BOID-ăl) **epithelium** cells are cubelike and look like dice. The **columnar** (kŏ-LŬM-năr) **epithelium** cells are tall and narrow, and look like columns.

Epithelial cells are arranged in either a single layer or multiple layers (see Figure 6-2). One layer of cells is

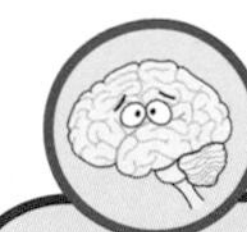

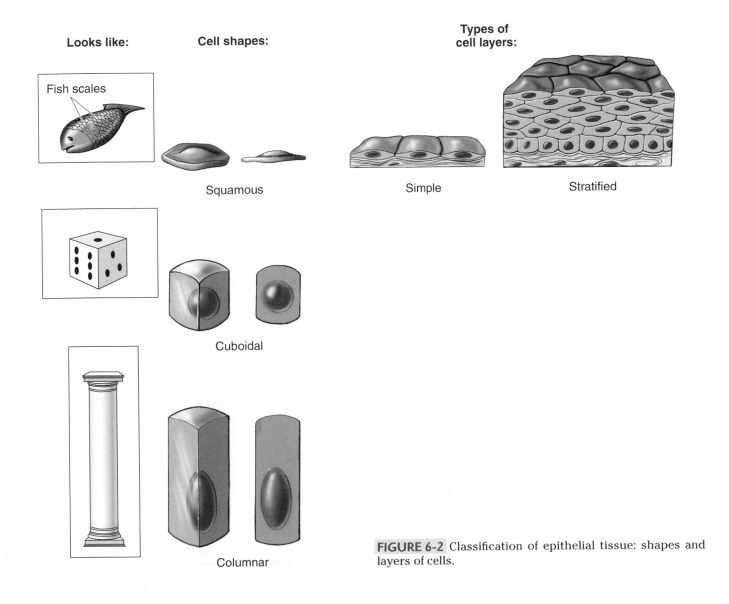

Do You Know...

What causes a pressure, or decubitus ("lying down"), ulcer?

A decubitus ulcer is another name for a bedsore or a pressure ulcer. The ulcer is caused by an interruption of the blood supply to a tissue. Decubitus ulcers often develop in patients who have been bedridden for long periods (decubitus comes from a Latin word meaning to lie down). They are caused by the weight of the body on the skin overlying a bony area (e.g., elbow, heel, hip). The weight of the body compresses, or squeezes, the blood vessels, cutting off the supply of blood to the tissues. Deprived of its blood supply, the tissue dies, forming an ulcer.

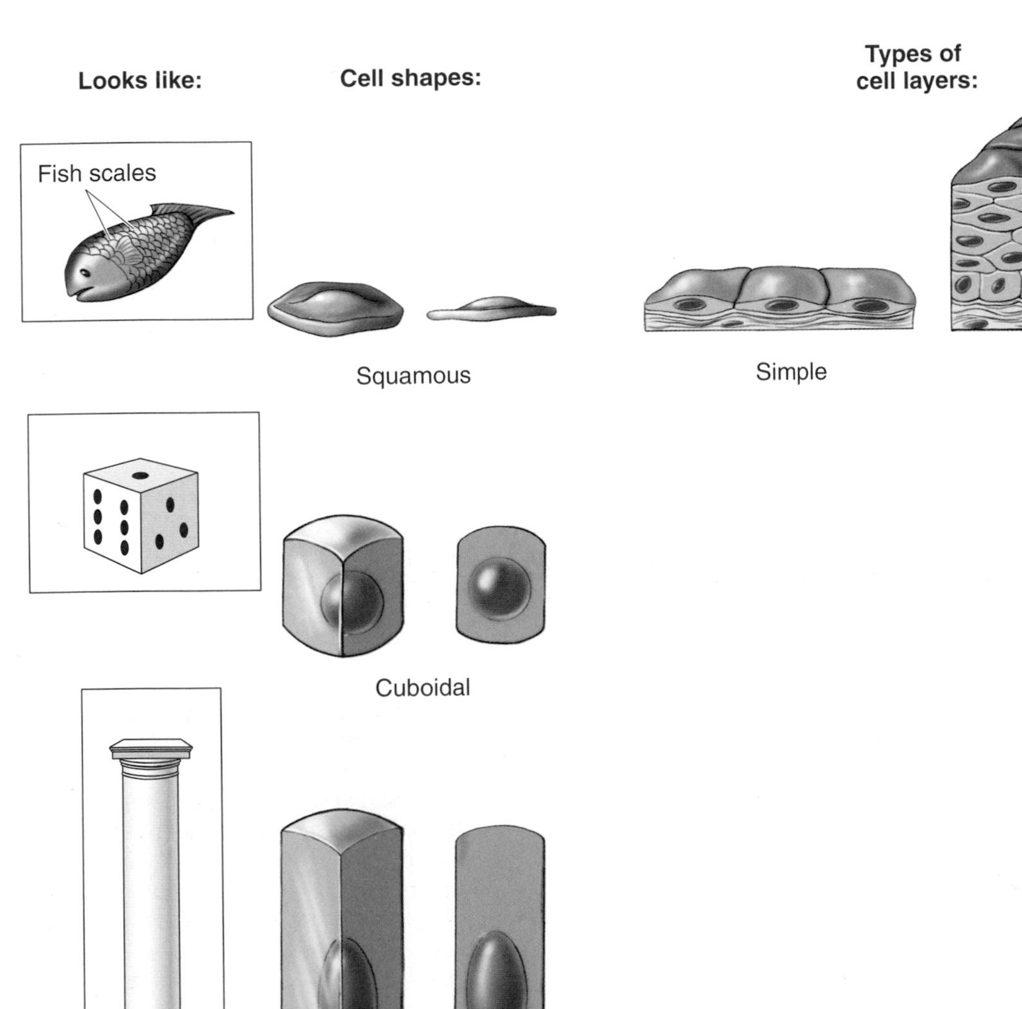

FIGURE 6-2 Classification of epithelial tissue: shapes and layers of cells.

a **simple epithelium.** Two or more layers of cells are a **stratified epithelium.**

Both the shape and the number of layers are used to describe the various types of epithelium. For instance, simple squamous epithelium refers to a single layer of squamous cells. Stratified squamous epithelium contains multiple layers of squamous cells. Note that Figure 6-2 shows stratified squamous epithelium but not stratified cuboidal or columnar tissue. Stratified cuboidal and stratified columnar epithelia are found in very few organs.

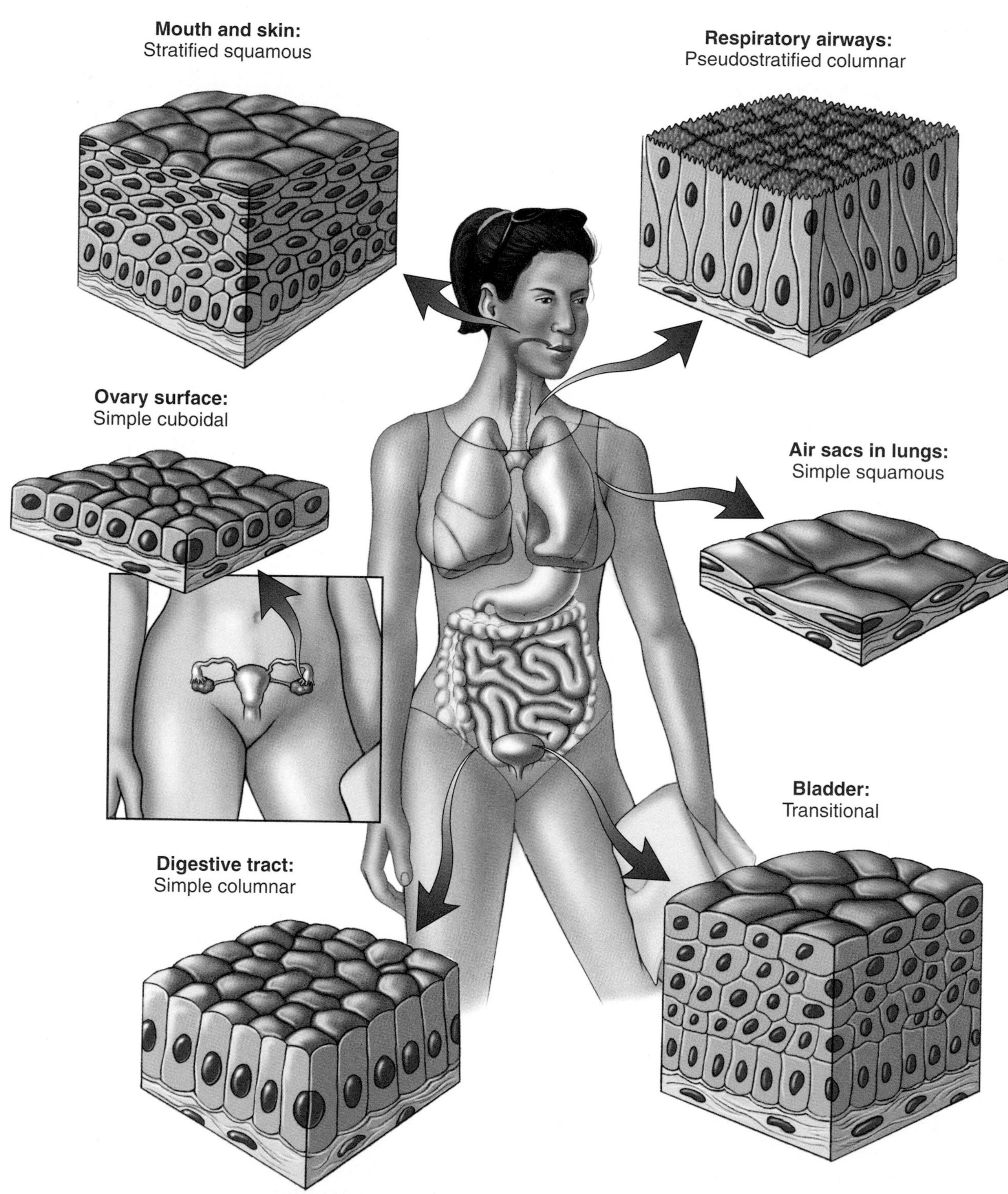

FIGURE 6-3 Types and location of epithelial tissue.

SIMPLE EPITHELIA

Because **simple epithelia** are so thin, they are concerned primarily with the movement, or transport, of various substances across the membranes from one body compartment to another (Figure 6-3).

Simple squamous epithelium is a single layer of squamous cells with an underlying basement membrane. Because this tissue is so thin, simple squamous epithelium is found where substances move by rapid diffusion or filtration. For instance, the walls of the capillaries (the smallest blood vessels) are composed of simple squamous epithelium. The walls of the alveoli (air sacs of the lungs) are also composed of simple squamous epithelium. This tissue allows the rapid diffusion of oxygen from the alveoli into the blood.

Simple cuboidal epithelium is a single layer of cuboidal cells resting on a basement membrane. This epithelial layer is most often found in glands and in the kidney tubules, where it functions in the transport and secretion of various substances.

Simple columnar epithelium refers to a single layer of columnar cells resting on its basement membrane. These tall, tightly packed cells line the entire length of the digestive tract and play a major role in the absorption of the products of digestion. Lubricating mucus is produced by **goblet cells,** which are modified columnar cells.

Pseudostratified columnar epithelium is a single layer of columnar cells. Because the cells are so irregularly shaped, they appear multilayered; hence the name pseudostratified, meaning falsely stratified. Their function is similar to the function of simple columnar cells: they facilitate absorption and secretion.

STRATIFIED EPITHELIA

Stratified epithelia are multilayered and are therefore stronger than simple epithelia. They perform a protective function and are found in tissue exposed to everyday wear and tear, such as the mouth, esophagus, and skin. Stratified squamous epithelium is the most common of the stratified epithelia.

Transitional epithelium is found primarily in organs that need to stretch such as the urinary bladder. This epithelium is called transitional because the cells slide past one another when the tissue is stretched. The cells appear stratified when the urinary bladder is empty (unstretched) and simple when the bladder is full (stretched).

GLANDULAR EPITHELIA

The function of glandular epithelium is secretion. A **gland** is made up of one or more cells that secrete a particular substance. Much of the glandular tissue is composed of simple cuboidal epithelium.

Two types of glands are the exocrine glands and the endocrine glands. The **exocrine** (ĕx-ŏ-krĭn) **glands** have ducts, or tiny tubes, into which the exocrine secretions are released before reaching body surfaces or body cavities. The exocrine secretions include mucus, sweat, saliva, and digestive enzymes. The ducts carry the exocrine secretions outside the body. For instance, sweat flows from the sweat glands through ducts onto the surface of the skin for evaporation (Figure 6-4).

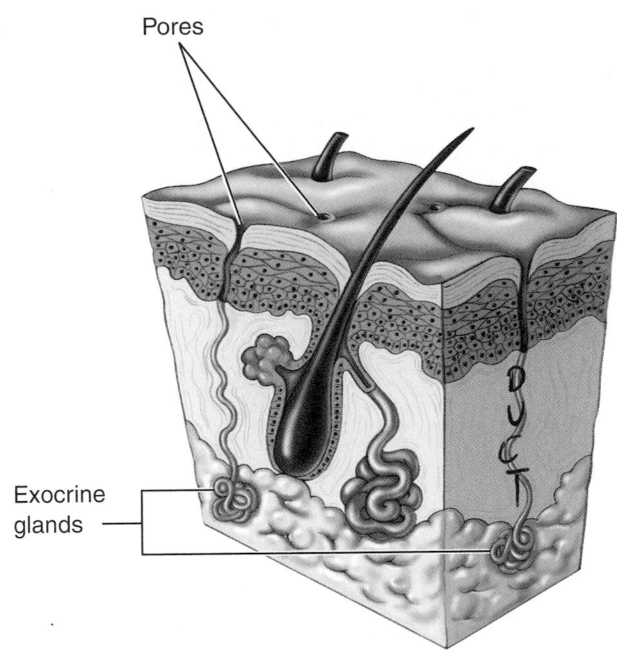

FIGURE 6-4 Exocrine gland; a sweat gland.

The **endocrine** (ĔN-dŏ-krĭn) **glands** secrete hormones, such as insulin. Endocrine glands do not have ducts and are therefore called ductless glands. Because endocrine glands are ductless, the hormones are secreted directly into the blood. The blood then carries the hormones to their sites of action.

CONNECTIVE TISSUE

WHERE IS IT FOUND?

Connective tissue is the most abundant of the four tissue types and is widely distributed throughout the body. Connective tissue is found in blood, under the skin, in bone, and around many organs. As the name suggests, connective tissue connects, or binds together, the parts of the body. Other functions include support, protection, fat storage, and transport of substances.

WHAT DOES IT LOOK LIKE?

Although connective tissue types may not resemble each other very closely, they share two characteristics. First, most connective tissue, with the exception of ligaments, tendons, and cartilage, has a good blood supply. Ligaments and tendons have a poor blood supply, and cartilage has no blood supply. As any athlete knows, an injury to these structures usually heals very slowly. The second characteristic shared by most connective tissue is an abundance of intercellular matrix.

The **intercellular matrix** is what makes the various types of connective tissue so different. The intercellular matrix is material located outside the cell. It fills the spaces between the cells (intercellular space). The cell makes the matrix and secretes it into the intercellular spaces. The hardness of the intercellular matrix varies from one cell type to the next. The intercellular matrix may be liquid as in blood; gel-like as in fat tissue; or hard, as in bone. The amount of matrix also varies from one cell type to the next. In fat tissue, the cells are close together, with little intercellular matrix. Bone and cartilage, however, have few cells and large amounts of intercellular matrix.

Also found in the matrix of most connective tissue are protein **fibers.** The fiber types include collagen, elastin , and reticular fibers (fine collagen). Collagen fibers are strong and flexible but are not easily stretched. Elastin fibers are not very strong, but they are stretchy, like a rubber band.

Recently, injections of collagen have been used cosmetically to remove unwanted lines and wrinkles. Collagen is obtained from cattle or, more often, from the patient's own hips, thighs, and abdomen. The collagen is then injected under the patient's skin. Acting as filler, the collagen smoothes out unwanted wrinkles, creating a surgical fountain of youth. Tex, here, could use some collagen filler.

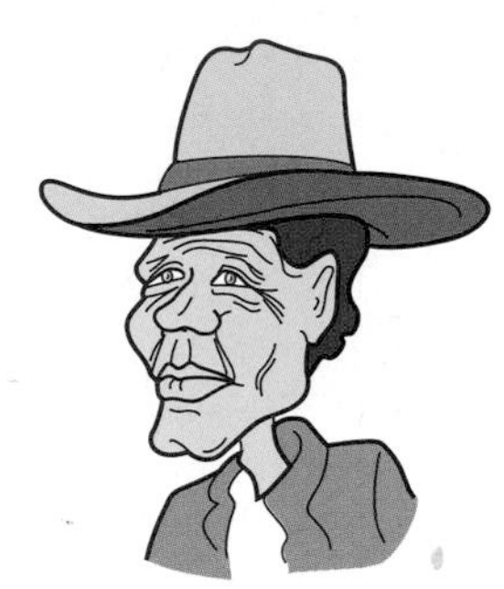

TYPES OF CONNECTIVE TISSUE

The many types of connective tissue are loose connective tissue, dense fibrous connective tissue, cartilage, bone, and the "liquid" connective tissue (blood and lymph) (Figure 6-5). Table 6-2 describes these types.

Table 6-2 Types of Connective Tissue

Type	Location	Function
Loose Connective		
Areolar	Beneath skin and most epithelial layers; between muscles	Binds together, protects, cushions; "tissue glue"
Adipose	Beneath skin (subcutaneous) Around kidneys and heart Behind eyeballs	Cushions, insulates, stores fat
Reticular	Lymphoid tissue such as lymph nodes, spleen, and bone marrow	Forms internal framework of lymphoid organs
Dense Fibrous Connective		
	Tendons, ligaments, capsules, and fascia Skin (dermis)	Binds structures together
Cartilage		
Hyaline	Ends of long bone at joints Connects ribs to sternum Rings in trachea of respiratory tract Nose Fetal skeleton	Supports, protects, provides framework
Fibrocartilage	Intervertebral discs (in backbone) Pads in knee joint Pad between pubic bones (symphysis pubis)	Cushions, protects
Elastic cartilage	External ear and part of larynx	Supports, provides framework
Bone	Bones of the skeleton	Supports, protects, provides framework
Blood	Blood vessels throughout the body	Transports nutrients, hormones, respiratory gases (oxygen and carbon dioxide), waste
Lymph	Lymphatic vessels throughout the body	Drains interstitial fluid; involved in immune response

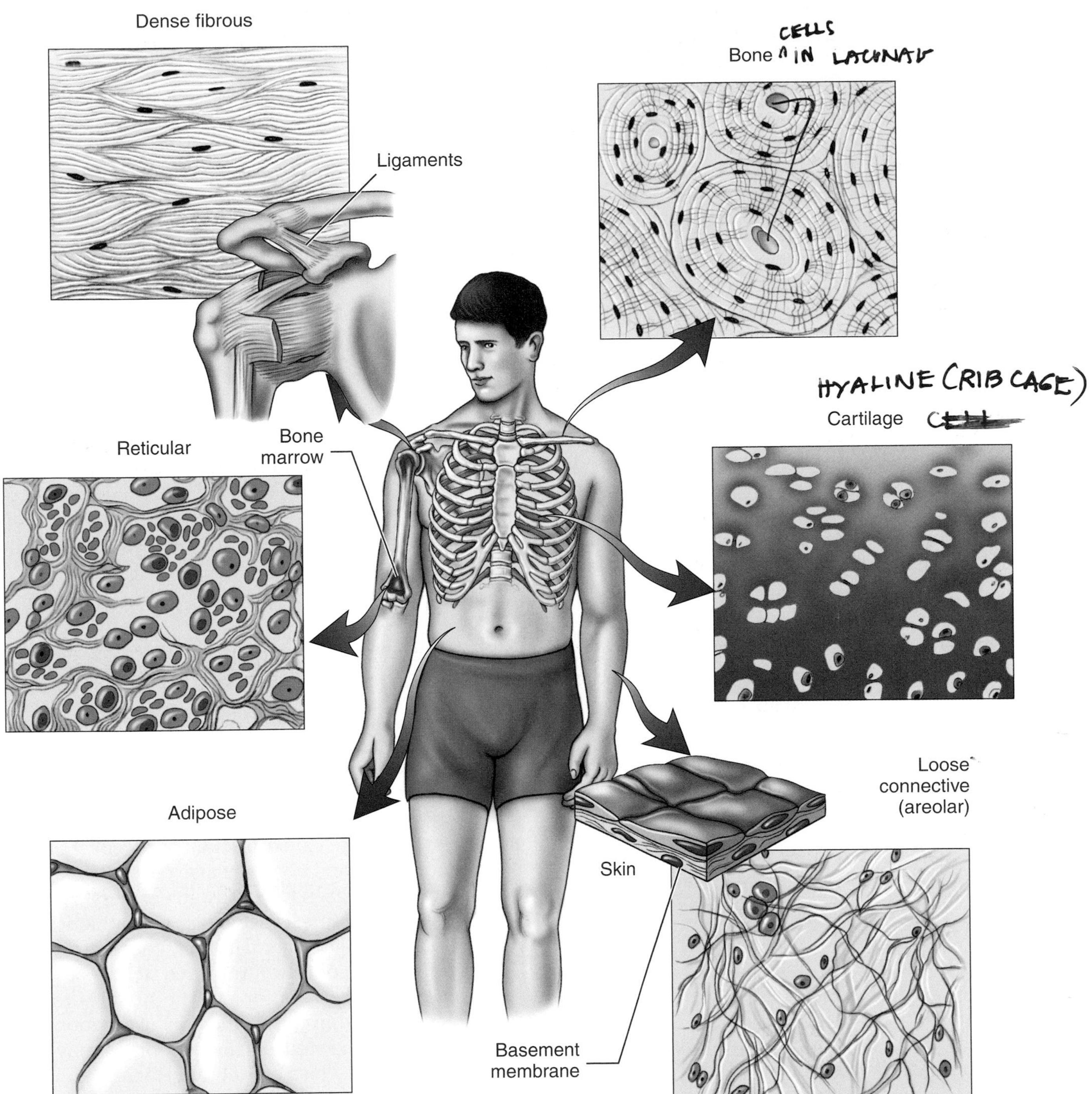

FIGURE 6-5 Types and location of connective tissue. (Blood and lymph are not shown.)

Loose Connective Tissue

Loose connective tissue contains fibers that are loosely arranged around cells. There are three types of loose connective tissue: areolar tissue, adipose tissue, and reticular connective tissue (see Figure 6-5).

Areolar (ă-RĒ-ō-lăr) **tissue** is made up of collagen and elastin fibers in a gel-like intercellular matrix. Areolar is soft and surrounds, protects, and cushions many of the organs. It acts like "tissue glue" because it holds the organs in position. It is the most widely distributed type of connective tissue.

Adipose (Ă-dĭ-pōs) **tissue** is a type of loose connective tissue that stores fat (adipose tissue is sometimes referred to as fat as well; see Figure 6-5). Adipose tissue

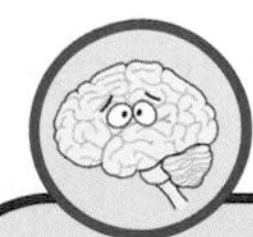

Do You Know...

Why an uptight tourniquet is "bad news"?

An uptight, too-tight tourniquet can cut off the flow of blood to a limb. If the blood supply to an area is stopped for too long, the tissue distal to the tourniquet is deprived of oxygen and dies. Tissue death (necrosis) due to diminished blood supply to an area is called gangrene.

forms the tissue layer underlying the skin, the subcutaneous layer. Because of its location, adipose tissue can insulate the body from extremes of outside temperature. For instance, in a cold environment, the adipose tissue prevents the loss of heat from the body. This protection is best appreciated in observing the fat content of animals living in arctic conditions. The walrus, for instance, has huge layers of fat tissue called blubber. Because of the insulating qualities of the blubber, the walrus can swim in deep, cold waters without freezing to death. Think of how long you could sit on an iceberg, even if you had a few extra pounds. Adipose tissue is also deposited around certain organs. The kidney, for instance, has a layer of fat tissue that helps hold it in place. In extremely thin individuals, this fat tissue may be absent, allowing the kidney to move around. This is called a floating kidney.

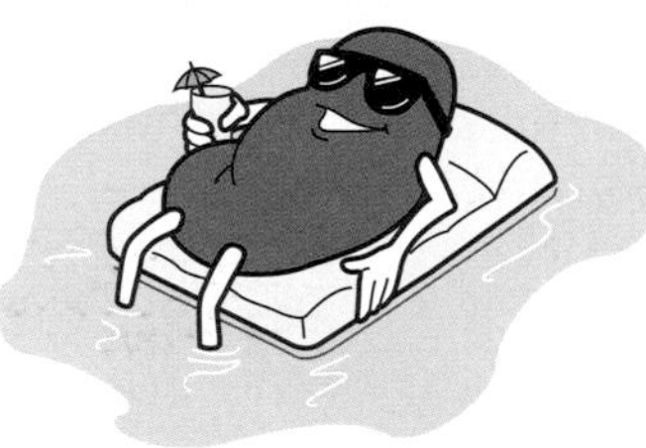

Reticular connective tissue is characterized by a network of delicately interwoven reticular (fine collagen) fibers. It forms the internal framework for lymphoid tissue such as the spleen, lymph nodes, and bone marrow.

Dense Fibrous Connective Tissue

Dense fibrous connective tissue is composed of an intercellular matrix that contains many collagen and elastic fibers. Collagen is the main type of fiber in dense fibrous tissue. The fibers form strong, supporting structures such as tendons, ligaments, capsules, and fascia.

Tendons are cordlike structures composed of dense fibrous connective tissue that attach muscles to bones. **Ligaments** are dense fibrous connective tissues that cross joints and attach bones to each other. Because ligaments contain more elastic fibers than tendons do, they stretch more easily. The ability to stretch is important; it prevents tearing of the ligaments when the joints bend. Dense fiber also forms tough **capsules** around certain organs such as the kidney and liver.

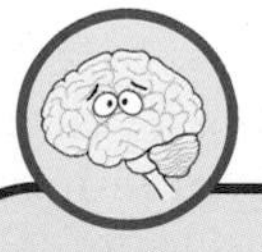

Do You Know...

Why overweight men and women "round out" into different shapes?

Overeating results in the storage of fat in adipose tissue. Because fat metabolism is affected by the sex hormones estrogen and testosterone, storage sites differ for males and females. In the male, excess fat is stored primarily in the abdominal region, whereas in the female, excess fat is stored around the breasts and hips. Excess adipose tissue, especially that which deposits in the abdominal region, becomes metabolically active and secretes hormones that adversely affect metabolism. The "spare tire" hormones increase blood glucose, increase resistance to insulin, and increase blood pressure, none of which is healthy.

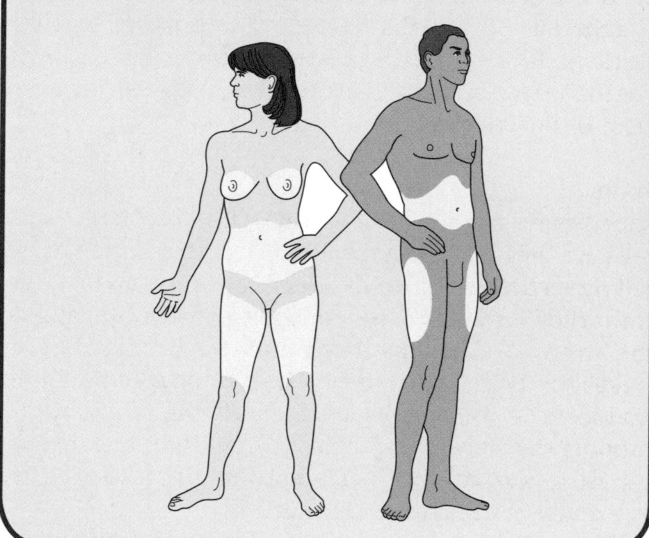

Lastly, dense fibrous connective tissue forms bands, or sheets, of tissue called **fascia.** Fascia covers muscles, blood vessels, and nerves; it also covers, supports, and anchors the organs to nearby structures.

If stretching is excessive, as with athletic injuries, tendons and ligaments can tear, causing severe pain and impaired mobility. A ruptured Achilles tendon, for example, is a serious injury. The Achilles tendon attaches the leg muscles to the heel of the foot. If excessive force is exerted on the tendon, it may snap or rupture, causing loss of foot movement.

Do You Know...

About Cooper's Droop?

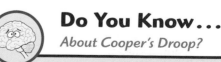

As we age the effects of gravity take over and some parts of the anatomy "head south." Breast tissue is anchored to the underlying structures by strands of connective tissue called suspensory ligaments (Cooper's ligaments). As we age, the tissue weakens and, sadly, sagging happens. The sorry saga of the sagging breasts is called Cooper's Droop.

Cartilage

Cartilage is formed by **chondrocytes** (KŎN-drō-sīts), or cartilage cells. The chondrocytes secrete a protein-containing intercellular matrix that is firm, smooth, and flexible. Although the matrix of cartilage is solid, it is not as hard as that of bone. Most cartilage is covered by **perichondrium,** a layer of connective tissue that carries blood vessels to the cartilage. The blood vessels supply oxygen and nutrients to the cartilage.

Types of Cartilage. Three types of cartilage are hyaline cartilage, elastic cartilage, and fibrocartilage. Hyaline cartilage is found in only a few places in the body: (1) the larynx, or voicebox; (2) the ends of long bones at joints; (3) the nose; and (4) the area between the breastbone and the ribs. Figure 6-5 illustrates the attachment of the ribs to the breastbone by hyaline cartilage. Hyaline cartilage is also found in large quantities in the fetal skeleton. As the fetus matures, however, most of the cartilage is converted to bone.

Bone

Bone tissue is also called **osseous** (ŎS-ē-ŭs) **tissue.** Bone cells are called osteocytes. Bone cells secrete an intercellular matrix that includes collagen, calcium salts, and other minerals. The collagen provides flexibility and strength; the mineral-containing matrix as a whole makes the bone tissue hard. The hardness of the bone enables it to protect organs such as the brain and to support the weight of the body for standing and moving. Bone also acts as a storage site for mineral salts, especially calcium (see Chapter 8).

When mineralization of bone tissue is diminished, as in osteoporosis, the bone is weakened and tends to break easily. Adequate dietary intake of calcium is essential for strong bones. Calcium is needed throughout the life cycle but is especially important during childhood, when bones are growing, and after menopause, when estrogen levels in women decline. Estrogen normally encourages the deposition of calcium in bone tissue. Exercise and weight-bearing activity also encourage the deposition of calcium within bones.

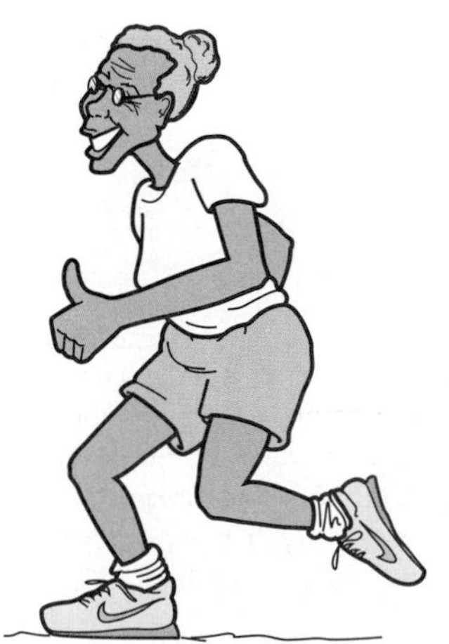

Blood and Lymph

Blood and **lymph** are two types of connective tissue that have a watery intercellular matrix; they form a "liquid" connective tissue. Blood consists of blood cells surrounded by a fluid matrix called **plasma.** Unlike other connective tissues, which contain collagen and elastin fibers in the intercellular matrix, plasma contains nonfibrous plasma proteins (see Chapter 15). Lymph is the fluid that is found in lymphatic vessels and is described in more detail in Chapter 20.

NERVOUS TISSUE

Nervous tissue makes up the brain, spinal cord, and nerves. Nervous tissue consists of two types of cells: neurons and neuroglia (Figure 6-6).

NEURONS

Neurons are nerve cells that transmit electrical signals to and from the brain and spinal cord. The neuron has three parts: (1) the dendrites, which receive information from other neurons, (2) the cell body, which contains the nucleus and is essential to the life of the cell; and (3) the single axon, which transmits information away from the cell body.

Neuroglia, or glia, are cells that support and take care of the neurons. The word glial means gluelike and refers to the ability of these cells to support, or stick together, the vast network of neurons. (Nervous tissue is described more fully in Chapters 10 to 13.)

MUSCLE TISSUE

Muscle tissue is composed of cells that shorten, or contract. In doing so, they cause movement of a body part. Because the cells are long and slender, they are called fibers rather than cells. The three types of muscle are skeletal, smooth, and cardiac (Figure 6-7).

SKELETAL MUSCLE

Skeletal muscle is generally attached to bone (the skeletal system). Because of the appearance of striations, or stripes, skeletal muscle is also called striated muscle. Skeletal muscles move the skeleton, maintain posture, and stabilize joints.

SMOOTH MUSCLE

Smooth muscle is generally found in the walls of the viscera, or organs, such as the stomach, intestines, and urinary bladder. It is also found in tubes such as the bronchioles (breathing passages) and blood vessels. The function of smooth muscle is related to the organ

Nervous Tissue

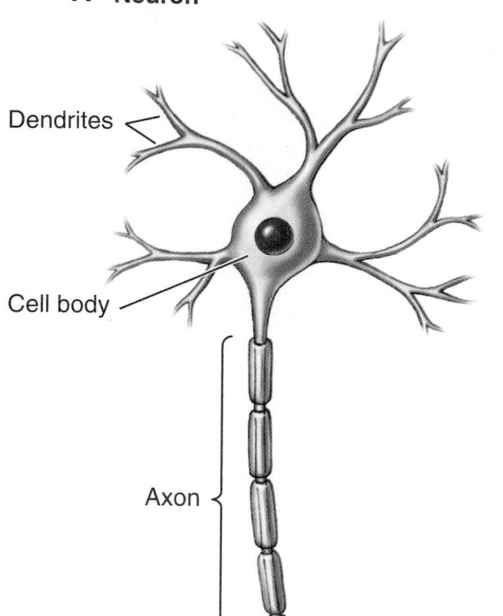

B Neuroglia (glia)

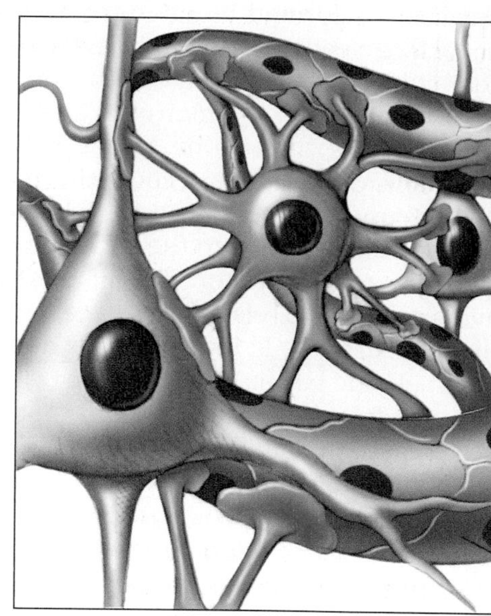

FIGURE 6-6 Two types of nervous tissue. **A,** Neuron. **B,** Neuroglia.

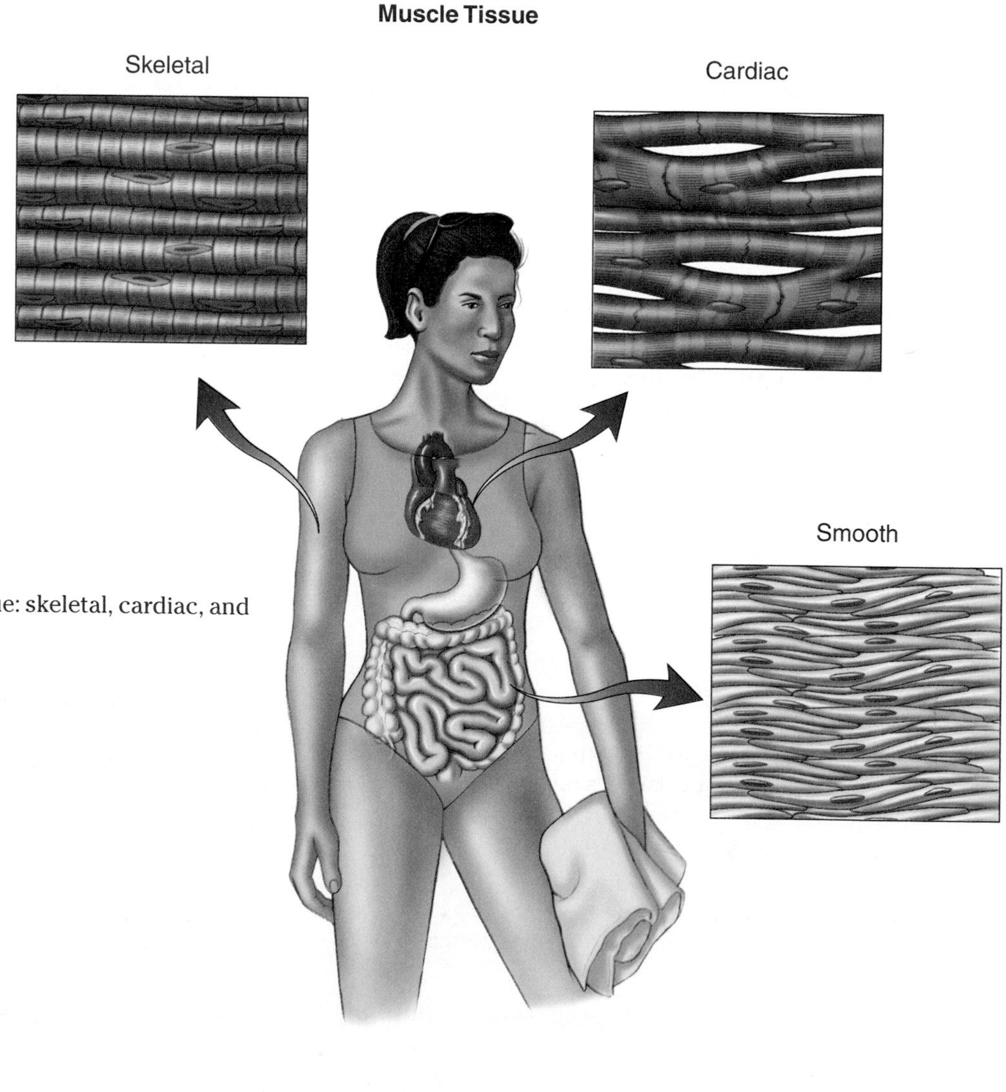

Muscle Tissue

Skeletal

Cardiac

Smooth

FIGURE 6-7 Types of muscle tissue: skeletal, cardiac, and smooth.

in which it is found. For instance, smooth muscle in the stomach helps to mash and churn food, while the smooth muscle in the urinary bladder helps to expel urine.

CARDIAC MUSCLE

Cardiac muscle is found only in the heart, where it functions to pump blood into a vast network of blood vessels. Cardiac muscle fibers are long branching cells that fit together tightly at junctions; this arrangement promotes rapid conduction of electrical signals throughout the heart.

TISSUE REPAIR

How does tissue repair itself after an injury? Two types of tissue repair are regeneration and fibrosis. Regeneration refers to the replacement of tissue by cells that are identical to the original cells. Regeneration occurs only in tissues whose cells undergo mitosis, such as the skin.

Fibrosis is the replacement of injured tissue by the formation of fibrous connective tissue, or scar tissue. The fibers of scar tissue pull the edges of the wound together and strengthen the area. Damaged skeletal muscle, cardiac muscle, and nervous tissue do not undergo mitosis and must be replaced by scar tissue. The steps involved in tissue repair are illustrated and described in Figure 6-8. The injured skin of some persons exhibit excessive fibrosis leading to the formation of keloids. Keloid scars develop most often on the upper trunk and earlobes and are of concern cosmetically. Unfortunately they tend to recur when surgically removed. Tribespeople practice scarification during which the skin is sliced in hopes of inducing keloid scar formation. The keloid scar pattern reflects a significant event or rite of passage in the person's life.

Sum It Up!

Tissues are groups of cells that are similar to each other in structure and function. The four types of tissues are epithelial, connective, nervous, and muscle. Epithelial tissue covers and lines; it is primarily concerned with the processes of secretion, filtration, and absorption. Connective tissue is the most widespread and diverse of the tissue types; it connects and binds together parts of the body. Nervous tissue is found in the brain, spinal cord, and nerves and is concerned with the transmission of information throughout the entire body. Muscle tissue is composed of cells that can contract and thus produce movement of body parts. The three types of muscle are skeletal, smooth, and cardiac.

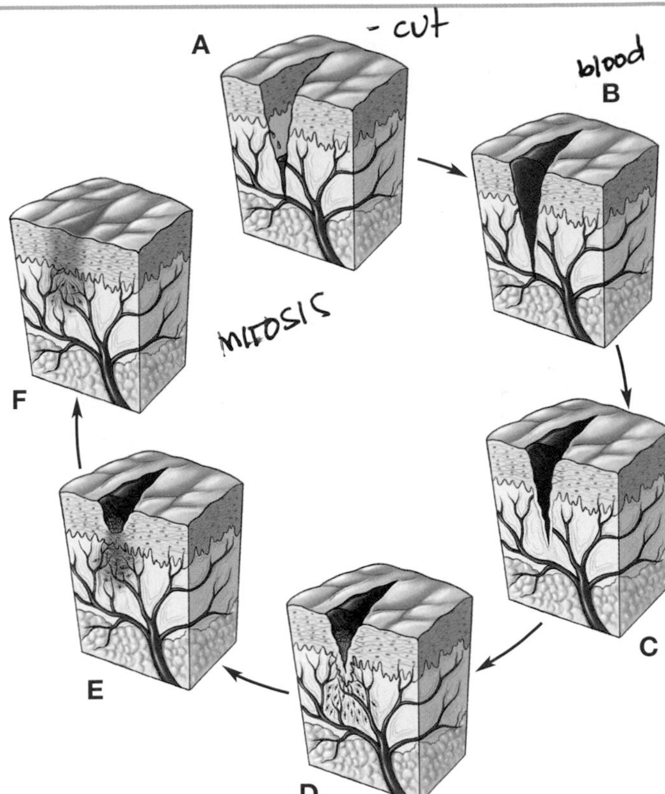

FIGURE 6-8 Steps in tissue repair. **A,** A deep wound to the skin severs blood vessels, causing blood to fill the wound. **B,** A blood clot forms, and as it dries, it forms a scab. **C** and **D,** The process of tissue repair begins. Scar tissue forms in the deep layers. **E,** At the same time, surface epithelial cells multiply and fill the area between the scar tissue and the scab. **F,** When the epithelium is complete, the scab detaches. The result is a fully regenerated layer of epithelium over an underlying area of scar tissue.

MEMBRANES

CLASSIFICATION OF MEMBRANES

Membranes are thin sheets of tissue that cover surfaces, line body cavities, and surround organs. Membranes are classified as epithelial or connective tissue (Table 6-3). (The connective tissue membranes are described in Chapters 8 and 10.)

EPITHELIAL MEMBRANES

The **epithelial membranes** include the cutaneous membrane (skin), the mucous membranes, and the serous membranes (Figure 6-9). Although called epithelial, these membranes contain both an epithelial sheet and an underlying layer of connective tissue.

Cutaneous Membrane

The **cutaneous membrane** is the skin. The outer layer of skin (epidermis) is stratified squamous epithelium. The underlying layer (dermis) is composed of fibrous connective tissue (see Chapter 7).

Table 6-3 Types of Membranes

Type	Location
Epithelial Membranes	
Cutaneous membrane	Skin (outer layer)
Mucous membrane	Digestive tract lining
	Urinary tract lining
	Reproductive tract lining
	Respiratory tract lining
Serous membrane	
Pleura	Thoracic cavity
Pericardium	Thoracic cavity around the heart
Peritoneum	Abdominal cavity
Connective Tissue Membranes	
Synovial	Lines joint cavities; secretes synovial fluid
Periosteum	Covers bone; contains the blood vessels that supply the bone
Perichondrium	Covers cartilage; contains capillaries that nourish the cartilage
Meninges	Covers brain and spinal cord
Fascia (various kinds)	Throughout body

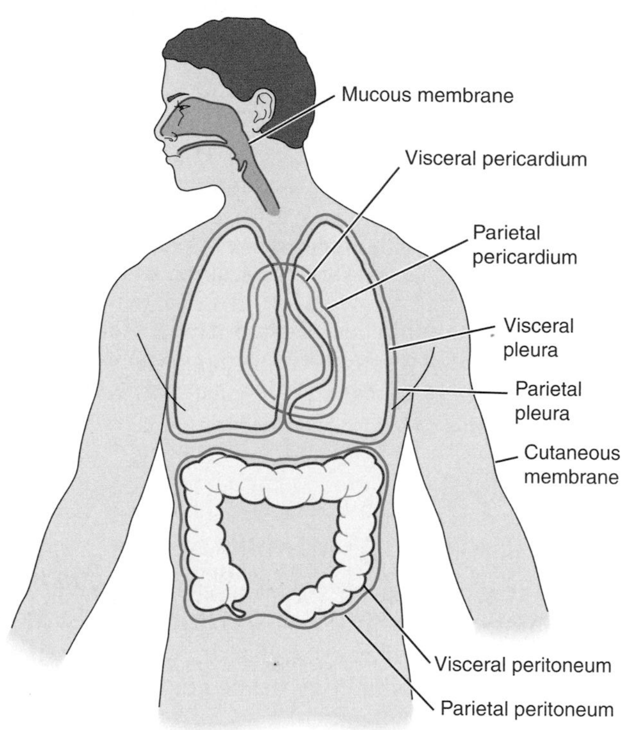

FIGURE 6-9 Epithelial membranes.

Mucous Membranes

Mucous membranes line all body cavities that open to the exterior of the body (see Figure 6-9). They include the digestive, urinary, reproductive, and respiratory tracts. For instance, the digestive tract opens to the exterior of the body at the mouth and anus, whereas the respiratory tract opens to the exterior at the nose and mouth. Mucous membranes usually contain stratified squamous epithelium or simple columnar epithelium. Most mucous membranes are adapted for absorption and secretion. Mucous membranes secrete mucus. The mucus keeps the membrane moist and also lubricates it. For instance, in the digestive tract, the mucus allows food to move through the tract with little friction.

Serous Membranes

Serous membranes line the ventral body cavities, which are not open to the exterior of the body. If you were to enter the abdominal or thoracic cavity surgically, you would be looking at serous membranes. Serous membranes secrete a thin, watery, serous fluid. The fluid allows the membranes to slide past one another with little friction.

A serous membrane is composed of simple squamous epithelium resting on a thin layer of loose connective tissue. Serous membranes line a cavity and then fold back onto the surface of the organs within that cavity. Thus part of the membrane lines the wall of the cavity, and the other part covers the organ or organs within that cavity. The part of the membrane that lines the walls of the cavity (like wallpaper) is the **parietal** (pă-RĪ-ĕ-tăl) **layer,** and the part of the membrane that covers the outside of an organ is the **visceral** (VĬS-ĕr-ăl) **layer.**

The three serous membranes are the pleura, pericardium, and peritoneum (see Figure 6-9). They are described as follows:

1. **Pleura** are found in the thoracic cavity. The parietal pleura line the wall of the thoracic cavity. The visceral pleura cover each lung. The space between the pleural layers is called the **pleural cavity;** the membranes are lubricated by pleural fluid. Why is pleurisy so painful? Pleurisy refers to an inflammation of the pleura and a decrease in serous fluid. As the inflamed and "dry" pleural membranes slide past one another during breathing movements, the person experiences pain.
2. The **pericardium** is found in the thoracic cavity and partially surrounds the heart. There is a

parietal and visceral pericardium that offers sling-like support to the heart. The space between the pericardial membranes is called the **pericardial cavity;** the membranes are lubricated by pericardial fluid. Pericardial structure is described further in Chapter 16.

3. The **peritoneum** is found within the abdominal cavity. The parietal peritoneum lines its walls, and the visceral peritoneum covers the abdominal organs (see Chapter 23).

Infection in the abdominal cavity often involves the peritoneum. For instance, a ruptured appendix allows the escape of intestinal contents, loaded with bacteria, into the peritoneal cavity. This leakage causes a life-threatening infectious condition called peritonitis. Aggressive treatment with antibiotics is required. Occasionally, the pus must be drained from the abdominal cavity. The pleural and pericardial membranes can also become inflamed or infected.

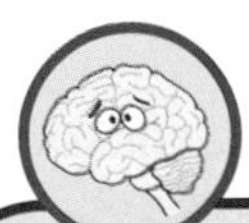

Do You Know...

How to name an -oma?

There are many -omas. -Oma at the end of a word means tumor or neoplasm. A lipoma is a neoplasm consisting of fatty tissue. -Omas are named for the tissues that form the tumors. An adenoma refers to a tumor consisting of glandular tissue. Carcinomas and sarcomas are malignant (cancerous) tumors. A carcinoma is a malignant tumor involving epithelial tissue, while a sarcoma involves connective tissue. All tumors should be biopsied. A biopsy refers to the removal of tumor tissue for microscopic examination. (Biopsy means to view with both eyes.) By viewing the tumor specimen under a microscope, the pathologist can determine whether the tumor is malignant (cancerous) or benign (noncancerous).

Sum It Up!

Membranes are sheets of tissue. Membranes cover surfaces, line body cavities, and surround organs. Membranes are classified as epithelial membranes or connective tissue membranes. The epithelial membranes include cutaneous (skin), mucous, and serous membranes. The location and functions of the epithelial and connective tissue membranes are summarized in Table 6-3.

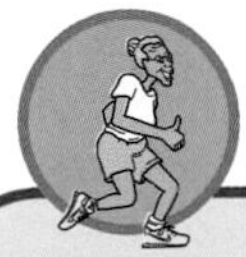

As You Age

1. Because tissues consist of cells, cellular aging alters the tissues formed by the cells. Alterations in tissues, in turn, affect organ function. For instance, by age 85, lung capacity has decreased by 50%, muscle strength has decreased by about 45%, and kidney function has decreased by 30%.
2. Collagen and elastin decrease in connective tissue. Consequently, tissues become stiffer, less elastic, and less efficient in their functioning.
3. Lipid and fat content of tissues change. In men, a gradual increase in tissue lipids and fat occurs until age 60, and then a gradual decrease follows. In women, lipids and fats accumulate in the tissues continuously; no decline occurs as in men.
4. The total amount of water in the body gradually decreases. The change in body fat and the decrease in water are major reasons that the elderly population responds differently to drugs than the younger population does.
5. Tissue atrophy causes a decrease in the mass of most organs.

Disorders of Tissues and Membranes

Adhesions	An abnormal joining of tissues by fibrous scar tissue. Adhesions may bind or constrict organs, causing decreased flexibility and obstruction, especially in the abdomen.
Cancer	Abnormal growth that can affect all types of tissues and membranes. Tumors are named according to the type of tissue involved. A carcinoma involves epithelial tissue (e.g., adenocarcinoma, a cancer arising from glandular tissue). A sarcoma involves connective tissue (e.g., osteosarcoma, a cancer involving bone).
Collagen diseases	For unknown reasons, collagen can be destroyed, causing damage to the connective tissue of the body. Because collagen is a main component of connective tissue, the effects of collagen diseases are widespread. Examples of collagen disease include rheumatoid arthritis, systemic lupus erythematosus (SLE), and scleroderma. Many of the collagen disease are autoimmune disorders, in which the patient's own immune system attacks and destroys collagen.
Gangrene	Death (necrosis) of the soft tissues of a body part such as the toes, fingers, or intestines. Gangrene occurs when the blood supply to the tissue is cut off. Diabetic patients experience gangrene of the toes when their arteries become clogged with fat deposits. Infection can also impede blood flow to a body part and therefore cause gangrene.
Neoplasm	A neoplasm (tumor) may be malignant (cancerous) or benign (noncancerous). Examples of benign connective tissue neoplasms include adenoma (glandular tissue); osteoma (bone); chondroma (cartilage); fibroma (fibroblasts); lipoma (fat tissue); and polyps (adenomas commonly found in vascular areas such as the nose, rectum, and uterus).

SUMMARY OUTLINE

Tissues are groups of cells similar to each other in structure and function. Membranes are thin sheets of tissue that cover surfaces, line body cavities, and surround organs.

I. Types of Tissue

A. Epithelial Tissue Types
1. Epithelial tissue covers surfaces, lines cavities, and engages in secretion/absorption and protective functions.
2. Epithelial tissue is classified according to cell shape (squamous, cuboidal, and columnar) and layers (simple and stratified).
3. The types and functions are summarized in Table 6-1.

B. Connective Tissue
1. The primary function of connective tissue is to bind together the parts of the body. Other functions include support, protection, storage of fat, and transport of substances.
2. Connective tissue has an abundant intercellular matrix that fills spaces between cells. The intercellular matrix may be liquid, gel-like, or hard. The matrix often contains protein fibers that are secreted by the cells.
3. There are three types of loose connective tissue: areolar, adipose, and reticular.
4. Dense fibrous connective tissue forms tendons, ligaments, capsules, and fascia, and is found in the skin (dermis).
5. Types of cartilage include: hyaline, elastic, and fibrocartilage.
6. Bone (osseous tissue) is connective tissue formed by osteocytes. Bone cells have a hard intercellular matrix that includes collagen, calcium salts, and other minerals.
7. Blood and lymph are types of connective tissue that have a watery intercellular matrix.

C. Nervous Tissue
1. Nervous tissue is found in the peripheral nerves, brain, and spinal cord.
2. The two types of nervous tissue are neurons, which transmit electrical signals, and neuroglia, which support and take care of the neurons.

D. Muscle Tissue
1. Muscle cells contract thereby causing movement.
2. The three kinds of muscle are skeletal, smooth, and cardiac.

II. Tissue Repair

A. Tissue Repair by Regeneration (replacement of tissue by cells that undergo mitosis).

B. Tissue Repair by Fibrosis (formation of scar tissue)

III. Membranes

A. Epithelial Membranes
1. The cutaneous membrane is the skin.
2. Mucous membrane is an epithelial membrane that lines all body cavities that open to the exterior of the body.
3. Serous membranes are epithelial membranes that line the ventral body cavities, which are not open to the exterior of the body.
4. Serous membranes form two layers: a parietal layer that lines the wall of the cavity and a visceral layer that covers the outside of an organ.
5. The three serous membranes are the pleura, the pericardium, and the peritoneum.

B. Connective Tissue Membranes
1. Synovial membranes are connective tissue membranes.
2. Other connective tissue membranes are listed in Table 6-3.

Review Your Knowledge

Matching: Tissues

Directions: Match the following words with their descriptions below. Some words may be used more than once.

a. epithelial
b. connective
c. muscle
d. nervous

1. ____ Important functions: secretion, absorption, excretion, and protection
2. ____ Blood, bone, cartilage, and adipose tissue
3. ____ Classified as squamous, cuboidal, or columnar
4. ____ Endocrine and exocrine glands arise from this type of tissue
5. ____ Binds together parts of the body; examples include tendons, ligaments, and fascia
6. ____ Skeletal, cardiac, and smooth
7. ____ Has the greatest amount of intercellular matrix
8. ____ Chondrocytes and osteocytes make up this tissue
9. ____ Intercellular matrix may be liquid, gel, or rigid
10. ____ Dendrites, axons, and glia

Matching: Membranes

Directions: Match the following words with their descriptions below.

a. visceral pleura
b. parietal peritoneum
c. connective tissue membranes
d. mucous membranes
e. parietal pleura

1. ____ Membranes lining all body cavities that open to the outside of the body
2. ____ Serous membrane that lines the walls of the thoracic cavity
3. ____ Serous membrane that lines the walls of the abdominopelvic cavity
4. ____ Serous membrane that covers each lung
5. ____ Synovial membrane, periosteum, and perichondrium

Multiple Choice

1. Which of the following is not characteristic of epithelial tissue?
   a. Arranged like floor tiles
   b. Simple, cuboidal, and columnar
   c. Large amount of mineral-containing intercellular matrix
   d. Gives rise to endocrine and exocrine glands
2. Adipose tissue is
   a. a type of connective tissue that stores fat.
   b. described as striated and voluntary.
   c. classified as endocrine and exocrine.
   d. classified as skeletal, cardiac, and smooth.
3. Osseous tissue
   a. contains hard mineral-containing intercellular fluid.
   b. contains osteocytes.
   c. is a type of connective tissue.
   d. All of the above.
4. With regard to the pleural membranes
   a. there is a visceral and parietal pleural membrane.
   b. they are connective tissues membranes.
   c. they are mucous membranes.
   d. they are located in the dorsal cavity.
5. The pleura, peritoneum, and pericardium
   a. are serous membranes.
   b. are located within the thoracic cavity.
   c. are located within the abdominal cavity.
   d. surround the lungs and the heart.

CHAPTER 7

Integumentary System and Body Temperature

KEY TERMS

Apocrine gland, p. 97
Ceruminous gland, p. 98
Conduction, p. 98
Convection, p. 98
Cutaneous membrane, p. 91
Dermis, p. 91
Eccrine gland, p. 97
Epidermis, p. 91
Evaporation, p. 99
Integument, p. 91
Keratin, p. 91
Melanin, p. 94
Radiation, p. 98
Sebaceous gland, p. 96
Stratum corneum, p. 92
Stratum germinativum, p. 91
Subcutaneous layer, p. 93
Sudoriferous gland, p. 97
Thermoregulation, p. 98

OBJECTIVES

1. Describe the two layers of skin: epidermis and dermis.
2. Define *stratum germinativum* and *stratum corneum.*
3. List the two major functions of the subcutaneous layer.
4. List the factors that influence the color of the skin.
5. Describe the accessory structures of the skin: hair, nails, and glands.
6. List six functions of the skin.
7. Describe how the skin helps to regulate temperature.
8. Explain four processes by which the body loses heat.

Oh no...a zit! How many times have you looked in the mirror only to see a pimple, rash, wrinkle, or unwanted hair? No other organ in the body is so scrutinized, scrubbed, lifted, and painted over as the skin. Yet year after year, the skin withstands the effects of harsh weather, the burning rays of the sun, constant bathing, friction, injury, and microorganisms that are constantly trying to penetrate its surface.

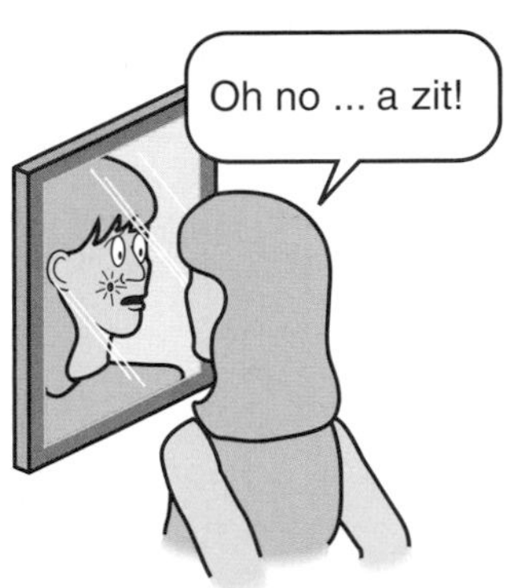

The skin, the accessory structures (sweat glands, oil glands, hair, and nails), and the subcutaneous tissue below the skin form the integumentary system. The **integumentary** (ĭn-tĕg-ū-MĔN-tăr-ē) **system** performs many roles, most of which protect the body from harm or act as a barrier against the external environment.

FUNCTIONS OF THE SKIN

The skin is a complex organ that performs many different functions. The skin performs the following functions:

- Keeps harmful substances out of the body and helps retain water and electrolytes.
- Protects the internal structures and organs from injuries due to blows, cuts, harsh chemicals, sunlight, burns, and pathogenic microorganisms.
- Performs an excretory function. Although excretion is a minor role, the skin is able to excrete water, salt, and small amounts of waste such as urea.
- Acts as a gland by synthesizing vitamin D. Skin cells contain a molecule that is converted to vitamin D when exposed to sunlight. Vitamin D is necessary for the absorption of calcium from the digestive tract.
- Performs a sensory role by housing the sensory receptors for touch, pressure, pain, and temperature. In this way, the skin helps to detect information about the environment.
- Plays an important role in the regulation of body temperature.

STRUCTURE OF THE SKIN

The skin is called the **integument** or **cutaneous** (kū-TĀN-ē-ŭs) **membrane** and is considered an organ. The skin has two distinct layers: the outer, or surface, layer is the **epidermis** (ĕp-ĭ-DĔR-mĭs) and the inner layer is the **dermis.** The dermis is anchored to a subcutaneous layer (Figure 7-1). The study of skin and skin disorders is referred to as **dermatology.**

LAYERS OF THE SKIN

Epidermis

The epidermis is the thin outer layer of the skin. The epidermis is composed of stratified squamous epithelium. Like all epithelial tissue, the epithelium is avascular; it has no blood supply of its own. Oxygen and nutrients, however, diffuse into the lower epidermis from the rich supply of blood in the underlying dermis. The epidermis can be divided into five layers. Two of the layers are the deeper stratum germinativum and the more superficial stratum corneum.

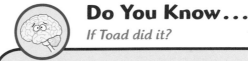

Do You Know...

If Toad did it?

Did Toad have anything to do with the wart on Helga's nose? No. A wart is an epidermal growth on the skin and is caused by a virus. Toad is innocent of this charge!

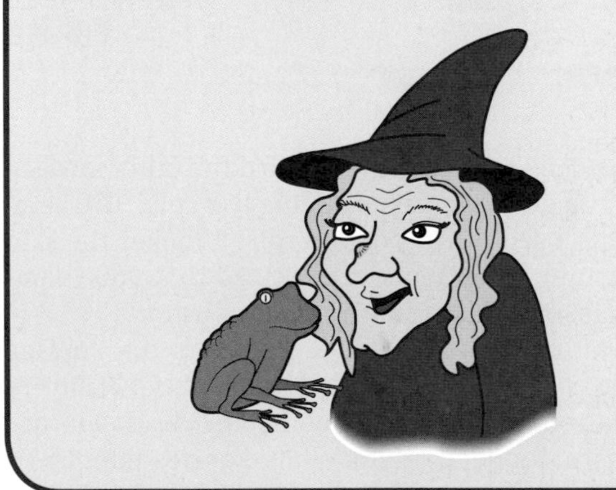

The **stratum germinativum** (jĕr-mĭ-NĀ-tĭv-ŭm) lies on top of the dermis and thus has access to a rich supply of blood. The cells of this layer are continuously dividing, producing millions of cells per day. As the cells divide, they push the older cells up toward the surface of the epithelium. As the cells move away from the dermis, two changes take place. First, as they move away from their source of nourishment, the cells begin to die. Second, the cells undergo a process of keratinization, whereby a tough protein, **keratin** (KĔR-ă-tĭn), is deposited within the cell. The keratin hardens and

Hair shaft
Pore
Stratum corneum
Epidermis
Stratum germinativum
Touch receptors
Sebaceous gland
Nerve ending
Pressure receptor
Free nerve endings
Dermis
Subcutaneous layer
Artery
Vein
Adipose tissue
Nerve (pain)
Sweat gland
Connective tissue

FIGURE 7-1 The skin.

flattens the cells as they move toward the outer surface of the skin. In addition to hardening the cells, the keratin performs a second important role: it makes the skin water-resistant. Have you ever noticed that your hand does not dissolve when you place it in water?

The **stratum corneum** (KŎR-nē-ŭm) is the surface layer of the epidermis. It is composed of about 30 layers of dead, flattened, keratinized cells. The dead cells are continuously sloughed off (exfoliated or desquamated) through wear and tear. The dead, sloughed cells are called dander; when dander is clumped together by the oil on the skull it is called dandruff. The sloughed cells are replaced by other cells that are constantly moving up from the deeper layers. Each month you have a new layer of epithelium.

Hanging You Out to Dry. About 500 ml/day of water is lost through the skin. This is called **insensible perspiration.** (Do not confuse insensible perspiration with sensible perspiration, which is due to the activity of the sweat glands.) If the epidermis is damaged, as in severe burns, the rate of insensible perspiration increases enormously; fluid loss is so great that the untreated patient dies from shock due to low volume (hypovolemic shock). The immediate needs of a severely burned patient are related to fluid replacement. Then there is the "water-logged" appearance of your hands (palms) and feet (soles)! When you immerse yourself in fresh water (hypotonic solution) your epithelial cells absorb water, increasing their volume and causing swelling.

Dermis

The dermis is located under the epidermis and is composed of dense fibrous connective tissue. It contains numerous collagen and elastin fibers that are surrounded

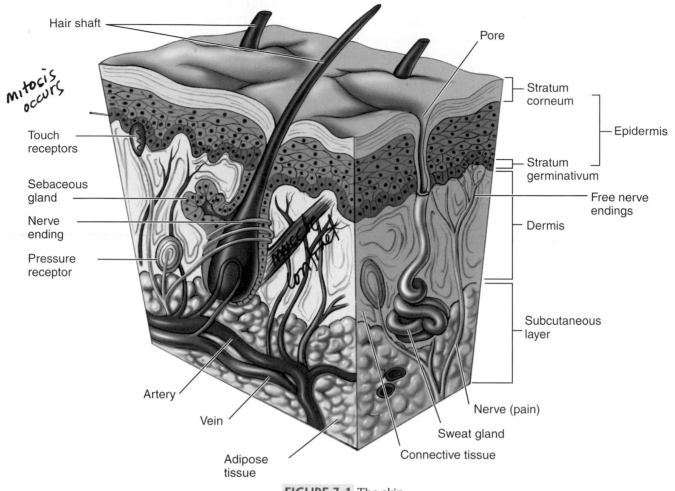

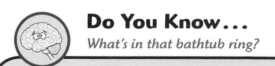

Do You Know...

What's in that bathtub ring?

The bathtub ring! What's in it? Dirt, grime ... and, yes, a piece of yourself: dead skin, or stratum corneum. How much dead skin? A person sheds about 1.5 lbs per year, or about 105 lbs over a lifetime. This means that you will scrape the equivalent of your entire body from the sides of your tub and watch it go down the drain.

by a gel-like substance. The fibers make the dermis strong and stretchable. Note how well the skin stretches during pregnancy and weight gain. Sometimes, however, excessive stretching of the skin causes small tears in the skin producing white lines. These lines are called stretch marks or striae. The thickness of the epidermis and dermis varies according to the location on the body. Look at the skin on the palms of your hands and the soles of your feet; it is much thicker here than it is over your inner arm or eyelids.

Although derived from the epidermis, the accessory structures such as the hair, nails, and certain glands are embedded within the dermis. Located within the dermis are blood vessels, nervous tissue, and some muscle tissue. Many of the nerves have specialized endings called sensory receptors that detect pain, temperature, pressure, and touch.

The Skin Tells a Story

- The skin reflects disease processes in the body. For example, a person with herpes zoster (shingles), an inflammation of nerves caused by the chickenpox virus, develops painful skin lesions along the path of the nerve. A person with a severe generalized staphylococcal infection may develop "scalded skin syndrome," a condition in which the skin appears scalded and peels off in layers.
- Drug reactions are often revealed by skin changes. For example, a person allergic to penicillin may develop hives or urticaria. Similarly, a person allergic to sulfa drugs may develop a generalized rash that can progresses to a lethal syndrome called Stevens-Johnson syndrome.
- The skin responds to chronic irritation. Epidermal cell growth increases in response to certain stimuli. For instance, constant irritation or rubbing of an area causes the rate of epidermal cell division to increase producing a thickened area called a callus. Constant rubbing of a toe by a poorly fitting shoe can also produce an overgrowth of epidermal cells arranged in a conical shape. This overgrowth is called a corn.
- The skin mirrors your stress level. How many times have you become stressed out and then broke out?
- The skin truly reveals on the outside what is going on inside!

Subcutaneous Layer

The dermis lies on the subcutaneous layer. This layer is not considered part of the skin; it lies under the skin and is therefore called the **subcutaneous layer** or the **hypodermis.** The subcutaneous layer is composed primarily of loose connective and adipose tissue. The subcutaneous tissue performs two main roles: it helps insulate the body from extreme temperature changes in the external environment, and it anchors the skin to the underlying structures. A few areas of the body have no subcutaneous layer; the skin anchors directly to the bone. Look at the skin over your knuckles. It is wrinkled and creased because it attaches directly to bone. Imagine what you would look like if all your skin were anchored directly to underlying bone. Drugs are often injected subcutaneously (SC) because the hypodermis has a rich supply of blood vessels; blood vessels absorb the drug and distribute it throughout the body.

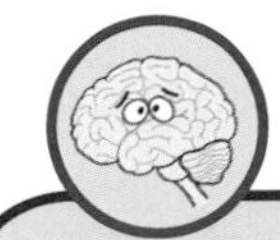

Do You Know...

How you inject a medication into the subcutaneous layer?

When injecting medication subcutaneously, you need to use a correctly sized needle and to insert the needle at the proper angle. The needle penetrates the epidermis and dermis so that the tip of the needle is located in the subcutaneous layer, where the medication is deposited.

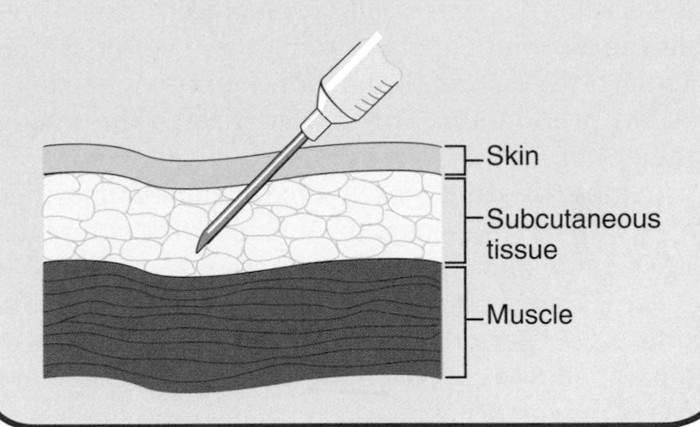

The Skin, Drugs, and Chemicals

The skin can absorb many chemicals. This is good news and bad news. The good news is concerned with drug absorption. Drugs can be placed on the surface of the skin and absorbed transdermally (across the skin) in order to achieve a systemic effect (within the body). For instance, nitroglycerine can be applied using an adhesive patch on the skin. The drug penetrates the skin, is absorbed by the dermal blood vessels, and is transported by the blood to the heart and blood vessels where it exerts its effects. The skin can also be used to detect allergies by injecting antigens (possible allergic substances) intradermally. An allergic response will appear as a skin reaction (redness, swelling, and itching). Lastly the subcutaneous route is a common way to inject drugs.

The bad news? Skin can absorb toxins; these include pesticides, dry cleaning fluid, the acetone in nail polish remover, mercury, and many other toxic chemicals that we encounter daily. Farm workers, exposed to chemical sprays, are commonly treated for pesticide poisoning. The sprayed pesticides saturate their clothing and are gradually absorbed across their skin. Hands in household chemicals? Wear gloves, and do not underestimate the ability of the skin to absorb toxins!

SKIN COLOR

Why are there different colors of skin? Skin color is determined by many factors: some genetic, some physiological, and some due to disease. When we think of skin color, we generally think of black, brown, yellow, and white, as well as the many shades in between! These skin colors are genetically determined.

Deep within the epidermal layer of the skin are cells called **melanocytes.** Melanocytes secrete a skin-darkening pigment called **melanin** (MĔL-ă-nĭn); the melanin stains the surrounding cells, causing them to darken. The more melanin secreted, the darker the skin color. Interestingly, we all have the same numbers of melanocytes. What determines our skin color is not the numbers of melanocytes but the amount of melanin secreted.

Can melanocytes increase their secretion of melanin? Yes! When exposed to the ultraviolet radiation of sunlight, the melanocytes secrete more melanin. The skin darkens in an attempt to protect the deeper layers from the harmful effects of radiation. Lighter-skinned persons often bake in the sun for hours trying to boost melanin production. This effort creates the famous summer tan.

A number of conditions involve malfunctioning melanocytes. What happens if the melanocytes completely fail to secrete melanin? In these persons, the skin, hair, and the colored part of the eye (iris) are white. This condition is referred to as albinism. Other persons develop a condition called vitiligo. This condition involves a loss of pigment (melanin) in certain areas of the skin, creating patches of white skin. Melanin can also stain unevenly. Freckles and moles are examples of melanin that becomes concentrated in local areas.

Moles are a normal occurrence; most people have 10 to 20 moles. Unfortunately, a mole may change, forming a malignant (cancerous) melanoma. A previously smooth mole that becomes darker and develops a rough or notched edge should be evaluated immediately. Malignant melanoma tends to metastasize (spread) very rapidly and is one of the cancers most difficult to treat. Exposure to sunlight increases the risk of malignant melanoma.

In addition to melanin, skin also contains a yellow pigment called carotene. The yellowish tint of carotene in most persons is hidden by the effects of melanin. Because people of Asian descent have little melanin in their skin, the carotene gives their skin a yellow tint. What accounts for the pinkish color of fair-skinned people? So little melanin is produced that the dermis is visible; it is the blood in the dermal capillaries that provides the pinkish tinge to the skin.

The ability of blood in the dermis to affect skin color also accounts for a number of other conditions. Poorly oxygenated blood causes the skin to look blue. This condition is called cyanosis. Embarrassment causes the blood vessels in the skin to dilate. This condition increases blood flow to the skin, causing the person to blush or flush. What about the saying, "He was white as a sheet!"? A person who is scared experiences a constriction of the blood vessels in the skin and a decrease in the amount of oxygenated blood. The resulting pale or ashen color is called pallor.

Skin color may also change in response to disease processes. Assessment of skin color provides valuable clues to underlying pathology. A person with liver disease is unable to excrete a pigment called bilirubin. This pigment is instead deposited in the skin, causing it to turn yellow, a condition known as jaundice. A person with a poorly functioning adrenal gland may deposit excess melanin in the skin and appear to be bronzed. A black-and-blue discoloration (bruise) indicates that blood has escaped from the blood vessels and clotted under the skin. A black-and-blue area is called an ecchymosis.

Lastly, skin color may also change in response to diet. For instance, it is possible to achieve a yellow tint to the skin by overeating carotene-rich vegetables such as carrots.

Sum It Up!

The integumentary system is composed of the skin and accessory organs (hair, nails, and glands). The skin is composed of two layers: the epidermis and the dermis. The dermis sits on a subcutaneous layer called the hypodermis. There are different colors of skin. Our natural skin color is genetically determined; we are light skinned, dark skinned, and many shades in between. The skin color changes in response to certain stimuli or underlying conditions; these changes include tanning, blushing, cyanosis, and jaundice. The skin can also reveal certain disease states, such as allergic responses, infections, and liver disease. The skin often announces on the outside what is happening on the inside.

ACCESSORY STRUCTURES OF THE SKIN

The skin is the home of several accessory structures, including the hair, nails, and glands.

HAIR

Thousands and thousands of years ago, we humans were a hairy lot. Like our furry pets, we depended on a thick crop of hair to keep us warm. Today, most of the hair covering our bodies is sparse and very fine, with the exception of the hair on our heads (and for some, that too is sparse). The main function of our sparse body hair is to sense insects on the skin before they can sting us. Some body parts are hairless. These include the palms of the hands, soles of the feet, lips, nipples, and parts of the external reproductive organs.

Some areas of hair perform important functions. For instance, the eyelashes and eyebrows protect the eyes from dust and perspiration. The nasal hairs trap dust and prevent it from being inhaled into the lungs. The hair of the scalp helps keep us warm and, of course, plays an important cosmetic role.

Hair growth is influenced by the sex hormones estrogen and testosterone. The onset of puberty is heralded by the growth of hair in the axillary and pubic areas in both males and females. In the male, the surge of testosterone also produces a beard and hairy chest. Estrogen, of course, does not have this effect. When a female has too much testosterone, excessive hair growth occurs, including facial hair. The excessive growth of hair is called hirsutism.

The chief parts of a hair are the shaft, the part above the surface of the skin, and the root, the part that extends from the dermis to the surface (Figure 7-2). Each hair arises from a group of epidermal cells that penetrate down into the dermis. This downward extension of epithelial cells forms the hair follicle. The epidermal cells at the base of the hair follicle receive a rich supply of blood from the dermal blood vessels. As these cells divide and grow, the older cells are pushed toward the surface of the skin. As they move away from their source of nourishment, the cells die. Like other cells that compose the skin, the hair cells also become keratinized. The hair that we brush, blow dry, and curl every day is a collection of dead, keratinized cells.

Hair color is genetically controlled and is determined by the type and amount of melanin. An abundance of melanin produces dark hair, whereas less melanin produces blond hair. With age, the melanocytes become less active; the absence of melanin produces white hair. Gray hair is due to a mixture of pigmented and nonpigmented hairs. Interestingly, red hair is due to a modified type of melanin that contains iron.

Curly, wavy, or straight, the shape of the hair shaft determines the appearance of the hair. A round shaft produces straight hair, whereas an oval shaft produces wavy hair. Curly and kinky hair are the result of flat hair shafts. One can make the hair curly by chemically flattening the hair shafts.

How does Frightened Kitty get her hair to stand on end? Attached to the hair follicle is a bundle of smooth muscle cells called the arrector pili muscles (see Figure 7-2). Contraction of these muscles causes the hair to stand on end. When frightened, the cat's brain sends its panic message along the nerves to these muscles. The muscles then contract and pull the hair into an upright position. Kitty looks more ferocious with her fur standing on end, and the "spiked look" helps frighten off her attackers. Her fur also stands on end when she is cold. The raised fur traps heat and helps keep her warm. Don't shave Kitty.

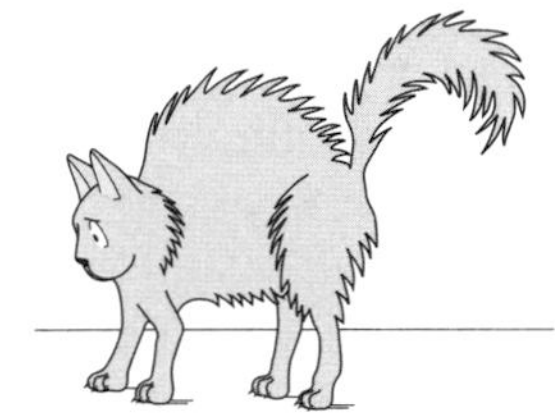

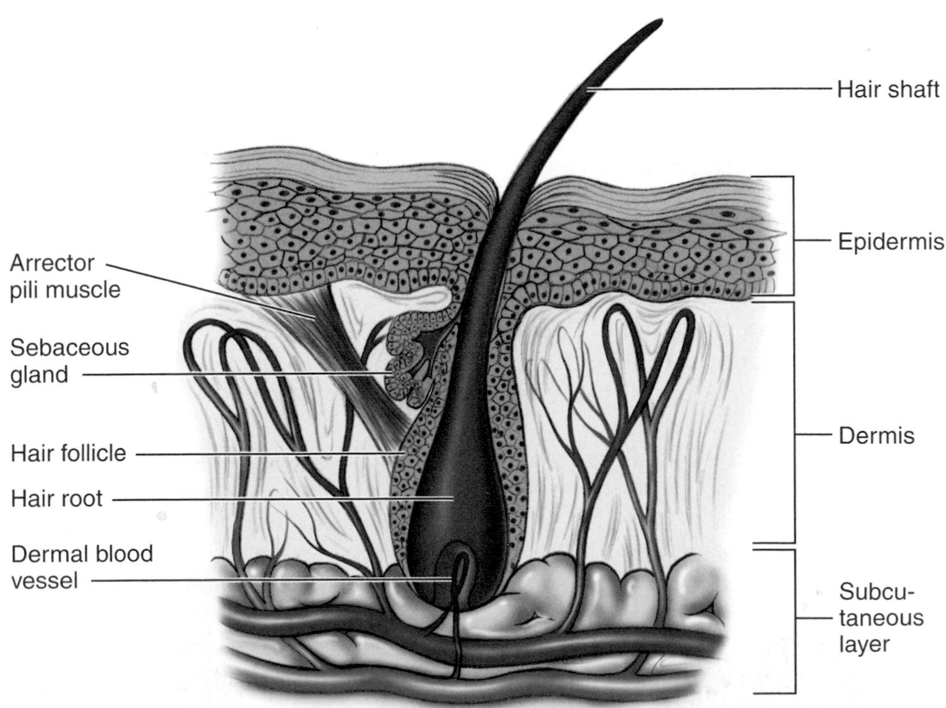

FIGURE 7-2 Hair follicle.

Although humans may not benefit as much from hair as do our furry friends, we respond to fear and cold in the same way. Contraction of the arrector pili muscles also causes our hair to stand on end. As the hair stands, it pulls the skin up into little bumps. This reaction is the basis of goose flesh, or goose bumps. Unlike Kitty, the erect human hair does not do much to trap heat; we must wear clothes instead.

Cosmetically, hair is important. Hair loss to the point of baldness is distressing. Enter the comb-over! The loss of hair is called alopecia. The most common type of baldness is male-pattern baldness. It is a hereditary condition characterized by a gradual loss of hair with aging. Hair today, gone tomorrow! A second common cause of hair loss is related to drug toxicity, as with chemotherapy or radiation therapy. Anticancer drugs are so toxic that they often destroy hair-producing cells. When drug therapy is terminated, the cells regenerate and start to grow hair again. Interestingly, the new hair may be a different color or texture from the original (predrug) hair. One more thing: apparently hair growth responds rather well to mind-body signals. The beards of men who have been stationed at sea experience a growth spurt of hair when told that they are going ashore!

Forensically, hair is a gold mine. For example, arsenic is called "inheritance powder," as it is a longtime favorite for dispatching wealthy family members. Chronic arsenic poisoning is difficult to detect medically, but analysis of the hair not only detects the presence of arsenic, it can also detect the time course of the poisoning.

NAILS

Nails are thin plates of stratified squamous epithelial cells that contain a very hard form of keratin (Figure 7-3). The nails are found on the distal ends of the fingers and toes and protect these structures from injury.

Each nail has the following structures: a free edge, a nail body (fingernail), and a nail root. The cells of the nail body develop and are keratinized in the nail root. The extent of nail growth is represented by the half-moon–shaped lunula, located at the base of the nail. As the nail body grows, it slides over a layer called the nailbed, a part of the epidermis. The pink color of nails is due to the blood vessels in the underlying dermal layer beneath the nail. The cuticle is a fold of stratum corneum that grows onto the proximal portion of the nail body.

Like the skin, the nails also tell stories. The assessment of the nails is important to determine not only their condition, but also evidence of systemic disease. Nails should be examined for shape, dorsal curvature, adhesion to the nail bed, color, and thickness. Some clinical observations include:

- Clubbing. Chronic lung and heart disease causes clubbing, a condition that indicates that the fingertips have received an insufficient supply of oxygenated blood over a period of time. Clubbing involves changes in the fingertips and nails. The fingertips enlarge and the nails become thick, hard, shiny, and curved at the free end. With severe clubbing the nail may detach from its base.
- In the Pink ... or Not. Nail color should be pink. Poor oxygenation makes the blood appear bluish-red (cyanosis) which, in turn, makes the nails appear bluish. Other color changes include pigment bands; these dark bands are normally seen in dark-skinned individuals. When present in light-skinned individuals the bands may indicate melanoma.
- Nail abuse. Trauma to the toenail, as in jogging, causes the nail to thicken or hypertrophy.
- Brittle. Nails may also be described as brittle; this is generally due to poor oxygenation and nutritional anemias.

GLANDS

Two major exocrine glands are associated with the skin. They are the sebaceous glands and the sweat glands (Figure 7-4).

Most **sebaceous** (sĕ-BĀ-shŭs) **glands,** or oil glands, are associated with hair follicles and are found in all

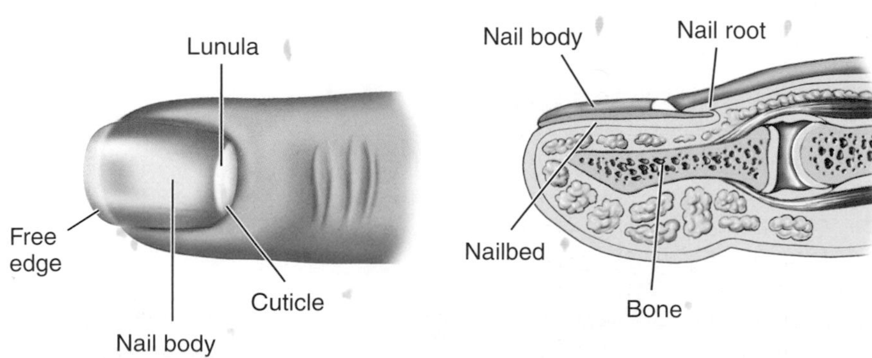

FIGURE 7-3 Nail.

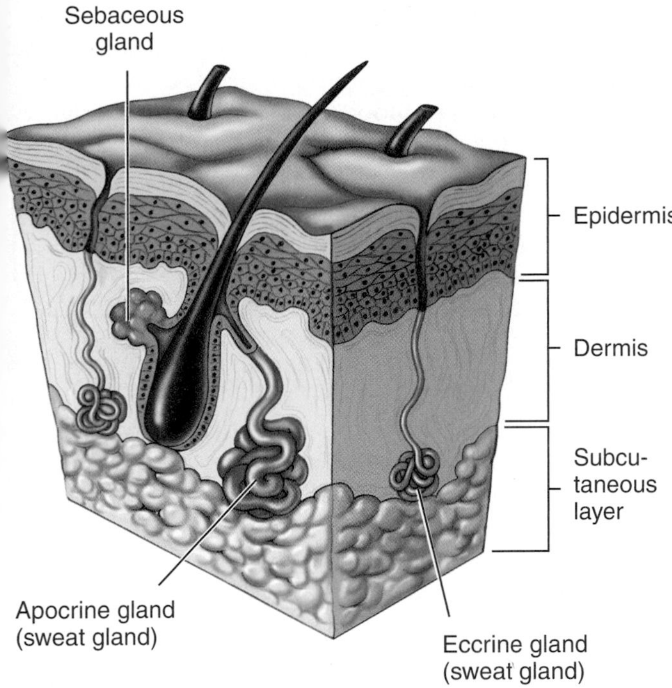

FIGURE 7-4 Skin glands: sebaceous glands and sweat glands.

areas of the body that have hair. They secrete an oily substance called **sebum** that flows into the hair follicle and then out onto the surface of the skin. A small number of sebaceous glands open directly onto the surface of the skin. The sebum lubricates and helps waterproof the hair and skin. The sebum also inhibits the growth of bacteria on the surface of the skin. With aging, sebum production gradually decreases. This change accounts, in part, for the dry skin and brittle hair seen in older persons. The sebaceous glands play a unique role in the fetus. Babies are born with a covering that resembles cream cheese. The covering is called the **vernix caseosa** and is secreted by the sebaceous glands.

Sometimes the sebaceous glands become blocked by accumulated sebum and other debris. When the sebum is exposed to the air and dries out, it turns black, forming a blackhead. When the blocked sebum becomes infected with staphylococci it is a pimple (pustule). You have seen the contents of a pimple. Blackhead and pimple formation is common among adolescents, because sebaceous gland activity responds to the hormonal changes associated with puberty. Baby too may have a problem with her sebaceous glands. The sebaceous glands on her scalp can oversecrete sebum, producing oily scales. Because this condition occurs during infancy, the cradle period, it is called cradle cap.

The **sweat glands,** or **sudoriferous** (sū-dŏ-RĬF-ĕr-ŭs) **glands,** are located in the dermis (see Figure 7-4). As the name implies, these glands secrete sweat; the sweat is secreted into a duct that opens onto the skin as a pore. An individual has approximately three million sweat glands.

Two types of sweat glands are the apocrine and the eccrine sweat glands. The **apocrine** (ĂP-ŏ-krĭn) **glands** are usually associated with hair follicles and are found in the axillary and genital areas. The apocrine glands respond to emotional stress and become active when the person is frightened, upset, in pain, or sexually excited. Because the development of these glands is stimulated by the sex hormones, they become more active during puberty. The sweat produced by these glands does not have a strong odor. If allowed to accumulate on the skin, however, the substances in sweat are degraded by bacteria into chemicals with a strong unpleasant odor. This is called body odor (BO) and is the reason we use deodorants.

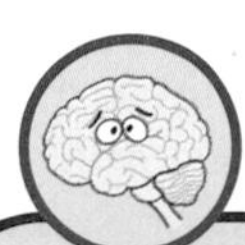

Do You Know...

'Bout them "apples"?

In some species of animals, the olfactory area of the brain, the "smell brain," is the largest part of the brain. The survival of these animals depends heavily on the sense of smell. Humans also have a smell brain that, although very small, plays a powerful role in our emotional responses and is responsible for some very strange responses. For instance, in Elizabethan times, lovers exchanged "love apples." And where did you get them? You made them. A woman peeled a common apple and placed it in her armpit until it was saturated with her perspiration (thanks to the apocrine glands). The sweat-soaked apple was then given to her lover to smell—at his leisure!

In animals, such as the dog (and us), some of these secretions act as sex attractants. Watch how eagerly Rover sniffs when a potential mate is in the immediate area! These sex attractants are called pheromones. The vaginal secretions of an ovulating female contain pheromones called copulines. The copulines can cause a testosterone surge (and an urge to merge) in the male.

The **eccrine** (ĔK-krĭn) **glands** are the more numerous and widely distributed of the sweat glands. They are located throughout the body and are especially numerous on the forehead, neck, back, upper lip, palms, and soles. Unlike apocrine glands, the eccrine glands are not associated with hair follicles.

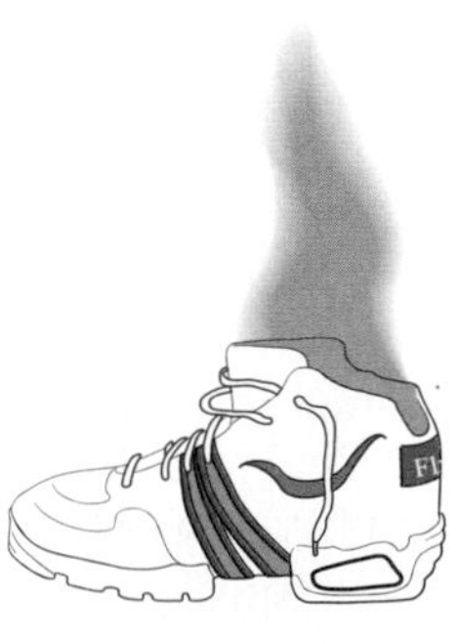

The sweat secreted by the eccrine glands plays an important role in temperature regulation. As sweat evaporates from the skin surface, heat is lost. These are the glands that make you sweat profusely on hot days or during periods of strenuous exercise. The eccrine glands are responsible for **sensible perspiration,** and, when operating maximally, can secrete 1 gallon of sweat per hour. Unlike the apocrine glands, which become active during puberty, the eccrine glands function throughout your entire lifetime. Eccrine secretion is composed primarily of water and a few salts.

Modified sweat glands include the mammary glands and the ceruminous glands. The mammary glands are located in the breasts; they secrete milk. (The secretion of milk is discussed further in Chapter 27.) The **ceruminous** (sĭ-RŪ-mĭ-nŭs) **glands** are found in the external auditory canal of the ear. They secrete **cerumen,** or ear wax. This yellow, sticky, wax-like secretion repels insects and traps foreign material. Silkworms and spiders use modified sweat glands to secrete silk and weave intricate webs.

Sum It Up!

The skin is the home of several accessory structures, including the hair, nails, and glands. There are two major exocrine glands, the sebaceous glands and the sweat glands (also called sudoriferous glands). There are two types of sweat glands: the eccrine glands and the apocrine glands. Modified sweat glands include the ceruminous glands, which secrete ear wax, and the mammary glands, which secrete milk.

BODY TEMPERATURE

The "normal" body temperature is said to be 98.6° F (although it can range from 97° F to 100° F). The temperature, however, fluctuates about 1.8° F in a 24-hour period, being lowest in the early morning and highest in the late afternoon. Body temperature also differs from one part of the body to another. The inner parts of the body (cranial, thoracic, and abdominal cavities) reflect the higher **core temperature.** The more surface areas (skin and mouth) reflect the cooler **shell temperature.** For instance, the rectal temperature measures core temperature and ranges between 99° F to 99.7° F, while the oral temperature is about one degree lower.

Body temperature is maintained by balancing heat production and heat loss. The mechanism whereby the body balances heat production and heat loss is called **thermoregulation.** Failure to thermoregulate causes body temperature to fluctuate; an excessive decrease in body temperature is called hypothermia while an excessive increase is called hyperthermia. Extreme changes in body temperature are often fatal.

Do You Know...

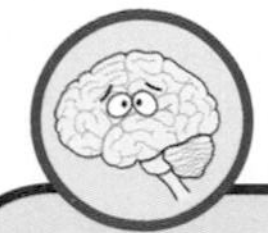

Why you shouldn't offer a hypothermic individual a rum punch?

While this is a thoughtful gesture, the alcohol in the rum causes dilation of the blood vessels in the skin, thereby increasing blood flow and the loss of heat. Mr. Hypothermia needs his heat. While he may prefer the rum punch, he is better served with a cup of hot tea.

BODY TEMPERATURE: HEAT PRODUCTION

Heat is thermal energy and is produced by the millions of chemical reactions occurring in the cells of the body. The heat produced by metabolizing cells is the basis of body temperature. In the resting state the greatest amount of heat is produced by the muscles, liver, and endocrine glands. The resting brain produces only about 15% of the heat. Interestingly, the studying brain does not produce much more heat.

The amount of heat produced can be affected by many factors: food consumption, the amounts and types of hormones that are secreted, and physical activity. With exercise, the amount of heat produced by the muscles may increase enormously. The hormonal effects on heat production is dramatically illustrated by persons with thyroid gland disease. The hypothyroid person generally has a lower than normal body temperature while the hyperthyroid person has an elevated temperature. In fact an extreme hyperthyroid state (thyroid storm) can elevate body temperature into a range that is potentially lethal. The heat produced in the cells is picked up and distributed throughout the body by the blood. Remember, the heat produced by the metabolizing cells is the basis of the body temperature.

BODY TEMPERATURE: HEAT LOSS

Most heat loss (80%) occurs through the skin. The remaining 20% is lost through the respiratory system (lungs) and in the excretory products (urine and feces). Heat loss occurs by four means: radiation, conduction, convection, and evaporation.

The amount of blood in the dermal blood vessels influences the amount of heat that can be lost or dissipated by radiation, conduction, and convection. **Radiation** means that heat is lost from a warm object (the body) to the cooler air surrounding the warm object. Thus a person loses heat in a cold room. **Conduction** is the loss of heat from a warm body to a cooler object in contact with the warm body. For example, a person (warm object) becomes cold when sitting on a block of ice (cooler object). Clinically, a cooling blanket may be used to reduce a dangerously high fever. The warm body of a feverish patient loses heat to the cooler object, the cooling blanket. **Convection** is the loss of heat by air currents moving over the surface of the skin. For example, a fan moves air across the surface of the skin, thereby constantly removing the layer of heated air next to the body.

Finally, heat may be lost through evaporation. **Evaporation** occurs when a liquid becomes a gas. For example, when liquid alcohol is rubbed on the skin, it evaporates and cools the skin. Likewise, during strenuous exercise, sweat on the surface of the skin evaporates and cools the body. Note that the evaporation of water is associated with a loss of heat. On a hot, humid day, water cannot evaporate from the surface of the skin. Hence, heat loss is diminished. This is why we feel the heat so intensely on a hot, humid day.

BODY TEMPERATURE: REGULATION

Normal body temperature is regulated by several mechanisms. The thermostat of the body is located in a part of the brain called the hypothalamus. The hypothalamus senses changes in body temperature and sends information to the skin (blood vessels and sweat glands) and skeletal muscle.

With exercise and temperature elevation, the blood vessels dilate, thereby allowing more blood to flow to the skin. This activity transfers heat from the deeper tissues to the surface of the body. Note how flushed our jogger is because of the blood coming to the surface (Figure 7-5). Temperature elevation also stimulates the activity of the sweat glands. As the sweat evaporates from the surface of the body, heat is lost. Under extreme conditions of heat, 12 liters (L) of sweat can be secreted in a 24-hour period. These two activities lower body temperature.

What about Mr. Ear Muffs in Figure 7-5? How does his body respond as his temperature decreases? First, the blood vessels constrict, reducing blood flow to the skin. This response traps the blood and heat in the deeper tissues, preventing heat loss. Second, the sweat glands become less active, also preventing heat loss. Third, skeletal muscles contract vigorously and involuntarily, causing shivering and an increase in the production of heat. These three activities raise body temperature to more normal levels. Contraction of the arrector pili muscles causes goose bumps, indicating a decline in body temperature, but contributes minimally to heat production. In furry animals the story is a little different; contraction of the arrector pili muscles pulls the fur upright, thereby trapping warm air. Not good to shave Rover in the winter!

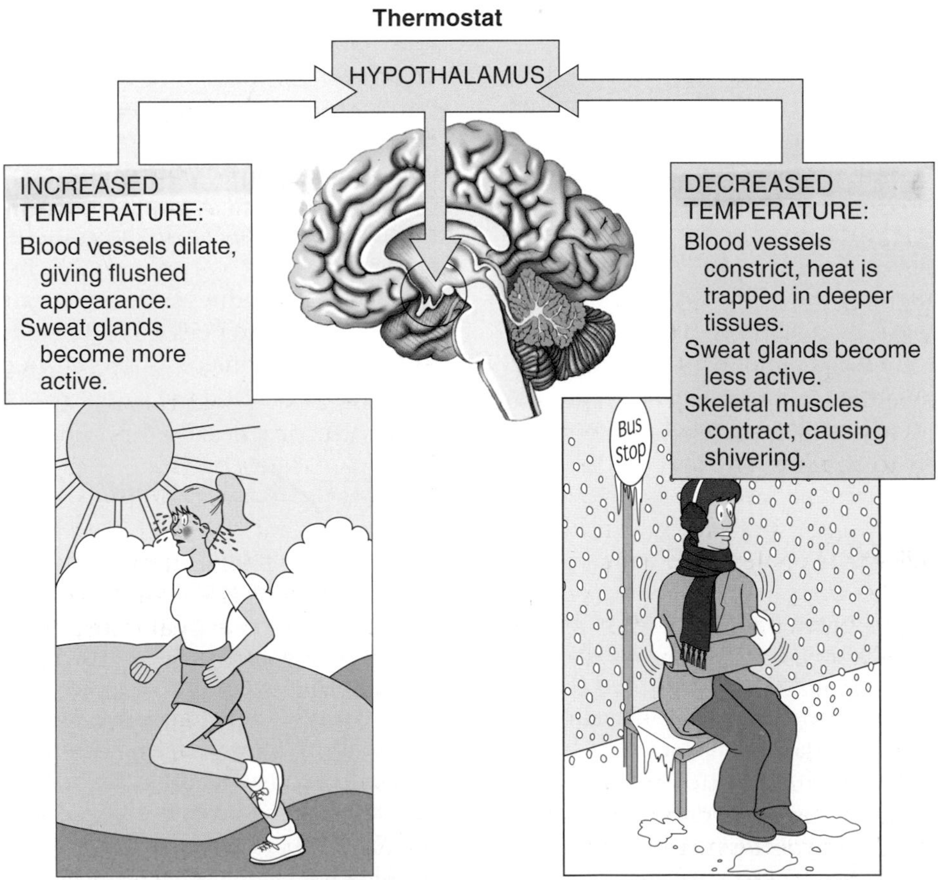

FIGURE 7-5 Temperature regulation.

Exposure to intense heat can cause a number of heat-related conditions: heat syncope (fainting), heat cramps, heat exhaustion, and finally heat stroke. Heat stroke is the most serious form of heat stress; it is a failure of the thermoregulatory mechanisms. Core temperature exceeds 104° F, and the patient experiences serious neurological symptoms including hallucinations and altered mentation. Heat stroke is a medical emergency. Hypothermia slows metabolism, enabling some people to survive very cold temperatures. If it's too cold (body temperature less than 95° F), however, the person may die as the heart develops fatal electrical abnormalities such as fibrillation.

Cold Baby Warmed by BAT! In the delivery room everyone is relieved when Baby takes her first breath and delivers her first wail: waa waa waa!. Next to establishing respiratory activity, however, is the infant's need to regulate body temperature. In short, the new baby (neonate) produces only about two thirds of the heat produced by an adult, but loses twice as much. There are several factors that contribute to the excess heat loss:

- the neonate generally has a large surface area that increases heat loss. (The curled up position of the infant decreases surface area and conserves heat. Don't unroll Baby.)
- the neonate generally has only a thin layer of subcutaneous fat. (Fat acts as an insulator preventing heat loss.)
- the neonate cannot shiver. (Shivering produces heat.)

Interestingly, the neonate, like a squirrel, produces heat by a process called **nonshivering thermogenesis.** A neonate has brown adipose tissue (BAT), or "brown fat," scattered throughout its body, especially around the neck and shoulder area. Metabolism of BAT generates more heat than does the metabolism of ordinary adipose tissue. The heat produced by BAT is picked up by the blood and dispersed throughout the body. BAT warms Baby.

While we are generally concerned about excessive heat loss in the neonate, we must also be concerned about excess heat. An infant has a very limited capacity to dissipate heat and is therefore at risk for hyperthermia. Do not leave Baby in a hot car!

WHEN SKIN IS BURNED

Large areas of skin are often lost because of burns. Burns are classified according to both the depth of the burn and the extent of the surface area burned (Figure 7-6, *A*). On the basis of depth, burns are classified as either partial-thickness burns or full-thickness burns. Partial-thickness burns are further divided into first-degree and second-degree burns. A first-degree burn is red, painful, and slightly edematous (swollen). Only the epidermis is involved. Sunburn is an example of a first-degree burn. A second-degree burn involves damage to both the epidermis and the dermis. With little damage to the dermis, the symptoms of a second-degree burn include redness, pain, edema, and blister formation. With greater damage to the dermis, the skin may appear red, tan, or white.

Full-thickness burns are also called third-degree burns. With a burn this severe, both the epidermis and the dermis are destroyed, often with destruction of the deeper underlying layers. Although first- and second-degree burns are painful, third-degree burns are painless because the sensory receptors have been destroyed. Third-degree burns may appear white, tan, brown, black, or deep cherry red.

The extent of the burn injury is initially evaluated according to the rule of nines (see Figure 7-6, *B*). In this system, the total body surface area is divided into regions. The assigned percentages are related to the number 9. For instance, the head and neck are considered 9% of the total body surface area. Each upper limb is 9%, whereas each lower limb is 18% (9×2). Note the percentages assigned to each specific body region. To determine proper treatment, the clinician needs to evaluate both the depth and the extent of the burn injury.

ESCHAR

Severe burns are associated with eschar formation. Eschar is dead burned tissue that forms a thick, inflexible scablike layer over the burned surface. Eschar is a problem for two reasons. First, it may surround an area, such as a leg, and act like a tourniquet thereby cutting off the flow of blood to the extremity. More seriously, if the eschar surrounds the chest, it prevents chest expansion and breathing. Second, eschar (which is initially sterile) becomes a breeding ground for bacteria and secretes toxins into the blood. These toxins adversely affect various organs in the body such as the lungs and kidneys. Because eschar can have such serious consequences it is often slit (escharotomy), so as to allow expansion of the burned area, or removed so as to rid the body of a source of toxin.

A NOTE ABOUT SKIN CARE

The skin is constantly exposed to all sorts of insults: the drying effects of soap and water, the damaging effects of the ultraviolet radiation of the sun, friction, numerous bumps, and exposure to sharp objects. While we cannot avoid normal wear and tear, we can protect the skin in several ways. For instance, we can lessen exposure of the skin to ultraviolet radiation. Sunbathing is deadly to the skin. Sun exposure both dries and irreversibly damages the skin. It also makes the skin leatherlike and increases the risk of skin cancer and malignant melanoma.

Skin care is particularly important in the elderly. The skin of an elderly person is normally drier, more easily

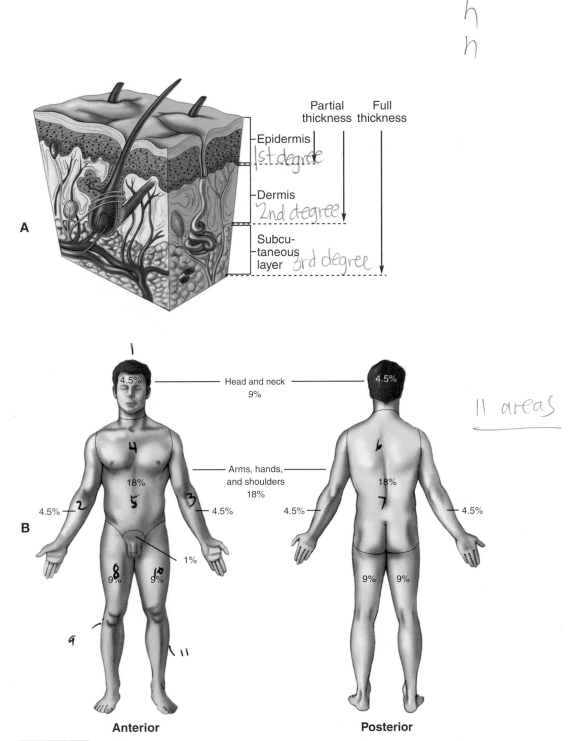

FIGURE 7-6 **A,** Parts of the skin damaged by burns. Partial-thickness (first- and second-degree burns) and full-thickness burns (third-degree burns). **B,** The rule of nines.

Do You Know...

What "vagabond syndrome" is and why it makes you "feel lousy"?

The skin of people who continuously harbor body lice becomes hardened and darkly pigmented; this condition is known as vagabond syndrome. Chronic infestation of lice also causes the person to feel tired and irritable, hence the term "feeling lousy."

injured, and slower to heal. Because the skin is so dry, excessive use of soap should be discouraged. Limiting the use of soaps and excessive bathing can help prevent additional drying of the skin. Moreover, maintaining the acid surface of the skin serves to discourage the growth of bacteria. In addition to becoming drier with aging, the skin changes in another important way. Both the dermis and the underlying subcutaneous layer become thinner. As a result, elderly people bruise more easily because the blood vessels are not as well protected. In addition, heat is lost from the blood vessels so that older people often feel cold.

Sum It Up!

The skin is a complex organ that performs many functions: it affords protection for the entire body, acts as a barrier, regulates temperature, detects sensations (touch, pressure, temperature, and pain), synthesizes vitamin D, and acts as an excretory organ. Thermoregulatory mechanisms balance heat production and heat loss. Because the skin protects us from and presents us to the external environment, we must take care of this marvelous organ.

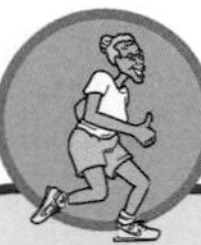

As You Age

1. Aging causes a generalized thinning of the epidermis; the epidermal cells reproduce more slowly and are larger and more irregular. These changes result in thinner, more translucent skin.
2. Melanocyte activity decreases, resulting in decreased protection from ultraviolet light and greater susceptibility to sunburn and skin cancer. Selected melanocytes increase melanin production, resulting in brown spots, or age spots, especially in areas exposed to the sun.
3. The dermis becomes thinner, with a decreased amount of collagen and decreased number of elastin fibers. The result is increased fragility of the skin, as well as increased wrinkles. The skin also heals more slowly.
4. Vascularity of the dermis decreases (a decreased number of blood vessels) with a slower rate of repair. This change causes the skin to become more susceptible to small hemorrhages and pressure ulcers.
5. Vascularity and circulation in the subcutaneous tissue decrease, so that drugs administered subcutaneously are absorbed more slowly.
6. The amount of adipose tissue in the subcutaneous layer decreases, resulting in folded and wrinkled skin that has a decreased ability to maintain body temperature. The person tends to feel cold.
7. Sebaceous gland activity decreases, resulting in dry, coarse, itchy skin.
8. Sweat gland activity decreases, resulting in decreased ability to regulate body temperature and intolerance to cold.
9. The rate of melanin production by the hair follicle decreases. As a result, hair may become lighter in color, turning gray or white. Hair does not replace itself as often and can become thinner.
10. Vascular supply to the nailbed decreases. Consequently, the nails can become dull, brittle, hard, and thick; growth rate also slows.

Disorders of the Integumentary System

Acne	A disorder of the skin in which the sebaceous glands oversecrete sebum. The most common form of acne occurring during adolescence is acne vulgaris.
Athlete's foot	A fungal infection characterized by vesicles, fissures, ulcers, and pruritus (itching). It most commonly affects the toes but may also involve the fingers, palms, and groin area.
Boil	Also called a furuncle; a localized collection of pus caused by staphylococcal infection of hair follicles and sebaceous glands. A carbuncle is multiple, interconnecting furuncles.
Cold sore	Also called a fever blister; a collection of watery vesicles caused by infection with the herpes simplex virus.
Cyst	Saclike structure containing fluid or semisolid material and surrounded by a strong capsule.
Dermatitis	Inflammation of the skin that may be caused by a variety of irritants such as chemicals, plants, and acids. Dermatitis is characterized by erythema (redness), papules (pimplelike lesions), vesicles (blisters), scabs, and crusts. Poison ivy is a form of contact dermatitis. Skin irritation occurs when contact is made with the irritating substance.

Disorders of the Integumentary System—cont'd

Eczema	From the Greek word meaning to erupt. Eczema is an inflammatory condition (atopic dermatitis) characterized by redness, papular and vesicular lesions, crusts, and scales.
Hives	Urticaria. Hives are due to an allergic reaction characterized by red patches (wheals) and generally accompanied by intense itching (pruritus).
Impetigo	A contagious infection of the skin generally caused by the staphylococcus bacterium.
Psoriasis	From the Greek word meaning to itch. Psoriasis is a chronic condition characterized by lesions that are red, dry, elevated, and covered by silvery scales.
Skin cancer	Several kinds of skin cancer are all related to excessive exposure to sun. The two most common types are basal cell carcinoma and squamous cell carcinoma. Basal cell carcinoma spreads locally and is successfully treated. The most serious and less successfully treated form of skin cancer is malignant melanoma, a cancer of the pigment-producing melanocytes.

SUMMARY OUTLINE

The integumentary system includes the skin; it covers the body, protects the internal organs, and plays an important role in the regulation of body temperature.

I. Structures: Organs of the Integumentary System

The integumentary system includes the skin, accessory structures, and subcutaneous tissue beneath the skin.

A. Skin
1. The skin is called the cutaneous membrane.
2. The skin has two layers, an outer layer called the epidermis and an inner layer called the dermis.
3. The epidermis has five layers. The stratum germinativum is the layer in which cell division takes place. The new cells produce keratin (waterproofing) and die as they are pushed toward the surface. The outer layer is the stratum corneum and consists of flattened, dead, keratinized cells.
4. The dermis lies on the subcutaneous tissue.
5. Skin color is determined by many factors: some genetic, some physiologic, and some due to disease. Melanin causes skin to darken. Carotene causes skin to appear yellow. The amount of blood in the skin affects skin color (e.g., flushing) as does the appearance of abnormal substances such as bilirubin (jaundice) and a low blood oxygen content (cyanosis).

B. Accessory Structures of the Skin
1. Hair is unevenly distributed over the skin. The location of the hair determines its function. Eyebrows and eyelashes protect the eyes from dust and perspiration.
2. The main parts of a hair are the shaft, root, and follicle.
3. Hair color is determined by the amount and type of melanin.
4. Nails are thin plates of stratified squamous epithelial cells that contain a hard form of keratin.
5. There are two major exocrine glands in the skin: the sebaceous glands and sweat glands.
6. The sebaceous glands (oil glands) secrete sebum. The sebum lubricates hair and skin. In the fetus, these glands secrete vernix caseosa, a cheeselike substance that coats the skin of a newborn.
7. The two types of sweat glands (sudoriferous glands) are the apocrine glands and the eccrine glands. The eccrine sweat glands play a crucial role in temperature regulation.
8. The mammary glands (which secrete milk) and the ceruminous glands (which secrete ear wax) are modified sweat glands.

C. Subcutaneous Tissue
1. Subcutaneous tissue anchors the dermis to underlying structures.

2. Subcutaneous tissue acts as an insulator; it prevents heat loss.

II. Regulation of Body Temperature

A. Heat Production
1. Heat produced by metabolizing cells constitutes the body temperature.
2. Most of the heat is produced by the muscles and the liver.

B. Heat Loss
1. Most of the heat (80%) is lost through the skin.
2. Heat loss occurs through radiation, conduction, convection, and evaporation.
3. Normal body temperature is set by the body's thermostat in the hypothalamus.
4. Heat is lost through sweating and vasodilation. Heat is conserved by vasoconstriction and produced by shivering.

III. When Skin Is Burned

A. Physiological Effects. These include short-term effects (fluid and electrolyte losses, shock, inability to regulate body temperature, infection) and long-term effects (scarring, loss of function, and cosmetic and emotional problems).

B. Classification of Burns
1. Classified according to the thickness of the burn (partial, full); also first, second, and third degree.
2. The rule of nines is a way to evaluate burns.

Review Your Knowledge

Matching: Skin

Directions: Match the following words with their descriptions below. Some words may be used more than once.

a. keratin
b. dermis
c. subcutaneous layer
d. epidermis

1. ____ Thin outer layer of skin
2. ____ Layer that sits on the hypodermis and supports the epidermis
3. ____ A protein that flattens, hardens, and makes the skin water resistant
4. ____ A layer of insulation
5. ____ Contains the stratum germinativum and stratum corneum

Matching: Glands

Directions: Match the following words with their descriptions below. Some words may be used more than once.

a. eccrine
b. sebaceous
c. ceruminous
d. mammary

1. ____ Oil glands
2. ____ Glands that secrete vernix caseosa
3. ____ Glands that play a crucial role in body temperature regulation
4. ____ Modified sweat glands that secrete ear wax
5. ____ Modified sweat glands that secrete milk

Matching: Colors

Directions: Match the following words with their descriptions below. Some words may be used more than once.

a. jaundice
b. cyanosis
c. melanin
d. vitiligo
e. ecchymosis

1. ____ Tanning pigment
2. ____ Condition in which the skin has a bluish tint because of poor oxygenation
3. ____ Yellowing of the skin because of bilirubin
4. ____ Patches of white skin due to loss of pigmentation
5. ____ Black and blue mark

Multiple Choice

1. Which of the following is most apt to increase body temperature?
   a. Dilation of the blood vessels in the skin
   b. Shivering
   c. Secretion of the eccrine glands
   d. Secretion of sebum
2. The stratum germinativum
   a. is a dermal layer.
   b. gives rise to epidermal cells.
   c. contains the blood vessels that nourish the epidermis.
   d. is part of the hypodermis.

3. The epidermis is nourished by the
   a. air in the environment that diffuses into the pores.
   b. blood vessels in the hair shafts.
   c. blood vessels in the underlying dermis.
   d. the oxygen and glucose in the sebum.
4. Which of the following is true of the stratum corneum?
   a. Continuously produces epidermal cells
   b. Secretes keratin for making the skin water resistant
   c. Is the dead layer that is sloughed off
   d. Continuously secretes bilirubin
5. Secretion of the eccrine glands
   a. “oils” the hair shafts.
   b. produces vernix caseosa that protects the skin of the fetus.
   c. lowers body temperature.
   d. tans the skin.
6. Cyanosis occurs when
   a. the blood in the cutaneous blood vessels is unoxygenated.
   b. bilirubin deposits in the skin and mucous membrane.
   c. cutaneous blood vessels dilate.
   d. sebum is exposed to air and changes color.

CHAPTER 8

Skeletal System

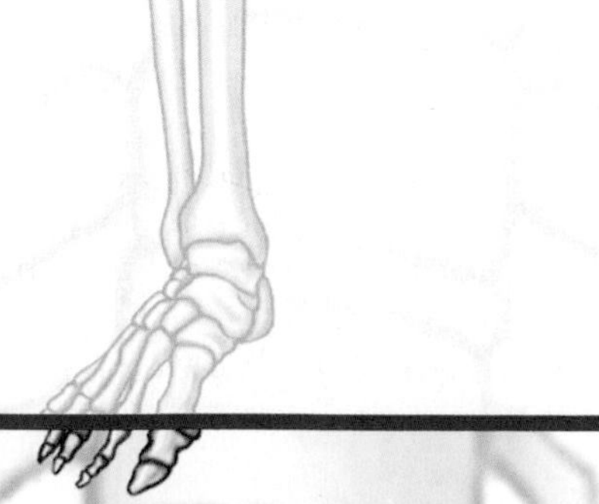

KEY TERMS

Abduction, p. 133
Adduction, p. 133
Appendicular skeleton, p. 114
Articulation, p. 127
Axial skeleton, p. 113
Diaphysis, p. 109
Epiphysis, p. 109
Extension, p. 133
Flexion, p. 133
Fontanel, p. 117
Haversian system, p. 107
Osteoblast, p. 111
Osteoclast, p. 112
Periosteum, p. 110
Synovial joint, p. 128

OBJECTIVES

1. List the functions of the skeletal system.
2. Describe the structure of a long bone.
3. Describe the roles of osteoblasts and osteoclasts.
4. List the bones of the axial skeleton.
5. List the bones of the appendicular skeleton.
6. Label important landmarks for selected bones on the skeleton.
7. List the main types and functions of joints.
8. Describe the types of joint movement.

The skeletal system consists of the bones, joints, and cartilage, and the ligaments associated with the joints. Bone tissue is living and metabolically active, but because it contains so much nonliving material such as calcium and phosphorus, it appears dead or dried up. In fact, the word skeleton comes from a Greek word meaning dried-up body.

The skeletal system, however, is anything but dead. It contains 206 bones that are very much alive and perform a number of important functions.

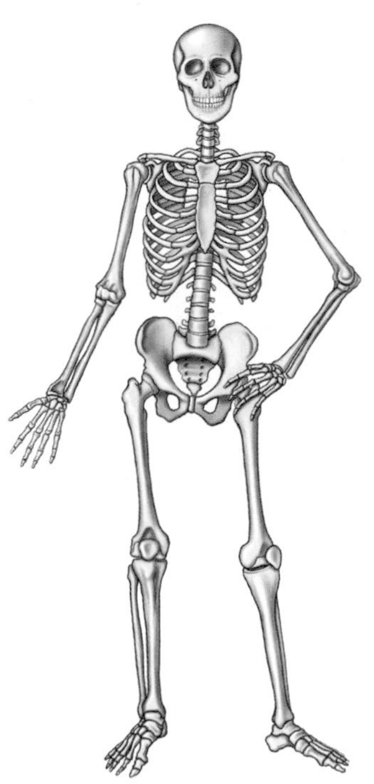

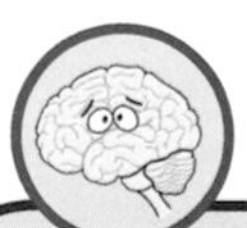

Do You Know...

About growing down with osteoporosis?

Osteoporosis is a common bone disorder, especially in postmenopausal women. Osteoporosis is characterized by a decline in bone-making activity and the loss of bone tissue. As tissue is lost, the bones weaken and break. Common sites of fracture due to osteoporosis are the hip, wrist, and vertebrae. Osteoporosis may also affect the vertebral column. As the vertebrae collapse, nerves may be pinched, causing severe pain. The collapsed vertebrae also cause a shortening of the vertebral column (growing down) and a change in its curvature. This change in shape, in turn, often impairs the functioning of organs such as the lungs.

ARRANGEMENT AND FUNCTIONS OF BONES

As you can see from Figure 8-1, the bones of the skeletal system are arranged to provide a framework for our bodies. The skeletal system gives us our basic shape. Imagine what you would look like without bones!

THE SKELETAL SYSTEM: WHAT IT DOES

In addition to shaping us up, the skeletal system performs other functions:

- The bones of the lower extremities support the weight of the body.
- The bones support and protect the soft body organs.
- With the assistance of muscles, the skeletal system enables the body to move about.
- Bones store a number of minerals, the most important being calcium and phosphorus.
- Red bone marrow produces blood cells.

MANY SIZES AND SHAPES OF BONES

Bones come in many sizes and shapes, from the pea-sized bones in the wrist to the 24-inch femur in the thigh. The size and shape of a bone reflect its function (Figure 8-2). The long, strong femur in the thigh, for instance, supports a great deal of weight and can withstand considerable force. Some of the skull bones, on the other hand, are thin, flat, and curved. Their function is to encase and protect the brain.

Bones are classified as follows:

- *Long bones:* Long bones are longer than they are wide. They are found in the arms and the legs.
- *Short bones:* Short bones are shaped like cubes and are found primarily in the wrists and ankles.
- *Flat bones:* Flat bones are thin, flat, and curved. They form the ribs, breastbone, and skull.
- *Irregular bones:* Irregular bones are differently shaped and are not classified as long, short, or flat. They include the hip bones, vertebrae, and various bones in the skull.

BONE TISSUE AND BONE FORMATION

Bone is also called **osseous tissue.** Bone cells, called **osteocytes,** secrete an intercellular matrix, containing calcium, other minerals, and protein fibers.

COMPACT AND SPONGY BONE

There are two types of bone: compact and spongy (Figure 8-3). **Compact bone** refers to dense, hard bone tissue found primarily in the shafts of long bones and on the outer surfaces of other bones. **Spongy,** or **cancellous, bone** is less dense. Spongy bone is located primarily at the ends of long bones and in the center of other bones.

Compact and spongy bone look different under the microscope. Compact bone is tightly packed, so that its density can provide a great deal of strength. The microscopic unit of compact bone is the **osteon,** or **haversian** (hă-VĔR-shăn) **system.** Each haversian system consists of mature osteocytes arranged in concentric

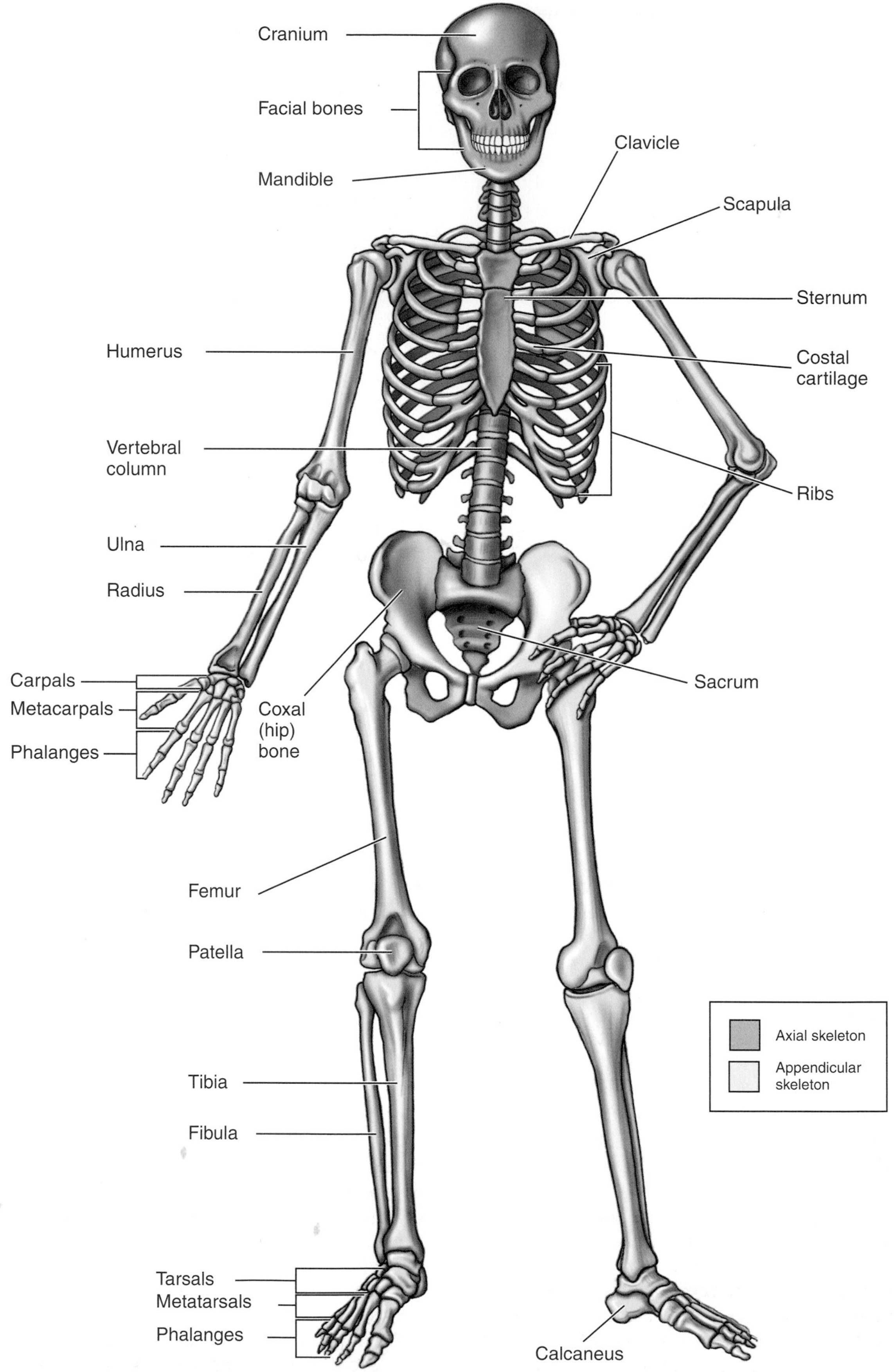

FIGURE 8-1 Skeleton. Axial skeleton *(red)* and appendicular skeleton *(brown)*.

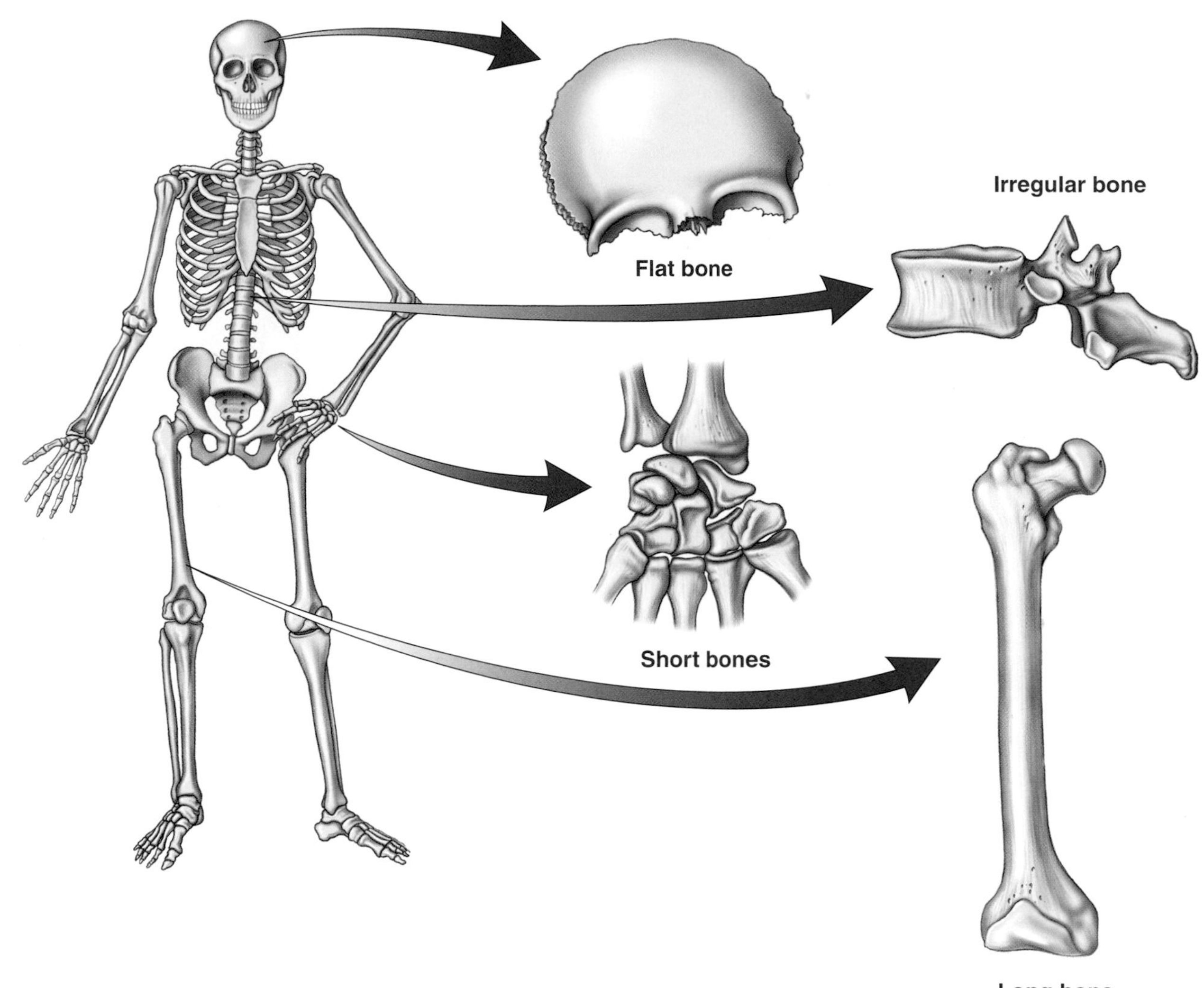

FIGURE 8-2 Types of bones.

circles around large blood vessels. The area surrounding the osteocytes is filled with protein fibers, calcium, and other minerals. The protein fibers provide elasticity while the minerals make bone tissue hard and strong. Each haversian system looks like a long cylinder.

Compact bone consists of many haversian systems running parallel to each other. Communicating blood vessels run laterally and connect the haversian systems with each other and with the periosteal lining that surrounds the bone. The network of blood vessels ensures that the bone tissue receives an adequate supply of blood. Blood supplies tissues with oxygen and nutrients.

Spongy, or cancellous, bone has a much different structure from compact bone (see Figure 8-3, *B*). Unlike compact bone, spongy bone does not contain haversian systems. In spongy bone, the bone tissue is arranged in plates called **trabeculae.** These bony plates are separated by holes that give spongy bone a punched-out "Swiss cheese" appearance. The holes are important for two reasons: (1) they decrease the weight of the bone, making it lighter, and (2) they contain red bone marrow. The red bone marrow richly supplies the spongy bone with blood and also produces blood cells for use throughout the body. Spongy bone is located in the short, flat, and irregular bones. It is also found in the ends of long bones.

LONG BONE

The arrangement of the compact and spongy tissue in a long bone accounts for its strength. Long bones also contain sites of growth and reshaping and structures associated with joints (see Figure 8-3, *A*). The parts of a long bone include the following:

- *Diaphysis:* The **diaphysis** (dī-ĂF-ĭ-sĭs) is the long shaft of the bone. It is composed primarily of compact bone and therefore provides considerable strength.
- *Epiphysis:* The enlarged ends of the long bone are the epiphyses. The **epiphysis** (ĕ-PĬF-ĭ-sĭs) of a bone articulates, or meets, with a second bone at

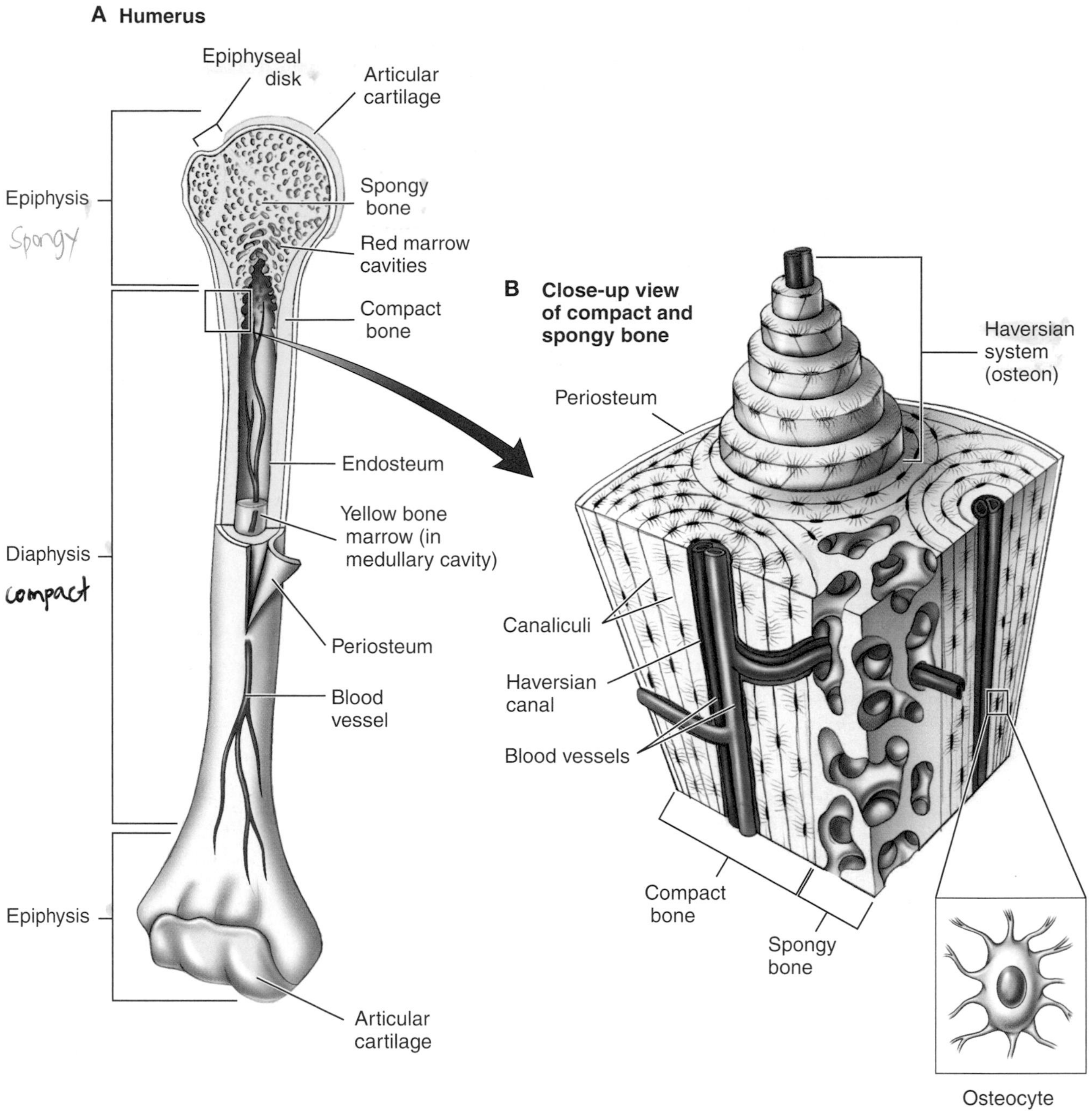

FIGURE 8-3 Bone. **A,** Anatomy of a long bone. **B,** Compact and spongy bone.

a joint. Each epiphysis consists of a thin layer of compact bone overlying spongy bone. The epiphyses are covered by cartilage.

- *Epiphyseal disc:* A growing long bone contains a band of hyaline cartilage located at each end, between the epiphysis and the diaphysis. This band of cartilage is the **epiphyseal disc,** or **growth plate.** It is here that longitudinal bone growth occurs.
- *Medullary cavity:* The **medullary cavity** is the hollow center of the diaphysis. In infancy, the cavity is filled with red bone marrow for blood cell production. In the adult, the medullary cavity is filled with yellow bone marrow and functions as a storage site for fat. The inside of the medullary cavity is lined with connective tissue called the **endosteum.**
- *Periosteum:* The **periosteum** (pĕr-ē-ŎS-tē-ŭm) is a tough fibrous connective tissue membrane that covers the outside of the diaphysis. It is anchored firmly to the outside of the bone on all surfaces except the articular cartilage. The periosteum protects the bone, serves as a point of attachment for muscle, and contains the blood vessels that nourish the underlying bone. Because the periosteum carries the blood supply to the underlying bone, any injury to this structure has serious

consequences to the health of the bone. Like any other organ, the loss of blood supply can cause its death.

- *Articular cartilage:* The **articular cartilage** is found on the outer surface of the epiphysis. It forms a smooth, shiny surface that decreases friction within a joint. Because a joint is also called an **articulation** (ăr-tĭk-ū-LĀ-shŭn), this cartilage is called articular cartilage.

OSSIFICATION

How does bone form? A 3-month-old fetus has an early skeleton-like frame composed of cartilage and connective tissue membrane (Figure 8-4). As the fetus matures, the cartilage and connective tissue change into bone. The formation of bone is called **ossification.** Ossification occurs in different ways in flat and long bones.

Ossification of Flat Bones

In the fetus, the flat bones (those in the skull) consist of thin connective tissue membranes. Ossification begins when **osteoblasts**, or bone-forming cells, migrate to the region of the flat bones. The osteoblasts secrete calcium and other minerals into the spaces between the membranes, thereby forming bone. This type of ossification involves the replacement of thin membrane with bone.

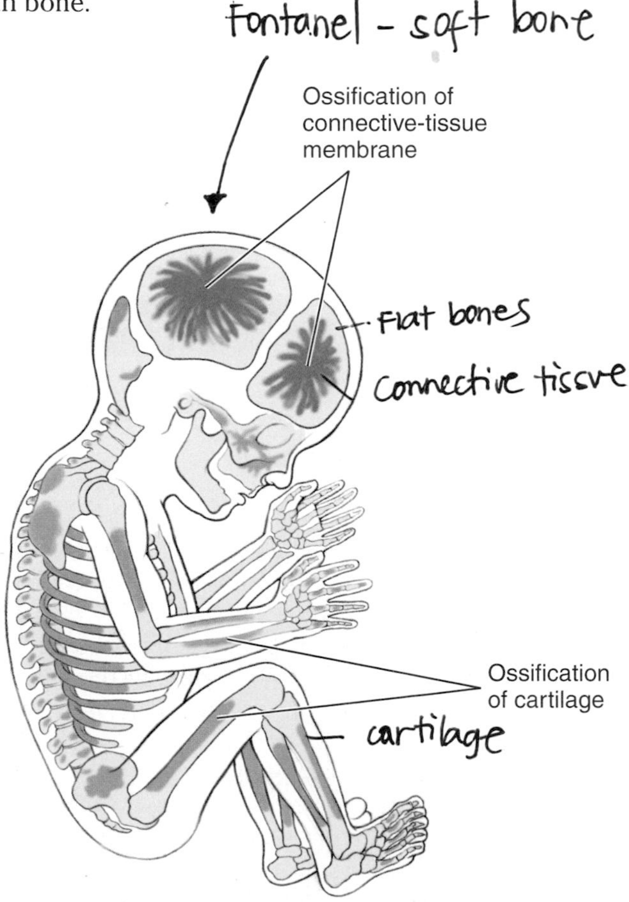

FIGURE 8-4 Ossification.

Ossification of Long Bones

Ossification of long bones occurs as bone tissue replaces cartilage. The fetal skeleton is composed largely of cartilage, and the layout of the cartilage in the fetus provides a model for bone formation (see Figure 8-4). As the baby matures, osteoblasts invade the cartilage and gradually replace the cartilage with bone. This process continues in each long bone until all but the articular cartilage and the epiphyseal disc have been replaced by bone. By the time the fetus has fully matured, most cartilage of the body has been replaced by bone. Only isolated pieces of cartilage, such as the bridge of the nose and parts of the ribs, remain.

GROWING BONES

Maturation from infancy to adulthood is characterized by two types of bone growth. Bones grow longitudinally and determine the height of an individual. Bones also grow thicker and become wider so as to support the weight of the adult body.

Growing Taller

Longitudinal bone growth occurs at the epiphyseal disc (also called the growth plate) (see Figure 8-3, *A*). The cartilage adjacent to the epiphysis continues to multiply and grow toward the diaphysis. The cartilage next to the diaphysis, however, is invaded by osteoblasts and becomes ossified. As long as the cartilage continues to form within the epiphyseal disc, the bone continues to lengthen. Longitudinal bone growth ceases when the epiphyseal disc becomes ossified and fused.

The epiphyseal disc is sensitive to the effects of certain hormones, especially growth hormone and the sex hormones. Growth hormone stimulates growth at the epiphyseal disc, making the child taller. The sex hormones estrogen and testosterone, however, cause the epiphyseal disc to fuse, thereby inhibiting further longitudinal growth. Because the epiphyseal disc is especially sensitive to the effects of the female hormone estrogen, girls tend to be shorter than boys. After puberty, which is associated with increasing plasma levels of sex hormones, longitudinal growth eventually ceases.

The What-Ifs of the Epiphyseal Disc

- What if there is an oversecretion or undersecretion of growth hormone? Giantism occurs with hypersecretion while a type of dwarfism develops with hyposecretion.
- What if the epiphyseal disc is injured? Longitudinal bone growth is impaired in the injured bone. A child who injures the disc in a leg bone, for instance, may end up with that leg considerably shorter than the noninjured leg.

Growing Thicker and Wider

Long after longitudinal bone growth has ceased, bones continue to increase in thickness and width. The bones are continuously being reshaped. Bone remodeling is accomplished by the combined actions of osteoblasts, which are bone-forming cells, and **osteoclasts,** which are bone-destroying cells. Osteoblasts on the undersurface of the periosteum continuously deposit bone on the external bone surface.

Figure 8-5 shows the way in which osteoblastic activity works like a bricklayer. While osteoblasts build new bone, osteoclasts, found on the inner bone surface surrounding the medullary cavity, break down bone tissue, thereby hollowing out the interior of the bone. Osteoclastic activity is like sculpting. The bricklayer and the sculptor gradually create a large, wide hollow bone that is strong but not too heavy.

The process whereby osteoclasts breakdown bone matrix is called **bone resorption** (not to be confused with the word reabsorption). Bone resorption not only widens bone, it also moves calcium from the bone to the blood. Bone resorption plays a crucial role in the regulation of blood calcium levels. The influence of parathyroid hormone on bone resorption is described in Chapter 14.

One of the factors that stimulates bone growth is weight-bearing. Exercise and weight-bearing keep calcium in the bone and increase bone mass. The bones of bedridden or sedentary people tend to lose bone mass and are easily broken when stressed. The weightlessness experienced by astronauts likewise causes a loss of bone mass and easily broken bones.

Bumps and Grooves

The surface of bone appears irregular and bumpy. This appearance is due to numerous ridges, projections, depressions, and grooves called bone surface markings.

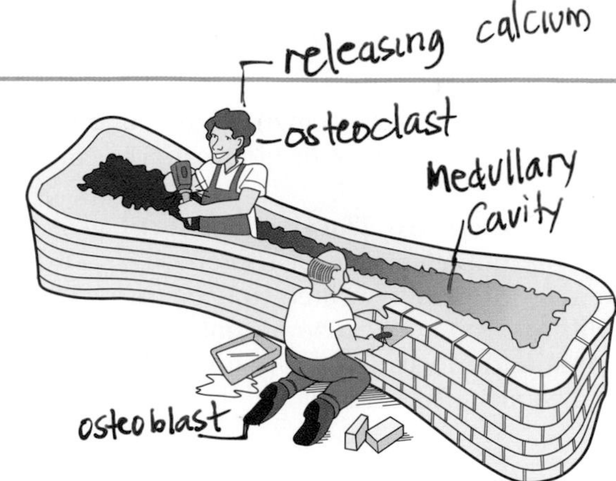

FIGURE 8-5 Bone remodeling. Osteoblasts (bricklayer) and osteoclasts (sculptor).

The projecting bone markings (the markings that stick out) serve as points of attachment for muscles, tendons, and ligaments. The grooves and depressions form the routes traveled by blood vessels and nerves as they pass over and through the bones and joints. The projections and depressions also help form joints. The head of the upper arm bone, for instance, fits into a depression in a shoulder bone, forming the shoulder joint. The specific bone markings are summarized in Table 8-1. Note the various markings on individual bones as they are described.

Broken Bones

Occasionally, a bone breaks, or fractures (Figure 8-6). A simple fracture is a break in which the overlying skin remains intact. Local tissue damage is minimal. A compound fracture is a broken bone that has also pierced the skin. The ends of the broken bone usually cause

Table 8-1 Bone Markings

Bone Markings	Definition
Projections/Processes	
Condyle	A large rounded knob that usually articulates with another bone
Epicondyle	An enlargement near or above a condyle
Head	An enlarged and rounded end of a bone
Facet	A small, flattened surface
Crest	A ridge on a bone
Process	A prominent projection on a bone
Spine	A sharp projection
Tubercle (tuberosity)	A knoblike projection
Trochanter	A large tubercle (tuberosity) found only on the femur
Depressions/Openings	
Foramen	An opening through a bone; usually serves as a passageway for nerves, blood vessels, and ligaments
Fossa	A depression or groove
Meatus	A tunnel or tubelike passageway
Sinus	A cavity or hollow space

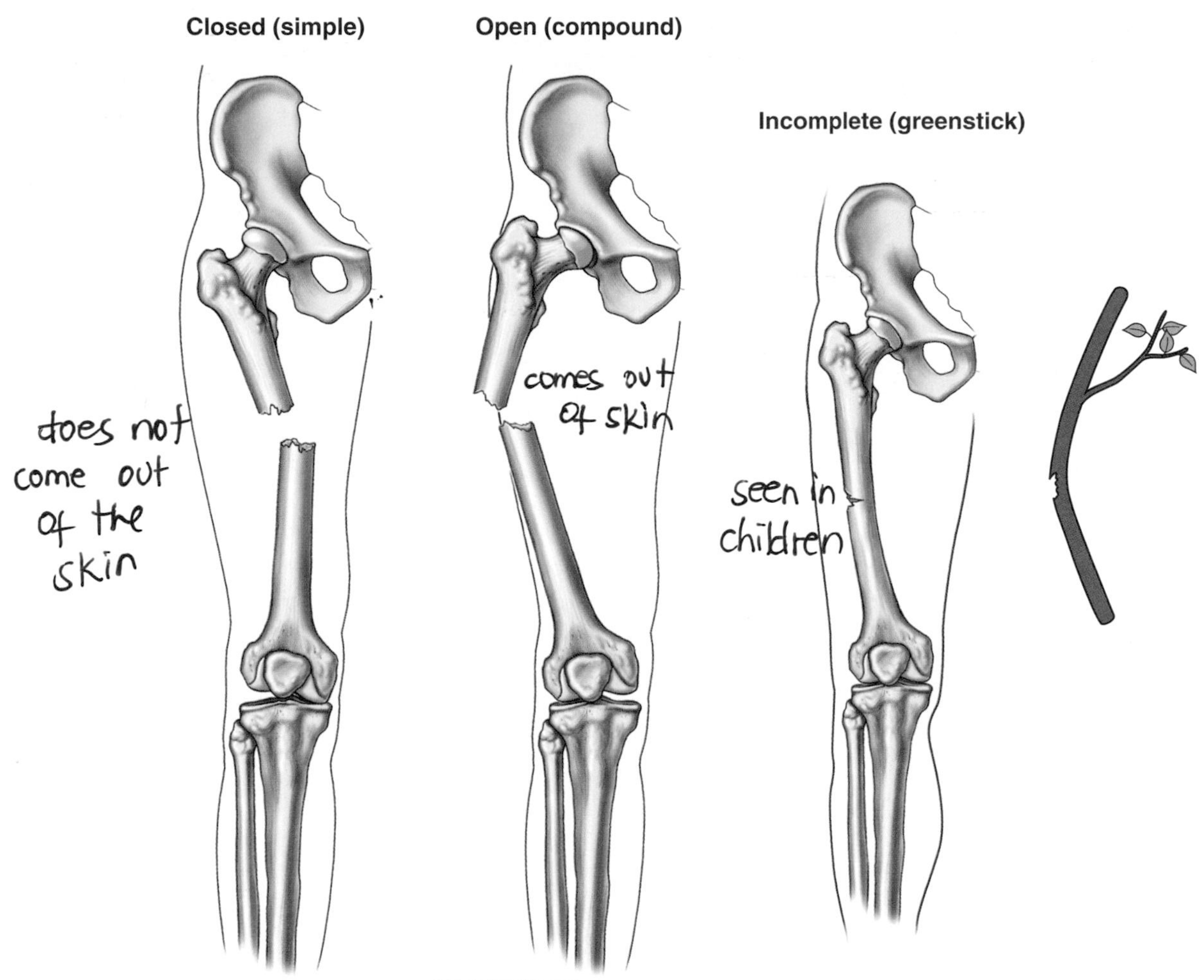

FIGURE 8-6 Common types of fractures.

extensive tissue damage. The risk of infection is a concern with a compound fracture.

A greenstick fracture is an incomplete break in the bone and usually occurs in children. Why is it called a greenstick fracture? If you were to bend a branch of a young tree, the branch would not snap and break apart completely. It would instead bend and perhaps break incompletely. The branch responds this way because it is young and pliable, much like a child's bone. Children's bones still have enough cartilaginous material to make them flexible.

There are many other types of bone fractures. For example, there is a spiral fracture in which the line of the fracture extends in a spiral direction along the diaphysis. It is caused when the bone is subjected to a twisting type of force. There is a comminuted fracture in which there are more than two bone fragments; the small fragments seem to be floating. An impacted fracture is a comminuted fracture in which the two parts of the broken bone have been jammed into each other. And the list of fractures goes on. Broken bones—many moans!

Sum It Up!

The skeletal system consists of bones, joints, cartilage, and ligaments found in and around the joints. Bones are composed of two types of osseous tissue: compact (dense bone) and spongy (cancellous bone). Bones come in a variety of sizes and shapes. They are classified as long, short, flat, or irregular. We begin life in the womb as a skeleton-like frame made of cartilage and thin connective tissue membrane. With maturation, the process of ossification replaces most of the cartilage and certain connective tissue membrane. As a person matures, the skeleton enlarges, and bones grow longer, wider, and thicker.

DIVISIONS OF THE SKELETAL SYSTEM

The skeleton is divided into the axial skeleton and the appendicular skeleton (see Figure 8-1). The **axial skeleton** includes the bones of the skull, hyoid bone, bones

Table 8-2 Bones of the Adult Skeleton

Bones	Number	Bones	Number
Axial Skeleton (80)		*Thoracic Cage (25)*	
Skull (28)		True ribs	14
Cranium (8)		False ribs	10
Frontal	1	Sternum	1
Parietal	2	*Appendicular Skeleton (126)*	
Temporal	2	*Pectoral Girdle (4)*	
Occipital	1	Scapula	2
Sphenoid	1	Clavicle	2
Ethmoid	1	*Upper Limbs (60)*	
Facial (14)		Humerus	2
Maxilla	2	Radius	2
Zygomatic	2	Ulna	2
Palatine	2	Carpals	16
Mandible	1	Metacarpals	10
Lacrimal	2	Phalanges	28
Nasal	2	*Pelvic Girdle (2)*	
Inferior concha	2	Coxal	2
Vomer	1	*Lower Limbs (60)*	
Middle-Ear Bones (6)		Femur	2
Malleus	2	Tibia	2
Incus	2	Fibula	2
Stapes	2	Patella	2
Hyoid Bone (1)		Tarsals	14
Vertebral Column (26)		Metatarsals	10
Cervical vertebrae	7	Phalanges	28
Thoracic vertebrae	12	**Total Number of Bones**	206
Lumbar vertebrae	5		
Sacrum	1		
Coccyx	1		

of the middle ear, vertebral column, and bony thorax. The **appendicular skeleton** includes the bones of the extremities (arms and legs) and the bones of the hip and shoulder girdles. The names of the 206 bones of the skeleton are listed in Table 8-2.

AXIAL SKELETON

Skull

The skull sits on top of the vertebral column and is formed by two groups of bones: the cranium and the facial bones (Figure 8-7).

Cranium. The **cranium** is a bony structure that encases and protects the brain. Your personal brain bucket is composed of eight bones.

- *Frontal bone:* The **frontal bone** forms the forehead, and the upper part of the bony structure surrounding the eyes.
- *Parietal bones:* The two **parietal bones** form the upper sides of the head, and the roof of the cranial cavity (top of the head).
- *Temporal bones:* The two **temporal bones** are on the sides of the head, close to the ears (commonly called the temples). Several important bone markings are found on the temporal bones. They include the **external auditory meatus,** an opening for the ear; the **zygomatic process,** which forms part of the cheekbone (do not confuse this with the zygomatic bones); the **styloid process,** a sharp projection used as a point of attachment for several muscles associated with the tongue and larynx; and the **mastoid process,** which forms a point of attachment for some of the muscles of the neck.

An interesting note about the temporal bone: *Tempor* is a Latin word meaning "time." As men

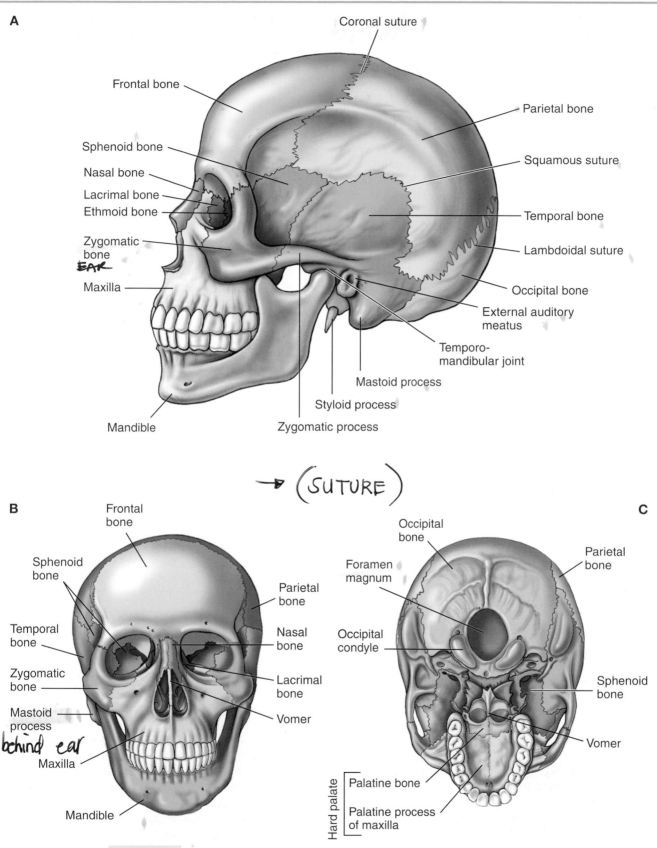

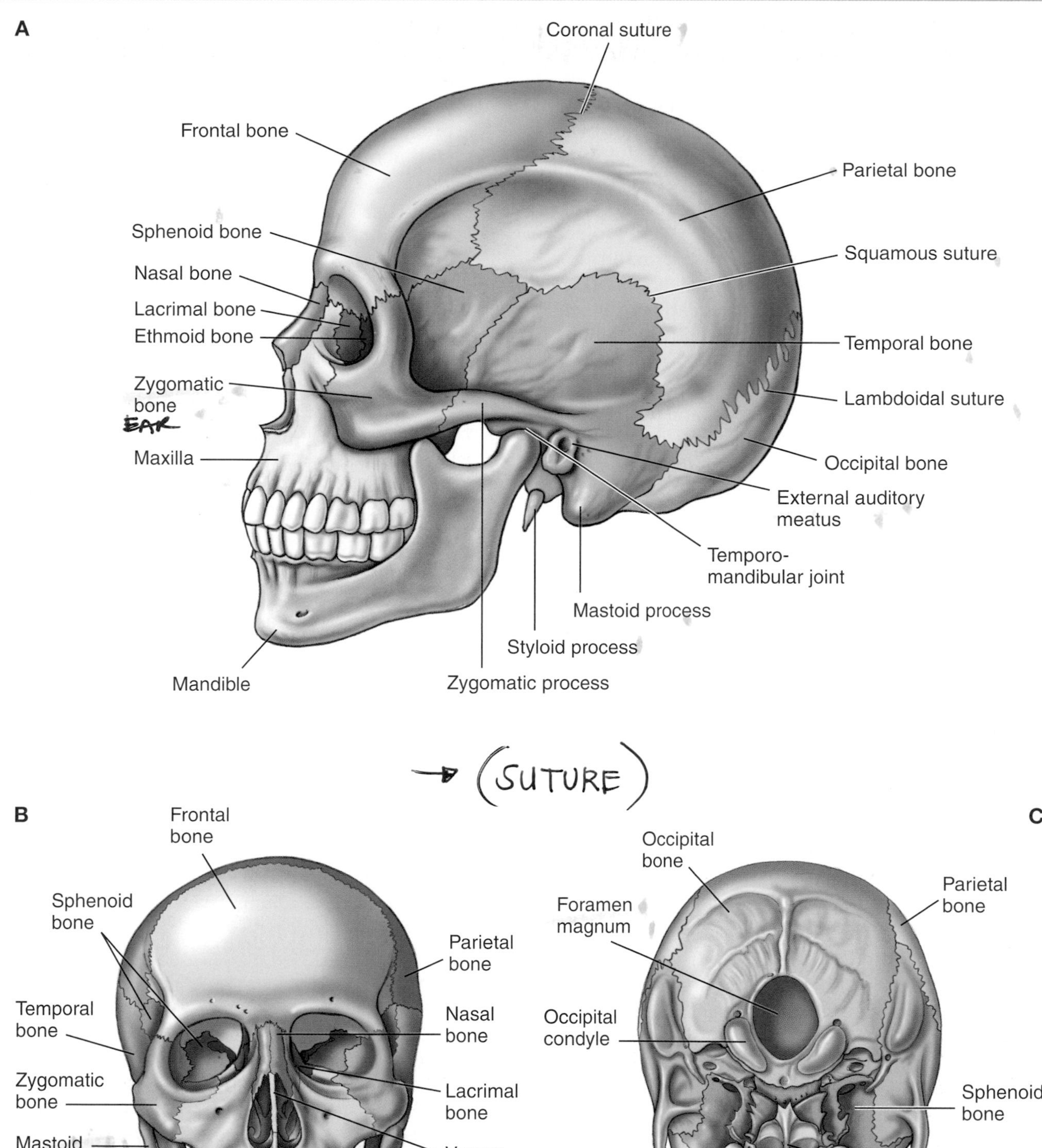

FIGURE 8-7 Bones of the skull. **A,** Side view. **B,** Front view. **C,** Base of the skull.

age, over time, they usually develop their first grey hairs over the temple area. The name of the temporal bone is an aging thing.

- *Occipital bone* (see Figure 8-7, *C*): The **occipital bone** is located at the back and base of the skull. The large hole in the occipital bone is called the **foramen magnum.** The foramen allows the brainstem to extend downward as the spinal cord. On either side of the foramen magnum are bony projections, called occipital condyles, that sit on the first vertebra of the vertebral column. Unfortunately, the foramen magnum can act as a deathtrap, since it provides the only major space in the cranium in the event that the brain swells. The increased intracranial pressure created by the swollen brain pushes the brain through the foramen magnum into the spinal region. The displacement or herniation of the brain exerts pressure on the brainstem, causing respiratory arrest and death.
- *Sphenoid bone:* The **sphenoid bone** is a butterfly-shaped bone that forms part of the floor and sides of the cranium (see Figure 8-7, *C*). The sphenoid bone also forms part of the orbits surrounding the eyes. In the midline of the sphenoid bone is a depression called the **sella turcica** (Turk's saddle); it forms the seat for the pituitary gland (not shown).
- *Ethmoid bone:* The **ethmoid bone** is an irregularly shaped bone located between the eye orbits; it helps form the bony structure of the nasal cavity. A projection of the ethmoid bone forms a point of attachment for the meninges. The meninges are membranes that surround the brain and contain cerebrospinal fluid. The location and shape of the ethmoid bone has important clinical implications. A sharp blow to the ethmoid bone can drive the pointed bone into the brain, causing severe brain injury and death. Because the shattered bone tears the meninges, cerebrospinal fluid leaks into the nasal passages. This type of injury also creates a direct opening into the brain for pathogens and subsequent infections of brain tissue. Watch that karate chop to the face! The impact of the face with the steering wheel during a car wreck can also drive the shattered ethmoid bone into the brain. Slow down!

Facial Bones. The face has 14 facial bones, most of which are paired (see Figure 8-7, *B*). Only the mandible and the vomer are single bones.

- *Mandible:* The **mandible,** the lower jaw bone, carries the lower teeth. The anterior portion of the mandible forms the chin. The mandible forms the only freely movable joint in the skull. Two posterior upright projections on the mandible have bony processes. These articulate with the temporal bones at the **temporomandibular joint (TMJ).** The TMJ can be felt as the depression immediately in front of the ear. Tension or stress often causes pain in the TMJ. This condition is often associated with tooth grinding (bruxism) during sleep. Bony processes on the mandible serve as points of attachment for chewing muscles.
- *Maxilla:* Two maxillary bones fuse to form the upper jaw. The **maxilla** carries the upper teeth. An extension of the maxilla, the palatine process, forms the anterior portion of the hard palate (roof) of the mouth (see Figure 8-7, *C*). These bones also form parts of the nasal cavity and the eye orbits.
- *Palatine bones:* Two **palatine bones** form the posterior part of the hard palate and the floor of the nasal cavity. Failure of the palatine and/or maxillary bones to fuse causes a cleft palate, making suckling very difficult for an infant. Fortunately, a cleft palate can be surgically repaired.
- *Zygomatic bones:* The **zygomatic bones** are the cheekbones. They also form a part of the orbits of the eyes.
- *Other facial bones:* Several other bones complete the facial structure. These bones include the lacrimal bones, the nasal bones, the vomer, and the inferior nasal conchae.

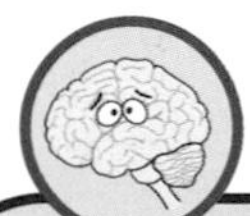

Do You Know...

How to fix a broken jaw?

Unlike a broken leg bone that can be immobilized by a cast, the mandible (lower jaw) can be immobilized only by wiring it to the maxilla (upper jaw). Can't talk, can't eat, can't vomit! In fact, people with wired jaws must have access to wire cutters in the event that they vomit. What about nutrition? Pureed food is delivered through a straw.

Sinuses. Sinuses are air-filled cavities located in several of the bones of the skull. They perform two important functions. First, they lessen the weight of the skull. Second, they increase the sound of the voice.

The four sinuses are called the **paranasal sinuses** because they surround and connect with the nasal structures (Figure 8-8). The names of the four sinuses reflect their location within the various skull bones: frontal sinus, ethmoidal sinus, sphenoidal sinus, and maxillary sinus.

Why Your Face Hurts. Because the sinuses connect with the nasal passages and the throat, infections may spread from the nose and throat into the sinuses. A sinus infection is called sinusitis and is characterized as stuffiness and pain in the overlying facial regions. Why do allergies sometimes make your face hurt?

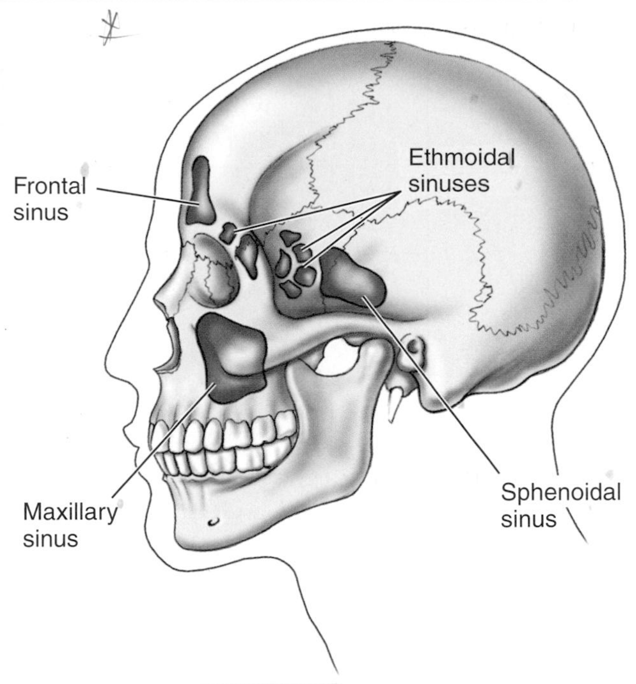

FIGURE 8-8 Sinuses.

Allergies often cause the membranes that line the facial sinuses to oversecrete mucus. The mucus forms an excellent medium for bacterial growth. As the mucus accumulates and the membranes swell, pressure and discomfort are often experienced in the facial region, which overlies the sinuses (around the eyes and nose).

How the Skull Bones Hold Together. The bones of the adult skull form a unique kind of joint called a **suture** (see Figure 8-7, *A*). The sutures join the bones of the skull much like a zipper. The major sutures include the coronal suture, the lambdoidal suture, and the squamosal suture. Unlike other bones in the body, no significant movement occurs between cranial bones.

The Infant Skull. The two major differences between the infant skull and the adult skull are fontanels and unfused sutures.

The infant skull has areas that have not yet been converted to bone. Instead, they are covered by fibrous membrane. Because these areas are soft to touch, they are called the baby's soft spots. Also, the rhythm of the baby's pulse can be felt in these soft spots, and so they are called **fontanels** (fŏn-tă-NĔLS), meaning "little fountains."

The two major fontanels are the larger, diamond-shaped anterior fontanel and the smaller, posterior, triangular occipital fontanel (Figure 8-9). By the time a child reaches 2 years of age, these fontanels have been gradually converted to bone and can no longer be felt.

The fontanels are one reason that the infant skull bones are more movable than those of the adult skull. Another reason is that the sutures of the infant skulls are not fused. Unfused sutures allow the skull to be compressed during birth. They also allow for the continued growth of the brain and skull after birth and throughout infancy. It also explains why your adorable newborn may look like a conehead. The fetal skull is too large to fit through the birth canal, so the movable bones overlap, thereby decreasing the diameter of the head. Fortunately, the pointy skull reshapes shortly after birth.

Occasionally, the sutures of the infant skull fuse too early, preventing the growth of the brain. This condition is called microcephalia and is characterized by a small skull and impaired intellectual functioning. Sometimes, the skull expands too much. For instance, if excessive fluid accumulates within the brain of an infant, the bones are forced apart, and the skull enlarges. This condition is called hydrocephalus (or what the layperson calls "water on the brain").

Observation of the fontanels can provide valuable information regarding brain swelling. What does a bulging or sunken fontanel indicate? If an infant suffers a head injury

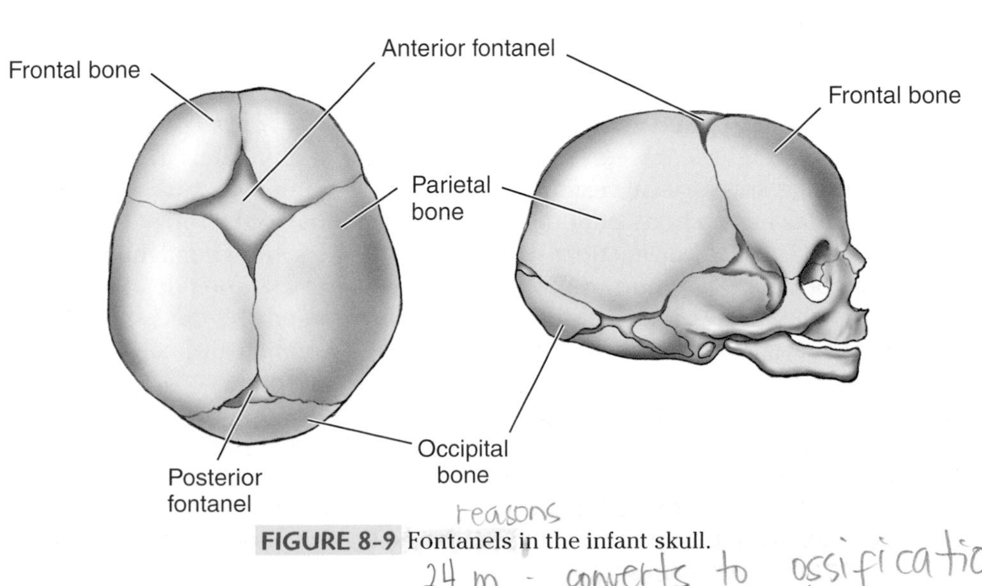

FIGURE 8-9 Fontanels in the infant skull.

or infection, the brain may swell. Because the fontanel is soft tissue, it will bulge outward in response to increasing pressure within the skull. Conversely, the fontanels may become sunken in the presence of dehydration.

Hyoid Bone. The **hyoid bone** is a U-shaped bone located in the upper neck. It anchors the tongue and is associated with swallowing. The hyoid bone is often fractured during strangulation. Watch for this on autopsy, you forensic sleuths!

Bones of the Middle Ear. Each ear contains three small bones called **ossicles** (see Chapter 13).

Vertebral Column

The Back and Its Stack of Bones. The **vertebral column,** also called the backbone, extends from the skull to the pelvis (Figure 8-10). The vertebral column consists of 26 bones, called vertebrae, stacked in a column. Sitting between each vertebra is a cartilaginous disc that acts as a shock absorber. The vertebral column performs four major functions: it forms a supporting structure for the head and thorax; it forms an attachment for the pelvic girdle; it encases and protects the spinal cord as the cord extends from the brain into the spinal cavity; and it provides flexibility for the body.

The vertebrae are named according to their location in the body. Seven cervical vertebrae (C1 to C7) are located in the neck region; if you run your hand down the cervical vertebrae you will feel a large bump. This large vertebra is C7 and is called the **vertebra prominens** (used as a landmark in assessing surface anatomy). Twelve thoracic vertebrae (T1 to T12) are located in the chest region; and the five lumbar vertebrae (L1 to L5) are located in the lower back region. If you place your hands on your hips, you are at the level of L4. In addition, five sacral vertebrae fuse into one **sacrum.** The sacrum forms the posterior wall of the pelvis. Four small vertebrae fuse into the tailbone. How did the sacrum get its name? The ancients thought the seat of the soul was located at the base of the spine and therefore dubbed the sacred area the "sacrum." The tailbone is called the **coccyx,** since it resembles the beak of a cuckoo bird.

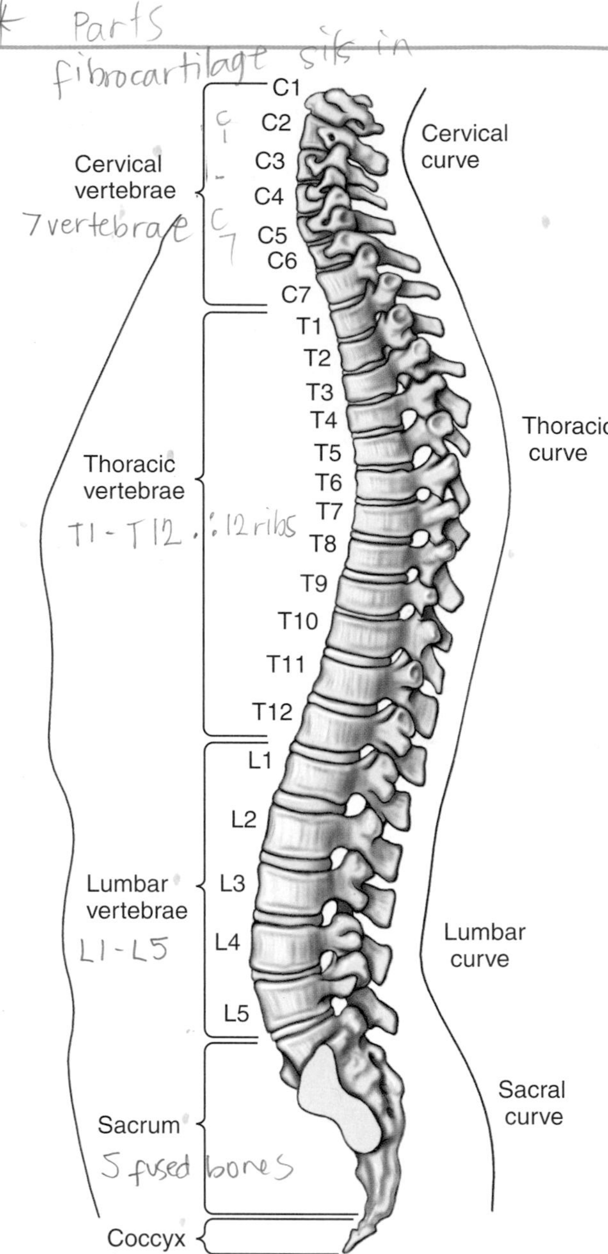

FIGURE 8-10 Vertebral column: cervical vertebrae (7), thoracic vertebrae (12), lumbar vertebrae (5), sacrum, and coccyx. Vertebral curves: cervical curve, thoracic curve, lumbar curve, and sacral curve.

Two Special Vertebrae: Atlas (C1) and Axis (C2). The first and second cervical vertebrae have several special features (Figure 8-11). The first cervical vertebra (C1) is called the **atlas.** The atlas has no body but does have depressions into which fit the bony projections of the occipital bone of the skull. The atlas supports the skull and allows you to nod "yes." The atlas is named after a figure in Greek mythology, Atlas, who carried the earth on his shoulders.

The second cervical vertebra (C2) is called the **axis.** The axis has a projection, called the dens (nicknamed for the toothlike odontoid process) that fits into the atlas and acts as a pivot or swivel for the atlas. The axis allows your head to rotate from side to side as you say "no." It is the "spin bone" in an otherwise no-spin zone. A strong blow to the top of the head can force the dens through the foramen magnum and into the base of the brain, causing sudden death. Not good! In children the fusion between the dens and the axis is incomplete. Shaking the child can easily dislocate the dens, causing injury to the spinal cord.

Characteristics of Vertebrae. The vertebra is an irregular bone that contains several distinct structures (see Figure 8-11). The body of the vertebra is padded by a cartilaginous disc, called an intervertebral disc, and supports the weight of the vertebra sitting on top of it. Some processes provide sites of attachment for ligaments,

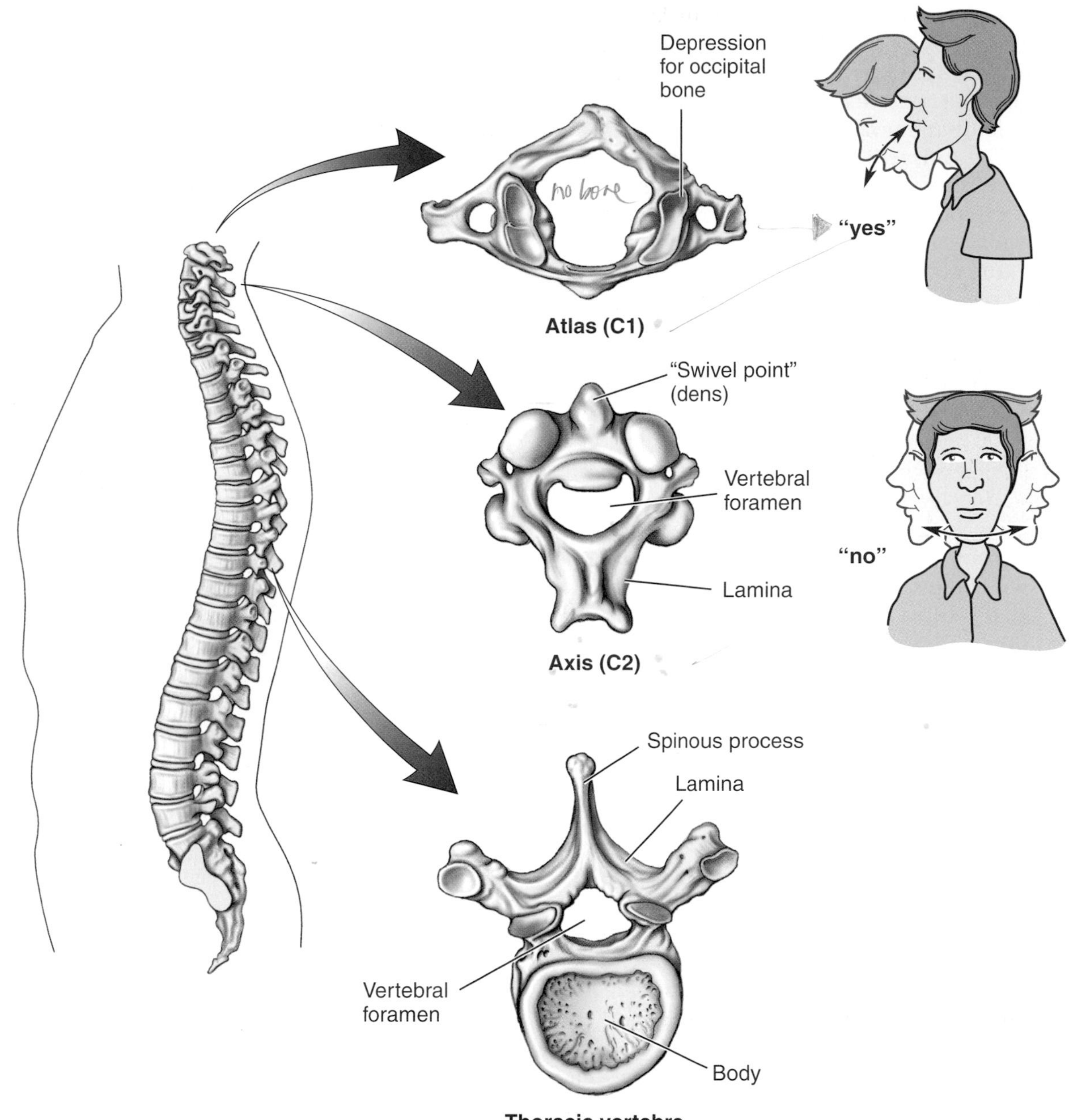

FIGURE 8-11 Anatomy of a vertebra: the atlas (C1); axis (C2); and thoracic vertebrae.

tendons, and muscles; other processes articulate with bones such as the ribs. The **vertebral foramen** is the opening for the spinal cord. The vertebrae are aligned so that if you run your hand down your back, you will feel the spinous processes. For this reason, the vertebral column is also called the **spine.** Note that the vertebrae become larger as the vertebral column descends. The larger lower vertebrae carry a heavier load.

Some Vertebral Column Concerns

- The vertebra has a barlike lamina. **Spina bifida** refers to the failure of the lamina to fuse during fetal development. The vertebral defect allows the spinal cord to protrude onto the surface of the back. Compression of the spinal cord then causes paralysis and loss of bladder and bowel control.
- A surgical procedure called a laminectomy may be performed to access the intervertebral disc; the opening allows the surgeon to remove a damaged or "slipped" disc. Occasionally several vertebrae are fused together to stabilize a part of the vertebral column. This procedure is called spinal fusion.
- Note that the spinal cord descends from the base of the brain through the vertebral foramen of the stack of vertebrae. Injury to the vertebral column at any point can compress or sever the spinal cord, causing paralysis. You must use extreme caution while treating a person with a spinal cord injury!

Curvatures. When viewed from the side, the vertebral column has four normal curvatures (see Figure 8-10): the cervical, thoracic, lumbar, and sacral curves. The directions of the curvatures are important. The cervical and the lumbar curvatures bend toward the front of the body. The thoracic and sacral curvatures bend away from the front of the body. These curves center the head over the body, thereby providing the balance needed to walk in an upright position.

The curvature of the fetal spine is different. Its single, C-shaped curvature bends away from the front of the body. Its shape reflects the curled-up position of the fetus during the nine months in the cozy, but cramped, uterine living quarters. The cervical curvature develops about 3 to 4 months after birth as infants start to hold up their heads. The lumbar curvature develops at about 1 year of age, when children begin walking.

Figure 8-12 illustrates several abnormal curvatures of the spine. **Scoliosis** refers to a lateral curvature, usually involving the thoracic vertebrae. If severe, a lateral curvature can compress abdominal organs. It can also diminish expansion of the rib cage and therefore impair breathing. **Kyphosis** is an exaggerated thoracic curvature. It is sometimes called hunchback. **Lordosis** is an exaggerated lumbar curvature and is sometimes called swayback. These abnormalities may be due to a genetic defect or may develop in response to disease or poor posture.

Thoracic Cage

The thoracic cage is a bony, cone-shaped cage that surrounds and protects the lungs, heart, large blood vessels, and some of the abdominal organs such as the liver and spleen (Figure 8-13). It plays a crucial role in breathing and helps to support the bones of the shoulder. The thoracic cage is composed of the sternum, ribs, and thoracic vertebrae.

Sternum. The **sternum,** or breastbone, is a dagger-shaped bone located along the midline of the anterior chest. The three parts are the manubrium, the body, and the xiphoid process. The xiphoid process is the tip of the sternum. It serves as a landmark for cardiopulmonary resuscitation (CPR). Note the suprasternal notch (also called the jugular notch), a depression on the upper part of the manubrium between the two clavicles; it is used as a landmark to locate other structures.

Ribs. Twelve pairs of ribs attach posteriorly to the thoracic vertebrae. Anteriorly, the top seven pairs of ribs attach directly to the sternum by costal cartilage. They are called **true ribs.** The next five pairs attach indirectly to the sternum or do not attach at all. They are called **false ribs.** The bottom two pairs of false ribs lack sternal attachment and are therefore called **floating ribs.** Because of their location and lack of sternal support, the floating ribs are easily broken. Note that the ribs are numbered. The numbering allows us to describe the location of thoracic structures. For instance, the heart is located between the 2nd and 6th ribs. You will spend a lot of time counting ribs as part of your clinical practice.

Other Thoracic Cage Structures. Located between the ribs are the intercostal muscles. Contraction of these muscles helps move the thoracic cage during breathing. If you put your hand on your chest and take a deep breath, you will feel your thoracic cage move up and out. The costal margins are the edges of the cartilage that form an angle as they converge near the xiphoid process. The costal angle should be less than 90 degrees. The costal angle can change size; for example,

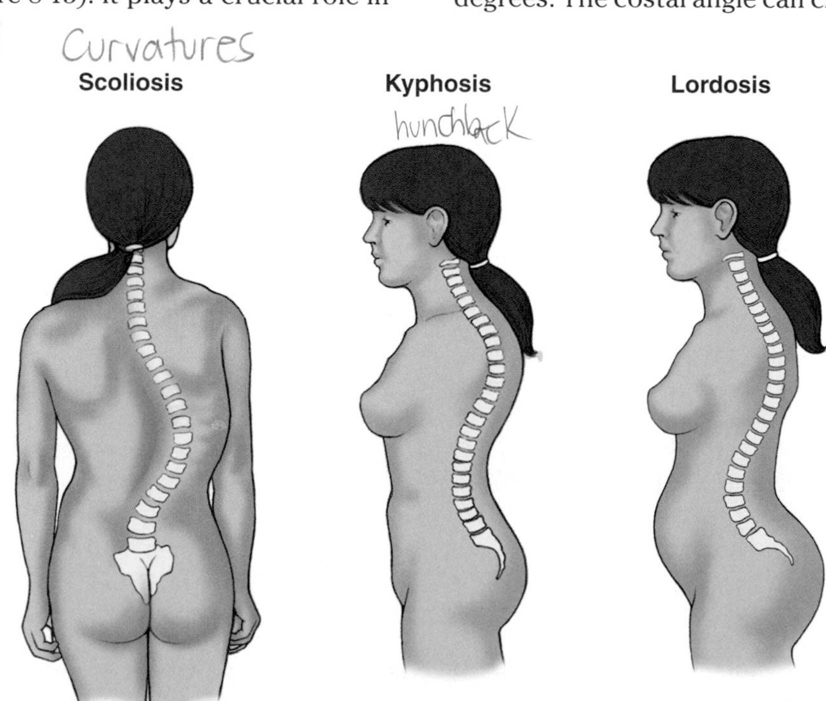

FIGURE 8-12 Abnormal curvatures of the vertebral column.

during pregnancy the angle increases. It also increases when the chest diameter expands with certain lung diseases such as emphysema. Another sternal landmark is the sternomanubrial junction, also called the angle of Louis. This landmark is used in counting ribs; it is at the level of the second rib.

APPENDICULAR SKELETON

The appendicular skeleton is composed of the bones of the shoulder girdle, upper limbs (arms), pelvic girdle, and lower limbs (thighs and legs) (see Figure 8-1).

Shoulder Girdle

The **shoulder girdle** is also called the **pectoral girdle.** Each shoulder contains two bones: one clavicle and one scapula (Figure 8-14). The shoulder supports the arms and serves as a place of attachment for the muscles. The shoulder girdle is designed for great flexibility; move your shoulder and upper arm around and note how many different movements you can make. Compare this with the limited movement you have at the elbow and the knee.

Clavicle. The **clavicle** is also called the collarbone. It looks like a long, slender, S-shaped rod and articulates

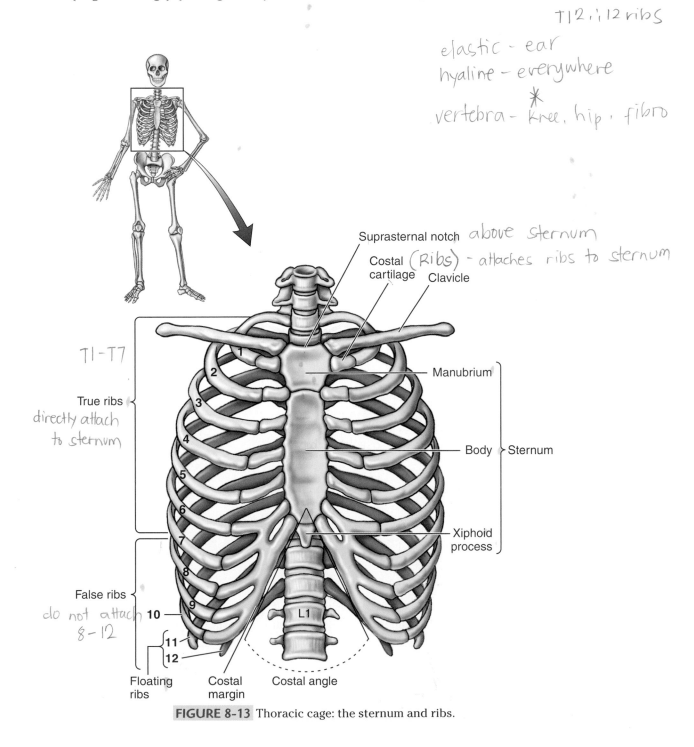

FIGURE 8-13 Thoracic cage: the sternum and ribs.

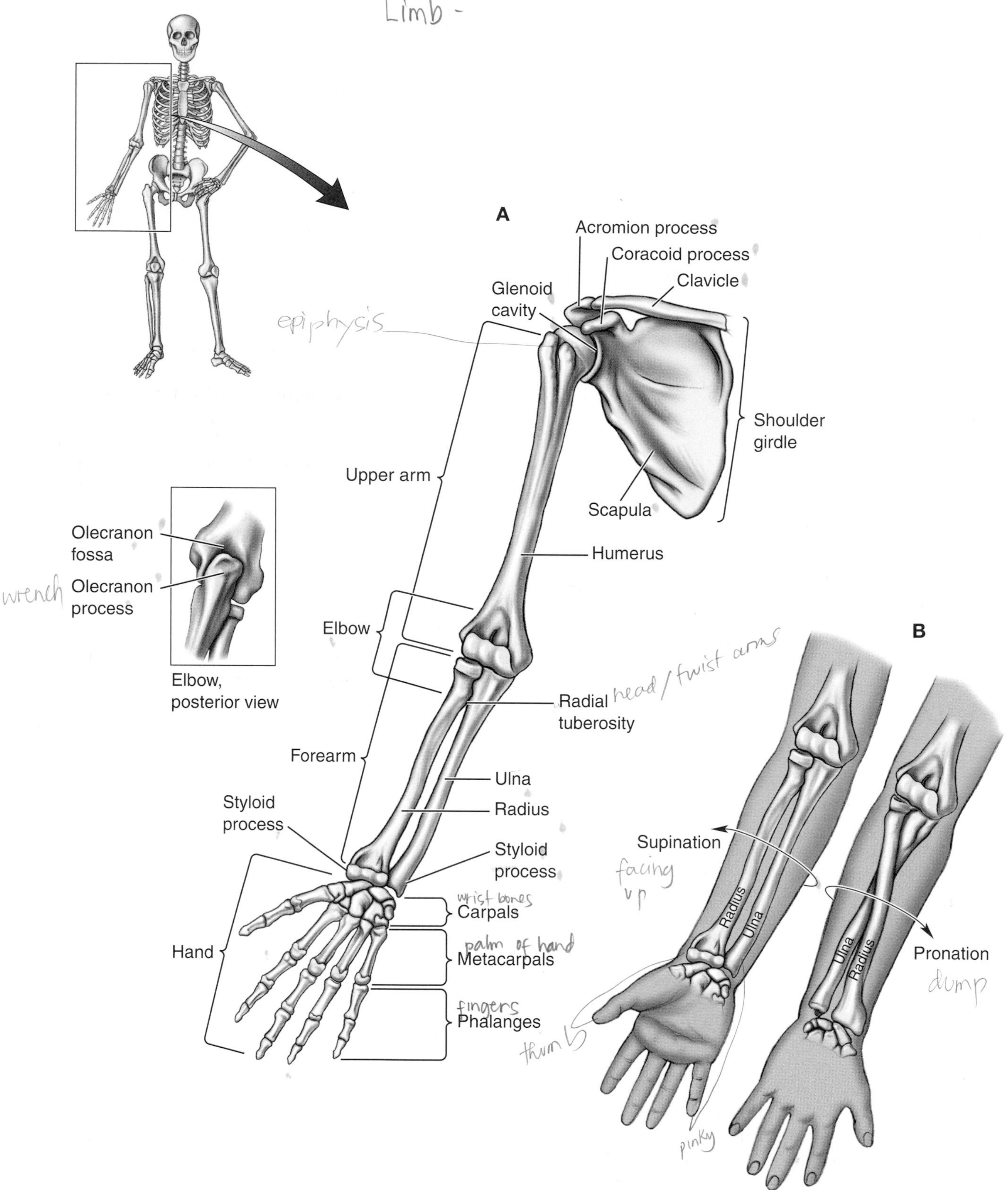

FIGURE 8-14 Bones of the upper limb. **A,** Shoulder girdle, upper arm, forearm, and hand. **B,** Position of the radius and ulna during supination and pronation.

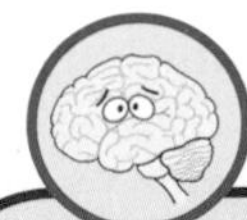

Do You Know...

About Xtreme Modeling and toe cleavage?

The saying, "You can never be too thin" (or off-balance) has taken on new meaning. In addition to a starvation diet, Xtreme Modeling has taken surgical aim at the skeletal system. It's called remodeling the model. How so? Surgeons have successfully shortened/removed toes, thereby allowing the foot to fit into the stylish "pointy pizza" shoes. More importantly, toe removal also creates revealing "toe cleavage." The toe is not the only osseous victim of this skeletal redesign. Removal of the lower floating ribs further slims the slim. When accompanied by high colonic irrigations (enemas) our "remodeled model" easily slips into the elusive size zero. Of obvious concern—the risk of general anesthesia, the loss of ribs that normally protect the kidneys, and the loss of toes that assist in walking, balance, and overall comfort! Go figure!

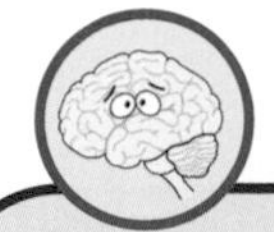

Do You Know...

Why hitting my funny bone doesn't feel funny?

When you hit your elbow and get that sharp pain that is associated with the "funny bone," you are actually hitting the ulnar nerve. The unprotected ulnar nerve lies over the distal end of the humerus and is therefore vulnerable to being bumped. Why do we call it "funny"? Maybe because of its location near the humerus, a "humorous" name for a bone.

with both the sternum and the scapula. The clavicle helps stabilize the shoulder. The attachment, however, is weak and easily dislocated or broken. The clavicle is the most frequently broken bone in the body.

Scapula. The **scapula,** also called the shoulder blade or wing bone, is a large, flat bone that is shaped like a triangle. The two scapulae are located on the posterior thorax. Two large processes on the scapula allow it to articulate with the clavicle and serve as points of attachment for arm and chest muscles. The **glenoid cavity** on the scapula is the site where the head of the **humerus** (upper arm bone) fits, thereby allowing you to rotate your arm at the shoulder. Note the **acromion process** and **coracoid process** on the scapula near the glenoid cavity. Both processes serve as points of attachment for ligaments and muscles. The acromion process forms the "pointy" part of the shoulder.

Upper Extremities (Arms)

The upper limb contains the bones of the upper arm (humerus); the forearm (ulna and radius); and the hand (carpals, metacarpals, and phalanges).

Humerus. The humerus is the long bone of the upper arm. The humerus contains a **head,** which fits into the glenoid cavity of the scapula, allowing the upper arm to rotate at the shoulder joint. At the other (distal) end of the humerus are several processes that allow it to articulate with the bones of the lower arm. The **olecranon fossa** is a depression of the humerus that holds the **olecranon process** of the ulna when the elbow is extended (arm is straight).

Radius. The **radius** is one of two bones of the forearm. It is located on the "thumb side" when the palm of the hand is facing forward. The head of the radius articulates with the humerus, ulna, and carpal bones. The radial tuberosity at the proximal end of the radius is the site of attachment for one of the muscles responsible for bending the forearm at the elbow.

Ulna. The **ulna** is the second bone of the forearm. The longer of the two bones, the ulna, is located on the little-finger side of the forearm. It has processes and depressions that allow it to articulate with the humerus, radius, and carpal bones. The **olecranon process** of the ulna is what you feel as the bony point of the elbow. Note that the distal ends of both the ulna and the radius have a pointed styloid process; the styloid processes can be felt at the wrist.

Also note the relationship of the radius to the ulna when the hand moves from a palm up (supination) to a palm down (pronation) position. When the palm is up, the two bones are parallel. When the palm is down, the two bones cross to achieve this movement.

Hand. The hand is composed of a wrist, palm, and fingers. The wrist contains eight bones called **carpal bones,** which are tightly bound by ligaments. Five **metacarpal bones** form the palm of the hand; each metacarpal bone is in line with a finger. The 14 finger bones are called **phalanges,** or digits. Note that each digit has three bones except the thumb (called the pollex), which has only two bones. The heads of the phalanges are prominent as the knuckles when a fist is made.

Pelvic Girdle

The **pelvic girdle** is composed of two coxal bones that articulate with each other anteriorly and with the sacrum posteriorly (Figure 8-15, *A*). The pelvic girdle performs three functions: it bears the weight of the body; it serves as a place of attachment for the legs; and it protects the organs located in the pelvic cavity, including the urinary bladder and the reproductive organs.

Pelvis. The **pelvis** is formed by the pelvic girdle, sacrum, and coccyx.

Male and Female Differences. The differences between the female and male pelvis are related to the child-bearing role of the female. In general, the female pelvis is broader and shallower than the male pelvis.

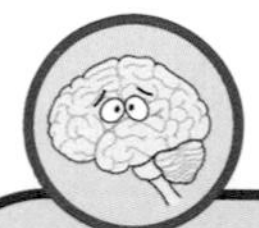

Do You Know...

About Dr. Pollex and Mr. Blackberry's thumb?

Mr. Blackberry presented to his family physician, Dr. Pollex, with a chief complaint of extreme pain in his left thumb. He writhed in pain and sobbed uncontrollably as he punched numbers into his cell and frantically dispatched text messages to everyone he had ever met. Dr. Pollex, however, was all over it. "Thumb abuse," he roared. He explained to Mr. Blackberry. "Your thumb (pollex) was not designed to click away 24/7; it's aching for relief. The sheath around your thumb is inflamed and swollen." The digit doc assured Mr. Blackberry that with rest and retraining he would soon be clicking away again. Other digits could be trained to share the clicking load. Thumb pain secondary to repetitive thumb-clicking marathons is called Blackberry thumb, a reference to the popular handheld device.

The male pelvis is narrow and funnel-shaped (see Figure 8-15, *C* and *D*).

Coxal Bone. The **coxal bone** is the hip bone (see Figure 8-15, *B*). Each coxal bone is composed of three parts: ilium, ischium, and pubis. The three bones join together to form a depression called the **acetabulum.** The acetabulum is important because it receives the head of the femur and therefore enables the thigh to rotate at the hip joint.

Ilium. The **ilium** is the largest part of the coxal bone. The ilium is the flared upper part of the bone and can be felt at the hip. The outer edge of the ilium is called the iliac crest. The ilium connects in the back with the sacrum, forming the sacroiliac joint. The greater sciatic notch is the site where blood vessels and the sciatic nerve pass from the pelvic cavity into the posterior thigh region. Like the sternum, the ilium produces blood cells and is a common site for bone marrow biopsy.

Ischium. The **ischium** is the most inferior part of the coxal bone. The ischium contains three important structures: ischial tuberosity, ischial spine, and lesser sciatic notch. The ischial tuberosity is the part of the coxal bone on which you sit. The ischial spine projects into the pelvic cavity and narrows the outlet of the pelvis. If the spines of a woman's two ischial bones are too close together, the pelvic outlet becomes too small to allow for the birth of a baby. The measurement of the distance between the two spines therefore provides valuable information as to the adequacy of the pelvis for childbearing.

Pubis. The **pubis** is the most anterior part of the coxal bone. The two pubic bones join together in front as the **symphysis pubis.** A disc of cartilage separates the pubic bones at the symphysis pubis. In women, the disc expands in response to the hormones of pregnancy, thereby enlarging the pelvic cavity to provide a bigger space for the growing fetus.

A large hole called the **obturator foramen** is formed as the pubic bone fuses with a part of the ischium. The obturator is the largest foramen in the body.

What is meant by the true and false pelvis? The **false pelvis** is the area surrounded by the flaring parts of the two iliac bones (see Figure 8-15, *C*). The **true pelvis** lies below the false pelvis and is much smaller. The true pelvis is a ring formed by the fusion of the pelvic bones; it is also called the **pelvic brim.** The true pelvis has an inlet and an outlet area. In women, the dimensions of these areas are important because they must be large enough to allow for the passage of an infant during childbirth.

Lower Extremities

The lower limb includes the bones of the thigh, kneecap, leg, and the foot (Figure 8-16).

Femur. The **femur** is the thighbone; it is the longest and strongest bone in the body. The femur articulates with the coxal bone to form the hip and with the bones of the lower leg to form the knee. The head of the femur sits in the acetabulum of the coxal bone and allows the thigh to rotate at the hip joint. The head of the femur continues as the neck. A number of bony processes are on the femur. The most important are the **greater** and **lesser trochanters.** These trochanters provide sites of attachment for many muscles.

In older persons, the neck of the femur is easily broken during a fall; this is known as a broken hip. Forced immobility (bedrest) often results in serious complications. For example, because of the weight of the injured leg, an immobile, bedridden person may experience an outward rotation of the hip. If allowed to develop, this outward rotation makes walking very difficult and therefore delays rehabilitation. Other hazards of immobility, such as blood clots and pneumonia, contribute to the seriousness of a fractured hip.

Patella. The **patella** is the kneecap. It is a triangular bone that is located within a tendon that passes over the knee. The patella articulates with both the femur and the tibia. An infant is born without kneecaps; somewhere between the ages of 2 and 6 years, in response to weight-bearing, a small sesamoid bone (one that looks like a sesame seed) in the patellar region enlarges, thereby forming the kneecap.

Tibia and Fibula. The tibia and the fibula form the leg. The **tibia** is the shinbone and articulates with the femur at the knee. The tibia is the larger weight-bearing bone of the leg. A protuberance called the **tibial tuberosity** is the site of attachment for the muscles and ligaments from the thigh. At the distal end of the tibia, a protuberance called the **medial malleolus** articulates with the inner ankle bones.

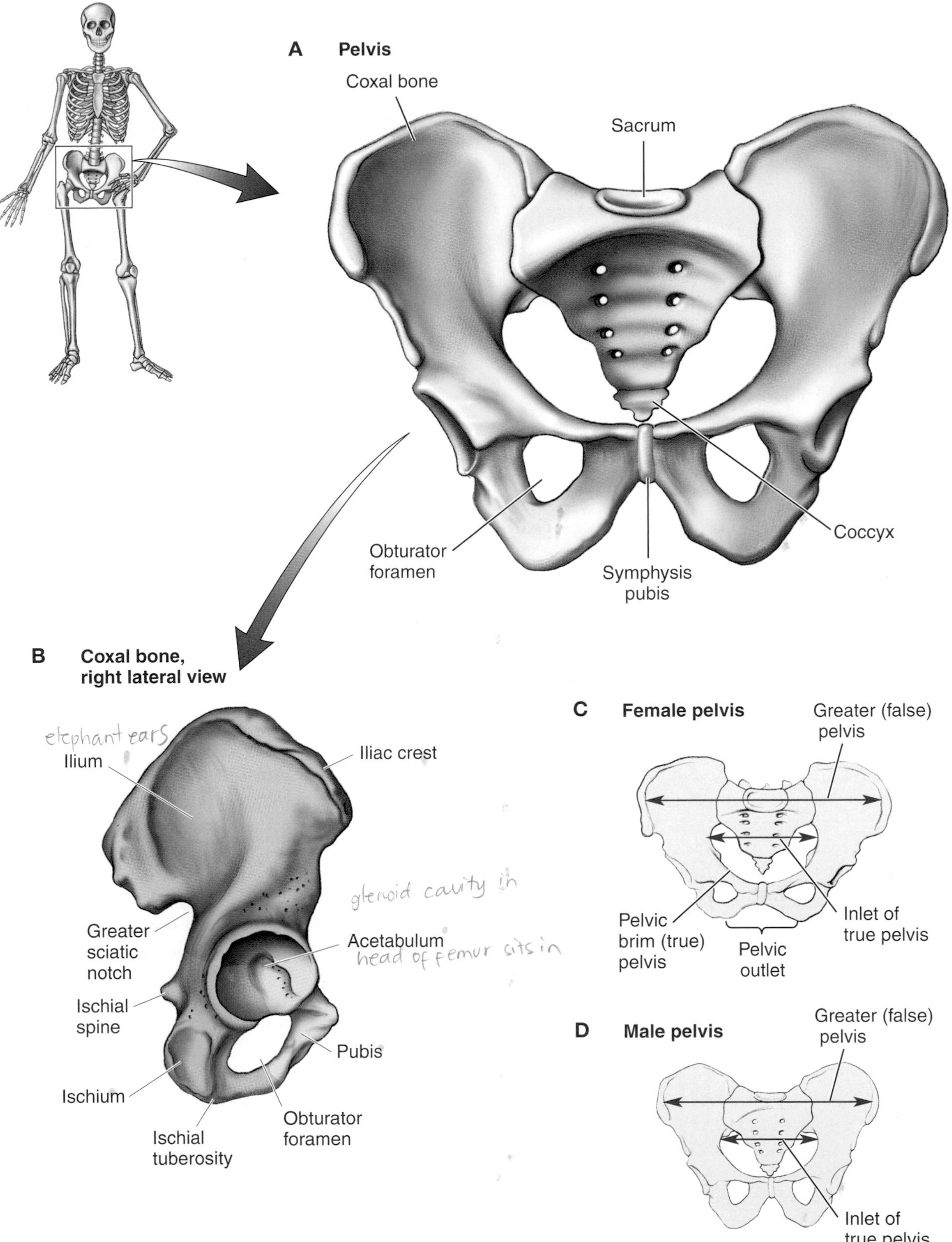

FIGURE 8-15 Pelvic cavity. **A,** Bones that make up the pelvic cavity. **B,** Coxal bone (ilium, ischium, and pubis). **C,** Female pelvis. **D,** Male pelvis.

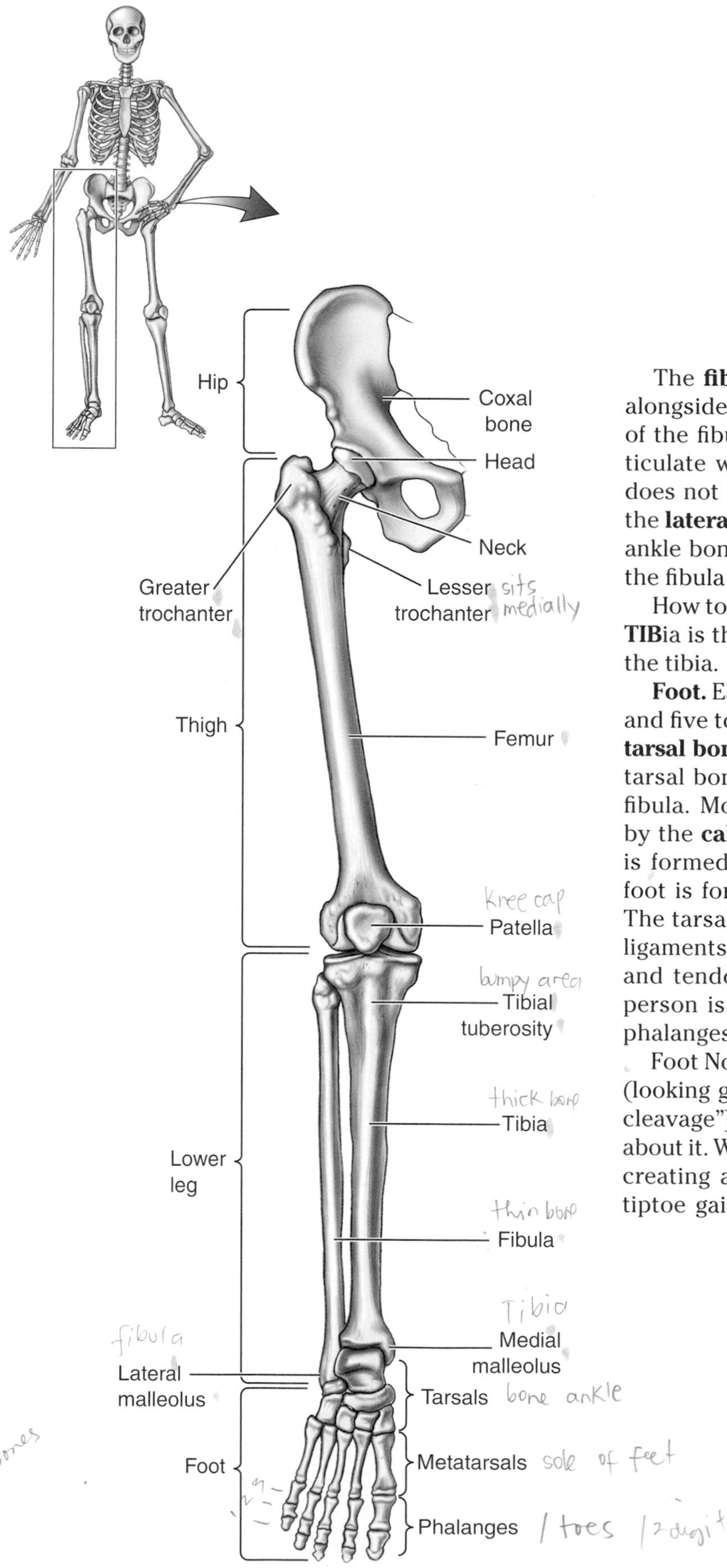

Hip
Coxal bone
Head
Neck
Greater trochanter
Lesser trochanter
Thigh
Femur
Patella
Tibial tuberosity
Tibia
Lower leg
Fibula
Medial malleolus
Lateral malleolus
Tarsals
Foot
Metatarsals
Phalanges

FIGURE 8-16 Bones of the lower limb: thigh, lower leg, and foot.

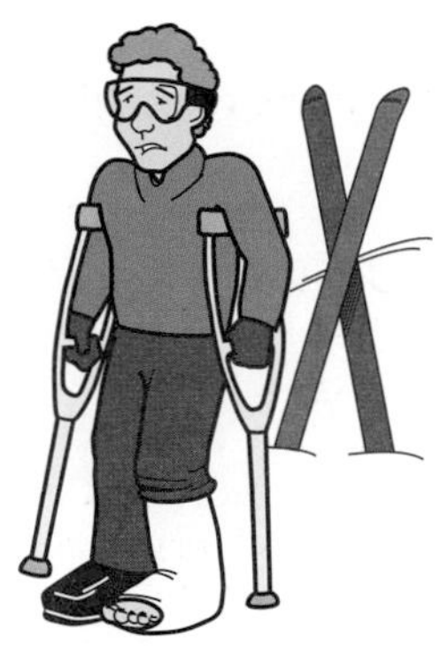

The **fibula** is a long thin bone positioned laterally alongside the tibia in the lower leg. The proximal end of the fibula articulates with the tibia. It does not articulate with the femur, is not part of the knee, and does not bear any body weight. The lower end forms the **lateral malleolus,** which articulates with the outer ankle bones. Skiers often twist their ankles and break the fibula at the lateral malleolus.

How to remember the position of the leg bones? The **TIB**ia is the ***T****hick* ***I****nner* ***B****one*; the fibu**LA** is ***LA****teral* to the tibia.

Foot. Each foot (Figure 8-17) has an ankle, an instep, and five toes. The great toe is called the **hallux.** Seven **tarsal bones** form the ankle. The most proximal of the tarsal bones, the **talus,** articulates with the tibia and fibula. Most of the weight of the body is supported by the **calcaneus** or heelbone. The instep of the foot is formed by five **metatarsal bones.** The ball of the foot is formed by the distal ends of the metatarsals. The tarsals, metatarsals, and associated tendons and ligaments form the **arches** of the foot. If the ligaments and tendons weaken, the arches can "fall," and the person is said to have flat feet. The toes contain 14 phalanges.

Foot Notes ... We all know about the thrill of victory (looking great in heels and flaunting the latest in "toe cleavage"). What about the "agony of de-feet"? Think about it. We jam our square feet into pointy pizza shoes, creating an unnatural, uncomfortable, and crippling tiptoe gait. The entire weight of the body is pushed

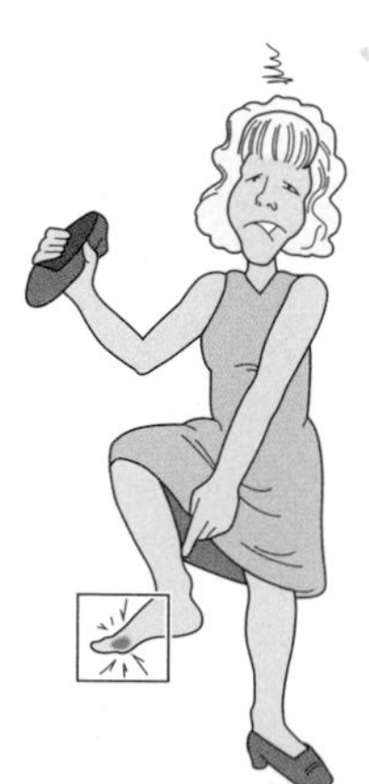

forward to the balls of the feet. What do we get for this effort?

- Bunions. Bunions develop in response to excessive force, whereby the big toe is compressed and forced toward the second toe. The joint becomes distorted, inflamed, and painful.
- Neuromas. The shift of body weight to the balls of the feet causes painful and debilitating nerve growths (neuromas) between the toes.
- Metatarsalgia. The shift of body weight causes metatarsalgia, pain in the ball of the foot.
- Shortening of the Achilles tendon. The tiptoe position causes contraction of the Achilles tendon; the shortened tendon makes the use of "flats" uncomfortable.
- Pump bump. Excess pressure of the heel of the shoe on the bone causes an enlargement (bump) on the heel bone. Pump bump is so common that it has its own medical name, Haglund's deformity.
- Knee pain. The shift in weight adds unnatural stress to the knee joint; knee joint replacement is more common in women and is often related to abusive footwear.
- Last but not least: There have been several documented cases of death associated with falling while wearing platform shoes.

What to do? Although it is done, the surgical removal of toes is not the answer. Instituting a fashion change is certainly less painful than redesigning the foot. In any event, heels are definitely an anatomic step in the wrong direction!

JOINTS (ARTICULATIONS)

A joint, or **articulation,** is the site where two bones meet. Joints perform two functions: they hold the bones together, and they provide flexibility to a rigid skeleton. Without joints, we would move around stiffly like robots. Think of how awkward a basketball player would

Do You Know...

What dripping "humours" have to do with gout?

The typical cartoon of a person experiencing gout is that of an elderly, red-faced, obese, well-to-do male. His elevated throbbing big toe fits the picture perfectly. Gout is due to an increase of uric acid in the blood. The uric acid deposits in joints where it forms tiny, sharp crystals (called tophi) that inflame the joint and cause intense pain. Foods high in uric acid can bring on an attack of gout. A diet of meat and alcohol (the rich man's diet) can cause it; hence, the caricature of a glutton—wealthy, obese, and red-faced—comes to mind. The term gout comes from *gutta,* a Latin word meaning "to drop." It was originally believed that gout was caused by unhealthy humours (fluids) or poisons that dropped or dripped into the joints, particularly the joint of the great toe. This disease was so common that the pubs often had "gout stools" for their portly porkers. Remember:

G great toe
O one joint, usually the great toe
U uric acid
T tophi
Y yikes! That hurts.

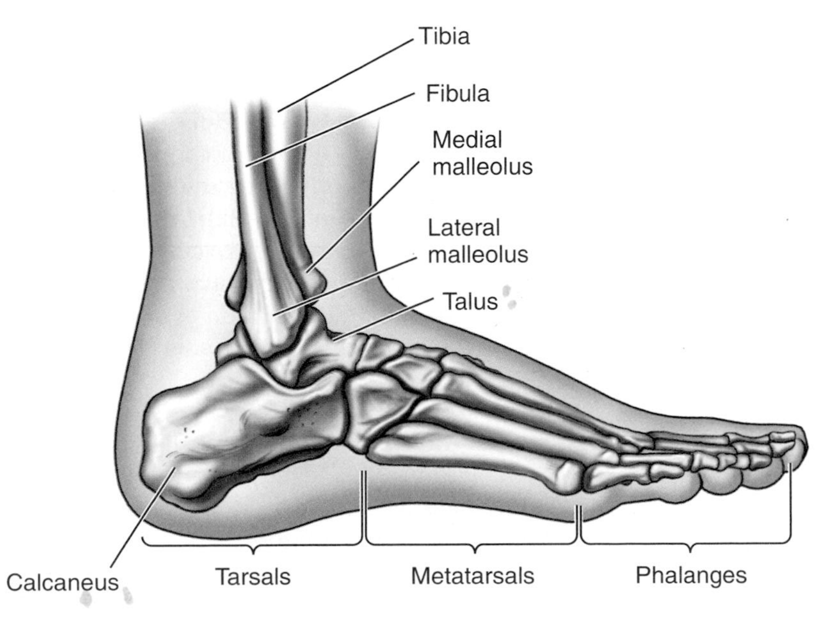

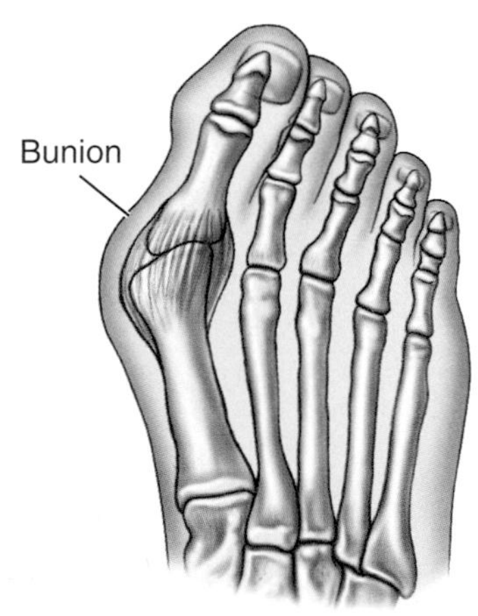

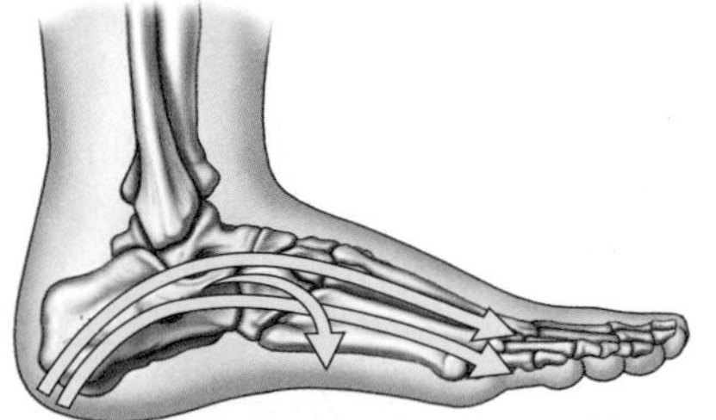

FIGURE 8-17 Foot: tarsals, metatarsals, and phalanges. Arches support the structure of the foot.

Table 8-3 Types of Joints

Type	Description	Example
Immovable	Suture/"zipper"	Cranial bones
Slightly movable	Disc of cartilage between two bones	Intervertebral discs; symphysis pubis
Freely movable	Ball and socket	Shoulder (scapula and humerus): hip (pelvic bone and femur)
	Hinge	Elbow (humerus and ulna): knee (femur and tibia); fingers
	Pivot	Atlas and axis; allows for rotation (side-to-side movement) of the head, indicating "no"
	Saddle	Thumb (carpometacarpal joint)
	Gliding	Carpals
	Condyloid	Temporal bone and mandible (jaw); knuckles

look if the entire skeleton were rigid! There is a branch of science that studies joints, called **arthrology.** The branch of medicine that studies disease of the joints is called **rheumatology.**

Joints can be classified into three groups according to the amount of movement: immovable, slightly movable, and freely movable (Table 8-3). Joints can also be classified according to the types of tissues (fibrous, cartilaginous, or synovial) that bind the bones at the joint.

IMMOVABLE JOINTS

Immovable joints permit no movement. The sutures in the skull are immovable joints. The sutures are formed as the irregular edges of the skull bones interlock and are bound by fibrous connective tissue. When fused they look like zippers.

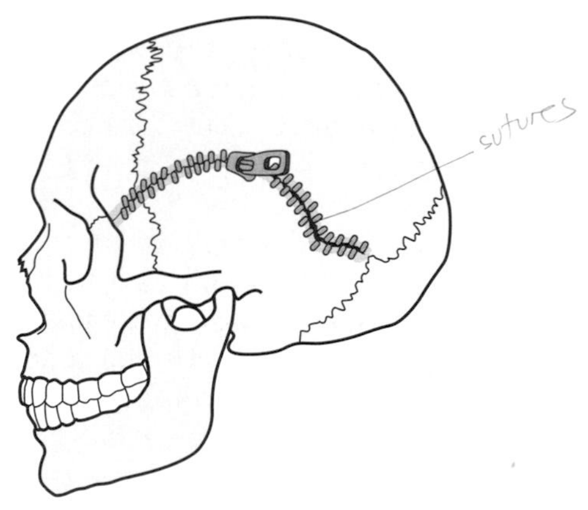

SLIGHTLY MOVABLE JOINTS

Slightly movable joints permit limited movement. Limited movement is usually achieved by bones connected by a cartilaginous disc. For instance, movement of the spinal column occurs at the intervertebral discs. Also, during pregnancy, the symphysis pubis allows the pelvis to widen.

FREELY MOVABLE JOINTS

Freely movable joints provide much more flexibility and movement than the other two types of joints. Most of the joints of the skeletal system are freely movable. All freely movable joints are **synovial** (sĭ-NŌ-vē-ăl) **joints** (Figure 8-18).

A typical synovial joint includes the following structures:

- *Articular cartilage:* The articulating surface of each of the two bones is lined with **articular cartilage,** forming a smooth surface within the joint.
- *Joint capsule:* The **joint capsule** is made of fibrous connective tissue. It encloses the joint in a strong, sleevelike covering.
- *Synovial membrane:* Lining the joint capsule is the **synovial membrane.** This membrane secretes synovial fluid into the joint cavity.
- *Synovial fluid:* **Synovial fluid** lubricates the bones in the joint, thereby decreasing the friction within the joint. Synovial fluid gets its name from an ovum or egg, because the thick consistency of the synovial fluid resembles the consistency of an egg white.
- *Bursae:* Many synovial joints contain **bursae** (singular: bursa). Bursae are small sacs of synovial fluid between the joint and the tendons that cross over the joint. Bursae permit the tendons to slide as the bones move. Excessive use of a joint may cause a painful inflammation of the bursae, called bursitis. Tennis elbow is bursitis caused by excessive and improper use of the elbow joint.
- *Supporting ligaments:* Surrounding the joint are **supporting ligaments.** These ligaments join the articulating bones together and stabilize the joint. Sometimes a ligament is stretched or torn, causing pain and loss of mobility.

NAMING JOINTS

The joints of the body are named so as to provide information about the articulating bones. The joints are named according to the bones they "connect." Refer to

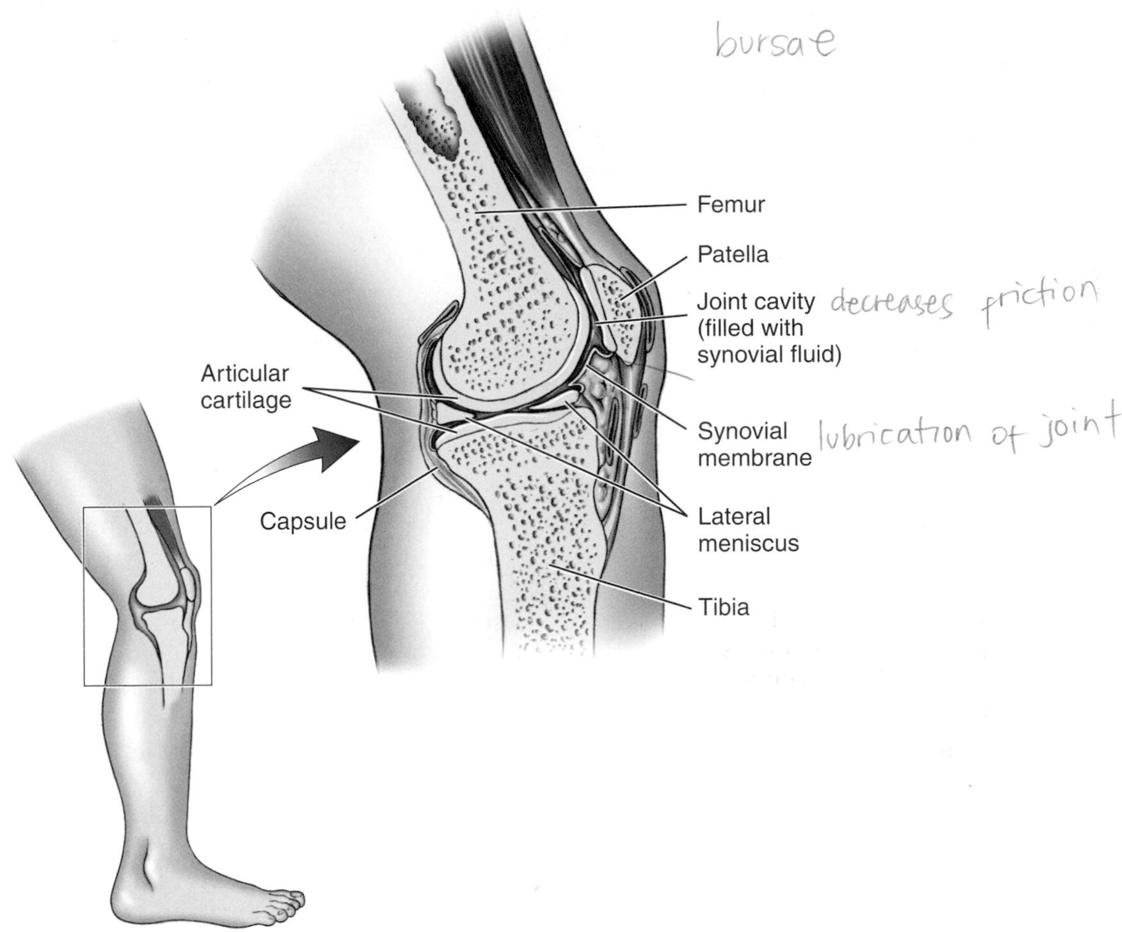

FIGURE 8-18 Synovial joint (knee): structure and contents.

Figure 8-19 as we identify several joints. The temporomandibular joint connects the temporal bone in the skull with the mandible (lower jaw). The tibiofemoral joint is the articulation between the tibia and the femur; it is also called the knee. The knuckles refer to the metacarpophalangeal joints. The name indicates that the metacarpal bone articulates with a phalange (finger). Some names specify the bony process rather than the bone. For instance, the glenohumeral joint names the glenoid cavity of the scapula and the humerus, the arm bone that "fits into" the glenoid cavity. The acromioclavicular joint is the articulation between the acromion process of the scapula and the clavicle. Lastly, locate the sternomanubrial joint (breastbone); it is a landmark used to count ribs.

FAVORITE SYNOVIAL JOINTS

Knee

The knee joint, called the tibiofemoral joint, is primarily a hinge joint. In addition to all the structures contained in a synovial joint, the knee joint contains extra cushioning in the form of pads of cartilage. These pads absorb the shock of walking and jumping. Two crescent-shaped pads of cartilage, the **medial meniscus** and the **lateral meniscus,** rest on the tibia. Like other synovial joints, the knee joint is reinforced and aligned by supporting ligaments, the cruciate ligaments in particular. There is an **anterior cruciate ligament** (ACL) and a **posterior cruciate ligament** (PCL).

Peas for the Knees and More Disease

- Knees are frequently sprained and strained. As every soccer mom knows, a bag of frozen peas is good first aid for injured knees and is consistent with the first aid treatment of strains and sprains, or RICE (**R**est, **I**ce, **C**ompression, and **E**levation).
- The cruciate ligaments, especially the ACL, are frequent victims of athletic events. The ACL prevents hyperextension of the knee and is torn when the knee is forcibly hyperextended. Torn cartilage is removed by arthroscopic surgery. An arthroscope is a viewing tube that allows the surgeon to see into the knee joint.
- As any football player knows, being tackled at the sides of the knees can put a fast end to one's career. A "clipping" penalty attests to the seriousness of knee injuries and is fully deserving of a 15-yard penalty.

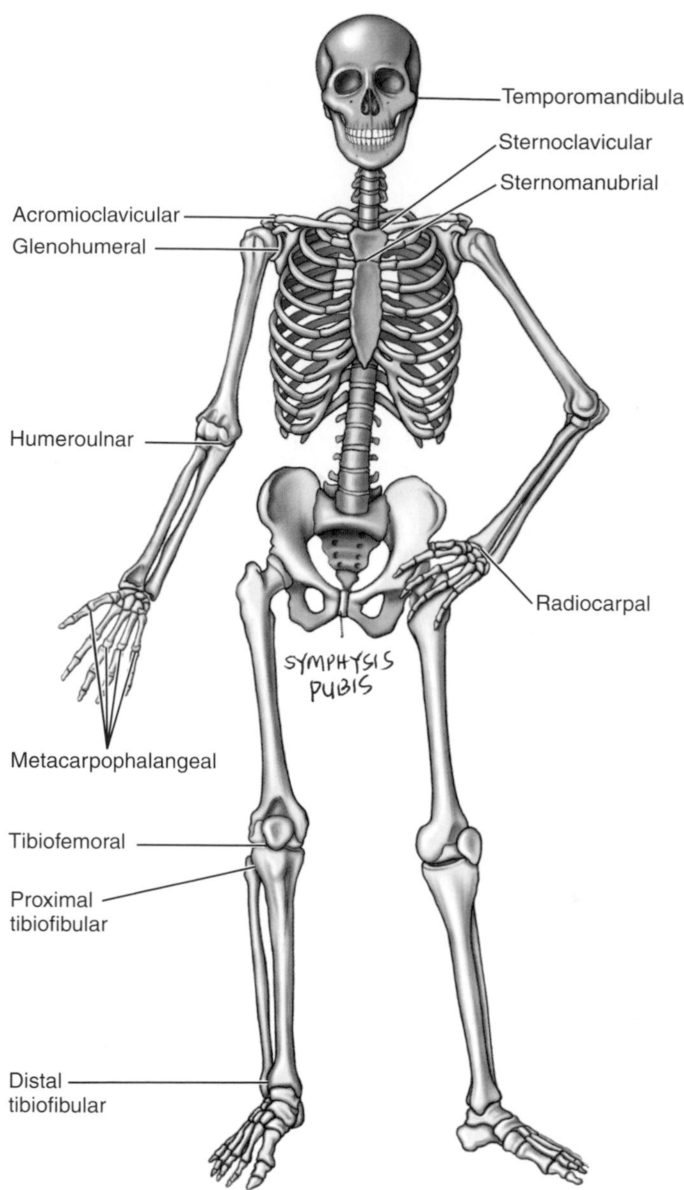

FIGURE 8-19 Naming joints.

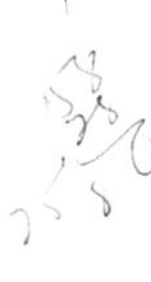

Shoulder

The shoulder joint is called the glenohumeral joint, indicating that the head of the humerus fits into the glenoid cavity of the scapula. The shoulder joint is a ball-and-socket joint and permits the greatest range of motion. The joint is stabilized by surrounding skeletal muscles, tendons, and ligaments. The rotator cuff muscles and tendons, in particular, hold the head of the humerus in the glenoid cavity. The shoulder joint is the most frequently dislocated joint.

Elbow

The elbow is called the humeroulnar joint; a lesser component is the humeroradial joint. The olecranon process of the ulna forms the pointy part of the elbow when it is flexed. The elbow is a hinge joint that is very stable; nonetheless, it can be injured. We have, for example, "nursemaid's" elbow caused by an impatient parent dragging a toddler by the arm. The upward twisting pull causes a partial dislocation of the child's elbow and possible damage to the growth plate (epiphyseal disc).

Hip

The hip, called the coxal joint, is a ball-and-socket joint that is formed where the head of the femur articulates with the acetabulum, the depression formed by the three coxal bones. The hip is strengthened by surrounding muscles, tendons, and ligaments. A fractured hip refers to a break in the neck of the femur.

MOVING SYNOVIAL JOINTS

The body contains many types of freely movable synovial joints. The type of motion and the degree of flexibility vary with each type of joint. For instance, if you move your elbow, your lower arm will move either up or down like two boards joined by a hinge. This motion is very different from the arm-swinging motion at the shoulder joint. Both the elbow and the shoulder joints are freely movable, but the types of movement differ.

Six types of freely movable joints are classified according to the type of movement allowed by the joint (Figure 8-20 and Table 8-3). Three of these joints are the hinge, the ball-and-socket, and the pivot joints.

Hinge Joint

The **hinge joint** allows movement similar to the movement of two boards joined together by a hinge. The hinge allows movement in one direction, where the angle at the hinge increases or decreases. Hinge joints include elbows, knees, and fingers. Move each of these joints to clarify the movement described here.

Ball-and-Socket Joint

A **ball-and-socket joint** is formed when the ball-shaped end of one bone fits into the cup-shaped socket of another bone, so that the bones can move in many directions around a central point. The shoulder and hip joints are ball-and-socket joints. The head of the humerus fits into the glenoid cavity of the scapula in the shoulder joint. The head of the femur fits into the acetabulum of the coxal bone in the hip joint.

Move your shoulder all around (as in pitching a softball) and note the freedom of movement. Compare this movement with the limited movement at the elbow or knee joints. The arrangement of the ball-and-socket joints allows for a wide range of movement, also allowing for easy displacement of the joint structures. When a strong force is applied to the shoulder, for instance, a dislocation may occur. Dislocations often occur when football players are thrown to the ground.

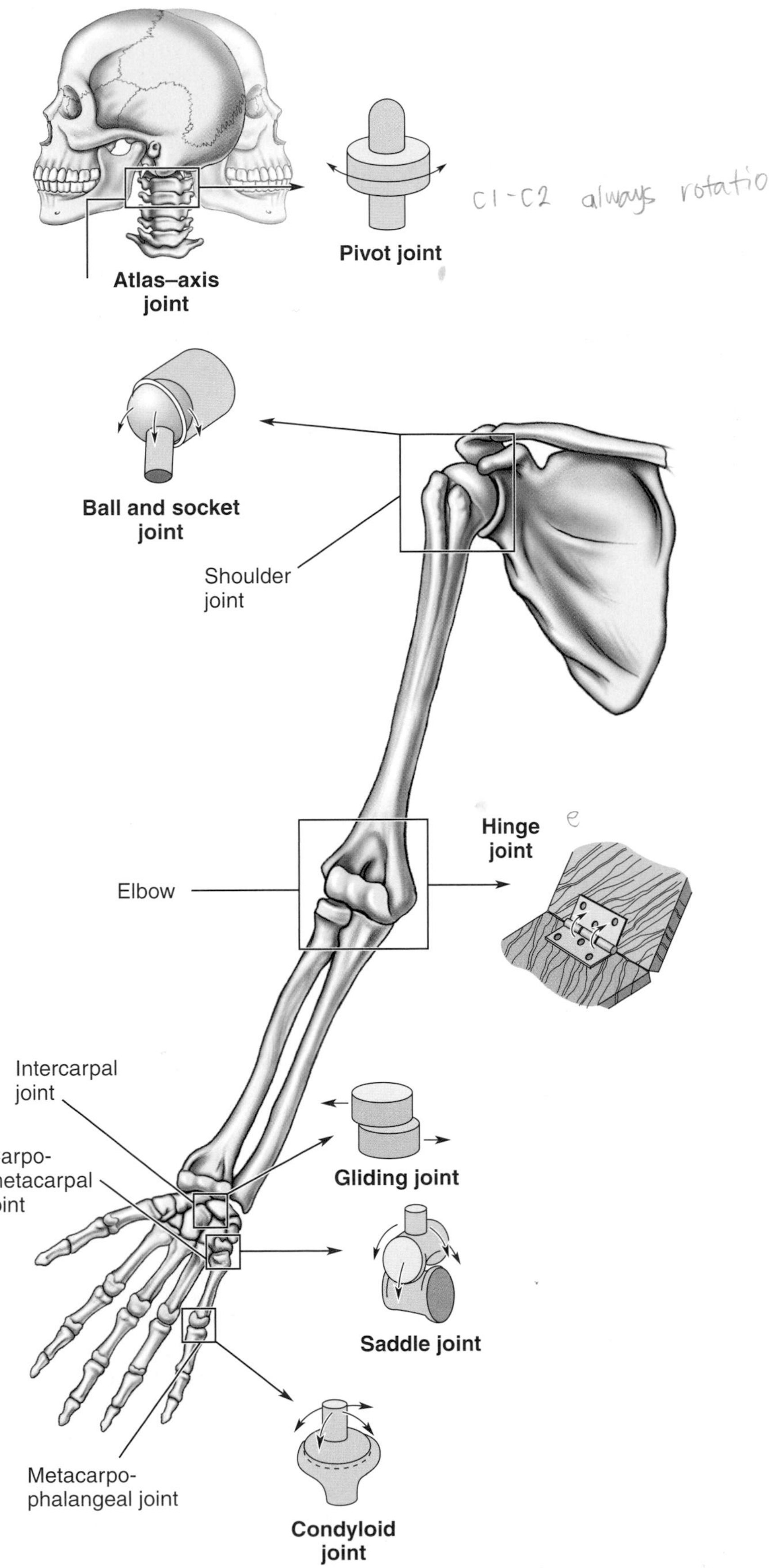

FIGURE 8-20 Freely movable joints.

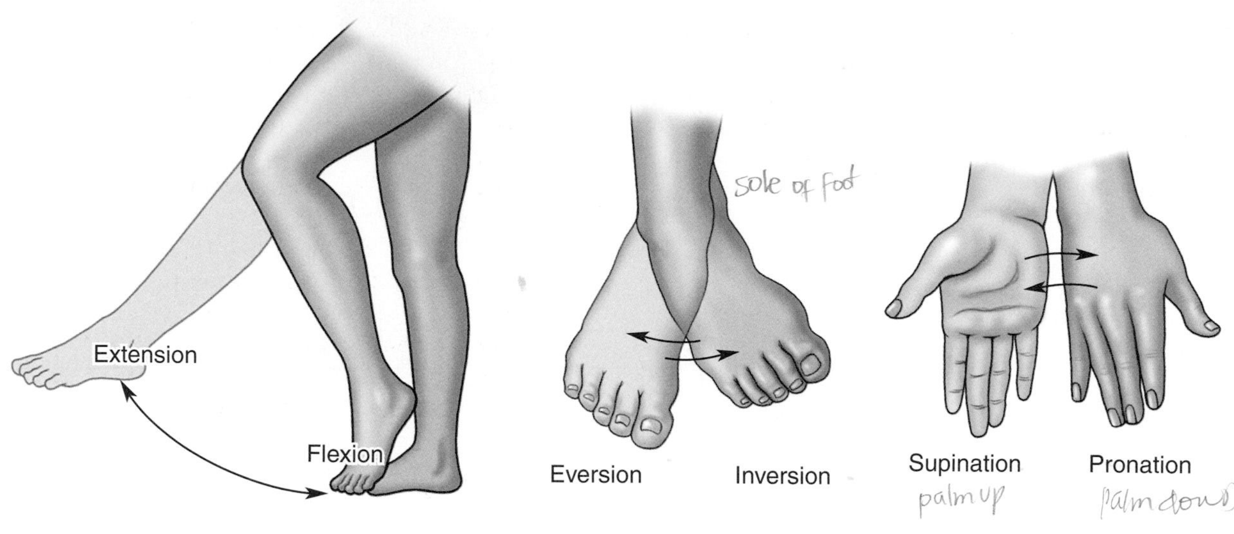

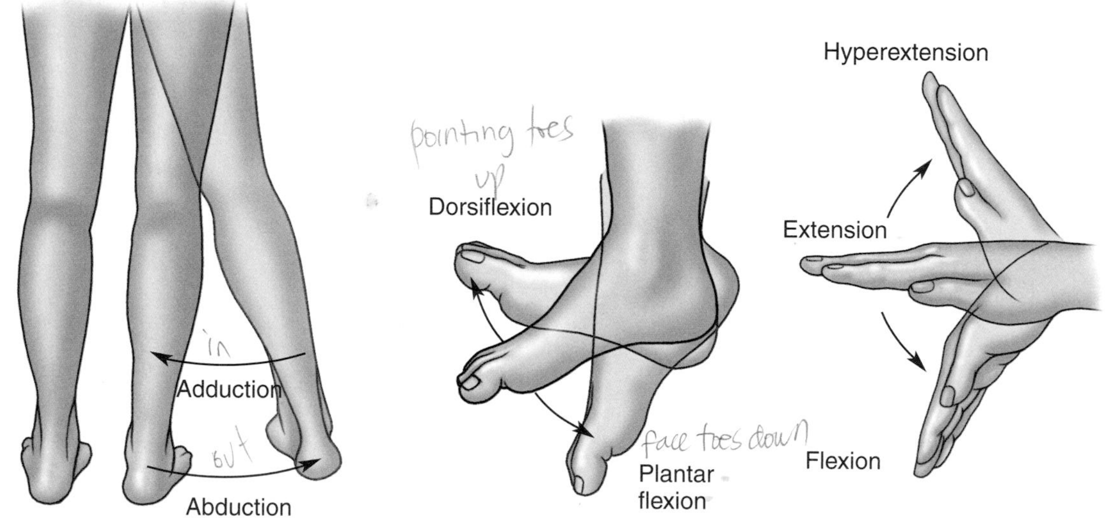

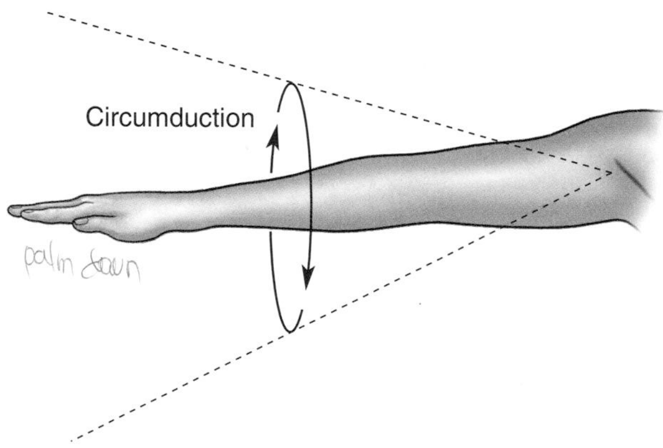

FIGURE 8-21 Types of movements at joints.

Pivot Joint

A **pivot joint** allows for rotation around the length of a bone. The pivot joint allows only for rotation. An example is the side-to-side movement of the head indicating "no." This rotation occurs as the atlas (first cervical vertebra) swivels around, or pivots, on the axis (second cervical vertebra).

ACHING JOINTS

A number of health problems affect joints, generally causing discomfort and impaired mobility. **Arthritis** refers to an inflammation of a joint. While there are over 25 types of arthritis, two types are of particular concern: osteoarthritis and rheumatoid arthritis. Osteoarthritis is called degenerative or "wear-and-tear" arthritis. It is the most common cause of arthritis and is most frequently seen in the elderly. It affects primarily the weight-bearing joints. The erosion of the cartilage causes pain and eventually bone-on-bone contact. In time the joint may deteriorate to the point where it needs to be replaced. Synthetic joints have been designed for replacement of most joints, including the hip, knee, shoulder, and elbow joints.

Rheumatoid arthritis (RA) is the most debilitating type of arthritis. It is an autoimmune disease characterized by inflammation of the joints and systemic symptoms such as fever, fatigue, and anemia. Joint disease progresses from thickening of joint tissue, called pannus formation, to cartilage destruction and finally deformity and fusion of the joints.

TYPES OF JOINT MOVEMENTS

Movements at freely movable joints occur when the muscles that lie across the joints contract and exert pressure on the attached bone. These movements are illustrated in Figure 8-21 and defined as follows:

- **Flexion:** the bending of a joint that decreases the angle between the bones (bending the leg at the knee or the fingers)
- **Extension:** the straightening of a joint so that the angle between the bones increases (e.g., straightening the leg at the knee or the fingers to open the hand)
- *Plantar flexion:* bending the foot down, as in toe dancing
- *Dorsiflexion:* bending the foot up toward the leg
- *Hyperextension:* overextending the joint beyond its normally straightened position, as in moving the hand toward the upper surface of the wrist
- **Abduction:** movement away from the midline of the body (move your leg sideways, away from your body)
- **Adduction:** movement toward the midline of the body (return your leg toward your body)
- *Inversion:* turning the sole of the foot inward so that it faces the opposite foot
- *Eversion:* turning the sole of the foot outward
- *Supination:* turning the hand so that the palm faces upward
- *Pronation:* turning the hand so that the palm faces downward
- *Circumduction:* a combination of movements, as in the circular arm movement that a softball pitcher makes while pitching the ball

Sum It Up!

A joint, or articulation, is the place where two or more bones meet. Three types of joints are immovable joints, slightly movable joints, and freely movable joints. Freely movable joints are also called synovial joints. Types of freely movable joints include hinge, ball and socket, and pivot joints. Because of the diverse types of joints, the skeleton is capable of various movements.

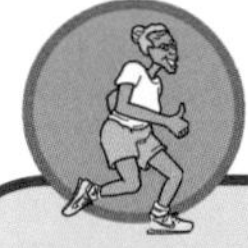

As You Age

1. Because of loss of calcium and organic material, bones are less strong and more brittle. Many older women develop osteoporosis. As a result, bones fracture more easily. Moreover, fractured bones heal incompletely and more slowly.
2. As sex hormones in the blood decrease, there is a decrease in new bone growth and in bone mass, increasing the susceptibility to osteoporosis.
3. Tendons and ligaments are less flexible. As a result, joints have a decreased range of motion. A thinning of the articular cartilage and bony overgrowths in the joints contributes to joint stiffness.
4. The intervertebral discs shrink. Because of the compressed discs and the loss of bone mass, body height decreases and the thoracic spine curves (causing kyphosis).

Disorders of the Skeletal System

Bursitis	Inflammation of one or more bursae, causing pain, swelling, and restriction of movement. Common forms include subacromial bursitis (painful shoulder), olecranon bursitis (miner's or tennis elbow); and prepatellar bursitis (housemaid's knee).
Cancer	Several types of cancer can occur in the skeletal system. Examples include osteosarcoma, a tumor of the bone, and chondrosarcoma, a tumor involving cartilage. The most common form of bone cancer is a myeloma, in which the malignant tumors in the bone marrow interfere with red blood cell production and cause destruction of bone.
Dislocation	Displacement, or luxation, of a bone from its joint with tearing of ligaments, tendons, and articular capsule. The shoulder joint is displaced more easily than other joints. The return of the bone into its joint is called a reduction. A partial dislocation is called a subluxation. When applied to the temporomandibular joint, a subluxation refers to the stretching of the capsule and ligaments that results in popping noises when the jaw moves.
Osteomalacia	Disease characterized by softening of the bones due to demineralization (loss of calcium and phosphorus). The demineralization is caused by vitamin D deficiency. The bone softening results in skeletal deformities. Osteomalacia in growing bones is called rickets.
Osteomyelitis	An inflammation of the bone and/or infection of the bone marrow most often caused by the *Staphylococcus* bacterium. Osteomyelitis often occurs as a complication of bone fractures and orthopedic surgery.
Osteoporosis	A loss of bone mass that makes the bones so porous that they crumble under the ordinary stress of moving about. Osteoporosis is related to loss of estrogen in older women, a dietary deficiency of calcium and vitamin D, and low levels of exercise.
Sprain	An injury to a joint caused by the twisting of the joint. A sprain causes pain, loss of mobility, swelling, and black-and-blue discoloration of the injured site. Ligaments may be torn, but no bone or joint damage occurs.
Strain	An injury to a muscle or tendon at a joint. A strain is due to overuse or overstretching and is less serious than a sprain.

SUMMARY OUTLINE

The skeletal system supports the weight of the body, supports and protects body organs, enables the body to move, acts as storage site for minerals, and produces blood cells.

I. Bones: An Overview

A. Sizes and Shapes

1. Bones are classified as long, short, flat, and irregular.
2. Bone markings function as sites of muscle attachments and passages for nerves and blood vessels.
3. A long bone has a diaphysis (shaft) and two epiphyses (ends). Articular cartilage is found on the outer surface of the epiphyses.
4. The diaphysis is composed of compact or hard bone. The epiphysis consists of spongy or soft bone; red marrow is found in the holes of spongy bone.

B. Bone Formation and Growth

1. Bones ossify in two ways. In the skull, osteoblasts replace thin connective tissue membrane, forming flat bones. Other bones form on hyaline cartilage models as osteoblasts replace cartilage with bone.
2. Bones grow longitudinally at the epiphyseal disc, to determine height; bones also grow thicker and wider to support the weight of the body.
3. Bone growth and reshaping occur throughout life and depend on many factors, including diet, exercise, and hormones.

II. Divisions of the Skeletal System

The names of the 206 bones of the skeleton are listed in Table 8-2.

A. Axial Skeleton

1. The axial skeleton includes the bones of the skull (cranium and face), hyoid bone, bones of the middle ear, bones of the vertebral column, and the thoracic cage.
2. The skull of a newborn contains fontanels, which are membranous areas that allow brain growth.
3. The skull contains air-filled cavities called sinuses.

4. The vertebral column is formed from 26 vertebrae, one sacrum, and one coccyx. The vertebrae are separated by cartilaginous discs. The vertebral column of the adult has four curvatures: cervical, thoracic, lumbar, and sacral.
5. The thoracic cage is a bony cone-shaped cage formed by the sternum, 12 pairs of ribs, and thoracic vertebrae.

B. Appendicular Skeleton
1. The appendicular skeleton includes the bones of the extremities (arms and legs), and the bones of the hip and shoulder girdles.
2. The shoulder girdle consists of the scapula and the clavicle.
3. The pelvic girdle is formed by the two coxal bones and is secured to the axial skeleton at the sacrum.

III. Joints

A joint or articulation is the site where two bones meet.

A. Types of Joints (based on the degree of movement)
1. Immovable joints.
2. Slightly movable joints.
3. Freely movable joints or synovial joints. Structures within a synovial joint (knee): articular cartilage, the joint capsule, synovial membrane, synovial fluid, bursae, and supporting ligaments.
4. The types of freely movable joints include hinge, ball and socket, pivot, gliding, saddle, and condyloid.

B. Joint Movement
1. Freely movable joints are capable of different types of movement.
2. Types of movements at freely movable joints include flexion and extension, abduction and adduction, inversion and eversion, supination and pronation, and circumduction.

Review Your Knowledge

Matching: Long Bone

Directions: Match the following words with their descriptions below.

a. epiphysis
b. spongy bone
c. epiphyseal disc
d. diaphysis
e. medullary cavity
f. haversian system
g. osteoblast
h. osteoclast
i. red bone marrow
j. periosteum

1. d Shaft of a long bone diaphysis
2. c Site of longitudinal bone growth
3. g A bone-building cell
4. i Site of blood cell production
5. j Tough outer covering of the bone
6. a Enlarged end of a long bone
7. b Cancellous bone
8. f Osteon
9. h A bone-eroding cell that helps in bone remodeling
10. e Hollow center of a long bone

Matching: Names of Bones

Directions: Match the following words with their descriptions below.

a. femur
b. scapula
c. mandible
d. ulna
e. sternum
f. coxal bone
g. tibia
h. calcaneus
i. frontal
j. phalanges

1. e Manubrium, body, xiphoid process
2. f Parts of this bone form the acetabulum
3. b Contains the glenoid cavity that holds the head of the humerus
4. d Contains the "pointy" olecranon process
5. g The thick inner bone of the leg
6. h Heel bone
7. j Fingers and toes
8. a The head of this bone that articulates with the acetabulum
9. c Lower jaw bone
10. i Forms the forehead

Matching: Joints and Joint Movement

Directions: Match the following words with their descriptions below. Some words may be used more than once.

a. ball-and-socket
b. adduction
c. flexion
d. pronation
e. dorsiflexion
f. circumduction
g. extension
h. plantar flexion
i. abduction
j. supination

1. ___ Type of joint movement at the elbow (angle decreases)
2. ___ Turning the forearm so that the palm of the hand "looks" at the sky
3. ___ Movement away from the midline of the body
4. ___ Toe dancing
5. ___ Movement of the ulna toward the humerus
6. ___ Type of joint at the shoulder and hip
7. ___ Shoulder movement as in pitching a softball
8. ___ Movement toward the midline of the body
9. ___ Turning the forearm so that the hand "looks" at the floor
10. ___ Straightening the bended knee

Multiple Choice

1. The epiphyseal disc
   a. is located in the medullary cavity.
   b. is composed of cartilage and is involved in the growth of long bone.
   c. is composed exclusively of osteoclasts.
   d. is the sight of blood cell formation.
2. Osteoclastic activity
   a. is responsible for longitudinal bone growth.
   b. lowers blood calcium levels.
   c. stimulates bone breakdown so as to increase blood calcium.
   d. regulates the production of blood cells.
3. Which of the following is not true of the acetabulum?
   a. Formed by the ilium, ischium, and pubis
   b. Receives the head of the femur
   c. Articulates with the greater trochanter
   d. Forms a ball and socket joint
4. The atlas and axis
   a. are pelvic bones.
   b. are processes located on the posterior scapula.
   c. form the glenoid cavity.
   d. are vertebrae that allow the head to move.
5. In order to determine the approximate length of the humerus you would measure from the
   a. olecranon process to the styloid process of the radius.
   b. acromion to the olecranon process.
   c. suprasternal notch to the ziphoid process.
   d. greater trochanter to the medial malleolus.
6. Depression of the red bone marrow
   a. causes a life-threatening decline in blood cells.
   b. stunts longitudinal bone growth.
   c. causes arthritis.
   d. causes loss of bone mineralization and osteoporosis.

CHAPTER 9

Muscular System

KEY TERMS

Acetylcholine, p. 141
Actin, p. 139
Antagonist, p. 146
Aponeurosis, p. 139
Belly, p. 139
Cardiac muscle, p. 139
Fascia, p. 139
Insertion, p. 146
Myosin, p. 139
Neuromuscular junction, p. 141
Origin, p. 146
Prime mover, p. 146
Recruitment, p. 145
Sarcomere, p. 139
Sarcoplasmic reticulum, p. 139
Skeletal muscle, p. 138
Smooth muscle, p. 138
Synergist, p. 146
Tetanus, p. 144
Tonus, p. 145

OBJECTIVES

1. Identify three types of muscle tissue.
2. Describe the sliding filament hypothesis of muscle contraction.
3. Describe the events that occur at the neuromuscular junction.
4. Explain the role of calcium and adenosine triphosphate in muscle contraction.
5. Identify the sources of energy for muscle contraction.
6. Trace the sequence of events from nerve stimulation to muscle contraction.
7. Define *twitch, tetanus,* and *recruitment.*
8. State the basis for naming muscles.
9. List the actions of the major muscles.

The word muscle comes from the Latin word *mus*, meaning little mouse. As muscles contract, the muscle movements under the skin resemble the movement of mice scurrying around. Thus the name mus, or muscle.

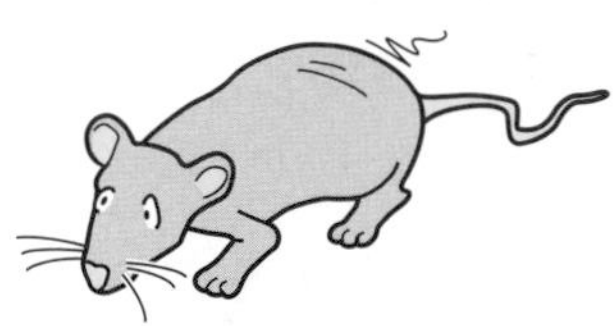

TYPES AND FUNCTIONS OF MUSCLES

The three types of muscles are skeletal, smooth, and cardiac (Figure 9-1). Smooth muscle is discussed throughout the book and cardiac muscle in Chapter 16. In this chapter, the focus is on skeletal muscle.

SKELETAL MUSCLE

Skeletal muscle is generally attached to bone. Because skeletal muscle can be controlled by choice (I choose to move my arm), it is also called **voluntary muscle.** The skeletal muscle cells are long, shaped like cylinders or tubes, and composed of proteins arranged to make the muscle appear striped, or **striated.** Skeletal muscles produce movement, maintain body posture, and stabilize joints. They also produce considerable heat and therefore help maintain body temperature.

SMOOTH MUSCLE

Smooth muscle is generally found in the walls of the viscera, such as the stomach, and is called **visceral muscle.** It is also found in tubes and passageways such as the bronchioles (breathing passages) and blood vessels. Because smooth muscle functions automatically, it is called **involuntary muscle.** Unlike skeletal muscles,

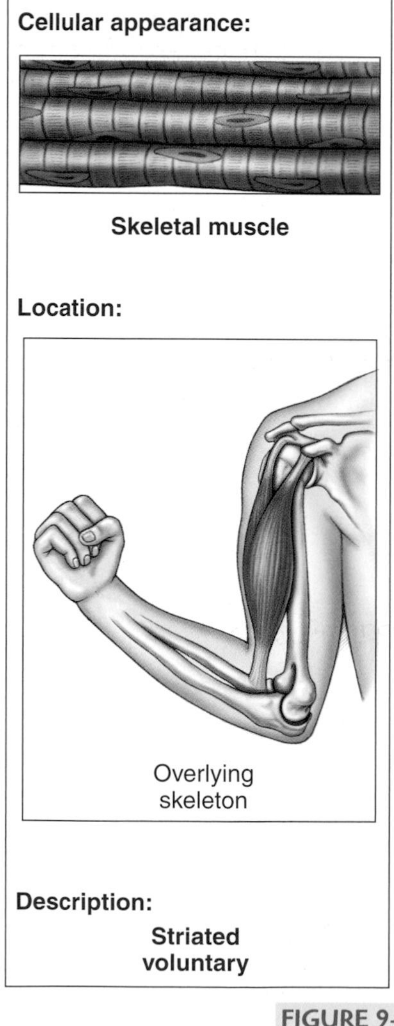

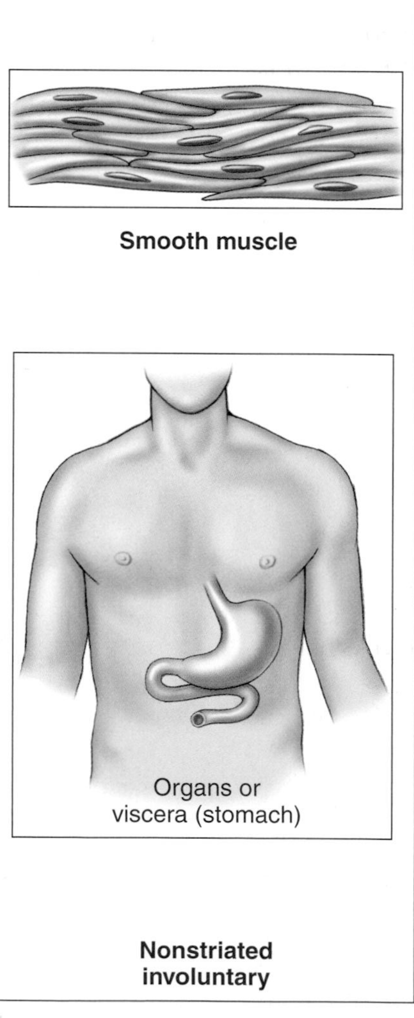

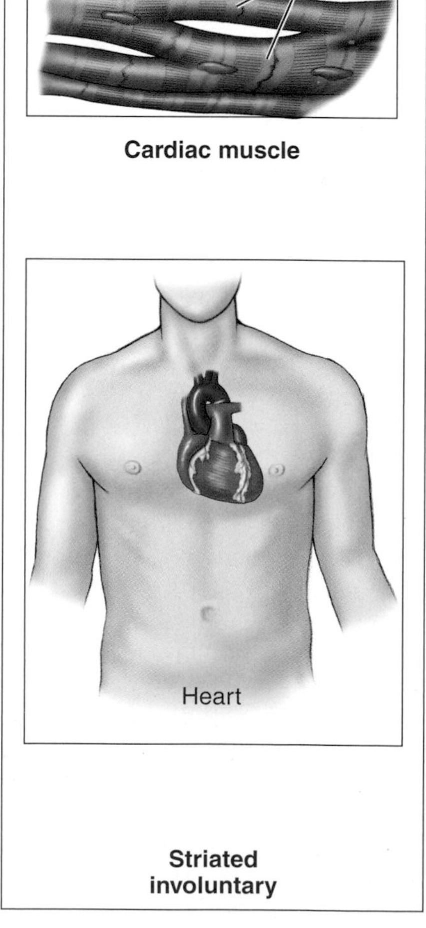

FIGURE 9-1 Three types of muscle: skeletal, smooth, and cardiac.

smooth muscle does not appear striped, or striated, and is therefore called **nonstriated muscle.**

The contraction of smooth muscle enables the viscera to perform their functions. Contraction of the stomach muscles, for instance, enables the stomach to mix solid food into a paste and push it forward into the intestine, where digestion continues.

CARDIAC MUSCLE

Cardiac muscle is found only in the heart, where it functions to pump blood throughout the body. Cardiac muscle cells are long branching cells that fit together tightly at junctions called **intercalated discs.** These tight-fitting junctions promote rapid conduction of electrical signals throughout the heart. Cardiac muscle is classified as striated and involuntary muscle.

STRUCTURE OF THE WHOLE MUSCLE

MUSCLE

If you touch your thigh, you will feel a large muscle. What you are actually feeling is the belly of the muscle; the **belly** refers to the enlarged fleshy body of the muscle between the slender points of attachment. This muscle is composed of thousands of muscle fibers (muscle cells).

LAYERS OF CONNECTIVE TISSUE

A large skeletal muscle is surrounded by layers of tough connective tissue called **fascia** (FĂSH-ē-ă) (Figure 9-2, *A*). This outer layer of fascia is called the **epimysium.** The fascia extends toward and attaches to the bone as a **tendon,** a strong cordlike structure. Another layer of connective tissue, called the **perimysium,** surrounds smaller bundles of muscle fibers. The bundles are called **fascicles.** Individual muscle fibers are found within the fascicles and are surrounded by a third layer of connective tissue called the **endomysium.**

In the limbs the extensive amount of fascia separates the muscles into isolated compartments. Each muscle compartment also receives blood vessels and nerves necessary for muscle function. With a severe "crush injury" the muscle is damaged; it becomes inflamed and leaks fluid into the compartment. Pressure within the compartment increases and compresses the nerves and blood vessels. Deprived of its oxygen and nourishment the muscle and nerves begin to die. This condition is called compartment syndrome or crush syndrome. The immediate treatment involves reduction of the compartment pressure by slicing the fascia lengthwise. Failure to restore blood flow to the muscle nerve results in permanent muscle and nerve damage.

MUSCLE ATTACHMENTS

Muscles form attachments to other structures in three ways. First, the tendon attaches the muscle to the bone. Second, muscles attach directly (without a tendon) to a bone or to soft tissue. Third, a flat, sheetlike fascia called **aponeurosis** (ăp-ō-nū-RŌ-sĭs) connects muscle to muscle or muscle to bone.

STRUCTURE AND FUNCTION OF A SINGLE MUSCLE FIBER

The muscle cell is an elongated muscle fiber (see Figure 9-2, *B*). The muscle fiber has more than one nucleus and is surrounded by a cell membrane called a **sarcolemma.** At several points the cell membrane penetrates deep into the interior of the muscle fiber, forming **transverse tubules (T tubules).** Within the muscle fiber is a specialized endoplasmic reticulum called the **sarcoplasmic reticulum** (săr-kō-PLĂZ-mĭK rĕ-TĬK-ū-lŭm).

Each muscle fiber is composed of long cylindrical structures called **myofibrils.** Each myofibril is made up of a series of contractile units called **sarcomeres** (SĂR-kō-mĭr) (see Figure 9-2, *C*). Each sarcomere extends from Z line to Z line and is formed by a unique arrangement of two contractile proteins, **actin** and **myosin.** The thin actin filaments extend toward the center of

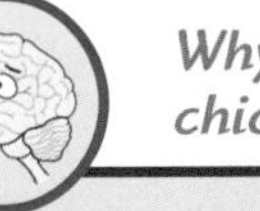

Do You Know...

Why beef is red and chicken meat is white?

Certain muscle fibers contain a reddish-brown pigment called myoglobin. The myoglobin stores oxygen in the muscle and gradually releases it when the muscle starts to work. Fibers that contain myoglobin are red because of the myoglobin pigment. This is the red meat of a steak. Fibers that do not contain myoglobin are white. This is the white meat in a chicken breast.

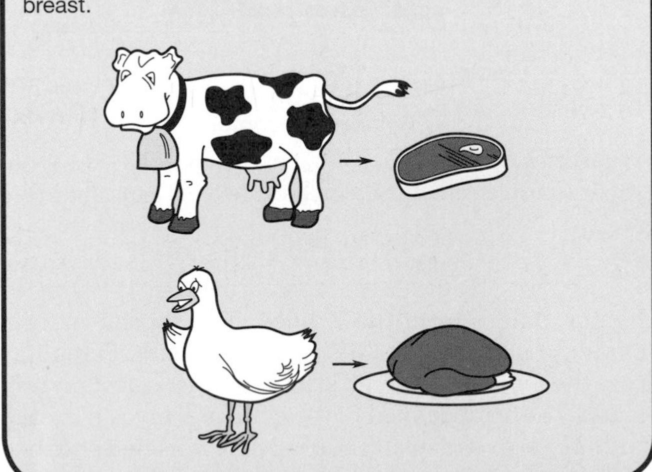

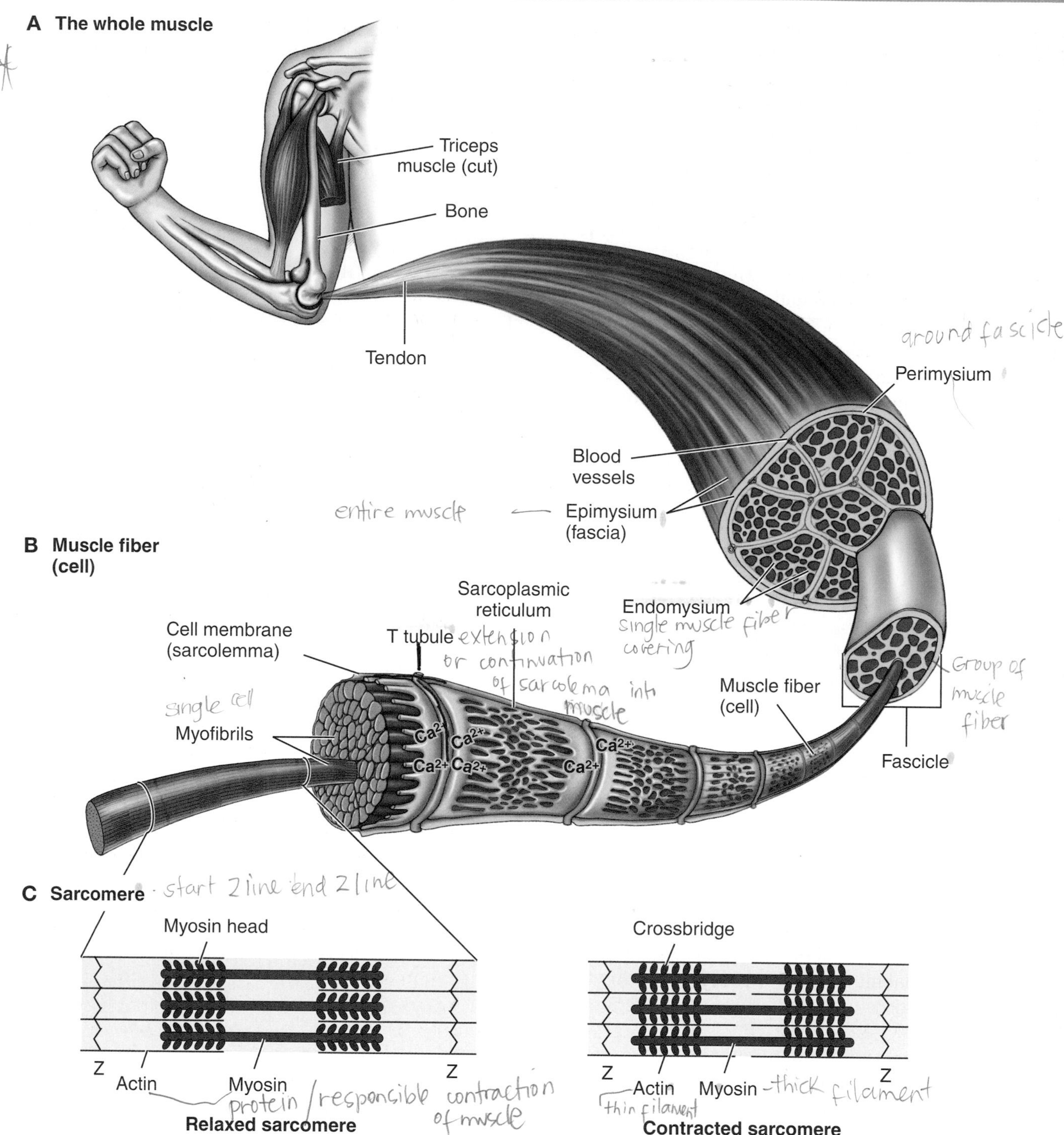

FIGURE 9-2 Muscle structure. **A,** Structure of a whole muscle attached to the bone by a tendon. **B,** Structure of a muscle fiber (muscle cell). **C,** Sarcomeres: relaxed and contracted.

the sarcomere from the Z lines. The thicker myosin filaments sit between the actin filaments. Extending from the myosin filaments are structures called **myosin heads.** The arrangement of the actin and myosin in each sarcomere gives skeletal and cardiac muscle its striped or striated appearance.

HOW MUSCLES CONTRACT

SLIDING FILAMENT THEORY

Muscles can only pull, not push! In order to pull, muscles contract. When muscles contract, they shorten. Muscles shorten because the sarcomeres shorten, and the sarcomeres shorten because the actin and myosin filaments slide past each other. Note how much shorter the contracted sarcomere appears (see Figure 9-2, *C*). How does the sarcomere shorten? When stimulated, the myosin heads make contact with the actin, forming temporary connections called **crossbridges.** Once the crossbridges are formed, the myosin heads rotate, pulling the actin toward the center of the sarcomere. The rotation of the myosin heads causes the actin to slide past the myosin. Muscle relaxation occurs when the crossbridges are broken and the actin and myosin return to their original positions. Because of this sliding activity of actin and myosin, muscle contraction is called the sliding filament theory of muscle contraction.

NOTE: The sarcomeres shorten not because the actin and myosin proteins shrink or shrivel up, but because the proteins slide past one another. The sliding is like a trombone. The trombone shortens because the parts slide past one another, not because the metal shrinks or shrivels. Actin and myosin do the same thing: they slide.

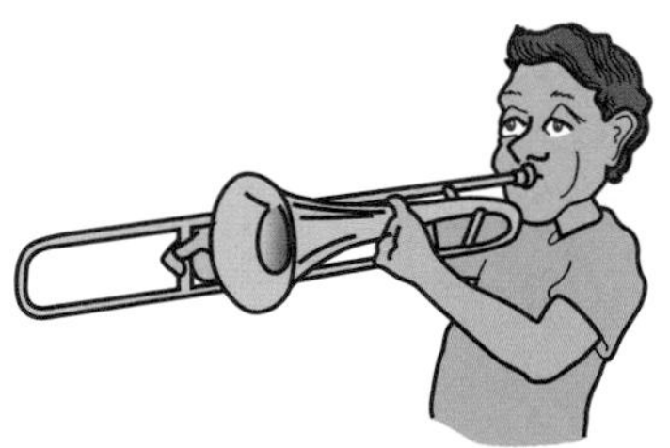

THE ROLE OF CALCIUM AND ATP

Adenosine triphosphate (ATP) and calcium play important roles in the contraction and relaxation of muscle. The ATP helps the myosin heads form and break crossbridges with the actin. The ATP, however, can perform its role only if calcium is present. When the muscle is relaxed, the calcium is stored in the sarcoplasmic reticulum (SR), away from the actin and myosin. When the muscle is stimulated, calcium is released from the SR and causes the actin, myosin, and ATP to interact. Muscle contraction then occurs. When calcium is pumped back into the SR, away from the actin, myosin, and ATP, the crossbridges are broken, and the muscle relaxes.

SKELETAL MUSCLES AND NERVES

SOMATIC MOTOR NEURON

Skeletal muscle contraction can take place only when the muscle is first stimulated by a nerve. The type of nerve that supplies the skeletal muscle is a **motor,** or **somatic nerve** (Figure 9-3, *A*). A motor nerve comes from the spinal cord and supplies several muscle fibers with nerve stimulation. The area where the motor nerve meets the muscle is called the **neuromuscular junction (NMJ)** (see Figure 9-3, *B*). Structures within the NMJ include the membrane at the end of the nerve, the space that exists between the nerve ending and muscle membrane, and the receptor sites on the muscle membrane.

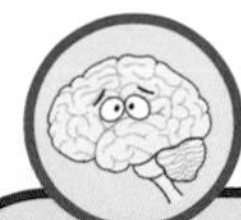

Do You Know...
What the "stiffness of death" is?

Both the formation of crossbridges (muscle contraction) and the detachment of crossbridges (muscle relaxation) depend on ATP. When a person dies, the production of ATP ceases. The deficiency of ATP prevents the detachment of the crossbridges, so muscles remain contracted and become stiff. This change is called rigor mortis, or "stiffness of death." An assessment of rigor mortis often helps determine the exact time of death. For instance, rigor begins 2 hours after death, peaks in 12 hours, and is over (subsides) in 36 hours. By assessing the degree of rigor, one can therefore determine the time of death. This fact has been used successfully in murder mysteries. By altering the environmental temperature, the murderer can alter the time course of rigor mortis and therefore make it difficult to determine the time of death.

THE NEUROMUSCULAR JUNCTION

What happens at the NMJ? The stimulated nerve causes the release of a chemical substance that diffuses across the NMJ and stimulates the muscle membrane. Four steps are involved in the transfer of the information from nerve to muscle at the NMJ (see Figure 9-3, *B*).

- Step 1: Stimulation of the nerve causes an electrical signal, or nerve impulse, to move along the nerve toward the nerve ending. Stored within the nerve ending are vesicles, or membranous pouches, filled with a chemical substance called a **neurotransmitter.** The neurotransmitter at the NMJ is **acetylcholine (ACh)** (ăs-Ē-tĭl-KŌ-lēn).
- Step 2: The nerve impulse causes the vesicles to move toward and fuse with the nerve ending. ACh is released from the vesicles into the space between the nerve ending and the muscle membrane.
- Step 3: ACh diffuses across the space and binds to the receptor sites on the muscle membrane.
- Step 4: The ACh stimulates the receptors and causes an electrical signal to develop along the muscle membrane. The ACh then unbinds the receptor site and is immediately destroyed by an enzyme that is found within the NMJ near the muscle membrane. The name of the enzyme is **acetylcholinesterase.** The free-binding sites are then ready for additional ACh when the nerve is stimulated again.

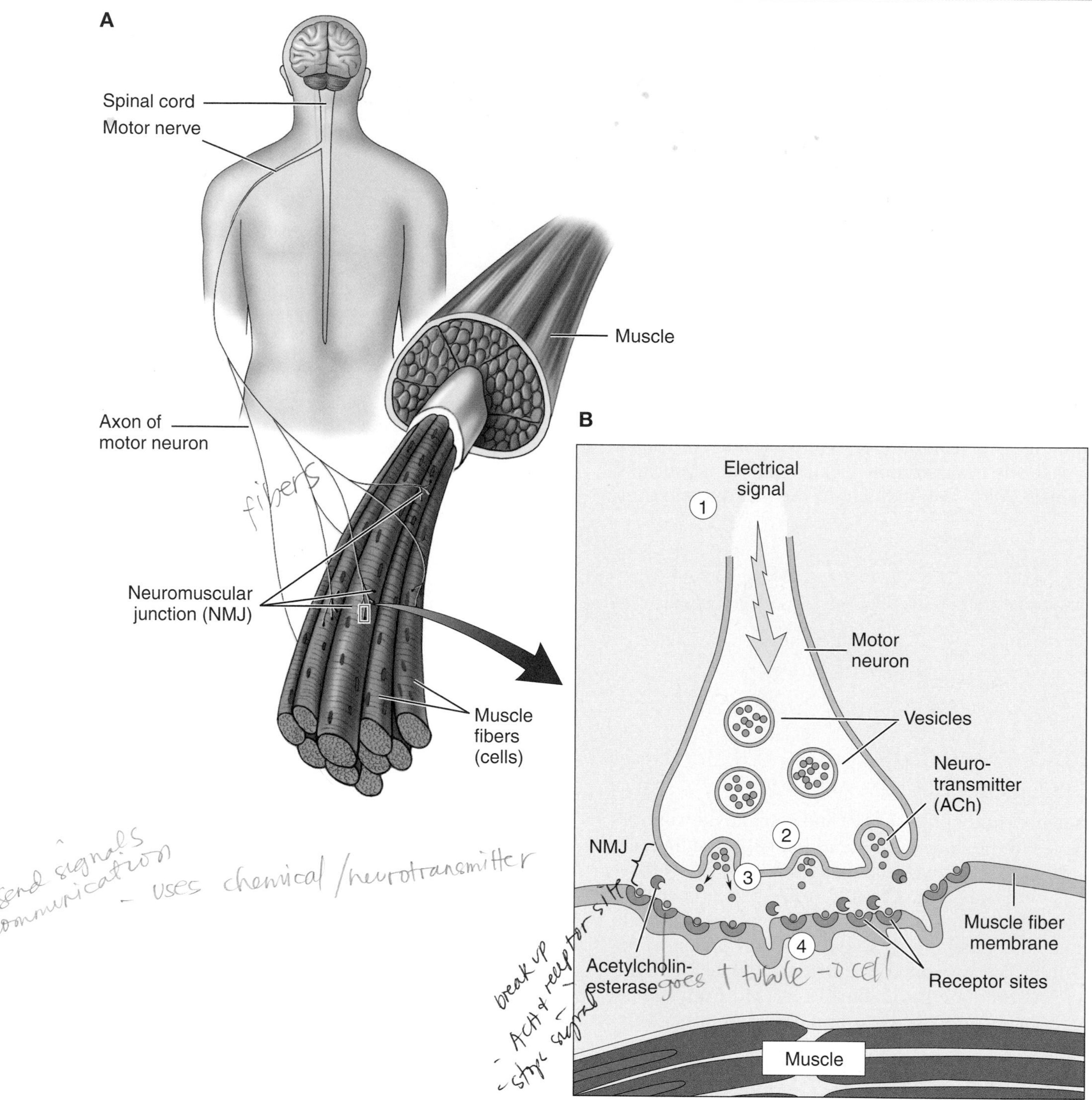

FIGURE 9-3 **A,** Muscle fibers and their motor neuron. **B,** The four steps in the transmission of the signal at the neuromuscular junction (NMJ).

The Stimulated Muscle Membrane

What happens to the electrical signal in the muscle membrane? It travels along the muscle membrane and triggers a series of events that result in muscle contraction (see Figure 9-2, *B*). Specifically, the electrical signal travels along the muscle cell membrane and penetrates into its interior through the T tubules. The electrical signal stimulates the sarcoplasmic reticulum to release calcium. The calcium floods the sarcomeres and allows for the interaction of actin, myosin, and ATP, producing muscle contraction. Eventually, the calcium is pumped back into the sarcoplasmic reticulum, away from the actin and myosin, causing muscle relaxation.

Disorders of the Neuromuscular Junction

Certain conditions can cause problems at the NMJ (Figure 9-4).

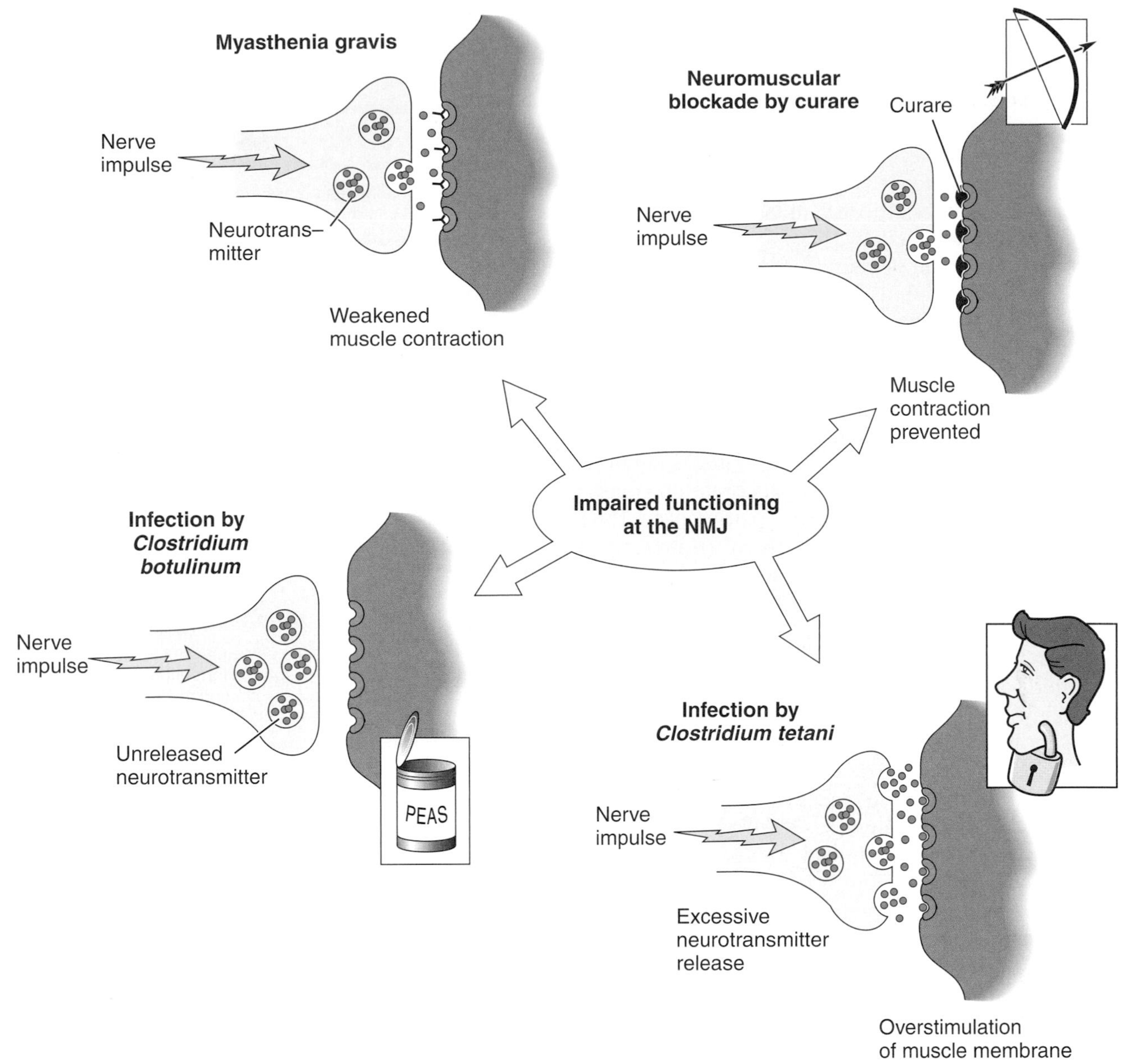

FIGURE 9-4 Abnormal functioning at the NMJ.

Myasthenia Gravis. Myasthenia gravis is a disease that affects the NMJ. The symptoms of the disease are due to damaged receptor sites on the muscle membrane. The receptor sites are altered so that they cannot bind ACh. Consequently, muscle contraction is impaired, and the person experiences extreme muscle weakness. (The word *myasthenia* means muscle weakness.) The muscle weakness becomes noticeable as low tolerance to exercise. As the disease progresses the person experiences difficulty in breathing since the breathing muscles are skeletal muscles.

Neuromuscular Blockade Caused by Curare. Curare is a drug classified as a skeletal muscle blocker. Skeletal muscle blockers are often used during surgery to promote muscle relaxation. Curare works by blocking the receptor sites on the muscle membrane. Because the receptors are occupied by the drug, the ACh cannot bind with the receptor sites, and muscle contraction is prevented.

Because the respiratory muscles are also affected by curare, the patient must be mechanically ventilated until the effects of the drug disappear. Otherwise, the patient stops breathing and dies. Historically, curare was used as a paralyzing drug in hunting animals. The tip of an arrowhead was dipped in curare. When the arrow pierced the skin of the animal, the curare was absorbed and eventually caused skeletal muscle blockade and paralysis.

Effects of Neurotoxins on Muscle Function. Neurotoxins are chemical substances that in some way disrupt normal function of the nervous system. Neurotoxins are produced by certain bacteria. For example, *Clostridium tetani* (a bacterium) secretes a neurotoxin that causes excessive firing of the motor nerves. This, in turn, causes excessive release of ACh, overstimulation of the muscle membrane, and severe muscle spasm and tetanic contractions. Hence the name **tetanus.** Because the muscles of the jaw are the first muscles affected, the disease is often called lockjaw.

A second neurotoxin is secreted by the bacterium *Clostridium botulinum.* This bacterium appears most often when food has been improperly processed and canned. Infection with this organism causes a disease known as botulism, a very serious form of food poisoning. The neurotoxin works by preventing the release of acetylcholine from the ends of the nerves within the NMJ. Without acetylcholine, the muscle fibers cannot contract, and the muscles, including the breathing muscles, become paralyzed. On a more positive note, the injection of small amounts of the "poison" (Botox) has been used successfully to treat severe muscle spasm (wryneck) and to erase muscle-induced wrinkles for cosmetic reasons.

Receptor Terminology. The somatic motor neuron is a cholinergic fiber and therefore secretes ACh as its neurotransmitter. The receptor on the muscle membrane is a cholinergic receptor; it is called a nicotinic receptor. Because it is located on the muscle membrane it is called a Nicotinic $_{\text{Muscle}}$ (N_M) receptor. There is a great deal of pharmacology that involves the N_M receptor. For instance, curare is a skeletal muscle blocker because it blocks the N_M receptor. Receptor blockade in turn prevents skeletal muscle contraction. What about a drug that activates the N_M receptor? It stimulates muscle contraction. For instance, neostigmine (Prostigmin) is a drug that inactivates cholinesterase (the enzyme that destroys ACh) thereby increasing the amount of ACh that can bind to the N_M receptors. (Because this drug inactivates cholinesterase it is called an anticholinesterase agent.) You can now understand why anticholinesterase agents improve the symptoms of myasthenia gravis and reverse postoperative sluggish intestinal activity.

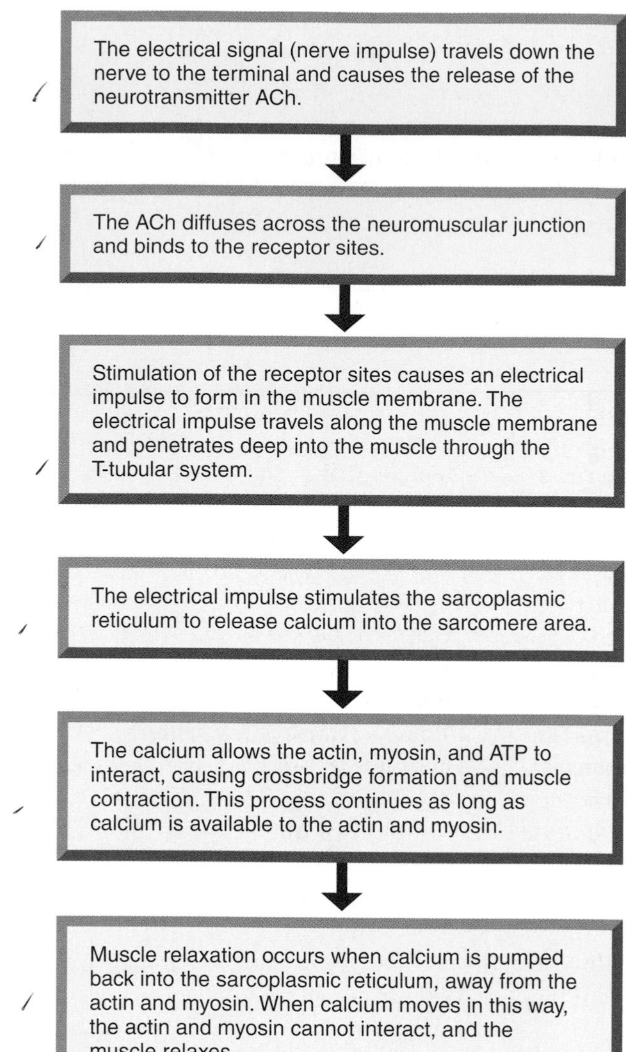

The electrical signal (nerve impulse) travels down the nerve to the terminal and causes the release of the neurotransmitter ACh.
The ACh diffuses across the neuromuscular junction and binds to the receptor sites.
Stimulation of the receptor sites causes an electrical impulse to form in the muscle membrane. The electrical impulse travels along the muscle membrane and penetrates deep into the muscle through the T-tubular system.
The electrical impulse stimulates the sarcoplasmic reticulum to release calcium into the sarcomere area.
The calcium allows the actin, myosin, and ATP to interact, causing crossbridge formation and muscle contraction. This process continues as long as calcium is available to the actin and myosin.
Muscle relaxation occurs when calcium is pumped back into the sarcoplasmic reticulum, away from the actin and myosin. When calcium moves in this way, the actin and myosin cannot interact, and the muscle relaxes.

FIGURE 9-5 Steps in contraction and relaxation of skeletal muscle.

Sum It Up!

The three types of muscle are skeletal, smooth, and cardiac. A whole muscle is composed of many muscle fibers (muscle cells) arranged in bundles. Each muscle fiber contains the contractile proteins actin and myosin, arranged into a series of sarcomeres. In accordance with the sliding filament theory, the interaction of the actin and myosin causes muscle contraction. Figure 9-5 summarizes the steps involved in the contraction and relaxation of skeletal muscle. Note the crucial role played by the motor nerve and the NMJ.

Do You Know...

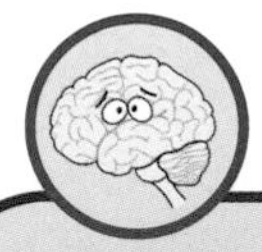

What the difference is between isometric contraction and isotonic contraction?

An isotonic muscle contraction is a muscle contraction that causes movement. Examples include jogging, swimming, and weight lifting. An isometric muscle contraction is a muscle contraction that does not cause movement. For example, if you try to lift a 1000-lb object, your muscles contract but do not move the object (it is too heavy).

As you sit reading this text, you can do isometric exercises. Tighten the muscle in your thigh. Hold the tension for 30 seconds and then relax the muscle. Repetition of this type of exercise can provide you with a mini-workout without leaving your desk.

RESPONSES OF A WHOLE MUSCLE

The sliding filament theory explains the contraction and relaxation of a single muscle fiber. A whole skeletal muscle, however, is composed of thousands of muscle fibers. The contractile response of a whole muscle differs from that of a single muscle fiber in a number of ways.

PARTIAL VERSUS ALL-OR-NOTHING RESPONSE

A single muscle fiber contracts in an all-or-nothing response. In other words, the single fiber contracts maximally (as strongly as possible), or it does not contract at all. It never partially contracts. A whole muscle, however, is capable of contracting partially; it can contract weakly or very strongly. For instance, only a small force of contraction is required to lift a pencil. A much greater force is required to lift a 100-lb weight.

How can a whole muscle vary its strength of contraction? Lifting the pencil may require the contraction of several hundred muscle fibers. These fibers contract in an all-or-nothing manner, but only a few fibers are contracting. Lifting a 100-lb weight, however, requires contraction of thousands of fibers, all contracting in an all-or-nothing manner. The greater muscle force is achieved by using, or recruiting, additional fibers. This process is called **recruitment.** Thus the strength of skeletal muscle contraction can be varied by recruitment of additional muscle fibers.

Twitch and Tetanus

Several important terms describe whole-muscle contraction. They include twitch and tetanus. Of the two, tetanus is the more important.

Twitch. If a single stimulus is delivered to a muscle, the muscle contracts and then fully relaxes. This single muscle response is termed a **twitch.** Twitches are not useful physiologically.

Tetanus. If the muscle is stimulated repeatedly, the muscle has no time to relax and remains contracted. Sustained muscle contraction is called **tetanus.** Tetanic muscle contractions play an important role in maintaining posture. If the muscles that maintain our upright posture merely twitched, we would be unable to stand and would instead twitch and flop around on the ground (not a pretty sight). Because the muscle is able to tetanize, we are able to maintain an upright posture. Fatigue occurs if the muscle is not allowed to rest. (Do not confuse the tetanus described in this section with the disease called tetanus, or lockjaw.)

MUSCLE TONE

Muscle tone, or **tonus,** refers to a normal, continuous state of partial muscle contraction. Tone is due to the contraction of different groups of muscle fibers within a whole muscle. To maintain muscle tone, one group of muscle fibers contracts first. As these fibers begin to relax, a second group contracts. This pattern of contraction and relaxation continues so as to maintain muscle tone. Muscle tone plays a number of important roles. For instance, the muscle tone of the smooth muscle in blood vessels helps to maintain blood pressure. If the muscle tone were to decrease, the person might experience a life-threatening decline in blood pressure.

ENERGY SOURCE FOR MUSCLE CONTRACTION

Muscle contraction requires a rich supply of energy (ATP). As ATP is consumed by the contracting muscle, it is replaced in three ways:

1. Aerobic metabolism: In the presence of oxygen, fuel such as glycogen, glucose, and fats can be completely broken down to yield energy (ATP).
2. Anaerobic metabolism: The body can also metabolize fuel in the absence of oxygen. When oxygen is not present, however, complete breakdown of the fuel is not possible, and **lactic acid** is produced. The accumulation of lactic acid may be responsible for some of the muscle soreness that accompanies heavy exercise.
3. Metabolism of creatine phosphate: Creatine phosphate contains energy that the body can use to replenish ATP quickly during muscle contraction. As a storage form of energy, creatine phosphate ensures that skeletal muscle can operate for long periods.

Do You Know...

What the good news is about oxygen debt?

Credit card debt—bad; oxygen debt—good! What's so great about oxygen debt? The payment of an oxygen debt means that you continue to expend energy and burn fat, long after you have come off the treadmill and have taken to your couch. In other words, you continue to exercise metabolically while recovering from your workout. This is how it works. When a person exercises strenuously, he or she burns fuel (fat). To do this, the body uses up available oxygen and borrows on the additional stores of oxygen found in the hemoglobin in blood and the myoglobin in muscles. When he or she stops exercising, the body requires an increased intake of oxygen to do some additional, exercise-induced metabolic work (to convert lactic acid to glucose), so 30 minutes of exercise is actually more than 30 minutes of exercise.

MUSCLE TERMS

ORIGIN AND INSERTION

The terms origin and insertion refer to the sites of muscle attachment. When muscle contracts across a joint, one bone remains relatively stationary or immovable. The **origin** of the muscle attaches to the stationary bone, while the **insertion** attaches to the more movable bone (Figure 9-6). For instance, the origin of the biceps brachii is the scapula, while the insertion is on the radius. On contraction of the biceps brachii, the radius (insertion) is pulled toward the scapula (origin).

PRIME MOVER, SYNERGIST, AND ANTAGONIST

Although most movement is accomplished through the cooperation of groups of muscles, a single muscle is generally responsible for most of the movement. The "chief muscle" is called the **prime mover.** Assisting the prime mover are "helper muscles" called **synergists** (SĬN-ĕr-jĭst). Synergists are said to work with other muscles. In contrast, **antagonists** are muscles that oppose the action of another muscle. For instance, contraction of the biceps brachii pulls the lower arm toward the shoulder. The triceps brachii (upper arm, posterior) is the antagonist. It opposes the action of the biceps brachii by pulling the lower arm away from the scapula (see Figure 9-6).

MUSCLE OVERUSE AND UNDERUSE TERMS

Hypertrophy

Overused muscles increase in size. This response to overuse is called hypertrophy. Athletes intentionally cause their muscles to hypertrophy. Weight lifters, for instance, develop larger muscles than do couch potatoes.

Like skeletal muscle, cardiac muscle can also hypertrophy. Cardiac hypertrophy is generally undesirable and usually indicates an underlying disease causing the heart to overwork. Hypertension, for instance, causes the heart to push blood into blood vessels that are very resistant to the flow of blood. This extra work causes the heart muscle to enlarge.

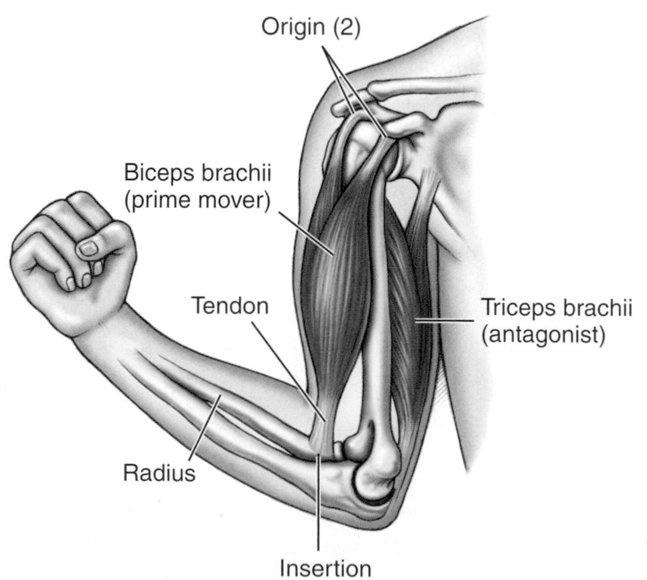

FIGURE 9-6 Origin and insertion/antagonists.

Atrophy

If muscles are not used, they will waste away, or decrease in size. A person with a broken leg in a cast, for instance, is unable to exercise that leg for several months. This lack of exercise causes the muscles of the leg to atrophy. When weight bearing and exercise are resumed, muscle size and strength can be restored.

Contracture

If a muscle is immobilized for a prolonged period, it may develop a contracture. A contracture is an abnormal formation of fibrous tissue within the muscle. It generally "freezes" the muscle in a flexed position and severely restricts joint mobility.

HOW SKELETAL MUSCLES ARE NAMED

The names of the various skeletal muscles are generally based on one or more of the following characteristics: size, shape, orientation of the fibers, location, number of origins, identification of origin and insertion, and muscle action.

SIZE

These terms indicate size: vastus (huge); maximus (large); longus (long); minimus (small); and brevis (short). Examples of skeletal muscles include vastus lateralis and gluteus maximus.

SHAPE

Various shapes are included in muscle names: deltoid (triangular); latissimus (wide); trapezius (trapezoid); rhomboideus (rhomboid); and teres (round). Examples include the trapezius muscle, the latissimus dorsi, and the teres major.

DIRECTION OF FIBERS

Fibers are oriented, or lined up, in several directions: rectus (straight); oblique (diagonal); transverse (across); and circularis (circular). Examples include rectus abdominis and the superior oblique.

LOCATION

The names of muscles often reflect their location in the body: pectoralis (chest); gluteus (buttock); brachii (arm); supra (above); infra (below); sub (underneath); and lateralis (lateral). Examples include biceps brachii, pectoralis major, and vastus lateralis.

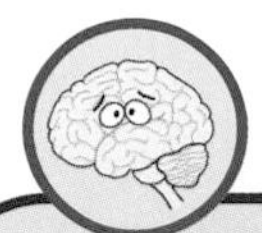

Do You Know...

What is wrong with bulking up?

Nothing is wrong with bulking up if it is done through weight lifting, exercise, and a healthy diet. Bulking up with the use of steroids, however, is dangerous. Steroids are thought to cause liver cancer, atrophy of the testicles in males, hypertension, and severe psychotic mood swings, among other health-related effects.

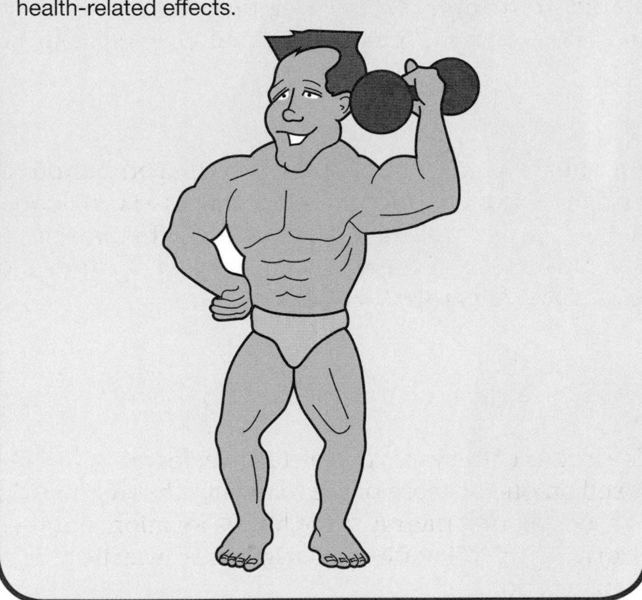

NUMBER OF ORIGINS

The muscle may be named according to the number of sites to which it is anchored: biceps (2); triceps (3); and quadriceps (4). Examples include the biceps brachii, triceps brachii, and quadriceps femoris.

ORIGIN AND INSERTION

Some muscles are named for sites of attachment both at the origin and insertion. The sternocleidomastoid, for example, has its origin on the sternum and clavicle and its insertion on the mastoid (temporal bone). This information allows you to determine the function of the muscle. The sternocleidomastoid flexes the neck and rotates the head.

MUSCLE ACTION

The action of the muscle may be included in the name. For instance, an abductor muscle moves the limb away from the midline of the body, while an adductor moves the limb toward the midline. In the same way, a flexor muscle causes flexion, while an extensor muscle straightens the limb. A levator muscle elevates a structure, and a masseter muscle enables you to chew. Examples include the adductor magnus, flexor digitorum, and levator palpebrae superioris.

MUSCLES FROM HEAD TO TOE

Figure 9-7 shows the major skeletal muscles of the body. Details of muscle location and function are summarized in Table 9-1.

MUSCLES OF THE HEAD

The muscles of the head are grouped into two categories: the facial muscles and the chewing muscles (Figure 9-8).

Facial Muscles

Many of the facial muscles are inserted directly into the soft tissue of the skin and other muscles of the face. When the facial muscles contract, they pull on the soft tissue. This kind of muscular activity is responsible for our facial expressions like smiling and frowning.

- Frontalis: The **frontalis** is a flat muscle that covers the frontal bone. It extends from the cranial aponeurosis to the skin of the eyebrows. Contraction of the muscle raises the eyebrows, giving you a surprised look. It also wrinkles your forehead.
- Orbicularis oculi: The **orbicularis oculi** is a sphincter muscle that encircles the eyes. A **sphincter** is a ring-shaped muscle that controls the size of an opening. Contraction of the muscle closes the eye and assists in winking, blinking, and squinting.
- Orbicularis oris: The **orbicularis oris** is a sphincter muscle that encircles the mouth. Contraction of this muscle assists in closing the mouth, forming words, and pursing the lips. It is sometimes called the kissing muscle.
- Buccinator: The **buccinator** is a muscle that inserts into the orbicularis oris and flattens the cheek when contracted. The buccinator is used in whistling and playing the trumpet. The buccinator is also considered a chewing muscle because on contraction, it helps position the food between the teeth for chewing.
- Zygomaticus: The **zygomaticus** is the smiling muscle; it extends from the corners of the mouth to the cheekbone.

Chewing Muscles

The chewing muscles are also called the muscles of **mastication** (chewing). All of them are inserted on the mandible, or lower jaw bone, and are considered some of the strongest muscles of the body (see Table 9-1).

Text continued on p. 152.

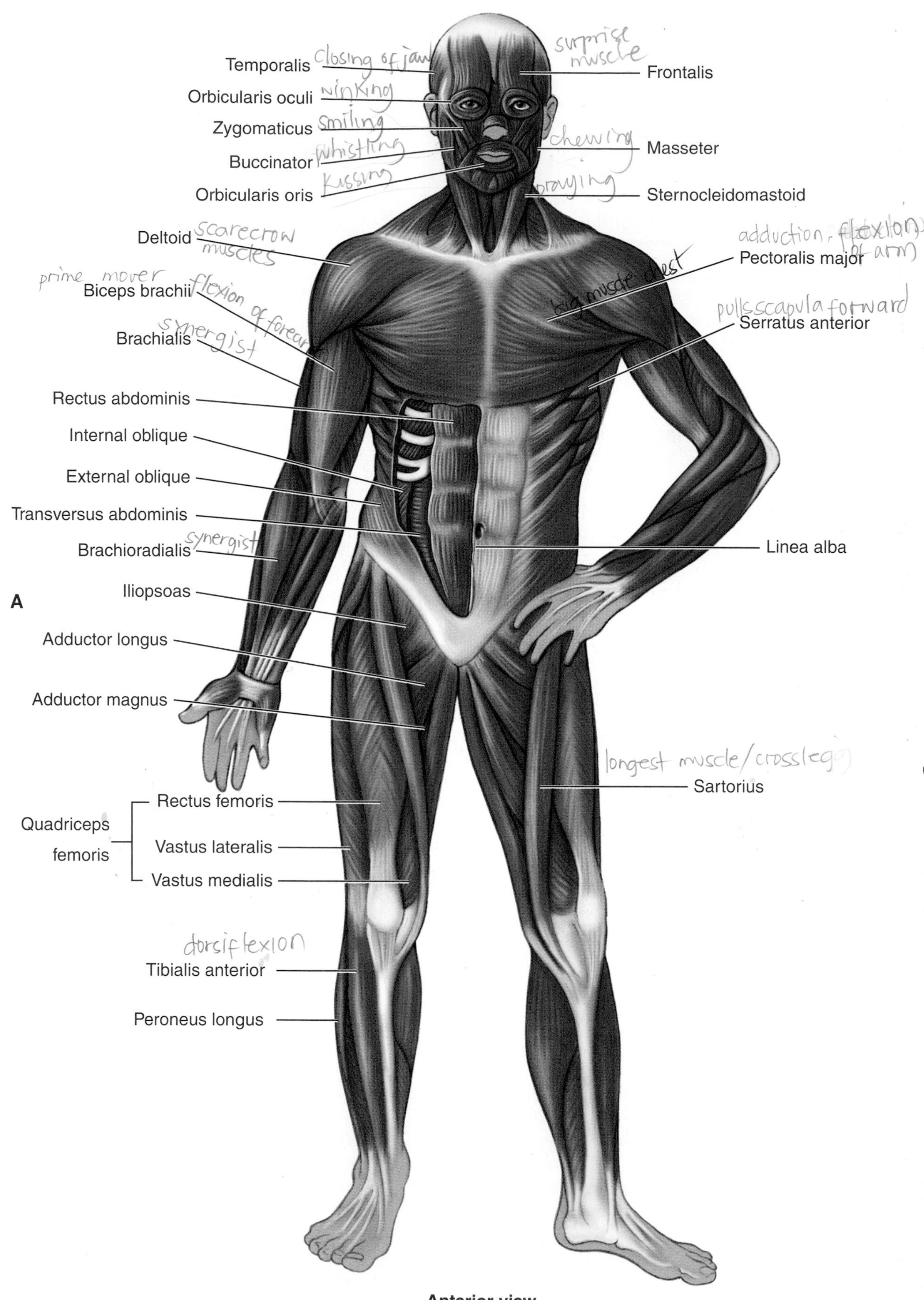

FIGURE 9-7 Major muscles of the body. **A,** Anterior view.

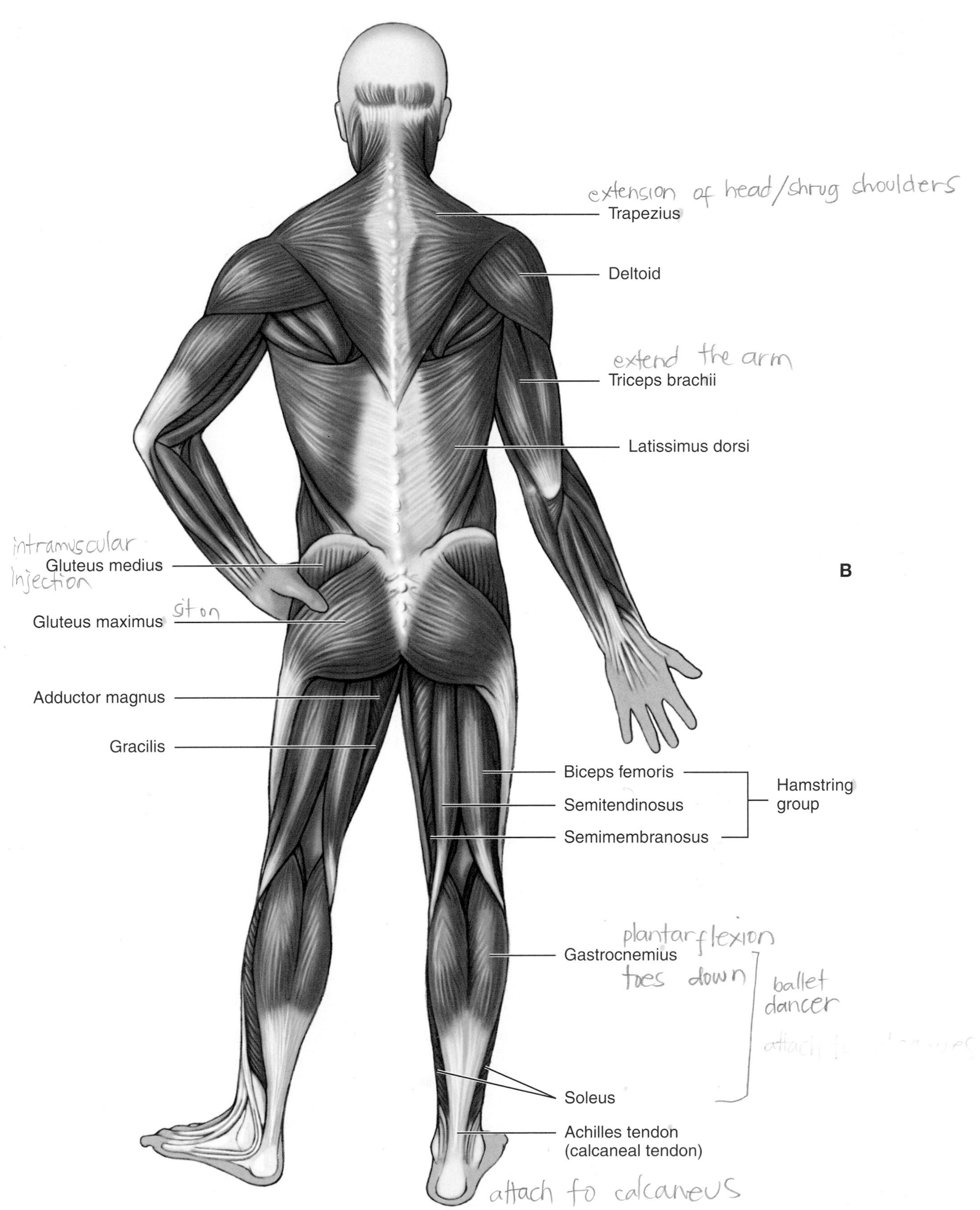

FIGURE 9-7, cont'd Major muscles of the body. **B,** Posterior view.

Table 9-1 Muscles of the Body

Muscle	Description	Function
Head		
Facial Muscles		
Frontalis	Flat muscle covering the forehead	Raises eyebrows; surprised look; wrinkles forehead
Orbicularis oculi	Circular muscle around eye	Closes eyes; winking, blinking, and squinting
Levator palpebrae superioris	Back of eye to upper eyelid	Opens eyes
Orbicularis oris	Circular muscle around mouth	Closes/purses lips; kissing muscle
Buccinator	Horizontal cheek muscle	Flattens the cheek; trumpeter's muscle; whistling muscle; helps with chewing
Zygomaticus	Extends from the corner of the mouth to cheekbone	Elevates corner of mouth; smiling muscle
Chewing Muscles		
Temporalis	Flat fan-shaped muscle over temporal bone	Closes jaw
Masseter	Covers the lateral part of the lower jaw	Closes jaw
Neck		
Sternocleidomastoid	Extends along the side of the neck; strong narrow muscle that extends obliquely from the sternum and clavicle to the mastoid process of the temporal bone	Flexes and rotates the head; praying muscle
Trapezius	Large, flat triangular muscle on the back of the neck and upper back to shoulders	Extends head so as to look at the sky; elevates shoulder and pulls it back; shrugs the shoulders
Trunk		
Muscles Involved in Breathing		
External intercostals	Intercostal spaces (between ribs)	Breathing (enlarges thoracic cavity)
Internal intercostals	Intercostal spaces (between ribs)	Breathing (decreases thoracic cavity in forced expiration)
Diaphragm	Dome-shaped muscle that separates the thoracic and abdominal cavities	Breathing: chief muscle of inspiration (enlarges thoracic cavity)
Muscles of abdominal wall External oblique Internal oblique Transversus abdominis Rectus abdominis	The muscles are arranged vertically, horizontally, and obliquely so as to strengthen the abdominal wall	As a group, the abdominal wall muscles compress the abdomen; the rectus abdominis also flexes the vertebral column
Muscles of the vertebral column	Muscles attached to the vertebrae	Movement of vertebral column
Muscles of the pelvic floor	Flat muscle sheets	Support pelvic viscera; assist in the function of the genitalia
Muscles That Move the Shoulder and Upper Arm		
Trapezius	Broad muscle on posterior neck and shoulder	Extends the head; looks at the sky Elevates shoulder and pulls it back; shrugs the shoulders
Serratus anterior	Forms the upper sides of the chest wall below the axilla	Pulls scapula forward; aids in raising arms
Pectoralis major	Large muscle that covers upper anterior chest	Adducts and flexes upper arm across chest Pulls shoulder forward and downward
Latissimus dorsi	Large broad flat muscle on mid and lower back	Adducts and rotates arm behind the back; "swimmer's muscle"
Deltoid	Thick muscle that covers the shoulder joint	Abducts arm as in "scarecrow" position
Rotator cuff muscles Supraspinatus Subscapularis Infraspinatus Teres minor	A group of four muscles that attaches the humerus to the scapula; tendons form a cuff over the proximal humerus	Rotate the arm at the shoulder joint

Table 9-1 Muscles of the Body—cont'd

Muscle	Description	Function
Muscles That Move the Forearm and Hand		
Biceps brachii	Major muscle on anterior surface of upper arm	Flexes and supinates forearm; muscle used to "make a muscle"; acts synergistically with brachialis and brachioradialis
Triceps brachii	Posterior surface of upper arm	Extends forearm; "boxer's muscle"
Brachialis	Deep to biceps brachii	Flexes forearm
Brachioradialis	Muscles of forearm	Flexes forearm
Flexor and extensor carpi groups	Anterior and posterior forearm to hand	Flex and extend hand
Flexor and extensor digitorum groups	Anterior and posterior forearm to fingers	Flex and extend fingers
Muscles That Move the Thigh		
Gluteus maximus	Largest and most superficial of the gluteal muscles; located on posterior surface of the buttocks	Forms the buttocks; extends the thigh; muscle for sitting and climbing stairs
Gluteus medius	Thick muscle partly behind and superior to the gluteus maximus	Abducts and rotates thigh; common site of intramuscular injections
Gluteus minimus	Smallest and deepest of the gluteal muscles	Abducts and rotates the thigh
Iliopsoas	Located on anterior surface of groin; crosses over hip joint to the femur	Flexes the thigh; antagonist to gluteus maximus
Adductor group	Medial inner thigh region	Adducts thigh; muscles used by horseback riders to stay on horse
Adductor longus		
Adductor brevis		
Adductor magnus		
Gracilis		
Muscles That Move the Leg		
Quadriceps femoris	Located on anterior and lateral surface of thigh; form a common tendon that inserts in tibia	Group used to extend the leg (e.g., kicking)
Rectus femoris		Rectus femoris can flex thigh at the hip joint
Vastus lateralis		Vastus lateralis is a common site for intramuscular injections in children
Vastus medialis		
Vastus intermedius		
Sartorius	Long muscle that crosses obliquely over the anterior thigh	Allows you to sit in crossed leg or lotus position
Hamstrings	Located on posterior surface of thigh; as a group they attach to the tibia and fibula	Flex leg; extend thigh; antagonistic to quadriceps femoris
Biceps femoris		
Semitendinosus		
Semimembranosus		
Muscles That Move the Ankle and Foot		
Tibialis anterior	Anterior leg	Dorsiflexes foot; inversion of foot
Peroneus longus	Lateral surface of leg	Plantar flexion; eversion of foot; supports arch
Gastrocnemius	Posterior surface of leg; large two-headed muscle that forms the calf	Plantar flexion of foot; toe-dancer muscle
Soleus	Posterior surface of leg	Plantar flexion of foot

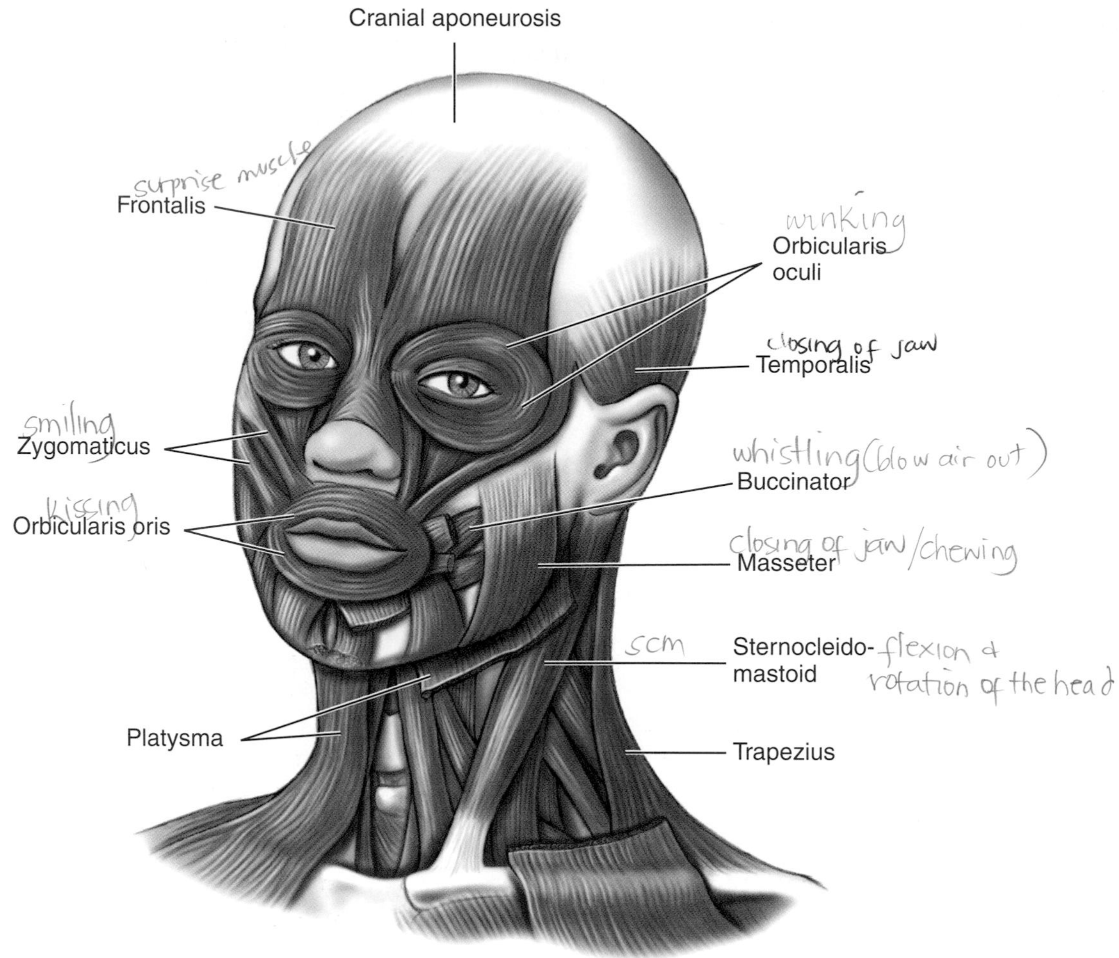

FIGURE 9-8 Muscles of the head and neck.

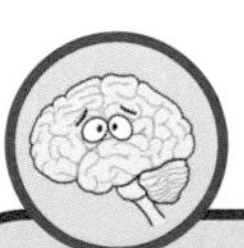

Do You Know...

About the "droops and drools" of Botox?

In the arsenal of antiaging drugs, Botox is a star. It is the wrinkle-remover par excellence. Beware of Botox blunders, however. Misplaced Botox around the eyelids can cause droopy lids. Similarly, poor aim around the mouth region can cause drooling. Mercifully, the effects of Botox gradually wear off, although there may be many weeks during which you sport the droop and drool look. Botched batches of Botox have also caused severe, long-term paralysis.

- Masseter: The **masseter** is a muscle that extends from the zygomatic process of the temporal bone in the skull to the mandible. Contraction of this muscle closes the jaw. It acts synergistically (works with) with the temporalis muscle to close the jaw.
- Temporalis: The **temporalis** is a fan-shaped muscle that extends from the flat portion of the temporal bone to the mandible. It works synergistically with the other chewing muscles.

MUSCLES OF THE NECK

Many muscles are involved in the movement of the head and shoulders and participate in movements within the throat.

Sternocleidomastoid

As the name implies, the **sternocleidomastoid** muscle extends from the sternum and clavicle to the mastoid process of the temporal bone in the skull. Contraction of both muscles on either side of the neck causes flexion of the head. Because the head bows as if in prayer, the muscle is called the praying muscle. Contraction of only one of the sternocleidomastoid muscles causes the head to rotate toward the opposite direction. A spasm of this muscle can cause torticollis, or wryneck. This condition is characterized by the twisting of the neck and rotation of the head to one side. Botox has been used successfully in the treatment of torticollis.

Trapezius

The **trapezius** has its origins at the base of the occipital bone in the skull and to the spine of the upper vertebral column (see Figure 9-7, *B*). Contraction of the trapezius allows the head to tilt back so that the face looks at the sky. The trapezius works antagonistically with the sternocleidomastoid muscle, which flexes and bows the head. The trapezius is also attached to and moves the shoulder.

MUSCLES OF THE TRUNK

The muscles of the trunk are involved in breathing, form the abdominal wall, move the vertebral column, and form the pelvic region.

Muscles Involved in Breathing

The chest, or thoracic, muscles include the intercostal muscles and the diaphragm. These muscles are primarily responsible for breathing (Figure 9-9). The **intercostal muscles** are located between the ribs and are responsible for raising and lowering the rib cage during breathing. External and internal intercostal muscles are attached to the rib cage; the ribs (bone appetít!) you barbecue are the intercostals.

The **diaphragm** is a dome-shaped muscle that separates the thoracic cavity from the abdominal cavity. The diaphragm is the chief muscle of inhalation, the breathing-in phase of respiration. Without the contraction and relaxation of the intercostal muscles and the diaphragm, breathing can not occur. The role of these muscles is described in Chapter 22.

Muscles That Form the Abdominal Wall

The abdominal wall consists of four muscles (see Figure 9-7, *A*) in an arrangement that provides considerable strength. The muscles are layered so that the fibers of each of the four muscles run in four different directions. This arrangement enables the muscles to contain, support, and protect the abdominal organs. Contraction of the abdominal muscles performs other functions. It causes flexion of the vertebral column and compression of the abdominal organs during urination, defecation, and childbirth.

The four abdominal muscles include the following:

- *Rectus abdominis:* As the name implies, the fibers of the **rectus abdominis** run in an up-and-down, or longitudinal, direction. They extend from the sternum to the pubic bone. Contraction of this muscle flexes, or bends, the vertebral column.
- *External oblique:* Abdominal muscles called the **external obliques** make up the lateral walls of the abdomen. The fibers run obliquely (slanted).
- *Internal oblique:* The **internal oblique** muscles are part of the lateral walls of the abdomen. They add to the strength provided by the external oblique muscles, as the fibers of the oblique muscles form a crisscross pattern.
- *Transversus abdominis:* The **transversus abdominis** muscles form the innermost layer of the abdominal muscles. The fibers run horizontally across the abdomen.

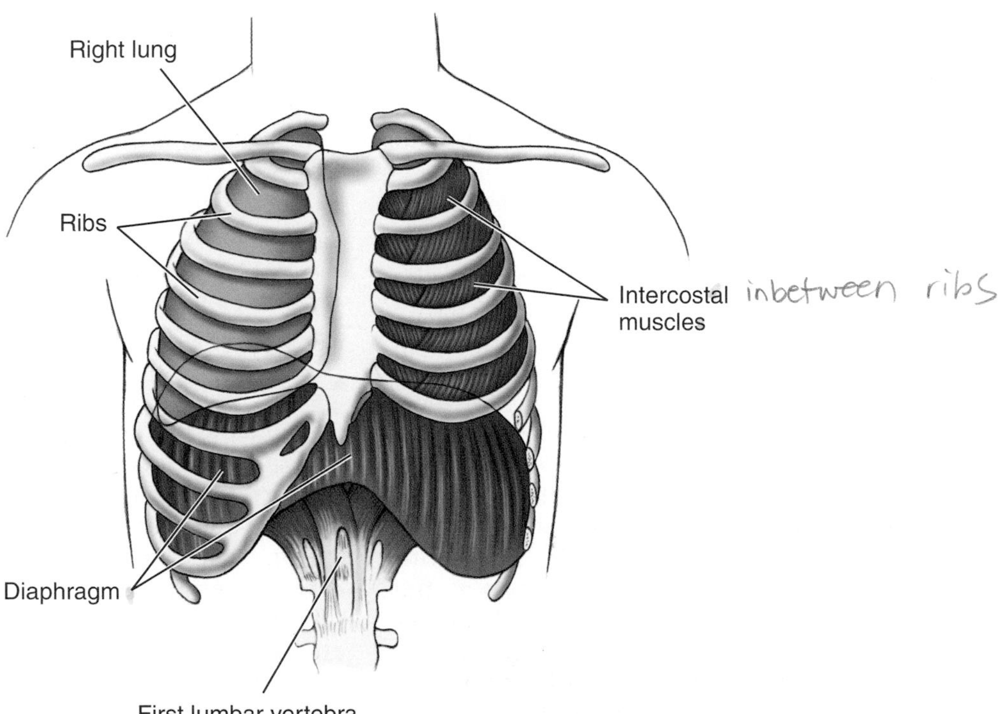

FIGURE 9-9 Breathing muscles. The intercostal muscles and the diaphragm.

To remember the abdominal muscles, think of that spare **TIRE.**

T transversus abdominis
I internal oblique
R rectus abdominis
E external oblique

The abdominal muscles are surrounded by fascia that forms a large aponeurosis along the midline of the abdominal wall. The aponeuroses of the abdominal muscles on opposite sides of the midline of the abdomen form a white line called the **linea alba.** The linea alba extends from the sternum to the pubic bone.

Muscles That Move the Vertebral Column

A group of muscles is attached to the vertebrae. These muscles assist in the movement of the vertebral column.

Muscles That Form the Pelvic Floor

The pelvic floor consists primarily of two flat muscle sheets and the surrounding fascia. These structures support the pelvic viscera and play a role in expelling the contents of the urinary bladder and rectum.

MUSCLES OF THE SHOULDER AND UPPER ARM

Many muscles move the shoulder and the upper arm. The most important are the trapezius, serratus anterior, pectoralis major, latissimus dorsi, deltoid muscles, and a group of muscles called the rotator cuff muscles (see Figure 9-7, *B*).

- Trapezius: The **trapezius** attaches to the base of the occipital bone (skull), thoracic vertebrae, and scapula (the wing bone or shoulder blade). When contracted, the trapezius shrugs the shoulders. The muscle gets its name because the right and left trapezius form the shape of a trapezoid.
- Serratus anterior: The **serratus anterior** is located on the sides of the chest and extends from the ribs to the scapula. The serratus muscle has a jagged shape, much like the jagged edge of a serrated knife blade. When the serratus anterior contracts, the shoulders are lowered, and the upper arm moves forward as if pushing a cart. The trapezius and the serratus anterior attach the scapula to the axial skeleton.
- Pectoralis major: The **pectoralis major** is a large, broad muscle that helps to form the anterior chest wall. It connects the humerus (upper arm) with the clavicle (collarbone) and structures in the anterior chest. Contraction of this muscle moves the upper arm across the front of the chest as in pointing to an object in front of you. Many gym exercises are designed to work the pecs.
- Latissimus dorsi: The **latissimus dorsi** is a large, broad muscle located in the middle and lower back region. It extends from the back structures to the humerus. Contraction of this muscle lowers the shoulders and brings the arm back as in pointing to an object behind you. This same backward movement occurs in swimming and rowing. The pectoralis major and the latissimus dorsi attach the humerus to the axial skeleton.
- Deltoid: The **deltoid** forms the rounded portion of the shoulder; your shoulder pad. The deltoid extends from the clavicle and scapula to the humerus. Contraction of the deltoid muscle abducts the arm, raising it to a horizontal position (the scarecrow position). Because of its size, location, and good blood supply, the deltoid is a common site of intramuscular injection.
- Rotator cuff muscles: The **rotator cuff muscles** are a group of four muscles that attach the humerus to the scapula. They include the subscapularis, supraspinatus, infraspinatus, and teres minor. The tendons of these muscles form a cap, or a cuff, over the proximal humerus, thus stabilizing the joint capsule. The muscles help to rotate the arm at the shoulder joint. What about the tennis buff and his rotator cuff? One of the most common causes of shoulder pain in athletes is known as impingement syndrome, or rotator cuff injury. It is caused by repetitive overhead motions and is commonly experienced by tennis players, swimmers, and baseball pitchers. The tendons are pinched and become inflamed resulting in pain. If the condition continues the inflamed tendon can degenerate and separate from the bone. The condition can be a career-ending sports injury.

MUSCLES THAT MOVE THE LOWER ARM

The primary muscles involved in the movement of the lower arm (forearm) are located along the humerus. They are the triceps brachii, biceps brachii, brachialis, and brachioradialis.

The **triceps brachii** lies along the posterior surface of the humerus; its ends attach to the scapula (origin) and the olecranon of the ulna (insertion). It is the prime mover of extension of the forearm. The triceps brachii is the muscle that supports the weight of the body when a person does push-ups or walks with crutches. It is also the muscle that packs the greatest punch for a boxer and is called the boxer's muscle (see Figure 9-7, *B*).

The **biceps brachii** is located along the anterior surface of the humerus; its ends attach to the scapula (origin) and the radius of the forearm (insertion). The biceps brachii acts synergistically with the **brachialis** and **brachioradialis** to flex the forearm. The biceps brachii and the brachialis are the prime movers for flexion of the forearm. When someone is asked to "make a muscle," the biceps brachii becomes most visible.

Pronation (palm down) is achieved by two pronator muscles located along the anterior forearm. The actions of the biceps brachii and a supinator muscle located along the posterior forearm causes supination (palm up).

MUSCLES THAT MOVE THE HAND AND FINGERS

More than 20 muscles move the hand and fingers. The muscles are numerous but small, making the hand and fingers capable of delicate movements. The muscles are generally located along the forearm and consist of **flexors** and **extensors.** The flexors are located on the anterior surface, and the extensors are located on the posterior surface. The tendons of these muscles pass through the wrist into the hand; contraction of the muscles (in the forearm) pull on the tendons thereby moving the fingers (like puppet strings). Imagine how fat your fingers would be if they were filled with muscle rather than tendons. Double or triple your ring size!

The flexors of the fingers are stronger than the extensors so that in a relaxed hand, the fingers are slightly flexed. If a person is unconscious for an extended period, the fingers remain in a flexed position. In response to inactivity, the tendons of the fingers shorten, thereby preventing extension of the fingers. This gives a claw-like appearance to the hand. This problem can be prevented by an exercise program that includes passive exercises of the hands and fingers.

The Carpal Tunnel

Most of the tendons of the muscles that supply the hand pass through a narrow tunnel created by transversely oriented carpal ligaments and the carpal (wrist) bones (Figure 9-10). The flexor tendons in the carpal tunnel are encased in tendon sheaths and normally slide back and forth very easily. However, repetitive motion of the hand and fingers can cause the tissues within the carpal tunnel to become inflamed and swollen. The swelling puts pressure on the median nerve, which is also located in the carpal tunnel. The irritated nerve causes tingling, weakness, and pain in the hand; the pain may radiate to the arm and shoulder. The condition is called carpal tunnel syndrome and is a major cause of disability in persons who must perform repetitive wrist motion (such as pianists, machinists, meat cutters, and keyboard operators).

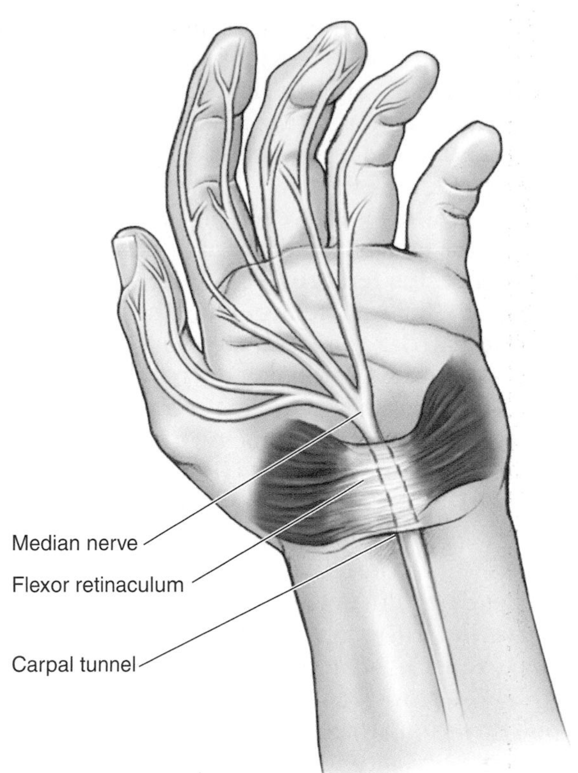

FIGURE 9-10 Carpal tunnel syndrome.

MUSCLES THAT MOVE THE THIGH, LEG, AND FOOT

The muscles that move the thigh, leg, and foot are some of the largest and strongest muscles in the body.

Muscles That Move the Thigh

The muscles that move the thigh all attach to some part of the pelvic girdle and the femur (thigh bone). These muscles include the gluteal muscles, the iliopsoas, and a group of adductor muscles. Contraction of these muscles moves the hip joint (see Figure 9-7).

The **gluteal muscles** are located on the posterior surface and include the **gluteus maximus, gluteus medius,** and **gluteus minimus.** The gluteus maximus is the largest muscle in the body and forms the area of the buttocks; it is the muscle you sit on.

The gluteus maximus straightens, or extends, the thigh at the hip, as you do while climbing stairs. It also produces the backswing of the leg while walking. In addition to hip extension, the gluteal muscles rotate and abduct the hip. The gluteus medius lies partly behind and superior to the gluteus maximus. Both gluteal muscles are commonly used sites for intramuscular injections.

The **iliopsoas** is located on the anterior surface of the groin. Contraction of this muscle flexes the thigh, making it antagonistic to the gluteus maximus.

The **adductor muscles** are located on the medial (inner) surface of the thigh. These muscles adduct the thighs, pressing them together. These are the muscles a horse rider uses to stay on the horse. The adductor muscles include the **adductor longus, adductor brevis, adductor magnus,** and **gracilis.**

Muscles That Move the Leg

The muscles that move the leg are located in the thigh. The extensor muscles lie along the anterior and lateral surfaces of the leg while the flexors lie along the posterior and medial surfaces. They include the quadriceps femoris, the sartorius, and the hamstring group.

The **quadriceps femoris** is the most powerful muscle in the body. It is located on the anterior thigh and is the prime mover of knee extension. The muscle has four heads (points of attachment), each of which has its own name: the **vastus lateralis, vastus intermedius, vastus medialis,** and **rectus femoris.** The muscle has its origins in the ilium (hip) and femur. The other end tapers and joins the patellar (kneecap) tendon. The muscle eventually attaches to the tibia by the patellar ligament at the tibial tuberosity. The "quads" straighten, or extend, the leg at the knee as in kicking a football.

Other Functions of the Quads. Because the rectus femoris originates on a pelvic bone, this muscle can also flex the thigh at the hip joint. The vastus lateralis is frequently used as an injection site for children because it is more developed than the gluteal muscles.

The **sartorius** is the longest muscle in the body. It is a straplike muscle located on the anterior surface of the thigh. The sartorius passes over the quadriceps in an oblique direction attaching to the hip bone (origin) and the tibial tuberosity (insertion); the muscle allows the legs to rotate so that you can sit cross-legged. At one time tailors used to sit cross-legged as they worked. The Latin word for tailor is *sartor,* so this muscle was named the sartorius.

The **hamstrings** are a group of muscles located on the posterior surface of the thigh. All the muscles extend from the ischium (pelvic bone) to the tibia. They flex the leg at the knee and are therefore antagonistic to the quadriceps femoris. Because these muscles also span the hip joint, they extend the thigh. The strong tendons of these muscles can be felt behind the knee. The tendons form the pit behind the knee called the **popliteal fossa.** These same tendons are found in hogs. Butchers used to use these tendons to hang the hams for smoking and curing, hence the name hamstrings. The hamstring muscles include the **biceps femoris, semimembranosus,** and **semitendinosus.**

An athlete often pulls a hamstring or experiences a groin injury. These injuries involve one or more of the hamstring muscles or their tendons.

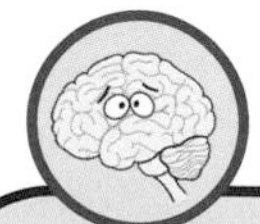

Do You Know...

What a wolf knows about the hamstrings?

Hungry wolves spot their prey—and the chase is on. The wolf will often attack the knee joint of its prey, severing the tendons of the hamstrings. Once the tendons are severed, the victim's legs are useless. Dinner is served!

Muscles That Move the Foot

The muscles that move the foot are located on the anterior, lateral, and posterior surfaces of the leg. The **tibialis anterior** is located on the anterior surface. It causes dorsiflexion of the foot. The **peroneus longus** muscle is on the lateral surface. It everts (turns outward) the foot, supports the arch of the foot, and assists in plantar flexion. The **gastrocnemius** and the **soleus** are the major muscles on the posterior surface of the leg and form the calf of the leg. They attach to the calcaneus (heel bone) by the **calcaneal tendon,** or **Achilles tendon** (the strongest tendon in the body). Contraction of these muscles causes plantar flexion. Plantar flexion aids in walking and allows a person to stand on tiptoes. For this reason the gastrocnemius is sometimes called the toe dancer's muscle.

Runners, especially sprinters, occasionally tear or rupture the Achilles tendon. Because the heel then cannot be lifted, this injury severely impedes the ability of the runner to perform.

Lastly, the toes. Like the fingers, some of the toes are "tugged on" by tendons whose muscles (flexors and extensors) lie in the leg. Other muscles have their origin in the tarsal and metatarsal bones.

Some muscles have acquired rather interesting names. Figure 9-11 shows the many interesting movements we are able to make.

Sum It Up!

The skeleton is stabilized and covered with muscle. The ability of the muscles to contract and relax allows the skeleton to move about and engage in all the activities that make life so enjoyable. The location and function of the major muscles of the body are summarized in Table 9-1.

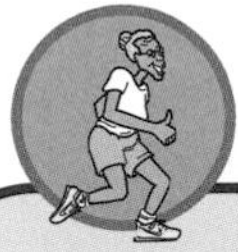

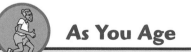

As You Age

1. At about the age of 40, the number and diameter of muscle fibers decrease. Muscles become smaller, dehydrated, and weaker. Muscle fibers are gradually replaced by connective tissue, especially adipose or fat cells. By the age of 80, about 50% of the muscle mass has been lost.
2. Mitochondrial function in muscles decreases, especially in muscles that are not exercised regularly.
3. Motor neurons are gradually lost, resulting in muscle atrophy.
4. These changes lead to decreased muscle strength and slowing of muscle reflexes.

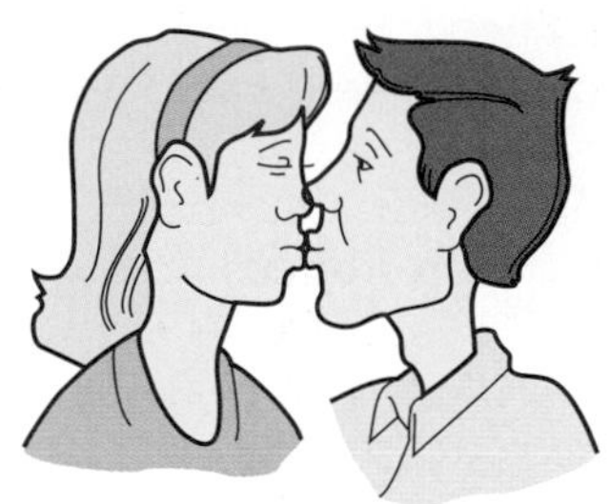

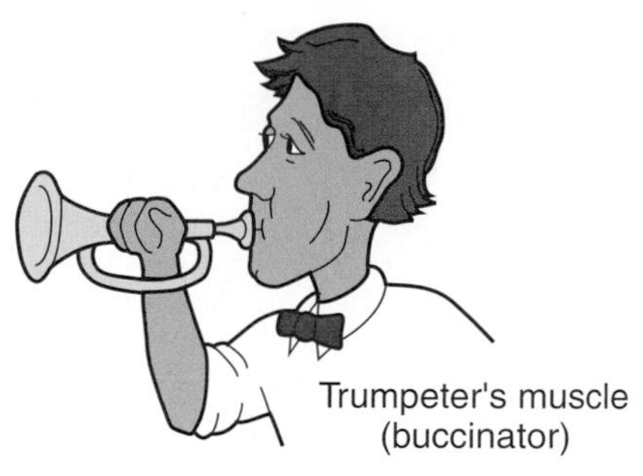

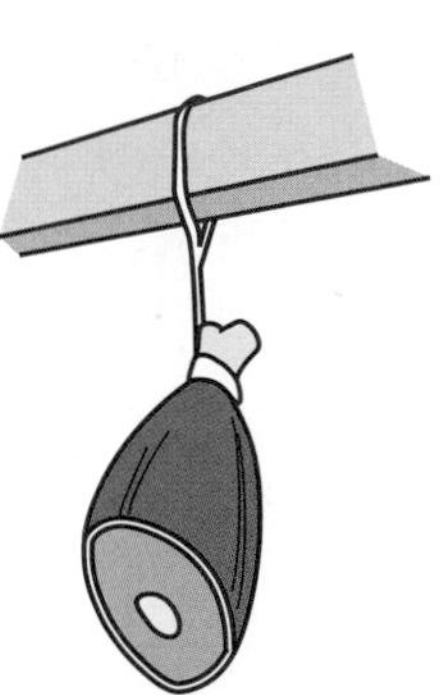

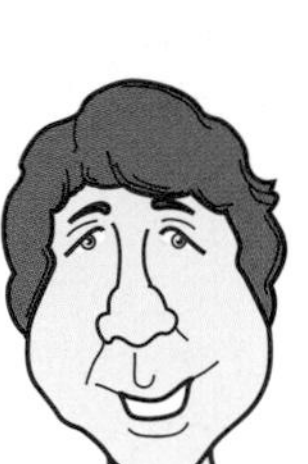

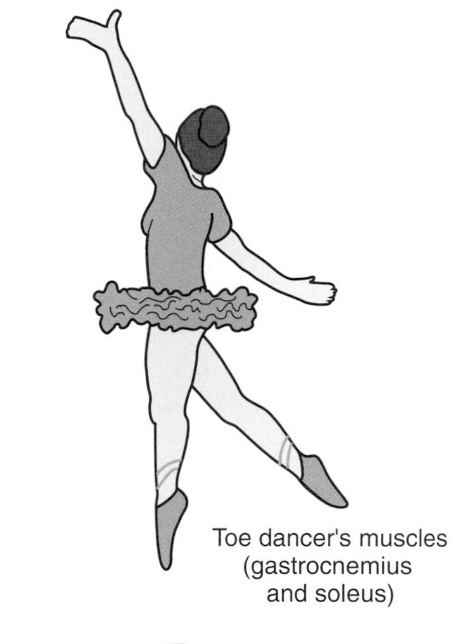

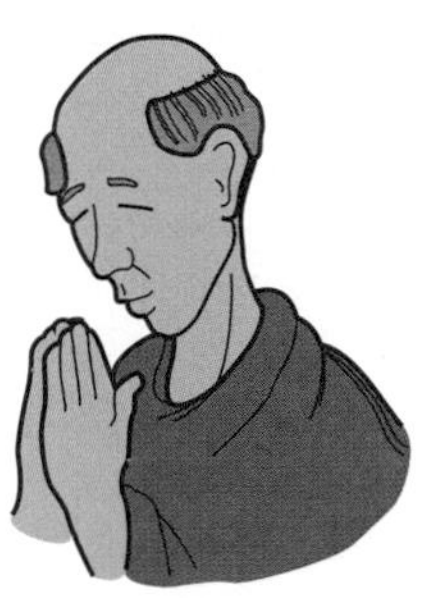

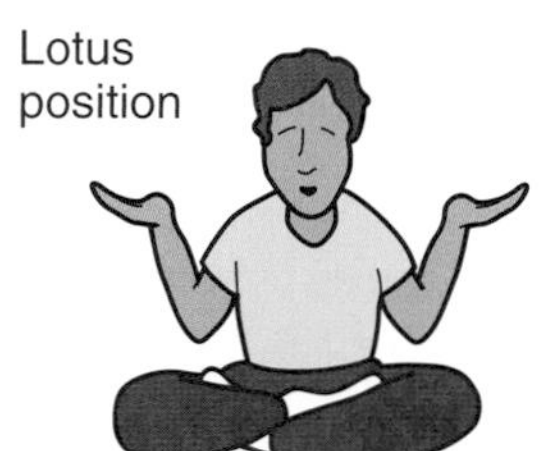

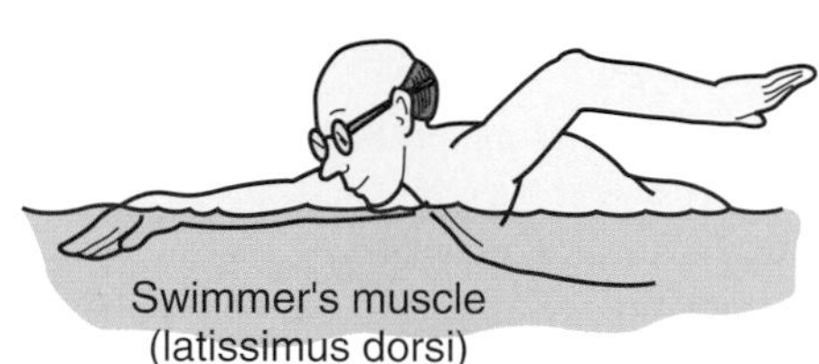

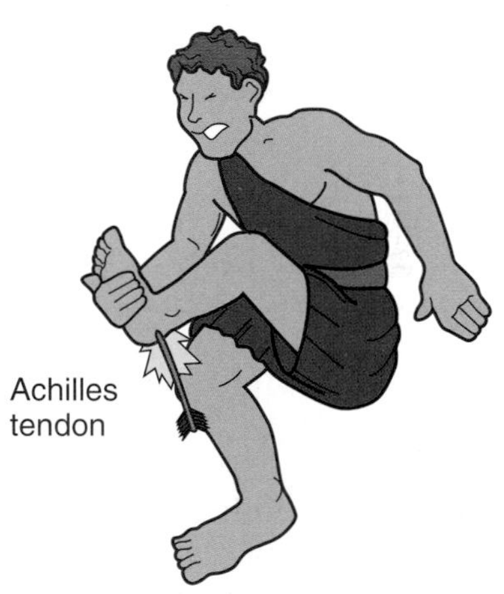

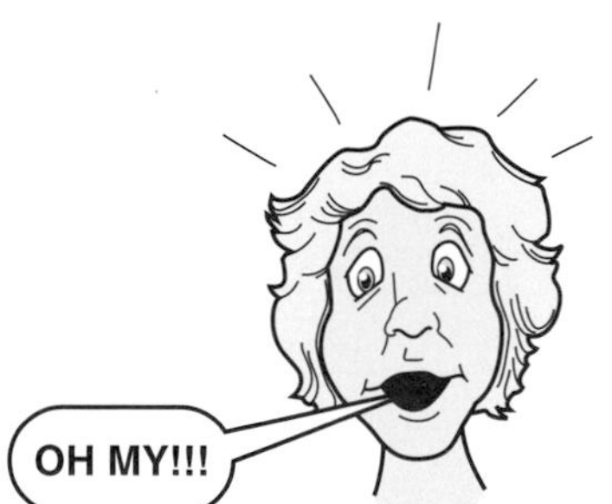

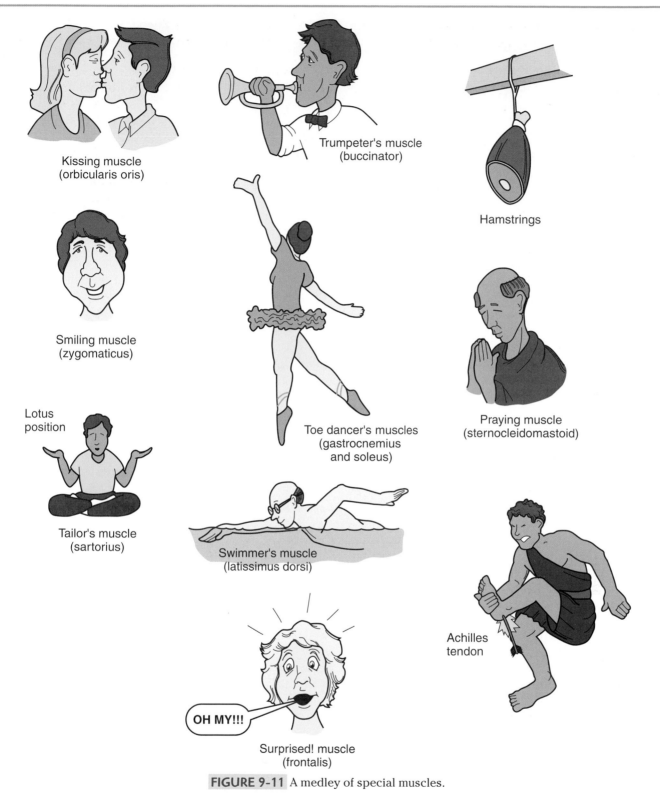

FIGURE 9-11 A medley of special muscles.

Disorders of the Muscular System

Atrophy (muscle)	Wasting of muscle tissue. The muscles become smaller. Disuse atrophy refers to muscle wasting due to lack of use in a muscle that has an intact nerve supply. Disuse atrophy is often seen in a casted extremity. Denervation atrophy refers to muscle wasting due to the lack of stimulation by the motor neurons that normally supply the muscle. It is seen in patients who have experienced spinal cord injury.
Cramp	A painful, involuntary skeletal muscle contraction.
Fibromyositis	Also called a charley horse. Fibromyositis refers to pain and tenderness in the fibromuscular tissue of the thighs usually due to muscle strain or tear.
Flatfoot	Abnormal flatness of the sole and the arch of the foot.
Frozen shoulder	Frozen shoulder is a condition in which the shoulder becomes stiff and painful, making normal movement difficult. It is often caused by disuse of the shoulder because of an injury or the pain associated with bursitis or tendonitis.
Hypertonia	Increased muscle tone causing spasticity or rigidity.
Hypotonia	Decrease in or absence of muscle tone, causing loose, flaccid muscles.
Myalgia	Pain or tenderness in the muscles. Fibromyalgia is a group of common rheumatic disorders characterized by chronic pain in muscles and soft tissues surrounding joints (affects the fibrous connective tissue portions of muscles, tendons, and ligaments).
Myopathy	Any disease of the muscles not associated with the nervous system. A dystrophy is a myopathy that is characterized by muscle degeneration. Muscular dystrophy refers to a group of diseases, usually inherited, in which there is progressive degeneration and weakening of the skeletal muscles. Deterioration of the muscle fibers causes decreased muscle function, atrophy, and motor disability.
Plantar fasciitis	Inflammation at the heel bone caused when the inflexible fascia in the heel is repeatedly stretched (as in running). The inflammatory response can produce spikelike projections of new bone called spurs (calcaneal spurs).
Shin splints	An exercise-related inflammatory condition involving the extensor muscles and surrounding tissues in the lower leg. Pain is generally experienced along the inner aspect of the tibia.
Torticollis	Also called wryneck. Torticollis refers to the twisting of the neck into an unusual position. It is caused by prolonged contraction of the neck muscles.

SUMMARY OUTLINE

The purpose of muscle is to contract and to cause movement.

I. Muscle Function: Overview

A. Types and Functions of Muscles

1. Skeletal muscle is striated and voluntary; its primary function is to produce movement.
2. Smooth (visceral) muscle is nonstriated and involuntary; it helps the organs perform their functions.
3. Cardiac muscle is striated and involuntary; it is found only in the heart and allows the heart to function as a pump.

B. Structure of the Whole Muscle

1. A large muscle consists of thousands of single muscle fibers (muscle cells).
2. Connective tissue binds the muscle fibers (cells) together (forming compartments in the limbs) and attaches muscle to bone and other tissue (by tendons and aponeuroses).

C. Structure and Function of a Single Muscle Fiber

1. The muscle fiber (cell) is surrounded by a cell membrane (sarcolemma). The cell membrane penetrates to the interior of the muscle as the transverse tubule (T tubule).

2. An extensive sarcoplasmic reticulum (SR) stores calcium.
3. Each muscle fiber consists of a series of sarcomeres. Each sarcomere contains the contractile proteins actin and myosin.

D. How Muscles Contract
1. Muscles shorten or contract as the actin and myosin (in the presence of calcium and ATP) interact through crossbridge formation, according to the sliding filament theory.
2. For skeletal muscle to contract, it must be stimulated by a motor nerve. The nerve impulse releases acetycholine (ACh) from the nerve terminal. ACh diffuses across the NMJ, binds to the muscle membrane and causes an electrical signal to form in the muscle membrane.
3. The electrical signal enters the T-tubular system and stimulates the SR to release calcium.
4. Actin, myosin, and ATP interact to form crossbridges, which cause sliding or shortening.
5. Calcium is pumped back into the SR and the muscles relax.

E. Responses of a Whole Muscle
1. A single muscle fiber contracts in an all-or-nothing response; a whole muscle can contract partially (i.e., not all-or-nothing).
2. A whole muscle increases its force of contraction by recruitment of additional muscle fibers.
3. Two terms describe the contractile activity of a whole muscle: twitch and tetanus. Tetanus refers to a sustained muscle contraction.
4. Energy for muscle contraction can be obtained from three sources: burning fuel aerobically, burning fuel anaerobically, and metabolizing creatine phosphate.

F. Terms That Describe Muscle Movement
1. Origin and Insertion: The attachments of the muscles.
2. Prime mover: The muscle most responsible for the movement achieved by the muscle group.
3. Synergist and Antagonist: works with, or has an opposing action.

II. Muscles from Head to Toe

A. Skeletal muscles are named according to size, shape, direction of fibers, location, number of origins, place of origin and insertion, and muscle action.

B. See Table 9-1 for a list of the body's muscles.

Review Your Knowledge

Matching: Muscle Terms

Directions: Match the following words with their descriptions below. Some words may be used more than once, others not at all.

a. origin
b. sarcoplasmic reticulum
c. smooth muscle
d. aponeurosis
e. actin
f. sarcomere
g. insertion
h. atrophy
i. synergist
j. skeletal muscle
k. myosin
l. tendon

1. ___ Cordlike structure that attaches muscle to bone
2. ___ Type of muscle that is classified as striated and voluntary
3. ___ Type of muscle that must be stimulated by a somatic motor nerve
4. ___ Flat, sheetlike fascia that attaches muscle to muscle or muscle to bone
5. ___ The head of this contractile protein binds to actin to form a crossbridge
6. ___ Calcium is stored within this muscle structure
7. ___ Series of contractile units that make up each myofibril: extends from Z line to Z line
8. _g_ The muscle attachment to the movable bone insertion
9. ___ Use it or lose it
10. _l_ A helper muscle synergist

Matching: Names of Muscles

Directions: Match the following words with their descriptions below. Some words may be used more than once, others not at all.

a. quadriceps femoris
b. gastrocnemius
c. masseter
d. hamstrings
e. triceps brachii
f. deltoid
g. pectoralis major
h. latissimus dorsi
i. gluteus maximus
j. biceps brachii
k. diaphragm

1. ____ A muscle of mastication
2. ____ The major breathing muscle
3. ____ Major muscle of the anterior chest; attaches to the humerus
4. ____ The shoulder pad; pulls the arm into the scarecrow position
5. ____ The muscle that flexes the arm at the elbow
6. ____ Muscles that lie along the anterior thigh; flexes the thigh at the hip and extends the leg
7. ____ The muscle group that lies along the posterior thigh; flexes the leg at the knee
8. ____ The large muscle on which you sit
9. ____ Contraction of this muscle causes plantar flexion
10. ____ This muscle attaches to the calcaneus by the Achilles tendon

Multiple Choice

1. When the electrical signal travels along the T tubule and stimulates the sarcoplasmic reticulum (SR)
   a. calcium is released causing crossbridge formation between actin and myosin.
   b. acetylcholine (ACh) is released into the neuromuscular junction (NMJ).
   c. calcium is pumped into the SR from the sarcomere.
   d. ACh binds to the receptor on the muscle membrane.
2. Which of the following does not occur within the neuromuscular junction (NMJ)?
   a. ACh is released from the motor nerve terminal.
   b. ACh diffuses across the junction.
   c. Actin and myosin "slide."
   d. ACh is inactivated by an enzyme.
3. When skeletal muscle is stimulated quickly and repetitively
   a. ACh within the NMJ is depleted.
   b. the muscle tetanizes.
   c. the sarcoplasmic reticulum is depleted of calcium and the muscle becomes flaccid.
   d. the muscle merely twitches.
4. Which of the following must occur in order to achieve flexion of the forearm?
   a. The triceps brachii contracts.
   b. The biceps brachii and brachialis contract.
   c. The brachioradialis relaxes.
   d. The deltoid and brachioradialis contract.
5. Which of the following does not characterize the quadriceps femoris?
   a. Has four heads, or points of attachment
   b. Is the prime mover for the extension of the leg
   c. Inserts on the proximal tibia at the tibial tuberosity
   d. Causes plantar flexion as in toe dancing
6. Which of the following is true of the hamstrings?
   a. Located on the anterior thigh
   b. Is the prime mover for flexion of the leg
   c. Acts synergistically with the gastrocnemius to cause dorsiflexion
   d. Attaches to the Achilles tendon and inserts on the calcaneus

CHAPTER 10

Nervous System: Nervous Tissue and Brain

KEY TERMS

Action potential, p. 166
Brain stem, p. 176
Cerebellum, p. 177
Cerebrospinal fluid, p. 179
Cerebrum, p. 171
Depolarization, p. 166
Frontal lobe, p. 173
Hypothalamus, p. 176
Limbic system, p. 177
Medulla oblongata, p. 177
Meninges, p. 178
Myelin, p. 164
Neuroglia, p. 163
Neuron, p. 163
Neurotransmitters, p. 170
Occipital lobe, p. 175
Parietal lobe, p. 175
Repolarization, p. 167
Reticular formation, p. 177
Synapse, p. 170
Temporal lobe, p. 175

OBJECTIVES

1. Define the two divisions of the nervous system.
2. List three general functions of the nervous system.
3. Compare the structure and functions of the neuroglia and neuron.
4. Explain the function of the myelin sheath.
5. Explain how a neuron transmits information.
6. Describe the structure and function of a synapse.
7. Describe the functions of the four major areas of the brain.
8. Describe the functions of the four lobes of the cerebrum.
9. Describe how the skull, meninges, cerebrospinal fluid, and blood-brain barrier protect the central nervous system.

THE NERVOUS SYSTEM: STRUCTURE AND FUNCTION

If you have ever listened to an orchestra warming up before a performance, you know something about the need for its conductor. Without the conductor, the sound is more like noise than music. The conductor coordinates, interprets, and directs the sound into the beautiful strains of a symphony. So it is with the nervous system. The various organ systems of the body need an interpreter to coordinate and direct them. This role is performed magnificently by the nervous system. The music of the body is every bit as beautiful as the strains of a symphony!

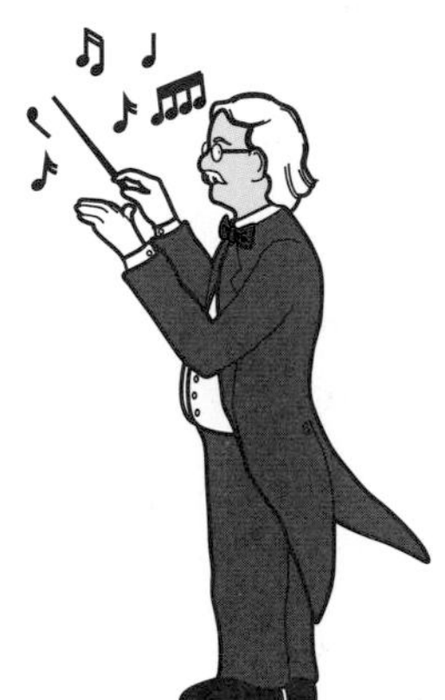

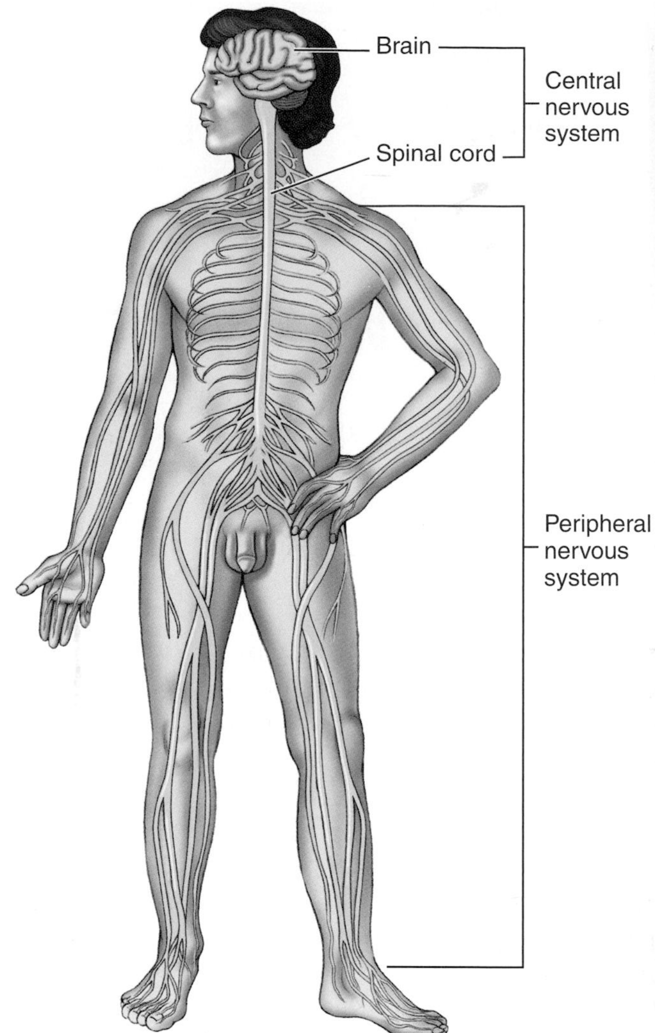

FIGURE 10-1 Nervous system: central nervous system and peripheral nervous system.

DIVISIONS OF THE NERVOUS SYSTEM

The structures of the nervous system are divided into two parts: the central nervous system and the peripheral nervous system. The **central nervous system (CNS)** includes the brain and the spinal cord. The CNS is located in the dorsal cavity. The brain is located in the cranium; the spinal cord is enclosed in the spinal cavity. The **peripheral nervous system** is located outside the CNS and consists of the nerves that connect the CNS with the rest of the body (Figure 10-1).

FUNCTIONS OF THE NERVOUS SYSTEM

As conductor, the nervous system performs three general functions: a sensory function, an integrative function, and a motor function (Figure 10-2).

Sensory Function

Sensory nerves gather information from inside the body and from the outside environment. The nerves then carry the information to the CNS. For instance, information about a cat is picked up by special cells in the eye.

Integrative Function

Sensory information brought to the CNS is processed or interpreted. The brain not only sees the cat but also does much more. It recalls very quickly how a cat behaves. It may determine that the cat is acting hungry or is distressed and ready to attack. The brain integrates, or puts together, everything it knows about cats and then makes its plan.

Motor Function

Motor nerves convey information from the CNS toward the muscles and glands of the body. Motor nerves carry out the plans made by the CNS. For instance, the person may decide to feed the hungry cat. Information must travel along the motor nerves from the CNS to all of the skeletal muscles needed to feed the cat. The motor nerve converts the plan into action.

CELLS THAT MAKE UP THE NERVOUS SYSTEM

Nervous tissue is composed of two types of cells: the neuroglia and the neurons.

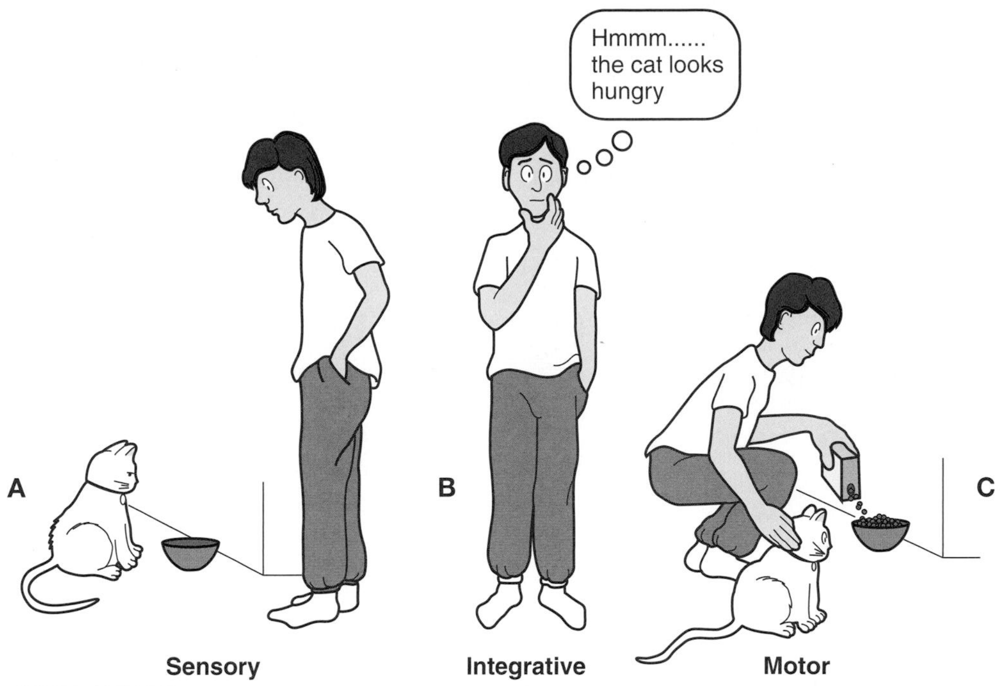

FIGURE 10-2 Three functions of the nervous system: **A,** Sensory function. **B,** Integrative function. **C,** Motor function.

NEUROGLIA

Neuroglia (nū-rō-GLĒ-ă), or **glial cells,** is the nerve glue. Neuroglia is the most abundant of the nerve cells; most glial cells are located in the CNS. Glial cells support, protect, insulate, nourish, and generally care for the delicate neurons. Some of the glial cells participate in phagocytosis; others assist in the secretion of cerebrospinal fluid. Glial cells, however, do not conduct nerve impulses.

Two of the more common glial cells are the astrocytes and the ependymal cells (Figure 10-3). The star-shaped **astrocytes** are the most abundant of the glial cells; they support the neurons and also form a protective barrier around the neurons of the CNS. This barrier helps prevent toxic substances in the blood from entering the nervous tissue of the brain and spinal cord. A second glial cell is the **ependymal cell.** These cells line the inside cavities of the brain and assist in the formation of cerebrospinal fluid. Other glial cells are listed in Table 10-1. Because glial cells undergo mitosis, most primary CNS tumors are composed of glial cells, such as astrocytomas.

NEURON

The second type of nerve cell is the neuron. Of the two types of nerve cells, the **neuron** (NŪ-rŏn) is most important in the transmission of information. The neuron enables the nervous system to act as a vast communication network. Neurons have many shapes and sizes. Some neurons are extremely short; others are very long, with some measuring 4 feet in length. Unlike glial cells, neurons are nonmitotic and therefore do not replicate nor replace themselves when injured. Because they are nonmitotic, neurons generally do not give rise to primary malignant brain tumors.

Table 10-1 Types of Neuroglia

Cell Name	Function
Astrocytes	Star-shaped cells present in blood-brain barrier; also anchor or bind blood vessels to nerves for support; act as phagocytes
Ependymal cells	Line the ventricles as part of the choroid plexus; involved in the formation of cerebrospinal fluid
Microglia	Protective role: phagocytosis of pathogens and damaged tissue
Schwann cells	Produce myelin sheath for neurons in the peripheral nervous system
Oligodendrocytes	Produce myelin sheath for neurons in the central nervous system

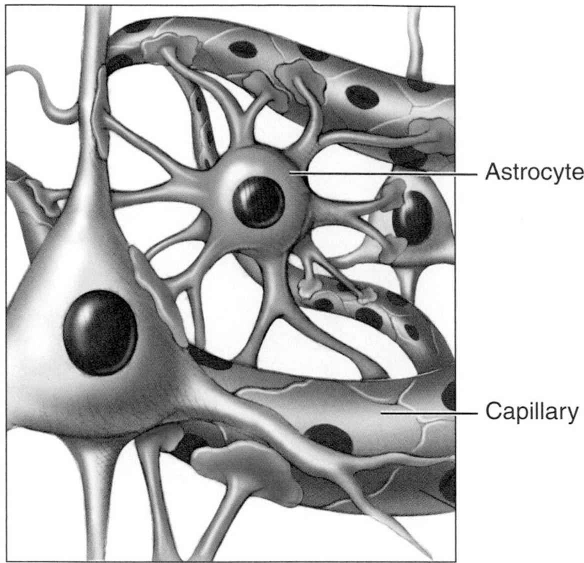

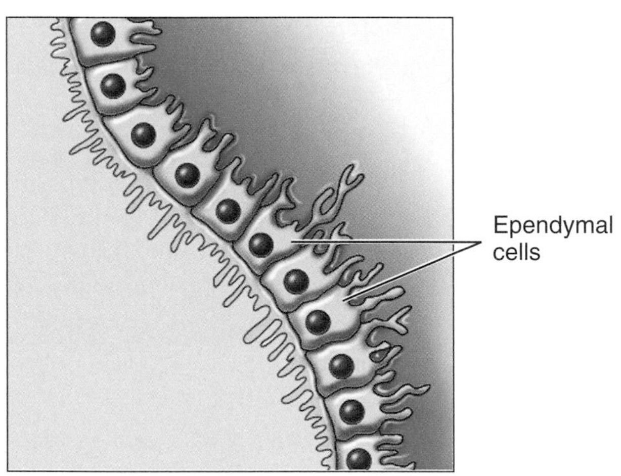

FIGURE 10-3 Neuroglia, or glia; astrocytes and ependymal cells.

Parts of a Neuron

Three Parts. The three parts of the neuron are the dendrites, cell body, and axon (Figure 10-4). **Dendrites** are treelike structures that receive information from other neurons and then transmit the information toward the cell body. One neuron may have thousands of dendrites. The **cell body** contains the nucleus and is essential for the life of the cell. The **axon** is a long extension that transmits information away from the cell body. The end of the axon undergoes extensive branching to form hundreds to thousands of axon terminals; it is within the **axon terminals** that the chemical neurotransmitters are stored. Information travels from the dendrite to the cell body to the axon. The arrow in Figure 10-4 indicates the direction in which information travels over the neuron.

The Axon: A Special Structure. What is so special about the axon? An enlarged view of the axon shows several unique structures: the myelin sheath, the neurilemma, and the nodes of Ranvier (see Figure 10-4). Most long nerve fibers of both the peripheral and central nervous systems are encased by a layer of white fatty material called the myelin sheath. **Myelin** (MĪ-ĕ-lĭn) protects and insulates the axon. Nerve fibers covered by myelin are said to be myelinated. Some neurons are not encased in myelin and are called unmyelinated neurons. Myelination begins during the fourth month of fetal life and continues into teenage years. Because some axons of immature motor neurons lack myelination, the movements of an infant are slower and less coordinated than those of an older child. Severely restricting the fat intake of an infant is unwise, since the child is still laying down myelin.

The formation of myelin sheath differs in the peripheral and central nervous systems. Surrounding the axon of a neuron in the peripheral nervous system is a layer of special cells called **Schwann cells.** The Schwann cells form the myelin sheath that surrounds the axon. The nuclei and cytoplasm of the Schwann cells lie outside the myelin sheath and are called the neurilemma. The neurilemma is important in the regeneration of a severed nerve.

In the CNS, the myelin sheath is formed not by Schwann cells but by **oligodendrocytes,** a type of glial cell (Table 10-1). As there are no Schwann cells, there is no neurilemma. The lack of the neurilemma surrounding the axons accounts, in part, for the inability of the CNS neurons to regenerate. Failure of the neurons of the CNS to regenerate, however, is not fully explained by the lack of neurilemma; other factors include the formation of scar tissue and the lack of critical growth factors. On a more positive note, there is evidence that stem cells are capable of forming new neurons. Despite the success of stem cell research, spinal cord injury can cause paralysis that is still considered permanent.

Nodes of Ranvier, areas not covered by myelin, appear regularly along the axon.

Types of Neurons

The three types of neurons are the sensory neuron, the motor neuron, and the interneuron. A **sensory neuron** carries information from the periphery toward the CNS. Sensory neurons are also called **afferent neurons.**

A **motor neuron** carries information from the CNS toward the periphery. Motor neurons are also called **efferent neurons.** Sensory and motor neurons are found in both the CNS and the peripheral nervous system.

Remember—what is the **SAME** about these fibers!

S sensory
A afferent
M motor
E efferent

The third type of neuron is the **interneuron;** it is found only in the CNS. Interneurons form connections between sensory and motor neurons. In the brain, interneurons play a role in thinking, learning, and memory.

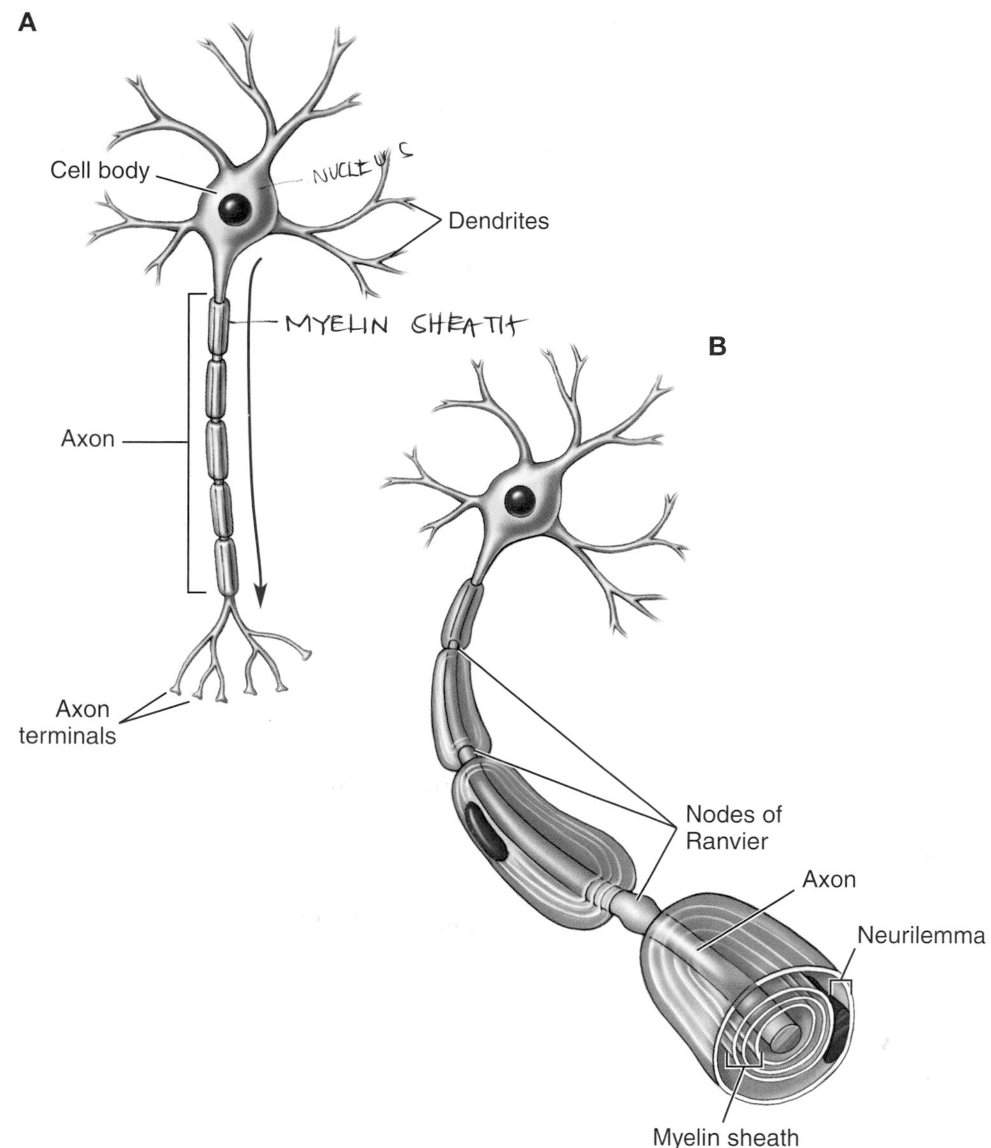

FIGURE 10-4 Structure of a neuron: **A,** Dendrites, cell body, axon, and axon terminals. **B,** Structure surrounding the axon, showing the myelin sheath, the nodes of Ranvier, and the neurilemma.

WHITE MATTER VERSUS GRAY MATTER

The tissue of the CNS is white and gray. White matter is white because of the myelin. Myelinated fibers are gathered together in the CNS in tracts. The gray matter is composed primarily of cell bodies, interneurons, and unmyelinated fibers.

Sometimes cell bodies appear in small clusters and are given special names. Clusters of cell bodies located in the CNS are generally referred to as **nuclei.** Small clusters of cell bodies in the peripheral nervous system are called **ganglia** (singular: **ganglion**). For instance, patches of gray called the **basal nuclei** are located in the brain. (Sometimes, these patches of gray are called basal ganglia, despite their location within the CNS.)

Sum It Up!

The nervous system plays a crucial role in allowing us to interact with our environment, both internal and external. The nervous system has two divisions: the central nervous system (CNS) and the peripheral nervous system. The nervous system performs three major functions: sensory, integrative, and motor. There are two types of nerve cells, the neuroglia and the neurons. The neuron is responsible for the rapid communication. The three parts of the neuron are the dendrites, cell body, and axon.

THE NEURON CARRYING INFORMATION

How do neurons carry information? Neurons allow the nervous system to convey information rapidly from one part of the body to the next. A stubbed toe makes itself known almost immediately. Think of how fast the information travels from your toe, where the injury occurred, to your brain, where the injury is interpreted as pain. Information is carried along the neuron in the form of a nerve impulse.

THE NERVE IMPULSE: WHAT IT IS

The **nerve impulse** is an electrical signal that conveys information along a neuron. A series of events causes the electrical charge inside the cell to move from its negative resting state (−) to its positive depolarized state (+) and back to its negative resting state (−). The nerve impulse is called the **action potential.** The action potential is a process of polarization, depolarization, and repolarization. Follow Figure 10-5 through the events of the action potential.

Polarization

Polarization characterizes the resting state of the neuron. When the neuron is polarized, the inside of the neuron is more negative than the outside. As long as the neuron is polarized, no nerve impulse is being transmitted. The cell is quiet, or resting.

Depolarization

When the neuron is stimulated, a change occurs in the cell's electrical state. In the resting (polarized) state, the inside of the cell is negative. When the cell is stimulated, the inside becomes positive. As the inside of the cell changes from negative to positive, it is said to **depolarize.**

Repolarization

Very quickly, however, the inside of the cell again becomes negative; in other words, it returns to its resting state.

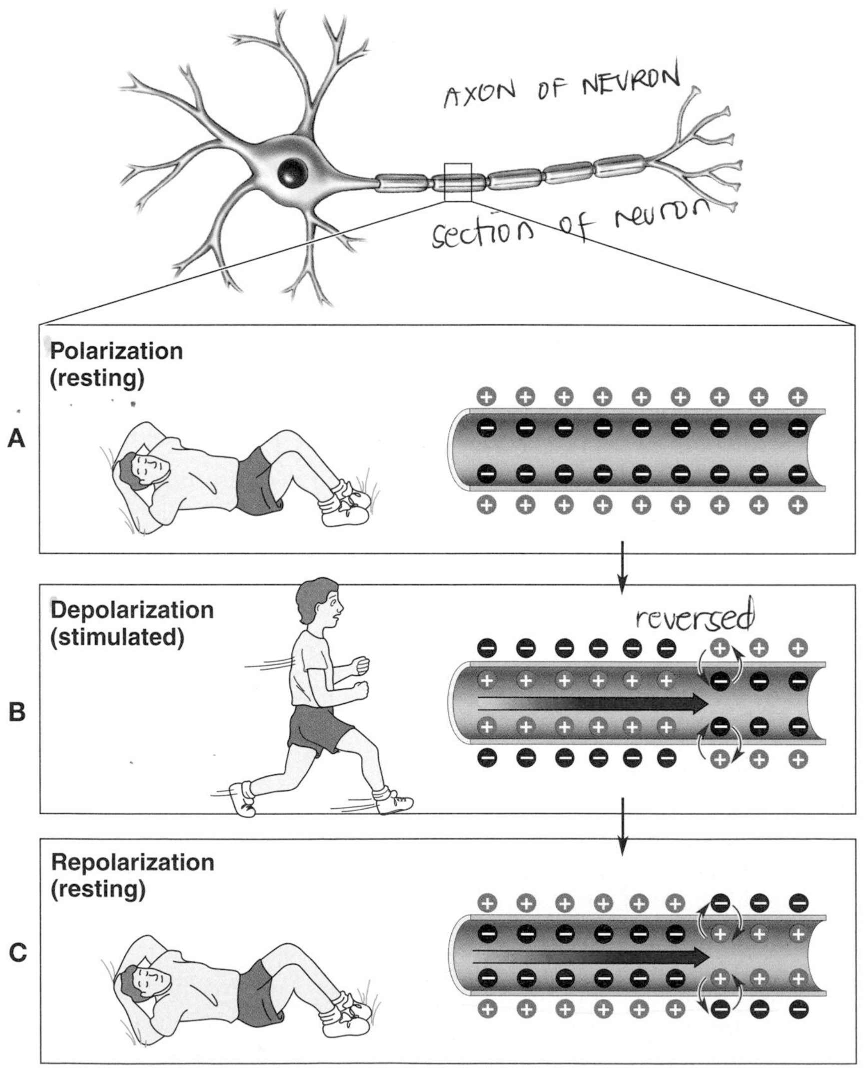

FIGURE 10-5 Nerve impulse (action potential): **A,** polarization, **B,** depolarization, and **C,** repolarization.

This return to the resting state is called **repolarization** (rē-pō-lăr-ĭ-ZĀ-shŭn). Unless the cell repolarizes, it cannot be stimulated again. The cell's inability to accept another stimulus until it repolarizes is called its **refractory period.** The refractory period is its unresponsive period.

THE NERVE IMPULSE: WHAT CAUSES IT

The changes associated with the action potential, or nerve impulse, are due to the movement of specific ions across the cell membrane of the neuron (Figure 10-6). Remember that the nerve impulse includes polarization, depolarization, and repolarization.

Polarization (Resting State)

What makes the inside of the cell negative in the resting state? The resting state is due to the numbers and types of ions located inside the neuron. The chief intracellular ions include the positively charged potassium ions (K^+) and several anions (negatively charged ions). How do these ions get into the cell in such high concentrations? They are pumped in by an ATP-driven pump in the cell membrane. In the resting state, the K^+ ions tend to leak out of the cell, taking with them the positive charge. The positive charge lost from the inside of the cell and the excess anions trapped in the cell make the inside of the cell negative.

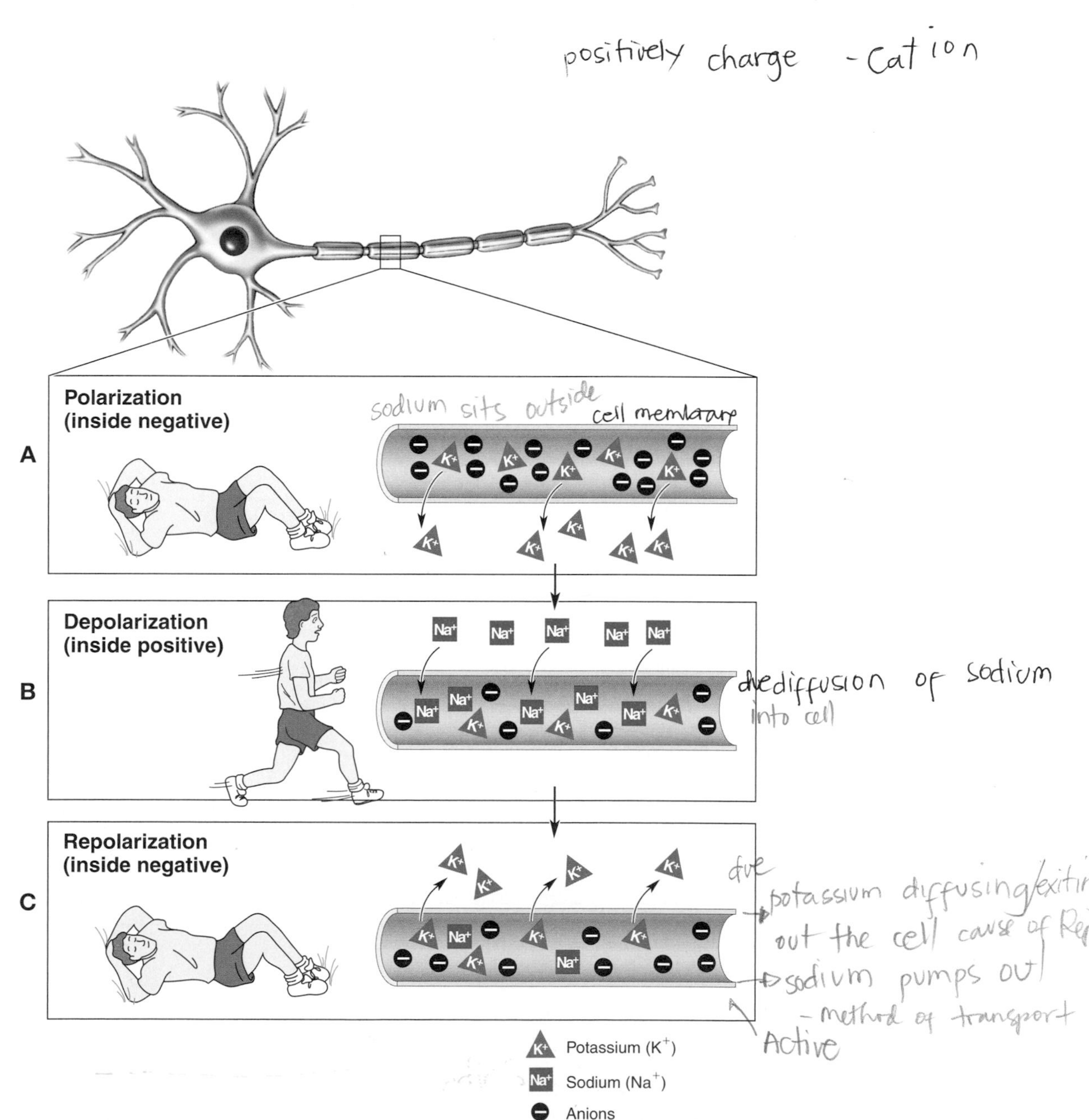

FIGURE 10-6 The cause of the nerve impulse (movement of ions): **A,** polarization, **B,** depolarization, and **C,** repolarization.

Depolarization (Stimulated State)

Why does the interior of the cell become positive when stimulated? When the neuron is stimulated, the neuronal membrane changes in a way that allows sodium ions (Na^+) to cross the membrane into the cell. Na^+ is the chief extracellular cation. With much more Na^+ outside the cell than inside, Na^+ diffuses into the cell, carrying with it a positive charge. This process makes the inside of the cell positive. Thus it is the inward diffusion of Na^+ that causes depolarization.

Repolarization (Return to Resting)

Why does the inside of the cell quickly return to its resting, negative state? Soon after the cell depolarizes, the neuronal membrane undergoes a second change. The change in the membrane does two things: it stops additional diffusion of Na^+ into the cell, and it allows K^+ to diffuse out of the cell. The outward movement of K^+ removes positive charge from the inside of the cell, leaving behind the negatively charged anions. Thus the outward movement of K^+ causes repolarization.

Eventually, the sodium will be removed from the neuron by pumps located in the neuronal membrane. (The pumps are ATP-driven pumps that help to maintain the sodium and potassium concentrations.) Note that the repolarizing phase of the nerve impulse is not due to the removal of Na^+ by the pump. Repolarization is due to the outward diffusion of K^+.

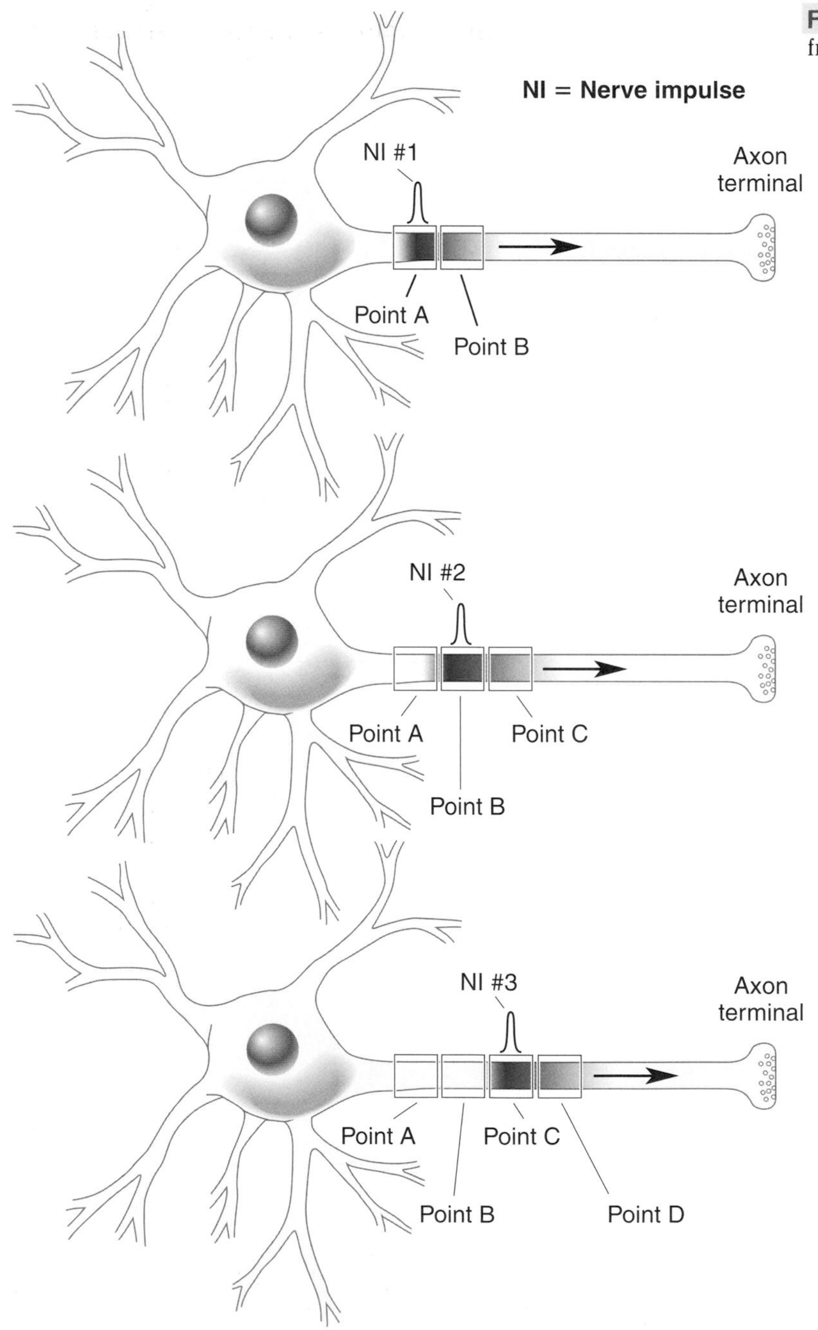

FIGURE 10-7 What causes the nerve impulse to move from the cell body to the axon terminals?

THE NERVE IMPULSE: WHAT CAUSES IT TO MOVE

To convey information, a nerve impulse must move the length of the neuron, from the cell body to the axon terminal. Figure 10-7 shows that when nerve impulse #1 forms at point A, it also depolarizes the next segment of the membrane (point B), causing nerve impulse #2 to form. Nerve impulse #2 then depolarizes the next segment of membrane at point C, causing the formation of nerve impulse #3.

Because of the ability of each nerve impulse to depolarize the adjacent membrane, the nerve impulse moves toward the axon terminal much like a wave. In addition to showing the movement of the nerve impulse, Figure 10-7 also shows that each nerve impulse fires in an all-or-nothing manner. The all-or-nothing firing means that the height of each nerve impulse is the same. This is important because it ensures that the nerve impulse does not weaken as it travels the length of a long axon.

THE NERVE IMPULSE: WHAT CAUSES IT TO MOVE QUICKLY

Myelination and speed. How does **myelination** affect the movement of the nerve impulse along the axonal membrane? Recall that the axons of most nerve fibers are wrapped in myelin, a fatty material. At the nodes of Ranvier, the axonal membrane is bare so that it is not covered with myelin.

The nerve impulse arrives at the axon but cannot develop on any part of the membrane covered with myelin. The nerve impulse can, however, develop at the nodes of Ranvier, the bare axonal membrane. Thus in a myelinated fiber, the nerve impulse jumps from node to node, much like a kangaroo, to the end of the axon (Figure 10-8). This "jumping" from node to node is called **saltatory conduction** (from the Latin word *saltare,* meaning to leap). Saltatory conduction increases the speed with which the nerve impulse travels along the nerve fiber. For this reason, myelinated fibers are considered fast-conducting nerve fibers.

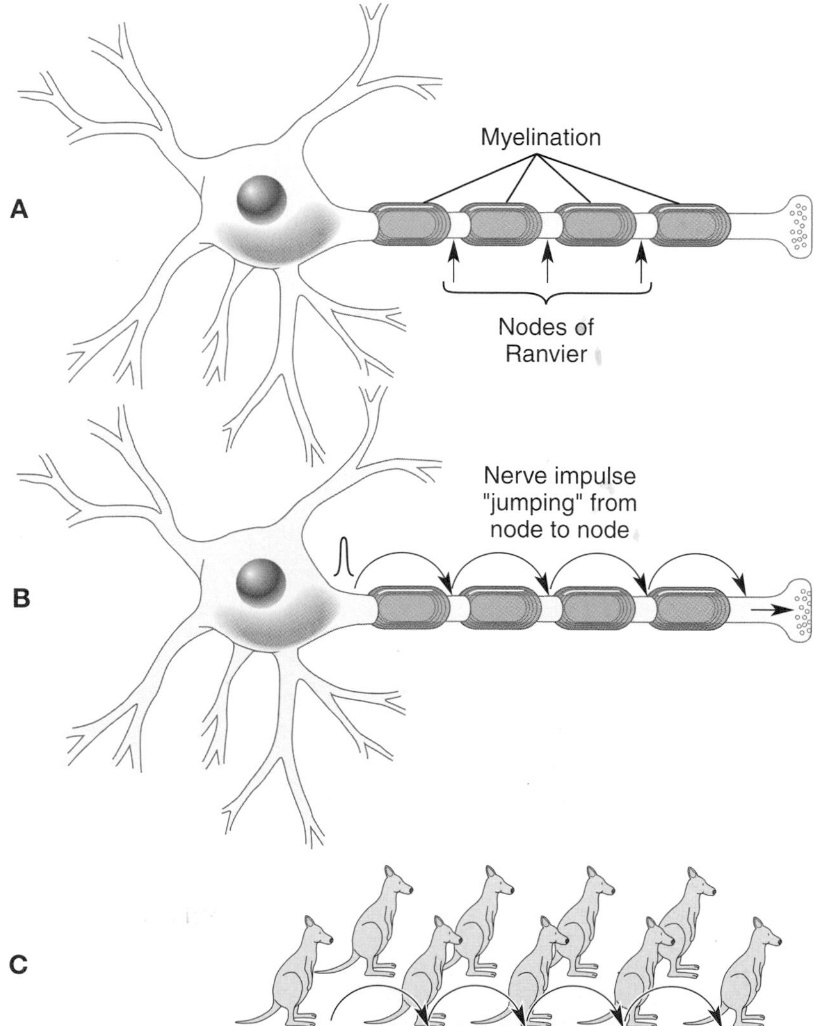

FIGURE 10-8 Jumping from node to node. **A,** A myelinated axon and the nodes of Ranvier. **B,** The nerve impulse jumps from node to node toward the axon terminal. **C,** The jumping of the nerve impulse resembles the jumping of a kangaroo.

SYNAPSE ACROSS NEURONS

A synapse helps information move from one neuron to the next. The big question is how.

PARTS OF A SYNAPSE

Synaptic Cleft

The **synapse** (SĬN-ăps) is a space. The space exists because the axon terminal of neuron A does not physically touch the dendrite of neuron B (Figure 10-9). The space is called the **synaptic cleft.**

Neurotransmitters

The axon terminal of neuron A contains thousands of tiny vesicles that store chemical substances called **neurotransmitters** (nū-rō-trăns-MĪ-tĕrs). The most common neurotransmitters are acetylcholine (ACh) and norepinephrine. Other CNS transmitters include epinephrine, serotonin, glutamate, gamma-aminobutyric acid (GABA), and endorphins.

Inactivators

Inactivators are substances that terminate the activity of the neurotransmitters when they have completed their task. For instance, the neurotransmitter ACh is terminated by acetylcholinesterase. Acetycholinesterase is an enzyme located in the same area as the receptor sites on neuron B. Once ACh has completed its task, it is inactivated by acetylcholinesterase.

Receptors

The dendrite of neuron B contains **receptor sites.** Receptor sites are places on the membrane to which the neurotransmitters attach, or bind. For instance, ACh binds to the receptors on dendrite B. Each receptor site has a specific shape and accepts only those neurotransmitters that "fit" its shape.

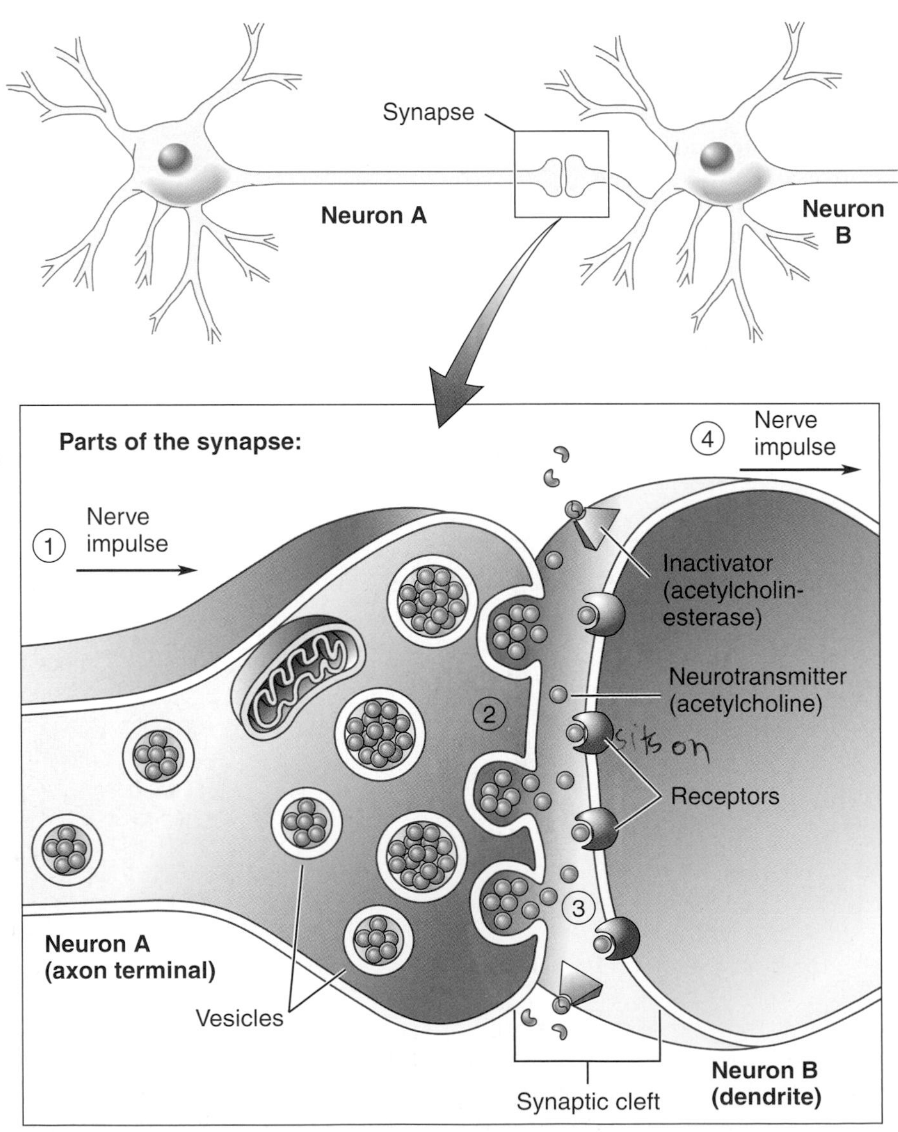

FIGURE 10-9 The synapse. Steps in the transfer of information across the synapse.

EVENTS AT THE SYNAPSE

The following details the events at the synapse (see Figure 10-9).

1. The nerve impulse travels along neuron A to its axon terminal.
2. The nerve impulse causes the vesicles to fuse with the membrane of the axon terminal. The vesicles open and release neurotransmitter into the synaptic cleft.
3. The neurotransmitter diffuses across the synaptic cleft and binds to the receptor sites. The binding of the neurotransmitter to the receptor sites causes a change in the membrane of the dendrite of neuron B. The membrane change is responsible for the formation of a new nerve impulse in the dendrite of neuron B.
4. This nerve impulse travels toward the cell body and axon of neuron B. What has happened at the synapse? Information from neuron A has been transmitted by chemicals (ACh) to neuron B.

Sum It Up!

The electrical signal that travels along the neuron is called the nerve impulse or action potential. The nerve impulse has three phases: polarization, depolarization, and repolarization. The phases of the nerve impulses are caused by the movement of ions, particularly Na^+ and K^+. Once the axon membrane is stimulated, the nerve impulse travels the length of the axon. Many of the axons are myelinated to increase the speed of the nerve impulse. The nerve impulse travels along the neuron from the dendrite to the end of the axon. The impulse stimulates the release of neurotransmitters into the synaptic cleft; the transmitter diffuses across the synaptic cleft, binds to the receptor, and stimulates the dendrites of the second neuron. This is the way that information is transmitted from one neuron to the next.

BRAIN: STRUCTURE AND FUNCTION

You read a book, listen to music, sing a song, laugh, rage, remember, learn, feel, move, sleep, awaken, and so much more. All these are functions of the brain!

The brain is located in the cranial cavity. It is a pinkish-gray, delicate structure with a soft consistency. The surface of the brain appears bumpy, much like a walnut. The "boss of it all" weighs but 3 lbs!

The blood supply to the brain is unique and is described in Chapter 18. Despite the fact that the brain weighs only 2% of total body weight, it requires 20% of the body's oxygen supply. The primary source of energy for the brain is glucose. When blood glucose levels get very low (hypoglycemia) the person experiences mental confusion, dizziness, convulsions, loss of consciousness, and death. No wonder that many of the body hormones are concerned with making glucose available to the brain.

The brain is divided into four major areas: the cerebrum, the diencephalon, the brain stem, and the cerebellum (Figure 10-10).

CEREBRUM

The **cerebrum** (sĕ-RĒ-brŭm) is the largest part of the brain. It is divided into the **right** and **left cerebral hemispheres.** The cerebral hemispheres are joined together by bands of white matter that form a large fiber tract called the **corpus callosum.** The corpus callosum allows the right and left sides of the brain to communicate with each other. Each cerebral hemisphere has four major lobes: frontal, parietal, temporal, and occipital (Figure 10-11). These four lobes are named for the overlying cranial bones.

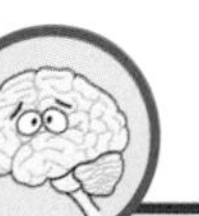

Do You Know...

If you are a left-brain or a right-brain person?

Some years ago a surgeon severed the corpus callosum in the brain of a patient with severe epilepsy. This surgical procedure eliminated all communication between the left and right cerebral hemispheres. From these and other experiments, neuroscientists learned that there is a left brain and a right brain, and that these two brains have different abilities. (The differences in function between the two cerebral hemispheres is called cerebral lateralization.) The left brain is more concerned with language and mathematical abilities; it is the reasoning and analytical side of the brain. The right side of the brain is far superior with regard to spatial relationships, art, music, and the expression of emotions. The right brain is intuitive; it is the poet and the artist. Many of us are predominantly left-brain or right-brain persons. How much richer our lives are when we use both sides of our brains!

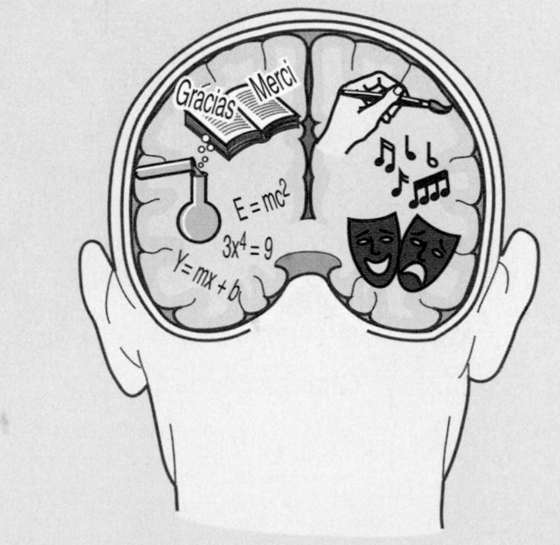

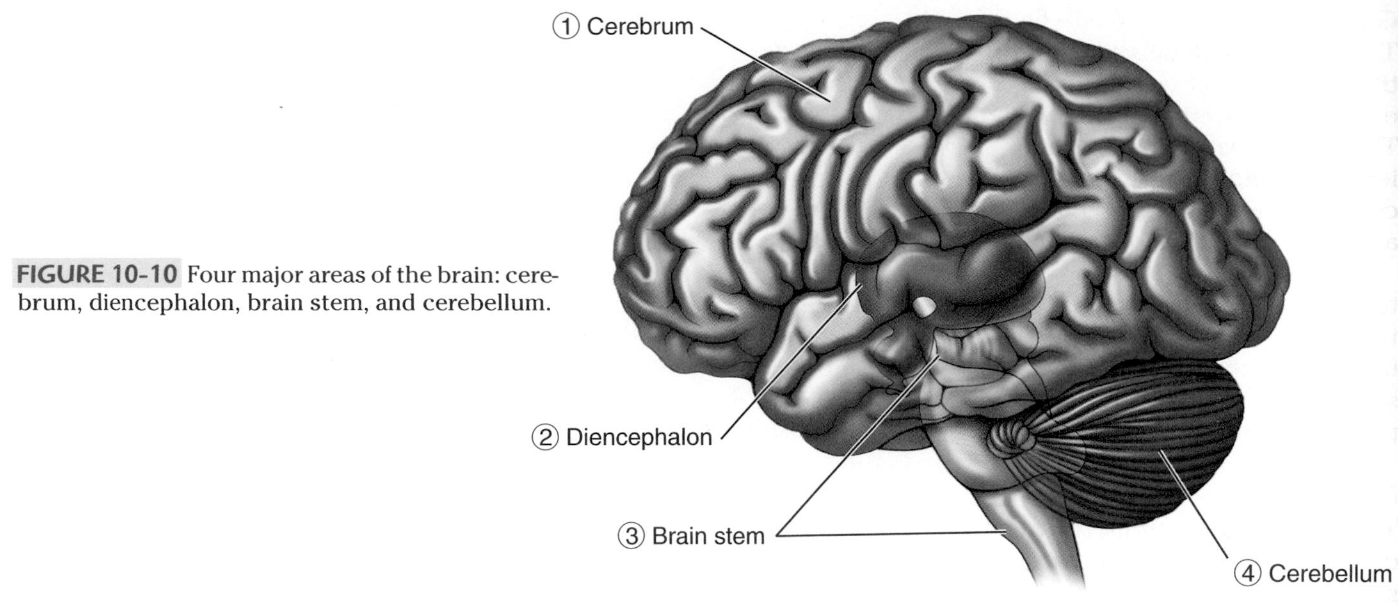

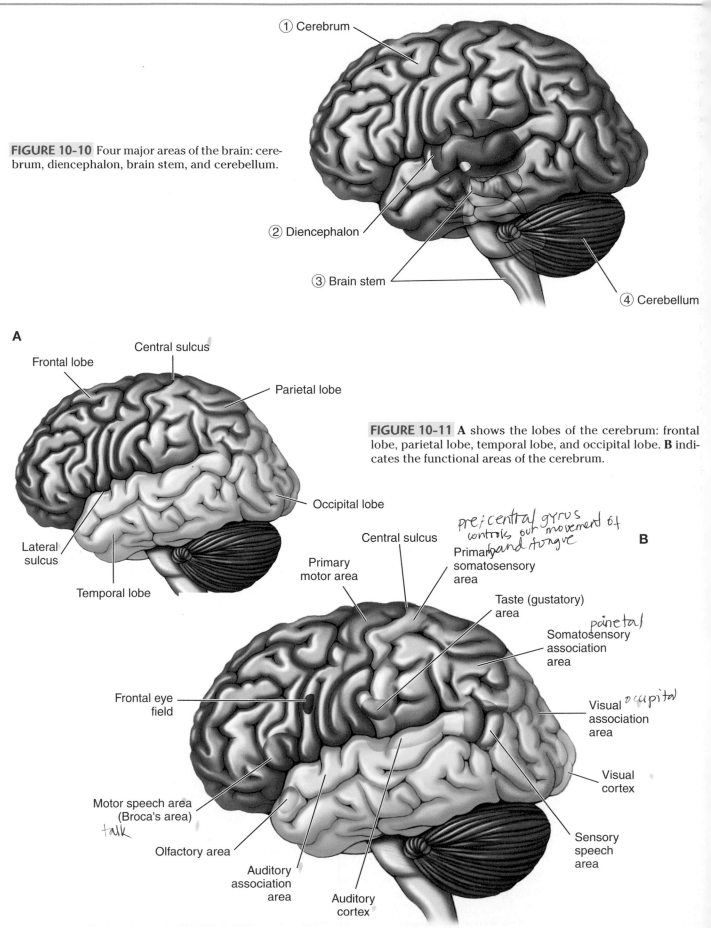

FIGURE 10-10 Four major areas of the brain: cerebrum, diencephalon, brain stem, and cerebellum.

FIGURE 10-11 **A** shows the lobes of the cerebrum: frontal lobe, parietal lobe, temporal lobe, and occipital lobe. **B** indicates the functional areas of the cerebrum.

Gray on the Outside, White on the Inside

The cerebrum contains both gray and white matter. A thin layer of gray matter forms the outermost portion of the cerebrum. This is called the **cerebral cortex.** The cerebral cortex is composed primarily of cell bodies and interneurons. The gray matter of the cerebral cortex allows us to perform higher mental tasks such as learning, reasoning, language, and memory.

The bulk of the cerebrum is composed of white matter located directly below the cortex. The white matter is composed primarily of myelinated axons that form connections between the parts of the brain and spinal cord. Scattered throughout the white matter are patches of gray matter called nuclei.

Markings of the Cerebrum

The lumpy bumpy surface of the cerebrum has numerous markings, or structures, with special names. The surface of the cerebrum is folded into elevations that resemble speed bumps on a road. The elevations are called **convolutions,** or **gyri** (singular: **gyrus**).

This extensive folding arrangement increases the amount of cerebral cortex, or thinking tissue. It is thought that intelligence is related to the amount of cerebral cortex and therefore to the numbers of convolutions or gyri. The greater the numbers of convolutions in the brain, the more intelligent is the species. For example, the cerebral cortex of the human brain has many more convolutions than does the brain of an elephant (except in the memory part of the brain). Big bumps, big thoughts.

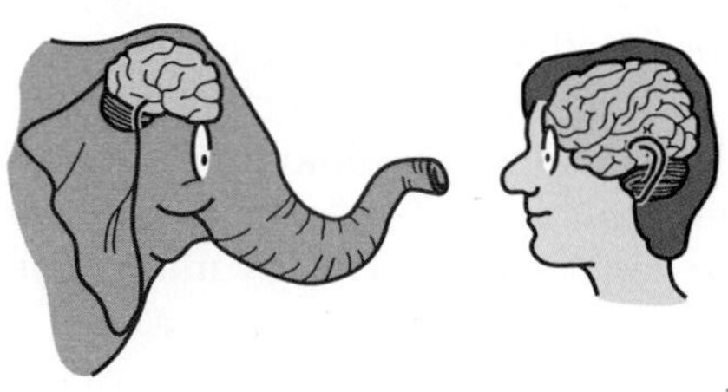

Gyri are separated by grooves called **sulci** (singular: **sulcus**). A deep sulcus is called a **fissure.** Sulci and fissures separate the cerebrum into lobes. Figure 10-11 illustrates two of the numerous sulci and fissures: the central sulcus and the lateral sulcus. (Identify each structure on the diagram as it is described in the text.)

The **central sulcus** separates the frontal lobe from the parietal lobe. The central sulcus is an important landmark, separating the precentral and postcentral gyri. The **precentral gyrus** is located in the frontal lobe, directly in front of the central sulcus, and the **postcentral gyrus** is located in the parietal lobe, directly behind the central sulcus. The **lateral fissure** separates the temporal lobe from the frontal and the parietal lobes. The **longitudinal fissure** separates the left and right cerebral hemispheres (not shown).

Lobes of the Cerebrum

What does each cerebral lobe do? The cerebral cortex is associated with specific functions (Table 10-2).

Frontal Lobe. The **frontal lobe** is located in the front of the cranium under the frontal bone (see Figure 10-11). The frontal lobe plays a key role in voluntary motor

Table 10-2 Brain Structure and Function

Structure	Functions
Cerebrum	
Frontal lobe	Motor area, personality; behavior; emotional expression; intellectual functions ("executive" functions); memory storage
Parietal lobe	Somatosensory area (especially from skin and muscle; taste; speech; reading)
Occipital lobe	Vision; vision-related reflexes and functions (reading, judging distances, seeing in three dimensions)
Temporal lobe	Hearing (auditory area); smell (olfactory area); taste; memory storage; part of speech area
Diencephalon	
Thalamus	Relay structure and processing center for most sensory information going to the cerebrum
Hypothalamus	Integrating system for the autonomic nervous system; regulation of temperature, water balance, sex, thirst, appetite, and some emotions (pleasure and fear); regulates the pituitary gland and controls endocrine function
Brain Stem	
Midbrain	Relays information (sensory and motor); associated with visual reflexes
Pons	Relays information (sensory and motor); plays a role in respiration
Medulla oblongata	Vital function (regulation of heart rate, blood flow, blood pressure, respiratory centers); reflex center for coughing, sneezing, swallowing, and vomiting
Cerebellum	Smoothes out and coordinates voluntary muscle activity; helps in the maintenance of balance and muscle tone
Other Structures	
Limbic system	Experience of emotion and behavior (emotional brain)
Reticular formation	Mediates wakefulness and sleep
Basal nuclei	Smoothes out and coordinates skeletal muscle activity

activity, personality development, emotional and behavioral expression, and the performance of high-level tasks such as learning, thinking, and making plans; these are sometimes called "executive functions." The frontal lobe contains the **primary motor cortex.** Nerve impulses that originate in the motor area control voluntary muscle movement. When you decide to move your leg, the nerve impulse originates in the precentral gyrus, or primary motor cortex, of the frontal lobe. The axons of these motor neurons form the voluntary motor tracts that descend to the spinal cord.

The function of the precentral gyrus of the frontal lobe is illustrated by a **homunculus,** meaning "little man" (Figure 10-12). The homunculus represents the amount of brain tissue that corresponds to a function of a particular body part. The homunculus shows two important points: each part of the body is controlled by a specific area of the cerebral cortex of the precentral gyrus, and the complicated nature of certain movements requires large amounts of brain tissue. (Locate the specific points for the toe, foot, leg, trunk, hand, and face.)

For instance, the movements of the hand are much more delicate and complicated than the movements of the foot. Therefore the amount of brain tissue devoted to hand and finger movement is much greater than the amount devoted to foot and toe movement. Consequently, the homunculus has huge hands and small feet. Note also the amount of brain tissue required to run your mouth.

In addition to its role in voluntary motor activity, the frontal lobe plays a key role in motor speech.

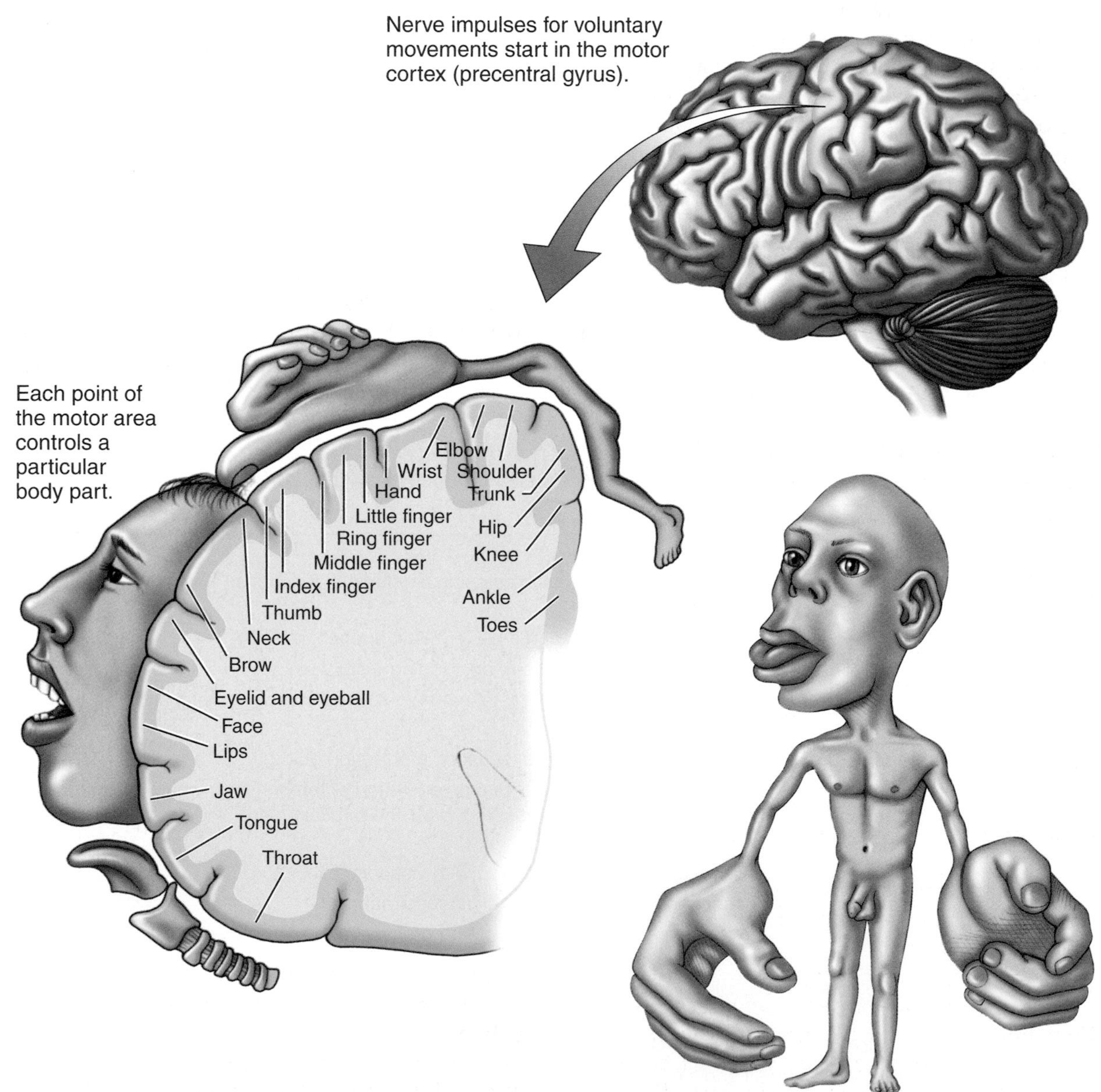

FIGURE 10-12 Motor area of the frontal lobe, illustrated with a homunculus.

Motor speech refers to the movements of the mouth and tongue necessary for the formation of words. The part of the frontal lobe concerned with motor speech is called **Broca's area.** In most persons, Broca's area is in the left hemisphere (see Figure 10-11). What happens when Broca's area is broken? If damaged, as happens with a stroke, the person develops a type of aphasia. The person knows what he or she wants to say, but can't say it. Just above Broca's area is an area called the **frontal eye field.** It controls voluntary movements of the eyes and the eyelids. Your ability to scan this paragraph is a function of this area.

Decussation. Why does damage to the left side of the brain cause paralysis of the right side of the body? The fibers that carry information from the motor area of the frontal lobe of the brain are crossed fibers. In other words, the fibers leave the motor area of the left frontal lobe, cross over, and innervate the right side of the body. The fibers from the right frontal lobe also cross over and innervate the left side of the body. The crossing over of fibers is called **decussation.**

Parietal Lobe. The **parietal lobe** is located behind the central sulcus (see Figure 10-11). The parietal lobe, particularly the postcentral gyrus, is primarily concerned with receiving general sensory information from the body. Because it receives sensations from the body, the parietal lobe is called the **primary somatosensory area.** This area receives information primarily from the skin and muscles and allows you to experience the sensations of temperature, pain, light touch, and proprioception (a sense of where your body is). The parietal lobe is also concerned with reading, speech, and taste.

Temporal Lobe. The **temporal lobe** is located inferior to the lateral fissure in an area just above the ear. The temporal lobe contains the **primary auditory cortex,** the area that allows you to hear. It receives sensory information from the ears. Damage to the temporal lobe causes cortical deafness. The temporal lobe also receives sensory information from the nose; this area is called the **olfactory area,** the area that controls smell. Sensory information from the **taste buds** in the tongue is interpreted in both the temporal and parietal lobes. **Wernicke's area** is a broad region that is located in the parietal and temporal lobes; it is concerned with the translation of thought into words. Damage to this area can result in severe deficits in language comprehension.

Occipital Lobe. The **occipital lobe** (ŏk-SĬP-ĭ-tăl) is located in the back of the head, underlying the occipital bone. The occipital lobe contains the **visual cortex.** Sensory fibers from the eye send information to the visual cortex of the occipital lobe, where it is interpreted as sight. The occipital lobe is also concerned with many visual reflexes and vision-related functions such as reading (through the visual association area). Damage to the occipital lobe causes cortical blindness.

Functions Involving Many Cerebral Lobes

Speech Area. Although specific functions can be attributed to each cerebral lobe, most functions depend on more than one area of the brain. The **speech area,** for instance, is located in an area that includes the temporal, parietal, and occipital lobes. In most people, the speech area is located in the left hemisphere. The speech area allows you to understand words, whether written or spoken. When you have gathered your thoughts Broca's area directs the muscles of the larynx, tongue, cheeks, and lips to speak.

Do You Know...

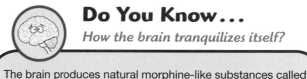

How the brain tranquilizes itself?

The brain produces natural morphine-like substances called endorphins (endogenous morphine) and enkephalins (meaning in the head). Like morphine, these substances bind to opiate receptors in the CNS, moderating pain, relieving anxiety, and producing a sense of well-being. The "high" experienced by joggers may be due to endorphins and enkephalins.

Other functions require input from more than one brain structure. The ability to read, for instance, requires interpretation of the visual information by the occipital lobe. It also requires understanding of the words and the coordination of the eyes as they scan the page. A vast amount of brain tissue beyond the occipital lobe is involved in vision and vision-related functions such as reading.

Association Areas

Large areas of the cerebral cortex are called association areas (see Figure 10-11). These areas are concerned primarily with analyzing, interpreting, and integrating information. For instance, a small area of the temporal lobe, called the primary auditory cortex, receives sensory information from the ear. The surrounding area, called the auditory association area, uses a large store of knowledge and experience to identify and give meaning to the sound. In other words, the auditory cortex hears the noise, and the auditory association area interprets the noise. The brain contains receiving and association areas for other sensations too (e.g., visual association area, somatosensory association area).

Patches of Gray

Scattered throughout the cerebral white matter are patches of gray matter called basal nuclei (sometimes called basal ganglia). The basal nuclei help regulate body movement and facial expression. The neurotransmitter dopamine is largely responsible for the activity of the basal nuclei.

A deficiency of dopamine within the basal nuclei is called Parkinson's disease. It is characterized by problems with movement: a shuffling and uncoordinated gait (walk), rigidity, slowness of speech, drooling, and a masklike facial expression. Because of the characteristic shaking (called tremors), Parkinson's disease is sometimes called shaking palsy. Dopamine or dopamine-like drugs are usually prescribed to treat this condition.

DIENCEPHALON

The **diencephalon** is the second main area of the brain. It is located beneath the cerebrum and above the brain stem. The diencephalon includes the thalamus and the hypothalamus (Figure 10-13).

The **thalamus** serves as a relay station for most of the sensory fibers traveling from the lower brain and spinal cord region to the sensory areas of the cerebrum. The thalamus sorts out the sensory information, gives us a "hint" of the sensation we are to experience, and then directs the information to the specific cerebral areas for more precise interpretation.

For instance, pain fibers coming from the body to the brain pass through the thalamus. At the level of the thalamus, we become aware of pain, but we are not yet aware of the kind of pain or the exact location of the pain. Fibers that transmit pain information from the thalamus to the cerebral cortex provide us with that additional information.

The **hypothalamus** is the second structure in the diencephalon. It is situated directly below the thalamus and helps regulate many body processes, including body temperature (thermostat), water balance, and metabolism. Because the hypothalamus helps regulate the function of the autonomic (involuntary) nerves, it exerts an effect on heart rate, blood pressure, and respiration.

Located under the hypothalamus is the pituitary gland. The pituitary gland directly or indirectly affects almost every hormone in the body. Because the hypothalamus controls pituitary function, the widespread effects of the hypothalamus are obvious.

BRAIN STEM

The **brain stem** connects the spinal cord with higher brain structures. It is composed of the midbrain, pons, and medulla oblongata (see Figure 10-13). The white matter of the brain stem includes tracts that relay both sensory and motor information to and from the cerebrum. Scattered throughout the white matter of the brain stem are patches of gray matter called nuclei. These nuclei exert profound effects on functions such as blood pressure and respiration.

Midbrain

The **midbrain** extends from the lower diencephalon to the pons. Like the rest of the brain stem structures, the midbrain relays sensory and motor information. The midbrain also contains nuclei that function as reflex centers for vision and hearing.

Pons

The **pons** (bridge) extends from the midbrain to the medulla oblongata. It is composed primarily of tracts that act as a bridge for information traveling to and from several brain structures. The pons also plays an important role in the regulation of breathing rate and rhythm.

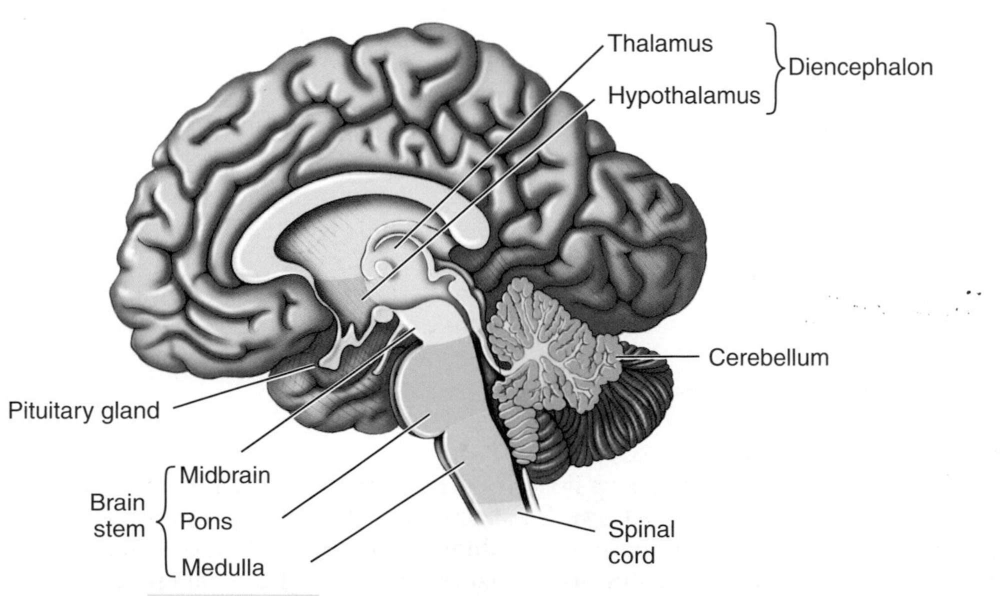

FIGURE 10-13 Diencephalon, brain stem, and cerebellum.

Medulla Oblongata

The **medulla oblongata** (mĕ-DŪL-ă ŏb-lŏn-GĂ-tă) connects the spinal cord with the pons. The medulla acts as a relay for sensory and motor information. Several important nuclei within the medulla control heart rate, blood pressure, and respiration. Because of its importance with regard to vital functions, the medulla oblongata is often called the **vital center.** Because these functions are vital to the body, you can understand the seriousness of a fracture at the base of the skull.

The medulla oblongata is also extremely sensitive to certain drugs, especially narcotics (specifically, opioids). An overdose of a narcotic causes depression of the medulla oblongata and thus death because the person stops breathing. This danger is the reason for counting the respiratory rate before giving a patient a narcotic. If the respiratory rate is less than 10 respirations per minute, the drug cannot be safely administered.

Vomiting Center

The medulla oblongata contains the vomiting center or emetic center (emesis refers to vomiting). The vomiting center can be activated either directly or indirectly. Direct activation includes stimuli from the cerebral cortex (fear), stimuli from sensory organs (distressing sights, bad odors, pain), and signals from the equilibrium apparatus of the inner ear (spinning). Indirect stimulation of the vomiting center comes from the chemoreceptor trigger zone (CTZ) located in the floor of the fourth ventricle. The CTZ can be stimulated by emetogenic compounds, such as anticancer drugs and narcotics. Signals from the digestive tract, especially the stomach send signals via the vagus nerve to the CTZ. The CTZ, in turn, activates the vomiting center. Antiemetic agents can work on both the CTZ and vomiting center to relieve nausea and vomiting. The pharmacologic management of vomiting is a common clinical problem.

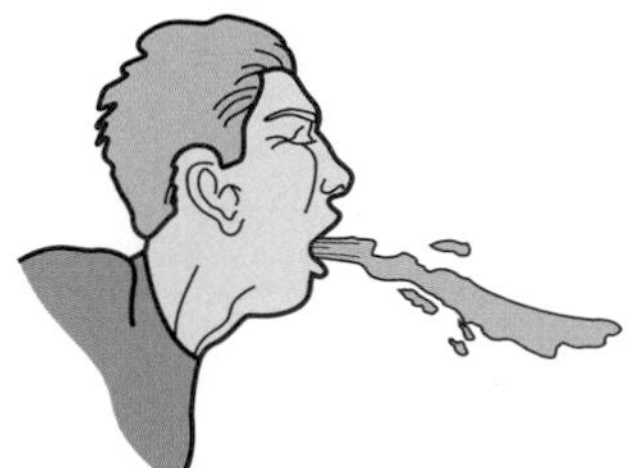

CEREBELLUM

The **cerebellum** (sĕr-ĕ-BĔL-ŭm), the fourth major area, is the structure that protrudes from under the occipital lobe at the base of the skull (see Figure 10-13). The cerebellum is concerned primarily with the coordination of voluntary muscle activity. Information is sent to the cerebellum from many areas throughout the body, including the eyes, ears, and skeletal muscles. The cerebellum integrates all of the incoming information to produce a smooth, coordinated muscle response.

Damage to the cerebellum produces jerky muscle movements, staggering gait, and difficulty maintaining balance or equilibrium. The person with cerebellar dysfunction may appear intoxicated. To diagnose cerebellar dysfunction, the physician may ask the person to touch the tip of his nose with his finger. Why? The cerebellum normally coordinates skeletal muscle activity. In attempting to touch his nose, a patient with cerebellar dysfunction may overshoot, first to one side and then to the other.

STRUCTURES ACROSS DIVISIONS OF THE BRAIN

Three important structures are not confined to any of the four divisions of the brain because they "overlap" several areas. These structures are the limbic system, the reticular system, and the memory areas.

Limbic System: The Emotional Brain

Parts of the cerebrum and the diencephalon form a wishbone-shaped group of structures called the limbic system. The **limbic system** functions in emotional states and behavior. For instance, when the limbic system is stimulated by microelectrodes, states of extreme pleasure or rage can be induced. Because of these responses, the limbic system is called the emotional brain.

Reticular Formation: Wake Up!

What keeps us awake? Why don't we slip into a coma when we go to sleep? Extending through the entire brain stem, with numerous connections to the cerebral cortex, is a special mass of gray matter called the **reticular formation.** The reticular formation is concerned with the sleep-wake cycle and consciousness. Signals passing up to the cerebral cortex from the reticular formation stimulate us, keeping us awake and tuned in.

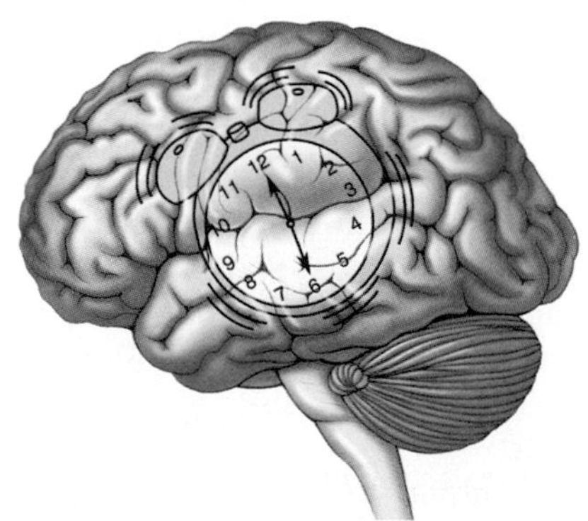

The reticular formation is very sensitive to the effects of certain drugs and alcohol. For example, the dangerous combination of benzodiazepines (tranquilizers) and alcohol can damage the reticular formation, causing permanent unconsciousness.

Consciousness, Sleep, and Coma. Consciousness is a state of wakefulness. Consciousness depends on the reticular activating system (RAS). The RAS continuously samples sensory information from all over the body and then selects and presents essential, unusual, and threatening information to the higher structures in the cerebral cortex. The different levels of consciousness include attentiveness, alertness, relaxation, and inattentiveness. **Sleep** occurs when the RAS is inhibited or slowed. What causes sleep? In the sixth century BC, it was believed that sleep was due to a temporary retreat of blood from the brain. Death was attributed to the permanent retreat of blood from the brain. As to the cause of sleep? We still do not know.

Coma is a sleeplike state with several stages, ranging from light to deep coma. In the lightest stages of coma, some reflexes are intact; the patient may respond to light, sound, touch, and painful stimuli. As the coma deepens, however, these reflexes are gradually lost, and the patient eventually becomes unresponsive to all stimuli. Damage to the reticular formation is associated with a state of deep coma, which can be permanent.

Many clinical conditions affect level of consciousness (LOC), often leading to coma. These include brain tumors, brain injury, drugs, toxins, hypoxia, hyperglycemia, acid-base imbalance, and electrolyte imbalance. As a clinician, you must be able to assess the patient's LOC.

Stages of Sleep. The two types of sleep are **non-rapid eye movements (NREM) sleep** and **rapid eye movement (REM) sleep.** The four stages of NREM sleep progress from light to deep. In a typical 8-hour sleep period, a person regularly cycles through the various stages of sleep, descending from light to deep sleep and then ascending from deeper sleep to lighter sleep. The person then ascends from NREM deep sleep to stage 2 (NREM) sleep to REM sleep. After a short period of REM sleep, the person descends again through the stages of NREM sleep. REM sleep totals 90 to 120 minutes per night.

REM sleep is characterized by fluctuating blood pressure, respiratory rate and rhythm, and pulse rate. The most obvious characteristic of REM sleep is rapid eye movements, for which the sleep segment is named. Most dreaming occurs during REM sleep. For unknown reasons, REM sleep deprivation is associated with mental and physical distress. Most sedatives and CNS depressants adversely affect REM sleep, perhaps accounting for a "hungover" feeling that often follows their use.

Memory Areas

Memory is the ability to recall thoughts and images. Many areas of the brain are concerned with memory: the frontal, parietal, occipital, and temporal lobes; the limbic system, and the diencephalon. There are two categories of memory: short-term and long-term memory. Short-term memory lasts for short period of time (seconds to a few hours). It allows you to recall bits of information, such as the price of those new jeans or a phone number that you looked up. Unfortunately, cramming for exams falls into this category: short-term memorization, five-second retention, and then—BLANK. Long-term memory lasts much longer: years or decades. If you continuously use the new address or phone number, you will enter that information into your long-term memory. The same effect is achieved when you study over a longer period of time.

PROTECTING THE CENTRAL NERVOUS SYSTEM

The tissue of the CNS (brain and spinal cord) is very delicate. Injury to CNS neuronal tissue cannot be repaired. Thus the CNS has an elaborate protective system that consists of four structures: bone, meninges, cerebrospinal fluid, and the blood-brain barrier.

BONE: FIRST LAYER OF PROTECTION

The CNS is protected by bone. The brain is encased in the cranium, while the spinal cord is encased in the vertebral column.

MENINGES: SECOND LAYER OF PROTECTION

Three layers of connective tissue surround the brain and spinal cord (Figure 10-14). These tissues are called the **meninges** (mĕ-NĬN-jēz). The outermost layer is a thick, tough, connective tissue called the **dura mater,** literally meaning "hard mother." Inside the skull, the dural membrane splits to form the dural sinuses. These sinuses are filled with blood. Beneath the dura mater is a small space called the subdural space. The middle layer is the **arachnoid** (meaning spiderlike) layer, so named because the membrane looks like a spiderweb.

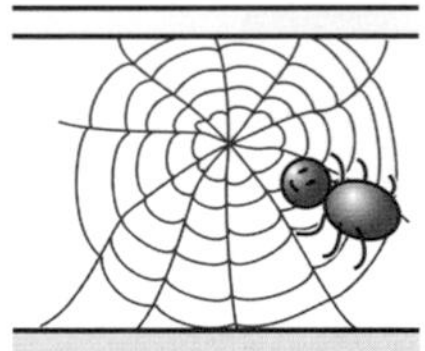

Do You Know...

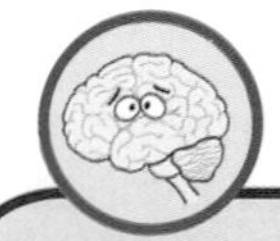

Why people in ancient times bored holes in the skull?

Trephination refers to the drilling of holes into the skull for the purpose of reducing intracranial pressure. It is performed in the operating room under sterile conditions. People in ancient times also performed trephination procedures. The patient sat on a log while the priest chipped a hole in the skull using a sharp stone. Ouch! It was thought that trephination could relieve headaches and release the devils of madness.

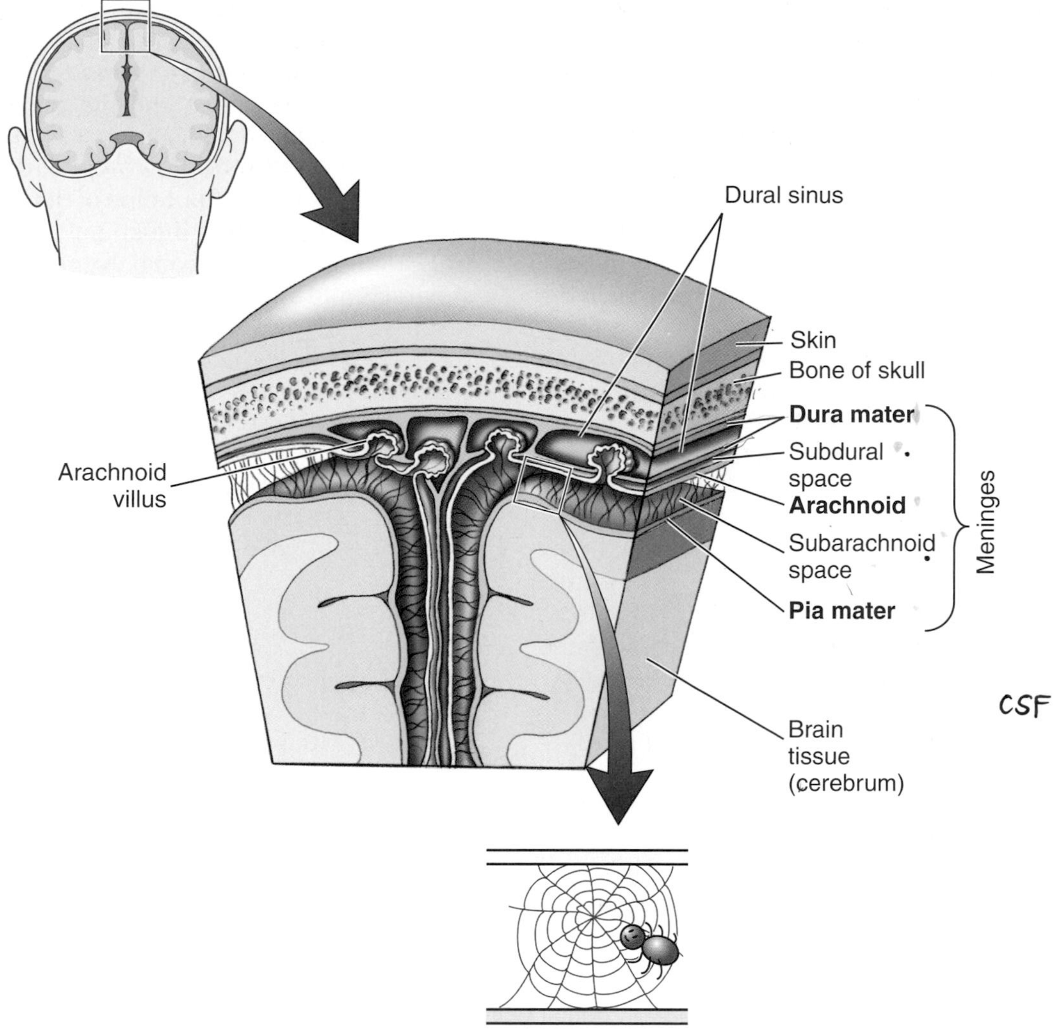

FIGURE 10-14 The three layers of meninges are the dura mater, arachnoid, and pia mater.

The **pia mater** is the innermost layer and literally means soft, or gentle, mother. The pia mater is a very thin membrane that contains many blood vessels and lies delicately over the brain and spinal cord. These blood vessels supply the brain with much of its blood. Between the arachnoid layer and the pia mater is a space called the **subarachnoid space.** A fluid called the **cerebrospinal fluid (CSF)** circulates within this space and forms a cushion around the brain and spinal cord. If the head is jarred suddenly, the brain first bumps into this soft cushion of fluid. Specialized projections of the arachnoid membrane, called the **arachnoid villi** (singular: villus), protrude up into the blood-filled dural sinuses.

Remember—The meninges form a **brain PAD** (noting that the brain is closer to Pia, the softer mother)!

P **p**ia mater
A **a**rachnoid
D **d**ura mater

The meninges can become inflamed or infected, causing meningitis. Meningitis is serious because the infection can spread to the brain, sometimes causing serious, irreversible brain damage. The bacterial or viral organism causing the meningitis can often be found in a sample of cerebrospinal fluid obtained by lumbar puncture.

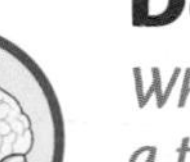

Do You Know...

Where and why there is a tent in your brain?

At several areas the dura mater forms rigid membranes that separate and support parts of the brain. One such membrane is the tentorium cerebelli; it forms a tentlike membrane over the cerebellum, separating it from the upper cerebral structures. The tentorium also functions as a common landmark in the brain. Brain tumors are classified according to their locations. Those that occur in structures located above the tentorium are called supratentorial brain tumors, while those occurring below the tentorium are called infratentorial brain tumors. An increase in intracranial pressure can force the brain downward past the tentorium, causing life-threatening symptoms. The displacement is called tentorial herniation.

CEREBROSPINAL FLUID: THIRD LAYER OF PROTECTION

The CSF forms a third protective layer of the CNS. CSF is formed from the blood within the brain. It is a clear fluid that looks like Sprite and is similar in composition to plasma. The CSF is composed of water, glucose, protein, and several ions, especially Na^+ and Cl^-. An adult circulates about 130 ml of CSF (500 ml is formed every 24 hours, so that CSF is replaced every 8 hours). In addition to its protective function, CSF also delivers nutrients to the CNS and removes waste.

Where is cerebrospinal fluid formed? CSF is formed within the ventricles of the brain by a structure called the **choroid plexus** (Figure 10-15, *A*). The four ventricles are two lateral ventricles, and a third and a fourth ventricle. The choroid plexus, a grapelike collection of blood vessels and ependymal cells (see Table 10-1), is suspended from the roof of each ventricle. Water and dissolved substances are transported from the blood across the walls of the choroid plexus into the ventricles (see Figure 10-15, *B*).

Where does the CSF flow? As CSF leaves the ventricles, it follows two paths. Some of the CSF flows through a hole in the center of the spinal cord called the **central canal.** The central canal eventually drains into the subarachnoid space at the base of the spinal cord. The rest of the CSF flows from the fourth ventricle laterally through tiny holes, or foramina, into the subarachnoid space that encircles the brain.

How does the CSF leave the subarachnoid space? Eventually, CSF flows into the arachnoid villi and drains into the blood within the dural sinuses. Blood flows

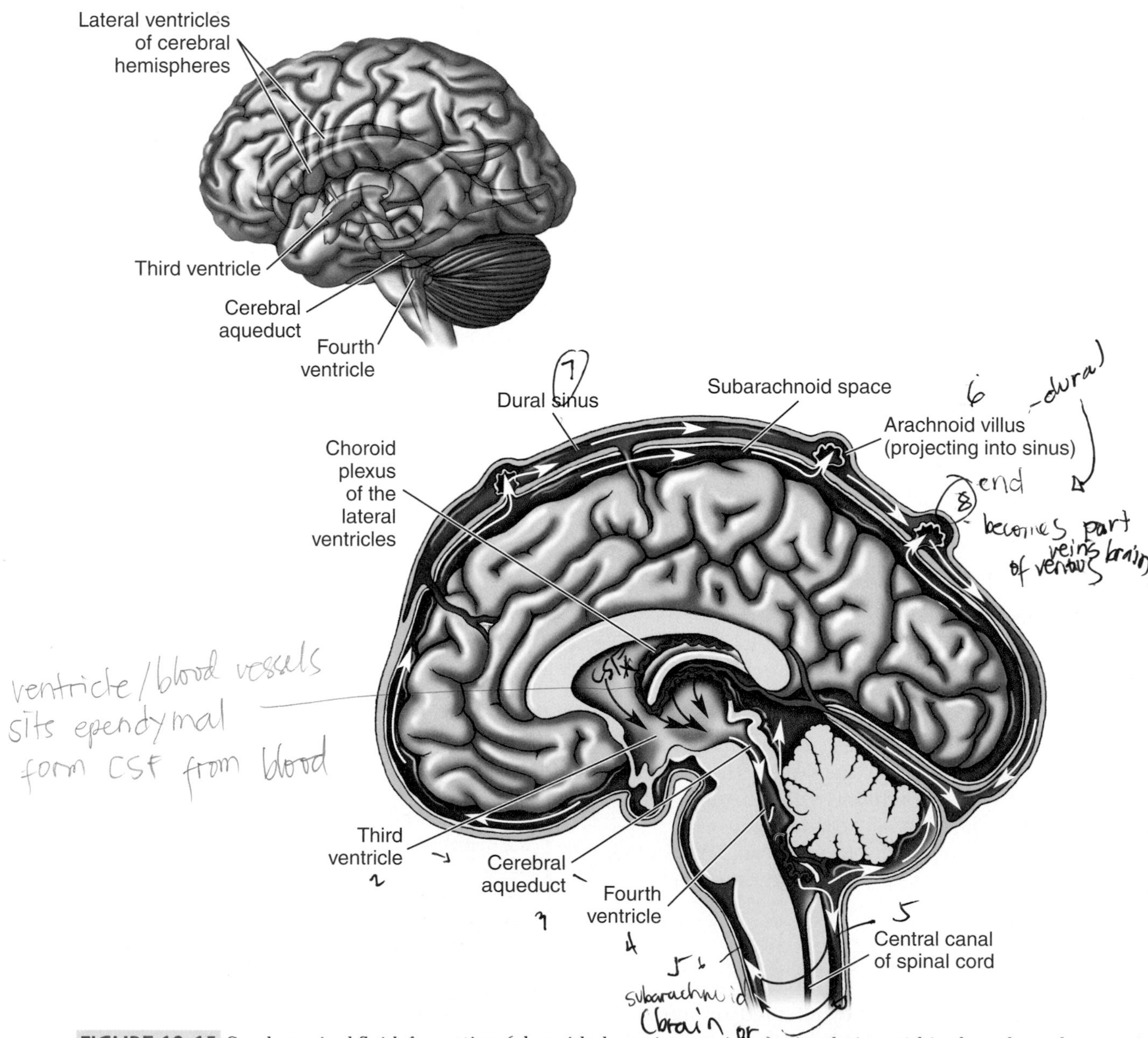

FIGURE 10-15 Cerebrospinal fluid: formation (choroid plexus in ventricles); circulation within the subarachnoid space; and drainage (arachnoid villus).

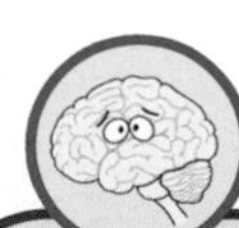

Do You Know...

What a little red worm's doing in your brain?

In the 1300s an anatomist claimed that mental function was controlled by a red worm. The worm referred to the fleshy choroid plexus of the ventricles of the brain. The plexi allegedly controlled brain functions by wiggling back and forth and modifying the flow of cerebrospinal fluid, which was supposed to contain the animal spirit. Several things have since been cleared up: mental function is due to neuronal activity and not to the flow of animal spirit; the choroid plexus secretes cerebrospinal fluid and does not wiggle and shake. There is, however, a little red worm—the choroid plexus—and it is located in the ventricles of your brain.

from the dural sinuses into the cerebral veins and back to the heart. Remember that the CSF is formed across the walls of the choroid plexus within the ventricles, circulates throughout the subarachnoid space around the brain and spinal cord, and then drains into the dural sinuses. The rate at which CSF is formed must equal the rate at which it is drained. If either excess CSF is formed or drainage is impaired, CSF will accumulate in the ventricles of the brain, increasing the pressure within the skull. The resulting increase in intracranial pressure can cause brain damage and death.

BLOOD-BRAIN BARRIER: FOURTH LAYER OF PROTECTION

The **blood-brain barrier** is an arrangement of cells, particularly the glial astrocytes, associated with the blood vessels that supply the brain and spinal cord. 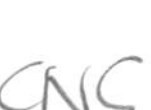 These cells select the substances allowed to enter the CNS from the blood. For instance, oxygen, glucose, and certain ions readily cross the membrane. However, if a potentially harmful substance is present in the blood, the cells of the blood-brain barrier prevent that substance from entering the brain and the spinal cord.

Although the blood-brain barrier is successful in screening many harmful substances, not all toxic substances are blocked. Alcohol, for instance, crosses the blood-brain barrier and affects brain tissue.

The blood-brain barrier may present a problem in the pharmacological treatment of infections within the CNS. Most antibiotics, for instance, cannot cross the blood-brain barrier and therefore cannot reach the site of infection. Given this problem, how is an infection of the CNS treated? The two options are to either select an antibiotic that does cross the blood-brain barrier or inject the antibiotic directly into the subarachnoid space.

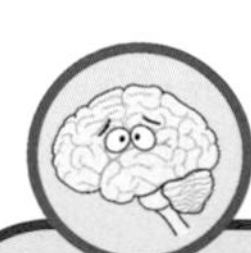

Do You Know...

Why an infant may develop water on the brain?

Occasionally, a newborn infant is born with a block (e.g., tumor) in the ventricular system of the brain. Cerebrospinal fluid (CSF) is formed at a normal rate but cannot be drained because of the block. The fluid accumulates within the ventricles, thereby increasing intracranial pressure and causing the skull to enlarge. This condition is called hydrocephalus (water on the brain). Head expansion in the infant is possible because the suture lines of the skull bones have not yet fused. If a block were to occur in an older child or adult, the intracranial pressure would increase. The skull, however, could not expand because of the fused sutures. Without surgical intervention or the use of a shunt that bypasses the block, the increased pressure would result in death.

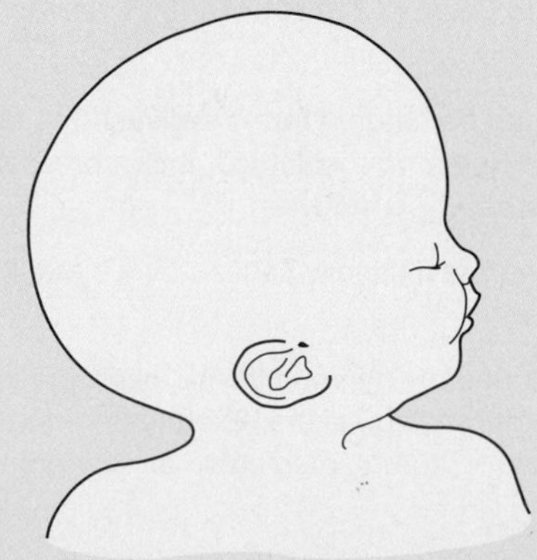

Sum It Up!

The CNS, especially the brain, performs eloquently as a conductor. It coordinates the various organ systems of the body efficiently, with fine precision. The brain makes us humans—that is, thinking, caring, feeling, remembering persons. The brain is divided into four regions: cerebrum, diencephalon, brain stem, and cerebellum. The cerebrum is the largest part of the brain and has four lobes: frontal, parietal, temporal, and occipital lobes. The diencephalon is composed of the thalamus and the hypothalamus. The brain stem is composed of the midbrain, pons, and medulla oblongata. The medulla is considered a vital structure in that it affects basic functions such as respiration, cardiac function, and blood vessel tone. Three other areas are the reticular formation, which keeps us awake, the limbic system (emotional brain), and the memory areas. Because of the crucial role played by the CNS, it is afforded excellent protection—that is, bone, three layers of meninges, a soft cushion of fluid, and a blood-brain barrier.

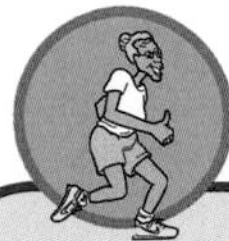

As You Age

1. Beginning at the age of 30, the number of neurons decreases. The number lost, however, is only a small percentage of the total number of brain cells and does not cause mental impairment. Although a decrease in short-term memory may cause some forgetfulness, most memory, alertness, intellectual functioning, and creativity remain intact. Severe alteration of mental functioning is generally due to age-related diseases such as arteriosclerosis.
2. Impulse conduction speed decreases along an axon; amounts of neurotransmitters are reduced; and the number of receptor sites decreases at the synapses. These changes result in progressive slowing of responses and reflexes.

Disorders of the Nervous Tissue and the Brain

Alcohol-induced neurotoxicity	Chronic and excessive ingestion of alcohol causing irreversible injury to the nervous system. The result is mental deterioration, loss of memory, inability to concentrate, irritability, and uncoordinated movement. Wernicke-Korsakoff syndrome is an alcohol-related type of encephalopathy.
Alzheimer's disease	A degenerative disease of the brain usually occurring in older persons. Alzheimer's disease is characterized by progressive loss of memory and impaired intellectual function. Evidence suggests brain atrophy, especially of the frontal and temporal lobes.
Cerebral palsy (CP)	A group of neuromuscular disorders that result from injury to an infant before, during, or shortly after birth. All forms of CP cause impairment of skeletal muscle activity. Mental retardation and speech difficulties may accompany the disorder.
Cerebrovascular accident (CVA)	Commonly called a stroke or "brain attack." A CVA is due to a sudden lack of blood, causing oxygen deprivation and brain damage. Depending on the location and severity of the brain damage, a CVA can result in loss of sensory and motor function (causing paralysis) and speech impairment. The major causes of CVA are thrombosis and cerebral hemorrhage. The hemorrhage may be due to a ruptured aneurysm, such as a Berry aneurysm (a congenital aneurysm of the circle of Willis, a collection of blood vessels at the base of the brain).
Concussion	A transient loss of consciousness, usually after head trauma.
Contusion	A bruise of the brain involving a torn cerebral or meningeal blood vessel.
Epilepsy	From the Greek word meaning to seize upon. Epilepsy refers to a group of symptoms that have many causes (such as brain tumor, toxins, trauma, or fever). Neurons in the brain fire suddenly and unpredictably. Grand mal (big illness) seizures occur when the motor areas fire repetitively, causing convulsive seizures and loss of consciousness. Petit mal (small illness) seizures occur when sensory areas are affected. Although a brief period of altered consciousness occurs, petit mal seizures are not accompanied by convulsions or prolonged unconsciousness.
Headache (migraine)	Severe, recurring headaches that usually affect only one side of the head. (The word migraine comes from the Latin *hemicranium,* meaning one side of the head.) A migraine may be preceded and accompanied by fatigue, nausea, vomiting, and a visual sensation of zigzag lines. Not all headaches are migraines. A simple tension headache may develop when a person is anxious or tense. Headaches may also develop in response to increased intracranial pressure, irritation of the meninges, and spasm of the cerebral blood vessels.
Hematomas	Refers to blood clots and generally caused by trauma. An epidural hematoma forms between the dura and the skull. A subdural hematoma forms under the dura mater. As the hematoma enlarges, it compresses the brain, elevates intracranial pressure, and can cause death unless the pressure is relieved.
Inflammations	Encephalitis and meningitis. Encephalitis is an inflammation of the brain usually caused by a virus. Meningitis is an inflammation of the meninges, caused by viruses and bacteria.
Tumors	Malignant and benign tumors in nervous tissue. The tumors can destroy nervous tissue, exert pressure on surrounding structures, and cause a life-threatening increase in intracranial pressure. Examples of tumors include gliomas (malignant tumors arising from glial tissue such as an astrocytoma); meningiomas (tumors arising from the meninges); and neuromas (tumors arising from the nerves).

SUMMARY OUTLINE

The purpose of the nervous system is to bring information to the central nervous system, interpret the information, and enable the body to respond to the information.

I. The Nervous System: Overview

A. Divisions of the Nervous System

1. The central nervous system (CNS) includes the brain and the spinal cord.
2. The peripheral nervous system includes the nerves that connect the CNS with the rest of the body.

B. Cells That Make Up the Nervous System

1. Neuroglia (glia) support, protect, and nourish the neurons.
2. Neurons conduct the nerve impulse.
3. The three parts of a neuron are the dendrites, cell body, and axon.

C. Types of Neurons

1. Sensory, or afferent, neurons carry information toward the CNS.
2. Interneurons are located in the CNS (make connections).
3. Motor, or efferent, neurons carry information away from the CNS toward the periphery.

D. White Matter and Gray Matter

1. White matter is due to myelinated fibers.
2. Gray matter is composed primarily of cell bodies, interneurons, and unmyelinated fibers.
3. Clusters of cell bodies (gray matter) are called nuclei and ganglia.

II. The Neuron Carrying Information

A. Nerve Impulse

1. The electrical signal is called the action potential or nerve impulse.
2. The nerve impulse is due to the following changes in the neuron: polarization, depolarization, and repolarization.
3. The nerve impulse is due to flow of ions: polarization (outward flux of K^+), depolarization (influx of Na^+), and repolarization (outward flux of K^+).
4. The refractory period is the unresponsive period of the neuron.
5. The nerve impulse jumps from node to node as it travels along a myelinated fiber. Myelination increases the speed of the nerve impulse.
6. The nerve impulse causes the release of the neurotransmitter.

B. Synapse

1. The synapse is a space between two neurons.
2. The nerve impulse of the first (presynaptic) neuron causes the release of neurotransmitter into the synaptic cleft. The neurotransmitter diffuses across the synaptic cleft and binds to the receptors on the second (postsynaptic) membrane. The activation of the receptors stimulates a nerve impulse in the second neuron.

III. Brain: Structure and Function

A. Cerebrum

1. The right and left hemispheres are joined by the corpus callosum.
2. The four main cerebral lobes are the frontal, parietal, temporal, and occipital lobes. Functions of each lobe are summarized in Table 10-2.
3. Large areas of the cerebrum, called association areas, are concerned with interpreting, integrating, and analyzing information.

B. Diencephalon

1. The thalamus is a relay station for most sensory tracts traveling to the cerebrum.
2. The hypothalamus controls many body functions such as water balance, temperature, and the secretion of hormones from the pituitary gland; it exerts an effect on the autonomic nervous system.

C. Brain Stem

1. Brain stem: midbrain, pons, and medulla oblongata.
2. The medulla oblongata is called the vital center because it controls the heart rate, blood pressure, and respirations (the vital functions).
3. The vomiting center is located in the medulla oblongata; it receives input directly and indirectly from activation of the chemoreceptor trigger zone (CTZ).

D. Cerebellum

1. The cerebellum is sometimes called the little brain.
2. The cerebellum is concerned primarily with the coordination of voluntary muscle activity.

E. Structures Involving More Than One Lobe

1. The limbic system is sometimes called the emotional brain.
2. The reticular formation is concerned with the sleep/wake cycle. It keeps us conscious and prevents us from slipping into a coma state.
3. The "memory areas" handle short-term and long-term memory.

IV. Protection of the CNS
A. Bone: cranium and vertebral column
B. Meninges: pia mater, arachnoid, and dura mater
C. Cerebrospinal fluid (CSF) that circulates within the subarachnoid space
D. Blood-brain barrier

Review Your Knowledge

Matching: Nerve Cells

Directions: Match the following words with their descriptions below.

a. efferent
b. ganglia
c. CNS
d. neuroglia
e. afferent
f. axon
g. nodes of Ranvier
h. Schwann cell
i. dendrite
j. myelin

1. ___ Also described as sensory neurons
2. ___ Nerve glue: astrocytes and ependymal cells
3. ___ Part of the neuron that carries the action potential away from the cell body
4. ___ Also described as motor neurons
5. ___ Composed of the brain and the spinal cord
6. ___ Clusters of cell bodies located outside of the CNS
7. ___ White insulating material that surrounds the axon; increases the speed that the signal travels along the axon
8. ___ Short segments of an axon that are not covered with myelin; allows for saltatory conduction
9. ___ A glial cell that makes myelin
10. ___ Treelike structure of the neuron that receives information from another neuron and transmits that information to the cell body

Matching: Brain

Directions: Match the following words with their descriptions below.

a. medulla oblongata
b. frontal
c. occipital
d. hypothalamus
e. temporal

1. ___ Cerebral lobe that performs the "executive functions" and contains the primary motor cortex
2. ___ Part of the brain stem that is called the vital center
3. ___ Part of the diencephalon that controls body temperature (thermostat) and endocrine function by its influence on the pituitary gland
4. ___ Cerebral lobe that contains the primary visual cortex
5. ___ Cerebral lobe that contains the primary auditory cortex

Multiple Choice

1. The precentral gyrus is
   a. located in the parietal lobe.
   b. the primary motor area.
   c. the primary visual cortex.
   d. a brain stem structure.
2. Which of the following is not descriptive of Broca's area?
   a. Located in the frontal lobe
   b. Concerned with motor speech
   c. Most often located in the left cerebral hemisphere
   d. Is the name of the frontal eye field area
3. Which of the following "brain claims" is true?
   a. The medulla oblongata is a cerebral structure.
   b. The hypothalamus is a brain stem structure.
   c. The medulla oblongata descends as the spinal cord.
   d. The midbrain, pons, and medulla oblongata are supratentorial structures.
4. Which of the following is not descriptive of the medulla oblongata?
   a. It is a brain stem structure.
   b. It is called the vital center.
   c. It is sensitive to the effects of narcotics (opioids).
   d. It performs the "executive" functions.
5. The postcentral gyrus
   a. is located in the parietal lobe.
   b. controls all voluntary motor activity.
   c. is the home of Broca's area.
   d. contains the primary visual cortex.

6. Cerebrospinal fluid (CSF)
   a. drains out of the subarachnoid space into the choroid plexus.
   b. circulates within the subarachnoid space.
   c. looks like blood.
   d. flows up the central canal into the fourth, third, and lateral ventricles.
7. Which of the following relationships is true?
   a. Temporal lobe: vision
   b. Frontal lobe: somatosensory (touch, pressure, pain)
   c. Occipital lobe: vision
   d. Parietal lobe: hearing
8. Neuroglia
   a. is classified as sensory and motor.
   b. include astrocytes, oligodendrocytes, Schwann cells, and ependymal cells.
   c. fire action potentials when stimulated.
   d. contain dendrites and axons.
9. Depolarization and repolarization
   a. are both due to the movement of Na^+ into the neuron.
   b. are phases of the action potential.
   c. occur only in the neuroglia.
   d. are both due to the movement of K^+ out of the neuron.

CHAPTER 11

Nervous System: Spinal Cord and Peripheral Nerves

KEY TERMS

Afferent neuron, p. 192
Cranial nerve, p. 194
Dermatome, p. 200
Efferent neuron, p. 192
Gray matter, p. 187
Mixed nerve, p. 189
Motor nerve, p. 193
Nerve tract, p. 187
Peripheral nervous system, p. 193
Plexus, p. 199
Reflex arc, p. 192
Sensory nerve, p. 189
Spinal nerve, p. 189
White matter, p. 187

OBJECTIVES

1. Describe the anatomy of the spinal cord and list its three functions.
2. List four components of the reflex arc.
3. List and describe the functions of the 12 pairs of cranial nerves.
4. Identify the classification of spinal nerves.
5. List the functions of the three major plexuses.

The brain, spinal cord, and peripheral nervous system work together as a vast communication system. The spinal cord continuously carries information to and from the brain. In the absence of spinal cord function, no sensory activity is present, and the person cannot feel. The person also lacks voluntary motor activity and cannot move. There is also the protective role of the nervous reflexes for those who operate dangerous equipment.

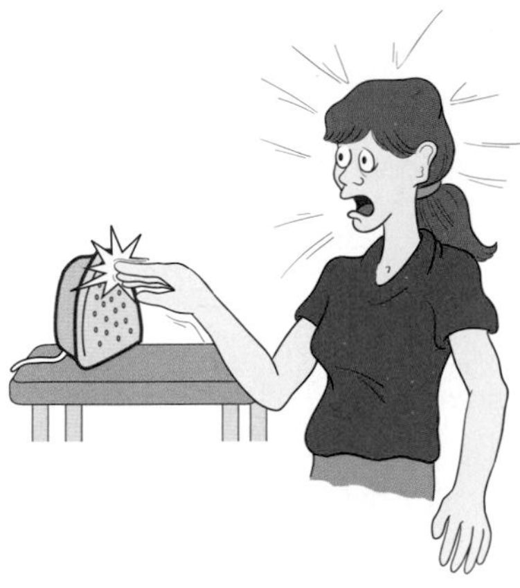

WHAT THE SPINAL CORD IS

LOCATION AND SIZE

The **spinal cord** is a continuation of the brain stem. It is a tubelike structure located within the spinal cavity. The diameter of the spinal cord is similar to the thickness of your thumb. The spinal cord is about 17 inches (43 cm) long and extends from the foramen magnum of the occipital bone to the level of the first lumbar vertebra (L1), just below the bottom rib. Like the brain, the spinal cord is well protected by bone (vertebrae), meninges, cerebrospinal fluid (CSF), and the blood-brain barrier (Figure 11-1).

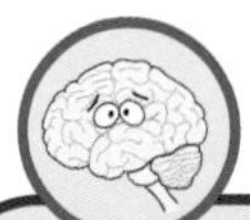

Do You Know...

Why a ruptured disc causes pain?

A ruptured disc is the herniation, or protrusion, of the central portion of the intervertebral disc into the spinal cavity. The herniated disc presses on a spinal nerve root, causing severe pain.

An infant's spinal cord extends the full length of the spinal cavity. As the infant grows, however, the spinal cavity grows faster than the cord. Because of the different rates of growth, the spinal cavity eventually becomes longer than the spinal cord, with the cord extending only to L1 in the adult. The meningeal membranes, however, extend the length of the spinal cavity.

This anatomical arrangement forms the basis for the site of a **lumbar puncture** (see Figure 11-1, *B* and *C*). In this procedure, a hollow needle is inserted into the subarachnoid space, between L3 and L4, at about the level of the top of the hip bone. A sample of CSF is withdrawn from the subarachnoid space. The CSF is then examined for pathogens, blood, or other abnormal signs. Because the spinal cord ends at L1, there is no danger of injuring the cord with the needle.

GRAY ON THE INSIDE, WHITE ON THE OUTSIDE

Gray Matter

A cross section of the spinal cord shows an area of gray matter and an area of white matter (Figure 11-2). The **gray matter** is located in the center and is shaped like a butterfly. It is composed primarily of cell bodies and interneurons. Two projections of the gray matter are the dorsal (posterior) horn and the ventral (anterior) horn. In the middle of the gray matter is the central canal. The **central canal** is an opening, or hole, that extends the entire length of the spinal cord. It is open to the ventricular system in the brain and to the subarachnoid space at the bottom of the spinal cord. CSF flows from the ventricles in the brain down through the central canal into the subarachnoid space at the base of the spinal cord. The CSF then circulates throughout the subarachnoid space surrounding the spinal cord and brain.

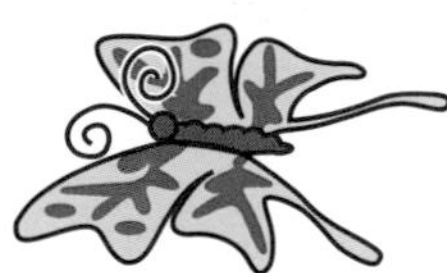

White Matter

The **white matter** of the spinal cord is composed primarily of myelinated axons. These neuronal axons are grouped together into **nerve tracts.**

Sensory tracts carry information from the periphery, up the spinal cord, and toward the brain (see Figure 11-2). They are therefore called **ascending tracts.** The spinothalamic tract is an example of an ascending tract. It carries sensory information for touch, pressure, and pain from the spinal cord to the thalamus in the brain. Note that the name of the tract (spinothalamic) often indicates its origin (spinal cord) and destination (thalamus).

Motor tracts carry information from the brain, down the spinal cord, and toward the periphery. They are called **descending tracts.** The major descending tracts are the pyramidal and extrapyramidal tracts. The **pyramidal tract,** also called the **corticospinal tract,** is the major motor tract, originating in the frontal lobe of the cerebrum. As its name (corticospinal) implies, motor

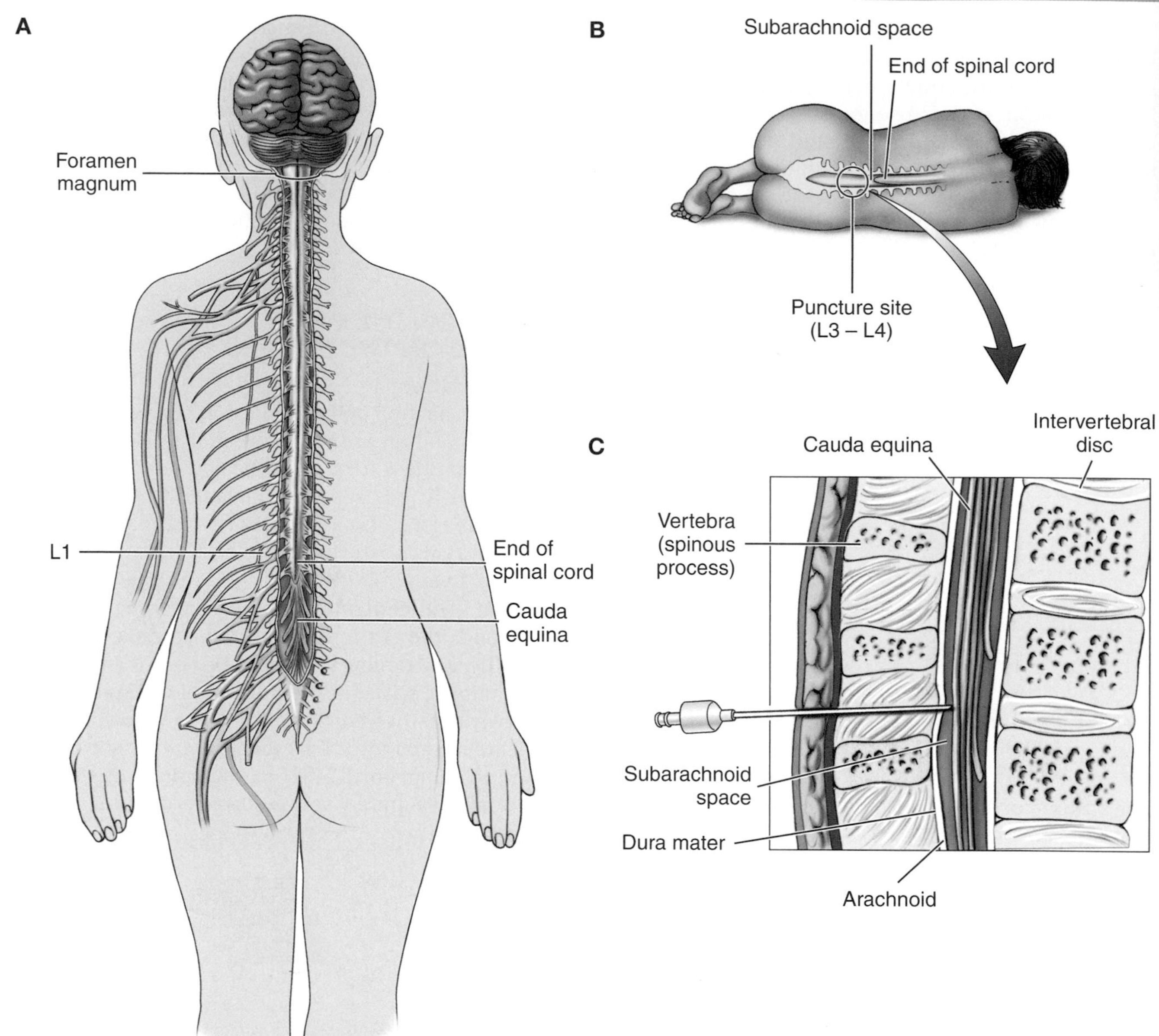

FIGURE 11-1 **A,** Location and length of the spinal cord. **B** and **C,** Lumbar puncture (spinal tap).

information is carried from the cortical region of the brain toward the spinal cord. Additional information concerning tracts and their functions is in Table 11-1.

Decussation. Most nerve tracts decussate or cross over from one side to the other. For instance, the corticospinal tract that originates in the left frontal lobe descends to the medulla oblongata, in the brain stem. The fibers then decussate, descend down the right side of the spinal cord, and innervate the right side of the body. Most motor tracts decussate at the level of the brain stem. Most sensory tracts decussate in the spinal cord and travel up the opposite side of the spinal cord to the brain.

Table 11-1 Major Spinal Cord Tracts

Tracts	Functions
Ascending	
Spinothalamic	Temperature; pressure; pain; light touch
Dorsal column	Proprioception; deep pressure; vibration
Spinocerebellar	Proprioception
Descending	
Pyramidal (corticospinal)	Skeletal muscle tone; voluntary muscle movement
Extrapyramidal	Skeletal muscle activity (balance and posture)

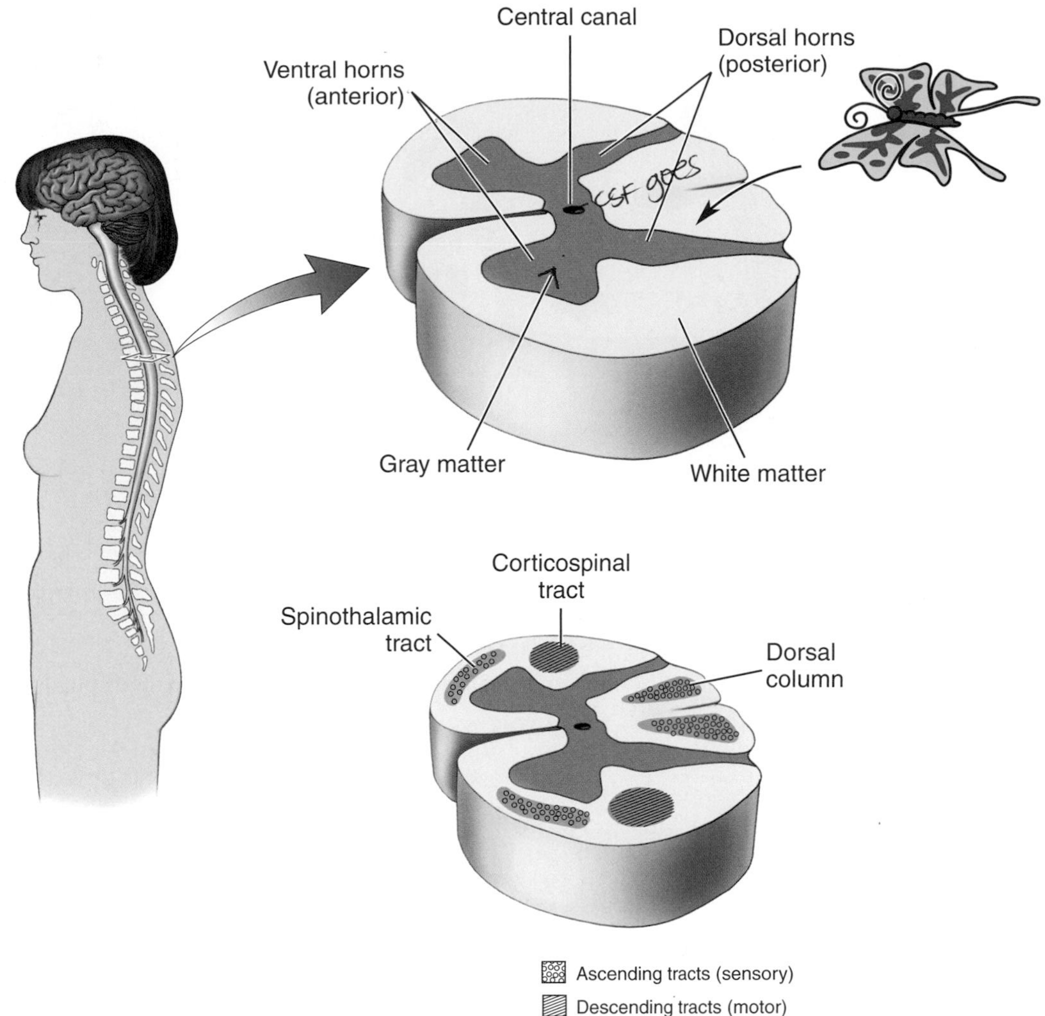

FIGURE 11-2 Cross section of the spinal cord showing the inner gray matter ("butterfly") and the outer white matter.

If injured, the neurons of the brain and spinal cord do not regenerate. If the neck is broken, the spinal cord might be severed. If the spinal cord is severed at the neck region, the trunk and all four extremities are paralyzed. This condition is called quadriplegia. This type of spinal cord injury is common in automobile and diving accidents in which the neck is either compressed or bent excessively (Figure 11-3). If the spinal cord injury is lower, involving only the lumbar region of the spinal cord, the person has full use of the upper extremities but is paralyzed from the waist down. Paralysis of the lower extremities is called paraplegia.

SPINAL NERVES ATTACHED TO THE SPINAL CORD

Attached to the spinal cord are the **spinal nerves.** Each nerve is attached to the spinal cord by two roots, the dorsal root and the ventral root (Figure 11-4). **Sensory nerve** fibers from the periphery travel to the cord through the **dorsal root.** The cell bodies of the sensory fibers are gathered together in the **dorsal root ganglia.** The **ventral root** is composed of motor fibers. These motor fibers are distributed to muscles and glands. The dorsal and ventral roots are packaged together to form a spinal nerve. Because spinal nerves contain both sensory and motor fibers, all spinal nerves are **mixed nerves.**

WHAT THE SPINAL CORD DOES

The spinal cord serves three major functions: sensory pathway, motor pathway, and reflex center.

- Sensory pathway: The spinal cord provides a pathway for sensory information traveling from the periphery to the brain. For instance, when you stick your finger with a sharp tack, sensory information travels from the finger toward the spinal cord. The information then ascends the spinal cord to

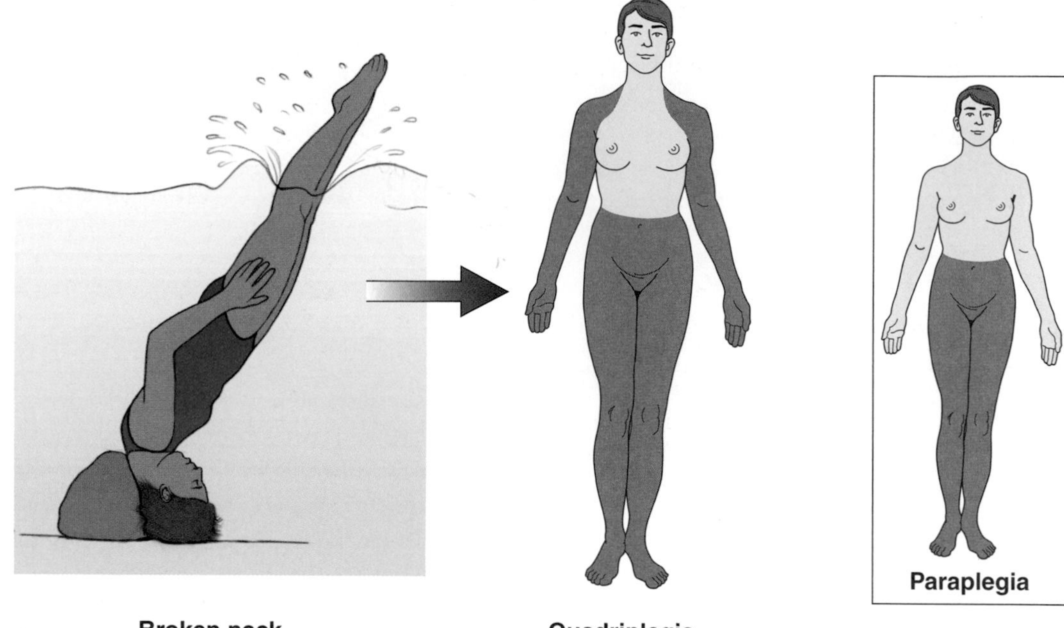

FIGURE 11-3 Spinal cord injuries. Diving into a shallow pool can result in a damaged spinal cord. Quadriplegia and paraplegia.

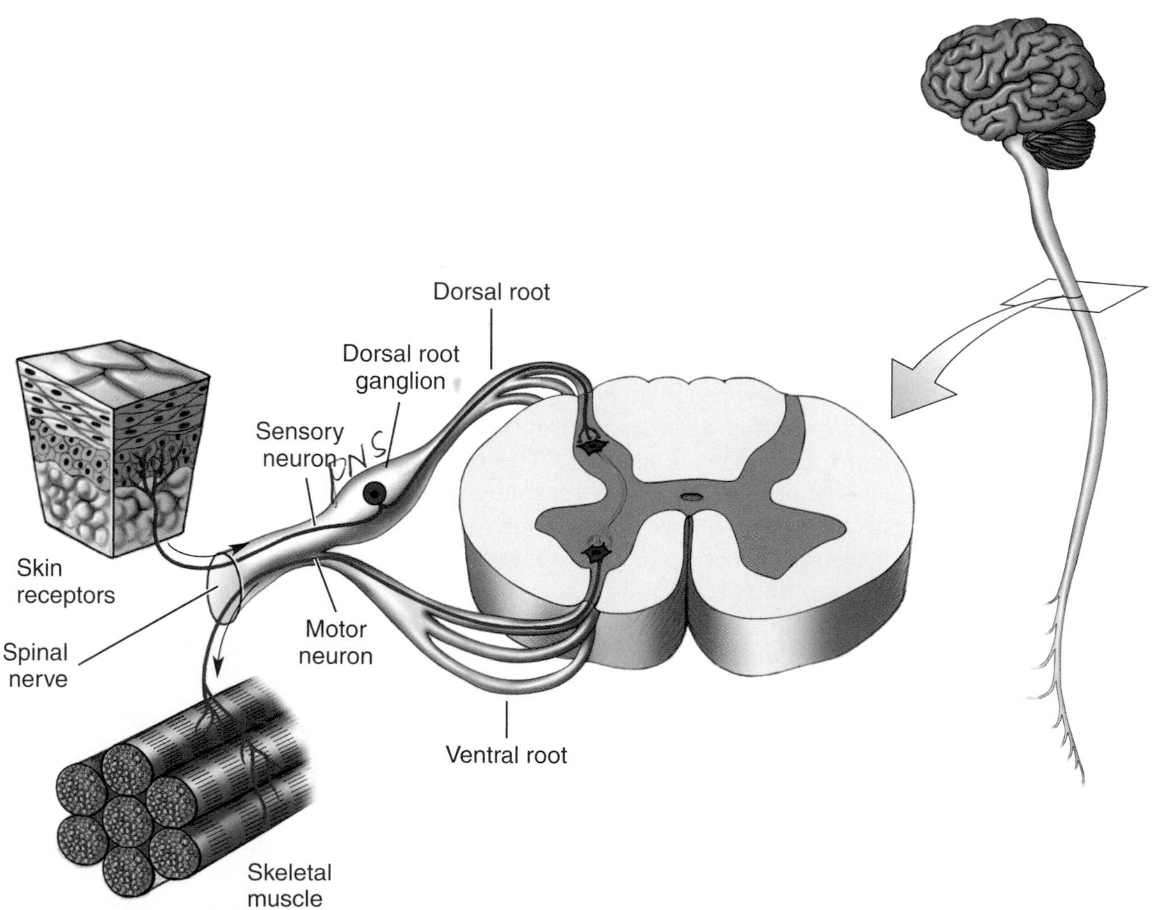

FIGURE 11-4 Attachment of the spinal nerves to the spinal cord.

the brain, where you experience the information as pain.

- Motor pathway: The spinal cord provides a pathway for motor information coming from the brain and going to the periphery. For instance, you decide to move your foot as in kicking a football. The information travels from the brain, down the spinal cord, and to the muscles of the leg and foot.
- Reflex center: The spinal cord acts as a major reflex center. For instance, when you stick your finger on a tack, you very quickly and automatically withdraw your finger from the source of injury. In other words, you reflexively remove your finger. The spinal cord, not the brain, performs this reflex for you.

REFLEXES

WHAT REFLEXES ARE

What is a reflex? Many of the activities that we engage in every day occur very rapidly and without any conscious control. In other words, they happen reflexively. Many of the reflexes occur at the level of the spinal cord. A **reflex** is an involuntary response to a stimulus. If you touch a hot surface, for instance, you very quickly remove your hand. Your hand is safely away from the source of injury long before you consciously say, "This is hot. I must remove my hand!" Similarly, your ability to walk and maintain your balance requires hundreds of reflex movements. You don't have to think about swinging your arms as you walk.

A typical reflex response is demonstrated by the **patellar,** or **knee-jerk reflex** (Figure 11-5). During a physical examination, the doctor taps the tendon below your kneecap. In response to the tap, your lower leg quickly and involuntarily pops up. The physician has elicited the patellar, or knee-jerk, reflex. How does this

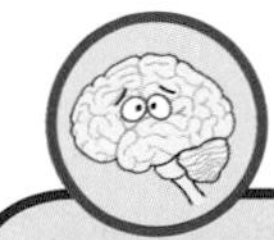

Do You Know...

How anesthesia affects the spinal cord?

Anesthetic agents such as novocaine may be injected into the subarachnoid space to achieve spinal anesthesia. When injected into the subarachnoid space, these drugs deaden, or anesthetize, the lumbar and sacral sensory nerves. Feelings of pain from the areas innervated by these deadened nerves are temporarily lost.

How is epidural anesthesia used in childbirth? During the last, uncomfortable phase of childbirth, anesthetic agents are continuously infused into the epidural space. The nerves that are deadened by the anesthesia supply the lower pelvic region of the body, thereby relieving the pain of childbirth.

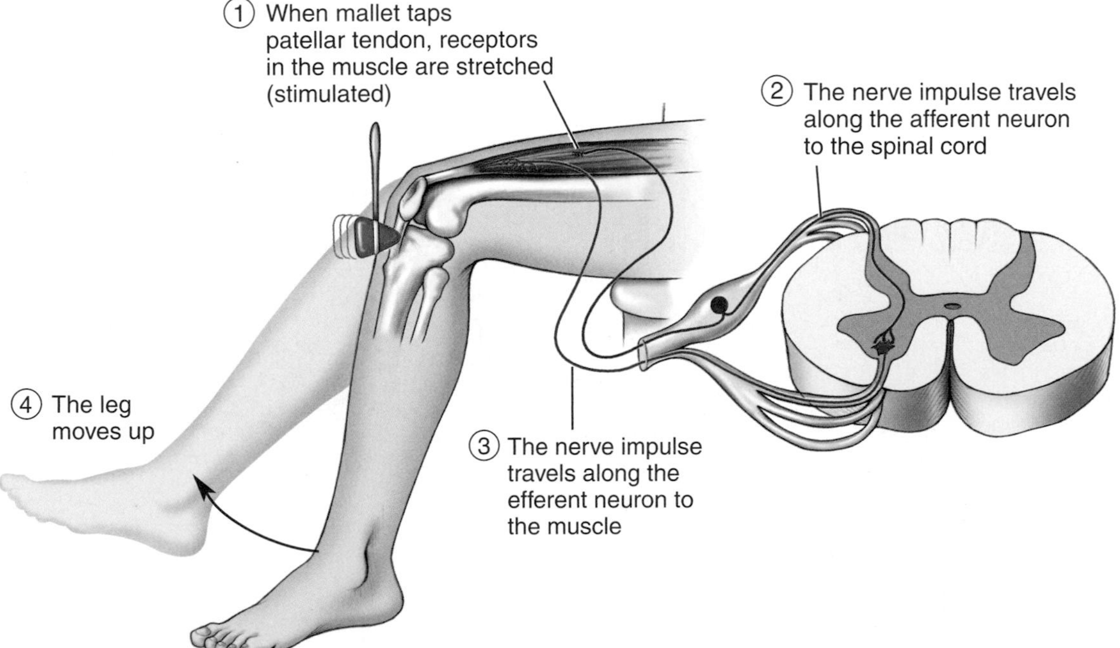
Knee-jerk reflex arc
1 When mallet taps patellar tendon, receptors in the muscle are stretched (stimulated)
2 The nerve impulse travels along the afferent neuron to the spinal cord
3 The nerve impulse travels along the efferent neuron to the muscle
4 The leg moves up

FIGURE 11-5 Reflex arc. The knee-jerk reflex illustrates the four components of the reflex arc.

reflex help you? If you are standing erect and your knee bends, even slightly, the patellar reflex is stimulated. In response to the bending, the quadriceps muscle in the thigh contracts, thereby straightening the lower leg and helping you maintain an upright position.

THE REFLEX ARC

The knee-jerk reflex illustrates the four basic components of the reflex arc (see Figure 11-5). The **reflex arc** is the nerve pathway involved in a reflex. The four basic components of the reflex arc include the following:

1. A **receptor.** By tapping the tendon, the mallet stimulates sensory receptors in the thigh muscles.
2. An **afferent** or sensory **neuron.** The nerve impulse is carried by the sensory neuron to the spinal cord.
3. An **efferent** or motor **neuron.** The nerve impulse is carried by a motor nerve to the muscles of the thigh.
4. An **effector organ.** The muscles of the thigh, specifically the quadriceps femoris, are effector organs. In response to the nerve impulse, the muscles contract and move the lower leg in an upward movement.

MANY, MANY REFLEXES

Ouch! The Withdrawal Reflex

The withdrawal reflex (Figure 11-6, *A*) helps protect you from injury. For instance, this reflex quickly moves your finger away from a hot iron, thereby preventing a severe burn. The "ouch" occurs after your finger is safely away from the hot iron.

Organ Reflexes. Reflexes also help regulate organ function. Figure 11-6 illustrates some of the reflexes that regulate body function. The **pupillary reflex,** for instance, regulates the amount of light that enters the eye. When a bright light is directed at the eye, the muscles that control pupillary size constrict. The size of the pupil diminishes, thereby restricting the amount of additional light entering the eye. Blood pressure is also under reflex control. When blood pressure changes, the **baroreceptor reflex** causes the heart and blood vessels to respond in a way that restores blood pressure to normal.

In addition to performing important physiological functions, some reflexes are used diagnostically to assess nerve function. Abnormal findings may indicate central nervous system (CNS) lesions, tumors, and

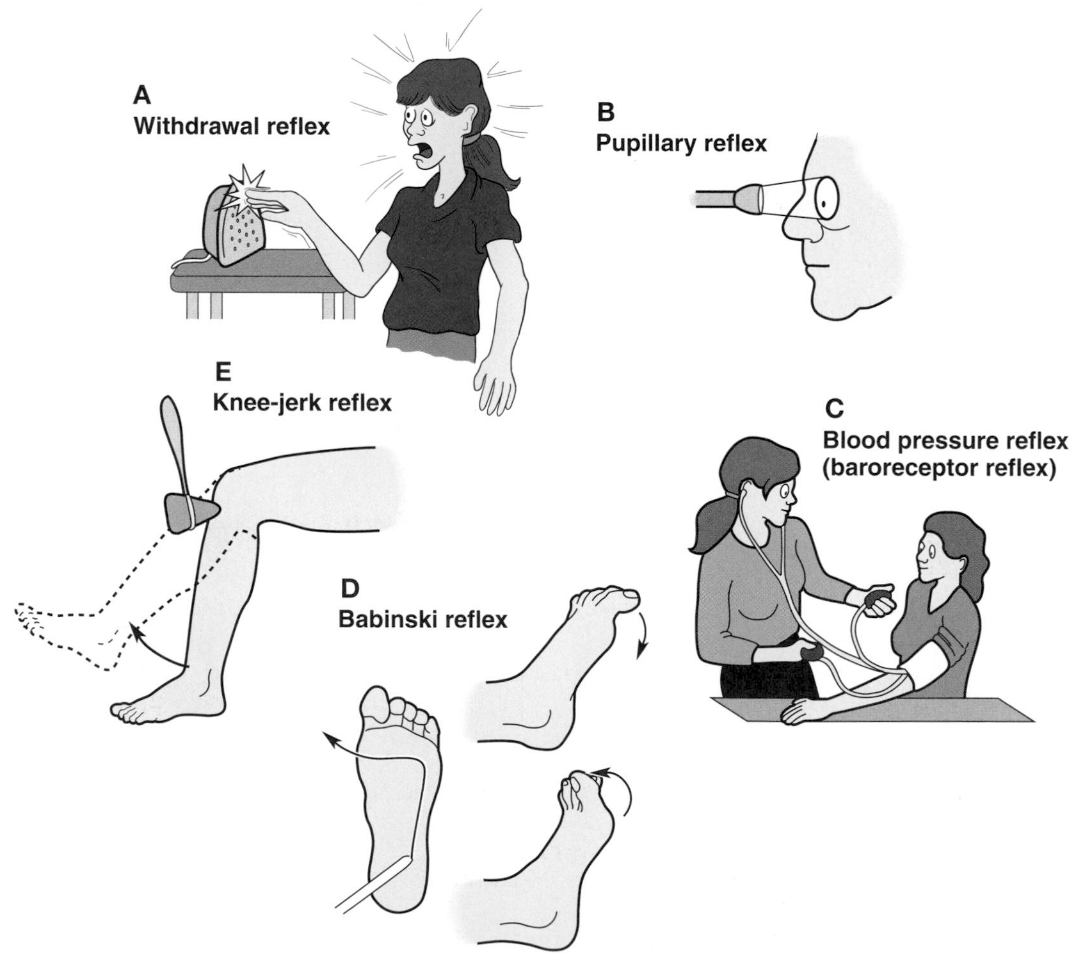

FIGURE 11-6 Many reflexes. **A,** Withdrawal reflex. **B,** Pupillary reflex. **C,** Blood pressure, or baroreceptor, reflex. **D,** Babinski reflex. **E,** Knee-jerk reflex.

other neurological diseases such as multiple sclerosis. You may have observed a physician elicit the **Babinski reflex** (Figure 11-6, *D*) by stroking the lateral sole of the foot in the direction of heel to toe with a hard blunt object. In the adult, the Babinski reflex is normal, or negative, if the response to the stroking is plantar flexion, a curling of the toes. An abnormal, or positive, Babinski reflex is dorsiflexion of the big toe, sometimes with fanning, the spreading of the other toes. An infant normally dorsiflexes the big toe, an indicator of the immaturity of the infant's nervous system. Some clinically significant reflexes and their functions are listed in Table 11-2.

Sum It Up!

The spinal cord and the peripheral nervous system allow the brain to communicate with the body and external environment. The spinal cord transmits information up and down the cord. Sensory information is brought to the brain from the lower cord region, whereas motor information is transmitted away from the brain, down the cord toward the periphery. In addition to providing pathways for the flow of information, the spinal cord acts as a center of reflex activity.

PERIPHERAL NERVOUS SYSTEM

The **peripheral nervous system** consists of the nerves and ganglia located outside the CNS.

NERVES

Before classifying the nerves, you need to differentiate between a nerve and a neuron (see Chapter 10). A neuron is a single nerve cell. The nerve contains many neurons bundled together with blood vessels and then wrapped in connective tissue (Figure 11-7). Nerves are located outside the CNS. Within the CNS, bundles of nerve fibers are called tracts. Nerves are classified as the following:

- **Sensory nerves,** composed only of sensory neurons
- **Motor nerves,** composed only of motor neurons
- **Mixed nerves,** containing both sensory and motor neurons. Most nerves are mixed and all spinal nerves are mixed.

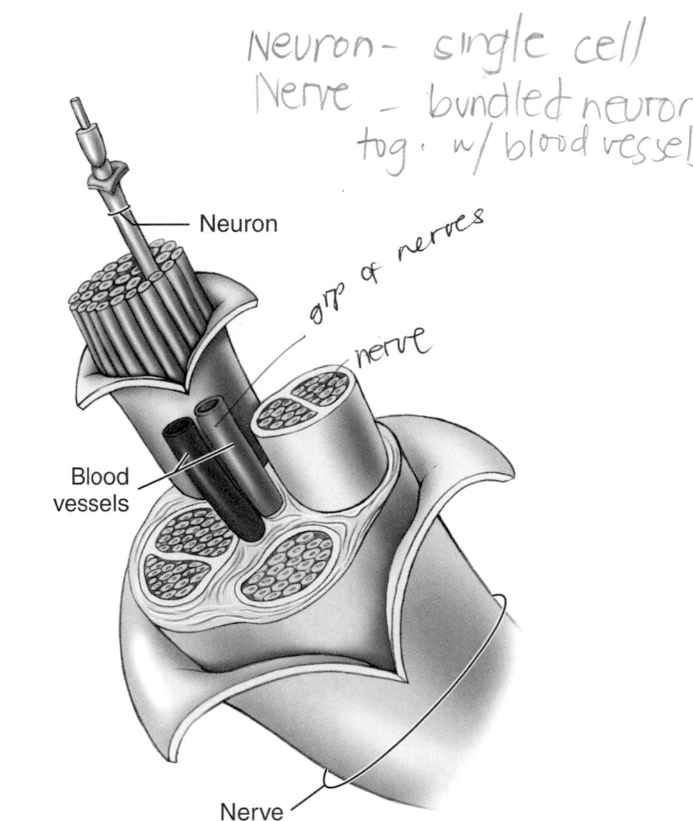

FIGURE 11-7 Difference between a neuron and nerve.

Table 11-2 Clinically Significant Reflexes

Reflex	Description	Meaning of Abnormal Response
Patellar (knee-jerk reflex)	A stretch reflex; the mallet strikes the patellar tendon below the knee—in response, the lower leg kicks up.	Impaired in damage to nerves involved in the reflex Impaired in damage to lumbar region of spinal cord Impaired in patients with diseases that affect the nerves and spinal cord (such as diabetes mellitus, neurosyphilis, and chronic alcoholism)
Achilles tendon (ankle-jerk reflex)	A stretch reflex; the mallet strikes the Achilles tendon, causing plantar flexion.	Impaired in damage to nerves involved in the reflex Impaired in damage to lower spinal cord (L5 to S2)
Abdominal	With stroking of the lateral abdominal wall, the abdominal wall contracts and moves the umbilicus toward the stimulus.	Impaired in lesions of peripheral nerves Impaired in lesions of spinal cord (thoracic) and in patients with multiple sclerosis
Babinski	With stroking of the lateral sole of the foot from heel to toe, the toes curl with slight inversion of the foot (see text).	Impaired in lesions/damage of the spinal cord In children less than 2 years of age, the Babinski reflex is positive

CLASSIFYING THE PERIPHERAL NERVOUS SYSTEM

The peripheral nervous system can be classified in two ways: structurally (by the parts) or functionally (according to what they do).

Structural Classification of the Peripheral Nervous System

The structural, or anatomical, classification of the peripheral nervous system divides the nerves into cranial and spinal nerves. The classification is based on the origin of the fiber (where it originates).

Cranial Nerves

Names and Numbers of Cranial Nerves. Twelve pairs of **cranial nerves** are shown in Figure 11-8. Each cranial nerve has a specific number, always designated by a Roman numeral, and a name. The numbers indicate the order in which the nerves exit the brain from front to back.

In general, the name of the nerve indicates the specific anatomical area served by the nerve. For instance, the optic nerve serves the eye. The cranial nerves primarily serve the head, face, and neck region, but one pair, the vagus, branches extensively and extends throughout the thoracic and abdominal cavities.

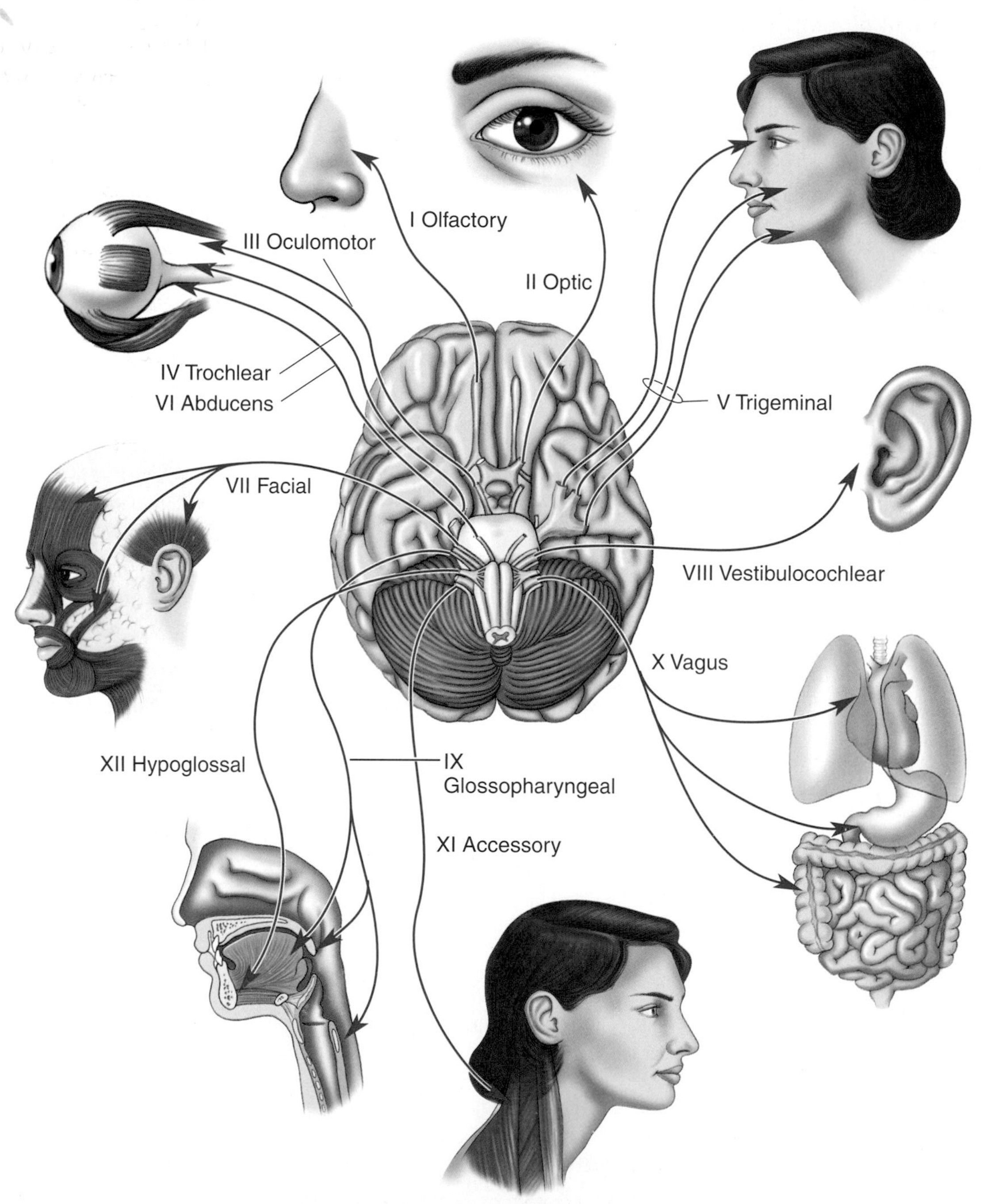

FIGURE 11-8 Cranial nerves.

A common mnemonic used to memorize the cranial nerves in proper order is shown in Table 11-3: On Old Olympus Towering Tops A Finn Viewed Germans Vaulting And Hopping. The first letter of each word is the same as the first letter of each cranial nerve. My personal mnemonic is Oh! Oh! Oh! Tough, Tricky Anatomy Final . . . Very Grave Vibes . . . Aching Head. Try to develop your own creative mnemonic.

Functions of Cranial Nerves. Cranial nerves perform four general functions. They carry

- sensory information for the special senses: smell, taste, vision, and hearing.
- sensory information for the general senses: touch, pressure, pain, temperature, and vibration.
- motor information that results in contraction of skeletal muscles.
- motor information that results in the secretion of glands and the contraction of cardiac and smooth muscle.

Cranial nerve function is summarized in Table 11-3. Locate each cranial nerve on Figure 11-8.

CN I, olfactory nerve: a sensory nerve that carries information from the nose to the brain. The olfactory nerve is concerned with the sense of smell. A person who damages the olfactory nerve may lose the sense of smell (anosmia). In addition, the person may complain of loss of taste because the appeal of food is determined by both taste and smell.

CN II, optic nerve: a sensory nerve that carries visual information from the eye to the brain, specifically the occipital lobe of the cerebrum. Damage to the optic nerve causes diminished vision or blindness in the affected eye.

CN III, oculomotor nerve: primarily a motor nerve that causes contraction of the extrinsic eye muscles, thereby moving the eyeball in the socket. The oculomotor nerve also raises the eyelid and constricts the pupil of the eye.

Because the oculomotor nerve is located close to the hard tentorium within the cranium, it is easily compressed by brain tumors or increased intracranial pressure. Compression of the nerve interferes with the ability of the pupil of the eye to respond to light (sluggish pupillary response). With more severe compression the pupils may become dilated and fixed. Compression of CN III also interferes with raising the eyelid; the person experiences ptosis of the eyelid. Observation of the eyes provides excellent clinical clues to neurological status.

CN IV, trochlear nerve: primarily a motor nerve that innervates one of the extrinsic muscles of the eyeball, thereby helping to move the eyeball. Damage may cause double vision and an inability to rotate the eye properly.

CN V, trigeminal nerve: a mixed nerve with three branches supplying the facial region. The two sensory branches carry information regarding touch, pressure, and pain from the face, scalp, eye, and teeth to the brain. The ophthalmic branch of the trigeminal nerve detects sensory information from the cornea. For instance, if you touch the surface of the cornea, the ophthalmic branch is stimulated and sends information to the brain. In response to the corneal irritation, motor fibers of the facial nerve (CN VII) respond by eliciting blinking and the secretion of tears. Thus, both the trigeminal and facial nerves participate in the corneal reflex. The motor branch innervates the muscles of mastication (chewing). Nerve damage causes a loss of sensation and impaired movement of the mandible (lower jaw).

Table 11-3 Cranial Nerves

Mnemonic	Nerve	Type	Function
On	I Olfactory	Sensory	Sense of smell
Old	II Optic	Sensory	Sense of sight
Olympus	III Oculomotor	Mixed (mostly motor)	Movement of eyeball, raising of eyelid; change in pupil size
Towering	IV Trochlear	Mixed (mostly motor)	Movement of eyeball
Tops	V Trigeminal	Mixed	Chewing of food; sensations in face, scalp, cornea (eye), and teeth
A	VI Abducens	Mixed (mostly motor)	Movement of eyeball
Finn	VII Facial	Mixed	Facial expressions; secretion of saliva and tears; taste; blinking
Viewed	VIII Vestibulocochlear	Sensory	Sense of hearing and balance
Germans	IX Glossopharyngeal	Mixed	Swallowing, secretion of saliva; taste; sensory for the reflex regulation of blood pressure; part of the gag reflex
Vaulting	X Vagus	Mixed	Visceral muscle movement and sensations, especially movement and secretion of the digestive system; sensory for reflex regulation of blood pressure
And	XI Accessory	Mixed (mostly motor)	Swallowing; head and shoulder movement; speaking
Hopping	XII Hypoglossal	Mixed (mostly motor)	Speech and swallowing

A person may experience an inflammation of the trigeminal nerve. This condition is called trigeminal neuralgia, or tic douloureux. It is characterized by bouts of severe facial pain. The pain may be triggered by such events as eating, shaving, and exposure to cold temperatures. In an effort to avoid these triggers, the patient often becomes a prisoner of the disease, refusing to eat, shave, or leave the house in cold weather.

CN VI, abducens nerve: primarily a motor nerve that, like the trochlear, controls eye movement by innervating only one of the extrinsic eye muscles. Nerve damage prevents a lateral rotation of the eye; at rest the eyes drift medially (toward the nose).

CN VII, facial nerve: a mixed nerve that performs mostly motor functions. It is called the nerve of facial expression; it allows you to smile, frown, and "make other faces." It also stimulates the secretion of saliva and tears. The facial nerve innervates the orbicularis oculi, the muscle involved in blinking. Blinking not only protects the eye from foreign objects, such as dust, it also washes tears over the cornea, thereby keeping the cornea moist and preventing corneal ulceration. Its sensory function is taste.

If the facial nerve is damaged, facial expression is absent on the affected side of the face. This condition is called Bell's palsy. Cosmetically, this condition is very distressing because one side of the face may smile and look alive while the other side of the face sags, drools, and is expressionless. Salivation and the secretion of tears are diminished, thereby requiring the use of eyedrops to protect the cornea. Fortunately Bell's palsy often responds well to steroid therapy.

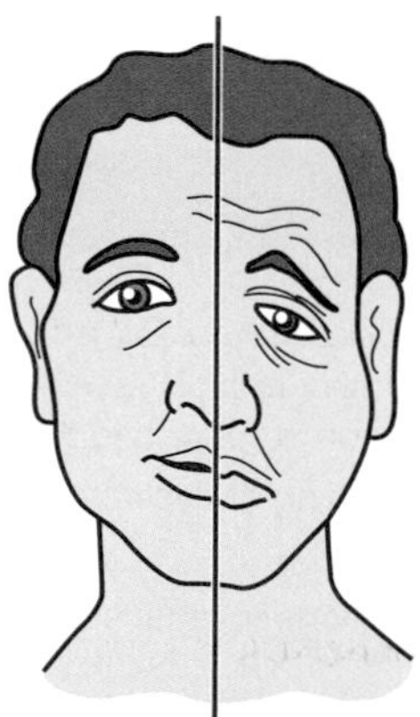

CN VIII, vestibulocochlear nerve: a sensory nerve that carries information for hearing and balance from the inner ear to the brain. The vestibular branch of this nerve is responsible for equilibrium, or balance, and the cochlear branch is responsible for hearing. Damage to this nerve may cause loss of hearing or balance or both (see Chapter 13).

CN IX, glossopharyngeal nerve: a mixed nerve that carries taste sensation from the posterior tongue to the brain. Motor fibers stimulate the secretion of salivary glands in the mouth. Other motor fibers innervate the throat and aid in swallowing. The glossopharyngeal nerve is also associated with the gag reflex. The gag reflex plays an important role in preventing food and water from entering the respiratory passages. Normally, when something goes down the wrong way, you gag and cough until the airway is cleared. Loss of the gag reflex places you at risk for choking. A second sensory function of this nerve involves the regulation of blood pressure (see Chapter 19).

CN X, vagus nerve: a mixed nerve that innervates the tongue, pharynx (throat), larynx (voicebox), and many organs in the thoracic and abdominal cavities (lungs, stomach, intestines). Nerve damage causes hoarseness or loss of voice, impaired swallowing, and diminished motility of the digestive tract. Damage to both vagus nerves can be fatal. The word vagus literally means wanderer; the name refers to the far-reaching distribution of this nerve. The sensory fibers of the vagus nerve also participate in the regulation of blood pressure (see Chapter 19).

CN XI, accessory nerve: primarily a motor nerve that supplies the sternocleidomastoid and the trapezius muscles, thereby controlling movement of the head and shoulder regions. Nerve damage impairs your ability to shrug your shoulders.

CN XII, hypoglossal nerve: primarily a motor nerve that controls movement of the tongue, thereby affecting

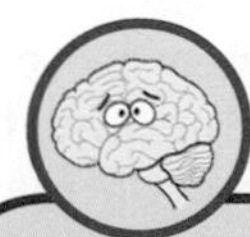

Do You Know...

Who has the "weakest blink"?

The facial nerve (CN VII) provides motor innervation to the orbicularis oculi, the eye muscle involved in blinking. Mr. Bell, who has a virally induced facial nerve paralysis, has the weakest blink. When told of his medical condition, he showed no expression.

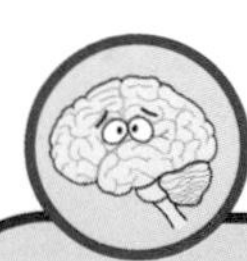

Do You Know...

About the "wandering" characteristics of the tenth cranial nerve?

Check the local jail, and you will find a couple of unsavory characters locked up on charges of vagrancy—the habit of wandering around and generally getting into trouble. The word *vagrant* means someone who wanders about (generally getting into trouble). The vagus nerve, the tenth cranial nerve, is also a wanderer. Unlike the other cranial nerves that are confined to the head and shoulder area, the vagus nerve leaves the head and wanders or makes its way throughout the thoracic and abdominal cavities. The vagus nerve is named for these vagrant or wandering characteristics.

speaking and swallowing activities. Nerve damage causes the tongue to deviate toward the injured side.

A neurological assessment includes simple procedures that test the ability of each cranial nerve to perform these functions. Table 11-4 illustrates simple methods used to test cranial nerve function. The table also includes common disorders and abnormal findings involving the cranial nerves.

Spinal Nerves

Names and Numbers of Spinal Nerves. Thirty-one pairs of spinal nerves emerge from the spinal cord (Figure 11-9). Each pair is numbered according to the level of the spinal cord from which it arises. The 31 pairs are grouped as follows: eight pairs of cervical nerves, 12 pairs of thoracic nerves, five pairs of lumbar nerves, five pairs of sacral nerves, and one pair of coccygeal nerves. The lumbar and sacral nerves at the bottom of the cord extend the length of the spinal cavity before exiting from the vertebral column. These nerves are called the **cauda equina** because they look like a horse's tail. The nerves exit from the bony vertebral column through tiny holes in the vertebrae called foramina.

Do You Know...

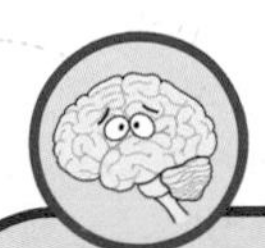

How to avoid hitting the sciatic nerve when giving an intramuscular (IM) injection into the buttock?

The buttock is divided into quadrants. The sciatic nerve runs through the inner quadrants. By administering IM injections into the gluteus medius, in the center of the upper outer quadrant, a clinician can avoid injury to the sciatic nerve.

Table 11-4 Cranial Nerves: Assessment and Disorders

Nerve	Assessment	Some Disorders
I Olfactory	Person is asked to sniff and identify various odors (e.g., vanilla).	Inability to smell (anosmia)
II Optic	Examination of the interior of the eye by ophthalmoscopic visualization. Use of eye charts and tests of peripheral vision.	Loss of vision
III Oculomotor	Test the ability of the eyes to follow a moving object. Examination of pupils for size, shape, and size equality. Pupillary reflex is tested with a penlight (the pupils should constrict). Test the ability of the eyes to converge.	Drooping upper eyelid (ptosis) Absence of pupillary reflex (e.g., dilated and fixed pupils that may indicate an increase in intracranial pressure) Difficulty in focusing eyes on an object
IV Trochlear	Test ability of the eyes to follow a moving object.	Inability to move eyeball in a particular direction
V Trigeminal	Sensations (pain/touch/temperature) are tested with sharp pin and hot/cold objects. Corneal reflex (sensory) is tested with a cotton wisp. Motor function is tested by asking the person to open the mouth (against resistance) and to move the jaw from side to side.	Loss of sensation (pain/touch); impaired corneal reflex Paresthesias (tingling, itching, and numbness) Difficulty in chewing Shift of jaw to side of lesion when opened
VI Abducens	Test ability of the eyes to follow a moving object.	Inability to move eyes laterally
VII Facial	Test anterior two thirds of tongue for sweet, salty, sour, and bitter taste. Person is asked to cause facial muscle movement (e.g., smile, close eyes, wrinkle forehead, whistle). Ability to secrete tears is tested by asking person to sniff ammonia fumes.	Bell's palsy (expressionless face, drooping mouth and drooling, inability to close eyes and blink) Loss of taste on anterior two thirds of tongue on side of lesion
VIII Vestibulocochlear	Hearing is checked by air and bone conduction (use of tuning fork).	Loss of hearing, noises in ear (tinnitus) Loss of balance (vertigo)
IX Glossopharyngeal	Check gag and swallowing reflex. Person is asked to speak and cough. Test posterior two thirds of tongue for taste.	Loss of gag reflex Difficulty in swallowing (dysphagia) Loss of taste on posterior two thirds of tongue Decreased salivation
X Vagus	Similar to testing for CN IX (because they both innervate throat).	Sagging of soft palate Hoarseness of voice due to paralysis of vocal fold
XI Accessory	Ask person to rotate head from side to side and to shrug shoulders (against resistance).	Drooping shoulders Inability or difficulty in rotating head (wryneck)
XII Hypoglossal	Person is asked to stick out tongue—note any deviation in position of the protruded tongue.	Some difficulty in speaking (dysarthria), chewing, and swallowing (dysphagia)

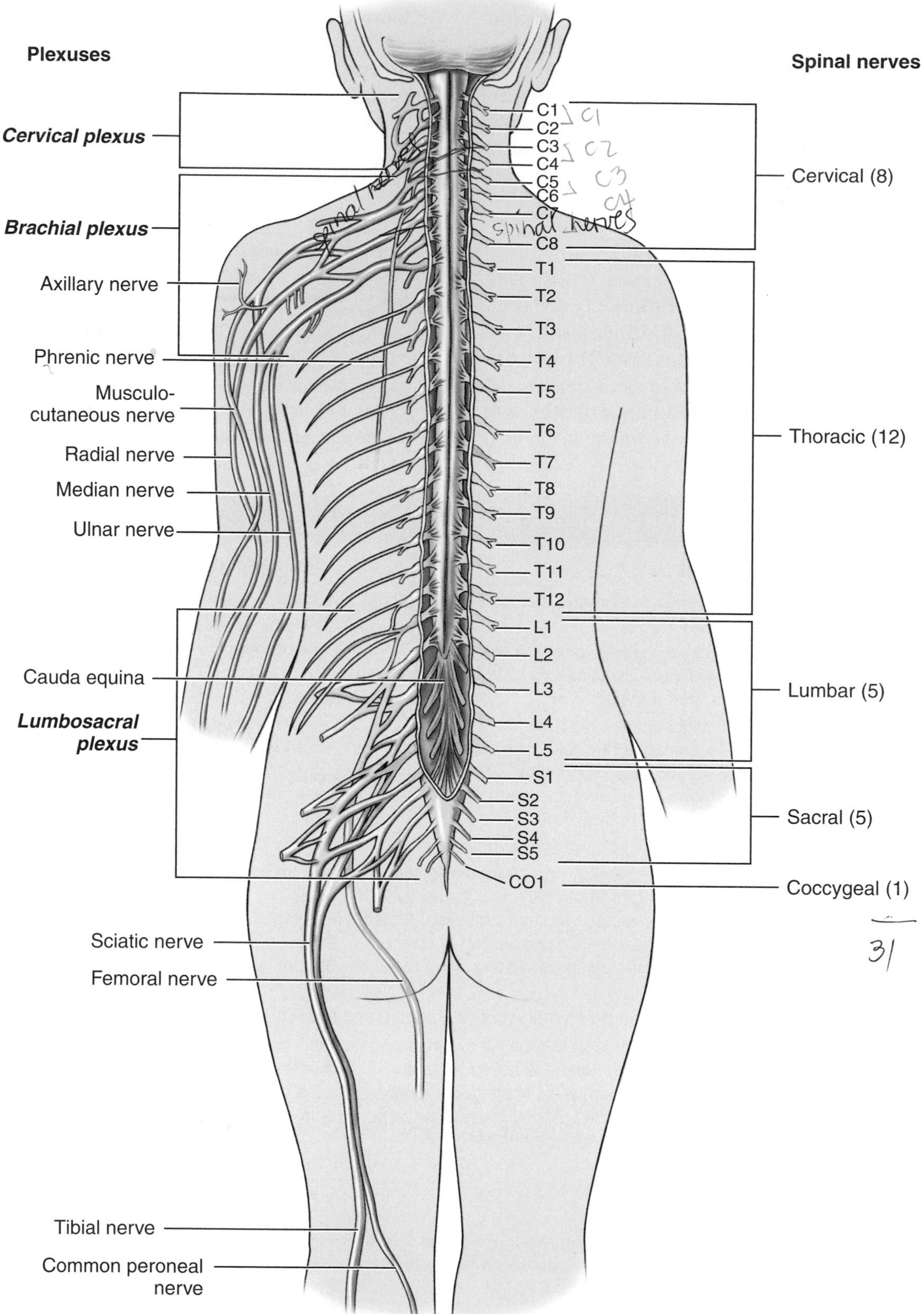

FIGURE 11-9 Spinal nerves: cervical, thoracic, lumbar, sacral, and coccygeal. Nerve plexuses: cervical, brachial, and lumbosacral.

Spinal Nerve Plexuses. As the spinal nerves exit from the vertebral column, they divide into many fibers. At various points, these nerve fibers converge, or come together again, into nerve **plexuses** (PLĔK-sŭs-ĕs), or networks. The three major nerve plexuses are the cervical plexus, the brachial plexus, and the lumbosacral plexus (see Figure 11-9). Each plexus sorts out the many fibers and sends them to a specific part of the body. The three plexuses and the major nerves that emerge from each plexus are listed in Table 11-5 and described below. The results of damage to major peripheral nerves are listed in Table 11-6.

Cervical plexus (C1 to C4): Fibers from the cervical plexus supply the muscles and skin of the neck. Motor fibers from this plexus also pass into the phrenic nerve. The phrenic nerve stimulates the contraction of the diaphragm, the major breathing muscle (see Figures 11-9 and 11-10).

If the spinal cord is severed below the C5 level, the person is paralyzed but can breathe. If the level of injury is higher, at C2, the phrenic nerve is injured, motor impulses to the diaphragm are interrupted, and the person cannot breathe normally. To breathe, the person generally needs the assistance of a ventilator.

Brachial plexus (C5 to C8, T1): the nerves that emerge from the brachial plexus supply the muscles and skin of the shoulder, arm, forearm, wrist, and hand. The axillary nerve emerges from this plexus and travels through the shoulder into the arm.

The axillary nerve in the shoulder region is susceptible to damage. For instance, a person using crutches should be taught to bear the weight of the body on the hands and not on the armpit, or axillary region. The weight of the body can damage the axillary nerve, causing crutch palsy.

The radial and ulnar nerves, which serve the lower arm, wrist, and hand, also emerge from the brachial plexus. Damage to the radial nerve can cause a wristdrop, and injury to the ulnar nerve causes the hand to appear clawlike; the person is unable to spread the fingers apart.

Lumbosacral plexus (T12, L1 to L5, S1 to S4): the lumbosacral plexus gives rise to nerves that supply the muscles and skin of the lower abdominal wall, external genitalia, buttocks, and lower extremities. The

Table 11-5 Spinal Nerve Plexuses

Plexus	Spinal Nerve Origin	Region Innervated	Major Nerves Emerging from Plexus
Cervical	C1 to C4	Skin and muscles of the neck and shoulder; diaphragm	Phrenic
Brachial	C5 to C8, T1	Skin and muscles of the upper extremities	Axillary Radial Median Musculocutaneous Ulnar
Lumbosacral	T12, L1 to L5 S1 to S4	Skin and muscle of lower torso and lower extremities	Femoral Obturator Sciatic Pudendal

Table 11-6 Major Peripheral Nerves: Results of Damage

Nerve	Body Area Served	Results of Nerve Damage
Phrenic	Diaphragm	Impaired breathing
Axillary	Muscles of shoulder	Crutch palsy
Radial	Posterior arm, forearm, hand; thumbs and first two fingers	Wristdrop (inability to lift or extend hand at wrist)
Median	Forearm and some muscles of the hand	Inability to pick up small objects
Ulnar	Wrist and many muscles in hand	Clawhand—inability to spread fingers apart
Intercostal	Rib cage	Impaired breathing
Femoral	Lower abdomen, anterior thigh, medial leg, foot	Inability to extend leg and flex hip
Sciatic	Lower trunk; posterior thigh and leg	Inability to extend hip and flex knee
Common peroneal	Lateral area of leg and foot	Footdrop—inability to dorsiflex foot
Tibial	Posterior area of leg and foot	Shuffling gait due to inability to invert and dorsiflex foot

CERVICAL PLEXUS

BRACHIAL PLEXUS

LUMBOSACRAL PLEXUS

Phrenic nerves

"Breathing muscles"

Damage to phrenic nerve

Damage to axillary nerve

Damage to median nerve

Irritation of sciatic nerve

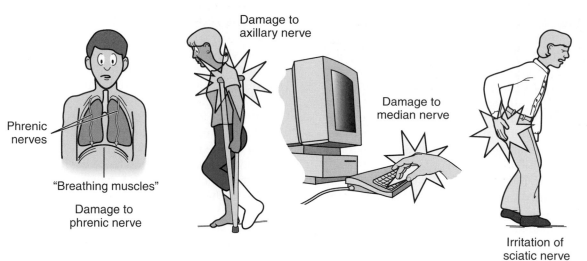

FIGURE 11-10 Examples of nerve damage.

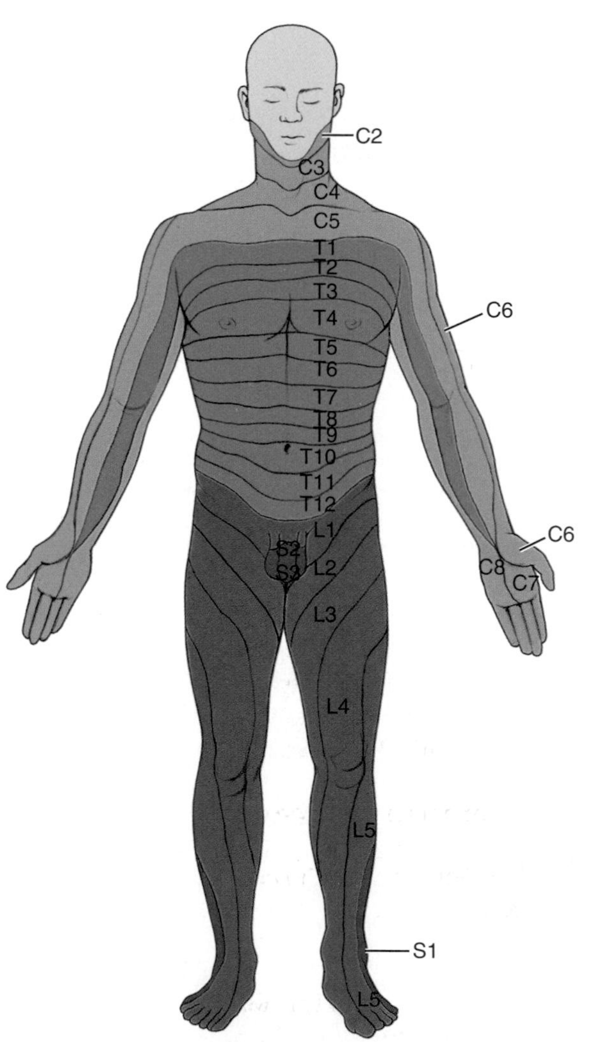

FIGURE 11-11 Dermatome.

sciatic nerve, the longest nerve in the body, arises from this plexus. The sciatic nerve supplies the entire musculature of the leg and foot. The sciatic nerve can become inflamed and cause intense pain in the buttock and posterior thigh region. A common cause of sciatica is a ruptured or herniated vertebral disc (Figure 11-10).

Do You Know...

What was on Dr. Herby Zoster's shingle?

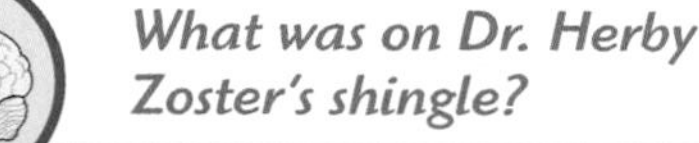

The doctor's shingle indicates that he specializes in chickenpox and shingles, both caused by the herpes zoster virus. Following a chickenpox infection the herpes virus "hides out" in nerves and often reactivates in later life causing shingles. Clusters of vesicles develop along cranial or spinal dermatomes. The painful lesions eventually crust over. The term *shingles* comes from a word meaning girdle, a reference to the usual appearance of lesions around the waist.

What a Dermatome Is. Each spinal nerve innervates a particular area of the skin; this distribution of nerves is called a **dermatome** (DĔR-mă-tōm). Figure 11-11 illustrates the dermatomes for the entire body. Each dermatome is named for the particular nerve that serves it. For instance, the C4 dermatome is innervated by the C4 spinal nerve. Dermatomes are useful clinically; for example, if the skin of the shoulder region is stimulated with the tip of a pin and the person cannot feel it, the clinician has reason to believe the C4 nerve is impaired.

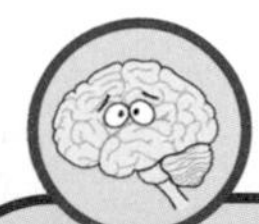

Do You Know...

About tingling thigh syndrome?

While tight, low-slung jeans are "in," your thigh nerves are on edge about this fashion craze. The snug jeans are compressing nerves in your thighs, causing a tingling sensation. The "tingling thigh syndrome" is easily cured, but the jeans have to go—or go higher.

Functional Classification of the Peripheral Nervous System

The functional classification explains where the nerves go and what they do. The functional classification for the peripheral nervous system includes the following:

- The somatic afferent nerves, which bring sensory information from the different parts of the body, particularly the skin and muscles, to the CNS (see Chapter 13).
- The somatic efferent nerves, which bring motor information from the CNS to the skeletal muscles throughout the body (Chapter 9).
- The autonomic nervous system (ANS) is composed of nerves that supply the organs (viscera) and glands. The ANS is the topic of Chapter 12.

Sum It Up!

The peripheral nervous system consists of the nerves and ganglia located outside the CNS. Nerves are sensory, motor, and mixed. Mixed nerves carry both sensory and motor neurons. The peripheral nervous system can be classified structurally and functionally. The structural classification divides the nerves into cranial and spinal nerves. The 12 pairs of cranial nerves contain fibers that originate in the brain (see Figure 11-8 and Table 11-3). There are 31 pairs of spinal nerves; their fibers originate in the spinal cord (see Figure 11-9, and Tables 11-5 and 11-6). The spinal nerve fibers converge into nerve plexuses, or networks. The three major nerve plexuses are the cervical plexus, brachial plexus, and lumbosacral plexus.

SUMMARY OUTLINE

The brain, spinal cord, and peripheral nervous system act as a vast communication system. The spinal cord transmits information to and from the brain. The peripheral nervous system brings information to the CNS (its sensory role) and delivers information from the CNS to the periphery (its motor role).

I. What the Spinal Cord Is

A. The spinal cord is a tubelike structure located in the spinal cavity, extending from the foramen magnum (occipital bone) to L1

B. Arrangement of Nervous Tissue

1. The gray matter is a butterfly-shaped area located centrally.
2. The white matter is composed of myelinated fibers arranged in tracts. Ascending tracts are sensory tracts. Descending tracts are motor tracts.
3. Spinal nerves are attached to the spinal cord. All spinal nerves are mixed (they contain sensory and motor fibers).
4. Sensory nerve fibers travel to the cord through the dorsal root. Motor nerve fibers travel in the ventral root.

II. What the Spinal Cord Does: Functions

A. The spinal cord relays both sensory and motor information.

B. The spinal cord acts as a major reflex center.

III. Reflexes

A. A reflex is an involuntary response to a stimulus

B. The four components to a reflex are a sensory receptor; an afferent (sensory) neuron; an efferent (motor) neuron; and an effector organ

IV. Peripheral Nervous System

A. Nerve

1. A nerve is a group of neurons, blood vessels, and connective tissue.
2. There are sensory nerves, motor nerves, and mixed nerves.

B. Structural Classification of Nerves

1. A classification of nerves on the basis of structure divides nerves into cranial nerves and spinal nerves. There are 12 pairs of cranial nerves (Table 11-3) and 31 pairs of spinal nerves (Table 11-6).
2. Spinal nerves are sorted out at nerve plexuses. The three major plexuses are the cervical plexus, the brachial plexus, and the lumbosacral plexus.
3. A dermatome is the area of skin innervated by each spinal nerve.

C. Functional Classification of Nerves

1. Somatic afferent nerves carry sensory information to the CNS.

2. Somatic efferent nerves carry motor information to skeletal muscles.

3. Autonomic nerves carry motor information to the organs (viscera).

Review Your Knowledge

Matching: Reflexes

Directions: Match the following words with their descriptions below.

a. gag reflex
b. baroreceptor reflex
c. withdrawal reflex
d. Achilles tendon reflex
e. pupillary reflex
f. patellar tendon reflex

1. ____ Helps you to maintain balance; also called the knee-jerk reflex
2. ____ Regulates blood pressure
3. ____ Controls the amount of light that enters the eye
4. ____ You pull your finger away from a sharp object
5. ____ Helps to prevent food and water from entering the respiratory passages
6. ____ Tapping of the calcaneal tendon causes plantar flexion

Matching: Nerves

Directions: Match the following words with their descriptions below. Some words may be used more than once.

a. oculomotor
b. optic
c. vagus
d. facial
e. sciatic
f. olfactory
g. phrenic
h. vestibulocochlear

1. ____ Innervates the skeletal muscles that move the eyeball
2. ____ Carries sensory information to the visual cortex of the occipital lobe
3. ____ Carries sensory information for hearing and balance
4. ____ Innervates the diaphragm, causing it to contract
5. ____ Innervates muscles of the thigh
6. ____ The "wanderer" nerve that is distributed throughout the thoracic and abdominopelvic cavities
7. ____ The "smell" nerve
8. ____ The nerve of facial expression
9. ____ Ototoxicity refers to this damaged nerve
10. ____ "Fixed and dilated" describes this injured nerve

Multiple Choice

1. Which of the following does not describe the oculomotor nerve?
   a. Is also CN III
   b. Innervates the skeletal muscles that move the eyeball
   c. Is the carrier of information to the visual cortex in the occipital lobe
   d. Innervates skeletal muscle that raises the eyelids
2. The trigeminal nerve
   a. is CN V.
   b. has both sensory and motor fibers.
   c. affects chewing.
   d. All of the above.
3. The sciatic nerve
   a. is a motor nerve that innervates thigh muscles.
   b. is a cranial nerve.
   c. enters the cervical plexus for distribution to the periphery.
   d. travels within the spinothalamic tract.
4. Which of the following is descriptive of the spinothalamic tract?
   a. Carries sensory information regarding touch, pressure, and pain
   b. Is the major motor tract
   c. Is also called the pyramidal tract
   d. Is a descending tract
5. Which of the following is least descriptive of the corticospinal tract?
   a. Descending tract
   b. Major motor tract
   c. Pyramidal tract
   d. Carries information from the spinal cord to the thalamus

CHAPTER 12

Autonomic Nervous System

KEY TERMS

Adrenergic fiber, p. 209
Autonomic nervous system, p. 204
Beta-adrenergic receptor, p. 210
Cholinergic fiber, p. 209
Craniosacral outflow, p. 208
Muscarinic receptor, p. 209
Nicotinic receptor, p. 209
Norepinephrine, p. 209
Parasympathetic nervous system, p. 206
Preganglionic fiber, p. 207
Postganglionic fiber, p. 207
Sympathetic nervous system, p. 205
Thoracolumbar outflow, p. 207

OBJECTIVES

1. Describe the function of the autonomic nervous system.
2. Identify the two divisions of the autonomic nervous system.
3. State the anatomical and functional differences between the sympathetic and parasympathetic nervous systems.
4. Define *cholinergic* and *adrenergic fibers.*
5. Name the major neurotransmitters of the autonomic nervous system.
6. Name and locate the cholinergic and adrenergic receptors.
7. Explain the terms used to describe the effects of drugs on autonomic receptors.

Throughout the day, you are busy doing things. You walk across a room, run up the stairs, write, tie your shoes, and chew your food. You perform all of these activities voluntarily and consciously. Your body, however, performs many more activities unconsciously and automatically. For instance, when you eat you don't consciously think, "I am eating. Therefore, I should increase the flow of my digestive enzymes and then increase the rate of contraction of my intestinal muscles in order to enhance the digestive process." Instead, your body automatically and unconsciously makes these decisions and carries them out for you. This automatic response is the function of the **autonomic nervous system.** Autonomic = automatic!

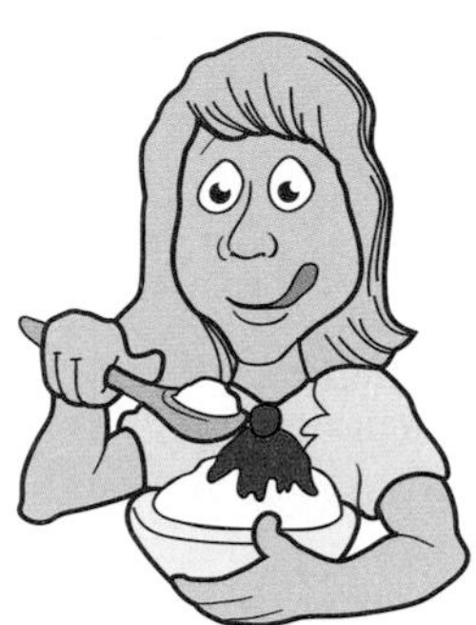

AUTONOMIC (VISCERAL) REFLEXES

WHAT THEY DO

Mention the word reflex and what comes to mind is the knee-jerk reflex. Tap the patellar tendon and up pops the knee. The knee-jerk reflex is mediated by somatic nerves. There are also visceral reflexes. They are mediated by the autonomic nervous system. As the name implies, visceral reflexes regulate organ function. Visceral reflexes control such things as heart rate, blood pressure, body temperature, digestion, airflow through respiratory passages, elimination and pupillary (eye) responses. Note the wide variety of functions controlled by autonomic activity. Takes a load off your mind.

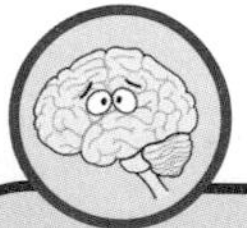

Do You Know...

What Pinocchio and your autonomic nervous system have in common?

While Pinocchio's nose was a dead giveaway to his lying ways, most of us do not do "the nose thing" in response to fibbing. But, fibbers beware! Your autonomic nervous system can act like the puppet's nose. Lying, even those little white lies, activates the sympathetic nervous system and causes physiologic responses that are readily captured by a polygraph machine. A modern-day Gepetto knew that we are generally unable to control the autonomic nervous system and so invented the lie detector.

PATHWAY

A visceral reflex is mediated in a manner similar to the knee-jerk reflex: activation of a receptor, transmission of sensory information to the CNS, the processing of the information by the CNS, and the motor response sent to the effector organ(s). For instance, a sudden decrease in blood pressure activates pressure receptors (baroreceptors). The information about the low blood pressure is carried to the medulla oblongata in the brain stem by sensory nerves. The medulla oblongata determines that the blood pressure is low and sends motor signals to the visceral effector organs (heart and blood vessels). The motor response results in changes in the heart and blood vessels that elevate blood pressure. What has been accomplished? A sudden decrease in blood pressure stimulates a visceral reflex that restores blood pressure to normal. All this has been accomplished without conscious input!

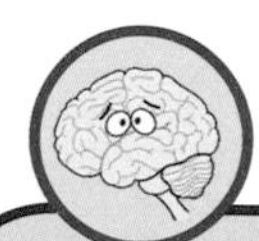

Do You Know...

Why 007 wears shades?

The autonomic nervous system is constantly adjusting our innards to environmental stresses. The adjustments are noticeable in our eye responses, particularly in the changes in pupil size. Bored, you say? Pupils constrict. Interested, excited, or scared? Pupils dilate. James Bond certainly doesn't want to give away any of his autonomic cues and therefore wears his shades—as do poker players.

ORGANIZATION AND FUNCTION OF THE AUTONOMIC NERVOUS SYSTEM

DIVISION OF THE AUTONOMIC NERVOUS SYSTEM (ANS)

The ANS is the part of the peripheral nervous system that supplies motor activity to the visceral effector organs: glands, smooth muscles within organs, and the heart.

The two divisions of the ANS are the sympathetic and parasympathetic nervous systems. The distribution of sympathetic and parasympathetic nerves to the viscera varies. A single organ most often receives fibers from both divisions of the ANS. This is referred to as **dual innervation.** In most instances, stimulation of one division of the ANS causes a specific effect, whereas stimulation by the other division causes an opposing effect. For instance, the cells of the heart that determine heart rate receive both sympathetic and parasympathetic fibers. Stimulation of the sympathetic fibers increases heart rate, whereas stimulation of the parasympathetic fibers decreases heart rate. There are exceptions to this arrangement. In a few organs that receive dual innervation, the effects of sympathetic and parasympathetic activity are complementary rather than opposite. For instance, in the male, erectile activity is regulated by the parasympathetics, while ejaculation is regulated by the sympathetics. The sympathetics and parasympathetics work in a complimentary way to achieve the desired effect, penetration of the female and ejection of the sperm. Finally, not all organs have dual innervation. For example, the blood vessels are innervated only by the sympathetic nervous system. Regulation of blood vessel diameter is achieved through an adjustment of sympathetic activity. Increased sympathetic activity causes constriction of the blood vessels, while decreased sympathetic activity causes the blood vessels to dilate.

Table 12-1 indicates the effects of sympathetic and parasympathetic stimulation on some major organs of the body.

Sympathetic Nervous System: Fight or Flight

In general, the **sympathetic nervous system** is activated during periods of stress or times when the person feels threatened in some way (Figure 12-1). For this reason the sympathetic nervous system is called the **fight or flight** division of the ANS. In other words, the sympathetic nervous system causes you to be prepared either to confront (fight) or remove yourself from the threatening situation (flight). Recall a time when you were frightened. Your heart raced and pounded in your chest. The pupils of your eyes opened wide. You breathed more quickly and more deeply. The palms of your hands became wet with perspiration, and your mouth became so dry you could hardly speak. The easiest way to remember the sympathetic responses is to recall your personal response to your own worst nightmare! You can check Table 12-1 to see if your responses matched the sympathetic column.

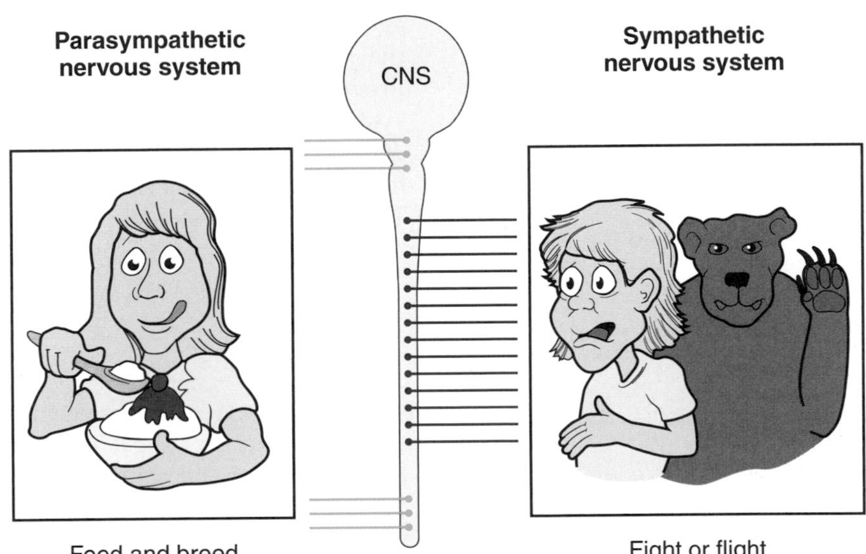

FIGURE 12-1 Autonomic nervous system: parasympathetic nervous system and sympathetic nervous system.

Table 12-1 Autonomic Nervous System: Organ Responses

Organ	Sympathetic Response	Parasympathetic Response
Heart	Increases rate and strength of contraction	Decreases rate: no direct effect on strength
Bronchial tubes	Dilates (↑ airflow)	Constricts (↓ airflow)
Iris of eye	Dilates (pupil enlarges)	Constricts (pupil becomes smaller)
Blood vessels	Constricts	No innervation
Sweat glands	Stimulates	No innervation
Intestine	Inhibits motility	Stimulates motility and secretion
Uterus	Relaxes muscle	No effect
Adrenal medulla	Stimulates secretion of epinephrine and norepinephrine	No effect
Salivary glands	Stimulates thick secretion	Stimulates watery secretion
Urinary system		
Bladder wall	No effect	Contracts muscle
Internal sphincter	No effect	Opens sphincter

While the sympathetic nervous system is activated during periods of stress, these periods are normally short-lived. If you keep yourself stressed out, however, the sympathetic nervous system keeps the body in a state of high alert. Over time, this state takes its toll on the body through stress-induced illnesses. Laughter, play, rest, and relaxation diminish sympathetic outflow and are good buffers against stress. So, relax and be happy!

Do You Know...

About the sympathetic nervous system gone wild?

There are several clinical conditions caused by out-of-control sympathetic activity. One condition is called autonomic dysreflexia. Autonomic dysreflexia is experienced by a person who has sustained a high cervical spinal cord injury (i.e., C4 transection and quadriplegia). This is what happens: The quadriplegic patient develops a distended urinary bladder, usually from a kinked urinary catheter. The distended bladder sends signals to the spinal cord, setting off massive thoracolumbar (sympathetic) discharge. The intense sympathetic activity severely elevates blood pressure, sometimes to the point of causing a cerebral hemorrhage (stroke). The sympathetic stimulation continues as long as the bladder remains distended. The autonomic nervous system cannot counteract the sympathetic firing because of the spinal cord injury. Immediate treatment is to remove the stimulus (distended bladder) which then lowers the blood pressure. Out of control sympathetic activity is life threatening and is always taken seriously.

Parasympathetic Nervous System: Feed and Breed

The **parasympathetic nervous system** is most active during quiet, nonstressful conditions. It has a calming effect on the body. The parasympathetic nervous system plays an important role in the regulation of digestion and in reproductive function. For this reason, it is sometimes referred to as the **feed and breed** division of the ANS. Another descriptive term for the parasympathetic nervous system is **resting and digesting.**

What is "paradoxical fear"? While the sympathetics are usually associated with fear reactions, the parasympathetics can be activated in situations that are perceived as hopeless and where fight or flight seems futile. The massive parasympathetic discharge can result in uncontrolled urination and defecation. It can also cause the heart rate to decrease so severely that the person faints or experiences a potentially lethal electrical disturbance of the heart. Clinically, this type of cardiac stress reaction is described as "bradying down," a reference to severe bradycardia (dangerously slow heart rate).

AUTONOMIC TERMINOLOGY, AUTONOMIC PHARMACOLOGY

Many drugs work by altering autonomic activity. Thus, many pharmacology terms refer to the autonomic nervous system. In fact you cannot understand pharmacology without knowing autonomic nervous system terminology. So get ready for some challenging words!

If a drug causes effects similar to the activation of the sympathetic nervous system it is called a **sympathomimetic** (as in mimicking) drug. A sympathomimetic agent increases heart rate, force of cardiac contraction, and blood pressure. If the drug causes effects that are similar to a situation where the sympathetic nervous system cannot be activated, the drug is called a **sympatholytic** (-lytic means inhibiting) drug. The administration of a sympatholytic drug prevents an increase in cardiac activity when the sympathetic nerves are fired.

If a drug causes effects similar to the activation of the parasympathetic nervous system, it is called a **parasympathomimetic** drug. A parasympathomimetic agent decreases heart rate and increases digestive activity. The administration of a **parasympatholytic** agent prevents activation of the parasympathetic nervous system. If an organ, such as the heart, is being driven excessively by the parasympathetic nervous system, heart rate becomes dangerously slow (bradycardia). The administration of a parasympatholytic drug, such as atropine, blocks the parasympathetic effect on the heart, thereby allowing heart rate to increase.

AUTONOMIC TONE AND VASOMOTOR TONE

The sympathetics and parasympathetics are active at the same time, creating a background (continuous, low-level) firing of the autonomic nervous system. This background autonomic activity is called **autonomic tone.** In the resting state, parasympathetic activity is generally stronger. For instance, parasympathetic tone maintains the resting heart rate around 72 beats per minute. When physical activity increases, however, the sympathetic nerves fire more intensely, while parasympathetic activity decreases. The shift to sympathetic discharge in exercise results in an increase in heart rate, thereby supplying more oxygen and energy to the exercising muscles. The balance between sympathetic and parasympathetic activity is maintained by the hypothalamus and parts of the brain stem.

A second example of autonomic tone involves the blood vessels. Blood vessels are innervated only by the sympathetic nerves; there is no parasympathetic innervation. Thus, the autonomic tone of the blood vessels is determined by the sympathetic nervous system. Background sympathetic firing keeps the blood vessels somewhat constricted. This sympathetically induced continuous state of blood vessel constriction is called **vasomotor tone.** Additional sympathetic firing causes blood vessels to constrict, thereby elevating blood pressure. A decrease in sympathetic firing causes blood vessels to dilate, thereby lowering blood pressure. A change in vasomotor tone is clinically very important; for instance, loss of vasomotor tone can dangerously lower blood pressure, plunging the person into a lethal shock.

Sum It Up!

The autonomic nervous system regulates visceral (organ) functions such as blood pressure. There are two divisions of the ANS: the sympathetic and parasympathetic nervous systems. Their functions are summarized as: sympathetic, or "fight or flight"; and parasympathetic, or "feed and breed." Background firing of the sympathetic nervous system to the blood vessels is responsible for vasomotor tone that, in turn, plays a crucial role in the maintenance of normal blood pressure.

AUTONOMIC NERVOUS SYSTEM NEURONS

NUMBERS AND GANGLIA

The numbers and arrangement of the neurons of the ANS are important. The pathways of the ANS use two neurons with a ganglion between each neuron (Figure 12-2, *A*) The cell body of neuron #1 is located in the CNS, in either the brain or the spinal cord. The axon of neuron number 1 leaves the CNS and extends to the ganglion (cell body of neuron number 2). The axon of neuron number 1 is called the **preganglionic fiber** (because it comes before—pre—the ganglion). The axon of neuron number 2 leaves the ganglion and extends to the organ. This axon is called the **postganglionic fiber** (because it comes after—post—the ganglion). Pay particular attention to the postganglionic fibers; they are key to understanding autonomic function. The postganglionic fibers of the sympathetic and parasympathetic nervous systems secrete different neurotransmitters. These different neurotransmitters account for the different effects caused by the sympathetic and parasympathetic nervous systems.

NEURONS OF THE SYMPATHETIC NERVOUS SYSTEM

The neurons of the sympathetic nervous system leave the spinal cord at the thoracic and lumbar levels (T1 to L2) (see Figure 12-2, *B*). The sympathetic nervous system is therefore called the **thoracolumbar outflow.** Most preganglionic sympathetic fibers travel a short distance and synapse within ganglia located close to

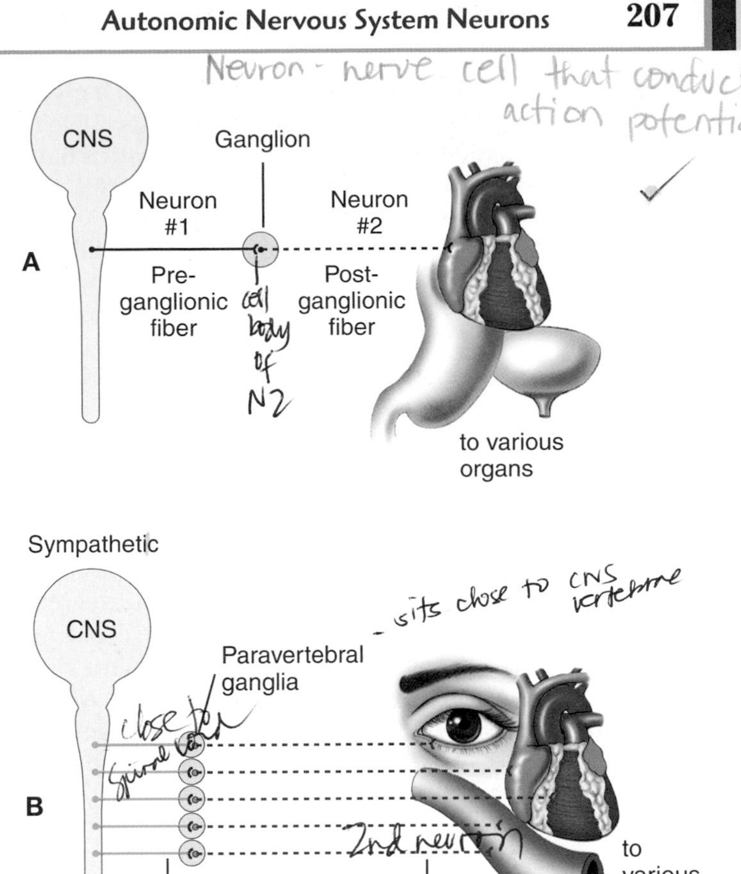

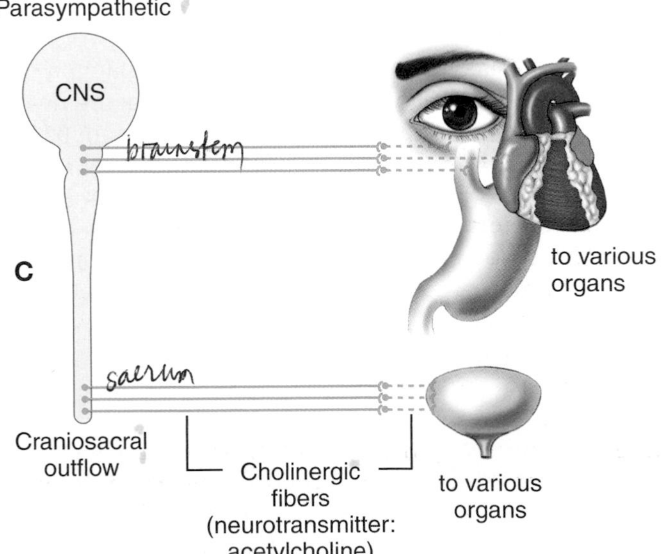

FIGURE 12-2 **A,** Arrangement of autonomic fibers. **B,** Sympathetic nervous system. **C,** Parasympathetic nervous system.

the spinal cord. The sympathetic ganglia form a chain that runs alongside the vertebral column. This chain is called the **paravertebral ganglia** or **sympathetic chain ganglia.** Postganglionic fibers leave the ganglia and extend to the various organs.

The location of the paravertebral ganglia is important. The paravertebral ganglia provide a site where each preganglionic fiber synapses with multiple postganglionic fibers. Why is this important? The firing of a single sympathetic neuron is capable of providing a generalized, widespread sympathetic response; many organs respond to sympathetic firing. This makes sense. If you are confronted with an emergency situation you want the entire body to respond immediately!

The adrenal gland (adrenal medulla) acts as a modified sympathetic ganglion. Preganglionic sympathetic fibers supply the adrenal medulla, causing it to secrete hormones (epinephrine and norepinephrine) that resemble the neurotransmitters of the sympathetic nervous system. These hormones circulate in the blood throughout the body. Thus the sympathetic nervous system and the adrenal medulla function together to achieve a sustained response.

NEURONS OF THE PARASYMPATHETIC NERVOUS SYSTEM

The neurons of the parasympathetic nervous system leave the CNS at the level of the brain stem and sacrum (S2 to S4) (see Figure 12-2, *C*). The parasympathetic nervous system is therefore called the **craniosacral outflow.**

Because the ganglia of the parasympathetic nervous system are located close to or within the target organs, the parasympathetic nerves do not have a chain of ganglia running alongside the spinal cord. The preganglionic fibers are long because the ganglia of the parasympathetic nervous system are located near the target organ. Short postganglionic fibers run from the ganglia to the smooth muscle or glands within the organ. Because of the location of the ganglia close to the target organs, parasympathetic activity generates a more localized response (as opposed to the generalized sympathetic response). Table 12-2 compares the anatomic arrangement of the sympathetic and parasympathetic nervous systems.

Running with Cranial Nerves (CNs)

Parasympathetic fibers travel from the brain stem with four cranial nerves: oculomotor (CN III), facial (CN VII), glossopharyngeal (CN IX), and vagus (CN X).

Oculomotor Nerve (CN III)

The oculomotor nerve innervates most of the extrinsic eye muscles (skeletal muscles) that move the eyeball. The oculomotor nerve also carries parasympathetic fibers to two intrinsic eye muscles: the constrictor muscle of the eye, which causes pupillary constriction, and the ciliary muscle, which controls the shape of the lens of the eye. Observation of pupillary reflexes is used clinically to observe for signs of increasing intracranial pressure and other neurologic disorders. In addition, many drugs alter parasympathetic activity of the intrinsic eye muscles and you will need to assess their clinical effects. You will have to do "eye checks"; pay close attention to the eye muscles and nerves of the eye.

Facial Nerve (CN VII)

The facial nerve carries parasympathetic fibers to the tear glands (eyes), salivary glands (mouth), and nasal glands (nose).

Glossopharyngeal Nerve (CN IX)

The glossopharyngeal nerve (with the assistance of the trigeminal nerve) carries parasympathetic fibers to the salivary glands in the mouth.

Vagus Nerve (CN X)

The vagus nerve (the "wanderer" nerve) carries over 80% of the parasympathetic fibers. It travels from the brain stem to organs within the thoracic and abdominal cavities.

Sum It Up!

The sympathetic nervous system is called the thoracolumbar outflow. The parasympathetic nervous system is called the craniosacral outflow. Each system has preganglionic and postganglionic fibers. The ganglia of the sympathetic nerves are located in the paravertebral ganglia, while the ganglia of the parasympathetics are located near the target organ. Parasympathetic fibers travel from the brainstem with four cranial nerves: oculomotor, facial, glossopharyngeal, and the vagus nerves.

Table 12-2 Autonomic Nervous System: Comparison

Characteristic	Sympathetic	Parasympathetic
Origin of fibers	Thoracolumbar	Craniosacral
Functions	Fight or flight	Feed and breed
Ganglia	Paravertebral ganglia	Located near or within target organ
Effects	Generalized/widespread	Localized
Neurotransmitter	Norepinephrine (postganglionic)	Acetylcholine

NAMING FIBERS AND NEUROTRANSMITTERS

The key to understanding autonomic function and autonomic pharmacology is based on knowledge of the autonomic neurotransmitters and their receptors. The two major neurotransmitters of the ANS are acetylcholine (ACh) and **norepinephrine** (NE).

The neurotransmitter is used to name the fibers of the ANS. For instance, a fiber that secretes NE as its neurotransmitter is called an **adrenergic fiber** (NE is also called nor*adrenaline*). A fiber that secretes ACh (acetyl*choline*) as its neurotransmitter is called a **cholinergic fiber.**

Now, here's the challenging part. Remember, we are concerned with four fibers (two preganglionic and two postganglionic fibers, sympathetic and parasympathetic). The preganglionic fibers secrete ACh and are therefore cholinergic fibers. The postganglionic fibers of the parasympathetic nervous system secrete ACh and are also cholinergic. The postganglionic sympathetic nervous system fibers, however, secrete NE and are called adrenergic fibers. Refer to Figure 12-2, *B* and *C*, and note the color-coding that differentiates the adrenergic from the cholinergic fibers. The cholinergic fibers are colored green, while the adrenergic fibers are colored red. You absolutely need this "fiber/ neurotransmitter" information embedded in your frontal lobe in order to learn autonomic pharmacology!

NEUROTRANSMITTERS: TERMINATION OF ACTIVITY

ACh is secreted by cholinergic fibers and diffuses to its receptor. After ACh exerts its effect on its receptor, it is quickly degraded by acetylcholinesterase (AChE), an enzyme found within the synapse.

NE is secreted by adrenergic fibers. The effects of NE are more prolonged because of the manner in which NE is terminated. Most of the NE is reabsorbed by the adrenergic nerve terminals themselves. The termination of NE is called "reuptake" (note that its termination differs from that of ACh). The NE that is taken up by the nerve terminal is processed in two ways. Most of the NE is simply reused. Excess NE can be degraded by an enzyme located within the adrenergic nerve terminal; the enzyme is called monoamine oxidase (MAO).

Do You Know...

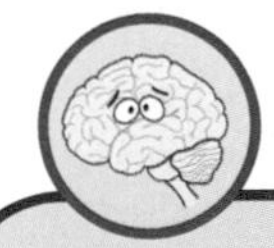

Why you might have to "hold the beer and sausage" if you are taking an MAO inhibitor?

Monoamine oxidase (MAO) is an enzyme that breaks down norepinephrine in the CNS. An MAO-inhibitor drug prevents the breakdown of NE and is used in the treatment of depression. While the drug relieves the depression by increasing NE within the CNS, it can also cause serious adverse effects such as a dangerously elevated blood pressure. Certain foods (beer, cheese, and sausage) contain an amino acid that is used in the synthesis of NE. The combination of the drugs and food increases NE and blood pressure and the possibility of a stroke. Some herbals such as St. John's Wort contain MAO-inhibitor activity and may also dangerously elevate blood pressure. Taking an MAO inhibitor? Hold the beer and sausage!

Sum It Up!

The two major neurotransmitters of the ANS are acetylcholine (ACh) and norepinephrine (NE). ACh is secreted by cholinergic fibers. The effects of ACh are short-lived, the ACh being degraded by acetylcholinesterase located within the synapse. NE is secreted by adrenergic fibers. The effects of the sympathetic nervous system are due primarily to NE. The effects of NE are more prolonged due to the manner in which NE is terminated (through reuptake). Excess NE is degraded by monoamine oxidase (MAO).

RECEPTORS OF THE AUTONOMIC NERVOUS SYSTEM

The neurotransmitters of the autonomic nervous system, ACh and NE, bind to receptors on target cells (cardiac muscle, smooth muscle, and glands). A receptor is any site on the cell to which a neurotransmitter binds, causing an alteration in cellular function. For instance, ACh binds to a receptor on a heart cell and causes the heart rate to decrease. NE binds to a different receptor on the heart cell and causes heart rate to increase. The autonomic nervous system has two receptor types, the cholinergic and the adrenergic receptors.

CHOLINERGIC RECEPTORS

There are two types of cholinergic receptors: **muscarinic receptors** and **nicotinic receptors.** The different types of cholinergic receptors explain the variety of effects of cholinergic receptor activation by ACh.

Where are these receptors located? Muscarinic receptors are located on the target organs (cardiac muscle, smooth muscle, and glands) of the parasympathetic nerves (Figure 12-3). Thus, activation of the parasympathetic nervous system releases ACh and stimulates muscarinic receptors. Refer to Table 12-3 and note several of the effects of muscarinic activation. For instance, activation of the muscarinic receptors on the constrictor muscle of the iris (pupil) causes pupil size to decrease. Activation of the muscarinic receptors in the heart (SA node) causes heart rate to decrease. Muscarinic activation of the urinary bladder

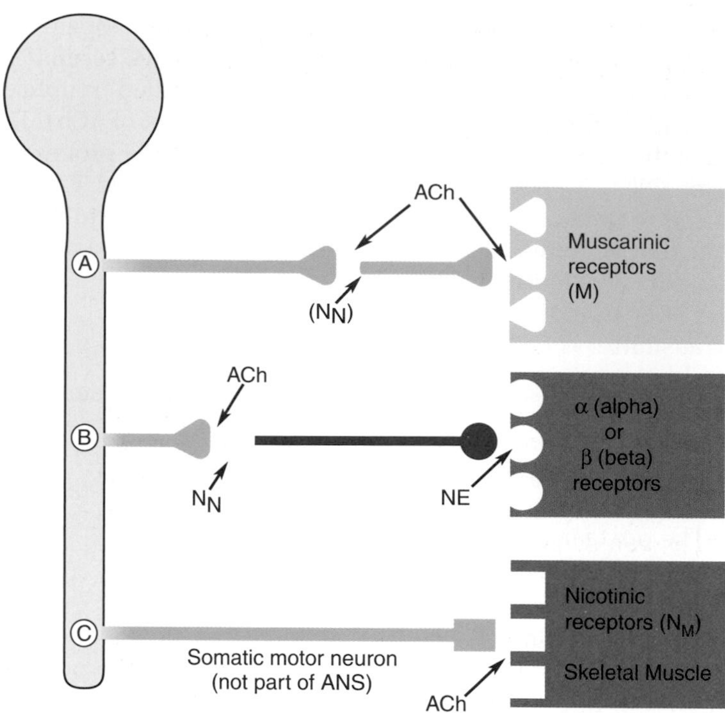

FIGURE 12-3 Receptors: adrenergic and cholinergic.

Table 12-3 Cholinergic Receptors and Responses*

Organ	Receptor	Activation Response
Heart	Muscarinic	Decreases heart rate
Bronchial tubes	Muscarinic	Constricts (↓ airflow)
Iris of eye	Muscarinic	Constricts (pupil becomes smaller)
Urinary system		
Bladder wall	Muscarinic	Contracts
Internal sphincter	Muscarinic	Relaxes and opens sphincter

*Table lists the most common muscarinic receptors targeted by pharmacological agents.

causes the bladder muscle to contract and the outlet sphincter muscle of the urinary bladder to relax; these coordinated muscarinic responses of the bladder promote urination.

There are two types of nicotinic receptors in the peripheral nervous system. The nicotinic-neural (N_N) receptors are located within the ganglia of the autonomic nervous system. Because these nicotinic receptors are located in both the sympathetic nervous system and the parasympathetic nervous system, the responses to nicotinic (N_N) activation are difficult to predict. Nicotinic receptors are also located outside of the ANS. For instance, the receptors located on skeletal muscles in the neuromuscular junction are nicotinic-muscle receptors (N_M). Activation of the N_M receptors in the neuromuscular junction causes skeletal muscle contraction. Remember, the N_N receptors are part of the autonomic nervous system; the N_M receptors are part of the somatic motor nervous system. The cholinergic receptor subtypes are important in pharmacology and are worthwhile learning; however, in this chapter we will refer only to the muscarinic receptors.

ADRENERGIC RECEPTORS

There are two main types of adrenergic receptors: alpha (α) and **beta** (β) **adrenergic** receptors. There are subtypes of the adrenergic receptors: alpha$_1$, alpha$_2$, beta$_1$, and beta$_2$ adrenergic receptors. Adrenergic receptors are located on the target organs of the sympathetic nerves, so that stimulation of the sympathetic nervous system causes activation of adrenergic receptors. See Table 12-4 for the effects of adrenergic receptor activation. Note that activation of the alpha$_1$ receptors of the

Table 12-4 Adrenergic Receptors and Responses*

Organ	Receptor	Activation Response
Heart	β_1	Increases heart rate and strength of contraction
Bronchial tubes	β_2	Dilates (↑ airflow)
Iris of eye	α_1	Dilates (pupil enlarges)
Blood vessels	α_1	Constricts
Uterus	β_2	Relaxes

*Table lists the most common adrenergic receptors targeted by pharmacological agents.
β = beta; α = alpha.

blood vessels of the mucous membrane causes constriction, thereby decreasing blood flow and "shrinking swollen membranes" to relieve the discomfort of a stuffy nose. Activation of the alpha$_1$ receptors on blood vessels causes vasoconstriction, thereby elevating blood pressure. These drugs are used in the treatment of conditions that involve low blood pressure, such as shock. Activation of the beta$_1$ receptors in the heart increases heart rate and the strength of cardiac muscle contraction. Activation of the beta$_2$ receptors dilates the breathing tubes, thereby increasing airflow; this action is the basis of the bronchodilators used in the treatment of asthma. Activation of the alpha$_1$ receptors in the iris (eye) causes the radial muscle to contract and the pupil to dilate. Finally, activation of the beta$_2$ receptors in the pregnant uterus causes the uterine muscles to relax, thereby preventing the premature delivery of the fetus. The adrenergic receptors can be activated by NE and other natural catecholamines such as epinephrine and dopamine.

There are a small number of dopamine receptors (also classified as adrenergic receptors) located in the blood vessels of the kidney. Activation of the dopamine receptors causes the blood vessels in the kidney to dilate, thereby increasing blood flow to the kidneys. Dopamine is often administered clinically to maintain blood flow to the kidneys during shock-like episodes that would normally diminish blood flow to the kidneys.

AUTONOMIC TERMINOLOGY: "DOING" AUTONOMIC PHARMACOLOGY

Autonomic pharmacology classifies drugs according to their receptors. For instance, a beta$_1$ adrenergic agonist is a drug that activates the beta$_1$ adrenergic receptors. (An **agonist** is a drug that directly activates receptors.) A beta$_1$-adrenergic antagonist is a drug that blocks the effect of beta$_1$-adrenergic activation. (An **antagonist** or **blocker** is a drug that prevents receptor activation.) A muscarinic agonist activates the muscarinic receptor, while a muscarinic antagonist blocks muscarinic receptor activation. The same terminology (agonist/antagonist) is applied to drugs that interact with the nicotinic receptors.

Using the autonomic receptor terminology and the information in the tables, let's see if you can figure out some autonomic physiology and pharmacology.

- Question 1. Mr. T was admitted to the ER experiencing respiratory distress caused by asthma. Why was he given a beta$_2$-adrenergic agonist (albuterol)? Check Table 12-4 for the respiratory effects of beta$_2$-adrenergic activation. Answer. Activation of the beta$_2$-adrenergic receptors on the bronchioles (airways) causes the airways to dilate (open up), thereby improving the flow of air and relieving the respiratory distress of asthma.
- Question 2. A very anxious Mr. Q was admitted with a rapid heart rate. Why was he given a beta$_1$-adrenergic blocker (propranolol)? Check Table 12-4 for the cardiac (heart) effects of beta$_1$-adrenergic response. Answer. Mr. Q's heart rate was elevated because of excess sympathetic stimulation (an anxiety effect). A beta$_1$-adrenergic blocker prevents activation of the beta$_1$-adrenergic receptors on the heart, thereby reducing heart rate.
- Question 3. A patient has had a heart attack and is experiencing a very slow heart rate caused by excessive parasympathetic (vagal) activity. Why was he given a muscarinic antagonist (atropine)? Check Table 12-3 for the effects of muscarinic activation on heart rate. Answer. Muscarinic activation (caused by excess parasympathetic activity) slows heart rate. By blocking muscarinic receptors with atropine, heart rate increases.
- Question 4. Ms. S is diagnosed with hypertension (high blood pressure). Why did her physician prescribe an alpha$_1$ adrenergic blocker? Check Table 12-4 for the effect of an alpha$_1$ adrenergic response on blood vessels. Answer. The alpha$_1$ adrenergic blocker blocks the alpha$_1$ receptors in the blood vessels causing them to dilate. Blood vessel dilation decreases blood pressure.
- Question 5. A postoperative patient is unable to urinate because of the anticholinergic drugs used during the perioperative period. Why was she given a muscarinic agonist such as bethanechol? Answer. Activation of the muscarinic receptors stimulates contraction of the urinary bladder and

relaxation of the bladder sphincter. Both actions facilitate urination.

- Question 6. A patient goes to his eye doctor for an eye exam. Why did the physician put anticholinergic eyedrops in his eyes? Answer. Activation of the muscarinic receptor on the pupillary muscles causes pupillary constriction. By using anticholinergic (antimuscarinic) eyedrops, the muscarinic receptors are blocked, and the pupil dilates. The dilated pupils facilitate the eye exam.

This is how you analyze autonomic function and "do" autonomic pharmacology. Learn the receptors and the consequences of receptor activation (agonist) and blockade (antagonist).

Sum It Up!

The neurotransmitters, ACh and NE, bind to receptors. There are two types of autonomic receptors: cholinergic and adrenergic. Cholinergic receptors are activated by ACh. There are two types of cholinergic receptors, muscarinic and nicotinic. The muscarinic receptors are located on the target organs of the parasympathetic nerves. The adrenergic receptors are activated by NE. There are two types of adrenergic receptors, alpha and beta adrenergic receptors. The adrenergic receptors are located on the target organs of the sympathetic nervous system.

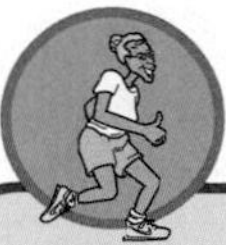

As You Age

1. Aging causes an increase in synaptic delay and a 5% to 10% decrease in the speed of nerve conduction. Consequently, nervous reflexes slow.
2. Aging causes a loss of the sense of vibration at the ankle after the age of 65. This change is accompanied by a decrease of the ankle-jerk reflex and may affect balance, increasing the chance of falling.
3. An aging autonomic nervous system causes many changes. For instance, a less efficient sympathetic nervous system may cause transient hypotension and fainting. A decreased responsiveness of the baroreceptor reflex contributes to the fainting episodes.
4. Decreased autonomic nerve activity supplying the eyes causes changes in pupil size and pupillary reactivity. There is some decline in function of the cranial nerves mediating taste and smell.

Disorders of the Spinal Cord and Peripheral Nerves

Multiple sclerosis	A progressive demyelination of the neurons and destruction of the oligodendrocytes. This degeneration impairs sensory and motor activity.
Peripheral neuropathy	Loss of sensation due to nerve damage. The loss is most severe in the hands and feet. Neuropathy can be caused by a number of conditions, but diabetes mellitus is a common cause.
Poliomyelitis	A contagious infection that affects the brain and the spinal cord. Specifically, the polio virus destroys the lower motor neurons in the brain stem and the spinal cord. As motor neurons are destroyed, paralysis occurs.
Sciatica	A form of neuritis characterized by sharp pains along the sciatic nerve and its branches. Pain usually radiates from the buttocks into the hip and thigh areas.
Shingles	Also called herpes zoster. Shingles is an acute inflammation of the dorsal root ganglia. Shingles develops when the dormant virus that caused childhood chickenpox is reactivated and attacks the root ganglia. Pain and rash progress along the course of one or more spinal nerves, usually the intercostal nerves (sometimes the trigeminal nerve). Painful lesions eventually develop along the affected nerves.
Spina bifida	A congenital defect in the wall of the spinal cavity. Spina bifida is generally accompanied by a meningocele (protrusion of meninges) or myelomeningocele (protrusion of the spinal cord and meninges).
Spinal cord injury	Any condition or event that damages the neurons of the spinal cord. Complete transection of the cord produces quadriplegia or paraplegia, depending on the level of injury. Immediately after the injury, the person experiences spinal shock that may last from several hours to several weeks.

SUMMARY OUTLINE

I. Autonomic or Visceral Reflexes
- A. What They Do: Autonomic nerves reflexly regulate organ function
- B. Pathway: The sequence is receptor activation, sensory input (→ CNS), motor neuron response, and effector response

II. Organization and Function of the Autonomic Nervous System
- A. Divisions of the ANS: There are two divisions.
  1. Sympathetic nervous system, called "Fight or Flight."
  2. Parasympathetic Nervous System, called "Feed and Breed."
- B. Autonomic Terminology and Autonomic Pharmacology
  1. Drugs that affect the sympathetic nervous system are called sympathomimetic and sympatholytic.
  2. Drugs that affect the parasympathetic nervous system are called parasympathomimetic and parasympatholytic.
- C. Autonomic Tone and Vasomotor Tone
  1. Background firing of the ANS causes autonomic tone.
  2. Background sympathetic stimulation of the blood vessels causes vasomotor tone.

III. ANS: Neurons
- A. Numbers and Ganglia
  1. Preganglionic fibers are fibers that extend from the CNS to the ganglia.
  2. Postganglionic fibers are fibers that extend from the ganglia to the effector organ.
- B. Neurons of the Sympathetic Nervous System
  1. The SNS is called the thoracolumbar outflow.
  2. The sympathetic ganglia are located in a chain close to the spinal cord; the chain is called paravertebral ganglia.
  3. The adrenal medulla secretes hormones that mimic the SNS.
- C. Neurons of the Parasympathetic Nervous System
  1. The parasympathetic nervous system is called the craniosacral outflow.
  2. Parasympathetic fibers travel with cranial nerves; most parasympathetics run with the vagus nerve CN X.
- D. Naming Fibers and Neurotransmitters
  1. Cholinergic fibers secrete acetylcholine (ACh).
  2. Adrenergic fibers secrete norepinephrine (NE).
- E. Neurotransmitters: Termination of Activity
  1. ACh is degraded immediately by acetylcholinesterase.
  2. NE activity is ended primarily by reuptake of the NE into the nerve terminal and by MAO activity within the nerve terminal.

IV. Receptors of the Autonomic Nervous System
- A. Cholinergic Receptors
  1. These are activated by ACh.
  2. There are two types: muscarinic and nicotinic (with subtypes).
- B. Adrenergic Receptors
  1. Activated by NE.
  2. There are two types: alpha and beta (with subtypes).
- C. Receptor activation and blockade can be determined by examining Tables 12-1, 12-3, and 12-4.
- D. Autonomic Receptors: "Doing Autonomic Pharmacology"
  1. Clinical examples where drugs target autonomic receptors.

Review Your Knowledge

Matching: Sympathetic or Parasympathetic

Directions: Indicate if the following statements describe the sympathetic nervous system (S) or the parasympathetic nervous system (P).

1. ____ Paravertebral ganglia
2. ____ Feed and breed function
3. ____ Thoracolumbar outflow
4. ____ Postganglionic fiber is adrenergic
5. ____ The target organs are stimulated by norepinephrine (NE)
6. ____ "Fight or flight" function
7. ____ The postganglionic fiber is cholinergic
8. ____ The target organs are stimulated by acetylcholine (ACh)
9. ____ Craniosacral outflow
10. ____ The effects of this system are more widespread and prolonged

Matching: Norepinephrine or Acetylcholine

Directions: Indicate if the statements are descriptive of norepinephrine (NE) or acetylcholine (ACh).

1. ____ Secreted by adrenergic fibers
2. ____ Causes activation of alpha adrenergic receptors
3. ____ Secreted by the postganglionic fibers of the parasympathetic nervous system
4. ____ Causes activation of muscarinic receptors
5. ____ Action is terminated by acetylcholinesterase, an enzyme located within the synapse
6. ____ Action is terminated by reuptake of the neurotransmitter and MAO
7. ____ Causes activation of beta adrenergic receptors
8. ____ Causes activation of nicotinic receptors, including the N_M receptors in the neuromuscular junction of skeletal muscle
9. ____ Mediates "fight or flight" (postganglionic)
10. ____ Mediates "feed and breed"

Multiple Choice

1. Which of the following is least related to the sympathetic nervous system?
   a. Includes the paravertebral ganglia
   b. Is also called the "fight or flight" response
   c. Is also called craniosacral outflow
   d. Uses norepinephrine as a transmitter
2. Which of the following is most related to the parasympathetic nervous system?
   a. Uses norepinephrine as a postganglionic transmitter
   b. Mediates feed and breed activities
   c. Is also called the "fight or flight" response
   d. The postganglionic fiber is adrenergic
3. What is the role of monoamine oxidase (MAO)?
   a. Destroys norepinephrine
   b. Activates the muscarinic receptors
   c. Activates the $beta_1$ adrenergic receptors
   d. Inactivates acetylcholine
4. Activation of the $beta_2$ adrenergic receptors
   a. is a response to the binding of ACh.
   b. causes wheezing.
   c. dilates the breathing passages.
   d. slows the heart rate.
5. Activation of the muscarinic receptors
   a. dilates the breathing passages.
   b. slows heart rate.
   c. dilates the pupil.
   d. is a response to norepinephrine.

CHAPTER 13

Sensory System

KEY TERMS

Chemoreceptor, p. 216
Cochlea, p. 233
Cornea, p. 223
Equilibrium, p. 233
Eustachian tube, p. 232
Mechanoreceptor, p. 216
Olfactory receptor, p. 220
Optic chiasm, p. 229
Ossicles, p. 232
Pain receptor, p. 216
Photoreceptor, p. 216
Proprioception, p. 220
Referred pain, p. 219
Refraction, p. 227
Retina, p. 225
Sclera, p. 223
Thermoreceptor, p. 216
Vestibule, p. 234

OBJECTIVES

1. State the functions of the sensory system.
2. Define the five types of sensory receptors.
3. Describe the four components involved in the perception of a sensation.
4. Describe the five general senses.
5. Describe the five special senses.
6. Describe the structure of the eye.
7. Explain the movement of the eyes.
8. Describe how the size of the pupils changes.
9. Describe the three divisions of the ear.
10. Describe the functions of the parts of the ear involved in hearing.
11. Explain the role of the ear in maintaining the body's equilibrium.

The sensory system allows us to experience the world. Senses let you see the trees, hear the voices of your friends and family, feel the heat of the sun, and taste your favorite foods. When the environment becomes threatening, the sensory system also acts as a warning system. For instance, if you place your hand on a hot surface, the sensory system experiences the episode as pain. The pain is a danger signal indicating that the body must make an adjustment to remove the harmful stimulus.

In addition to sensing outside information, the sensory system also allows us to keep track of what is happening within our bodies. For instance, when the stomach fills with food, sensory information is carried to the central nervous system (CNS). In response to this information, the stomach is told to digest the food.

RECEPTORS AND SENSATION

CELLS THAT DETECT STIMULI

Sensory neurons transmit information to the CNS (Table 13-1). A **receptor** is a specialized area of a sensory neuron that detects a specific stimulus. For instance, the receptors in the eye respond to light, whereas the receptors on the tongue respond to chemicals in food. The five types of sensory receptors are as follows:

- **Chemoreceptors** (KĒ-mō-rĕ-SĔP-tŏr): receptors stimulated by changes in the chemicals such as H^+, calcium, and food
- **Pain receptors** or **nociceptors:** receptors stimulated by tissue damage or distension
- **Thermoreceptors:** receptors stimulated by changes in temperature
- **Mechanoreceptors** (mĕ-KĂN-ō-rĕ-SĔP-tŏr): receptors stimulated by changes in pressure or movements of body fluids
- **Photoreceptors:** receptors stimulated by light

WHAT SENSATION IS

A **sensation** is the conscious awareness of incoming sensory information. "Ouch," for example, indicates that you have become aware of a painful stimulus.

EXPERIENCING A SENSATION

Four Components

Four components are involved in the perception of a sensation. Using the sense of sight as an example, these four components are illustrated in Figure 13-1 and described as follows:

- **Stimulus:** Light is the stimulus for the sense of sight. In the absence of light, you cannot see.
- **Receptor:** Light waves stimulate the photoreceptors in the eye, producing a nerve impulse.
- **Sensory nerve:** The nerve impulse is conducted by a sensory nerve to the occipital lobe of the brain.
- **Special area of the brain:** The sensory information is interpreted as sight in the occipital lobe of the brain. This is an important point; the sensation is experienced by the brain and not by the sensory receptor. For instance, you see an object, hear a voice, or feel pain because the sensory information has stimulated a part of the brain.

As you study each sensation, identify the stimulus, type of receptor, name of the sensory nerve, and specific area of the brain that interprets the sensation.

Two Characteristics of Sensation

Two important characteristics of sensation are projection and adaptation. **Projection** describes the process by which the brain, after receiving a sensation, refers that sensation back to its source. You see with your eyes, hear with your ears, and feel pain in your injured finger because the cortex of your brain receives the sensation and projects it back to its source. Projection answers the question, "If pain is experienced by the brain, why does my injured finger hurt?" (Figure 13-2, *A*).

The experience of "phantom limb" pain is another example of projection. If a leg is amputated, the person may still feel pain in the amputated leg (see Figure 13-2, *B*). The missing leg often throbs with pain. What is the cause of phantom limb sensation? The severed nerve endings of the amputated leg continue to send sensory information to the parietal lobe of the brain. The brain interprets the information as pain and projects the feeling back to the leg area. For most amputees the phantom limb pain diminishes as the severed nerves

Table 13-1 Types of Sensory Receptors

Receptor	Stimulus	Example
Chemoreceptors	Changes in chemical concentrations of substances	Taste and smell
Pain receptors (nociceptors)	Tissue damage	Pain
Thermoreceptors	Changes in temperature	Heat and cold
Mechanoreceptors	Changes in pressure or movement of fluids	Hearing and equilibrium
Photoreceptors	Light energy	Sight

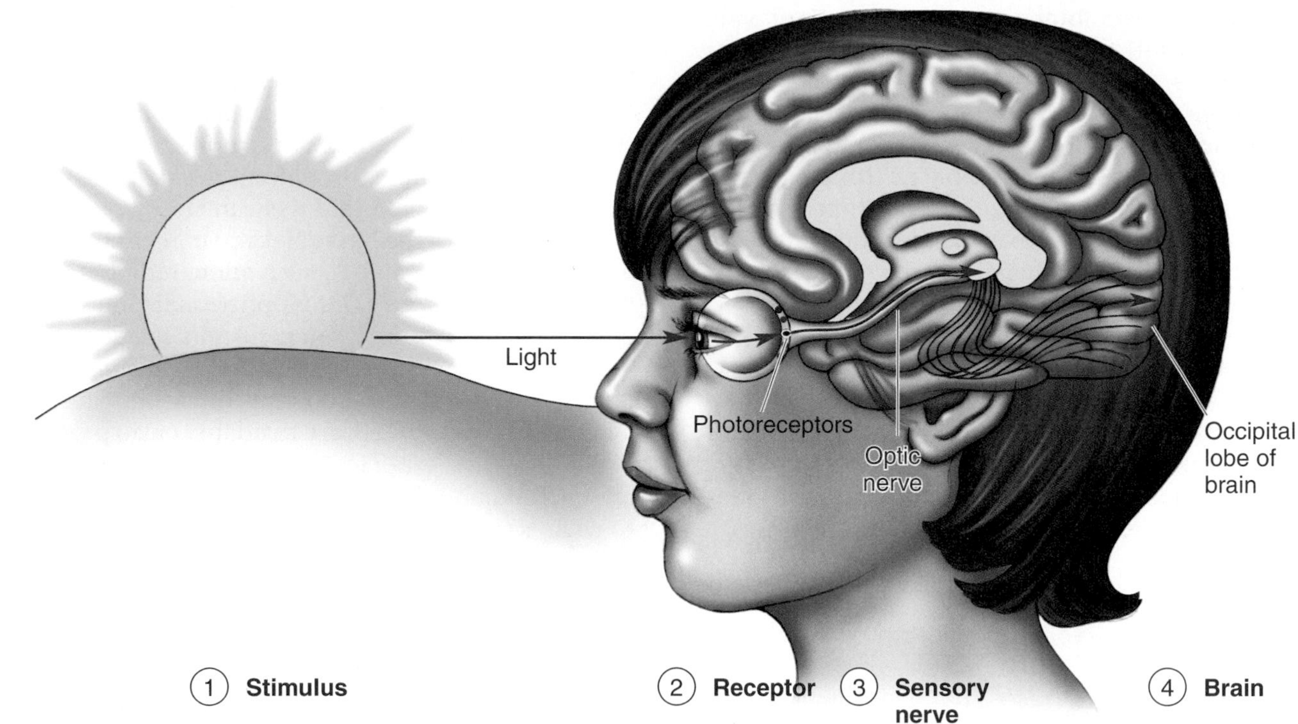

FIGURE 13-1 Four components of sensation.

heal, but the person often experiences a phantom limb presence. The leg still feels as though it is attached. There is some good news about phantom limb pain: the sensation often "locates" the amputated limb and helps a patient learn to use an artificial limb.

Sensory **adaptation** is another characteristic of sensation. It is illustrated by the sense of smell. When you enter a room with a strong odor, the odor at first seems overwhelming. After a short period, however, the odor becomes less noticeable. The sensory receptors in the nose have adapted. When continuously stimulated, these receptors send fewer signals to the area of the brain that interprets sensory information as smell.

Receptors vary in their ability to adapt. Pain receptors do not adapt, whereas receptors for pressure and touch adapt rapidly. Receptors that determine body

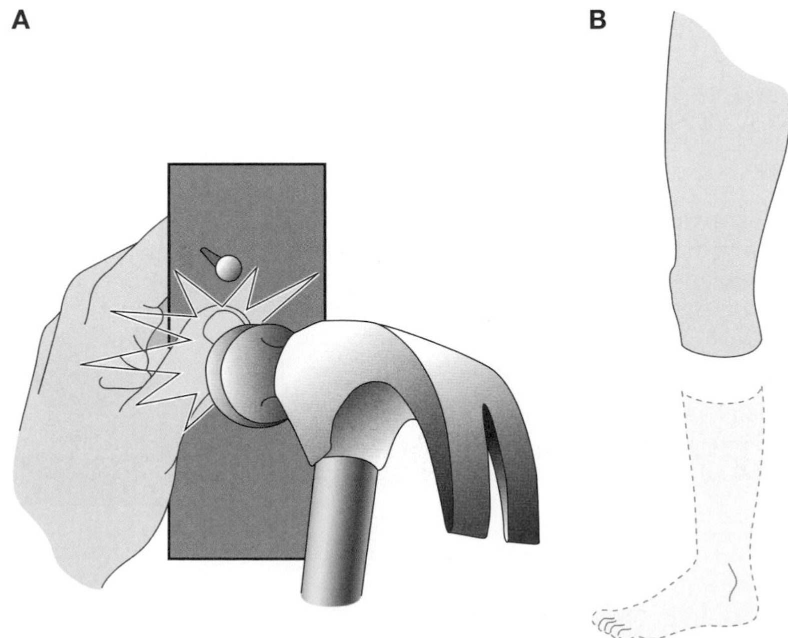

FIGURE 13-2 **A,** Projection ... ouch! **B,** Phantom limb. The dashed line represents the amputated part.

position and detect blood chemistries adapt very slowly because they are important in maintaining homeostasis.

Two groups of senses are general and special senses. **General senses** are called general, or somatic, because their receptors are widely distributed throughout the body. The **special senses** are localized within a particular organ in the head. The special senses include taste, smell, sight, hearing, and balance.

THE GENERAL SENSES

General senses include pain, touch, pressure, temperature, and proprioception (Figure 13-3). Receptors for the general senses are widely distributed and are found in the skin, muscles, joints, and viscera.

PAIN

The receptors for pain (nociceptors) consist of free nerve endings that are stimulated by tissue damage. Pain receptors do not adapt and may continue to send signals after the stimulus is removed. Pain receptors are widely distributed throughout the skin, the visceral organs, and other internal tissues. Oddly enough, the nervous tissue of the brain lacks pain receptors. There is no pain in the brain. Tissues surrounding the brain, like the meninges and the blood vessels, however, do contain pain receptors. You can feel a headache.

Pain serves a protective function. Being unpleasant, pain motivates the person to remove its cause. The failure of the pain receptors to adapt is also protective. For instance, if a person is admitted to the ER with abdominal pain, the pain is used as a valuable clue as to what is wrong. Once the diagnosis is made, then the

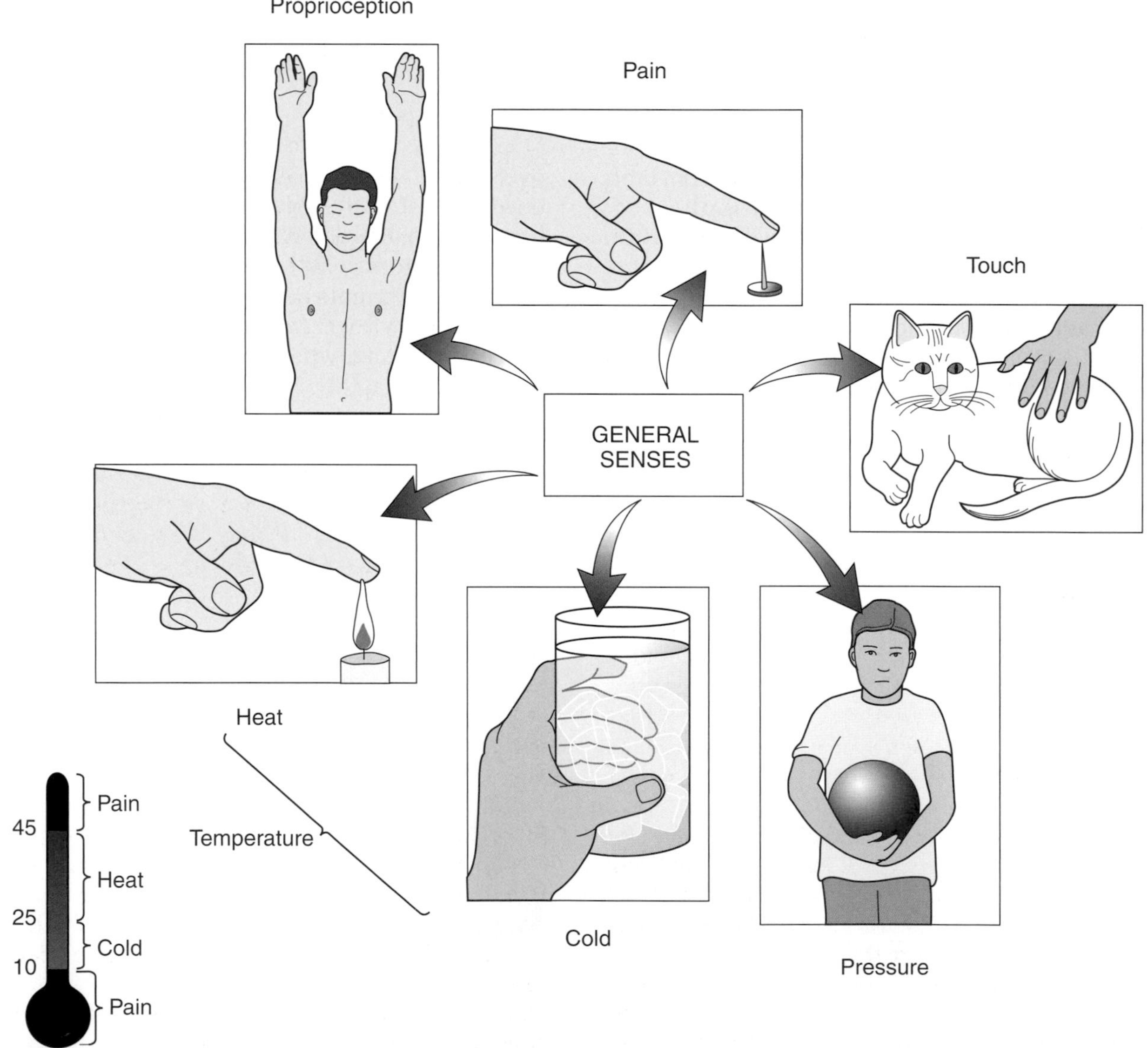

FIGURE 13-3 General senses.

pain is treated. Although unpleasant and undesirable, pain serves the body well.

Some patients are at risk because of a diminishment in the sensation of pain. Patients with diabetes mellitus, for instance, often develop nerve damage in their legs and feet; the nerve damage is called diabetic neuropathy. Patients with neuropathy may develop blisters on their feet because of poorly fitting shoes. Because they cannot feel the pain, the blister is ignored. The injured site continues to expand and eventually becomes infected and gangrenous, necessitating amputation. This is a common experience among diabetic persons and is the reason for meticulous attention to foot care.

What stimulates the pain receptors? The specific signals that stimulate pain are not well understood. Three pain triggers have been identified. First, tissue injury promotes the release of certain chemicals that stimulate pain receptors. Second, a deficiency of oxygen stimulates pain receptors. For instance, if the blood supply to a visceral organ is diminished (a condition called ischemia), the tissue is deprived of oxygen, and the person experiences pain. The pain of a heart attack is due in part to the oxygen deprivation experienced by the cardiac muscle. The administration of oxygen helps to relieve pain. Third, pain may be experienced when tissues are stretched or deformed. It appears that the stimulus is mechanical (distention, distortion) rather than chemical. For instance, if the intestine becomes distended, the person will often experience a severe cramping pain.

Why is pain originating in the heart often experienced in the shoulder and left arm? When pain feels as if it is coming from an area other than the site where it originates, it is called **referred pain** (Figure 13-4). Patients with heart disease often complain of pain or an aching sensation that starts in the shoulder region and moves down the left arm into the fourth and fifth fingers. In other words, stimulation of pain receptors in the heart causes pain that is experienced as being outside the heart.

What is the explanation for referred pain? The occurrence of referred pain is due to shared sensory nerve pathways. The nerve pathways that carry information from the heart are the same pathways that carry information from the shoulder and left arm. As a result, the brain interprets heart pain as shoulder and arm pain.

Once the pain receptors are stimulated, where does the information go? Pain impulses for most of the body travel up the spinal cord in a sensory nerve tract called the spinothalamic tract. The information is then transmitted to the thalamus, where the person first becomes aware of the pain, and then to the cerebral cortex of the parietal lobe. The cerebral cortex can identify the source of the pain and judge its intensity and other characteristics. In other words, the parietal lobe will determine the origin of pain and if the pain is sharp or dull, deep or superficial.

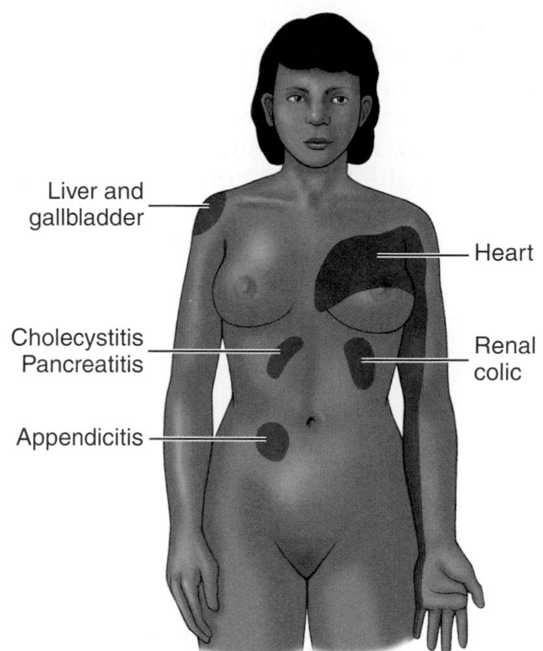

FIGURE 13-4 Sites of referred pain.

There are many types and intensities of pain, and you will spend much time trying to relieve pain. Drugs called **analgesics,** including aspirin, acetaminophen, ibuprofen, and opioids (morphine), can relieve pain. Pain is such a huge clinical problem that clinics have been designed to specifically manage pain.

TOUCH AND PRESSURE

The receptors for touch and pressure are mechanoreceptors; they respond to forces that press, move, or deform tissue. Touch receptors are also called **tactile receptors** and are found mostly in the skin; they are what allows us to feel a cat's soft fur (see Figure 13-3). They are particularly numerous in the lips and the tips of the fingers, toes, tongue, penis, and clitoris. Receptors for heavy pressure are located in the skin, subcutaneous tissue, and the deep tissue. Pressure receptors are stimulated by the heavy ball in the boy's arms in Figure 13-3.

Touch is the first sensory system to develop in the fetus and is essential to its growth and development. Simply stated, if an infant is not touched, it does not thrive and will likely die. An appreciation of touch in the health of a preterm infant forms the basis of kangaroo care (KC). The tiny, diaper-clad infant is placed in the blouse or shirt of its parent. The warmth and physical contact with the parent causes many neurobiological changes that calm the infant, stabilize its temperature, and improve feeding. Touch is life sustaining!

TEMPERATURE

The two types of thermoreceptors are heat and cold receptors. Thermoreceptors are found in free nerve endings, as well as in other specialized sensory cells beneath the skin, and are scattered widely throughout the body. Note the temperature scale in Figure 13-3. The **cold receptors** are stimulated at between 10° C (50° F) and 25° C (76° F). **Heat receptors** are stimulated between 25° C (76° F) and 45° C (112° F). At both ends (extremes) of the temperature scale, pain receptors are stimulated, producing either a freezing or burning sensation. Both heat and cold thermoreceptors display adaptation so that the sensation of heat or cold fades rapidly.

Immerse your hand in warm water and note how quickly the feeling of warmth disappears, even though the temperature of the water has not decreased. Your heat receptors have adapted. Remember that pain receptors do not adapt. If you place your hand in boiling water, you will feel intense continuous pain. Sensory information regarding temperature is sent to the parietal lobe. What about the cooling effects of menthol? Menthol anesthetizes the heat receptors. Thus the only thermoreceptors that can be activated are the cold receptors.

PROPRIOCEPTION

Proprioception (prō-prē-ō-SĔP-shŭn) is the sense of orientation, or position. This sense allows you to locate a body part without looking at it. In other words, if you close your eyes, you can still locate your arm in space; you do not have to see your arm to know that it is raised over your head (see Figure 13-3). Proprioception plays an important role in maintaining posture and coordinating body movement.

The receptors for proprioception, called **proprioreceptors,** are located in muscles, tendons, and joints. Proprioreceptors are also found in the inner ear, where they function in equilibrium. The cerebellum, which plays a major role in coordinating skeletal muscle activity, receives sensory information from these receptors. Sensory information regarding movement and position is also sent to the parietal lobe of the cerebrum.

Sum It Up!

The sensory system is designed to detect information from within and outside the body and to convey that information to the CNS for interpretation. Receptors located on sensory neurons respond to specific stimuli. Senses are classified as either general or special. The general senses include pain, touch, pressure, temperature, and proprioception.

THE SPECIAL SENSES

The five special senses are smell, taste, sight, hearing, and balance (Table 13-2). The receptors of the special senses are located in the head.

SENSE OF SMELL: THE NOSE

The sense of smell, **olfaction,** is associated with sensory structures located in the upper nose (Figure 13-5). These **olfactory** (ŏl-FĂK-tĕr-ē) **receptors** are classified as chemoreceptors, meaning that they are stimulated by chemicals that dissolve in the moisture of the nasal tissue. Once the olfactory receptors have been stimulated, the sensory impulses travel along the olfactory nerve (CN I). The sensory information is eventually interpreted as smell within the olfactory area of the temporal lobe. Olfactory receptors adapt quickly.

What a Smell Can Tell

Some odors (chemicals) also stimulate the pain receptors of the trigeminal nerve (CN V). For instance, since ammonia fumes activate the trigeminal nociceptors, these "smelling salts" quickly and uncomfortably revive a semiconscious person.

Olfactory input to different parts of the brain can trigger visceral and emotional responses. For instance, putrid odors can stimulate the vomiting (emetic) reflex, while an odor associated with childhood memories can trigger a variety of emotions attached to the memories.

Table 13-2 Special Senses

Type of Sense	Organ	Specific Receptor	Stimulus	Receptor
Smell	Nose	Olfactory cell	Changes in chemical concentrations of substances	Chemoreceptor
Taste	Tongue	Gustatory cell	Changes in chemical concentrations of substances	Chemoreceptor
Sight	Eye	Rods and cones	Light energy	Photoreceptor
Hearing	Inner ear: cochlea	Organ of Corti (hair cells)	Movement of fluids	Mechanoreceptor
Balance	Inner ear: vestibular apparatus	Hair cells	Movement of fluids	Mechanoreceptor

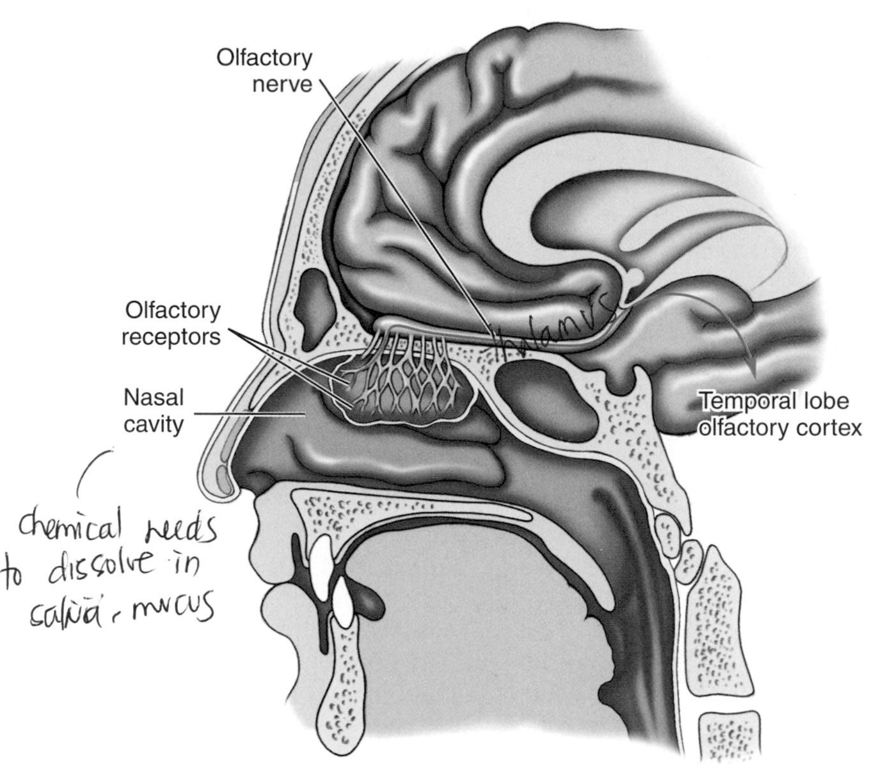

FIGURE 13-5 Sense of smell: olfactory receptors, olfactory nerve, and the temporal lobe of the cerebrum.

Do You Know...

That you can smell your way to better grades?

It is generally agreed that odors are stored in long-term memory; in other words, you don't easily forget odors. The question, then, is since odors are so easily learned, can olfactory cues enhance the learning of other information? According to one investigator, when children were given olfactory (smell) information along with a word list, the list was recalled much more easily and better retained in memory than when given without the olfactory cues. So—smell your way to better grades. How about a scratch-'n-sniff anatomy book!

Food odors, especially when you are hungry, can stimulate the digestive tract secretions, literally getting you to drool.

Some persons experience an olfactory aura, meaning that they smell an odor that is not present. Olfactory auras most often occur prior to seizure activity or to the onset of a migraine headache. The person may "smell" chicken soup, bleach, rotting flesh, or worse. Sometimes the aura is a distortion of an odor. For instance, a person may experience body odor as a smell of beer. These strange "smell events" are sometimes called olfactory hallucinations.

SENSE OF TASTE: THE TONGUE

The sense of taste is also called the **gustatory sense** or **gustation. Taste buds** are the special organs of taste. The taste receptors are located on the tongue and are classified as chemoreceptors, meaning that they are sensitive to the chemicals in our food. The four basic taste sensations are salty, sweet, sour, and bitter. Each sensation is concentrated on a particular area of the tongue, as illustrated in Figure 13-6. The tip of the tongue is most sensitive to sweet and salty substances. Sour sensations are found primarily on the sides of the tongue, while bitter substances are most strongly tasted on the back part of the tongue.

When the taste receptors are stimulated, the taste impulses travel along three cranial nerves (facial, glossopharyngeal, and vagus nerves) to various parts of the brain, eventually arriving in the parietal and temporal lobes of the cerebral cortex. Note that since the taste sensation is carried by three cranial nerves, when assessing cranial nerve function you will be asking the patient to detect specific tastes and stimulating only parts of the tongue. For instance, a person with damage to the facial nerve may experience loss of taste only on the anterior two thirds of the left side of the tongue.

Some Tasteful Comments

- The salty receptors can trigger a "salt craving." For instance, as the blood volume expands during

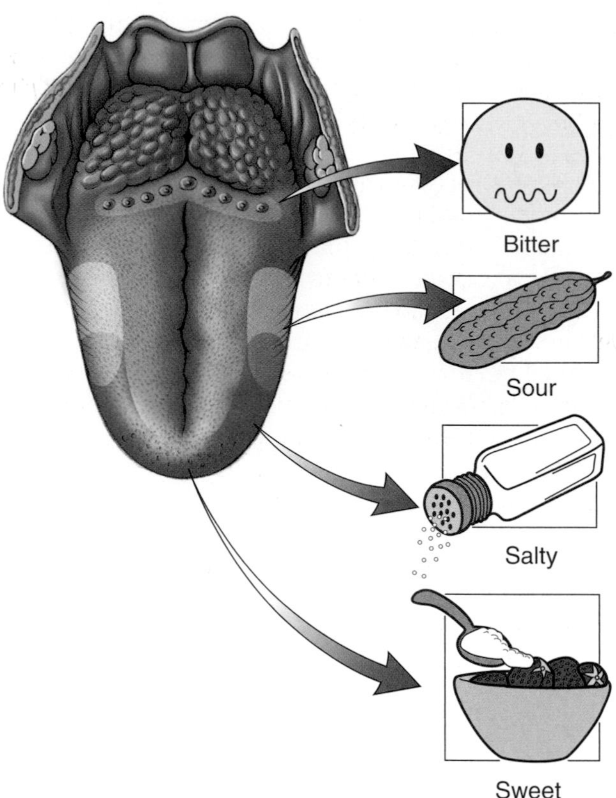

FIGURE 13-6 Sense of taste. Four taste sensations: bitter, sour, salty, and sweet.

pregnancy, the woman's taste buds may sense a decrease of salt in her blood, causing her to increase her intake of salt. Since salt plays a crucial role in blood volume regulation, the "salt craving" performs an important survival role. Ever notice the gathering of deer around a "salt lick"?

- Taste receptors seem especially sensitive to bitter-tasting substances. This sensitivity serves a protective role because the poisonous substances in plants are often bitter.
- Food often tastes differently when you have a cold. The senses of taste and smell are closely related. When interpreted in the cerebral cortex, information from both senses may combine to produce a different taste sensation. Therefore food often tastes different when you have a cold or stuffy nose.
- The sense of taste can be lost or altered. Drugs and radiation used in the treatment of cancer often change or destroy the sensation of taste. Obviously, the loss of taste affects appetite and nutrition.
- Two other tastes have been suggested. A metallic taste has been attributed to the effects of certain drugs. A second taste has been described by a Japanese word, *umami. Umami* means yummy or delicious and refers to a meaty flavor.
- There is also some evidence that the tongue can taste the texture and shape of the food.

SENSE OF SIGHT: THE EYE

The sense of sight (vision) is one of our most cherished senses. Think of all that you see that brings so much joy to your life—the smiles of children, the faces of your friends, and the beautiful colors of the trees and flowers. The eyes are the organs of vision; they contain the visual receptors. Assisting the eyes in their function and protecting them from injury are the visual accessory organs. The study of the eye is called **ophthalmology.**

Visual Accessory Organs

The **visual accessory organs** include the eyebrows, eyelids, conjunctiva, eyelashes, lacrimal apparatus, and extrinsic eye muscles (Figure 13-7).

Eyebrows. The **eyebrows,** patches of hair located above the eyes, perform a protective role. They keep perspiration out of the eyes and shade the eyes from glaring sunlight. Eyebrows also participate in facial expression, as in the "raised eyebrow" look.

Eyelids. The **eyelids,** or **palpebrae,** protect the eyes. They prevent the entrance of foreign objects; the eyelids also wash tears over the surface of the eye. The upper and lower eyelids meet at the corners of the eyes. The corners are called the **medial (inner) canthus** and **lateral (outer) canthus.** The eyelids are composed of four layers: skin, skeletal muscle (orbicularis oculi), connective tissue, and an inner lining called the conjunctiva. The margin of the eyelids contain tarsal glands that secrete an oil that coats the surface of the eye and reduces evaporation of the tears. Skeletal muscles open and close the eyelids. The **levator palbebrae superioris** muscle (*levator* means to raise, like an elevator)

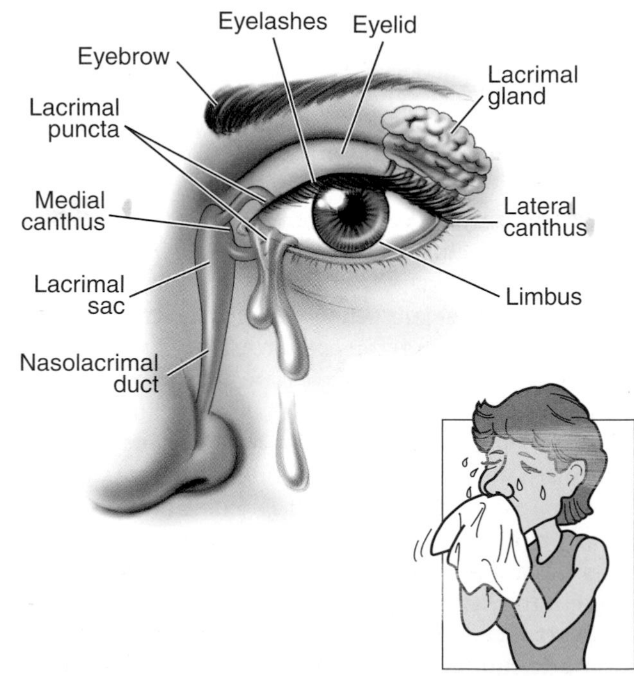

FIGURE 13-7 Visual accessory organs.

is attached to the eyelid and the upper bony orbit; contraction of the muscle opens the eye. Contraction of the **orbicularis oculi** muscle closes it.

Look in the mirror. Lid levels matter. Your eyelid normally covers a small part of the iris (colored part of your eye); it should not cover the pupil (hole). Sometimes a patient is unable to lift the eyelid completely and the person has a sleepy look. This condition is called ptosis of the eyelid. The upper eyelid of a person with an overactive thyroid may appear to be pulled up too high, thereby exposing the white sclera above the iris. This is called lid lag. Thus the eyelids often provide diagnostic clues to underlying diseases or disorders. As long as you are looking in the mirror, pull down your lower lid and note its inner lining; it forms a sac (called the conjunctival sac). Eyedrops are temporarily held in this sac until the blinking eyelids wash the medication over the surface of the eye.

Conjunctiva. The **conjunctiva** is a thin mucous membrane that lines the inner surface of the eyelid. The conjunctiva also folds back to cover a portion of the sclera on the anterior surface of the eyeball; this part of the sclera is called the white of the eye. The conjunctiva does not cover the cornea. The conjunctiva secretes a substance that moistens the surface of the eye. The anterior surface of the eye must be kept moist, otherwise it will ulcerate and scar. (Figure 13-7 identifies the limbus, the meeting place of the white of the eye with the cornea that overlies the colored iris.)

The conjunctiva is very vascular, meaning that it has many blood vessels. Evidence of its rich vascularity is the "bloodshot" appearance when the blood vessels are dilated. Eyedrops that claim to "get the red out" cause the blood vessels of the conjunctiva to constrict, thereby decreasing the amount of blood. "Pink eye," also associated with dilated blood vessels, is a highly contagious bacterial conjunctivitis (or inflammation of the conjunctiva). It is commonly seen among groups of children for whom it is difficult to maintain good hygienic conditions. Conjunctivitis can also be caused by irritation and allergies.

Eyelashes. Eyelashes line the edges of the eyelid and help trap dust. Touching the eyelashes stimulates blinking—a mascara challenge! Interestingly, the camel has three eyelids and two layers of eyelashes in order to deal with its sandy environment. Imagine how long it would take to get out of the house with so many lids and lashes to paint!

Occasionally, a hair follicle at the edge of the lid becomes infected, usually by *Staphylococcus.* This infection is called a sty, or hordeolum; it is red, swollen, and painful.

Lacrimal Apparatus. The **lacrimal apparatus** is composed of the lacrimal gland and a series of ducts called tear ducts (see Figure 13-7). The **lacrimal gland** is located in the upper lateral part of the orbit. The lacrimal gland secretes tears, which flow across the surface of the eye toward the nose. The tears drain through small openings called **lacrimal puncta** and then into the **lacrimal sac** and **nasolacrimal ducts.** The nasolacrimal ducts eventually empty into the nasal cavity. Normally tears flow to the back of the throat and are swallowed. If the secretion of tears increases, as in crying, the nose begins to run. The excess tears may overwhelm the drainage system and spill onto the cheeks. The nasolacrimal ducts can become swollen and close when a person has a cold. The tears cannot drain and thus spill out onto the cheeks.

Tears perform several important functions. They moisten, lubricate, and cleanse the surface of the eye. Tears also contain an enzyme called **lysozyme,** which helps destroy and prevents infection. Blinking stimulates lacrimation and helps spread the tears over the surface of the eye. Routine use of eyewashes may do more harm than good by washing away natural antibacterial secretions.

Extrinsic Eye Muscles. Extrinsic eye muscles also function as visual accessory organs (see Muscles of the Eye later in this chapter).

The Eyeball

The **eyeball** has a spherical shape and is approximately ¾ to 1 inch (2 to 3 cm) in diameter (Figure 13-8, *A*). Most of the eyeball sits within the bony orbital cavity of the skull, partially surrounded by a layer of orbital fat. Thus the eyeball is well protected. The eyeball is composed of three layers: the sclera, the choroid, and the retina.

Sclera. The outermost layer is called the **sclera** (SKLĔ-ră). The sclera is a tough fibrous connective tissue that covers most of the eyeball. The sclera helps contain the contents of the eye; it also shapes the eye and is the site of attachment for the extrinsic eye muscles. The sclera extends toward the front of the eye. The anterior sclera is covered by conjunctiva and is called the white of the eye. A transparent extension of the sclera is called the **cornea** (KŎR-nē-ă). The cornea covers the area over the iris (the colored portion of the eye).

The cornea is avascular (contains no blood vessels) and transparent, meaning that light rays can go through this structure. Because light enters the eye first through the cornea, it is called the window of the eye. The cornea has a rich supply of sensory nerve fibers and is therefore sensitive to touch. If the surface of the cornea is touched lightly, the eye blinks to remove the source of irritation. This response is called the **corneal reflex.** It serves a protective function.

Name the nerves. The corneal reflex involves two cranial nerves. A branch of the trigeminal nerve (CN V) provides sensory fibers to the surface of the cornea. The facial nerve (CN VII) provides motor fibers that result in blinking. Think of how your eye responds to a piece of dust—through blinking, tearing, and pain.

Choroid. The middle layer of the eye is the **choroid.** The choroid layer is highly vascular and is attached to

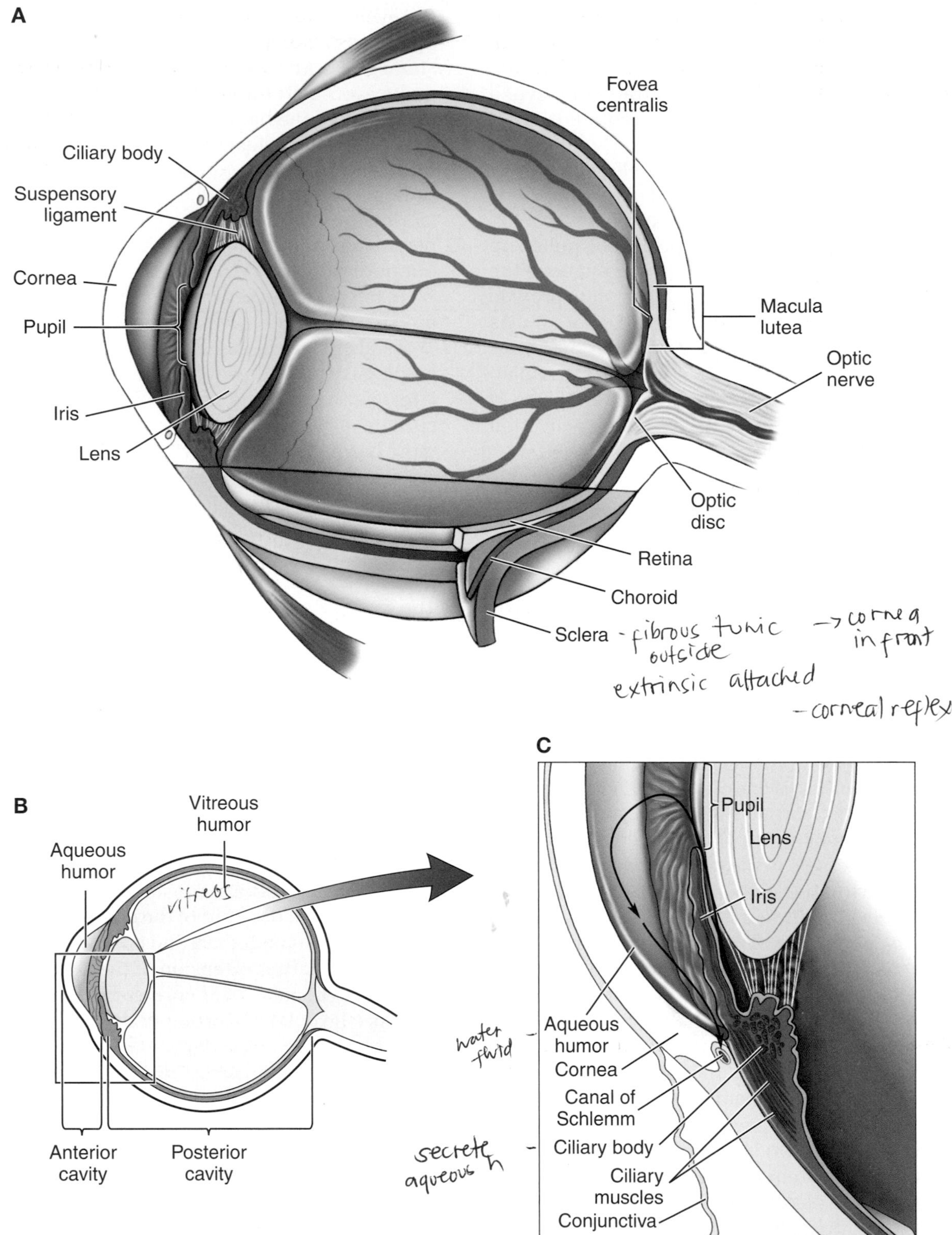

FIGURE 13-8 **A,** Structure of the eyeball. **B,** Cavities and fluids. **C,** Flow of aqueous humor from the ciliary body to the canal of Schlemm *(arrow)*.

the innermost layer, the retina. The choroid performs two functions. First, it provides the retina with a rich supply of blood. Second, dark pigments located in the choroid absorb any excess light to prevent glare.

The choroid extends toward the front of the eyeball to form the ciliary body and the iris. The **ciliary body** secretes a fluid called aqueous humor, and it gives rise to a set of intrinsic eye muscles, called the **ciliary muscles.** The most anterior portion of the choroid is the **iris,** the colored portion of the anterior eye. The song "Beautiful Brown Eyes" is a serenade to the iris.

The opening, or hole, in the middle of the iris is called the **pupil.** The size of the pupil is determined by two sets of intrinsic eye muscles located in the iris. The iris regulates the amount of light entering the eye.

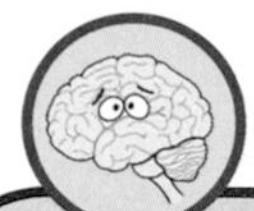

Do You Know...

Why the "beautiful lady" can't see?

A group of drugs, including atropine and scopolamine (muscarinic receptor antagonists), belong to a drug classification called belladonna, or "beautiful lady." Why so beautiful? When belladonna is placed in the eyes of the young lady, the pupils dilate, becoming wide and very seductive. Dilated pupils may indeed be beautiful, but they do not help acute vision. "Beautiful lady" may be beautiful, but she needs an escort because she certainly cannot see.

Today, belladonna drugs are still used, primarily for their mydriatic and cycloplegic effects in eye examinations and surgical procedures. Interestingly, atropine is still used by photographers to create photographs of "beautiful ladies."

Retina. The innermost layer of the eyeball is the **retina** (RĔT-ĭ-nă). It lines the posterior two thirds of the eyeball. The retina is the nervous layer containing the visual receptors, which are sensitive to light and are therefore called photoreceptors. The two kinds of photoreceptors are rods and cones. The **rods** are scattered throughout the retina but are more abundant along its periphery. The **cones** are most abundant in the central portion of the retina. The area of the retina that contains the highest concentration of cones is called the **fovea centralis,** an area in the center of a yellow spot called the **macula lutea** (see Figure 13-8, *A*). Because the fovea centralis contains so many cones, it is considered the area of most acute vision.

A second small circular area of the retina is in the back of the eye. The neurons of the retina converge there to form the optic nerve; it contains no rods or cones. This area is called the **optic disc.** Because there are no photoreceptors on the optic disc, images that focus on this area are not seen. The optic disc is therefore called the **blind spot.**

You can locate your own blind spot. Draw a rectangle with a small X on the left side and a dot on the right. Using only one eye (cover the second eye), look at the X as you move it closer to your eye. At some point you will not be able to see the dot on the right when it focuses on your blind spot.

Another interesting fact about the optic disc! A head-injured person may develop increased intracranial pressure. This increased pressure pushes the optic disc forward. The bulging optic disc seen on ophthalmic examination is described as a choked disc or papilledema. The eyes can provide a wealth of information about a patient with a head injury.

Cavities and Fluids. The two cavities in the eyeball are the posterior and anterior cavities (see Figure 13-8, *B*). The **posterior cavity** is larger and is located between the lens and the retina. The posterior cavity is filled with a gel-like substance called the **vitreous humor.** The vitreous humor gently pushes the retina against the choroid layer, thereby ensuring that the retina receives a good supply of blood.

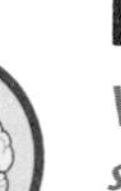

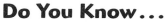

Do You Know...

Why we sometimes see spots in front of our eyes?

The spots are called floaters or muscae volitantes, meaning flying flies. They are either particles or red blood cells that have escaped from the capillaries in the eye. These substances float through the vitreous humor, occasionally getting in our line of vision. The presence of these substances is usually considered normal and harmless. However, the sudden appearance of floaters or an increase in the number of floaters may indicate that a hole has formed in the retina. The development of a retinal tear often precedes retinal detachment and demands immediate professional attention.

The **anterior cavity** is located between the lens and the cornea. The anterior cavity is filled with a watery fluid called **aqueous humor.** Aqueous humor is produced by the ciliary body and circulates through the pupil into the space behind the cornea (see Figure 13-8, *B*). The aqueous humor performs two functions: it maintains the shape of the anterior portion of the eye, and it provides nourishment for the cornea. The aqueous humor leaves the anterior cavity by way of tiny canals located at the junction of the sclera and the cornea. These outlet canals are called **venous sinuses** or the **canals of Schlemm** (see Figure 13-8, *C*).

Drainage of aqueous humor through the canal of Schlemm may become impaired. Consequently, aqueous humor accumulates in the eye and elevates the pressure in the eye. An elevated intraocular pressure is called glaucoma. Glaucoma is serious because the elevated pressure compresses the choroid, thereby choking off the blood supply to the retina. Glaucoma is a leading cause of retinal damage and blindness. Treatment of glaucoma is aimed at decreasing the formation of aqueous humor and improving the drainage of aqueous humor through the canal of Schlemm.

Muscles of the Eye

The two groups of muscles associated with the eye are the extrinsic and intrinsic eye muscles. The **extrinsic eye muscles** move the eyeball in its bony orbit. The **intrinsic eye muscles** move structures within the eyeball.

Extrinsic Eye Muscles. How do you move your eyes? The extrinsic eye muscles are skeletal muscles located outside the eye (Figure 13-9, *A*). Six extrinsic eye muscles attach to the bone of the eye orbit and the sclera, the tough outer connective tissue layer of the eyeball. There are four rectus muscles and two oblique muscles.

The extrinsic eye muscles move the eyeball in various directions. You can move your eyes up, down, and sideways because of the rectus muscles. You can also roll your eyes because of the oblique muscles. The extrinsic eye muscles are innervated by three cranial nerves, the most important being the oculomotor nerve (CN III). Then there is LR_6SO_4, which sounds like a nasty chemical formula. However, it helps you to remember that the lateral rectus muscle is innervated by the abducens (CN VI) while the superior oblique muscle is innervated by the trochlear nerve (CN IV).

Back to the mirror. Note that both eyes move together in a coordinated way; when one eye moves, the other eye moves. In the event of a traumatic injury to an eye you may want to immobilize the injured eye, usually by applying a loose covering over the eye. Because both eyes move in a coordinated way, if you want to immobilize the injured eye you must cover both eyes. Then it is off to the ophthalmologist for treatment.

Occasionally, the eyeballs are not aligned so as to focus on a desired point. This condition is called strabismus (Figure 13-10). If the eye deviates medially toward the nasal side, the eyes look crossed. Hence the term cross-eyed. This condition is called convergent strabismus. Eyes can also deviate laterally so that one eye appears to be looking off to the side. This condition is called divergent strabismus. If uncorrected, strabismus not only presents a serious cosmetic problem but can also lead to loss of vision.

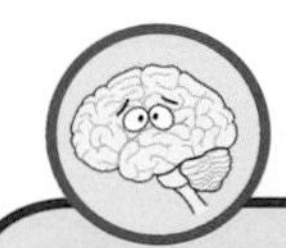

Do You Know...

About lazy eye?

Normally both eyes work together and focus on one object; in response, the brain forms a single image. Sometimes both eyes do not focus on the same object usually because the muscles of one eye are weak (lazy) and therefore unable to move the affected eye into position. The occipital lobe is then presented with different information from each eye. The occipital lobe, however, can't process both signals; it receives information from one eye and suppresses information from the lazy eye. If uncorrected the "lazy" eye will become nonfunctional (blind). Lazy eye is also called suppression amblyopia. It is common and treatable; treatment, however, must begin early.

Intrinsic Eye Muscles. The intrinsic muscles are smooth muscles located in the eyeball, specifically in the iris and the ciliary body. There are three intrinsic eye muscles.

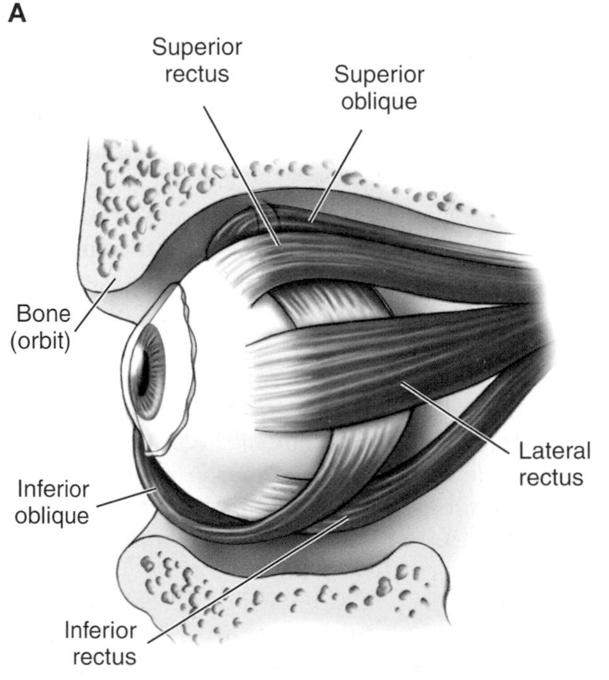

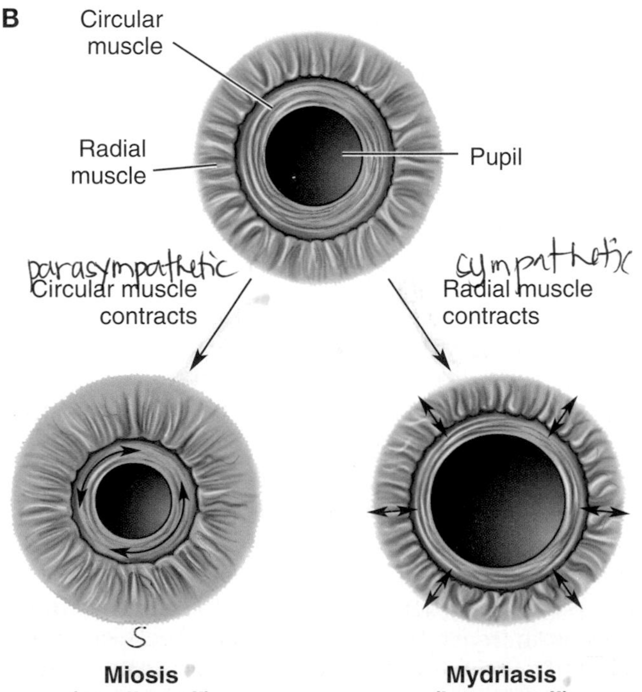

FIGURE 13-9 **A,** Extrinsic muscles: rectus muscles and two oblique muscles (only five are shown). **B,** Intrinsic eye muscles: circular muscle and radial muscle.

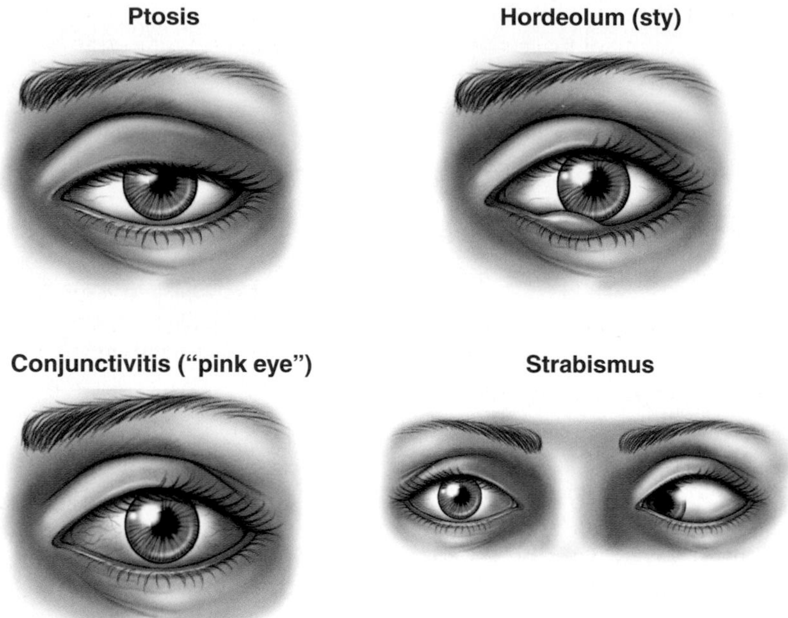

FIGURE 13-10 Conditions of the eye and visual accessory structures.

Muscles of the Iris. The iris contains two eye muscles, the radial muscle and the circular muscle (see Figure 13-9, *B*). These muscles control the size of the pupil and therefore regulate the amount of light that enters the eye. The muscle fibers of the radial muscle are arranged like the spokes of a wheel. Just as the spokes radiate from the center of the wheel, the radial muscle fibers radiate from the area of the pupil. Contraction of the radial muscle causes the pupil to dilate, thereby increasing the amount of light entering the eye. Sympathetic nerve fibers supply the radial muscles. Thus sympathetic nerve stimulation causes pupillary dilation, or **mydriasis.** Drugs that dilate the pupil are called **mydriatic agents.**

The second muscle located in the iris is the circular muscle. Its fibers are arranged in a circular fashion. Contraction of the **circular muscles** causes the pupil to constrict, thereby decreasing the amount of light entering the eye. The circular muscle is supplied by parasympathetic nerve fibers in the oculomotor nerve (CN III). Parasympathetic nerve stimulation causes pupillary constriction, or **miosis** (see Figure 13-9, *B*). Drugs that constrict the pupils are called **miotic agents.** Some drugs, such as opioids (narcotics), constrict the pupils so intensely that the pupils are described as pinpoint. (An easy way to remember the difference between mydriasis and miosis is that the words ***d**ilate* and *my**d**riasis* both contain the letter **d.**)

Photopupillary Reflex. When one eye is exposed to light, the pupil immediately constricts, thereby restricting the amount of light entering the eye. This response is called the **photopupillary reflex.** The pupil of the other eye also constricts even if no light is directed at it. The second eye is said to constrict consensually; it consents to constrict when the photopupillary reflex is stimulated in the opposite eye. Both these effects are assessed when an eye exam is performed.

Who is PERRLA? Pupillary function is evaluated by noting the size, shape, and reactivity to light. PERRLA is an assessment term for pupillary function: Pupils Equal, Round, React to Light, and Accomodation.

Ciliary Muscle. The third intrinsic eye muscle is the ciliary muscle. The **ciliary muscles** arise from the ciliary body. The ciliary muscles attach to the suspensory ligaments which, in turn, tug on the lens, causing the lens to change its shape. Why tug? Read on.

Refraction and Accommodation

For us to see, the light waves must enter the eye and bend so as to focus on the retina. The bending of light waves is called **refraction.**

Let's see how this happens. While the cornea and aqueous humor are all capable of refracting light, the lens can change its shape and its refracting abilities. Refraction by the lens is illustrated in Figure 13-11, *A*. In the top panel, the light waves are shown traveling in a straight line toward the retina. Unless light waves 1 and 3 are bent, they will not focus on point X.

How does the lens bend light waves (Figure 13-11, *B*)? The bottom part of light wave #1 hits the lens first and

A

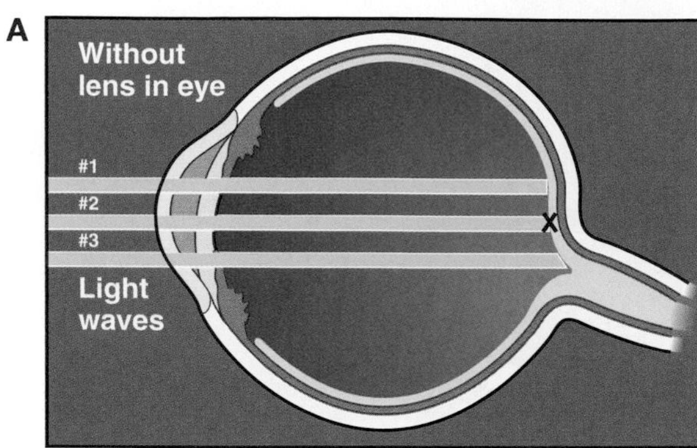

B

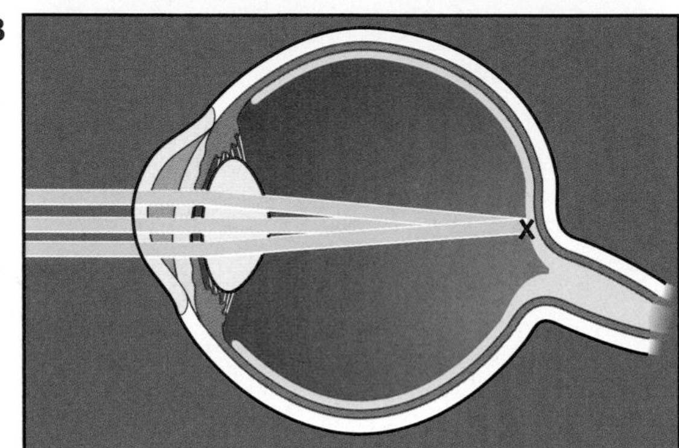

FIGURE 13-11 Refraction. **A,** Path that the light waves travel (without lens). **B,** Refraction of the first and third light waves.

is slowed before penetrating it. The top of the light wave continues to travel until it hits the lens. For a split second, the top of the light wave travels faster than the bottom. The light wave therefore bends. The bottom panel illustrates how the lens bends several light waves. For sharp vision, light waves must be refracted to focus on one particular area of the retina.

Why and how does the lens change its shape? The **lens** can change its shape, becoming fatter or thinner. The lens is an elastic structure held in place by the **suspensory ligaments** attached to **ciliary muscles** (see Figure 13-8, *A*). When the ciliary muscles contract and relax, the tension on the lens causes the changes in the shape of the lens. The lens either flattens out or becomes rounder. The change in shape affects how much the light is bent. For instance, if the lens becomes rounder or fatter, the light wave is bent at a sharper angle. If the lens flattens, the degree of refraction lessens and the light wave is not bent as much.

The ability of the lens to change its shape allows the eye to focus objects close up or at a distance. For instance, if you hold a pencil 6 inches in front of your eyes, you will be able to see it clearly. The focusing of the close-up object (pencil) on the retina is due primarily to the lens. The lens becomes rounder and bends the light waves more acutely so as to focus them on the retina. This ability of the lens to change its shape

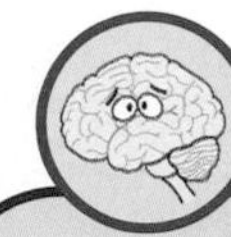

Do You Know...

What is meant by 20/20 vision?

The ability of the eye to focus an image on the retina is assessed by use of the Snellen chart. This chart is composed of lines of letters arranged in decreasing size. The person is placed at a distance 20 feet away from the chart and is asked to cover one eye and read a line of letters. A score of 20/20 means that the person is able to see at 20 feet what a person with normal eye function can see. Thus, 20/20 vision is considered normal. A score of 20/40 means that a person can see at 20 feet what a person with normal vision can see at 40 feet. Thus, 20/40 vision is less perfect than 20/20 vision. A score of 20/200 indicates severely impaired vision, and the person is considered legally blind.

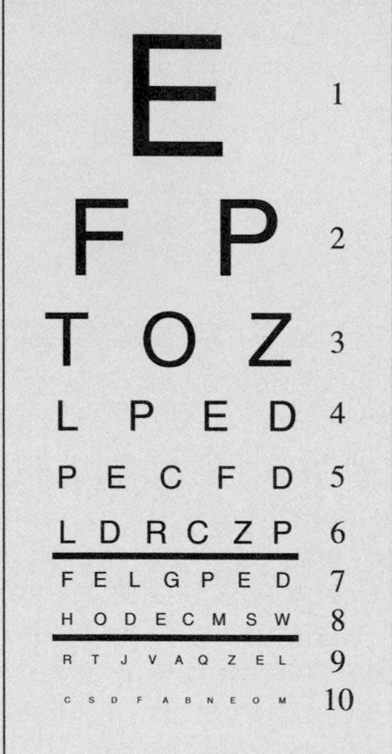

to focus on a close object is called **accommodation.** A professional who assesses the ability of the eyes to refract light is called an **optometrist.** Optometrists prescribe lenses to correct the errors of refraction. (Do not confuse ophthalmologist with optometrist.)

Accommodation is accompanied by pupillary constriction and by **convergence,** the movement of the eyes inward (medially toward the nose). Accommodation, pupillary constriction, and convergence all work together to focus both eyes on one object.

Emmetropia refers to the normal eye; it is the ability of the eye to refract light without the assistance of a corrective lens. With advancing age, the lens loses some of its ability to change shape, thereby diminishing the ability to accommodate for close objects. This condition, which is often evident after age 40, is called presbyopia (*presbyter* means an elderly person). Persons with presbyopia have difficulty adjusting to close objects. Presbyopia accounts for the tendency of older persons to hold the newspaper at arm's length. You may have heard elderly people comment good naturedly on how their arms have shortened with age.

Stimulation of the Photoreceptors

Once the light penetrates the various eye structures, it must stimulate the photoreceptors (rods and cones). Why do you see black and white at night and color during daylight?

Night Vision. The rods are widely scattered throughout the retina but are more abundant in the periphery. Rods are sensitive to dim light and provide us with black and white vision. The image produced by the stimulation of rods is somewhat fuzzy. Because rods respond to dim light, stimulation of rods is often called night vision. A vitamin A–dependent chemical is involved in night vision. Thus a vitamin A deficiency can cause night blindness.

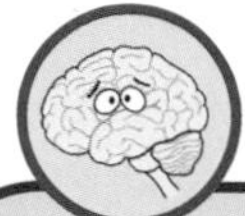

Do You Know...

What night blindness is?

Stimulation of the rods (night vision photoreceptors) by light waves causes the breakdown of a chemical substance called rhodopsin. This breakdown, in turn, stimulates nerve impulses. As nerve impulses are formed, the amount of rhodopsin is used up and must be replaced. The synthesis of additional rhodopsin requires vitamin A. Because night vision depends on an adequate supply of rhodopsin, a deficiency of vitamin A can cause night blindness.

Color Vision. Cones are the photoreceptors for color vision. Cones are most abundant in the central portion of the retina, especially in the macula lutea. The image produced by the stimulation of cones is colored and sharp. There are three types of cones, each with a different visual pigment (a light-sensitive chemical). One type of cone produces a green color, another produces blue, and a third produces red. Stimulation of combinations of these cones produces the many different colors and shades of colors we enjoy.

Informing the Brain: The Visual Pathway

Nerve impulses that arise from the photoreceptors leave the eye by way of the optic nerve (CN II). The nerve impulses travel along the fibers of the optic nerve to the occipital lobe of the brain. This pathway from the eye to the brain is called the **visual pathway.**

Figure 13-12 illustrates the pathways of the optic nerves as each leaves the eye. Note that half of the fibers from the left eye cross over and travel to the right side of the brain, and half of the fibers from the right eye cross over and travel to the left side of the brain. The crossing over of the fibers allows the occipital lobe to integrate the information from both eyes and produce only one image. The point at which the fibers from the left and right eyes crisscross is called the **optic chiasm** (KĪ-azm). The optic chiasm is located directly in front of the pituitary gland. An enlargement of the pituitary gland can therefore cause visual disturbances as the tumor presses on the optic chiasm and interferes with the transmission of the nerve impulse to the occipital lobe.

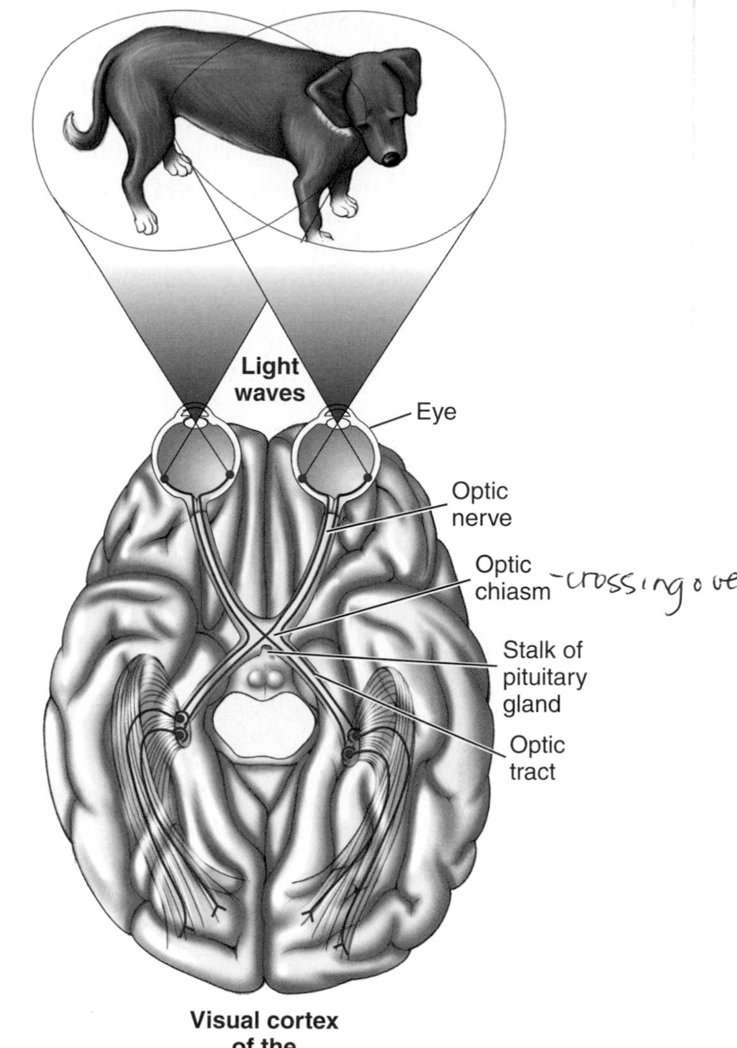

FIGURE 13-12 Visual pathway. Note the optic chiasm and the pituitary gland (behind the optic chiasm).

Seeing Happens When...

When all of the parts of the eye, visual pathway, and brain are working correctly, you can see. Light waves enter your eye, are refracted, and are focused on the photoreceptors of the retina. The photoreceptors translate the light signal to a nerve impulse, which is then transmitted from the retina, along the optic nerve, and finally to the occipital lobe of the brain, where you experience vision.

Seeing Doesn't Happen When...

When the parts of the eye do not work normally, the person may experience diminished vision or blindness. Any defect along this pathway from the cornea to the brain can interfere with vision. Certain conditions may prevent the entrance of light into the eye. For instance, a scarred cornea or a cloudy lens (cataract) may block the entrance of light, thereby preventing the stimulation of the rods and cones. Errors of refraction, such as nearsightedness, farsightedness, and astigmatism, can adversely affect the focusing of light on the retina (Figure 13-13). While these conditions can diminish vision, they are generally treatable. The more serious and often untreatable conditions affect the retina:

- Increased intraocular pressure (glaucoma) may squeeze the blood vessels of the choroid, depriving the retina of an adequate blood supply. The cells of the retina then die and blindness results.
- The photoreceptors of the macula lutea can degenerate, causing macular degeneration and a loss of vision.
- A person with diabetes often experiences severe damage of the retinal blood vessels. The blood vessels develop microaneurysms. The aneurysms rupture, causing bleeding and scar formation throughout the retina. This is called diabetic retinopathy.
- Another type of retinal damage includes a detached retina (the retina falls away from the choroid, its blood supply).
- Certain conditions or injuries can destroy the optic nerve. For instance, a tumor on the optic nerve or at the optic chiasm can interfere with the transmission of the nerve impulse along the nerve to the brain.
- Finally, tumors, blood clots, or trauma can damage the occipital lobe of the brain, causing cortical blindness (a blindness due to the loss of cortical brain tissue).

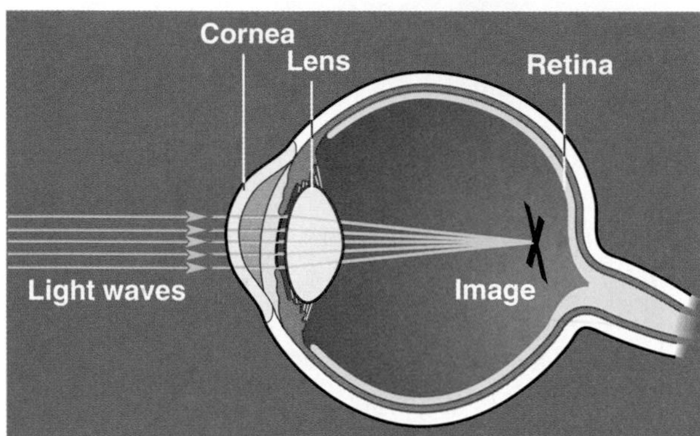

Myopia (nearsightedness)

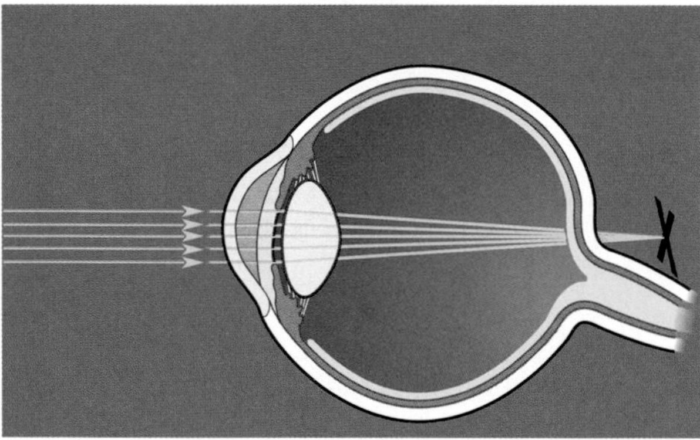

Hyperopia (farsightedness)

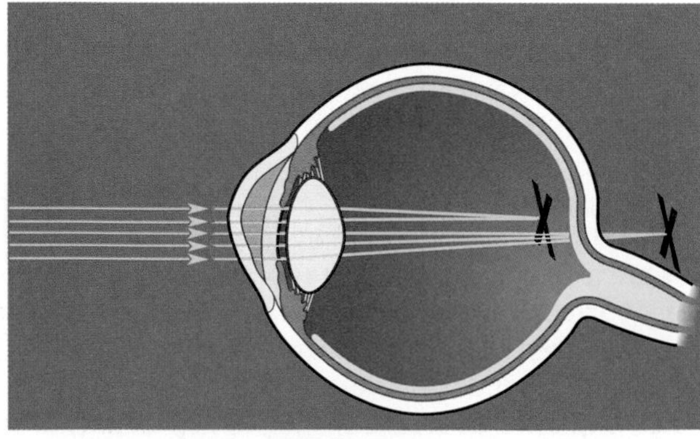

Astigmatism

FIGURE 13-13 Errors of refraction.

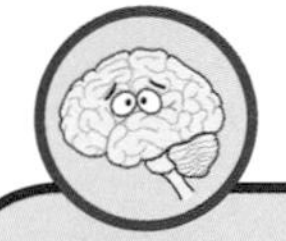

Do You Know...

About high concentrations of oxygen and blindness?

The administration of oxygen is generally beneficial and often lifesaving. Oxygen therapy, however, must be delivered with care, particularly in preterm infants. In "premies" less than 32 weeks' gestation, the administration of very high concentrations of oxygen can cause blindness. The oxygen is usually administered to a severely hypoxemic infant. While relieving the hypoxemia the high concentration of O_2 also causes constriction of the developing blood vessels of the retina. Deprived of its blood supply, the retina dies and is replaced by a retrolental membrane of fibrous tissue. The O_2-induced blindness is called retrolental fibroplasia or the retinopathy of prematurity.

SENSE OF HEARING: THE EAR

Listen to the sounds around you! Perhaps some of it is background noise that you mostly ignore. Other sounds provide you with information. Most importantly, you hear sounds that you enjoy, such as the voices of friends and sounds of music. The ear is the organ of the sense of hearing.

Structure of the Ear

The ear is divided into three parts: the external ear, the middle ear, and the inner ear (Figure 13-14).

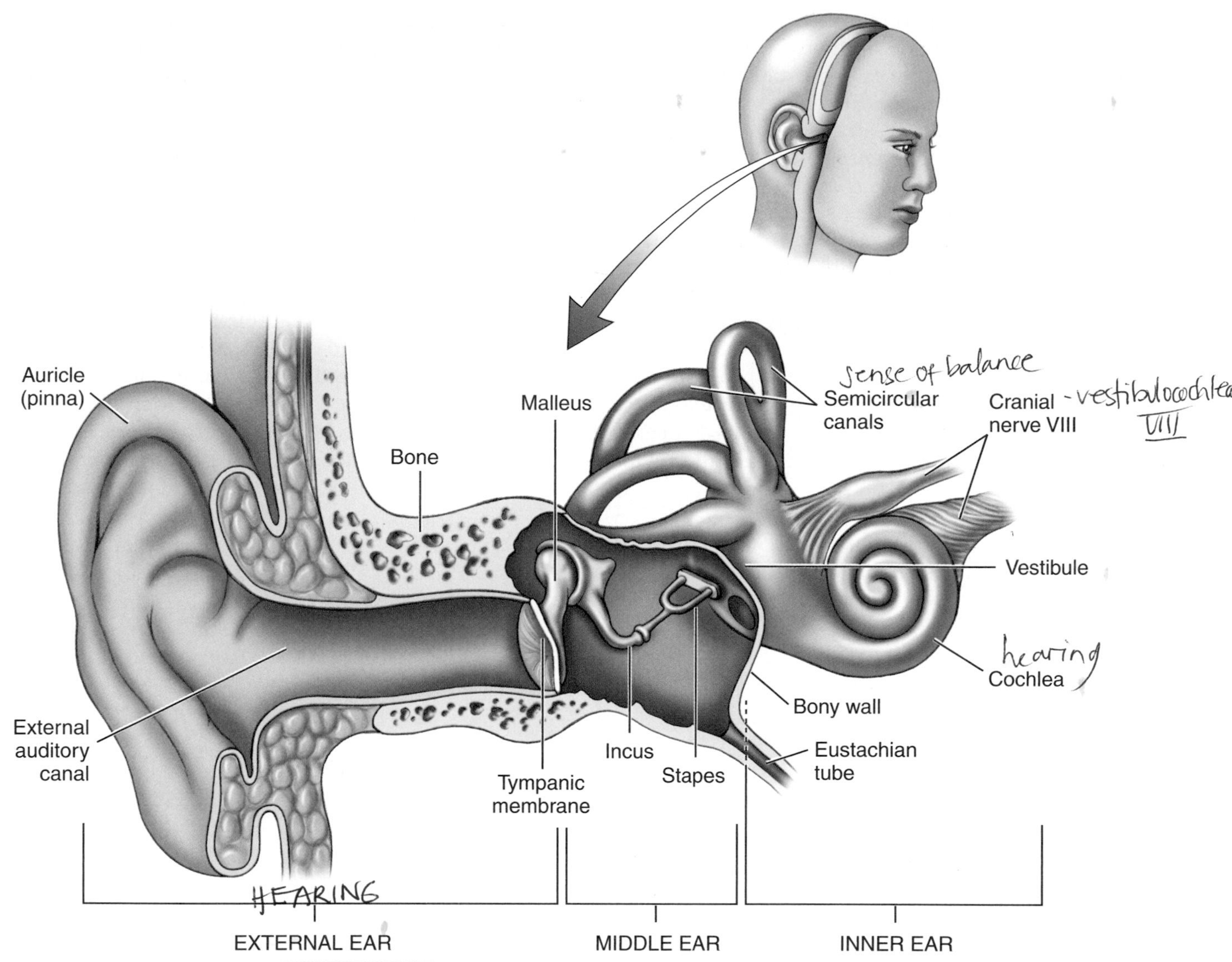

FIGURE 13-14 Structure of the ear: the three divisions.

External Ear. The **external ear** is the part of the ear you can see. It is composed of the auricle and the external auditory canal. The **auricle, or pinna** (Latin for wing), is composed of cartilage covered by a layer of loose-fitting skin. The auricle opens into the **external auditory canal.** This canal provides a passageway for sound waves to enter the ear. The external auditory canal is hollowed out of the temporal bone. It is about 1 inch long (2.5 cm) and ½ inch (1.25 cm) wide and extends to the **tympanic membrane, or eardrum.** The tympanic membrane separates the external ear from the middle ear.

The external auditory canal is lined with tiny hairs and glands that secrete **cerumen,** a yellowish, waxy substance also known as earwax. The hairs and cerumen help prevent dust and other foreign objects from entering the ear. Cerumen tends to be a victim of our cleanliness fetish; we insert hairpins, toothpicks, and other sharp objects into the canal in an attempt to dig out the wax. These objects may damage the tympanic membrane. Cotton-tipped applicators, while appearing safer, actually remove very little wax and can push any accumulated wax up against the eardrum. It is best not to insert any objects into the ear canal. This is more common than you think. A young child may insert an object such as a bean into the external canal; over time the bean accumulates moisture and swells, making it difficult to remove. Off to the ear doctor for bean removal!

Middle Ear. The **middle ear** is a small, air-filled chamber located between the tympanic membrane at one end and a bony wall at the other end (see Figure 13-14). The middle ear contains several structures: the tympanic membrane, three tiny bones, and the eustachian tube.

The tympanic membrane is composed primarily of connective tissue and has a rich supply of nerves and blood vessels. The tympanic membrane vibrates in response to sound waves entering the ear through the external auditory canal. The vibration of the tympanic membrane is passed on to the tiny bones in the middle ear.

The middle ear contains three tiny bones, or **ossicles.** These are the tiniest bones in the body. The names of the bones are the **malleus** (hammer); **incus** (anvil); and **stapes** (stirrup). The ossicles transmit vibration from the tympanic membrane to the ossicles (malleus → incus → stapes) and to the oval window, a membranous structure that separates the middle ear from the inner ear.

The middle ear has a passageway connecting it to the pharynx, or throat. This passageway is called the **auditory tube,** or the **eustachian** (ū-STĀ-shŭn) **tube.** The purpose of the tube is to equalize the pressure on both sides of the tympanic membrane by permitting air to pass from the pharynx into the middle ear. If the pressures across the membrane become unequal, the tympanic membrane bulges. As the tympanic membrane is stretched, pain receptors are stimulated. Pain caused by stretched tympanic membranes is the reason your ears sometimes hurt when you take off and land in an airplane.

Inner Ear. The **inner ear** consists of an intricate system of tubes, or passageways, hollowed out of the temporal bone. This coiled network of tubes is called a **bony labyrinth** (Figure 13-15). Inside the bony labyrinth is a similarly shaped **membranous labyrinth.** The bony labyrinth is filled with a fluid called **perilymph.** The membranous labyrinth is surrounded by perilymph and is itself filled with a thick fluid called **endolymph.** The perilymph and the endolymph form the fluid of the inner ear. The inner ear has three parts: the vestibule, the semicircular canals, and the cochlea. The cochlea is concerned with hearing. The **vestibule** and the **semicircular canals** are concerned with balance.

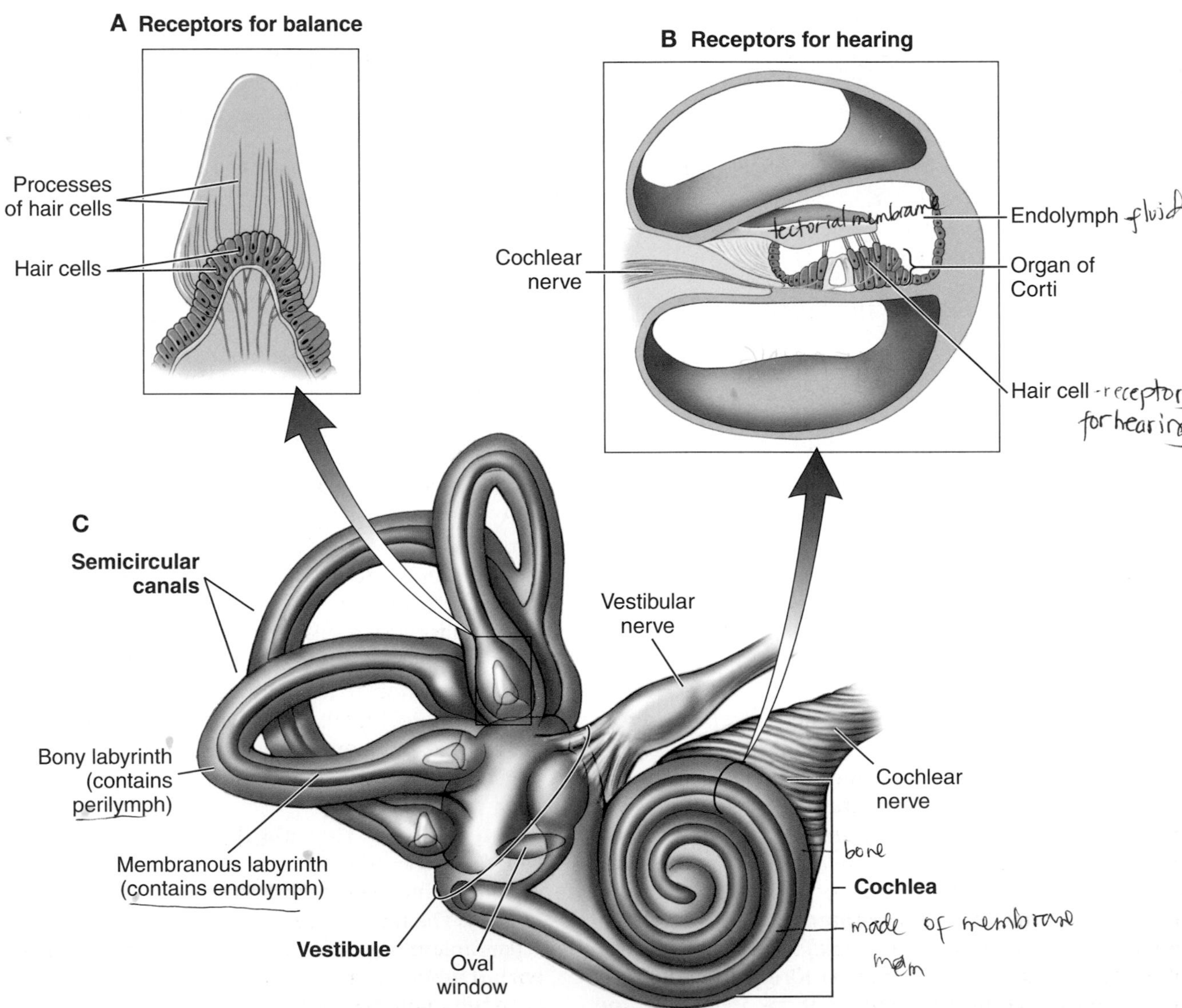

FIGURE 13-15 Inner ear. **A,** The receptors for balance. **B,** The receptors for hearing (organ of Corti) are located within the cochlea. **C,** Structures of the inner ear.

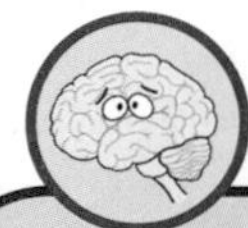

Do You Know...

Why children tend to outgrow ear infections?

The size and position of the eustachian tube in a child are different than in an adult. The eustachian tube of a child is shorter and lies in a more horizontal position than the adult eustachian tube. The child who develops a cold will often sniffle, thereby forcing the nasal drainage from the throat region into the eustachian tubes and middle ear. This drainage results in a middle ear infection called otitis media.

As the child grows, the eustachian tube grows longer and becomes less horizontal. There is less chance for bacteria to enter the middle ear from the throat. In this sense, children are said to outgrow ear infections.

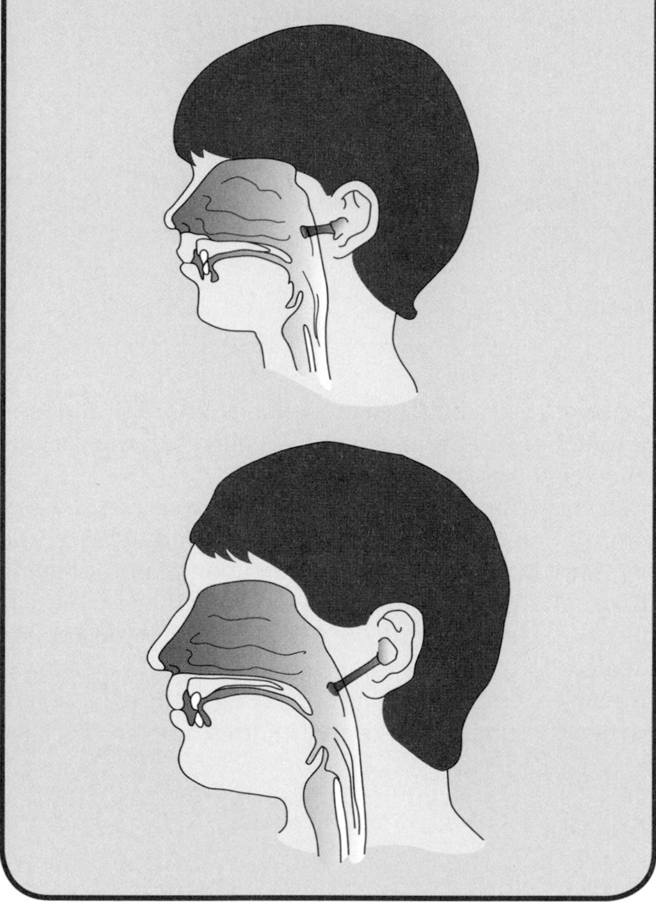

The **cochlea** (KŎK-lē-ă) is a snail-shaped part of the bony labyrinth. Sitting on a membrane within the cochlea and immersed in endolymph are the receptors for hearing (see Figure 13-15, *B*). The receptors are cells that contain tiny hairs and are called the **organ of Corti.** When the hairs on the receptor cells are bent, a nerve impulse is sent by the cochlear branch of the vestibulocochlear nerve (CN VIII) to the primary auditory cortex of the temporal lobe of the brain, where the sensation is interpreted as hearing. Note that the receptors are stimulated by the bending of the hairs; hence, the receptors are classified as mechanoreceptors.

Hearing Happens When...

Hearing is accomplished by structures within the external, middle, and inner ears. How do we hear the sounds of music? As Figure 13-16 illustrates, the vibrating guitar strings disturb the air, causing sound waves. The sound waves travel through the external auditory canal and hit the tympanic membrane, causing the tympanic membrane to vibrate. This vibration, in turn, causes the middle ear bones (malleus, incus, and stapes) to vibrate. The stapes, sitting within the oval window, then causes the fluid in the inner ear to move. Because the hairs (organ of Corti) are sitting within the fluid, movement of the fluid causes the hairs to bend. The bending of the hairs triggers a nerve impulse carried by the cochlear branch of the vestibulocochlear nerve (CN VIII) to the brain. The temporal lobe of the cerebrum interprets the impulses as sound.

Hearing Doesn't Happen When...

What happens when the parts do not work? Following the steps listed in Figure 13-16, consider the number of ways our hearing may become impaired. For example, the vibration of the tympanic membrane may become blunted if a plug of cerumen (earwax) becomes lodged against the tympanic membrane. The sound waves may then be unable to vibrate the eardrum. The tiny ossicles may also become fused to one another. This condition diminishes the ability of the bones to transmit vibration from the tympanic membrane to the oval window. This problem often develops in children who have experienced repeated middle ear infections.

Another problem is that the stapes may become glued, or fixed, to the oval window. This condition diminishes the transmission of vibration to the inner ear. The cochlear branch of cranial nerve VIII may also be damaged. The damaged nerve cannot conduct nerve impulses from the ear to the brain. This condition develops in persons exposed to prolonged periods of loud noise. For example, "rock and roll deafness" is hearing loss associated with loud music. Nerve damage also occurs in response to certain drugs, especially antibiotics. Drugs that cause damage to the vestibulocochlear nerve are called ototoxic agents. Nerve conduction deafness is commonly experienced by the elderly. Lastly, the temporal lobe that interprets the nerve impulse as hearing may be damaged. The person will then experience a cortical deafness.

SENSE OF BALANCE: THE EAR

We all appreciate our ears as organs of hearing, but we may not realize that our ears play an important role in **equilibrium** or balance. Damage to certain parts of the ear, for instance, may make it impossible for us to stand without losing balance.

The receptors for balance are mechanoreceptors. These cells contain hairlike projections immersed in

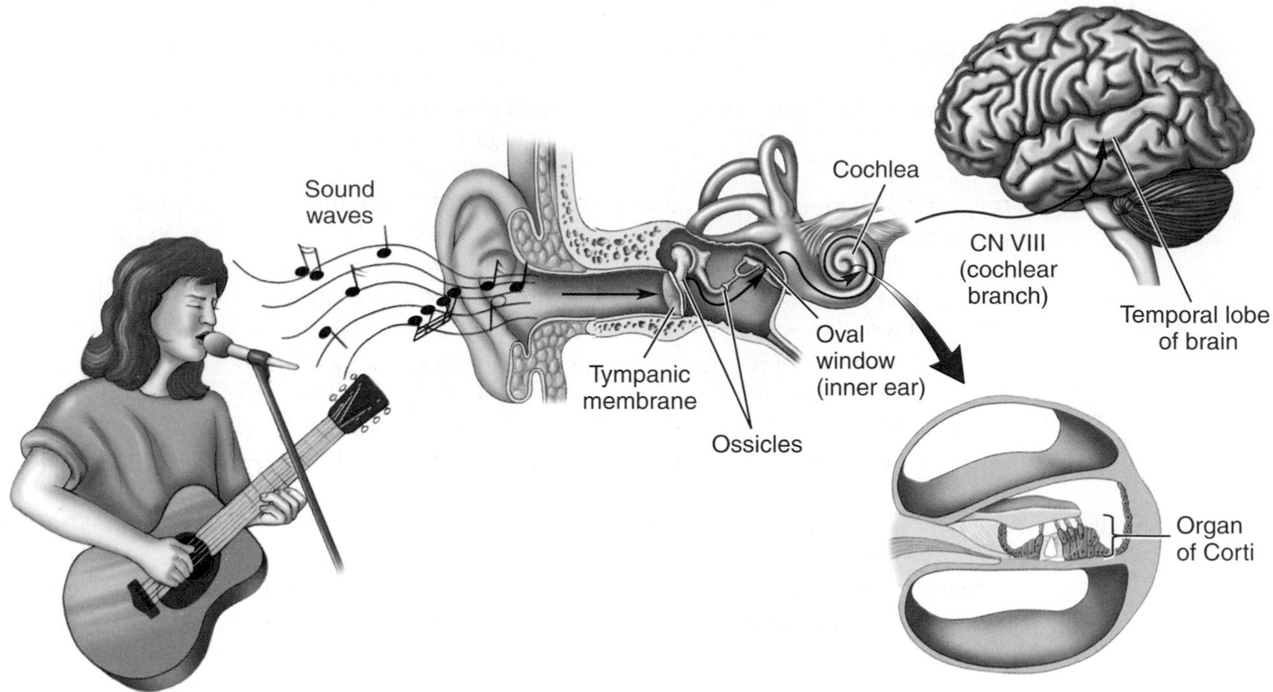

FIGURE 13-16 Steps in hearing.

the fluid of the inner ear. The receptors are located within the vestibule and the semicircular canals of the inner ear (see Figure 13-15). The **vestibule** contains the receptors that provide information about the position of the head at rest. The receptors in the **semicircular canals** provide information about the position of the body as it moves about. These receptors sense the changing positions of the head. When the positions change, the hairs are bent, and the receptor cells send nerve impulses through the vestibular branch of the vestibulocochlear nerve (CN VIII) to several parts of the brain, including the cerebellum, midbrain, and temporal lobe. The brain dispatches signals to the various muscles to restore balance.

Because the vestibulocochlear nerve carries sensory information concerning both hearing and balance, the person with an ear infection may complain of feeling dizzy. The person should be assured that as the ear infection clears, the dizzy feeling will also disappear. Ménière's disease, an inner ear disease, is characterized by nausea, tinnitis (ringing or buzzing in the ear), severe vertigo (dizziness), fall-related injuries, and hearing loss.

Do You Know...

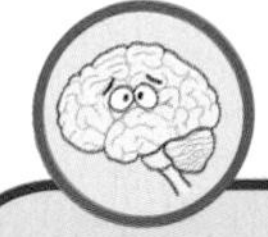

Why rocks in your head keep you balanced?

Tiny hairs on the inner ear cells concerned with balance (vestibule and the semicircular canals) bend in response to movement of the head. The tiny hair receptors contain little stones called otoliths. The stones make the hairs much more sensitive to a change in head position. So otoliths, the rocks in your head, keep you balanced. Notably, sharks have elaborate otoliths. Ask any Great White about his otoliths and he will quickly tell you that the rocks in his head keep him balanced, coordinated, and fine tuned for Xtreme fishing. He would quickly starve without his array of otoliths.

Sum It Up!

The special senses include smell, taste, sight, hearing, and balance. The nose and tongue are the organs of smell and taste, respectively. The eye, the organ of sight, includes a number of visual accessory organs. Sight requires light, which focuses on the retina, stimulating the photoreceptors and causing nerve impulses. The nerve impulses go to the occipital lobe of the brain and are interpreted as vision. The ear is an organ containing structures that stimulate nerve impulses that the brain perceives as sound. The ear is also the organ that senses balance.

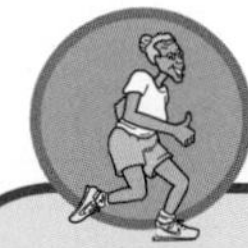

As You Age

1. In general, the senses diminish with age. A decrease in the number and sensitivity of sensory receptors, dermatomes, and neurons result in dulling of pain, touch, and tactile sensation.
2. A gradual loss in taste and smell begins around the age of 50 years.
3. Cumulative damage to hair cells in the organ of Corti occur after the age of 60. Older adults can lose the ability to hear high-pitched sounds and the consonants *ch, f, g, s, sh, t, th,* and *z.* 25% of older adults are hearing impaired.
4. Vision diminishes by the age of 70, primarily because of a decrease in the amount of light that reaches the retina and impaired focusing of the light on the retina.
5. The muscles of the iris become less efficient, so the pupils remain somewhat constricted most of the time.
6. The lacrimal glands become less active, and the eyes become dry and more susceptible to bacterial infection and irritation.

Disorders of the Sensory System

Amblyopia	Also called lazy eye. Amblyopia is the loss of vision in an eye that is not used.
Corneal abrasion	A scratching of the cornea causing pain and tearing; commonly caused by a speck of dust or contact lenses.
Deafness	Loss of hearing. Conduction deafness is due to impaired conduction of sound caused by impacted ear wax or fused middle ear ossicles. Sensorineural deafness is due to damage of the nervous structures associated with hearing.
Detached retina	Retina detached from the choroid, its nutritive supply. The result is retinal damage and blindness.
Keratitis	Inflammation of the cornea.
Macular degeneration	Deterioration of the macula lutea of the retina, causing loss of central vision.
Ménière's disease	A disorder of the inner ear resulting in vertigo (dizziness), tinnitus (ringing or buzzing in the ear), and hearing loss.
Motion sickness	Also called car sickness and seasickness. Motion sickness is characterized by vertigo, nausea, vomiting, and drowsiness that occurs in response to excessive stimulation of the equilibrium receptors in the inner ear.
Retinopathy	Irreversible damage to the retina usually caused by hypertension or diabetes mellitus. Retinopathy causes loss of vision and even blindness.
Ruptured eardrum	Eardrum rupture as a result of direct injury with a sharp object (including the use of a hairpin to remove earwax), trauma, or infection such as otitis media (middle ear infection). Repeated infection and tearing of the eardrum may cause hearing loss. Sometimes tubes are placed through the eardrum so as to drain fluid from the middle ear, thereby preventing rupture of the eardrum. This procedure is called a myringotomy.

SUMMARY OUTLINE

The sensory system allows us to experience the world through a variety of sensations: touch, pressure, pain, proprioception, temperature, taste, smell, vision, hearing, and equilibrium.

I. Receptors and Sensation

A. Receptor
1. A receptor is a specialized area of a sensory neuron that detects a specific stimulus.
2. The five types of receptors are chemoreceptors, pain receptors (nociceptors), thermoreceptors, mechanoreceptors, and photoreceptors.

B. Sensation
1. A sensation is a conscious awareness of incoming sensory information.
2. There are four components of a sensation.

3. The two characteristics of sensation are projection and adaptation.

II. General Senses

A. Pain
1. Pain receptors (nociceptors) are free nerve endings.
2. The stimuli for pain are tissue damage, lack of oxygen, and stretching or distortion of tissue.

B. Touch and Pressure
1. Receptors are mechanoreceptors and respond to forces that press, move, or deform tissue.
2. The receptors for pressure are located in the skin, subcutaneous tissue, and the deep tissue.

C. Temperature
1. There are thermoreceptors for heat and cold.
2. Thermoreceptors are found in free nerve endings and in other specialized sensory cells beneath the skin.

D. Proprioception
1. Proprioreceptors are located primarily in the muscles, tendons, and joints.
2. Proprioreceptors sense orientation or position.

III. Special Senses

A. Sense of Smell: The Nose
1. Olfactory receptors are chemoreceptors.
2. Sensory information travels along the olfactory nerve to the temporal lobe.

B. Sense of Taste: The Tongue
1. Taste buds contain chemoreceptors for taste.
2. There are four basic taste sensations: sweet, salty, sour, and bitter.
3. Sensory information travels along the facial and glossopharyngeal nerves to the gustatory cortex in the parietal lobe.

C. Sense of Sight: The Eye
1. The visual accessory organs include the eyebrows, eyelids, eyelashes, lacrimal apparatus, and extrinsic eye muscles.
2. The eyeball has three layers: the sclera, choroid, and retina (contains the photoreceptors, rods, and cones).
3. The eyeball has two cavities. One is a posterior cavity filled with vitreous humor, the other is an anterior cavity filled with aqueous humor.
4. There are two sets of eye muscles: extrinsic and intrinsic eye muscles.
5. The extrinsic eye muscles move the eyeball.
6. The intrinsic eye muscles control the size of the pupil and shape of the lens for refraction.
7. Light stimulates the photoreceptors.
8. The electrical signal is carried to the occipital lobe via the visual pathway.
9. Steps in seeing are summarized in Figure 13-1.

D. Sense of Hearing: The Ear
1. There are three parts of the ear: the external ear, middle ear, and the inner ear.
2. The middle ear contains the ossicles.
3. The inner ear structure concerned with hearing is the cochlea. It contains the hearing receptors and organ of Corti.
4. Hearing information is carried by the cochlear nerve to the temporal lobe.
5. Steps in hearing are summarized in Figure 13-16.

E. Sense of Balance: The Ear
1. The receptors are mechanoreceptors located in the vestibule and the semicircular canals of the inner ear.
2. The receptors are activated when the head changes position.
3. Balance information travels along the vestibular nerve to many areas of the brain (cerebellum, midbrain, and temporal lobe).

Review Your Knowledge

Matching: Senses

Directions: Match the following words with their descriptions below. Some words may be used more than once.

a. sight
b. taste
c. smell
d. hearing
e. balance

1. ____ Involves rods and cones, the retina, and CN II
2. ____ Involves the organ of Corti and CN VIII
3. ____ Is the olfactory sense; uses chemoreceptors
4. ____ Uses mechanoreceptors; sensory information transmitted by the vestibular branch of CN VIII
5. ____ Gustatory sensation
6. ____ From receptors to the occipital lobe
7. ____ From receptors to the auditory cortex

Matching: Structures of the Eye

Directions: Match the following words with their descriptions below. Some words may be used more than once.

a. choroid
b. vitreous humor
c. lens
d. cornea
e. iris
f. aqueous humor
g. conjunctiva
h. retina

1. ____ The layer of the eyeball that contains the photoreceptors
2. ____ The colored muscle portion of the eye that determines the size of the pupil
3. ____ The shape of this structure is determined by the ciliary muscles; refracts light
4. ____ Layer of the eyeball that provides the blood supply for the retina
5. ____ Secreted by the ciliary body and drained by the canal of Schlemm
6. ____ Gel-like substance in the posterior cavity; maintains the shape of the eye and helps hold the retina in place
7. ____ Contains the radial and circular muscles; mydriasis and miosis.
8. ____ The window of the eye; an avascular structure
9. ____ Includes the macula lutea
10. ____ Inner lining of the lids; "pink eye"

Matching: Structures of the Ear

Directions: Match the following words with their descriptions below. Some words may be used more than once.

a. external ear
b. middle ear
c. inner ear

1. ____ Contains the malleus, incus, and stapes
2. ____ Connected to the pharynx by the eustachian tube
3. ____ Home of cerumen
4. ____ Location of the organ of Corti and CN VIII
5. ____ Cochlea, semicircular canals, and vestibule
6. ____ Endolymph and perilymph; mechanoreceptors
7. ____ Separated from the middle ear by the tympanic membrane
8. ____ Separated from the inner ear by the oval window
9. ____ Bone conduction deafness
10. ____ Nerve conduction deafness

Multiple Choice

1. The retina
   a. refracts light.
   b. contains rods and cones.
   c. covers the optic disc, the area of most acute vision.
   d. secretes vitreous humor.
2. What is the consequence of diminished blood flow to the choroid?
   a. Aqueous humor cannot be formed and the intraocular pressure increases.
   b. Light cannot be refracted.
   c. The retina dies.
   d. The pupil constricts.
3. A drug or effect that is described as mydriatic
   a. decreases intraocular pressure.
   b. dilates the pupil.
   c. increases the secretion of aqueous humor.
   d. increases the numbers of cones.
4. Which of the following does not describe the middle ear?
   a. Contains the malleus, incus, and stapes
   b. Connects with the pharynx by the eustachian tube
   c. Is the home of the organ of Corti
   d. Is concerned with bone conduction
5. The organ of Corti
   a. is the receptor for hearing.
   b. refers to the ossicles within the middle ear.
   c. leans up against the tympanic membrane and "feels" its vibration.
   d. activates CN II.
6. Touch, pressure, pain, and temperature are
   a. mediated through mechanoreceptors.
   b. classified as general senses.
   c. interpreted in the precentral gyrus.
   d. general senses that are interpreted in the occipital lobe.

CHAPTER 14

Endocrine System

KEY TERMS

Adenohypophysis, p. 243
Adrenal gland, p. 251
Catecholamine, p. 251
Endocrine gland, p. 239
Hormone, p. 239
Neurohypophysis, p. 246
Pancreas, p. 254
Parathyroid gland, p. 249
Pineal gland, p. 257
Steroid, p. 251
Thymus gland, p. 257
Thyroid gland, p. 247

OBJECTIVES

1. List the functions of the endocrine system.
2. Define *hormone.*
3. Explain negative feedback control as a regulator for hormone levels.
4. Describe the relationship of the hypothalamus to the pituitary gland.
5. Describe the location, hormones, and regulation of the pituitary gland.
6. Identify the major endocrine glands and their hormones.
7. Explain the effects of hyposecretion and hypersecretion of the major endocrine glands.

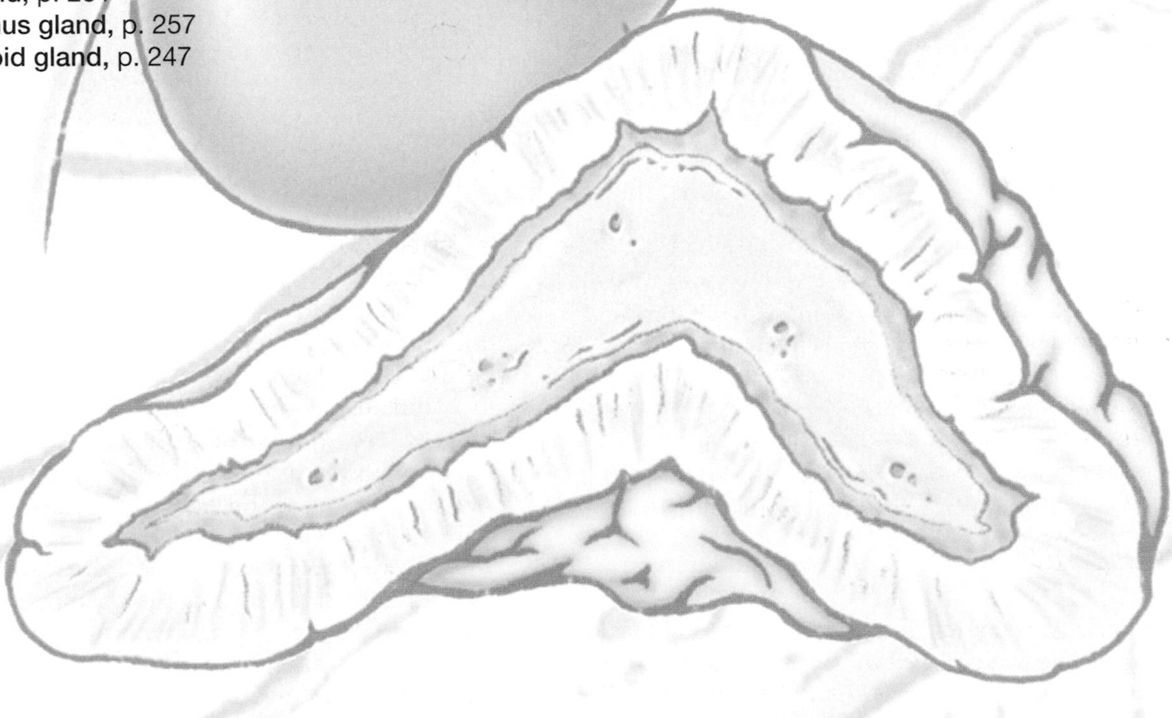

While performing his mating ritual, Rooster is dancing out the meaning of the word hormone, the main focus of the endocrine system. It is a Greek term meaning "to arouse or to set into motion." Rooster's testosterone has truly set him in motion. It has him prancing and dancing his mating ritual and has both him and Hen aroused.

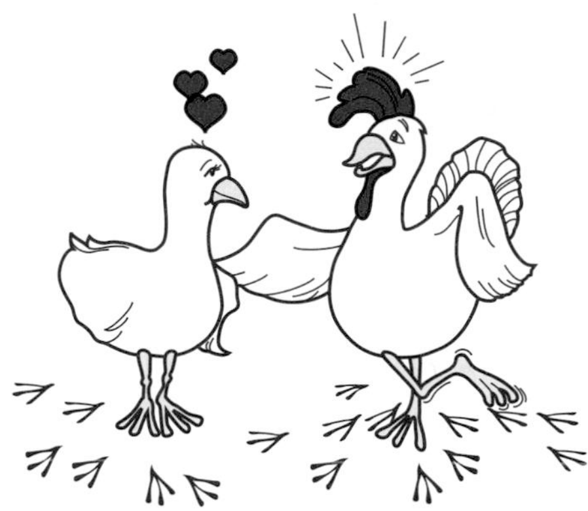

The nervous system and the endocrine system are the two chief communicating and coordinating systems in the body. They regulate nearly all organ systems. Although the nervous and endocrine systems work together closely, they have several differences. The nervous system communicates through electrical signals called nerve impulses. Nerve impulses communicate information rapidly and generally achieve short-term effects. The endocrine system, in contrast, communicates through chemical signals called hormones. The endocrine system responds more slowly and generally exerts longer-lasting effects.

ENDOCRINE GLANDS

The endocrine system is composed of endocrine glands that are widely distributed throughout the body (Figure 14-1). **Endocrine glands** secrete the chemical substances called hormones. Endocrine glands are ductless glands—that is, they secrete the hormones directly into the blood and not into ducts. For instance, the pancreas secretes the hormone insulin into the blood, which then delivers the insulin to cells throughout the body.

HORMONES

A **hormone** is a chemical messenger that influences or controls the activities of other tissues or organs. In general, the endocrine system and its hormones help regulate metabolic processes involving carbohydrates, proteins, and fats. Hormones also play an important role in growth and reproduction and help regulate water and electrolyte balance. When you become hungry, thirsty, hot, or cold, your body's response includes secretion of hormones. Lastly, hormones help your body meet the demands of infection, trauma, and stress. The study of the endocrine system is called **endocrinology.**

CLASSIFICATION OF HORMONES

Chemically, hormones are classified as either proteins (and protein-related substances) or steroids. With the exception of secretions from the adrenal cortex and the sex glands all hormones are protein or protein-related. The adrenal cortex and the sex glands secrete steroids.

TARGETS

Each hormone binds to a specific tissue, called its **target tissue** or **organ** (Figure 14-2, *A*). The target tissue may be located close to or at a distance from the endocrine gland. Some hormones, such as thyroid hormone and insulin, have many target tissues and therefore exert more widespread, or generalized, effects. Other hormones, such as parathyroid hormone, have fewer target tissues and therefore exert fewer effects.

HORMONE RECEPTORS

Hormones interact with the receptor sites of the cells of their target tissues. The two types of receptors are those located on the outer surface of the cell membrane (membrane receptors) and those located within the cell (intracellular receptors).

How do hormones recognize their target tissues? The hormone and its receptor can be likened to a lock and key. The key must fit the lock. The same is true for the hormone and receptor; a part of the hormone (key) "fits into" its receptor (lock) on the target. Unless the match is perfect, the hormone cannot lock into and stimulate the receptor. For example, the hormone insulin circulates throughout the body in the blood and is therefore delivered to every cell in the body. Insulin, however, can only stimulate the cells that have insulin receptors. The lock-and-key theory guarantees that a particular hormone affects only certain cells. The hormone-receptor relationship insures **specificity,** meaning that there is a specific hormone for each receptor.

Protein hormones generally combine with the receptor sites located on the cell membrane (see Figure 14-2, *B*). The interaction of the hormone with its receptor stimulates the production of a **second messenger** such as cyclic adenosine monophosphate (cAMP). The cAMP, in turn, helps activate the enzymes in the cell. For instance, when epinephrine stimulates its receptors on the heart, cAMP is formed and then stimulates the heart itself.

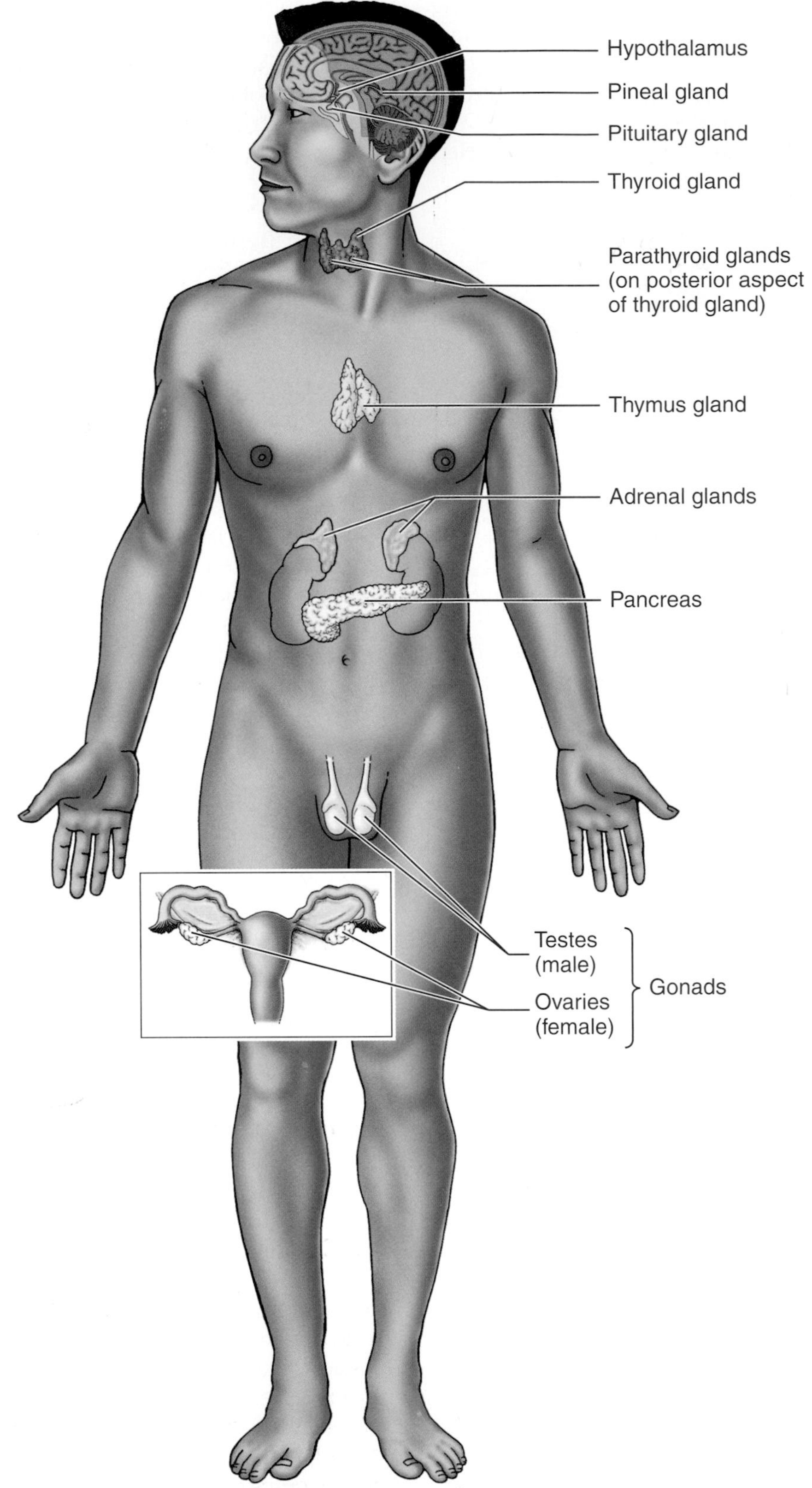

FIGURE 14-1 Major endocrine glands of the body.

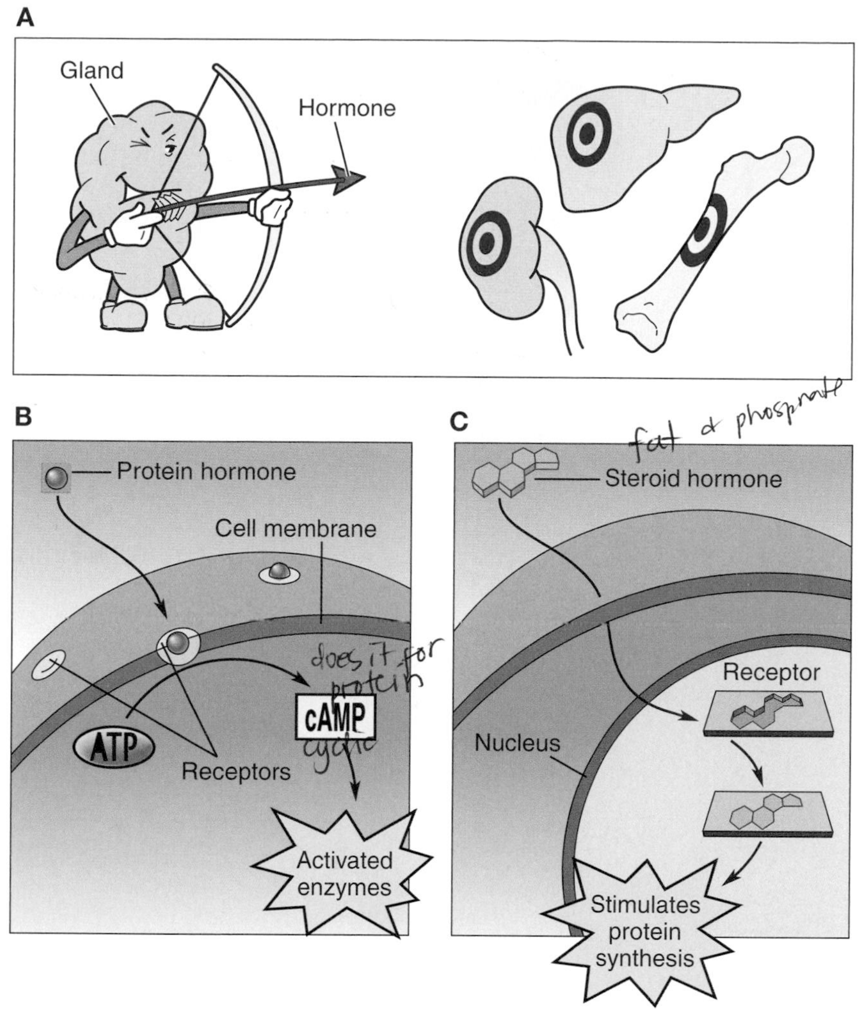

FIGURE 14-2 What hormones do. **A,** Hormones are aimed at target tissues or target organs. **B,** Protein hormones and membrane receptors. **C,** Steroid hormones and intracellular receptors.

The second type of receptor is located intracellularly (see Figure 14-2, *C*). Steroid hormones, which are lipid-soluble, pass through the plasma membrane of the target cell and bind to receptors in the nucleus. The steroid-receptor complex then stimulates protein synthesis. The newly synthesized protein alters cellular function.

CONTROL OF HORMONE SECRETION

Three mechanisms control the secretion of hormones. They are negative feedback control, biorhythms, and control by the central nervous system (CNS).

Negative Feedback, or "Enough Is Enough"

Normal endocrine function depends on normal plasma levels of hormones. Life-threatening complications develop when the glands either hypersecrete or hyposecrete hormones. For instance, if too much insulin is secreted, the amount of blood glucose decreases to dangerous levels. On the other hand, if the secretion of insulin is inadequate, the blood glucose levels increase and cause serious problems. So how does the pancreas, the insulin-secreting gland, know when it has secreted enough insulin?

Many of the endocrine glands maintain normal plasma levels of their hormones through a mechanism called **negative feedback** (Figure 14-3). With negative feedback, information about the hormone or the effects of that hormone is fed back to the gland that secretes the hormone. The pattern of insulin secretion is one example of negative feedback. When blood levels of glucose increase after eating, insulin is released from the pancreas. Insulin causes glucose to move from the blood into the cell. As the glucose enters the cells, the blood levels of glucose decrease. As blood glucose levels decrease, the stimulus for insulin secretion also decreases.

What information was fed back to the gland? It was the decrease in blood glucose. What was the gland's response? The gland decreased its secretion of insulin. Negative feedback is a common means of control within the endocrine system.

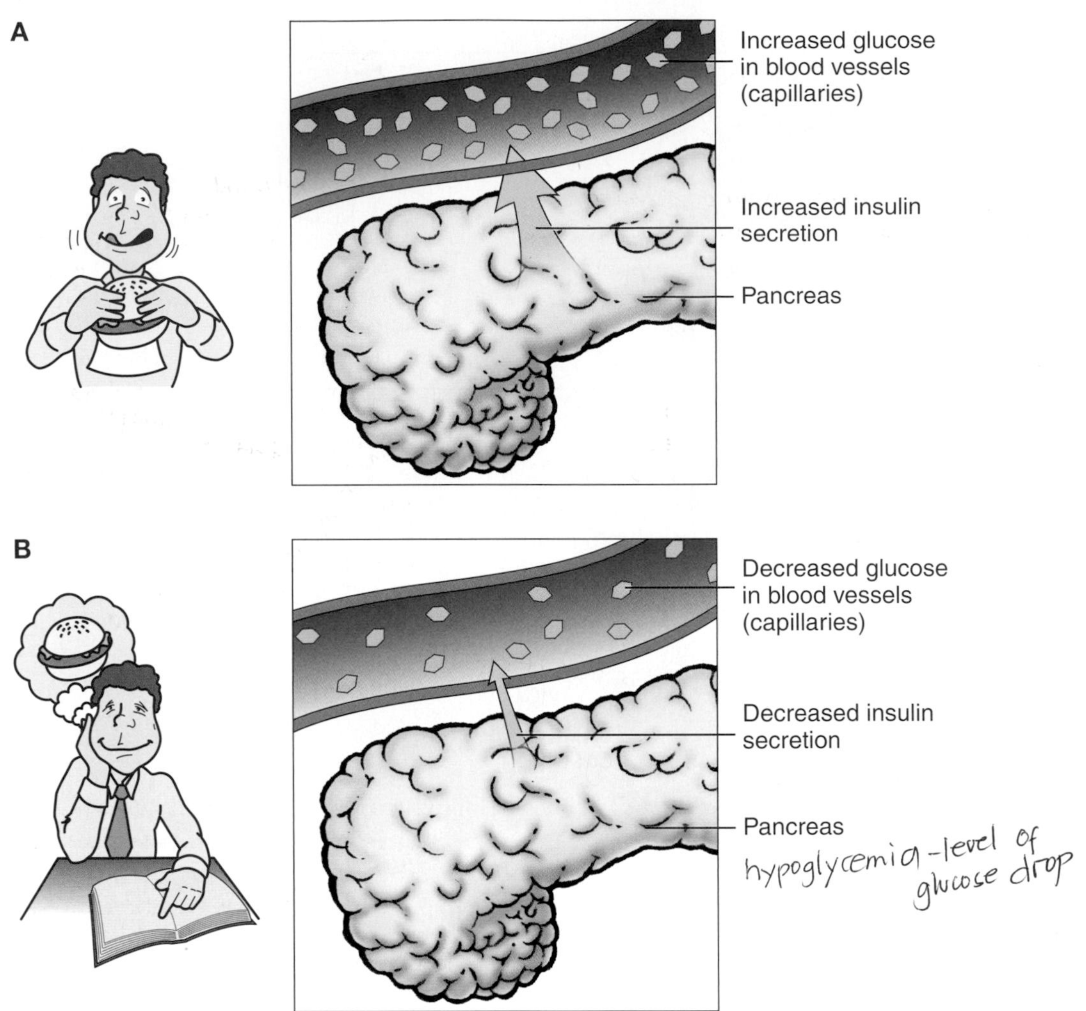

FIGURE 14-3 Negative feedback control. **A,** Increased blood glucose levels trigger the release of insulin from the pancreas. **B,** Decreased blood glucose levels cause the pancreas to decrease its secretion of insulin.

Biorhythms

Blood levels of most hormones are also controlled by **biorhythms.** A biorhythm is a rhythmic alteration in a hormone's rate of secretion. Some hormones, such as cortisol, are secreted in a circadian rhythm. A **circadian rhythm** (*circa* means around; *dian* means day) is a 24-hour rhythm; its pattern repeats every 24 hours. Because of its circadian rhythm, cortisol secretion is highest in the morning hours (peak at 8 AM) and lowest in the evening hours (lowest at midnight). The female reproductive hormones represent another biorhythm. They are secreted in a monthly pattern, hence the monthly menstrual cycle.

Unfortunately, biorhythms can be disturbed by travel and alterations in sleep patterns. For instance, jet lag and the symptoms of fatigue experienced by persons who work the night shift are related to alterations of biorhythms. The problem has become so acute that some hospitals have developed staffing schedules based on biorhythms.

Sometimes drugs are administered on a schedule that mimics normal biorhythms. For instance, steroids are administered in the morning, when natural steroid levels are highest. Coordinating with the natural rhythms increases the effectiveness of the drug and causes fewer side effects. The effect of biorhythms is so important on drug effects that a branch of pharmacology addresses this issue; it is called **chronopharmacology.**

Control by the Central Nervous System

The CNS helps control the secretion of hormones in two ways: activation of the hypothalamus and stimulation of the sympathetic nervous system. Think about this: the CNS exerts a powerful influence over the endocrine system. Because the CNS is also the center for our emotional life, it is not surprising that our emotions, in turn, affect the endocrine system.

For instance, when we are stressed out, the CNS causes several of the endocrine glands to secrete stress hormones, thereby alerting every cell in the body to the threat. Many women have experienced the effect of stress on the menstrual cycle. Stress can cause the menstrual period to occur early or late; it may even cause the cycle to skip a month. These effects illustrate the power of emotions on our body. In fact, the functions of the nervous system and the endocrine system are so closely related that the word **psychoneuroendocrinology** is used.

Sum It Up!

The endocrine system is composed of endocrine glands widely distributed throughout the body. The endocrine glands secrete hormones. Hormones stimulate target tissues by binding to cell receptors. The receptors are located either on the cell membrane or within the cell. Three control mechanisms regulate the secretion of hormones: negative feedback, biorhythms, and CNS activity.

Do You Know...

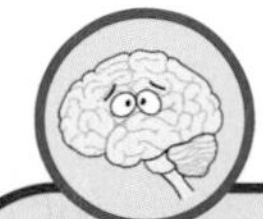

Why the pituitary gland is "uppity" but not snotty?

The pituitary gland is also known as the master gland. A pretty important gland it is! When first discovered, however, the pituitary gland was relegated to the lowly role of mucus secretion (*pituita* is the Greek word for mucus). The gland was credited with secreting mucus as a cooling agent. After cooling the body, mucus was then eliminated through the nose. But this is not true. Mucus is secreted by the mucous membrane that lines the nasal passages and does not act as a coolant. Mucus merely does the nasal housework—it traps the dust and gets blown out your nose. The pituitary gland, on the other hand, has more important things to do. It secretes many hormones and controls much of the endocrine function of the body. Unfortunately, this master gland is stuck with the name pituitary (mucus-making). Its other name, hypophysis, isn't much more flattering; it means undergrowth (referring to its location under the brain). Mucus and undergrowth—humbling for a master!

THE PITUITARY GLAND

THE PITUITARY GLAND AND THE HYPOTHALAMUS

The pituitary gland, also called the **hypophysis,** is a pea-sized gland located in a depression of the sphenoid bone. It is attached to the undersurface of the hypothalamus by a short stalk called the infundibulum. The pituitary contains two main parts: the anterior pituitary gland and the posterior pituitary gland. The major hormones and their target glands are illustrated in Figure 14-4, *A*.

The secretion of the anterior pituitary gland is controlled by the hypothalamus. Although it is part of the brain, the hypothalamus secretes several hormones and is therefore considered to be an endocrine gland. These hormones are called **releasing hormones** and **release-inhibiting hormones.** They either stimulate or inhibit the secretion of anterior pituitary hormones. For instance, prolactin-releasing hormone, secreted by the hypothalamus, stimulates the pituitary gland to secrete prolactin. Prolactin-inhibiting hormone (PIH), secreted by the hypothalamus, inhibits the secretion of prolactin by the anterior pituitary gland.

How do the hypothalamic hormones reach the anterior pituitary gland? The hypothalamus secretes its hormones into a network of capillaries (tiny blood vessels) that connect the hypothalamus with the anterior pituitary gland (see Figure 14-4, *B*). These connecting capillaries are called the **hypothalamic-hypophyseal portal system.** Thus hormones secreted by the hypothalamus flow through the portal capillaries to the anterior pituitary.

ANTERIOR PITUITARY GLAND

The anterior pituitary gland is composed of glandular epithelial tissue and is also called the **adenohypophysis** (ăd-ĕ-nō-hī-PŎF-ĭ-sĭs) (*adeno-* means "glandular"). The anterior pituitary secretes six major hormones (see Figure 14-4, *A,* and Table 14-1). These hormones control other glands and affect many organ systems. In fact, the anterior pituitary affects so many other glands that it is often called the master gland. You must understand the command of the grand gland!

The hormones of the anterior pituitary include thyroid-stimulating hormone (TSH); adrenocorticotropic hormone (ACTH); growth hormone (GH); the gonadotropins; and prolactin (PRL).

Remember!

PRO	Prolactin
ATHletes	ACTH
Got	Gonadotropins (FSH, LH)
To	TSH
GROW	Growth Hormone

Growth Hormone

Growth hormone (GH) is also called **somatotropin** or **somatotropic hormone.** Its primary effects are on the growth of skeletal muscles and the long bones of the body, thereby determining a person's size and height. GH also exerts powerful metabolic effects. It causes amino acids to be built into proteins and fats to be broken down and used for energy. It also stimulates the conversion of protein to glucose, especially during periods of fasting between meals. GH thus causes blood glucose levels to rise. GH is secreted during periods of exercise, sleep, and hypoglycemia. Like your mother

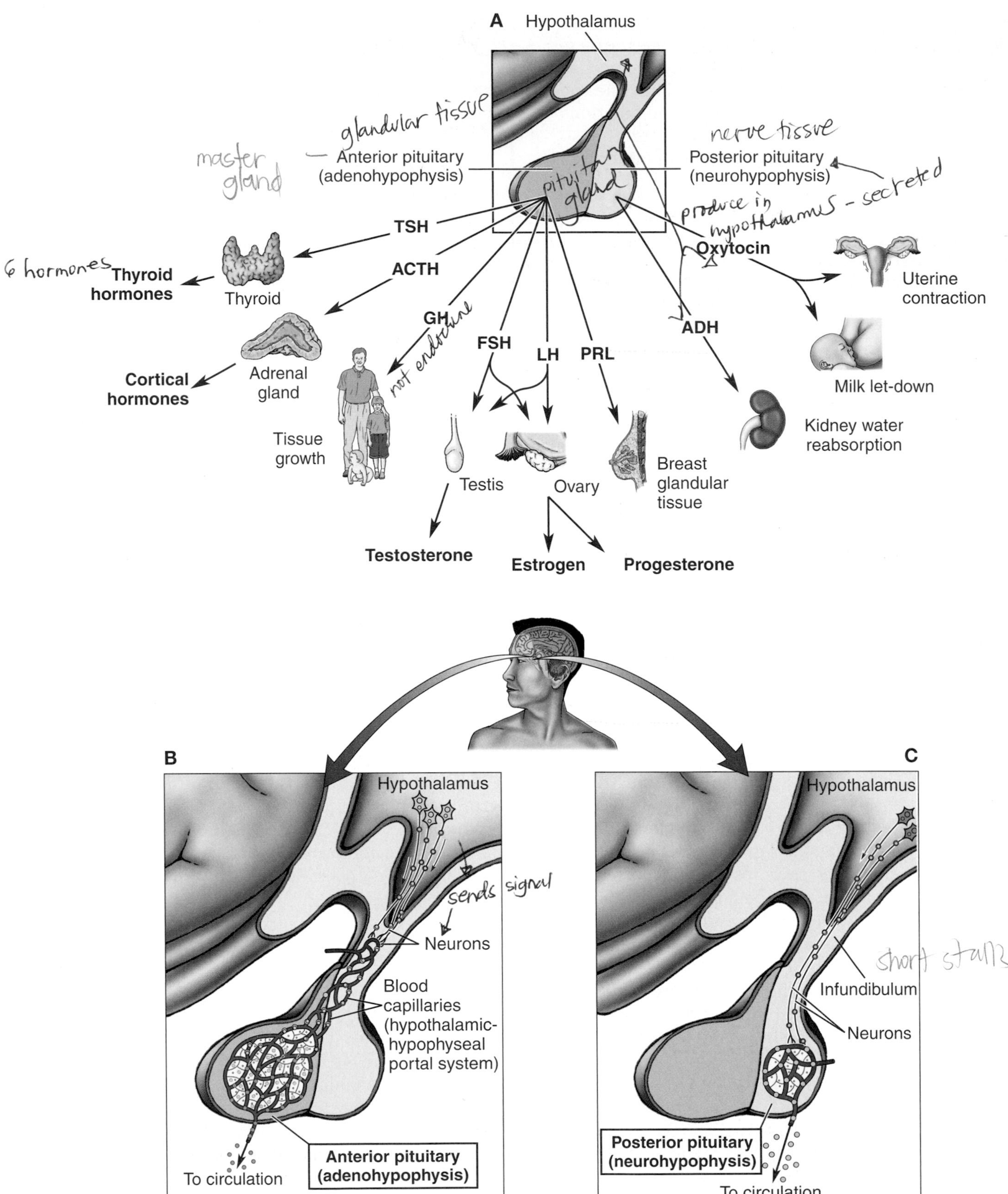

FIGURE 14-4 Pituitary gland. **A,** Hormones of the anterior and posterior pituitary glands; also shows the target organs. **B,** Effect of the hypothalamus on the anterior pituitary gland. **C,** Effect of the hypothalamus on the posterior pituitary gland.

Table 14-1 Hormones and Their Functions

Hormone	Functions
Anterior Pituitary Gland	
Growth hormone (GH)	Stimulates the growth of bone and soft tissue; stimulates the synthesis of glucose during periods of fasting
Prolactin	Stimulates the breast to develop and produce milk
Thyroid-stimulating hormone (TSH)	Stimulates the thyroid gland to produce thyroid hormones (T_3 and T_4)
Adrenocorticotropic hormone (ACTH)	Stimulates the adrenal cortex to secrete steroids, especially cortisol
Gonadotropic hormones	Relay structure and processing center for most sensory information going to the cerebrum
Follicle-stimulating hormone (FSH)	Stimulates the development of ova and sperm
Luteinizing hormone (LH)	Causes ovulation in women and stimulates the secretion of progesterone in women and testosterone in men
Posterior Pituitary Gland	
Antidiuretic hormone (ADH)	Stimulates water reabsorption by the kidney; also constricts blood vessels
Oxytocin	Contracts uterine muscle during labor; releases milk from the mammary glands (breast-feeding)
Hormones of the Thyroid and Parathyroid Glands	
Thyroid hormones (T_3, T_4)	Triiodothyronine (T_3) and tetraiodothyronine (T_4, or thyroxine) are secreted by the thyroid gland; control metabolic rate and regulate growth and development
Calcitonin	Secreted by the thyroid gland; decreases plasma levels of calcium
Parathyroid hormone (PTH)	Secreted by the parathyroid glands: increases plasma calcium
Hormones of the Adrenal Gland	
Catecholamines: epinephrine and norepinephrine	Stimulates the "fight or flight" response
Steroids	
Cortisol	A glucocorticoid that helps regulate glucose, fat, and protein metabolism; is part of the stress response
Aldosterone	A mineralocorticoid that causes the kidneys to reabsorb sodium and water and to excrete potassium; helps regulate fluid and electrolyte balance
Sex hormones	Especially the androgens (testosterone); helps develop the secondary sex characteristics in the female and male
Hormones of the Pancreas	
Insulin	Secreted by the beta cells of the islets of Langerhans; helps regulate the metabolism of carbohydrates, proteins, and fats; lowers blood glucose
Glucagon	Secreted by the alpha cells of the islets of Langerhans; raises blood glucose
Other Hormones	
Estrogens and progesterone	Secreted by the ovaries Stimulates the development of the ova (eggs) and development of the secondary sex characteristics in the female
Testosterone	Secreted primarily by the testes The chief male androgen; stimulates the development of sperm and the secondary sex characteristics in the male
Thymosins	Stimulates the maturation of the T-lymphocytes
Melatonin	Secreted by the pineal gland and helps set the biorhythms
Melanocyte-stimulating hormone (MSH)	Stimulates the secretion of melanin; causes darkening of the skin

said, "Plenty of rest and exercise makes you grow big and strong." (And you thought she didn't know her physiology!)

As its name implies, GH exerts a profound effect on growth. A person who hypersecretes GH as a child develops gigantism and will grow very tall, often achieving a height of 8 or 9 feet. If hypersecretion of GH occurs in an adult after the epiphyseal discs of the long bones have sealed, only the bones of the jaw, the eyebrow ridges, the nose, the hands, and the feet enlarge. This condition is called acromegaly. GH deficiency in childhood causes the opposite effect, a pituitary dwarfism. With this condition, body proportions are normal, but the person's height is very short.

Prolactin

Prolactin (PRL) is also called **lactogenic hormone.** As its name suggests (*pro-* means "for"; *-lact-* means "milk"),

PRL promotes milk production in women. PRL stimulates the growth of the mammary glands and stimulates the mammary glands to produce milk after childbirth. Got milk? As long as the lactating mother continues to breastfeed, PRL levels remain high and milk is produced. (PRL is discussed in more detail in Chapter 27.) The role of PRL in males is not known.

Tropic Hormones

The remaining hormones of the anterior pituitary gland are **tropic hormones.** Tropic hormones are aimed at and control other glands. The names of tropic hormones usually end in tropin, or tropic, as in thyrotropin or adrenocorticotropic hormone. The tropic hormones include:

- Thyrotropin, or thyroid-stimulating hormone (TSH): The target gland for **thyroid-stimulating hormone** is the thyroid gland. TSH stimulates the thyroid gland to secrete two thyroid hormones.
- Adrenocorticotropic hormone (ACTH): The target gland for **adrenocorticotropic hormone** is the adrenal cortex. ACTH stimulates the adrenal cortex to secrete steroids.
- Gonadotropic hormones: The target glands for the **gonadotropic hormones** are the gonads, or sex glands (ovaries and testes). The two gonadotropins are **follicle-stimulating hormone (FSH)** and **luteinizing hormone (LH).** FSH stimulates the development of ova (eggs) in the female and sperm in the male. LH causes ovulation in the female and causes the secretion of sex hormones in both the male and the female. LH in the male is also called **interstitial cell–stimulating hormone (ICSH)** because it stimulates the interstitial cells in the testes to synthesize and secrete testosterone. (These hormones are described further in Chapter 26.)

POSTERIOR PITUITARY GLAND

The posterior pituitary gland is an extension of the hypothalamus (see Figure 14-4, *C*). The posterior pituitary is composed of nervous tissue and is therefore called the **neurohypophysis** (nū-rō-hī-PŎF-ĭ-sĭs). The two hormones of the posterior pituitary gland are produced in the hypothalamus and transported to the gland where they are stored until needed. The two hormones are antidiuretic hormone and oxytocin.

Antidiuretic Hormone

Antidiuretic hormone (ADH) is released from the posterior pituitary gland in an attempt to conserve water. The primary target organ for ADH is the kidney. ADH causes the kidney to reabsorb water from the urine and return it to the blood. By doing so, the amount of urine the kidney excretes decreases; hence the term antidiuretic hormone (*anti-* means "against"; *diuresis* means "urine production").

What is the signal for the release of ADH? ADH is released in response to a concentrated blood, as occurs in dehydration. Blood concentration is increased when either blood volume decreases or the amount of solute in the blood increases. Other triggers for the release of ADH are stress, trauma, and drugs such as morphine. Alcohol, in contrast, inhibits ADH secretion—hence the excessive urination that accompanies beer-drinking!

In the absence of ADH, a profound diuresis occurs, and the person may excrete up to 25 liters of dilute urine per day. This ADH-deficiency disease is called diabetes insipidus and should not be confused with the more common diabetes mellitus, which is an insulin deficiency. (The effect of ADH on the kidney is described in Chapter 24.)

Antidiuretic hormone also causes the blood vessels to constrict, thereby elevating blood pressure. Because of this blood pressure–elevating effect, ADH is also called **vasopressin.** (A vasopressor agent is one that elevates blood pressure.)

Oxytocin

The target organs of **oxytocin** are the uterus and the mammary glands (breasts). Oxytocin stimulates the muscles of the uterus to contract and plays a role in labor and the delivery of a baby. The word oxytocin literally means "swift birth," and an oxytocic drug is one that causes uterine contractions and hastens delivery. You have probably heard of the use of IV "pit" (Pitocin) to initiate labor. Oxytocin also plays a role in breast-feeding. When the baby suckles at the breast, oxytocin is released and stimulates contraction of the smooth muscles around the mammary ducts within the breasts, thereby releasing breast milk. The release of milk in response to suckling is called the milk let-down reflex (this is discussed further in Chapter 27). Oxytocin has recently been dubbed the bonding or relationship hormone; it seems that a high blood level of oxytocin generates feelings of goodwill and an urge to be cooperative, protective, and friendly. Get that in a pill!

A TINY THIRD LOBE

Melanocyte-Stimulating Hormone

While the pituitary gland is divided into two main parts, the anterior and the posterior pituitary, there is a small, third lobe that secretes **melanocyte-stimulating hormone (MSH).** MSH stimulates the melanocytes in the skin, thereby darkening skin color. When MSH is oversecreted, skin color darkens. Exposure to sunlight releases MSH causing the famous summer tan. Adrenal cortical insufficiency also causes a hypersecretion of MSH, causing the person to appear bronzed.

Sum It Up!

The pituitary gland is called the master gland because it controls many other endocrine glands. The anterior pituitary gland (adenohypophysis) is controlled by hypothalamic hormones, called releasing hormones. These hormones are secreted by the hypothalamus into the hypothalamic-hypophyseal portal system. The anterior pituitary gland secretes six major hormones. The posterior pituitary gland is an extension of the hypothalamus and is called the neurohypophysis. The posterior pituitary gland secretes two hormones. Melanocyte-stimulating hormone (MSH) is secreted by a small, third lobe of the pituitary gland.

THYROID GLAND

The **thyroid gland** is the largest of the endocrine glands and is located in the anterior neck; it is situated on the front and sides of the trachea (Figure 14-5, *A*). The thyroid gland is butterfly-shaped and has two lobes connected by a band of tissue called the **isthmus.** The thyroid gland contains two types of cells: the follicular cells, located within the thyroid follicle, and the parafollicular cells, located between the follicles. Each type of cell secretes a particular hormone (Table 14-1).

THYROID FOLLICLE

The thyroid gland is composed of many secretory units called **follicles.** The cavity in each follicle is filled with a clear, viscous substance called **colloid.** Follicular cells secrete two thyroid hormones, **triiodothyronine (T_3)** and **tetraiodothyronine (T_4, or thyroxine).**

WHAT THYROID HORMONES (T_3 AND T_4) DO

The thyroid hormones T_3 and T_4 have similar functions, although T_3 is the more potent. Thyroid hormones regulate all phases of metabolism and are necessary for the proper functioning of all other hormones. Thyroid hormones are necessary for the normal maturation of the nervous system and for normal growth and development. If you were a tadpole, you would require adequate thyroid hormone before you could develop into a frog.

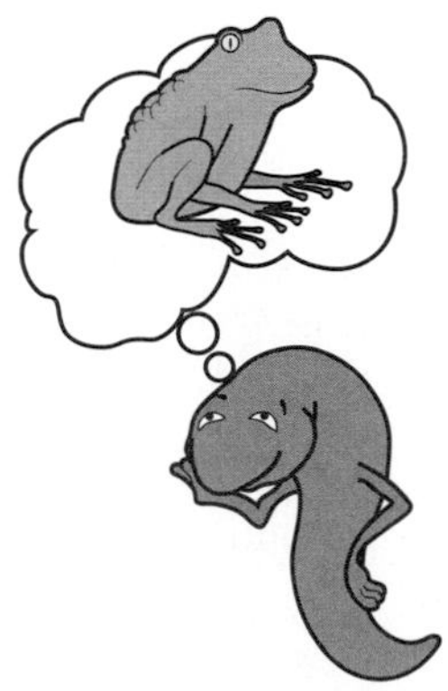

Perhaps the best way to demonstrate the importance of thyroid hormones is to observe the effects of thyroid hormone deficiency (hypothyroidism) and excess (hyperthyroidism).

Hypothyroidism

Hypothyroidism in an adult results in a condition called myxedema. Myxedema is a slowed-down metabolic state characterized by a slow heart rate, sluggish peristalsis resulting in constipation, a low body temperature, low energy, loss of hair, and weight gain. The skin becomes thick and puffy because of the accumulation of a thick fluid under the skin; hence the name myxedema (*myx* means "mucus").

If an infant is born with no thyroid gland, a condition called cretinism develops. An infant with cretinism fails to develop both physically and mentally. The child will be short and stocky with abnormal skeletal development and severe mental retardation. Early diagnosis and prompt treatment with thyroid hormone can prevent further developmental delay.

Hyperthyroidism

An excess of thyroid hormones produces hyperthyroidism, a sped-up metabolic state. A common type of hyperthyroidism is Graves' disease. It is characterized by an increase in heart rate, an increase in peristalsis resulting in diarrhea, elevation in body temperature (heat intolerance), hyperactivity, weight loss, and wide emotional swings. The hyperthyroid person exhibits an increased sensitivity to the effects of catecholamines (epinephrine) and is at risk for the development of rhythm (fast) disorders of the heart. Graves' disease is also characterized by bulging eyes, a condition known as exophthalmia. In exophthalmia, the eyes are thought to bulge because the fat pads behind the eyeballs enlarge, pushing the eyeballs forward in the eye socket. Severe exophthalmia may make it difficult for the patient to close his eyelids over the cornea of the eye; the exposed cornea may then dry out, ulcerate, and scar, leading to a loss of vision.

REGULATION OF SECRETION

The regulation of thyroid gland activity is illustrated in Figure 14-5, *B*. The hypothalamus secretes a releasing hormone, which stimulates the anterior pituitary to secrete TSH. TSH stimulates the thyroid gland to secrete T_3 and T_4. When the plasma levels of the thyroid hormones increase sufficiently, negative feedback prevents further secretion of TSH.

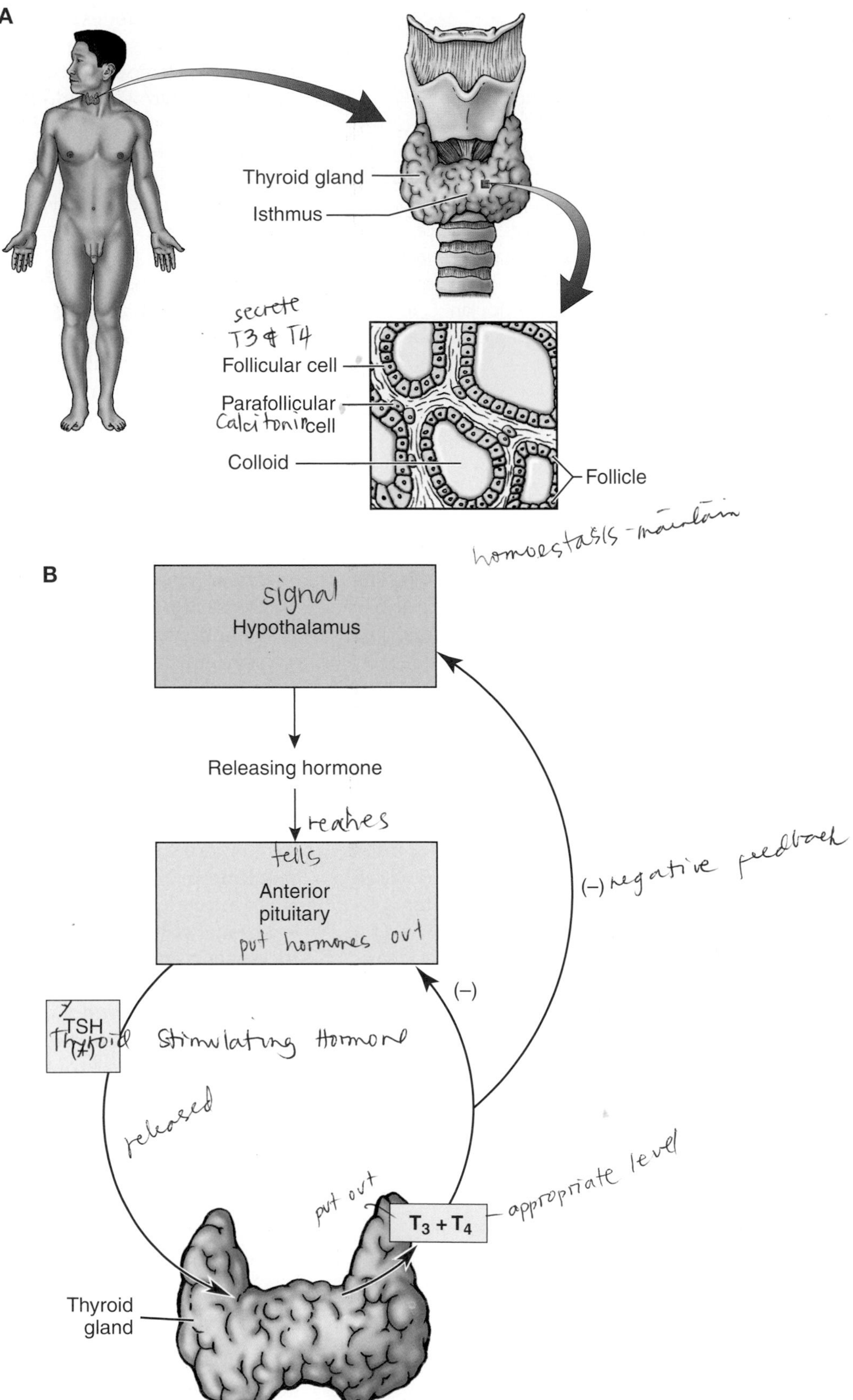

FIGURE 14-5 Thyroid gland. **A,** Location; the thyroid follicle. **B,** Control of the secretion of T_3 and T_4.

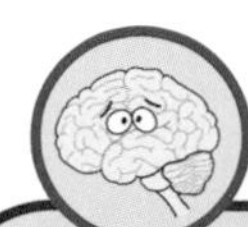

Do You Know...

Why an overactive thyroid gland is hot stuff?

An overactive thyroid gland secretes excess thyroid hormones. Thyroid hormones increase the utilization of oxygen by most cells of the body. As oxygen is used, excess heat is made by the working or metabolizing cells and body temperature rises. The heat-producing effect of the thyroid hormones is called the calorigenic effect and is responsible for the higher body temperature of the hyperthyroid person. Hot stuff, that thyroid disease!

THE NEED FOR IODINE

Synthesis of Thyroid Hormone

The synthesis of T_3 and T_4 requires iodine. The iodine in the body comes from dietary sources. Most of the iodine in the blood is actively pumped into the follicular cells of the thyroid gland, where it is used in the synthesis of the thyroid hormones. Tetraiodothyronine, or thyroxine, contains four iodine atoms and therefore is called T_4. Triiodothyronine contains three iodine atoms and is called T_3.

Iodine Deficiency

Why does an iodine-deficient diet cause the thyroid gland to enlarge? In an iodine-deficient state, the amount of T_3 and T_4 production decreases because iodine is necessary for the synthesis of the thyroid hormones. With insufficient iodine, thyroid hormones cannot be made in quantities great enough to shut off the secretion of TSH through negative feedback. Persistent stimulation of the thyroid gland by TSH causes the thyroid gland to enlarge; an enlarged thyroid gland is called a goiter.

Clinical assessment of thyroid function makes use of the iodine-pumping activity of the gland. For instance, if a patient drinks radioactive iodine (^{131}I) the thyroid gland will pump the radioactive iodine from the blood into the gland. The rate of iodine uptake by the thyroid gland can be determined by a gamma-ray scanner placed over the thyroid gland. Increased iodine uptake is observed in hyperthyroid and iodine-deficient patients, while a decrease in iodine uptake is noted with hypothyroid patients. Larger therapeutic doses of ^{131}I can be used to destroy thyroid tissue in the hyperthyroid state.

CALCITONIN

The parafollicular cells of the thyroid gland secrete a hormone called calcitonin. Although calcitonin is a thyroid hormone, its effects are very different from T_3 and T_4. Calcitonin helps regulate blood levels of calcium. Read on.

PARATHYROID GLANDS

Four tiny **parathyroid glands** lie along the posterior surface of the thyroid gland (Figure 14-6). The parathyroid glands secrete **parathyroid hormone (PTH).** The stimulus for the release of PTH is a low blood level of calcium. PTH has three target organs: bone, digestive tract (intestine), and kidneys. The overall effect of PTH is to increase plasma calcium levels. PTH elevates blood calcium in three ways:

- PTH increases the release of calcium from bone tissue (called resorption). It does so by stimulating osteoclastic (bone-breakdown) activity. In response, calcium moves from the bone to the blood.
- PTH stimulates the kidneys to reabsorb calcium from the urine. At the same time, PTH causes the kidneys to excrete phosphate. The excretion of phosphate by the kidneys is called its phosphaturic effect. The urinary excretion of phosphate is important because of the inverse relationship of phosphate and calcium in the blood. The inverse relationship means that as phosphate levels decrease, calcium levels increase; when phosphate levels increase, calcium levels decrease. Thus, in order to raise blood calcium it is necessary to lower blood phosphate.
- Working with vitamin D, PTH increases the absorption of calcium by the digestive tract (intestine). Thus a vitamin D deficiency can decrease the dietary absorption of calcium.

BLOOD CALCIUM: REGULATION BY PTH AND CALCITONIN

Blood calcium concentration is also regulated by calcitonin. The thyroid gland secretes calcitonin in response to elevated blood levels of calcium. Calcitonin decreases blood calcium primarily by stimulating osteoblastic (bone-making) activity in the bones, thereby moving calcium from the blood into the bone. Calcitonin also increases the excretion of calcium in the urine. In general, calcitonin acts as an antagonist to PTH. Blood calcium levels control the secretion of calcitonin and PTH through negative feedback control. High blood calcium levels stimulate secretion of calcitonin and inhibit secretion of PTH. Low blood calcium levels inhibit secretion of calcitonin and stimulate secretion of PTH.

HYPOSECRETION AND HYPERSECRETION

Hypocalcemia

What is the hand in Figure 14-7 doing? The hand and wrist muscles are contracted and cannot relax, thereby producing a carpal spasm. What causes the

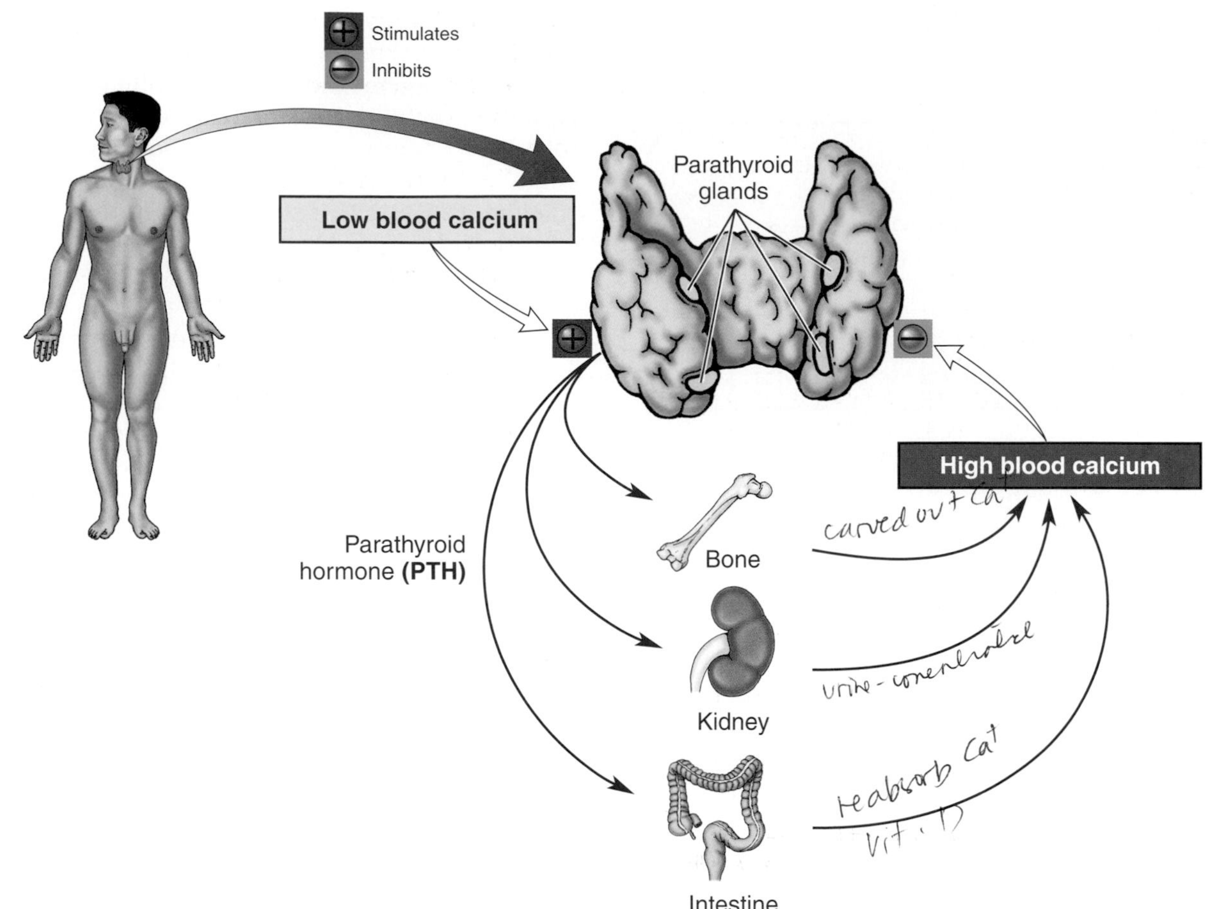

FIGURE 14-6 Parathyroid glands and the three target organs of PTH.

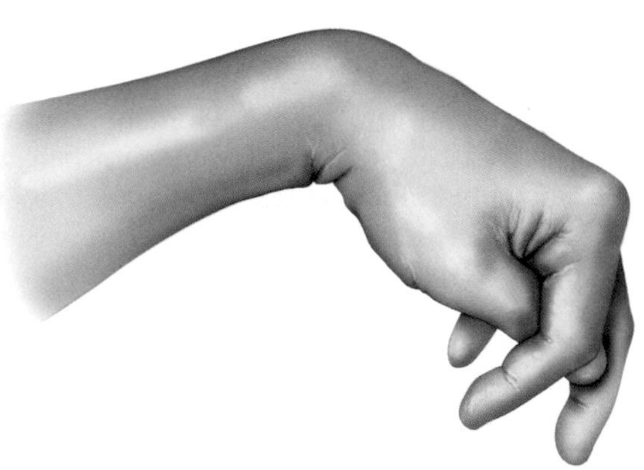

FIGURE 14-7 Carpal spasm.

carpal spasm? Calcium normally stabilizes nerve and muscle membranes. In the absence of sufficient calcium (hypocalcemia) the nerve and muscle membranes become unstable and continuously fire electrical signals, causing the muscles to remain contracted. Sustained skeletal muscle contraction is referred to as tetany. Hypocalcemic tetany not only contorts the wrist; more seriously, it causes sustained contractions of the muscles of the larynx (laryngospasm) and the breathing muscles. Inability of these muscles to relax causes asphyxiation and death. Hypocalcemia is life threatening!

Hypercalcemia

The clinical effects of hypercalcemia are best summarized as: Bones, Stones, Moans, and Groans. The patient develops hyperparathyroidism in response to a tumor in the parathyroid gland. The PTH stimulates osteoclastic activity in the bones, thereby moving calcium from the bones to the blood and causing hypercalcemia. Bone pain results from persistent osteoclastic activity (bones and groans). Hypercalcemia causes excess calcium to be filtered into the urine, causing hypercalciuria; the excess calcium in the urine precipitates out as kidney stones (bones, stones, and groans). Hypercalcemia also depresses the nervous, cardiac, and gastrointestinal systems causing a variety of symptoms including depression (moans), fatigue, bradycardia, anorexia, and constipation. The Groan Zone, indeed!

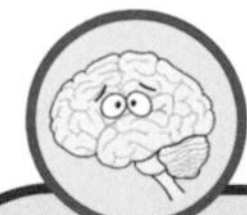

Do You Know...

Why Mr. Graves's face is a-twitching?

Mr. Graves just had a thyroidectomy. As part of his postsurgical care, his nurse periodically tapped the area over the facial nerve. "He is twitching," thought his nurse and immediately reported this observation as a (+) Chvostek's sign. Hyperirritability of the facial nerve occurs when the plasma levels of calcium decrease. Sometimes the parathyroid glands, which are embedded in the thyroid gland, are mistakenly removed or injured during thyroid surgery. If the parathyroid glands are removed, plasma calcium levels decrease because there is no PTH. The nerves become so irritable that they fire continuously, causing continuous muscle contraction (tetany). Unless treated with intravenous calcium, the person may develop a fatal hypocalcemic tetany.

Sum It Up!

The thyroid gland and the parathyroid glands are located in the anterior neck region. The thyroid gland secretes two iodine-containing hormones, T_3 and T_4. These hormones regulate the body's metabolic rate. Excess secretion of T_3 and T_4, called hyperthyroidism, increases the body's metabolic rate. Hypothyroidism causes a hypometabolic state. The thyroid gland also secretes calcitonin, which decreases blood levels of calcium. The parathyroid glands secrete PTH. PTH increases blood calcium levels through its effect on three target organs: bone, kidneys, and digestive tract.

ADRENAL GLANDS

The two small glands located above the kidneys are called **adrenal glands** (*ad* means near; *renal* means kidney) (Figure 14-8, *A*). An adrenal gland consists of two regions: an inner medulla and an outer cortex. The medulla and the cortex secrete different hormones (see Table 14-1).

ADRENAL MEDULLA

The **adrenal medulla** is the inner region of the adrenal gland and is considered an extension of the sympathetic nervous system. Remember that the sympathetic nervous system is called the "fight or flight" system. Chromaffin cells in the adrenal medulla secrete two hormones: epinephrine (adrenaline) and norepinephrine.

Epinephrine and norepinephrine, classified as **catecholamines,** are secreted in emergency or stress situations. You may have heard the expression, "I can feel the adrenaline flowing"; it is another way of saying, "I'm ready to meet the challenge." The catecholamines help the body respond to stress by causing the following effects:

- Elevating blood pressure
- Increasing heart rate
- Converting glycogen to glucose in the liver, thereby making more glucose available to the cells
- Increasing metabolic rate of most cells, thereby making more energy
- Causing bronchodilation (opening up of the breathing passages) to increase the flow of air into the lungs
- Changing blood flow patterns, causing dilation of the blood vessels to the heart and muscles and constriction of the blood vessels to the digestive tract

Occasionally, a person develops a tumor of the adrenal medulla and displays signs and symptoms that resemble sympathetic nervous system excess. The tumor is called a pheochromocytoma; it causes life-threatening high blood pressure. Immediate treatment is directed at lowering the blood pressure. Long-term treatment involves surgical removal of the tumor.

ADRENAL CORTEX

The **adrenal cortex,** the outer region of the adrenal gland (see Figure 14-8, *A*), secretes hormones called steroids. **Steroids** are lipid-soluble hormones made from cholesterol. The adrenal cortex secretes three steroids: glucocorticoids, mineralocorticoids, and sex hormones. Adrenal cortical hormones are essential for life. If the adrenal cortex is removed or its function is lost, death will occur unless steroids are administered. An easy way to remember the functions of the adrenal-cortical steroids is that they regulate sugar, salt, and sex.

Glucocorticoids	**Sugar**
Mineralocorticoids	**Salt**
Sex hormones	**Sex**

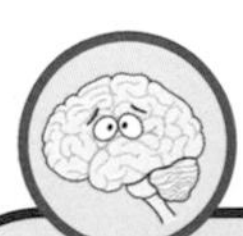

Do You Know...

About 'roid rage?

Bulking up with steroids ("'roids") is costly, physically, emotionally, and socially. Particularly scary is the ability of steroids to foster uncontrollable aggressive behavior, hence the term 'roid rage. 'Roid rage has been implicated in many cases of serious sports-related injuries. The 'roids have also sent many a steroid abuser to prison for fighting, scrapping, brawling, and mauling. Not a pretty picture.

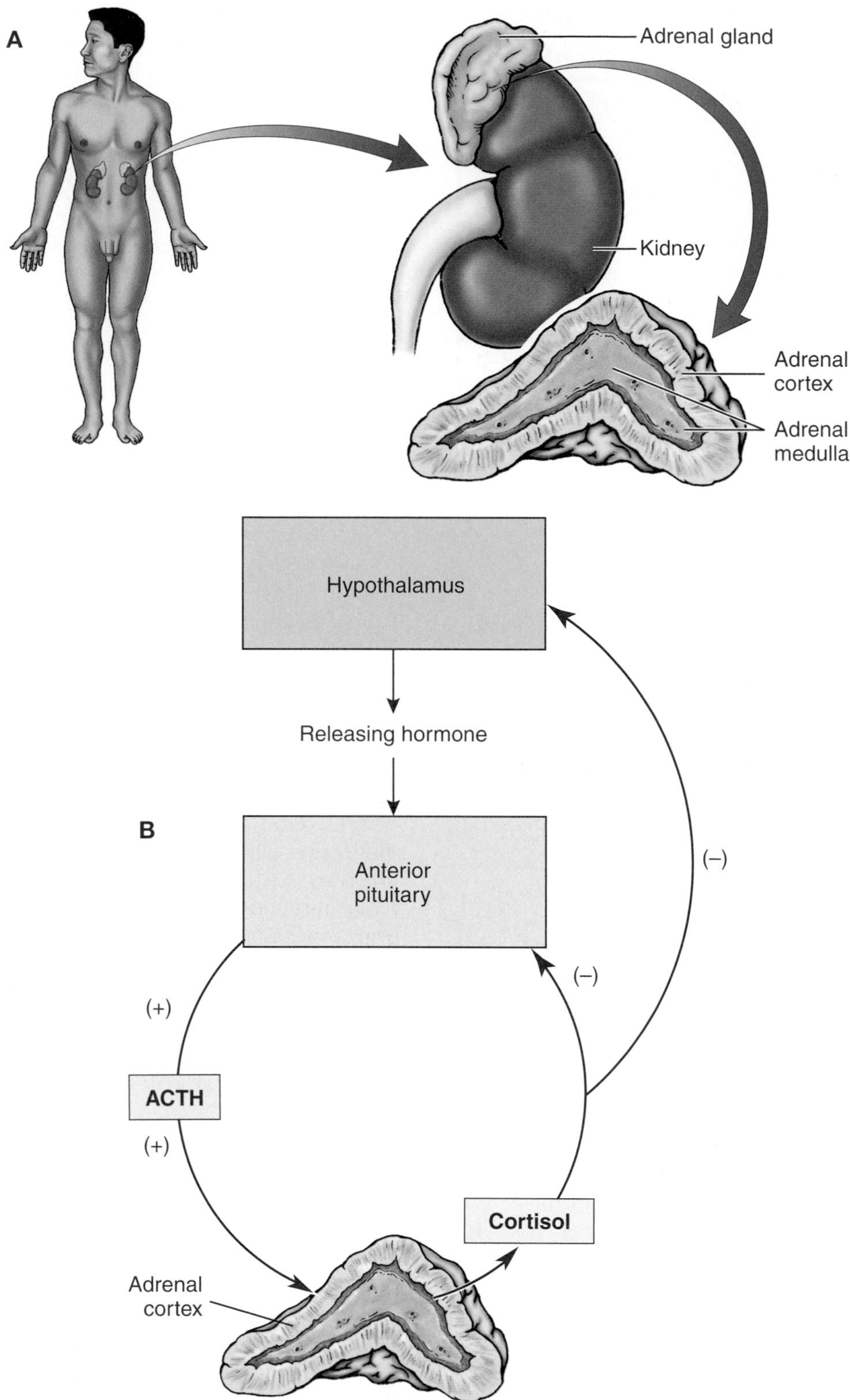

FIGURE 14-8 **A,** The adrenal glands: adrenal medulla and adrenal cortex. **B,** Control of the secretion of cortisol.

Glucocorticoids

As their name implies, the **glucocorticoids** affect carbohydrates. They convert amino acids into glucose (gluconeogenesis) and help maintain blood glucose levels between meals. This action ensures a steady supply of glucose for the brain and other cells. Glucocorticoids also affect protein and fat metabolism, burning both substances as fuel to increase energy production.

The chief glucocorticoid is cortisol. **Cortisol** is a stress hormone in that it is secreted in greater amounts during times of stress. (Stress means physiological stress such as disease, physical injury, hemorrhage, infection, pregnancy, extreme temperature, and emotional stress such as anger and worry.) Cortisol also has an antiinflammatory effect. In other words it prevents injured tissues from responding with the classic signs of inflammation: redness, heat, swelling, and pain. For this reason, cortisol (a cortisol-like drug is prednisone) is used as a drug to prevent inflammation in the treatment of arthritis and severe allergic responses.

Control of Cortisol Secretion. The secretion of cortisol involves the hypothalamus, anterior pituitary gland, and adrenal gland (see Figure 14-8, *B*). The hypothalamus secretes a releasing hormone, which then stimulates the anterior pituitary gland to secrete ACTH. ACTH, in turn, stimulates the adrenal cortex to secrete cortisol. Through negative feedback, the cortisol inhibits the further secretion of ACTH. This process decreases the secretion of cortisol.

Mineralocorticoids

The chief **mineralocorticoid** is **aldosterone.** Aldosterone plays an important role in the regulation of blood volume and blood pressure and in the concentration of electrolytes, especially salt (NaCl). Aldosterone is often called the salt-retaining hormone. The primary target organ of aldosterone is the kidney. Aldosterone reabsorbs sodium and water and eliminates potassium in the urine. The role and regulation of aldosterone is described in Chapter 24.

Sex Hormones

The sex hormones, secreted in small amounts, include the female hormones called estrogens and male hormones called androgens (primarily testosterone). The sex hormones of the ovaries usually mask the effects of the adrenal sex hormones. In females, the masculinizing effects of the adrenal androgens, such as increased body hair, may become evident after menopause, when levels of estrogens from the ovaries decrease.

What's with the cat? His name is Steroid **CAT.** Steroid **CAT** secretes **C**ortisol, **A**ldosterone, and **T**estosterone.

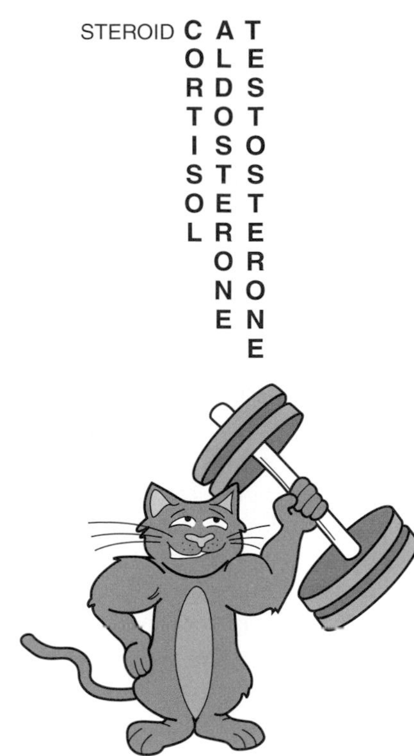

Hyposecretion and Hypersecretion

Hyposecretion. In some persons the adrenal gland fails to secrete adequate amounts of adrenal cortical hormones. This condition is called adrenal cortical insufficiency, or Addison's disease. It is characterized by generalized weakness, muscle atrophy, a bronzing of the skin, and severe loss of fluids and electrolytes. Left untreated, adrenal insufficiency progresses to low blood volume, shock, and death. Adrenal insufficiency is life threatening and must be treated with steroids and replacement of fluids and electrolytes.

Hypersecretion. More commonly, some persons have an excess of adrenal cortical hormones. This condition may be caused by a hypersecretion of either ACTH by the anterior pituitary gland or cortisol by the adrenal cortex. Most often, however, elevated levels of cortisol are due to the administration of steroids as drugs such as prednisone. Elevated blood levels of steroids cause a condition called Cushing's syndrome. It is characterized by trunkal obesity, a rounded facial appearance (moon face), excess fat deposition between the shoulders (buffalo hump), masculinizing effects (virilization), facial hair (hirsutism), thin skin that bruises easily, bone loss, and muscle weakness. Salt and water retention cause blood volume and blood pressure to increase. Prolonged use of steroids causes many harmful effects, particularly in young athletes who take steroids to improve their athletic performance. The price of enhanced athletic performance is high. Severe and irreversible health problems, such as cancer, osteoporosis (bone softening), gonadal atrophy, sterility, and mental illness are possible complications. Don't do it!

The Case of the Lazy Gland. The effects of steroid drugs on adrenal cortical function provide a dramatic example of negative feedback control. Consider this situation: a patient is given prednisone (cortisol) as a drug for the treatment of arthritis. As blood cortisol levels rise, the secretion of ACTH is inhibited by negative feedback. In the absence of ACTH, the adrenal gland becomes "lazy" and stops its production of cortisol. As long as the person continues to take the prednisone, blood cortisol levels remain high. If, however, the person suddenly discontinues the drug, the "lazy" adrenal gland no longer produces cortisol, and the person eventually develops acute adrenal insufficiency and will die unless treated. (Remember! Steroids are essential for life.) Because of lazy adrenal function, steroid drugs are never discontinued abruptly; dosage is tapered off over an extended period. This gradual reduction in drug dose gives the lazy gland time to recover and regain its ability to respond to ACTH.

Sum It Up!

The adrenal glands are composed of the medulla and the cortex; both secrete stress hormones. The adrenal medulla is an extension of the sympathetic nervous system ("fight or flight") and secretes two catecholamines called epinephrine (adrenaline) and norepinephrine. The adrenal cortex secretes three steroids: the glucocorticoids (cortisol); the mineralocorticoids (aldosterone); and the sex hormones. The adrenal cortex is controlled by a hypothalamic-releasing hormone and ACTH from the anterior pituitary gland. The functions of the adrenal cortex are concerned with the regulation of sugar, salt, and sex.

PANCREAS

The **pancreas** (PĂN-krē-ăs) is a long, slender organ that lies transversely across the upper abdomen, extending from the curve of the duodenum to the spleen (see Figure 14-1). The pancreas functions as both an exocrine gland and an endocrine gland. (Its exocrine function is concerned with the digestion of food and is discussed in Chapter 23.)

The pancreas secretes two hormones, insulin and glucagon. Consult Ms. PIG in Figure 14-9; she will help remind you the **p**ancreas secretes **i**nsulin and **g**lucagon. The hormone-secreting cells of the pancreas are called the **islets of Langerhans.** The islets of Langerhans have two types of cells: the **alpha cells,** which secrete glucagon, and the **beta cells,** which secrete insulin. Both insulin and glucagon help regulate blood glucose levels.

INSULIN

Secretion and Effects

Figure 14-9 illustrates the relationship of the blood glucose to the pancreatic hormones. **Insulin** is released in response to increased blood levels of glucose as occurs following a meal. The secretion of insulin decreases as blood levels of glucose decrease. Insulin has many target tissues and therefore exerts widespread effects.

- Insulin helps transport glucose into most cells. Without insulin, glucose remains outside the cells, thereby depriving the cell of its fuel. (The liver and brain do not require insulin for glucose transport.)
- Insulin helps control carbohydrate, protein, and fat metabolism in the cell. Insulin stimulates the breakdown of glucose (glycolysis) for energy and stimulates the liver and skeletal muscles to store excess glucose as glycogen (glycogenesis). Insulin also increases the transport of amino acids into cells and then stimulates the synthesis of protein from the amino acids. Lastly, insulin promotes the making of fats from fatty acids.

Insulin and Blood Glucose

Insulin decreases blood glucose levels for two reasons. First, insulin increases transport of glucose from the blood into the cells. Second, insulin stimulates the cells to burn glucose as fuel. **Insulin is the only hormone that lowers blood glucose.** All other hormones increase glucose levels.

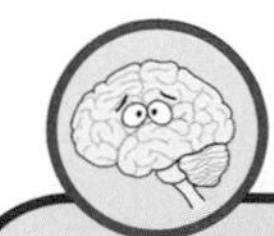

Do You Know...

Why some diabetic persons require an injection of insulin while others can take a pill?

Some diabetic persons require insulin injections, and others control their diabetes with a pill. The difference is that the pancreas of a person with severe diabetes produces no insulin, so this person must receive insulin injections. These people have insulin-dependent diabetes. In contrast, the pancreas of a person with another form of diabetes may still be able to produce some insulin. This person may not require insulin injections and may benefit from oral medication. Some diabetic pills work by stimulating the person's pancreas to produce more insulin. Others work by preventing the hepatic (liver) synthesis of glucose. A person with diabetes who does not require insulin injections is considered to have non–insulin-dependent diabetes.

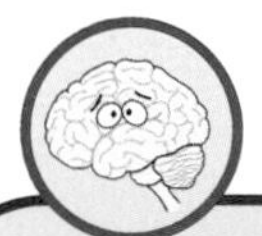

Do You Know...

How one rebounds with Somogyi?

A diabetic person takes insulin to lower his or her blood glucose. If too much insulin is taken, blood glucose becomes too low (hypoglycemia). The hypoglycemia, in turn, stimulates the secretion of glucose-elevating hormones such as glucagon and cortisol; this causes hyperglycemia. The hyperglycemia requires additional insulin to lower blood glucose. The additional insulin causes hypoglycemia. A vicious cycle of hypoglycemia and hyperglycemia occurs. The Somogyi effect is a rebound phenomenon where hypoglycemia is followed by hyperglycemia as a result of an overreaction to the low blood sugar.

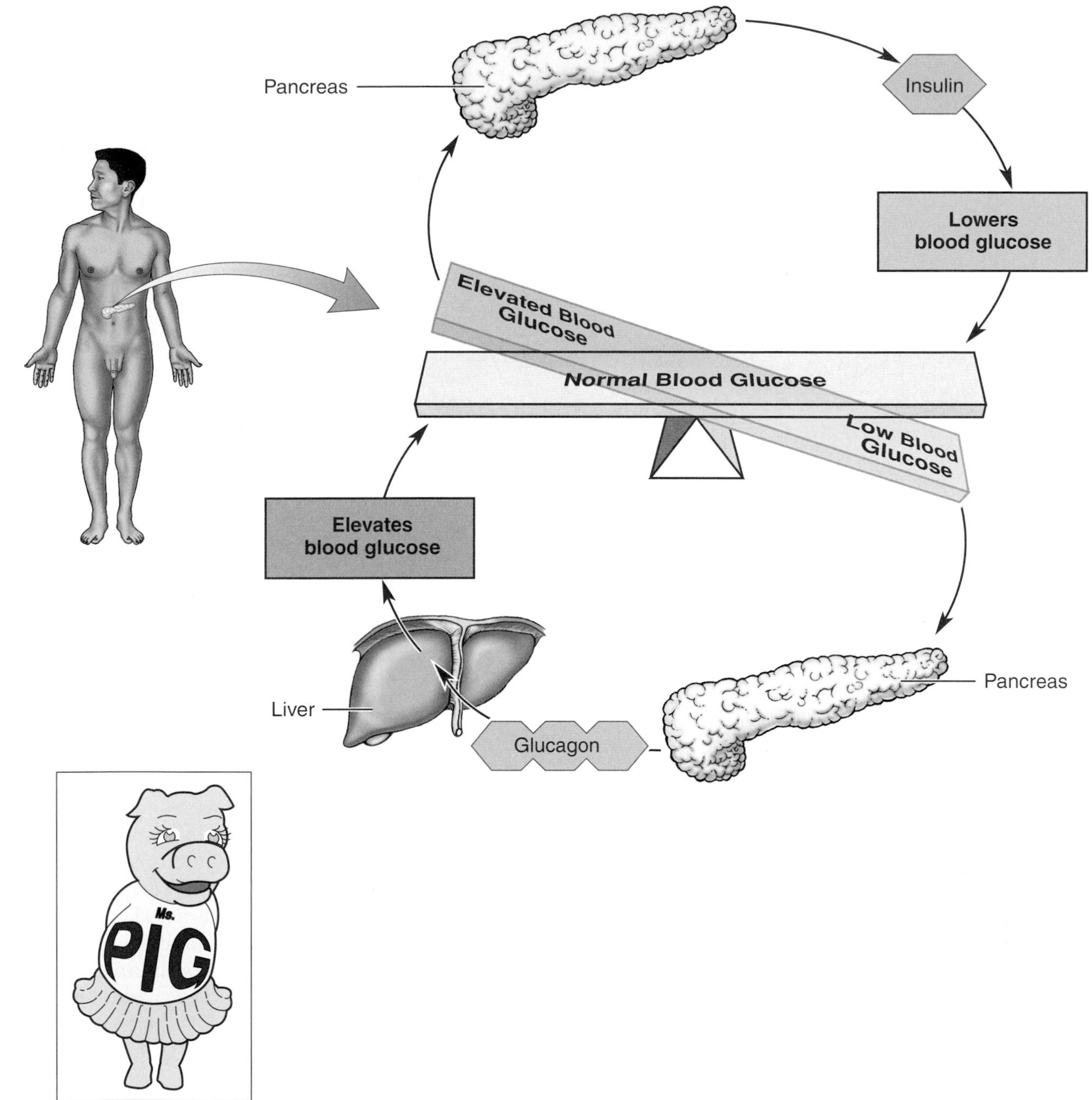

FIGURE 14-9 Regulation of blood glucose by the pancreas: insulin and glucagon.

Diabetes Mellitus: "A Melting Down of the Flesh and Limbs into Urine"

Because insulin plays such an important role in the metabolism of all types of foods (carbohydrates, proteins, and fats), a deficiency of insulin causes severe metabolic disturbances. Insulin deficiency or insulin ineffectiveness is called diabetes mellitus. Before insulin therapy was discovered, diabetes mellitus was described as a "melting down of the flesh and the limbs into urine." This description attests to the devastating effects of untreated juvenile-onset diabetes mellitus. The child took one year to literally "melt away." Read on to understand the physiologic effects of insulin deficiency; note specifically the three "polys" of diabetes mellitus: polyuria, polydipsia, and polyphagia.

- Hyperglycemia: Excess glucose in the blood is called hyperglycemia. This condition is due to two factors. The first is the inability of glucose to enter the cells, where it can be burned for energy. Failure to move the glucose into the cells causes it to accumulate in the blood. The second is the making of additional glucose. In the absence of insulin, the body makes glucose from protein (gluconeogenesis). The excess glucose cannot be used by the cells and therefore accumulates in the blood. In essence, the diabetic body converts its tissue to glucose that it cannot burn as fuel and then eliminates it in the urine. The body is "starving in the midst of plenty" (of glucose).

- Glucosuria or glycosuria: Glucose in the urine is called glucosuria or glycosuria. The hyperglycemia causes more glucose to be eliminated in the urine.
- Polyuria: Excretion of a large volume of urine is called polyuria. Whenever the kidney excretes a lot of glucose, it must also excrete a lot of water. Glucosuria therefore causes polyuria.
- Polydipsia: Excessive thirst is called polydipsia. Polyuria causes an excessive loss of body water, thereby stimulating the thirst mechanism in an attempt to replace the water lost in the urine.
- Polyphagia: Polyphagia refers to excessive eating. Despite plenty of glucose in the blood, the cells cannot use it; instead, the diabetic eats excessive amounts of food to fuel the cells.
- Acidosis: An excess of H^+ in the blood causes acidosis. Because the cells cannot burn glucose as fuel, they burn fatty acids instead. The rapid, incomplete breakdown of fatty acids produces strong acids (H^+) called ketoacids. This process causes a condition called diabetic ketoacidosis.

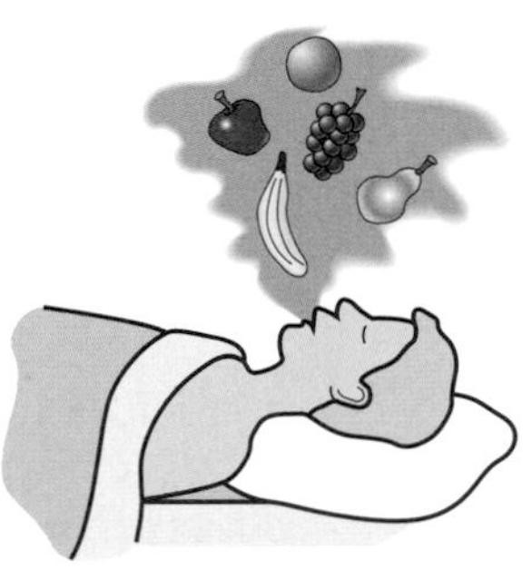

- Fruity odor to the breath: The rapid, incomplete breakdown of fatty acids causes the formation of acetone, a ketone body. Acetone smells fruity and makes the patient's breath smell like rotten apples. A fruity odor is a sign of ketoacidosis. Treatment of diabetic ketoacidosis requires the prompt administration of insulin and the correction of the fluid and electrolyte disturbances.

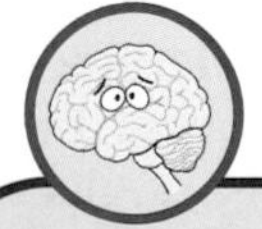

Do You Know...

Why your diabetic patients may soon be taking "lizard spit"?

The saliva of some lizards contains a blood glucose–lowering substance. If this substance can be turned into a pill, it will almost certainly be used as a hypoglycemic agent in the treatment of diabetes mellitus.

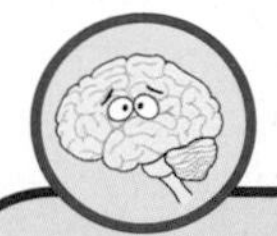

Do You Know...

Why you don't die of hypoglycemia between meals?

After you eat a meal, the blood level of glucose rises as the food products are absorbed from the digestive tract into the blood. The increased blood glucose level signals the release of insulin; the insulin then causes the blood glucose level to decrease. As the blood glucose levels decrease, however, insulin secretion decreases and other hormones such as growth hormone, epinephrine, and cortisol are secreted. These other hormones antagonize the effects of insulin by increasing blood glucose and preventing fatal hypoglycemia. Thus you can fast for several weeks and not become hypoglycemic! Chances are that you will not die from fasting—it will only feel as if you are dying!

Insulin Receptors and the Diabetic State

As indicated above, diabetes mellitus can be caused by a lack of insulin. Some diabetics (called adult-onset, or type 2 diabetes mellitus), however, have excess insulin (hyperinsulinemia) and are still hyperglycemic. What's that about? Under normal conditions, insulin binds to the insulin receptors on the cell membrane. What if:

- The insulin receptors are damaged? The damaged receptors cannot respond to the insulin and the person becomes hyperglycemic. The hyperglycemia then triggers the release of additional insulin and the person becomes hyperinsulinemic.
- There is a diminished number of receptors? The number of insulin receptors on the membrane can increase or decrease. Obesity and lack of exercise can cause the number of insulin receptors to decrease. This means that obese people can secrete plenty of insulin, but their cells cannot respond to that insulin. The good news is that weight loss and exercise increase the number of insulin receptors, thereby improving the insulin response and relieving the symptoms of diabetes.
- Excess fat (adipose) tissue secretes hormones that oppose the effects of insulin? The cytokines, especially resistin, antagonize insulin, causing a state of insulin resistance.

Needless to say, there is a strong link between insulin resistance, obesity, and diabetes. A new term, metabolic syndrome, addresses this issue.

GLUCAGON

Glucagon, a second pancreatic hormone, is secreted by the alpha cells of the islets of Langerhans. Its primary action is to increase blood glucose levels (Figure 14-9). Glucagon raises blood glucose in two ways: by stimulating the conversion of glycogen to glucose in the liver and by stimulating the conversion of proteins into glucose (gluconeogenesis). Both these processes ensure a supply of glucose for the busy cells. Because of its effect on blood glucose, glucagon is used clinically to treat hypoglycemia, low blood glucose. The stimulus for the release of glucagon is a decrease in blood levels of glucose.

Do You Know...

Who is Dawn and what is her phenomenon?

Dawn refers to the early morning hours, as in sunrise. Diabetics are often hyperglycemic in the early morning hours (at dawn), despite insulin therapy and the lack of food intake during the night. This is what happens. Throughout the night the person secretes growth hormone (GH). GH increases blood glucose (gluconeogenesis) and accounts for the early morning hyperglycemia. An adjustment in the timing of insulin therapy corrects the dawn phenomenon.

Glucagon, Infection, and Diabetes. A patient with diabetes is prone to infection. Infection increases glucagon secretion as well as the secretion of all stress hormones, including epinephrine, cortisol, and growth hormone. All of these hormones elevate blood glucose, causing hyperglycemia. Thus diabetic people with an infection always have difficulty in controlling their blood glucose; they require frequent blood glucose monitoring and additional insulin.

Sum It Up!

A number of hormones, particularly those secreted by the pancreas, regulate blood glucose levels. Insulin works in two ways to decrease blood glucose levels: first, it increases the transport of glucose from the blood into the cells, and second, it stimulates the cells to burn glucose as fuel. Glucagon antagonizes the effects of insulin by increasing blood glucose levels. Note: Insulin is the only hormone that decreases blood glucose levels.

GONADS

The **gonads** are the sex glands and refer to the **ovaries** in the female and to the **testes** in the male. The gonads not only produce ova (eggs) and sperm but also secrete hormones. The gonads are therefore glands. The ovaries secrete two female sex hormones: estrogen and progesterone. A female appears female (i.e., size, hair, and fat distribution) primarily because of estrogen. The testes secrete testosterone; a male appears male primarily because of testosterone. (Reproductive anatomy and physiology are discussed in Chapters 26 and 27.)

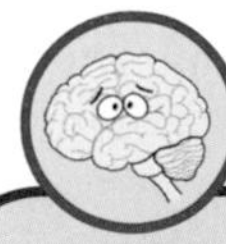

Do You Know...

When diabetes is called "insipidus"?

"Yuck! This urine is tasteless . . . it's insipid!" growled the physician as he sipped his patient's urine. What is going on here? This patient has diabetes insipidus, a condition that is due to a deficiency of antidiuretic hormone (ADH) and characterized by the excretion of a large amount of pale dilute urine.

In the good old days, physicians commonly tasted the patient's urine as a way to diagnose disease. The pale, dilute urine of ADH deficiency is tasteless, in contrast to the sweet-tasting urine of a patient with insulin deficiency, or "sugar" diabetes. The word *diabetes* refers to diuresis (increased flow of urine), whereas the words *insipidus* and *mellitus* refer to the taste of the urine. Fortunately, and none too soon, the "Taste Bud Assay" has given way to modern lab tests.

THYMUS GLAND

The **thymus gland** lies in the thoracic cavity behind the sternum. The thymus gland is much larger in a child than in an adult. The gland involutes, or becomes smaller, as the child enters puberty. The thymus gland secretes hormones called **thymosins,** which play a role in the immune system (described in Chapter 21).

PINEAL GLAND

The **pineal** (pĭ-NĒ-ăl) **gland** is a cone-shaped gland located close to the thalamus in the brain. It has been called the body's "biological clock," controlling many of the biorhythms. The pineal gland secretes a hormone called **melatonin.** Melatonin affects the reproductive cycle by influencing the secretion of hypothalamic-releasing hormones. In general, melatonin plays an important role in sexual maturation.

Melatonin is also thought to play a role in the sleep-wake cycle. The amount of melatonin secreted is related to the amount of daylight. Melatonin secretion is lowest during daylight hours and highest at night. As melatonin levels increase, the person becomes sleepy. Melatonin is therefore said to have a tranquilizing effect. Persons who work night shifts and sleep during the day have a reversed cycle of melatonin production. The reversal of the melatonin cycle is related to the fatigue experienced by night-shift workers. Elevated melatonin levels have also been implicated in a type of depression called seasonal affective disorder (SAD). This condition occurs primarily in parts of the world where daylight hours are short in the winter, usually in areas far north and far south.

OTHER HORMONES

ORGAN-SPECIFIC HORMONES

The glands identified in Figure 14-1 make up the endocrine system, but numerous hormone-secreting cells are scattered throughout the body. These hormones usually control the activities of a particular organ. For instance, hormone-secreting cells in the digestive tract secrete cholecystokinin and gastrin. These hormones help regulate digestion. The kidneys secrete erythropoietin, which helps regulate red blood cell production. (These hormones are described in later chapters.)

PROSTAGLANDINS

The **prostaglandins** are hormones derived from a fatty acid called arachidonic acid. The prostaglandins are produced by many tissues and generally act near their site of secretion. The prostaglandins play an important role in the regulation of smooth-muscle contraction and the inflammatory response. Prostaglandins are also thought to increase the sensitivity of nerve endings to pain. Drugs such as aspirin and ibuprofen block the synthesis of prostaglandins and are therefore useful in relieving pain and inflammation.

ADIPOSE TISSUE HORMONES

Excess adipose tissue acts as a gland—a very nasty gland—that secretes hormones called cytokines. First, a word about fat; there is bad fat and worse fat. How so? There's the bad fat that collects around the thighs, giving the person a pear-shaped appearance. There's also a worse fat that collects around the abdominal area ("ab flab") creating an apple shape. The apple shape is also associated with excess visceral fat (surrounding the organs).

The Tab of Ab Flab

It's high, with regard to heart disease, diabetes mellitus, cancer, and joint disease. Read on!

Heart and Blood Vessels. Most believe that obesity is a risk for heart disease merely because excess weight overburdens the heart. While this is true, excess adipose tissue, through its cytokines, affects the heart and blood vessels in other ways. For instance, adipose tissue contains many narrow blood vessels; in fact, miles of additional blood vessels may be required to carry blood throughout the excess fat. The additional narrowed blood vessels increase blood pressure and strain the heart. Adipose tissue secretes many chemicals, called cytokines, that cause the blood vessels to become even more narrow. The cytokines also stimulate the immune system, causing inflammation, an important risk factor for heart disease. In fact, inflammation plays a larger role in heart attacks than does the narrowing of the coronary (heart) arteries by cholesterol. The cytokines also stimulate blood clotting. Blood clots, in turn, impair blood flow to the heart and brain, thereby predisposing the obese person to heart attack and stroke.

Diabetes Mellitus. Adipose tissue secretes several cytokines that adversely affect glucose metabolism and predispose the person to type 2 diabetes mellitus. First, the cytokines oppose the action of insulin, thereby decreasing the transport of glucose into the cells. Secondly, the cytokines stimulate the liver to make excess glucose. Both these actions increase blood glucose, causing hyperglycemia, a hallmark of diabetes mellitus. In short, cytokines make the obese person insulin resistant.

Cancer. Fat cells secrete estrogen, a hormone that has been linked to several types of cancer, especially breast cancer.

Joint Disease. The added body weight puts additional stress on joints such as the knees. The joints simply cannot support the extra weight.

So, lose the potato chips, get off the couch, and exercise!

Sum It Up!

The gonads are glands that include the ovaries in the female and the testes in the male. The ovaries secrete estrogens and progesterone. The testes secrete testosterone. Other endocrine glands include the thymus and the pineal gland. The thymus gland plays an important role in the immune response. The pineal gland is thought to be the body's "biological clock," affecting reproduction and biorhythms. Other hormone-secreting cells are scattered throughout the body. Prostaglandins are chemical mediators of pain and inflammation. Excess adipose tissue functions as a nasty endocrine gland that contributes to the development of heart disease, diabetes, cancer, and joint disease.

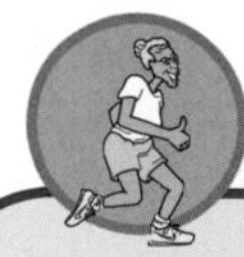

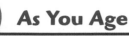

As You Age

1. In general, age-related endocrine changes include an alteration in the secretion of hormones, the circulating levels of hormones, the metabolism of hormones, and the biological activity of hormones.
2. Although most glands decrease their levels of secretion, normal aging does not lead to deficiency states. For instance, while adrenal cortical secretion of cortisol decreases, negative feedback mechanisms maintain normal plasma levels of the hormones, thereby preserving water and electrolyte homeostasis.
3. Changes in the thyroid gland cause a decrease in the secretion of thyroid hormones, thereby decreasing metabolic rate.
4. Decreased secretion of growth hormone causes a decrease in muscle mass and an increase in storage of fat.
5. A diminishment of circadian control of hormone secretion occurs.

Disorders of the Endocrine System

Acromegaly	Excess secretion of growth hormone in the adult.
Addison's disease	A deficiency of adrenal cortical hormones. If untreated, the patient may develop life-threatening adrenal shock.
Cretinism	A deficiency of thyroid hormone during fetal development, causing a profound physical and mental developmental delay.
Cushing's syndrome	Excess secretion of adrenal cortical hormones. Cushing's syndrome is also present in patients who take steroids as a medication.
Diabetes insipidus	A deficiency of antidiuretic hormone (ADH), causing the patient to urinate approximately 5 to 6 L of pale, dilute urine per day.
Diabetes mellitus	A deficiency of insulin. The deficiency affects carbohydrate, protein, and fat metabolism. If untreated, the patient develops diabetic ketoacidosis, profound dehydration, and shock. There are several types of diabetes mellitus (DM) and millions of cases; it is epidemic in the United States. Type 1 DM, also called juvenile-onset diabetes, usually develops in children and must be treated with insulin. Type 2 DM is called adult-onset diabetes. The typical adult-onset diabetic is older, obese, and sedentary. Type 2 DM is often treated with oral hypoglycemic agents but may require insulin injections. Gestational diabetes mellitus refers to the appearance of diabetic symptoms only during pregnancy. The symptoms usually subside when the baby is delivered. Unfortunately, in the United States type 2 is developing in children. The development of MODY (maturity-onset diabetes in youth) is related to lifestyle (diet, exercise, obesity).
Gigantism	Excess secretion of growth hormone in a child, usually caused by a pituitary tumor. A deficiency of growth hormone in a child causes pituitary dwarfism.
Goiter	An enlargement of the thyroid gland. A toxic goiter is an enlargement that secretes excess thyroid hormones and produces symptoms of hyperthyroidism. A nontoxic goiter or iodine-deficiency goiter does not produce excess thyroid hormones and therefore is not accompanied by symptoms of hyperthyroidism.
Graves' disease	A form of hyperthyroidism. The hypersecretion of thyroid hormones, T_3 and T_4 causes an increase in metabolism. A severe episode of hyperthyroidism is called thyroid storm, a condition that can exhaust the body and cause the heart to fail.
Metabolic syndrome	A cluster of symptoms that occur primarily in obese and sedentary persons. The signs and symptoms include insulin resistance/hyperglycemia, hypertension, and decreased "good" cholesterol.
Myxedema	A deficiency of thyroid hormone in adults. The deficiency causes a decrease in metabolism.
Tetany	A deficiency of parathyroid hormone (PTH) that results in low plasma levels of calcium. The hypocalcemia, in turn, causes neuromuscular hyperactivity and sustained muscle contraction (tetanus).

SUMMARY OUTLINE

The endocrine system and the nervous system are the two major communicating and coordinating systems in the body. The endocrine system communicates through chemical signals called hormones.

I. Hormones

A. Classification of Hormones
1. Hormones are secreted by endocrine glands directly into the blood.
2. Hormones are classified as proteins (protein-related substances) and steroids.

B. Hormone Receptors
1. Hormones are aimed at receptors of target organs.
2. Receptors are located on the outer surface of the membrane or inside the cell.
3. Hormone secretion is controlled by three mechanisms: negative feedback control, biorhythms, and control by the central nervous system.

II. Pituitary Gland

A. Hypothalamic-Hypophyseal Portal System
1. The portal system is a system of capillaries that connects the hypothalamus and the anterior pituitary.
2. The portal system transports releasing hormones from the hypothalamus to the anterior pituitary gland.

B. Hormones of the Anterior Pituitary Gland
1. Growth hormone stimulates growth and maintains blood glucose during periods of fasting.
2. Prolactin (lactogenic hormone) stimulates milk production by the breasts.
3. Tropic hormones stimulate other glands to secrete hormones. These include thyrotropin, adrenocorticotropic hormone, and the gonadotropins.
4. Thyroid-stimulating hormone stimulates the thyroid gland.
5. Adrenocorticotropic hormone (ACTH) stimulates the adrenal cortex.
6. The gonadotropic hormones stimulate the gonads (ovaries and testes).

C. Hormones of the Posterior Pituitary Gland
1. Antidiuretic hormone (ADH) stimulates the kidney to reabsorb water.
2. Oxytocin stimulates the uterine muscle to contract for labor and stimulates the breast to release milk during suckling (milk let-down reflex).

D. A tiny, third lobe secretes melanocyte-stimulating hormone.

III. Other Endocrine Glands

A. Thyroid Gland
1. The follicular cells synthesize triiodothyronine (T_3) and tetraiodothyronine, or thyroxine (T_4). T_3 and T_4 regulate metabolic rate.
2. The parafollicular cells secrete calcitonin. Calcitonin lowers blood calcium.

B. Parathyroid Glands
1. The parathyroid glands secrete parathyroid hormone (PTH).
2. PTH stimulates the bones, kidneys, and intestines to increase blood calcium levels.

C. Adrenal Gland
1. The adrenal medulla secretes the catecholamines epinephrine and norepinephrine and causes the “fight or flight” response.
2. The adrenal cortex secretes the steroids: glucocorticoids, mineralocorticoids, and sex hormones.

D. Pancreas
1. The pancreas secretes insulin and glucagon.
2. Insulin lowers blood glucose while glucagon increases blood glucose.

E. Gonads
1. The ovaries are stimulated by the gonadotropins and secrete estrogens and progesterone.
2. The testes are stimulated by the gonadotropins and secrete testosterone.

F. Thymus Gland: plays an important role in the immune response

G. Pineal Gland: houses the “biological clock” and secretes melatonin

H. Other hormones include organ-specific hormones (cholecystokinin), prostaglandins, and hormones of adipose tissue.

Review Your Knowledge

Matching: Glands

Directions: Match the following words with their descriptions below. Some words may be used more than once.

a. pancreas
b. adrenal cortex
c. anterior pituitary gland
d. adrenal medulla
e. thyroid gland
f. parathyroid glands
g. posterior pituitary gland
h. hypothalamus

1. ____ Contains the beta cells of the islets of Langerhans
2. ____ Secrete glucocorticoids, mineralocorticoids, and androgens
3. ____ Its hormonal secretion is controlled by ACTH
4. ____ Secretes iodine-containing hormones
5. ____ Secretes releasing hormones
6. ____ Secretes ACTH, TSH, prolactin, growth hormone, and the gonadotropins
7. ____ Its hormone moves calcium from the bone to the blood
8. ____ Secretes both insulin and glucagon
9. ____ Part of the "fight or flight" system; secretes catecholamines
10. ____ The neurohypophysis; secretes ADH and oxytocin

Matching: Hormones

Directions: Match the following words with their descriptions below. Some words may be used more than once.

a. aldosterone
b. insulin
c. prolactin
d. growth hormone
e. parathyroid hormone
f. epinephrine
g. T_3 and T_4
h. oxytocin
i. ACTH
j. ADH

1. ____ Stimulates osteoclastic activity to increase blood calcium
2. ____ Regulates metabolic rate
3. ____ Lowers blood glucose
4. ____ Cortisol is released in response to this hormone
5. ____ Stimulates the breast to produce milk
6. ____ Catecholamine that participates in the "fight or flight" response
7. ____ The neurohypophyseal hormone that controls water balance
8. ____ Prednisone (Cortisol) shuts down the secretion of this adenohypophyseal hormone
9. ____ Also called somatotropic hormone
10. ____ The mineralocorticoid that is called the salt-retaining hormone

Multiple Choice

1. Which of the following is true about cortisol?
   a. It is a catecholamine.
   b. It is secreted by the adrenal cortex in response to ACTH.
   c. It stimulates the secretion of ACTH.
   d. It is released by the adrenal medulla in response to sympathetic nerve stimulation.
2. Aldosterone is
   a. a mineralocorticoid secreted by the adrenal cortex.
   b. the primary regulator of blood glucose.
   c. an adenohypophyseal hormone that stimulates the adrenal cortex to secrete cortisol.
   d. a neurohypophyseal hormone that causes the kidneys to reabsorb water.
3. The pancreas
   a. secretes steroids that are concerned with sugar, salt, and sex.
   b. is controlled by a hormone secreted by the anterior pituitary gland.
   c. secretes both insulin and glucagon.
   d. secretes hormones that only lower blood glucose.
4. Which of the following best describes the function of insulin?
   a. Regulates blood volume
   b. Stimulates cells to make glucose (gluconeogenesis)
   c. Causes ketone body formation and acidosis
   d. Lowers blood glucose
5. As plasma levels of calcium decrease
   a. insulin is secreted.
   b. the parathyroid glands secrete calcitonin.
   c. the kidneys excrete calcium and phosphorus.
   d. PTH is secreted, thereby stimulating osteoclastic activity.
6. Hypocalcemic tetany is
   a. a consequence of a deficiency of PTH.
   b. caused by calcitonin deficiency.
   c. a consequence of osteoclastic activity.
   d. of concern because it causes osteoporosis.

CHAPTER 15

Blood

KEY TERMS

Albumin, p. 263
Anemia, p. 264
Basophil, p. 271
Coagulation, p. 273
Eosinophil, p. 271
Erythrocyte, p. 264
Erythropoietin, p. 267
Fibrin, p. 273
Hematocrit, p. 264
Hematopoiesis, p. 264
Hemoglobin, p. 266
Hemolysis, p. 277
Hemostasis, p. 273
Leukocyte, p. 264
Lymphocyte, p. 264
Monocyte, p. 264
Neutrophil, p. 269
Plasma, p. 263
Platelet, p. 264
Red blood cell, p. 264
Reticulocyte, p. 266
Serum, p. 264
Thrombocyte, p. 264
White blood cell, p. 264

OBJECTIVES

1. Describe three functions of blood.
2. Describe the composition of blood.
3. Describe the three types of blood cells: erythrocytes, leukocytes, and thrombocytes.
4. Explain the formation of blood cells.
5. Explain the breakdown of red blood cells and the formation of bilirubin.
6. Identify the steps of hemostasis.
7. Describe the four blood types.
8. Describe the Rh factor.

Long before modern medicine, blood was viewed as the part of the body that possessed the life force. This belief arose from the observation that severe bleeding episodes often ended in death, suggesting that the life force flowed out of the body with the blood. Blood was also credited with determining personality traits and emotions. For instance, the wealthy were called bluebloods. Feuding groups often attributed the cause of the troubled relationship to bad blood. Anger was said to cause the blood to boil, while fear could generate blood-curdling screams. The qualities of blood seemed so magical that a sharing of a few drops of blood could make one's friend a blood brother. Although we no longer speak of blood in such terms, we do recognize that an adequate blood supply is essential for life. We are still fascinated by blood and have a fancy word for its study: **hematology.**

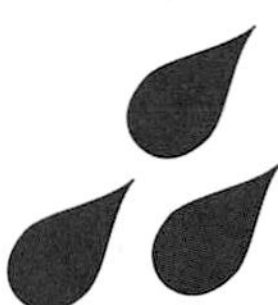

Blood flows through a closed system of blood vessels. The force that pushes the blood through the vessels is the pumping action of the heart (see Chapter 16).

WHAT BLOOD DOES

Blood performs three general functions: transport, regulation, and protection. First, the blood transports many substances around the body. For instance, blood delivers oxygen from the lungs to every cell in the body. Blood picks up waste material from the cells and delivers the waste to organs that eliminate it from the body. Nutrients, ions, hormones, and many other substances use blood as the vehicle for movement throughout the body. Second, blood participates in the regulation of fluid and electrolyte balance, acid-base balance, and body temperature. Third, blood helps protect the body from infection. Blood also contains clotting factors, which help protect the body from excessive blood loss.

COMPOSITION OF BLOOD

CHARACTERISTICS

Blood is a type of connective tissue that has a liquid intercellular matrix. The color of blood varies from a bright red to a darker blue-red. The difference in color is due to the amount of oxygen in the blood. Well-oxygenated blood is bright red, whereas oxygen-poor blood is blue-red. The amount of blood varies depending on body size, gender, and age. The average adult has 4 to 6 L of blood.

Do You Know...

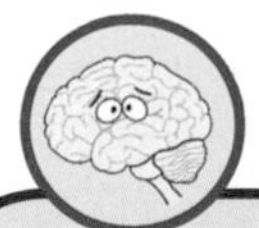

Why George Washington's nine pints of blood went down the drain?

You probably remember George Washington for chopping down the cherry tree, his penchant for truth, and for being the first president, but here is something you probably didn't know about George's medical history. George had been quite ill with a long winter cold, pneumonia, and throat infection. Despite many home remedies and much attention, the infection lingered and worsened. Enter the "quacks"! Immediately before his death George was bled of 9 pints of blood in an attempt to rid his body of disease. This commonly used procedure was called bloodletting.

The practice of bloodletting had been around since before the days of Hippocrates (a long, long time ago). Bloodletting grew out of the belief that health was due to a balance of the four body humours (fluids): blood, phlegm, black bile, and yellow bile. Disease was therefore attributed to an imbalance of the humours. By draining George's blood, the bloodletter hoped to balance George's unbalanced humours. Not funny! The fact that George died immediately after being drained of 9 pints is not surprising. At a time when he needed all the help he could get from his blood, he was literally drained and probably plunged into a state of low volume circulatory shock. Although the practice of bloodletting has been discredited, a friendly reminder of our past is the barbershop pole.

Barbers and surgeons were the early bloodletters, and the pole advertised their trade. The barbershop pole is striped red and white. Red represents blood, white represents the tourniquet, and the pole itself represents the stick that the patient squeezed to dilate the veins for easy puncturing. Fortunately, today's barbers go for your hair and not your jugular.

Other characteristics of blood include pH (7.35 to 7.45) and viscosity. Blood **viscosity** refers to the ease with which blood flows through the blood vessels. Viscosity is best demonstrated by comparing the flow of water and molasses. If water and molasses are poured out of a bottle, the molasses flows more slowly. Molasses is said to be more viscous, or thicker, than water. Blood is normally three to five times more viscous than water. Although blood viscosity does not normally fluctuate widely, an increase in viscosity can thicken the blood so much that it puts an extra burden on the heart, thereby causing the pumping action of the heart to fail.

BLOOD HAS TWO PARTS

Blood is composed of two parts: the plasma and the blood cells.

The **plasma** is a pale yellow fluid composed mostly of water. The plasma also contains proteins, ions, nutrients, gases, and waste. The plasma proteins consist of **albumin** (ăl BŪ-mĭn), various clotting factors, antibodies, and complement proteins. In general, the plasma proteins help regulate fluid volume, protect the body from pathogens, and prevent excessive blood loss in the event of injury. **Serum** is the plasma minus the clotting proteins.

The blood cells include the following:

- **Red blood cells (RBCs),** are also called **erythrocytes** (ĕ-RĬTH-rō-sīts) (from *erythro,* meaning red). RBCs are primarily involved in the transport of oxygen to all body tissues.
- **White blood cells (WBCs),** are also called **leukocytes** (LOO-kō-sīts) (from *leuko,* meaning white). WBCs protect the body from infection.
- **Platelets** (PLĀT-lĕts) are also called **thrombocytes** (THRŎM-bō-sīts). They protect the body from bleeding.

The two parts of blood (plasma and blood cells) can be observed in a test tube. If a sample of blood is collected in a tube and spun, two phases appear. The heavier blood cells appear at the bottom of the tube, whereas the lighter plasma accumulates at the top.

The separation of blood into two phases forms the basis of a blood test called the **hematocrit** (hē-MĂT-Ăō-krĭt) (Figure 15-1). The hematocrit (Hct or 'crit) is the percentage of blood cells in a sample of blood. A sample of blood is normally composed of 45% blood cells and 55% plasma. The blood cells are composed mainly of RBCs. A small layer of cells between the plasma and the RBCs is called the buffy coat and consists of WBCs and platelets. Because the buffy coat is so thin, any change in the Hct is generally interpreted as a change in the numbers of RBCs. For instance, a person with a low Hct is considered to be anemic, with a lower-than-normal number of RBCs.

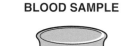

BLOOD SAMPLE

Plasma 55%

Buffy coat

Red blood cells (RBCs; erythrocytes)

Formed elements 45%

FIGURE 15-1 Hematocrit.

ORIGIN OF BLOOD CELLS

Where are the blood cells made? The three types of blood cells (RBCs, WBCs, and platelets) are made in hematopoietic tissue. The process of blood cell production is called **hematopoiesis** (hē-măt-ō-poi-Ē-sĭs). The two types of hematopoietic tissue in the adult are the red bone marrow and the lymphatic tissue, which is found in the spleen, lymph nodes, and thymus gland. Red bone marrow is found primarily in the ends of long bones, such as the femur, and in flat and irregular bones, such as the sternum, cranial bones, vertebrae, and bones of the pelvis.

Hematopoiesis and Red Bone Marrow

How does the red bone marrow produce three different kinds of blood cells? The three types of blood cells are produced in the red bone marrow from the same cell, called a **stem cell.** Under the influence of specific growth factors, the stem cell differentiates into a RBC, a WBC, or a platelet. Note the stem cell in Figure 15-2. In line 1, the stem cell differentiates into the RBC (erythrocyte). In lines 2, 3, and 4, the stem cells form five different WBCs (leukocytes). The **lymphocytes** and **monocytes** originate in the bone marrow; some of the lymphocytes mature and reproduce in the lymphatic tissue. In line 5, the stem cell differentiates into a **megakaryocyte,** a large blood cell that breaks up into tiny fragments. The fragments of the megakaryocytes are called platelets (thrombocytes).

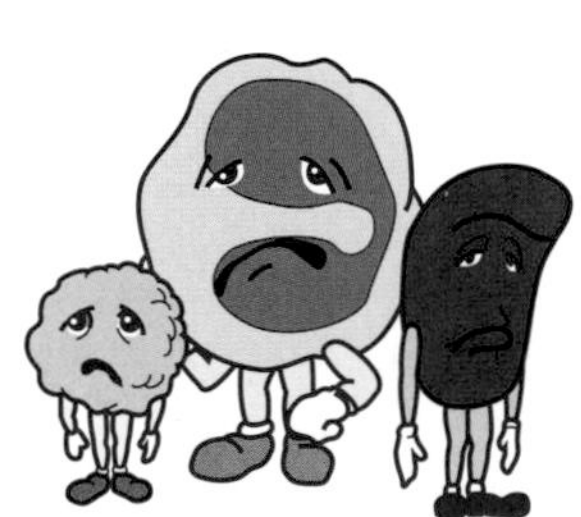

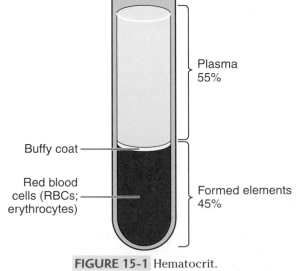

BONE MARROW MISERY

Bone Marrow Depression

Cheer up! Even bone marrow gets depressed! Under certain conditions, the bone marrow cannot produce enough blood cells. Bone marrow depression is called **myelosuppression** (from the Greek word *myelo,* meaning marrow). What happens if the bone marrow is depressed? Depressed bone marrow leads to a severe deficiency of RBCs, causing a serious form of **anemia** called aplastic anemia. Myelosuppression can also cause a deficiency of WBCs (leukocytes) called **leukopenia.** The leukopenic person is defenseless against infection and may die from a common cold. Depressed bone marrow may also produce inadequate numbers of platelets, or thrombocytes. This condition is called **thrombocytopenia.** The thrombocytopenic person is at high risk for hemorrhage. Why the concern for bone marrow

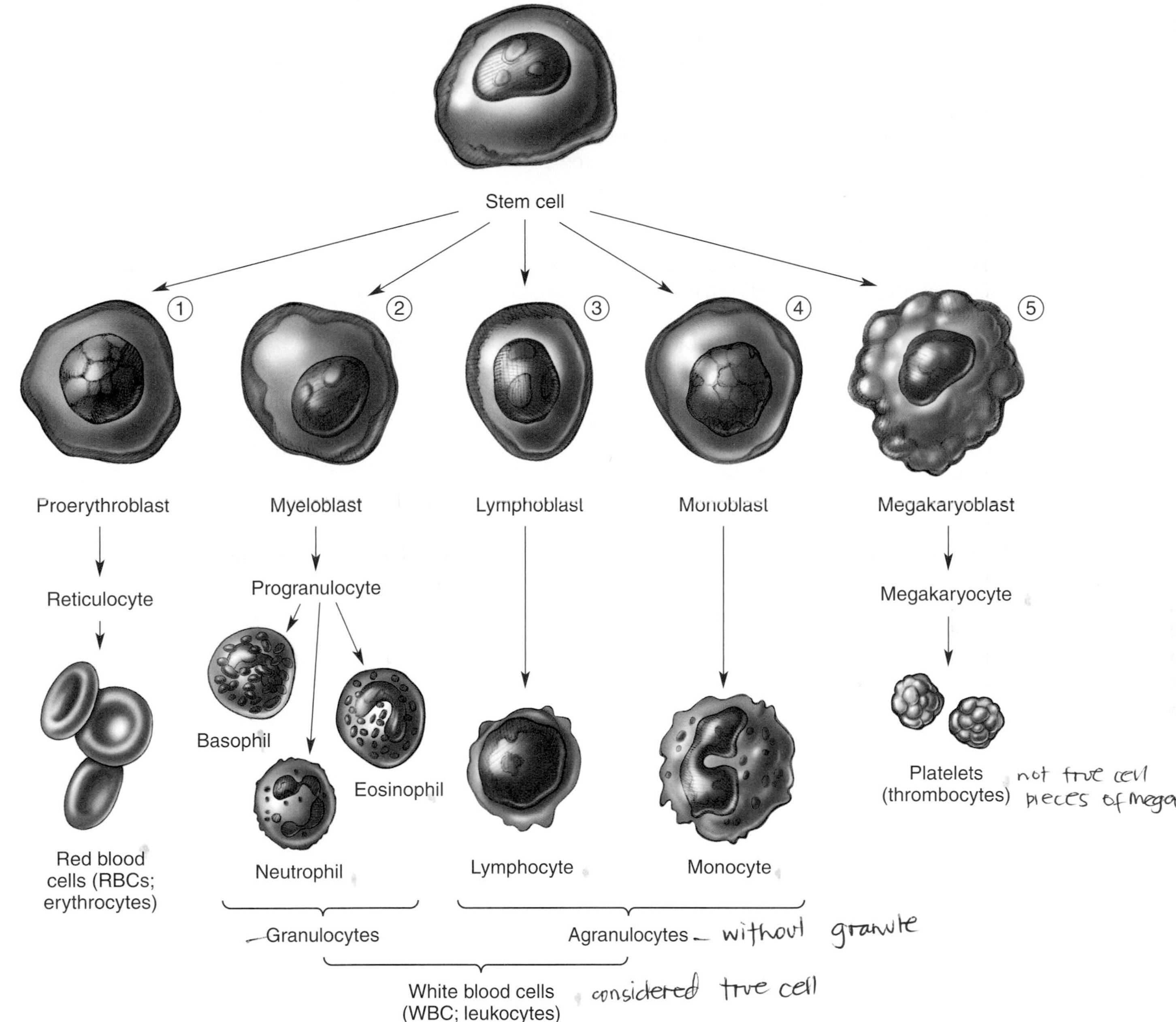

FIGURE 15-2 Differentiation of a stem cell into RBCs, WBCs, and platelets.

depression? Because many drugs and certain procedures, such as radiation, depress the bone marrow, a person exposed to any of these therapies must be monitored for symptoms of myelosuppression. Clinically, this is huge.

Bone Marrow Overactivity

Then there is my buddy, Bloody Ruddy. Bloody Ruddy suffers from polycythemia vera. That's bone marrow gone wild—the overactivity and the excess production of RBCs. The excess thickened blood (increased viscosity) burdens the heart, overwhelms the clotting system, and produces a beet-red, ruddy face. To help his condition, Ruddy may be given a drug that depresses the bone marrow. He may also require phlebotomy in order to remove and discard excess blood.

BLOOD CELLS

RED BLOOD CELLS

The red blood cells (RBCs), or erythrocytes, are the most numerous of the blood cells. Between 4.5 and 6.0 million RBCs are in one microliter of blood. The rate of production by the red bone marrow is several million RBCs per second. RBCs are primarily concerned with the transport of oxygen.

"Retics"

The immature RBC is called a **reticulocyte** (clinical nickname: retics; see Figure 15-2). The number of reticulocytes in blood is normally very small (0.5%-1.5%). Why measure the reticulocyte count? A high reticulocyte count may indicate blood loss or another iron-deficient state. Why? A loss of blood stimulates the bone marrow to make more RBCs. The greater the bone marrow activity, the higher the number of reticulocytes prematurely added to the circulation. Conversely, a low reticulocyte count might indicate that the patient is unable to make RBCs as in myelosuppression or severe iron deficiency. Hence, changes in the reticulocyte count can provide valuable diagnostic clues.

Shape

What do RBCs look like? First, RBCs are large. Because of their size they stay within the blood vessels and do not roam around the tissue spaces as do the WBCs. Second, RBCs are disc-shaped cells that have a thick outer rim and a thin center (Figure 15-3). The RBC can bend and therefore squeeze its way through tiny blood vessels. This flexibility allows the RBC to deliver oxygen to every cell in the body. The RBC's ability to bend is important. If the RBC were not able to bend, it would not fit through the tiny blood vessels, and tissue cells would be deprived of oxygen and die. Decreased oxygenation and cell death occur in a condition known as sickle-cell disease. Instead of bending, the RBCs assume a C-shape or sickle shape and block blood flow through the tiny blood vessels.

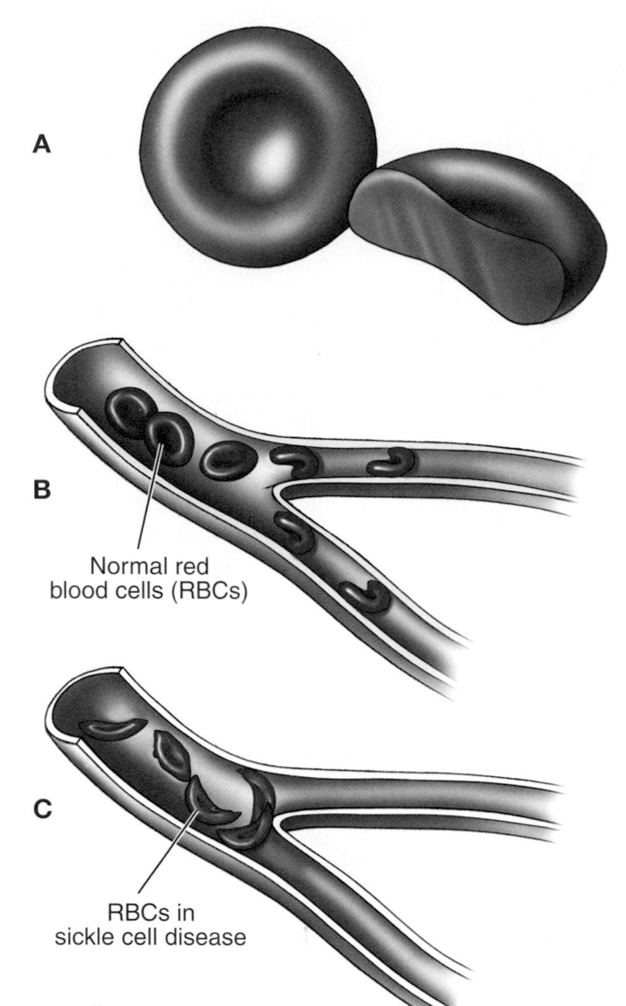

FIGURE 15-3 **A,** The RBCs are large and doughnut-shaped. **B,** The RBCs must bend to fit through the blood vessel. **C,** Sickled RBCs blocking the flow of blood through the blood vessel.

Hemoglobin

Red blood cells are filled with a large protein molecule called **hemoglobin** (HĒ-mō-GLŌ-bĭn) (Figure 15-4). Hemoglobin consists of two parts, globin (protein) and heme, an iron-containing substance. Hemoglobin contains four globin chains with each globin having a heme group. The hemoglobin molecule is responsible for RBC function.

What is so important about heme? As the RBCs circulate through the blood vessels in the lungs, oxygen (O_2) attaches loosely to the iron atom in the heme. The oxygenated hemoglobin is referred to as **oxyhemoglobin.** Then, as the blood flows to the various tissues in the body, the oxygen detaches from the hemoglobin. The unloaded oxygen diffuses from the blood to the cells, where it is used during cellular metabolism.

The globin portion of hemoglobin also plays a role in gas transport. Globin transports some of the carbon dioxide (CO_2) from its site of production (the metabolizing cells) to the lungs, where it is excreted. The CO_2-hemoglobin complex is called **carbaminohemoglobin.**

Why Blood Changes Its Color

The color of blood changes from bright red to blue-red. When hemoglobin is oxygenated, blood appears bright red. When hemoglobin is unoxygenated, blood assumes a darker blue-red color. Thus blood coming from the lungs is well oxygenated and appears red. Blood leaving the cells has given up its oxygen and appears blue-red. When a person is deprived of oxygen, the blood is a blue-red color, causing the skin to look blue, or cyanotic. **Cyanosis** is a sign of hypoxemia, a deficiency of oxygen in the blood.

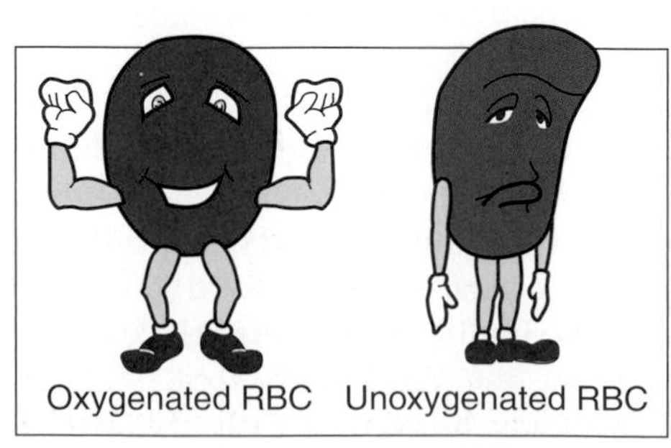

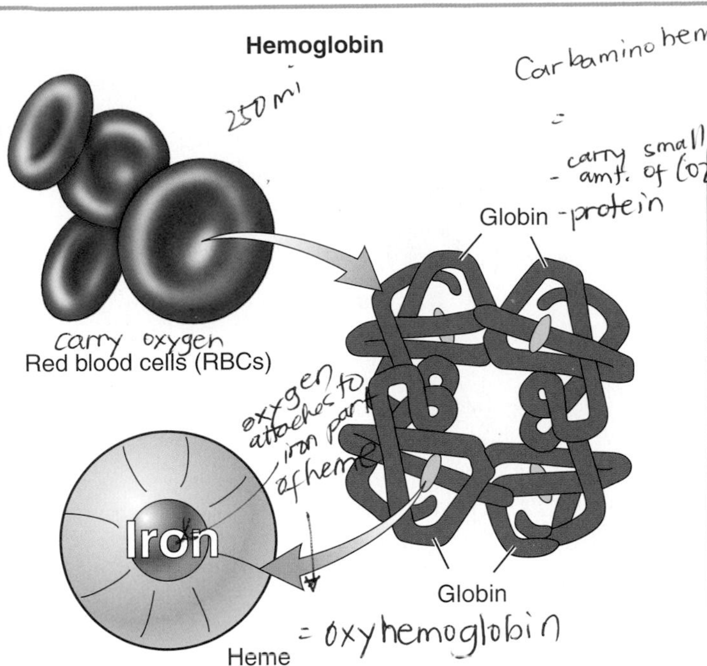

FIGURE 15-4 Hemoglobin and iron.

Do You Know...

Why there is a needle in this hip bone?

Because the red bone marrow is the site of blood cell production, certain abnormalities of blood cells can be detected through a bone marrow biopsy. In this procedure, a needle is inserted into the red bone marrow, usually at the iliac crest (hip bone) or the sternum (breastbone). A sample of bone marrow is withdrawn, or aspirated, and then microscopically studied. The analysis includes numbers and types of blood cells and the specific characteristics of each cell type.

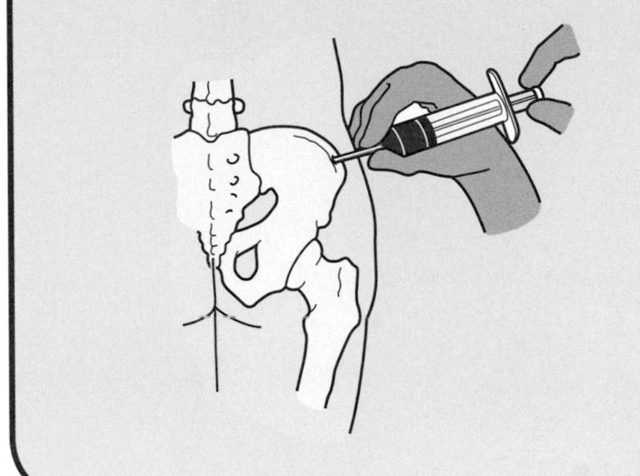

Why can a person have cherry red blood and be hypoxic at the same time? Blood is bright red when the hemoglobin is saturated with oxygen. Carbon monoxide, like oxygen, binds to the iron and also makes the blood appear bright cherry red. When carbon monoxide occupies the iron site, however, no oxygen can be carried by the hemoglobin. Therefore, the person with carbon monoxide poisoning can be both cherry red and hypoxic.

Substances Essential for Hemoglobin Production

What does the body need to make adequate amounts of hemoglobin? In addition to healthy bone marrow, the body requires certain raw materials. Iron, vitamin B_{12}, folic acid, and protein are essential for hemoglobin synthesis. Recall that the heme, the oxygen-carrying component of hemoglobin, contains iron. A diet deficient in iron can result in inadequate hemoglobin synthesis and a condition called iron-deficiency anemia. As you might expect, young women are more prone to iron-deficiency anemia than are young men. Women not only are more apt to get caught up in rigorous and unhealthy dieting, but they also tend to lose more iron because of the blood loss associated with menstruation. Persons with low incomes also have a higher incidence of iron-deficiency anemia because iron-rich foods such as meat are expensive.

A deficiency of other raw materials can cause other specific anemias. A deficiency of folic acid, for instance, causes folic acid deficiency anemia. Besides adequate dietary intake, raw materials must be absorbed from the digestive tract. Absorption of some of the raw materials requires special transport proteins. Adequate absorption of vitamin B_{12}, for instance, requires a transport protein called intrinsic factor. Intrinsic factor is normally secreted by the lining of the stomach. The inability to secrete adequate intrinsic factor in some persons results in inadequate absorption of vitamin B_{12}. This condition results in a form of anemia called pernicious anemia.

Regulation of RBC Production

New RBCs are constantly added to the circulation, and old, worn-out RBCs are constantly removed from the circulation. The steps for RBC release appear in Figure 15-5. When the oxygen in the body tissues starts to decrease, the kidneys sense the need for additional oxygen and secrete a hormone called **erythropoietin** (ĕ-rĭth-rō-PŌ-ĕ-tĭn). The erythropoietin (EPO) stimulates the bone marrow to release RBCs into the circulation. The increase in the number of RBCs causes an increase in the amount of oxygen transported to the tissues. As tissue oxygen increases, the stimulus for EPO release diminishes, and the bone marrow slows its rate of RBC production.

Three clinical thoughts about EPO:

- Note what happens in a person who is chronically hypoxic, such as a person with emphysema. The low oxygen in the blood stimulates the secretion of excess EPO causing additional RBC production. Thus a person with emphysema often has polycythemia (excess RBCs) secondary to chronic lung disease.
- Patients with bone marrow depression may be given EPO as a drug to increase RBC production. On a less upbeat note, athletes sometimes use

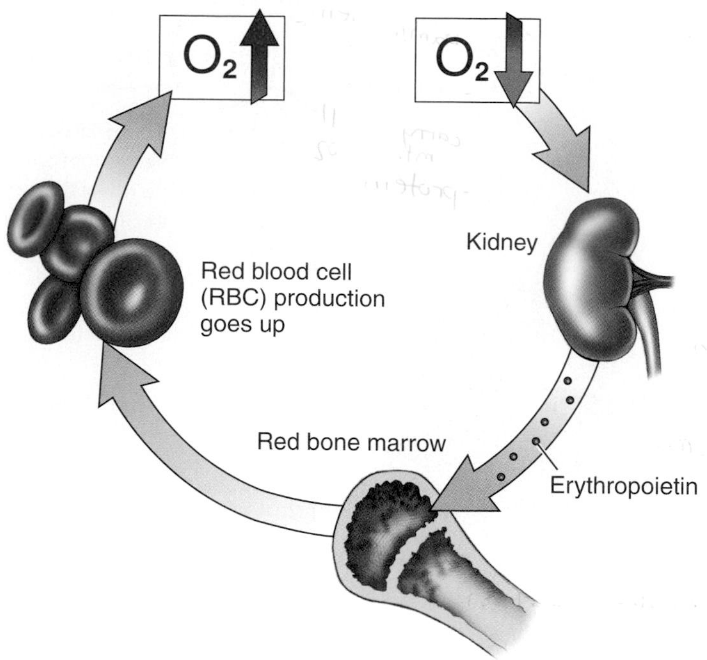

FIGURE 15-5 Regulation of RBC production by erythropoietin.

EPO illegally. The drug increases RBC production, thereby increasing the amount of oxygen delivered to exercising muscle.

- Patients with declining kidney function do not produce enough EPO and therefore become anemic. This type of anemia is called the anemia of chronic renal (kidney) failure. It is treated with the administration of EPO.

Removal and Breakdown of RBCs

How does the body know when an RBC needs to be removed from the circulation? The life span of the RBC is 120 days. Because the mature RBC has no nucleus, it cannot reproduce and must be replaced as it wears out. With time, as it performs its job, the RBC eventually gets misshapen, ragged around the edges, and fragile; the poor thing looks worn out! The ragged RBC membrane is detected by the macrophages that line the spleen and liver. The macrophages, or big eaters, remove the RBCs from the circulation and phagocytose them. Sometimes the RBCs are broken down very rapidly (hemolysis), exceeding the rate of RBC replacement. This results in hemolytic anemia—decreased RBCs and jaundice.

Recycle!

As the old, worn-out RBC is dismantled, its components are recycled. The hemoglobin is broken down into globin and heme (Figure 15-6). The globin is broken down into various amino acids that are later used in the synthesis of other proteins. The heme is further broken down into

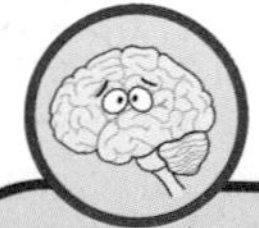

Do You Know...

About the cause of jaundice: is it blood sludge or vile bile?

Jaundice is caused by an elevation of bilirubin in the blood (hyperbilirubinemia). The hyperbilirubinemia can be caused by excessive blood cell destruction (hemolysis) or the reduction in the elimination of bilirubin from the blood (via the liver and bile). When jaundice is present, it is essential to determine the cause of the hyperbilirubinemia. Is it the blood ("blood sludge") or the bile ("vile bile")?

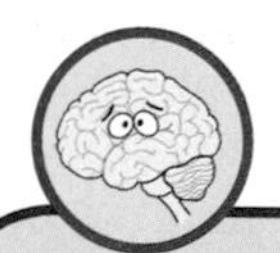

Do You Know...

Who this little yellow bird called icterus is?

In the event of excessive breakdown of RBCs (hemolysis), the amount of bilirubin released into the circulation increases. Increasing levels of bilirubin cause the bilirubin to enter the tissues, staining the tissue yellow. The person is described as jaundiced, or icteric. The word *icterus* comes from the name of a little yellow bird.

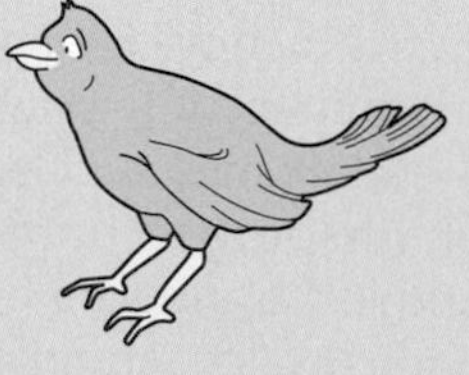

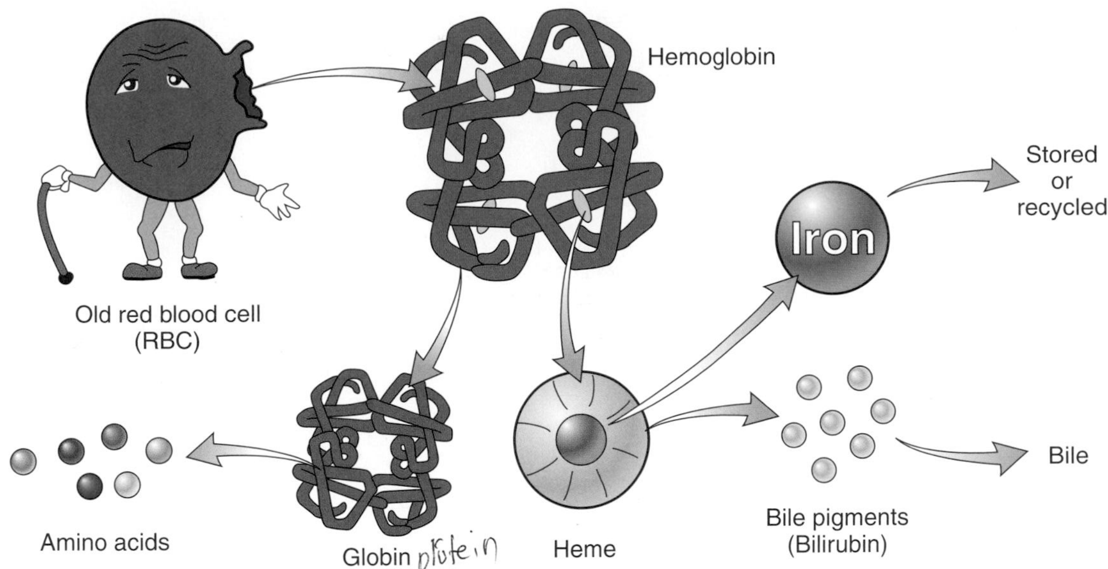

FIGURE 15-6 Breakdown of old RBCs. Note the recycling of amino acids and iron and the excretion of bilirubin.

iron and bile pigments. The iron is stored in the liver until it is needed by the bone marrow for the synthesis of new hemoglobin. The liver removes bile pigments, especially bilirubin, from the blood and excretes them into the bile. Bile eventually flows into the intestines and is excreted from the body in the feces.

Sum It Up!

Blood is composed of plasma and blood cells (red blood cells, white blood cells, and platelets). Most of the cells are formed in the red bone marrow. Normal red blood cells are formed only in the presence of adequate raw materials, normal genetic information that directs hemoglobin synthesis, and healthy bone marrow. RBC production is regulated by erythropoietin, which, in turn, responds to tissue levels of oxygen. Hemoglobin is broken down into globin and bilirubin. The iron is recycled and the bilirubin is excreted in the bile. Figure 15-7 on p. 270 summarizes RBC formation and function through the various anemias.

WHITE BLOOD CELLS

White blood cells (WBCs), or leukocytes, are large round cells that contain nuclei. WBCs lack hemoglobin and are less numerous than RBCs. Normally, a microliter of blood contains between 5,000 and 10,000 WBCs (Table 15-1). WBCs function primarily to protect the body by destroying disease-producing microorganisms (pathogens) and remove dead tissue and other cellular debris by **phagocytosis.** When an infection is present in the body, the numbers of WBCs generally increase. This increase in the number of WBCs is called **leukocytosis.**

Unlike RBCs, which normally circulate within the blood vessels, WBCs can leave the blood vessels. The WBCs squeeze through the cells of the blood vessel walls and move toward the site of infection, where they destroy the pathogens and remove cellular debris (Figure 15-8).

Kinds of White Blood Cells

Each of the five kinds of WBCs has a different name, appearance, and function (Table 15-2). How do we tell the difference? WBCs are classified according to granules in their cytoplasm. WBCs that contain granules are called **granulocytes.** Other WBCs do not have granules within their cytoplasm and are called **agranulocytes,** meaning without granules. Granulocytes are produced in the red bone marrow. Three types of granulocytes are neutrophils, basophils, and eosinophils.

Neutrophils

The **neutrophil** (NŪ-trō-fĭl) is the most common granulocyte. Neutrophils account for 55% to 70% of the total WBC population and usually remain in the blood for a short time (about 10 to 12 hours). The neutrophil's most important role is phagocytosis. These cells quickly move to the site of infection, where they phagocytose pathogens and remove tissue debris. The battle between the neutrophils and the pathogens at the site of infection leaves behind a collection of dead neutrophils, parts of cells, and fluid. This collection is called pus.

Sometimes the body can wall off the collection of pus from the surrounding tissue, forming an abscess. Abscess formation is one of the ways that the body has of preventing the spread of infection. The neutrophil plays such an important role in the defense of the body that a deficiency of neutrophils (neutropenia or granulocytopenia) is considered life-threatening. Unless resolved, the person may die from an overwhelming infection.

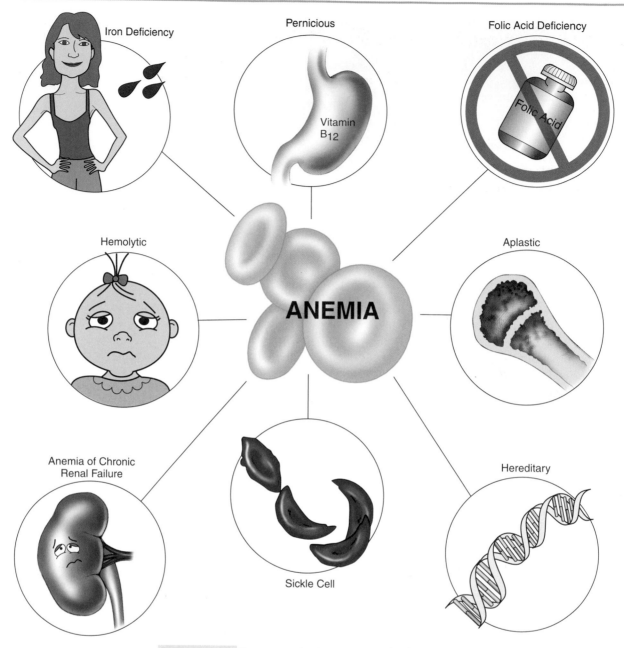

FIGURE 15-7 Summary: RBC formation and anemias.

Naming the Neutrophil. Because it plays such an important role in protecting the body from infection, the neutrophil is often the center of attention. Depending on its appearance and what it is doing at the moment, the neutrophil has many nicknames.

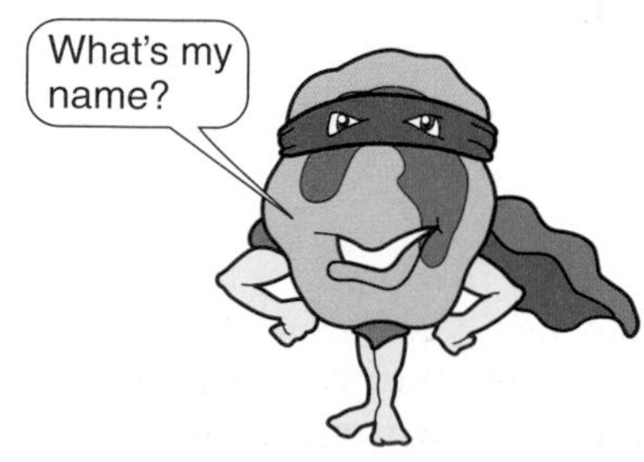

Polys, Polymorphs, or Polymorphonuclear Leukocytes. The neutrophil is a round cell that contains a nucleus. The nucleus can have many shapes and different sizes. Because of the many-shaped (polymorphic) nucleus, neutrophils are called polymorphs or **polymorphonuclear leukocytes,** or **PMNs.** Sometimes they are simply called polys.

Segs. The nucleus of the mature neutrophil appears segmented when viewed under a microscope. Neutrophils are therefore called **segs.**

Band Cells, Staff Cells, and Stab Cells. The nucleus of the immature neutrophil looks like a thick, curved band, hence the name **band cells.** Because the band resembles the shape of a staff, the band cells are also called **staff cells.** Neutrophils are also called **stab cells.**

Table 15-1 Types and Functions of Blood Cells

Cell Type	Normal Range	Primary Function
Red blood cells (RBCs)	4.5–6.0 million mm^3	Transport oxygen and carbon dioxide
Hemoglobin (Hgb)	12–18 g/dL	
Hematocrit (Hct)	38%–54%	
Reticulocytes	0.5%–1.5%	
White blood cells (WBCs)*	5000–10,000 mm^3	Protect the body from infection
Platelets (thrombocytes)	150,000–450,000 mm^3	Help control blood loss from injured blood vessels

mm^3, Microliter.
*See Table 15-2 for the white blood cell differential count.

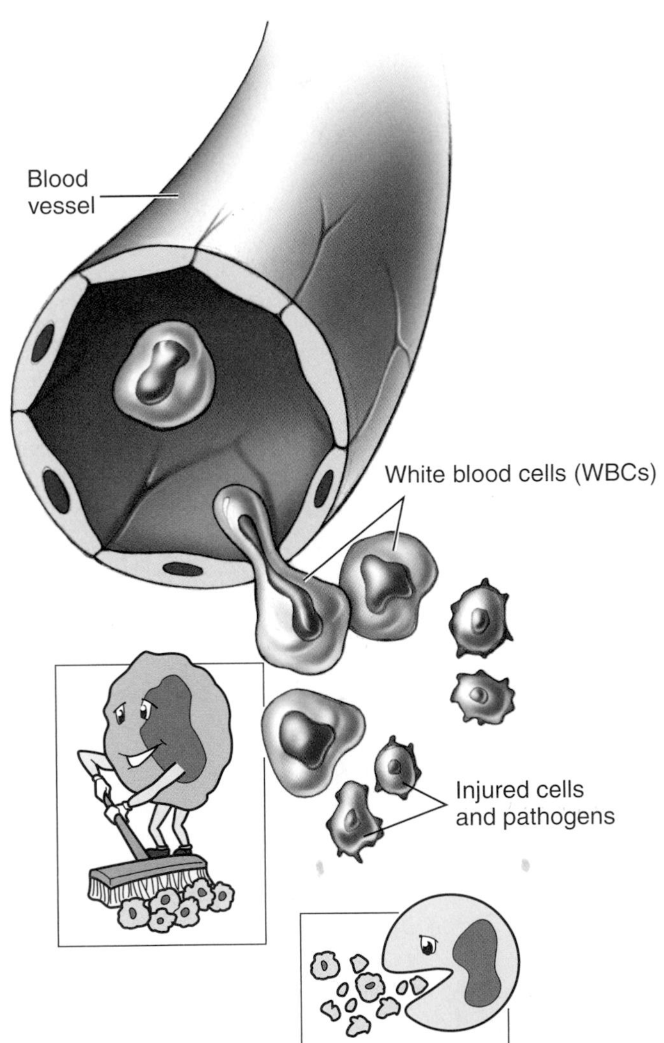

FIGURE 15-8 White blood cells: traveling, housekeeping, and eating.

What Is a Shift to the Left? As the body tries to mount an attack against a pathogen, it needs more neutrophils. The production of the neutrophils may be so rapid that the time for cells to mature is inadequate. A greater proportion of the neutrophils are therefore immature and appear banded. Infection? The bands march in! When immature neutrophils (bands) become prominent in the differential WBC count, the condition is called a shift-to-the left. The term derives from early studies that used tabular headings to report the numbers of each cell type. The cell types were listed across the top of the page, starting with bands on the left and the more mature neutrophils on the right. Thus a shift to the left indicates an infection.

Differential Count. A differential white blood cell count indicates the percentage of each type of white blood cell (see Table 15-2). The differential count provides valuable diagnostic information because it indicates which WBC is involved. For instance, one infection may cause an elevation primarily in the numbers of neutrophils, but a different infection may cause an elevation in the monocytes.

Basophils

The second type of granulocytic WBCs, **basophils** (BĀ-sō-fĭl), are normally present in small numbers. Basophils make up less than 1% of the WBCs. The basophil plays a role in the inflammatory response, primarily through its release of histamine. The basophil also releases **heparin,** an anticoagulant. Because basophils are found in abundance in areas with large amounts of blood (lungs and liver), the release of heparin is thought to reduce the formation of tiny blood clots.

Eosinophils

The third type of granulocytic WBC is the **eosinophil** (ē-ō-SĬN-ō-fĭl). Eosinophils are present in small numbers, constituting only 1% to 3% of the WBCs. They are involved in the inflammatory response, secreting chemicals that destroy certain parasites, engage in phagocytosis, and become elevated in persons with allergies. A person with a parasitic infection or allergic reaction generally has an elevated eosinophil count.

Different-Colored Granulocytes

The three granulocytes stain different colors. The colors are used to name the granulocytes. Neutrophils do not stain deeply; they are relatively neutral with regard

Table 15-2 White Blood Cells (Leukocytes)*

Type of WBC	Percent of Total WBC Count	Function of Cell
Granulocytes		
Neutrophils	55–70	Phagocytosis
Eosinophils	1–3	Inflammatory responses; parasitic infection; allergies
Basophils	0–1	Inflammatory responses; release of heparin
Agranulocytes		
Lymphocytes	25–38	Immunity
Monocytes	3–8	Phagocytosis

*A differential white blood cell count indicates the percentage of each type of white blood cell.

to staining characteristics. For this reason they are called neutrophils. The other two granulocytes stain deeply and are named for the color stain each absorbs. The eosinophil stains a bright pink, and the basophil stains a dark blue.

Agranulocytes

The two kinds of agranulocytes are lymphocytes and monocytes. The lymphocytes are produced in the red bone marrow; some mature and reproduce in the lymphoid tissue (lymph nodes, liver, spleen). Lymphocytes constitute 25% to 38% of the WBCs and perform an important role in the body's immune response. (Immunity will be discussed further in Chapter 21.) Monocytes are the second type of agranulocyte. Like the neutrophil, the monocyte is phagocytotic. Although the neutrophils are more abundant (55% to 70% of the WBCs), the monocytes (3% to 8% of the WBCs) are more efficient phagocytes.

Monocytes differentiate, or change, into macrophages. These **macrophages** become either wandering or fixed. Wandering macrophages travel or wander about the body, patrolling for pathogens and cleaning up debris. Wandering macrophages are particularly abundant under the mucous membrane and the skin, where they destroy pathogens that gain entrance through cuts and abrasions. In contrast, fixed macrophages are fixed in a particular organ, such as the liver, spleen, lymph nodes, or red bone marrow. As blood or lymph flows through these organs, the fixed macrophages phagocytose any pathogens. These same macrophages also phagocytose worn-out RBCs, thereby helping remove them from circulation.

Good News, Bad News

The bad news is that clinically, you must know the names and classifications (granulocytes, agranulocytes) of the WBCs. The good news is that you can use the monkey business in Figure 15-9. "**N**aughty **L**ittle **M**onkeys **E**at **B**ananas," says **GRAN**pa **BEN.** Do the capital letters. "Naughty Little Monkeys Eat Bananas" identifies the types of WBCs: neutrophils, lymphocytes, monocytes, eosinophils, and basophils. GRANpa BEN indicates that the granulocytes are basophils, eosinophils, and neutrophils.

PLATELETS

Platelets are the tiniest blood cells. Normally, each microliter of blood contains between 150,000 and 450,000 platelets. They are produced in the red bone marrow

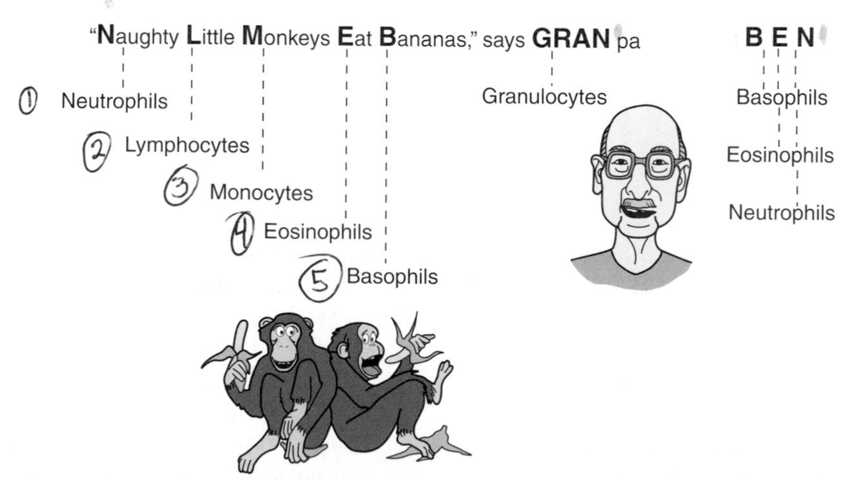

FIGURE 15-9 Naming WBCs.

from the large megakaryocyte (see Figure 15-2) and have a life span of 5 to 9 days.

Platelets prevent blood loss. Failure of the bone marrow to replace platelets (thrombocytes) at an adequate rate results in a deficiency called thrombocytopenia. This condition is characterized by petechiae, little pinpoint hemorrhages under the skin, and abnormal, potentially lethal bleeding episodes.

COMPLETE BLOOD COUNT

A **complete blood count (CBC)** is a laboratory test that provides information about the composition of the blood. A CBC provides the normal range of the numbers of RBCs, WBCs, and platelets. In addition to the numbers of blood cells, the CBC provides information specific to each cell type. Relative to the RBC, the CBC indicates the normal hemoglobin (Hgb) content of the RBC, the normal hematocrit (Hct), and the percentage of the reticulocytes (the immature RBCs). With regard to information concerning the WBCs, a CBC indicates the percentage of each type of WBC (WBC differential count).

Sum It Up!

The WBCs (leukocytes) protect the body by destroying pathogens and removing dead tissue and other cellular debris by phagocytosis. The five kinds of WBCs are granulocytes (neutrophils, basophils, and eosinophils) and agranulocytes (lymphocytes and monocytes). Platelets (thrombocytes) play a key role in the prevention of blood loss.

HEMOSTASIS: PREVENTION OF BLOOD LOSS

Injury to a blood vessel causes bleeding. Bleeding usually stops spontaneously when the injury is minor. What causes the bleeding to stop? The process that stops bleeding is called **hemostasis** (hē-mō-STĀ-sĭs). The word literally means that the blood *(hemo)* stands still *(stasis)*. Hemostasis involves three events: blood vessel spasm, the formation of a platelet plug, and blood clotting (Figure 15-10). (Do not confuse the words *hemostasis* and *homeostasis.*)

BLOOD VESSEL SPASM

When a blood vessel is injured, the smooth muscle in the blood vessel wall responds by contracting. This process is called **vascular spasm.** Vascular spasm causes the diameter of the blood vessel to decrease, thereby decreasing the amount of blood that flows through the vessel. In the tiniest of vessels, vascular spasm stops the bleeding completely. In the larger vessels, vascular spasm alone may slow bleeding but is generally insufficient to stop bleeding.

FORMATION OF A PLATELET PLUG

When a blood vessel is torn, the inner lining of the vessel activates the platelets. The platelets become sticky and adhere to the inner lining of the injured vessel and to each other. By sticking together, they form a **platelet plug.** The plug diminishes bleeding at the injured site. Over several minutes, the plug will be invaded by activated blood-clotting factors and will eventually evolve into a stable, strong blood clot. In addition to forming a plug, the platelets also release chemicals that further stimulate vascular spasm and help activate the blood-clotting factors. Thus the platelets participate in all three phases of hemostasis. Good news! Exercise decreases platelet stickiness and the formation of deadly blood clots. However, stress increases platelet stickiness. Chill!

Aspirin and Bleeding

Aspirin slows vascular spasm and exerts an antiplatelet effect. Aspirin is commonly used to suppress hemostasis. A baby aspirin a day keeps the heart doctor away. Excess aspirin therapy, however, can cause serious bleeding episodes, especially in a person who is thrombocytopenic or is taking anticoagulant drugs.

BLOOD CLOTTING

Vascular spasm and a platelet plug alone are not sufficient to prevent the bleeding caused by a large tear in a blood vessel. With a more serious injury to the vessel wall, bleeding stops only if a blood clot forms. **Blood clotting,** or **coagulation,** is the third step in the process of hemostasis. A blood clot is formed by a series of chemical reactions that result in the formation of a netlike structure. The net is composed of protein fibers called **fibrin** (FĪ-brĭn). As blood flows through the fibrin net, large particles in the blood, such as RBCs and platelets, become trapped within it. The structure formed by the fibrin net and the trapped elements is called a **blood clot.** The blood clot seals off the opening in the injured blood vessel and stops the bleeding.

Formation of the Blood Clot

How does the clot form? The clot is the result of a series of chemical reactions in which a number of clotting factors are activated. Follow the three stages of blood coagulation identified in Figure 15-11.

- *Stage I:* Injury to the blood vessel wall activates various clotting factors. These clotting factors normally circulate in the blood in their inactive form. When activated, the clotting factors produce a substance called **prothrombin activator (PTA).**

Spasm

Injured vessel

Platelet

Red blood cells (RBCs)

A

Formation of platelet plug

B

Blood clotting at the site of the injury.

Red blood cells (RBCs)

Fibrin threads

C

FIGURE 15-10 Hemostasis: steps. **A,** Blood vessel spasm. **B,** Formation of the platelet plug. **C,** Blood clotting (coagulation).

Do You Know...

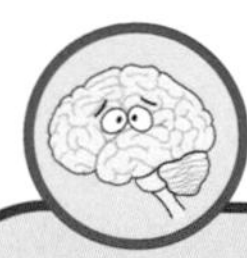

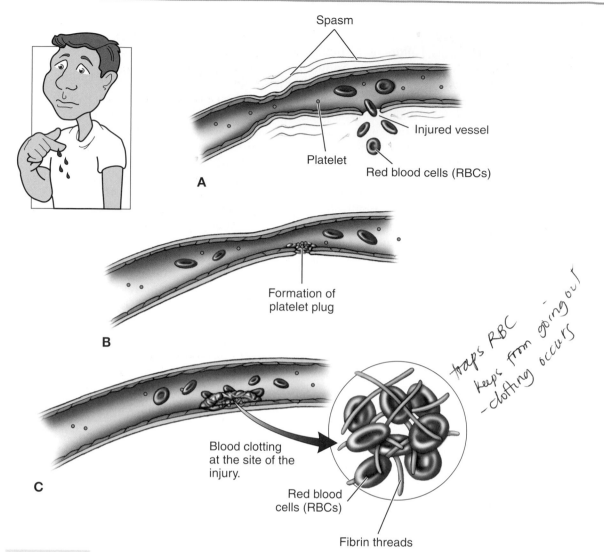

What Queen Victoria, the "royal disease," and factor VIII have in common?

Hemophilia is a bleeding disorder caused by the deficiency of a clotting factor called factor VIII, or the hemophilic factor. Hemophilia was common in the royal families of Europe; hence it was called the "royal disease." Why was hemophilia so prevalent in the royal families? Hemophilia is genetically transmitted. Because of the tendency of the royals to intermarry (e.g., cousin marrying cousin), the gene carrying hemophilia was kept in the family and expressed frequently in the royal offspring. Queen Victoria of England carried the gene for hemophilia. Victoria, being both prolific and politically astute, placed a descendent on every throne in Europe. As each descendent married and intermarried, the incidence of hemophilia increased.

- *Stage II:* In the presence of calcium, platelet chemicals, and PTA, **prothrombin** is activated to form **thrombin.**
- *Stage III:* Thrombin activates **fibrinogen.** Activated fibrinogen forms the fibrin fibers, or net. The net traps other blood cells and particles to form the clot. Other factors then stabilize and strengthen the clot.

Anticoagulants

Although the body must be able to stop bleeding, it is equally essential for it to prevent excessive clot formation. Several mechanisms prevent clot formation. Two of the most important mechanisms are a smooth inner lining (endothelium) of the blood vessels and the secretion of heparin, an anticoagulant.

Endothelium. The inner lining (endothelium) of the blood vessels is smooth and shiny and allows blood to flow easily along its surface. If the surface of the

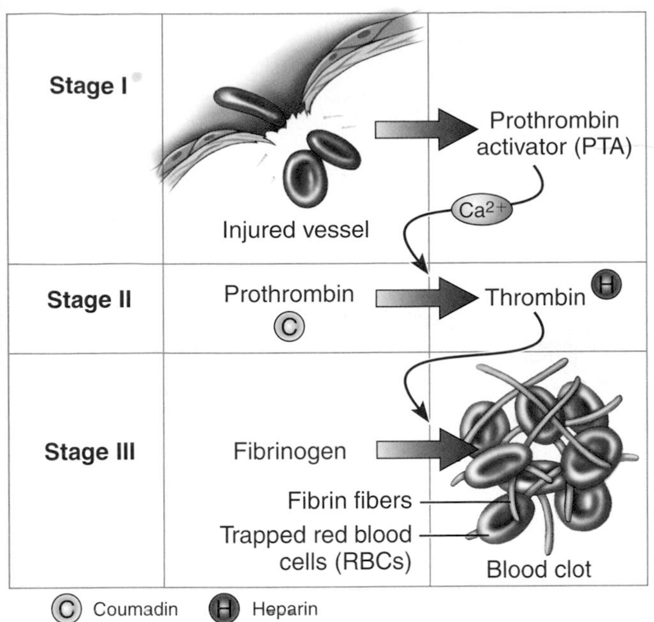

FIGURE 15-11 Blood clotting: three stages. The sites of Coumadin (C) and heparin (H) activity are indicated.

endothelium becomes roughened, however, coagulation factors are activated and blood clots are apt to form.

Secretion of Heparin. Heparin is secreted by mast cells. Mast cells are basophils that are concentrated in and around the liver and lungs. These are sites where the blood is rather stagnant and therefore apt to clot easily. Heparin acts as an anticoagulant by removing thrombin from the clotting process. In other words, heparin is an antithrombin agent. Note in Figure 15-11 that the formation of thrombin in stage II is crucial for clot formation (the conversion of fibrinogen to fibrin).

Anticoagulant Medications. At times, the administration of anticoagulant drugs may be necessary. Anticoagulants are administered in an attempt to prevent the formation of a blood clot. The blood clot is called a **thrombus;** the process of blood clot formation is called thrombosis. A piece of the thrombus may break off and travel through the blood to the lungs. The traveling thrombus is called an **embolus.** The danger is that the embolus may lodge in the blood vessels of the lungs, causing a fatal pulmonary embolus.

Thrombosis may be prevented by the administration of two types of anticoagulants: heparin and coumadin. Heparin, designated H in Figure 15-11, acts as an antithrombin agent. Another anticoagulant, called Coumadin (warfarin), also prevents clot formation. Like heparin, Coumadin interferes with the clotting scheme but does so at a different step. Coumadin, designated C in Figure 15-11, decreases the hepatic (liver) utilization of vitamin K in the synthesis of prothrombin, causing hypoprothrombinemia (a diminished amount of prothrombin in the blood). Less prothrombin means less thrombin. Less thrombin means that blood clotting is diminished.

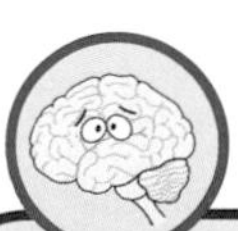

Do You Know...

Why this toe needs this leech?

This toe was accidentally severed from its owner. In reattaching the toe to the foot, the surgeon recognized that the toe graft would be successful only if the blood supply to the toe was good. Frequently after surgery of this type, blood clots develop at the graft site, resulting in a decrease in blood flow. Leeches, or bloodsuckers, may be applied to the site of the graft. As the leech attaches to the skin to feed, it injects a potent anticoagulant. The leech anticoagulant prevents blood clotting at the graft site, thereby maintaining a good blood flow and improving the chances for successful grafting.

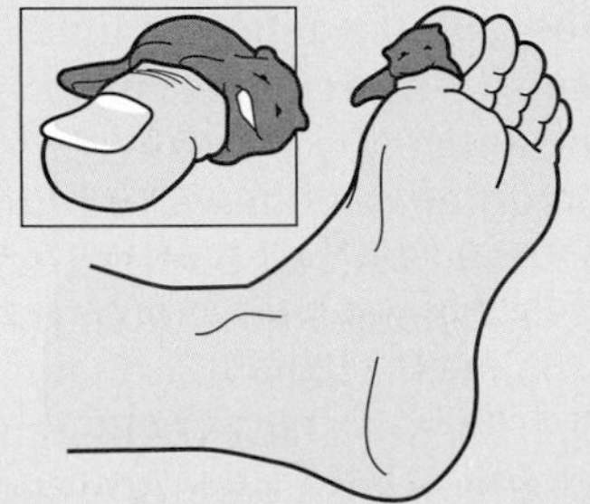

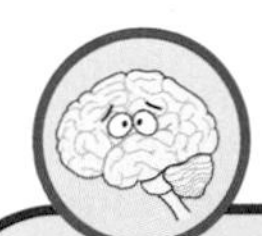

Do You Know...

About Harry Clotter and his spinach salad?

Harry was diagnosed with deep vein thrombosis (DVT) after a 15-hour nonstop flight on his broomstick. After a 3-day stay in the hospital with heparin therapy, he was discharged on Coumadin (warfarin) and directed not to eat spinach. Why no spinach? The drug Coumadin works by blocking the utilization of vitamin K in the hepatic synthesis of prothrombin. Because spinach contains a lot of vitamin K, it reduces the effectiveness of Coumadin, thereby reversing its anticoagulant effects. So leave the spinach to Popeye, Harry. (Harry was also advised to lose the stick and walk.)

Clot Retraction

What happens to the clot after it forms? After the clot forms, it becomes smaller as water is squeezed out. This process is called **clot retraction.** As the clot retracts, the edges of the injured blood vessels are also pulled together. This pulling together slows bleeding and sets the stage for repair of the blood vessel.

Clot Busting and the Vampire Bat

After the clot accomplishes its task, it is dissolved by a process called **fibrinolysis** (Figure 15-12). A substance called **plasmin** dissolves the clot. Plasmin is formed from its inactive form, **plasminogen,** which normally

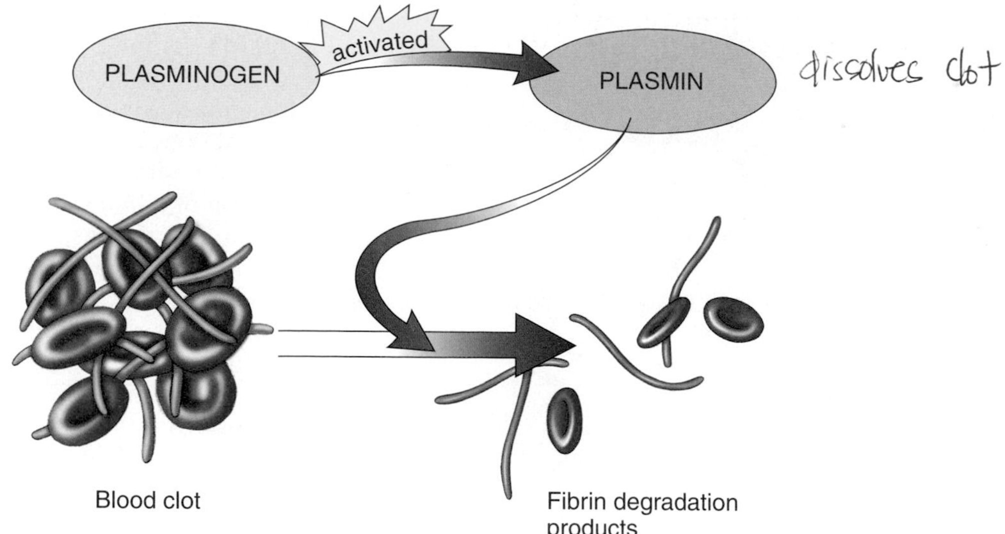

FIGURE 15-12 Fibrinolysis: "clot busting."

circulates within the blood. **Tissue plasminogen activator (TPA),** formed by injured tissue, activates plasminogen.

Recently, TPA has been administered as a drug to persons with life-threatening conditions caused by clots. TPA and related substances form a classification of drugs called clot busters. These drugs have revolutionized the treatment of myocardial infarction (heart attacks caused by blood clots in the blood vessels of the heart) and strokes (blood clot in the blood vessels of the brain). Long before we started injecting clot-busting drugs, the vampire bat had figured out plasmin physiology and had perfected the technique. Vampire bat saliva contains a TPA-like substance that dissolves clots.

Sum It Up!

The process that stops bleeding after injury is called hemostasis. Hemostasis involves three events: blood vessel spasm, the formation of a platelet plug, and blood clotting (coagulation). Clotting occurs when thrombin causes the conversion of fibrinogen into a fibrin clot. Blood clots are eventually dissolved by plasmin.

BLOOD TYPES

Medicine has seen attempted blood transfusions since its earliest days. While some were successful, others were medical disasters. The earliest physicians recognized that a severely wounded person was in need of blood. They did not realize, however, that blood from one person cannot always be mixed with blood from another. These physicians unknowingly demonstrated by disaster the presence of different blood types.

Do You Know...

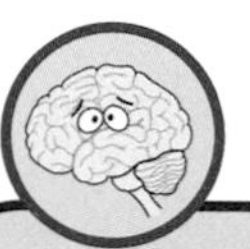

About Miss Muffet, her curds, whey, and blood clot?

As you know, little Miss Muffet sat on her tuffet eating her curds and whey—that is, her soured milk. The lumps in soured milk are called curds, and the watery part is called whey. So much for Muffet's diet. What does this have to do with blood? Thrombosis (blood clotting) is from a Greek word meaning to curdle, as in the curdling of milk. Serum is from a Latin word that refers to whey or the watery residue left after milk has curdled. Miss Muffet didn't really have a blood clot, but her diet inspired blood-clotting vocabulary. Her tuffet and arachnophobic personality are another story!

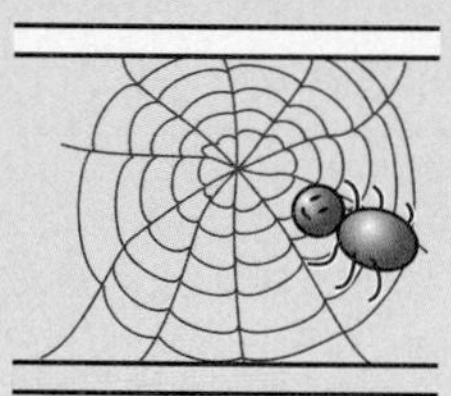

ANTIGENS AND BLOOD TYPES

Blood is classified according to specific antigens on the surface of the RBC. An antigen is a genetically determined substance that the body recognizes as foreign. As a foreign substance, an antigen stimulates an antigen-antibody response. This response is designed to attack and destroy the antigen.

The **ABO grouping** contains four blood types: A, B, AB, and O. The letters A and B refer to the antigen on the RBC. Table 15-3 shows what it means to be type A, B, AB, or O. A person with type A blood has the A antigen on the RBC. A person with type B blood has a B antigen on the RBC. A person with type AB blood has both A and B antigens on the RBC. A person with type O blood

Table 15-3 ABO Blood Groups

Blood Type	Antigen (RBC Membrane)	Antibody (Plasma)	Can Receive Blood From	Can Donate Blood To
A (40%)	A antigen	Anti-B antibodies	A, O	A, AB
B (10%)	B antigen	Anti-A antibodies	B, O	B, AB
AB* (4%)	A antigen B antigen	No antibodies	A, B, AB, O	AB
O† (46%)	No antigen	Both anti-A and anti-B antibodies	O	O, A, B, AB

*Type AB: universal recipient.
†Type O: universal donor.

has neither A nor B antigen on the RBC. Remember: the antigen is located on the RBC membrane.

ANTIBODIES AND BLOOD TYPE

In addition to the antigens on the RBCs, specific **antibodies** are found in the plasma of each blood type (see Table 15-3). Antibodies bind to specific substances and inactivate them. A person with type A blood has anti-B antibodies in the plasma. A person with type B blood has anti-A antibodies in the plasma. A person with type AB blood has neither anti-A nor anti-B antibodies in the plasma. The person with type O blood has both anti-A and anti-B antibodies in the plasma.

ANTIGEN-ANTIBODY INTERACTION

Table 15-3 indicates that type A blood contains the A antigen and anti-B antibodies. What would happen if a person had the A antigen on his RBCs and anti-A antibodies in his plasma? The A antigen and the anti-A antibody would cause a clumping reaction much like the curdling seen when milk and vinegar are mixed together.

This clumping of the antigen-antibody interaction is called **agglutination.** Agglutination reactions cause the RBCs to burst or lyse, a process called **hemolysis.** If rapid hemolysis were to occur within the circulation, hemoglobin would be liberated from the RBCs, eventually clogging the kidneys and possibly causing death.

COMPATIBILITY AND INCOMPATIBILITY OF BLOOD TYPES

The curdling, or agglutination, reaction has important implications for blood transfusions. Some blood types mix without undergoing agglutination reactions; they are said to be **compatible blood groups.** Other blood groups agglutinate, causing severe hemolysis, kidney failure, and death. These blood groups are **incompatible.** To avoid giving a person incompatible blood, donor blood is first typed and cross-matched.

What do blood typing and cross-matching mean? First, the blood type (A, B, AB, or O) is determined. Then a sample of donor blood (blood from the person who is donating it) is mixed (cross-matched) with a sample of recipient blood (blood from the person who is to receive the donated blood). Any evidence of agglutination indicates that the donor blood is incompatible with the recipient's blood.

Suppose a recipient of a blood transfusion has type A blood. She then can be given type A blood and type O blood (see Table 15-3). No antigen-antibody reaction (agglutination) would occur because type A donor blood has the A antigen and the recipient has only anti-B antibodies (plasma). The type O donor blood does not cause agglutination because that person's RBC has neither the A nor the B antigen. Type A and type O blood are therefore compatible with type A blood.

Note what happens, however, if the type A recipient receives type B blood (see Table 15-3). Type B donor blood has the B antigen on each RBC surface. The plasma antibodies of the recipient are anti-B antibodies. The B antigen and the anti-B antibodies cause agglutination, thus type B blood is incompatible with type A blood. What happens if the type A recipient is given type AB blood? In this case, the RBC contains both A and B antigens. The plasma of the recipient contains anti-B antibodies. Thus when types A and AB are mixed, an agglutination reaction occurs; these blood groups are incompatible. The administration of incompatible blood groups forms the basis of hemolytic blood transfusion reactions. The presence or absence of antibodies dictates the compatibility/incompatibility characteristics of the four blood groups (see Table 15-3).

Note in Table 15-3 that type O blood can be given to all four blood groups. Type O blood is therefore called the **universal donor.** For this reason blood banks stock a large supply of type O blood. Note also that type AB blood can receive all four types of blood; it is called the **universal recipient.** Recipients can receive their own blood types. In other words, a type A recipient can receive type A blood. The type B recipient can receive type B blood. The same is true for types AB and O. Table 15-3 also indicates the prevalence of the four blood types. Type A blood occurs in 40% of the population. Ten percent of the population has type B. Four percent has type AB, and 46% has type O. Thus type O is the most common while type AB is the least common. What blood type are you? You should have that information.

RH CLASSIFICATION SYSTEM

Blood is also classified according to the Rh factor. The **Rh factor** is an antigen located on the surface of the RBC. The Rh factor was named for the Rhesus monkey, in which it was first detected. If an RBC contains the Rh factor, the blood is said to be Rh-positive (+). If the RBC lacks the Rh factor, it is said to be Rh-negative (−). Thus, A^+ blood refers to type A blood that also has the Rh factor, while A^- blood is type A blood that does not have the Rh factor. Approximately 85% of the population is Rh-positive (+).

Plasma does not naturally carry anti-Rh antibodies. In two conditions however, the plasma of an Rh-negative (−) person can develop anti-Rh antibodies.

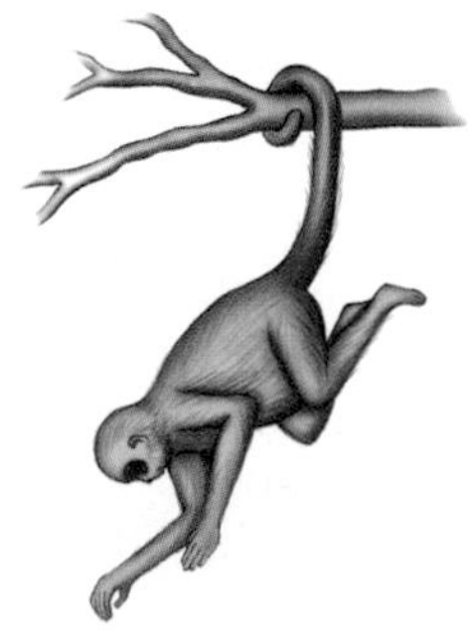

The first condition involves the administration of Rh-positive (+) blood to an Rh-negative (−) person. If Rh-positive (+) blood from a donor is administered to an Rh-negative (−) person (the recipient), the Rh antigen of the donor stimulates the recipient to produce anti-Rh antibodies. The recipient is now said to be sensitized. If the Rh-negative (−) person is later given a second transfusion of Rh-positive (+) blood, the anti-Rh antibodies in the plasma of the recipient will attack the Rh antigen of the Rh-positive (+) donor blood, causing agglutination and hemolysis.

The Rh factor may cause a serious problem in a second condition, that of an Rh-negative (−) pregnant mother who is carrying an Rh-positive (+) fetus (Figure 15-13). During this first pregnancy, the baby grows to term and is delivered uneventfully. During childbirth, however, some of the baby's Rh-positive (+) blood crosses the placenta and enters the mother's blood. The Rh antigen stimulates the mother's immune system to produce anti-Rh antibodies. In other words, the mother has become sensitized by her first baby. If the mother becomes pregnant for a second time with an Rh-positive (+) baby, the anti-Rh antibodies move from the mother's circulation into the baby's circulation. These anti-Rh antibodies attack the baby's RBCs, causing agglutination. In response, the baby becomes jaundiced and anemic as the RBCs undergo hemolysis.

This hemolytic condition is called erythroblastosis fetalis. The hemolysis causes a rapid rise in plasma levels of bilirubin. The hyperbilirubinemia (increased bilirubin in the blood), in turn, causes severe jaundice and a condition called kernicterus. Kernicterus, caused by the staining of a part of the brain with bilirubin, is characterized by severe retardation in mental development.

Erythroblastosis fetalis can be prevented by the administration of the drug RhoGAM. RhoGAM is administered to the mother during pregnancy and within 72 hours after delivery. RhoGAM surrounds, or coats, the baby's Rh-positive (+) antigens, thereby preventing them from stimulating the development of anti-Rh antibodies by the mother.

Sum It Up!

Blood is classified according to the antigens on the surface of the RBC. The ABO grouping contains four blood types: A (A antigens); B (B antigens); AB (A and B antigens); and O (neither A nor B antigens). An antigen-antibody reaction, called agglutination, occurs when blood is mismatched. Type AB blood is the universal recipient blood. Type O blood is the universal donor blood. The Rh factor is another type of antigen on the RBC. Rh-positive blood has the Rh factor on the RBC, whereas Rh-negative blood does not contain the Rh factor.

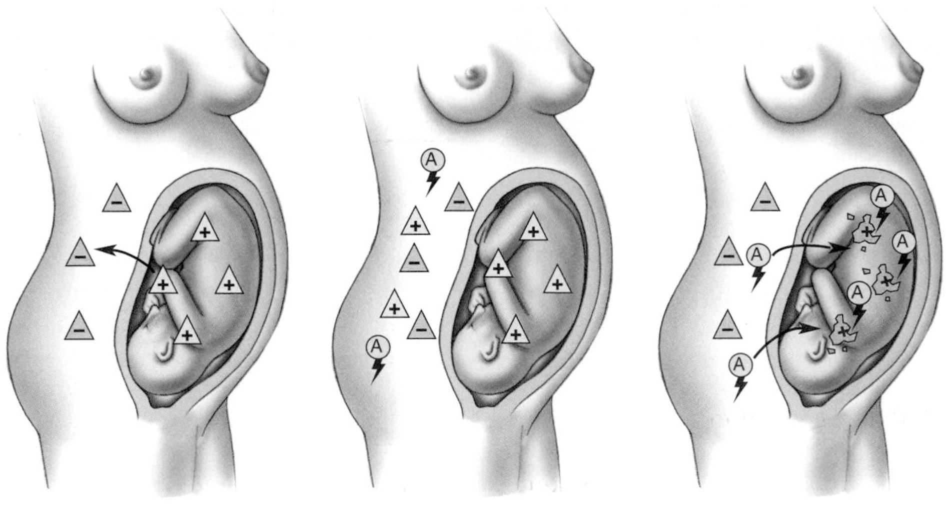

 Rh– Red blood cell (RBC) of mother

 Rh+ RBC of fetus with Rh antigen on surface

 Anti–Rh antibody made against Rh+ RBC

Hemolysis of Rh+ RBC

FIGURE 15-13 Hemolysis: erythroblastosis fetalis.

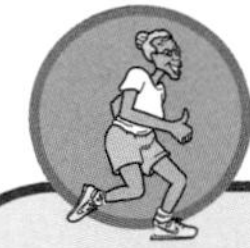

As You Age

1. The volume and composition of blood remain constant with age, so most laboratory values remain normal. Alterations in laboratory values for blood usually indicate alterations in other organ systems. For instance, the fasting blood glucose level increases with aging. This alteration is not the result of changes in the blood, however. Rather, it is the result of age-related changes associated with insulin. The same is true regarding serum lipids. Serum lipids increase 25% to 50% after the age of 55, but the increase is due to an altered metabolism and not to changes of the blood and blood-forming organs.
2. The amount of red bone marrow decreases with age. The total number of blood cells remains normal, but older persons do take longer to form new blood cells and hence recover more slowly from bleeding episodes (hemorrhages).
3. An age-related decline occurs in white blood cell (WBC) activity. Although WBC activity still increases in response to infection, it does so more slowly.

Disorders of the Blood

Anemia	A condition in which the number of red blood cells (RBCs) decreases or the amount of hemoglobin decreases. There are many types of anemia. Hemorrhagic anemia is due to loss of blood. Aplastic anemia is a decrease in RBCs because of impaired bone marrow activity. Hemolytic anemia develops in response to excess RBC destruction. Anemias may develop when necessary substances are not present. For instance, a dietary deficiency of iron causes iron-deficiency anemia. A dietary deficiency of folic acid causes folic aciddeficiency anemia. An inability to absorb vitamin B_{12} is called pernicious anemia.
Blood poisoning	Also called septicemia from the Greek word meaning rotten blood. Blood poisoning refers to the presence of harmful substances such as bacteria and toxins in the blood.
Ecchymosis	Also called a bruise. Blood leaks into the tissue after injury. As the hemoglobin breaks down, it forms breakdown products, which first color the skin black and blue and then dull yellow-brown.

Continued

Disorders of the Blood—cont'd

Hemophilia	A hereditary deficiency of factor VIII, or the hemophilic factor, resulting in an impaired ability to clot blood and severe bleeding episodes. There are many other hereditary bleeding disorders. Christmas disease is a deficiency of factor IX, and von Willebrand's disease is a deficiency of a protein that affects factor VIII function.
Leukemia	Called cancer of the blood and characterized by uncontrolled leukocyte production. The abnormal leukocytes invade the bone marrow and impair normal blood cell production. As with other cancers, malignant cells metastasize through the body.
Polycythemia	Means many cells in the blood. Polycythemia vera (meaning true polycythemia) is due to the overproduction of blood cells (usually red blood cells) by the bone marrow. Secondary polycythemia refers to an increase in blood cell production in response to a condition that interferes with oxygenation, such as lung disease.

SUMMARY OUTLINE

Blood has three main functions: it delivers oxygen to all cells; it helps regulate body functions, such as body temperature; and it protects the body from infection and bleeding.

I. Blood

II. Composition and Characteristics of Blood

A. Blood is composed of plasma and blood cells.

B. The blood cells originate in the bone marrow and lymphoid tissue.

III. Blood Cells

A. Red Blood Cells (RBCs) or Erythrocytes

1. RBCs are filled with hemoglobin.
2. Oxyhemoglobin transports oxygen, and carbaminohemoglobin transports carbon dioxide.
3. RBC production is regulated by erythropoietin (senses oxygen).

B. White Blood Cells (WBCs)

1. WBCs are classified as granulocytes and agranulocytes.
2. The granulocytes are neutrophils, basophils, and eosinophils.
3. The nongranulocytes are the lymphocytes and monocytes.

C. Platelets

1. Platelets are thrombocytes.
2. Platelets are involved in hemostasis.

IV. Hemostasis

A. Stages of Hemostasis

1. The three stages of hemostasis are blood vessel spasm, formation of a platelet plug, and blood coagulation.
2. The three stages of blood coagulation are summarized in Figure 15-11.

B. Dissolving Clots and Preventing Clot Formation

1. Eventually the clot dissolves by a process called fibrinolysis; clot dissolution is achieved primarily by plasmin.
2. Natural anticoagulant mechanisms include a smooth endothelial lining and heparin.

V. Blood Types

A. ABO Blood Types

1. There are 4 types of blood: type A, B, AB, and O.
2. The A and B antigens are on the membrane of the RBC.
3. Blood plasma contains anti-A and anti-B antibodies.
4. Blood antigen and antibodies are summarized in Table 15-3.

B. Rh Factor

1. An Rh-positive person has the Rh antigen on the RBC membrane; an Rh-positive person does not have anti-Rh antibodies in the plasma.
2. The Rh factor must be considered when blood is transfused; an Rh (−) person cannot receive Rh (+) blood.
3. An Rh-negative mother carrying an Rh-positive baby may give birth to a baby with erythroblastosis fetalis.

Review Your Knowledge

Matching: Blood Cells

Directions: Match the following words with their descriptions below. Some words may be used more than once.

a. platelets
b. white blood cells
c. red blood cells

1. ____ Contains the antigens A and B
2. ____ Requires erythropoietin for production
3. ____ The reticulocyte is an immature cell of this type
4. ____ Includes the neutrophil, eosinophil, and basophil
5. ____ A deficiency causes petechiae and bleeding
6. ____ Stickiness and plug both describe the functional role of this cell type
7. ____ Primarily concerned with infection
8. ____ Measured as the hematocrit
9. ____ Classified as granulocytes and agranulocytes
10. ____ Primarily concerned with the delivery of oxygen

Matching: Blood Clots

Directions: Match the following words with their descriptions below. Some words may be used more than once.

a. embolus
b. plasmin
c. heparin
d. warfarin (Coumadin)
e. thrombus

1. ____ A blood clot in the leg
2. ____ Drug that interferes with the hepatic utilization of vitamin K in the synthesis of prothrombin
3. ____ A traveling or moving blood clot
4. ____ Enzyme that dissolves clots
5. ____ An anticoagulant that works by removing thrombin (antithrombin activity)

Matching: Blood Types

Directions: Match the following blood types with their descriptions below. Some may be used more than once.

a. A
b. B
c. AB
d. O

1. ____ The blood cells that contain neither the A antigen nor the B antigen
2. ____ The universal donor
3. ____ This blood type can receive type B and type A blood
4. ____ This blood type contains only anti-B antibodies
5. ____ This blood type contains both anti-A and anti-B antibodies

Multiple Choice

1. The erythrocyte
   a. is phagocytic.
   b. contains hemoglobin and transports oxygen.
   c. initiates blood coagulation.
   d. produces antibodies that are involved in the immune response.
2. The neutrophil
   a. is a T lymphocyte.
   b. is a granulocytic phagocyte.
   c. secretes antibodies.
   d. activates plasmin.
3. Thrombin
   a. activates fibrinogen.
   b. is responsible for the formation of the platelet plug.
   c. is inactivated by vitamin K.
   d. is inactivated by prothrombin.
4. What statement is true regarding the administration of type A^+ blood to an O^- recipient?
   a. The blood types are compatible; no hemolytic reaction is expected.
   b. Persons with O^- blood are allergic to type A^+ blood.
   c. The administration of type A^+ blood to a type O^- recipient causes hemolysis.
   d. Persons with type O^- blood can safely receive type A^+ blood.
5. Erythropoietin
   a. is synthesized by the kidneys.
   b. stimulates the bone marrow to make RBCs.
   c. is released by the kidney in response to hypoxia.
   d. All of the above.
6. Which of the following is most likely to cause jaundice?
   a. Anemia
   b. A deficiency of erythropoietin
   c. A deficiency of intrinsic factor
   d. Hemolysis

CHAPTER 16

Anatomy of the Heart

KEY TERMS

Atrium, p. 285
Bicuspid valve, p. 289
Cardiology, p. 283
Chordae tendineae, p. 288
Endocardium, p. 283
Epicardium, p. 283
Mitral valve, p. 289
Myocardium, p. 283
Pericardium, p. 283
Precordium, p. 283
Purkinje fibers, p. 293
Semilunar valve, p. 288
Tricuspid valve, p. 289
Ventricle, p. 285

OBJECTIVES

1. Describe the location of the heart.
2. Name the three layers and covering of the heart.
3. Explain the function of the heart as two separate pumps.
4. Identify the four chambers of the heart.
5. Explain the functions of the four heart valves.
6. Describe blood flow through the heart.
7. List the vessels that supply blood to the heart.
8. Identify the major components of the heart's conduction system.

Throughout history, many functions have been attributed to the heart. Some philosophers have called it the seat of the soul. The ancient Egyptians, for instance, weighed the heart after a person's death because they believed that the weight of the heart equaled the weight of the soul. The heart has also been described as the seat of wisdom and understanding; accordingly, it thinks and makes plans. More often than not, however, history has portrayed the heart as the seat of the emotions. An overly compassionate person is described as soft-hearted, a generous person has a heart of gold, and a grief-stricken person is broken-hearted. Every Valentine's Day card displays hearts, hearts, and more hearts. These cards celebrate love. None focus on the heart as an efficient pump. Enter the modern day heart specialist and the science of **cardiology,** the study of the heart.

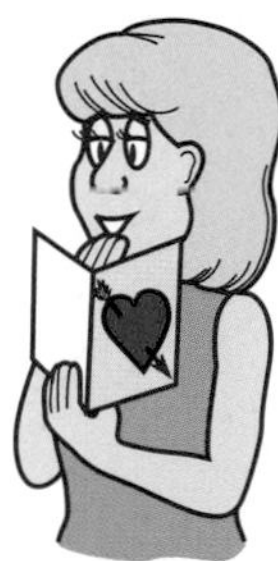

FUNCTION, LOCATION, AND SIZE OF THE HEART

The heart is a hollow, muscular organ. Its primary function is to pump and force blood through the blood vessels of the body, providing every cell in the body with vital nutrients and oxygen. The heart pumps an average of 72 times each minute for your entire lifetime. If you live until you are 75, your heart will beat in excess of 3 billion times. Puts the Energizer Bunny to shame!

The adult heart is about the size of a closed fist and weighs less than 1 pound. The heart sits in the chest within the mediastinum, between the two lungs (Figure 16-1). Two thirds of the heart is located to the left of the midline of the sternum, and one third is located to the right. The upper, flat portion of the heart, called the **base,** is located at the level of the second rib. The lower, more pointed end of the heart is the **apex;** it is located at the level of the fifth intercostal space. The **precordium** refers to the area of the anterior chest wall overlying the heart and great vessels. You need to know the precise location of the heart, because you will be asked to evaluate different heart sounds, accurately position electrodes for an electrocardiogram, and provide life-saving cardiopulmonary resuscitation (CPR).

THE HEART'S LAYERS AND COVERINGS

The heart is made up of three layers of tissue: endocardium, myocardium, and epicardium (Figure 16-2).

ENDOCARDIUM

The **endocardium** is the heart's innermost layer. The endocardium also lines the valves and is continuous with the blood vessels that enter and leave the heart. The smooth and shiny surface allows blood to flow over it easily.

MYOCARDIUM

The **myocardium** is the middle layer of the heart. It is the thickest of the three layers. The myocardium is composed of cardiac muscle that contracts and pumps blood through the blood vessels. (Review muscle contraction in Chapter 9, especially the "sliding" of actin and myosin.)

EPICARDIUM

The **epicardium** is the thin, outermost layer of the heart. The epicardium also helps forms the pericardium.

PERICARDIUM

The heart is supported by a slinglike structure called the **pericardium.** The pericardium attaches the heart to surrounding structures, such as the diaphragm and the large blood vessels that attach to the heart. The pericardium has three layers. The innermost layer (closest to the heart) is the epicardium, also called the visceral pericardium. At the base of the heart, the visceral pericardium folds back and becomes the parietal pericardium. The parietal pericardium attaches to the outer fibrous pericardium that anchors the heart to its surrounding structures. Between the visceral pericardium and parietal pericardium is a space called the **pericardial space,** or **pericardial cavity.** The pericardial membranes are serous membranes that secrete a small amount of slippery, serous fluid (10 to 30 ml) into the pericardial space. The pericardial fluid lubricates the surfaces of the membranes and allows them to slide past one another with little friction or rubbing.

At times, the pericardial membranes become inflamed; this condition is called pericarditis and is characterized by pain and a sound called a friction rub. The friction rub is similar to the sound of scratchy sandpaper and is best heard when the stethoscope is placed over the left sternal border near the apex of the heart. The inflamed pericardial membranes also secrete excess serous fluid into the pericardial space. This collection of fluid in the pericardial space (called

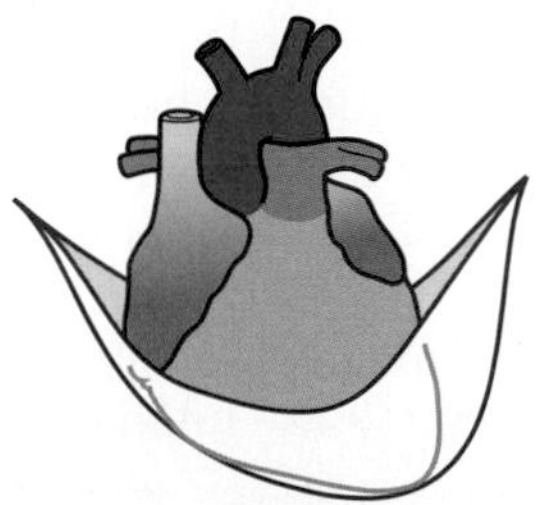

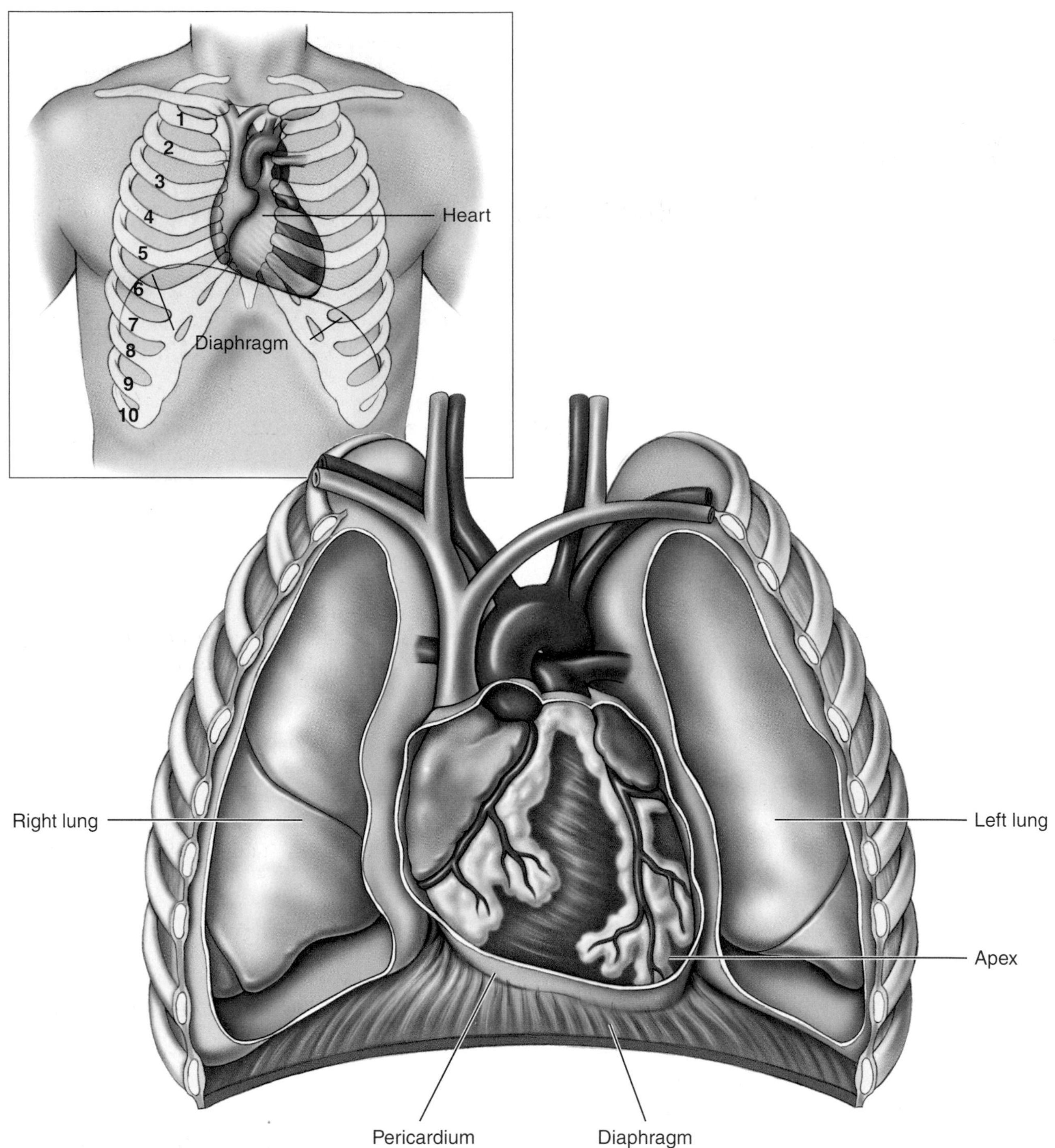

FIGURE 16-1 Location of the heart within the mediastinum.

pericardial effusion) may compress the heart externally, making it difficult for the heart to relax and fill with blood. Consequently, the heart is unable to pump a sufficient amount of blood to the body. This life-threatening condition is called cardiac tamponade. Cardiac tamponade may be treated by inserting a long needle into the pericardial space and aspirating (sucking out) the serous fluid through the needle.

A DOUBLE PUMP AND TWO CIRCULATIONS

The myocardium enables the heart to pump blood. The heart is a double pump that beats as one. The pumps are the **right heart** and the **left heart** (Figure 16-3). The right heart receives unoxygenated blood from the superior and inferior venae cavae, large veins that collect blood from all parts of the body. The right heart is

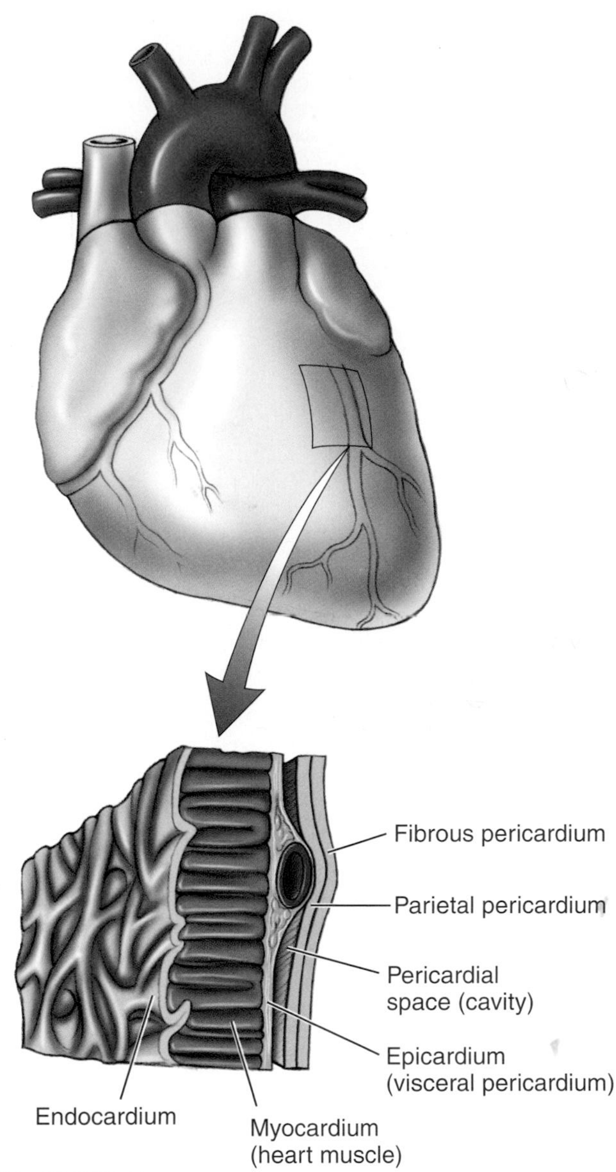

FIGURE 16-2 Layers of the heart and the pericardium.

colored blue because it contains unoxygenated blood. The right heart pumps blood to the lungs, where the blood is oxygenated.

The path that the blood follows from the right side of the heart to and through the lungs and back to the left side of the heart is called the **pulmonary circulation.** The only function of the pulmonary circulation is to pump blood through the lungs in order to pick up oxygen and get rid of carbon dioxide. Oxygen diffuses from the lungs into the blood for delivery to the tissues, while carbon dioxide diffuses from the blood into the lungs for excretion.

The left heart receives the oxygenated blood from the lungs and pumps it to all the organs of the body. The left heart is colored red because it contains oxygenated blood. The path that the blood follows from the left heart to all the organs of the body and back to the right heart is called the **systemic circulation.** The systemic circulation is the larger of the two circulations.

THE HEART'S CHAMBERS AND GREAT VESSELS

The heart has four chambers: two atria and two ventricles (Figure 16-4). The **atria** (singular: **atrium**) are the upper chambers and receive the blood into the heart; the **ventricles** (VĔN-trĭ-k'lz) are the lower chambers and pump blood out of the heart. The right and left hearts are separated from one another by a septum. The interatrial septum separates the two atria; the interventricular septum separates the two ventricles.

RIGHT ATRIUM

The right atrium is a thin-walled cavity that receives unoxygenated (blue) blood from the superior and inferior venae cavae. The **superior vena cava** collects blood from the head and upper body region while the **inferior vena cava** receives blood from the lower part of the body.

RIGHT VENTRICLE

The right ventricle receives unoxygenated blood from the right atrium. The primary function of the right ventricle is to pump blood through the pulmonary arteries to the lungs.

LEFT ATRIUM

The left atrium is a thin-walled cavity that receives oxygenated (red) blood from the lungs through four pulmonary veins.

LEFT VENTRICLE

The left ventricle receives oxygenated blood from the left atrium. The primary function of the left ventricle is to pump blood into the systemic circulation. Blood leaves the left ventricle through the aorta, the largest artery of the body. Note the thickness of the myocardial layer of the ventricles as compared to the thinner atrial muscle. The thick muscle is needed to create enough force to pump blood out of the heart. Note also that the left ventricular myocardium is thicker than the right ventricular myocardium. This difference is due to the greater amount of force required to pump blood into the systemic circulation (aorta).

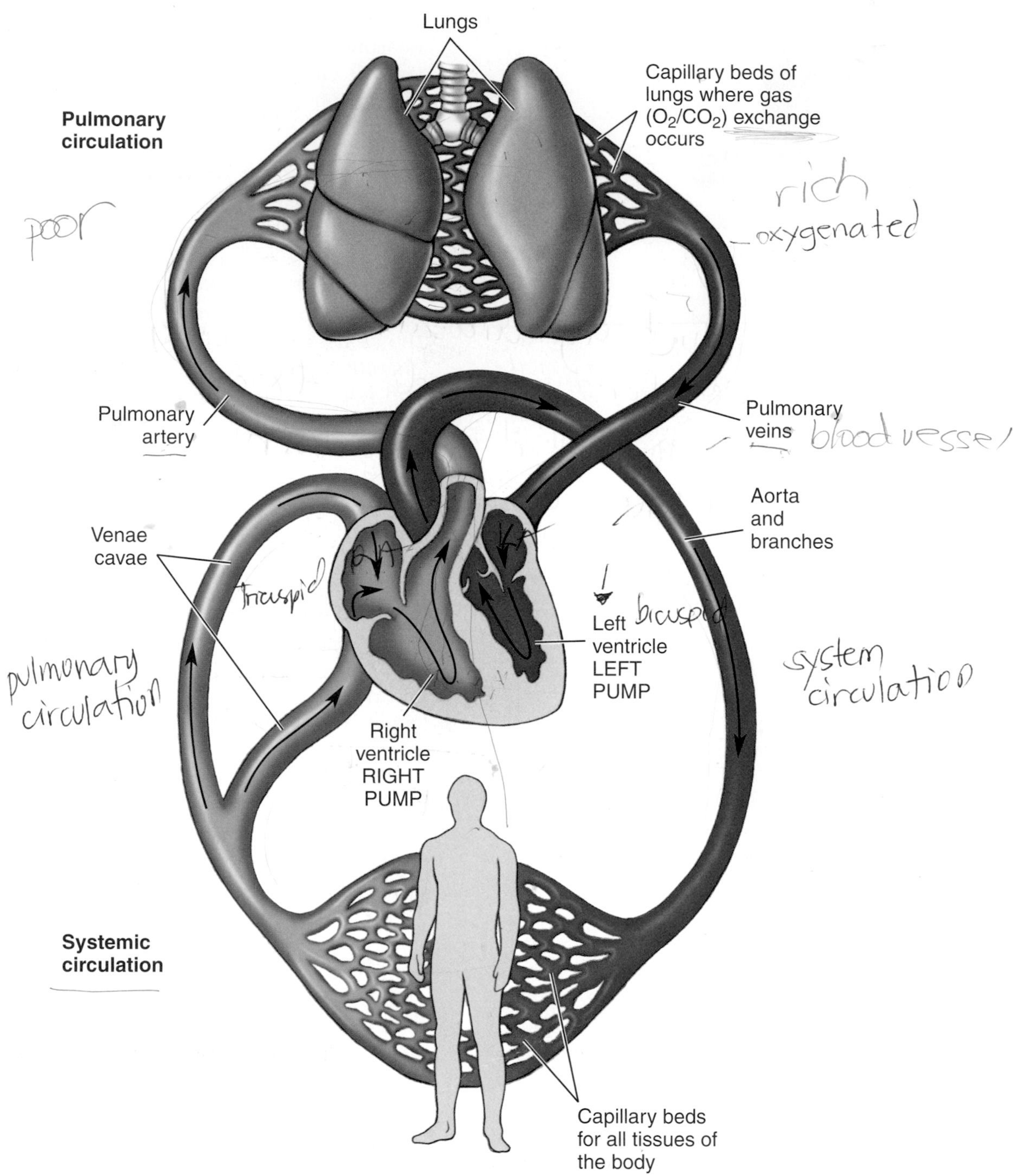

FIGURE 16-3 A double pump and two circulations (pulmonary and systemic circulations).

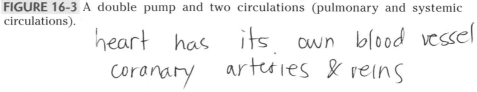

As previously noted, the thickness of the myocardium reflects the amount of work performed by the myocardium. If a ventricle is forced to overwork it will eventually enlarge, a condition called ventricular hypertrophy. For example, a chronically hypertensive (high blood pressure) person generally develops left ventricular hypertrophy. Why? The high blood pressure (in the aorta) makes it more difficult for the left ventricle to pump blood into the aorta. The left ventricle works harder and therefore enlarges or hypertrophies. If the

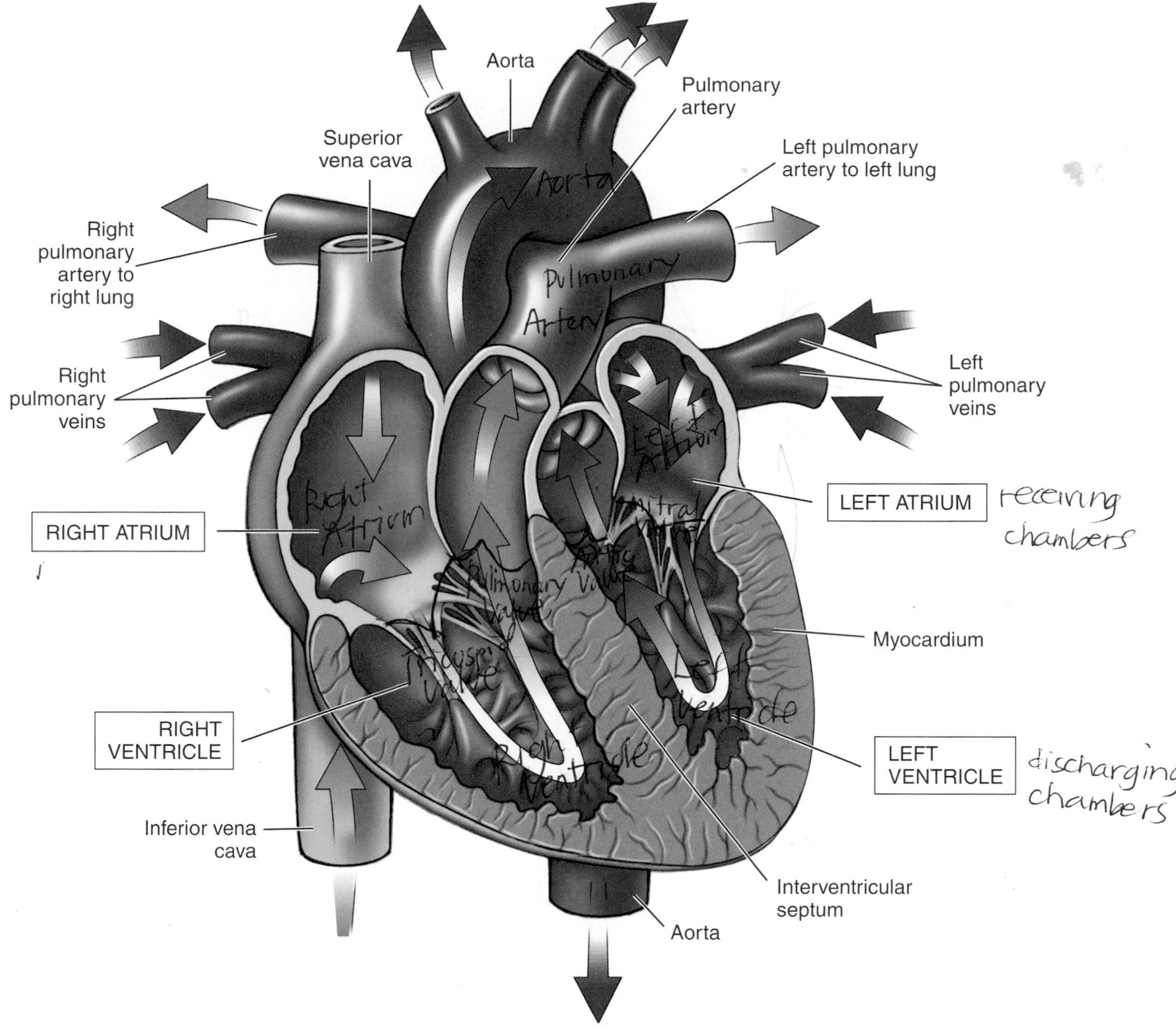

FIGURE 16-4 Chambers of the heart and the great vessels; arrows indicate the blood flow through the heart.

blood pressure is not lowered, the left ventricle will eventually weaken and fail as a pump. For the same reason, a person with pulmonary artery hypertension develops right ventricular hypertrophy and right heart failure.

GREAT VESSELS OF THE HEART

The large blood vessels attached to the heart are called the **great vessels.** They include the superior and inferior venae cavae, pulmonary artery, four pulmonary veins, and the aorta.

Sum It Up!

The heart, a hollow muscular organ that pumps blood, is located within the mediastinum of the thoracic cavity. The heart is a double pump; the right heart pumps blood to the pulmonary circulation while the left heart pumps blood to the systemic circulation. The heart has three layers: endocardium, myocardium, and epicardium. It is supported and anchored by a slinglike pericardium. The heart has four chambers: two atria and two ventricles. The upper atria are receiving chambers while the lower ventricles are pumping chambers. The great blood vessels carry blood to and from the heart.

HEART VALVES

The heart has four valves (Figures 16-5 and 16-6). The purpose of the heart valves is to keep the blood flowing in a forward direction. The valves lie at the entrance and exit of the ventricles. Two of the valves are called **atrioventricular valves,** or **AV valves.** They are located between the atria and the ventricles. Blood flows from the atria through the atrioventricular valves into the ventricles. Atrioventricular valves are entrance valves because they allow blood to enter the ventricles.

The other two valves are classified as **semilunar valves,** so named because the flaps of the valves resemble a half moon (*semi-* means half, *lunar* means moon). The semilunar valves control the outflow of blood from the right and left ventricles and are therefore exit valves.

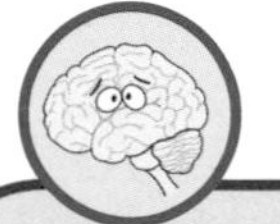

Do You Know...

Why a decline in heart rate can cause a person to faint?

Since blood pressure is determined by heart rate, stroke volume, and peripheral vascular resistance, a decline in any of the three can lower blood pressure. If blood pressure is lowered too much, blood flow to the brain declines and the person faints (syncope). Good news and bad news regarding the faint. The good news: By dropping to the floor the person assumes a horizontal position, restores cerebral blood flow, and "comes to." The downside? Injury on impact (with the floor). People with a history of fainting should be assessed for an underlying cardiac condition.

ATRIOVENTRICULAR VALVES

The AV valves are located between the atria and the ventricles on each side of the heart. The AV valves have cusps, or flaps (see Figure 16-5). When the ventricles are relaxed, the cusps hang loosely within the ventricles; in this position the valves are open and permit the flow of blood from the atria into the ventricles.

What closes the AV valves? Pressure! When the ventricles contract, the heart muscle compresses and squeezes the blood in the ventricles. The blood then gets behind and pushes the cusps upward toward the atria, into a closed position. The closed AV valves prevent the backward flow of blood from the ventricles to the atria.

Why are the cusps not pushed completely through the openings, into the atria, as the pressures within the ventricles increase during muscle contraction? The cusps are attached to the ventricular wall by tough, fibrous bands of tissue called **chordae tendineae** (KŎR-dē tĕn-DĬN-ē-ē). As blood pushes the cusps into a closed position, the chordae tendineae are stretched to their full length. The stretched chordae tendineae hold onto the cusps and prevent them from "blowing" through into the atria, like an umbrella.

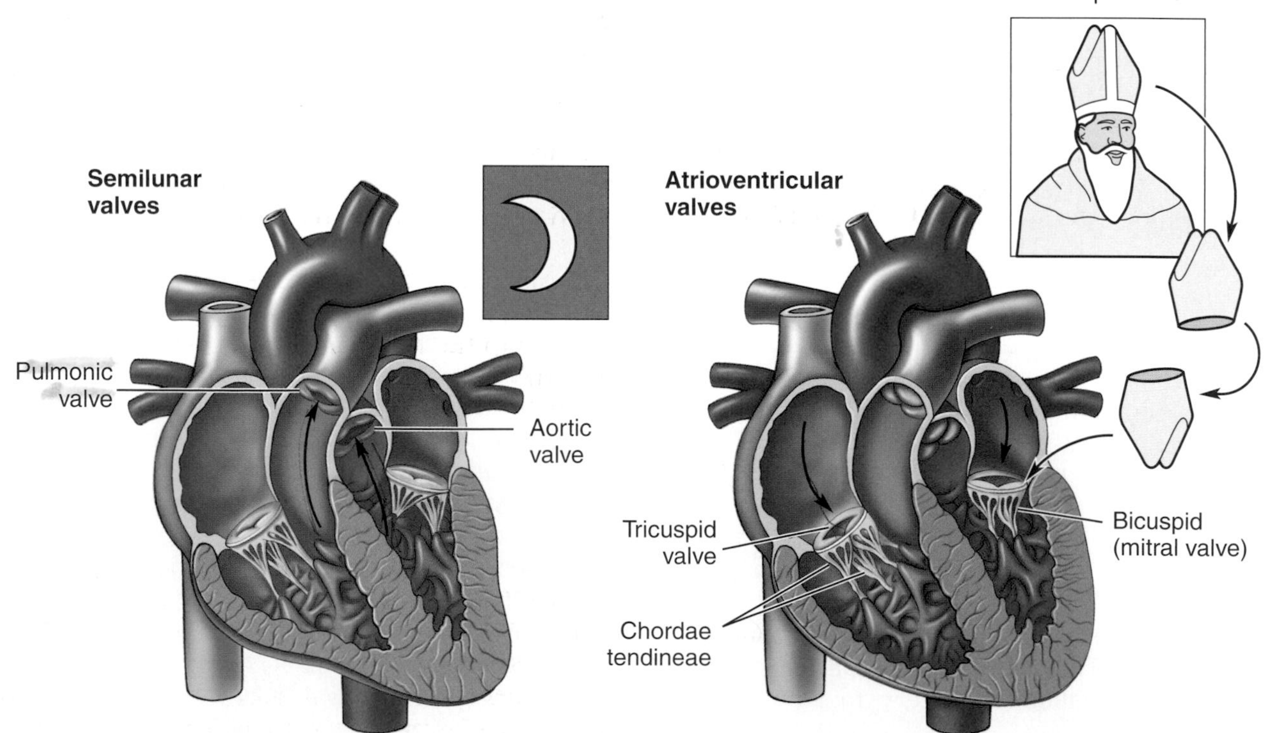

FIGURE 16-5 Valves of the heart: semilunar valves and atrioventricular (AV) valves.

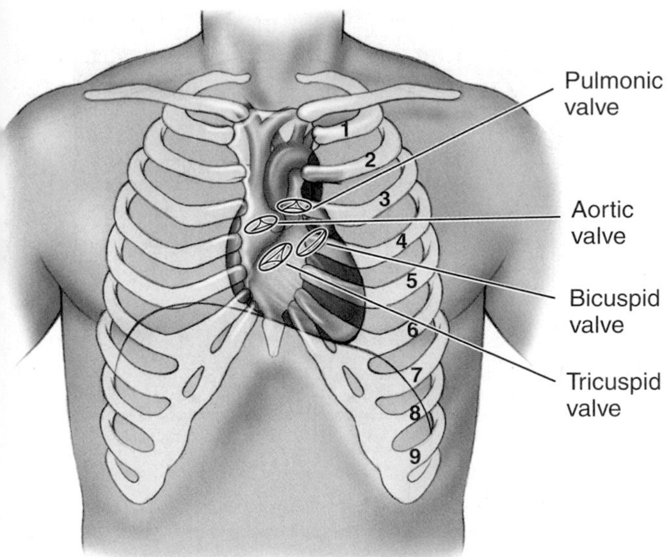

FIGURE 16-6 Location of heart valves.

The **right atrioventricular (AV) valve** is located between the right atrium and the right ventricle. The right AV valve is also called the **tricuspid** (trī-KŬS-pĭd) **valve** because it has three cusps. When the tricuspid valve is open, blood flows freely from the right atrium into the right ventricle. When the right ventricle contracts, however, the tricuspid valve closes and prevents blood from flowing back into the right atrium. The valve ensures a forward flow of blood.

The **left atrioventricular (AV)** valve is located between the left atrium and the left ventricle. The left AV valve is also called the **bicuspid** (bī-KŬS-pĭd) **valve** because it has two cusps. It is also known as the **mitral** (MĪ-trăl) **valve** because it resembles a bishop's mitre, a hat with two flaps. When the mitral valve is open, blood flows from the left atrium into the left ventricle. When the left ventricle contracts, the mitral valve closes and prevents the flow of blood from the left ventricle back into the left atrium.

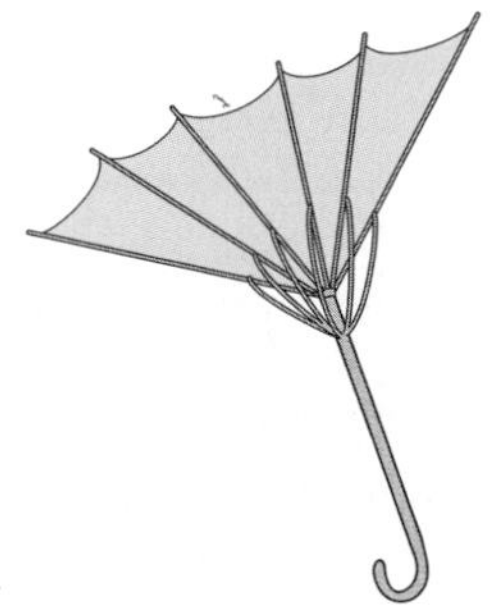

SEMILUNAR VALVES

The two semilunar valves (exit valves) are the pulmonic and aortic valves (see Figure 16-5).

Pulmonic Valve

The **pulmonic semilunar valve** is also called the **right semilunar valve.** It is located between the right ventricle and the pulmonary artery. When the right ventricle relaxes, the valve is in a closed position. When the right ventricle contracts, blood from the ventricle forces the pulmonic valve open. Blood then flows into the pulmonary artery, the large vessel that carries the blood from the right ventricle to the lungs. When the right ventricle relaxes, the pulmonic valve snaps closed and prevents any blood from returning to the right ventricle from the pulmonary artery.

Aortic Valve

The **aortic semilunar valve** or the **left semilunar valve** is located between the left ventricle and the aorta. When the left ventricle relaxes, the valve is in a closed position. When the left ventricle contracts, blood from the ventricles forces the aortic valve open and flows into the aorta. When the left ventricle relaxes, the aortic valve snaps closed and prevents any backflow of blood from the aorta into the ventricle.

How and why do the semilunar valves close? Pressure! The semilunar valves close when the pressure in the pulmonary artery and the aorta becomes greater than the pressure in the relaxed ventricles. The blood in these large blood vessels gets behind the flaps of the valves, snapping them closed. The closed semilunar valves prevent the backward flow of blood from the pulmonary artery and aorta into the ventricles. Repeat! Valves open and close in response to the changing pressures within the heart chambers.

Valves are sometimes defective; they can become narrow or incompetent. Narrowing of the valve is called stenosis. A stenotic valve makes it difficult for the heart chamber to force blood through the valve, thereby increasing the work of the pumping chamber. Thus, aortic valve stenosis increases the work of the left ventricle, causing left ventricular hypertrophy and failure of the left ventricle as a pump. What happens when a heart valve becomes leaky? A leaky, or incompetent, valve allows blood to leak back into the chamber from which it has just been pumped. For instance, an incompetent aortic valve allows blood that has been pumped into the aorta to leak back into the left ventricle. The left ventricle must then pump the same blood again. Over time stenotic and leaky valves impair cardiac function and damage the heart; they are surgically repaired or replaced.

HEART SOUNDS

The heart sounds ("lubb-dupp, lubb-dupp") are made by the vibrations caused by the closure of the valves. When valves become faulty, the heart sounds change. Abnormal heart sounds are called murmurs.

The heart sounds can be heard through a stethoscope placed over the chest wall. The first heart sound (the "lubb") is called S_1. S_1 is due to the closure of the AV valves at the beginning of ventricular contraction; it is best heard over the apex. The second heart sound (the "dupp") is called S_2. S_2 is due to the closure of the semilunar valves at the beginning of ventricular relaxation. S_2 can be heard best at the base of the heart. Listening to S_1 and S_2 is like the sound made by drumming two fingers on a table. Sometimes extra sounds can be heard; they are due to vibrations caused by the rapid flow of blood into the ventricles. The extra sounds are called S_3 and S_4. When both S_3 and S_4 occur, a "gallop rhythm" is heard (sounds like a galloping horse).

Sum It Up!

The purpose of the heart valves is to keep blood flowing forward. There are four heart valves: two atrioventricular valves and two semilunar valves. The heart sounds are due to the closure of the valves.

PATHWAY OF BLOOD FLOW THROUGH THE HEART

The arrows in Figure 16-4 indicate the pathway of blood as it flows through the heart. Unoxygenated (blue) blood enters the right atrium from the superior and inferior venae cavae. The blood flows through the tricuspid valve into the right ventricle. From the right ventricle, the blood flows through the pulmonic valve into the pulmonary artery. The right and left pulmonary arteries carry unoxygenated blood to the lungs for gas exchange. The blood releases carbon dioxide as waste and picks up a fresh supply of oxygen.

The oxygenated (red) blood flows through four pulmonary veins from the lungs into the left atrium. From the left atrium, the blood flows through the bicuspid, or mitral, valve into the left ventricle. Left ventricular contraction forces blood through the aortic valve into the aorta for distribution to the systemic circulation. The pathway of blood flow through the heart and pulmonary circulation is summarized in Figure 16-7.

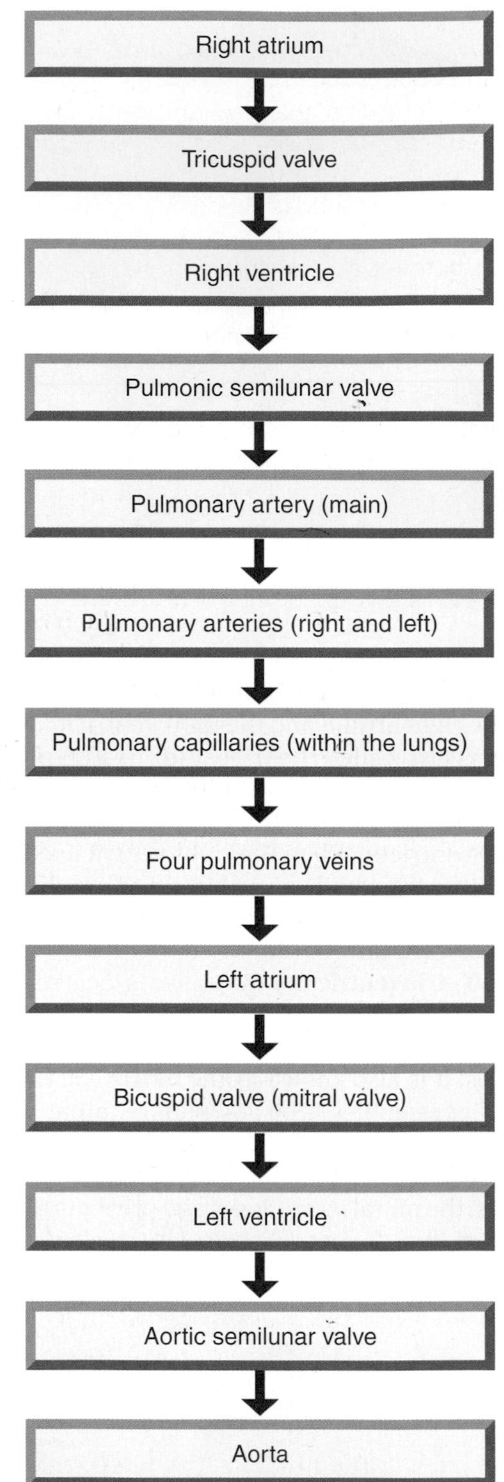

FIGURE 16-7 Blood flow through the heart and pulmonary circulation.

WHOOPS AND DETOURS

Normally blood flows through four separate chambers, from the right side of the heart, to the lungs, and back to the left side of the heart. Congenital heart defects often detour or shunt blood so that the normal circulatory path is disrupted. Let's see how this happens. Keep in mind the following points as we analyze the effects of shunts:

- The right and left hearts are separated by the interatrial and interventricular septa.
- Blood flows in response to a pressure gradient (from a high pressure to a low pressure).
- Pressure is higher in the left heart than in the right heart.
- Blood in the left heart is oxygenated and is bright red while blood in the right heart is unoxygenated and is bluish-red.

Shunts

A shunt is a passageway that diverts blood from its normal circulatory path. There are two types of shunts: a left-to-right shunt and a right-to-left shunt.

Left-to-Right Shunt

A left-to-right shunt can be illustrated by a child with a hole in his interventricular septum. The ventricular septal defect (VSD) causes the left ventricle to do two things. It pumps blood into the aorta, and it also pumps blood into the right ventricle through the hole in the septum. Because blood is shunted from the left heart to the right heart it is called a left-to-right shunt. The child is not cyanotic because the left ventricle is pumping oxygenated blood to the systemic circulation. A VSD is thus described as a left-to-right shunt that is acyanotic.

Right-to-Left Shunt

A right-to-left shunt is illustrated by a child who has a VSD and a stenotic (narrowed) pulmonic valve. The stenotic pulmonic valve increases the pressure within the right ventricle. The elevated right ventricular pressure pumps blood into the left ventricle. Since blood is shunted from the right heart to the left heart it is called a right-to-left shunt. Note that the left ventricle now contains unoxygenated blood. The left ventricle pumps unoxygenated blood into the systemic circulation and the child appears cyanotic. This is an example of a cyanotic right-to-left shunt. Note that a VSD can be either acyanotic or cyanotic depending on other complicating factors.

There are numerous congenital heart defects that result in shunting of blood. You must be able to analyze the defect(s) in terms of the direction (pressure gradients) of the shunt and its implication for blood oxygen content (oxygen saturation).

BLOOD SUPPLY TO THE MYOCARDIUM

Although blood constantly flows through the heart, this blood does not nourish the myocardium. The blood supply that nourishes and oxygenates the myocardium is provided by the **coronary arteries** (Figure 16-8). The arteries supplying the myocardium are called coronary arteries because they resemble a crown encircling the heart. The coronary arteries arise from the base of the aorta just beyond the aortic semilunar valve.

The two main coronary arteries are the **left** and the **right coronary arteries.** The right coronary artery nourishes the right side of the heart, especially the right ventricle. The left coronary artery branches into the **left**

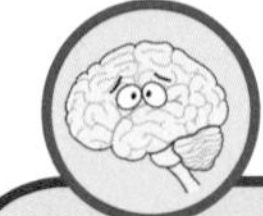

Do You Know...

Why the LAD is called the "widow-maker"?

The LAD is the left anterior descending coronary artery. It supplies blood to a large part of the left ventricle. If the LAD becomes blocked the blood supply to the left ventricle is cut off, causing extensive myocardial damage and death.

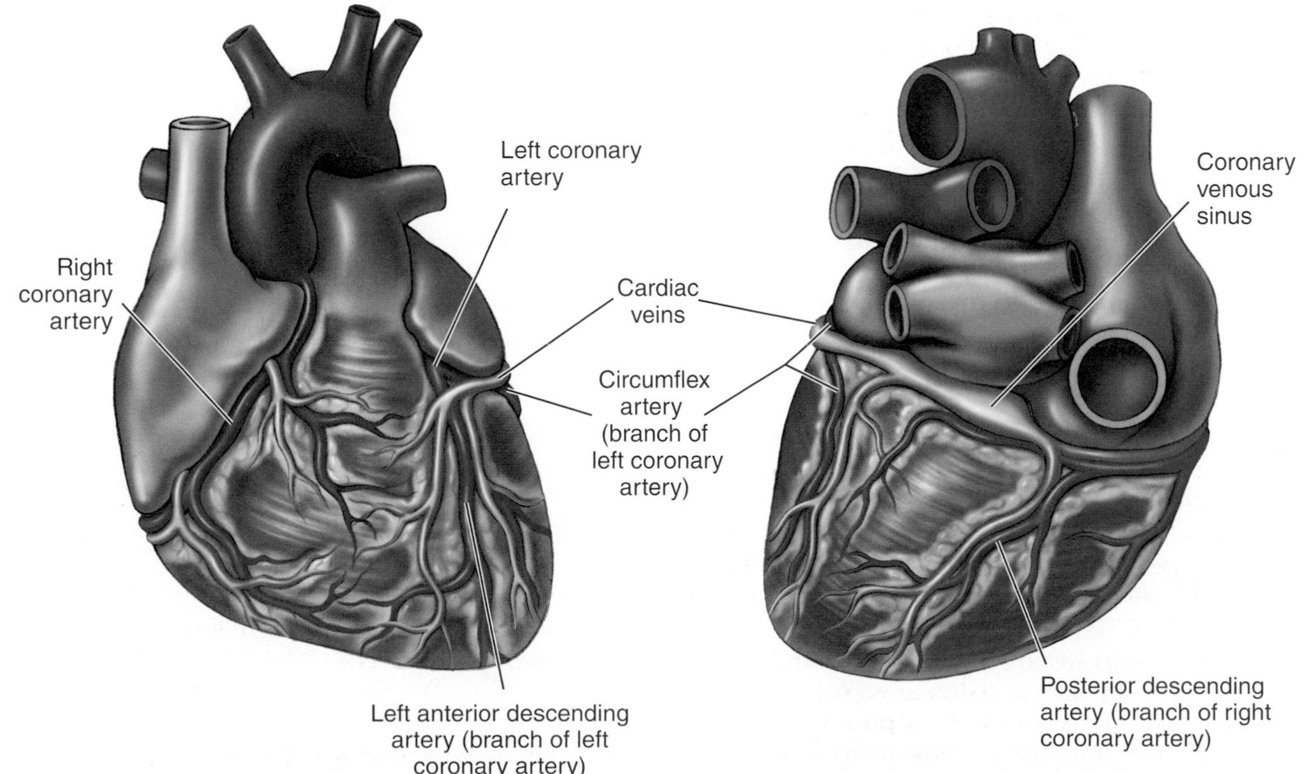

FIGURE 16-8 Blood supply to the myocardium: coronary blood vessels.

anterior descending (LAD) artery and the **circumflex artery.** These arteries carry blood to the left side of the heart, especially the left ventricular wall. The **coronary veins** collect the blood that nourishes the myocardium. The coronary veins carry the blood to the **coronary sinus,** which empties the blood into the right atrium.

There are three important characteristics of coronary blood flow:

- Coronary blood flow can increase. The heart must have a constant supply of oxygenated blood. Under resting conditions the heart muscle removes almost all of the oxygen from the blood flowing through the coronary arteries. Thus, if the heart needs more oxygen, coronary blood flow must increase. With exertion coronary blood flow can increase up to four to five times in the normal heart. However, coronary arteries that have severe fatty plaque buildup are usually maximally dilated at rest. With exertion coronary blood flow cannot increase and the myocardium experiences oxygen deprivation. Thus patients with coronary artery disease will often experience pain with exertion.

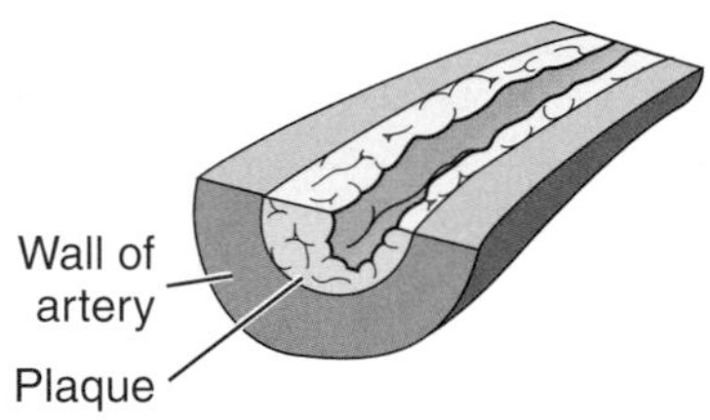

- Coronary blood flow is greatest during myocardial relaxation. Why? Because contraction of the myocardium compresses or squeezes the coronary vessels, thereby cutting off blood flow. When the heart muscle relaxes, the coronary blood vessels open, thereby restoring blood flow. Thus, when the relaxation phase is shortened, as in a "racing heart," coronary blood flow is decreased and the myocardial cells may experience signs of oxygen deprivation, causing chest pain.
- Coronary arteries can form anastomoses, multiple connections between the arteries. An anastomosis allows blood to flow around an artery that is blocked. Additional collateral blood vessels develop in response to diminished coronary blood flow as often occurs with aging and chronic coronary artery disease. For this reason older persons often experience less myocardial damage from a heart attack than do younger persons.

Do You Know...

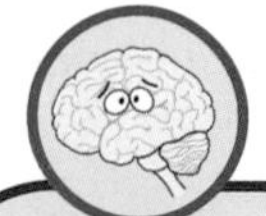

Why heart attacks are treated with clot busters?

A blood clot may block the flow of blood through a coronary artery, causing myocardial damage. The prompt administration of a new class of drugs called clot busters, or thrombolytics, dissolves the clot and restores coronary blood flow, thereby preventing further myocardial damage.

THE "ACHY BREAKY" HEART

If coronary blood flow diminishes, the myocardium experiences oxygen deprivation (ischemia) and soon informs its owner of the situation. For instance, a coronary artery may become partially occluded by fatty plaque (or blood vessel spasm), thereby diminishing coronary blood flow. The person experiences chest pain (angina) that often radiates to the left shoulder and down the left arm into the fingers. Pain at the pump? Think angina. Angina is often relieved by rest and the administration of drugs such as nitroglycerin that decrease the work of the heart.

Do You Know...

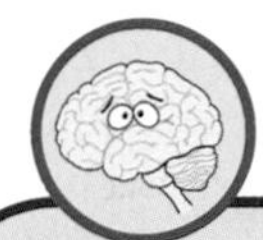

What that balloon is doing in Anne Gyna's chest?

Angina (chest pain) is most often due to the accumulation of fatty plaque within the coronary arteries. Coronary artery occlusion is often treated with balloon therapy. A deflated balloon is inserted into the coronary artery. It is then inflated against the fatty plaque, flattening the plaque against the arterial wall and restoring coronary blood flow. The same effect can be achieved by the insertion of a stent, a small hollow wire-mesh cylinder (looks like a tiny Slinky), into the occluded coronary artery. Improved cardiac blood flow improves myocardial oxygenation, reduces chest pain, and prevents myocardial damage.

Sometimes the coronary artery occlusion worsens when a platelet-containing fatty plaque ruptures and completely blocks coronary blood flow. The oxygen-deprived myocardial cells die, causing a myocardial infarction (MI) or heart attack. An adult male having a heart attack often experiences nausea and vomiting, diaphoresis (profuse sweating), and severe crushing chest pain. With a fist clenched over his heart, the person may complain that the pain feels as though an elephant is sitting on his chest. Moan he will! **MOAN** is a good way for you to remember the emergency treatment for MI:

M morphine (pain and anxiety)
O oxygen (pain and myocardial oxygenation)
A aspirin (antiplatelet effects): chew and swallow
N nitroglycerin (drug that decreases cardiac work)

Elders and women who experience an MI may present a much different clinical picture. For instance, many do not experience crushing chest pain and diaphoresis. They often complain of fatigue and digestive symptoms such as heartburn and upset stomach. Depending on the severity and location of the infarction the person may recover uneventfully or experience a lethal electrical disturbance, cardiogenic shock, or heart failure.

CARDIAC ENZYMES AND LEAKY CELLS

The dead myocardial cells leak enzymes into the blood, causing plasma elevations of cardiac enzymes: creatine phosphokinase (CPK), aspartate aminotransferase (AST), and lactic dehydrogenase (LDH). A regulator myocardial protein, called troponin, also leaks out of the necrotic myocardium into the blood. Thus, plasma elevations of CPK, AST, LDH, and troponin are indicative of MI. The leaked enzymes thus provide a valuable diagnostic tool for heart attacks.

Sum It Up!

Blood flows from the right atrium to the right ventricle, where it is pumped to the lungs for oxygenation (pulmonary circulation). Oxygenated blood returns to the left atrium and then to the left ventricle where it is pumped into the aorta and systemic circulation. The myocardium (pump) is nourished by the coronary blood vessels. Coronary blood flow must be maintained if the heart is to function normally. Occlusion of the coronary arteries is a major cause of disability and death.

CARDIAC CONDUCTION SYSTEM

How does the heart know when to contract (pump) and when to relax? The heart's conduction system initiates an electrical signal and then moves that signal along a special pathway through the heart. The cardiac conduction system not only provides the stimulus (cardiac impulse) for muscle contraction but also coordinates the pumping activity of the atria and ventricles. First, both atria must contract forcing blood into the relaxed ventricles. Then the ventricles contract. The cardiac conduction system gets it going and keeps it organized!

PARTS OF THE CARDIAC CONDUCTION SYSTEM

The conduction system is located within the walls and septum of the heart. The conduction system consists of the following structures: the sinoatrial node, the atrial conducting fibers, the atrioventricular node, and the His-Purkinje system (Figure 16-9).

Sinoatrial Node (SA Node)

The **sinoatrial (SA) node** is located in the upper posterior wall of the right atrium. An electrical signal originates within the SA node. The electrical signal is called the action potential or the **cardiac impulse.** In this text, we use the term cardiac impulse.

The SA node fires a cardiac impulse 60 to 100 times per minutes (average 72 times). Because the firing of the SA node sets the rate at which the heart beats, or contracts, the SA node is called the **pacemaker** of the heart. Heart rate is set by this pacemaker just as the speed of a race is set by the pace car.

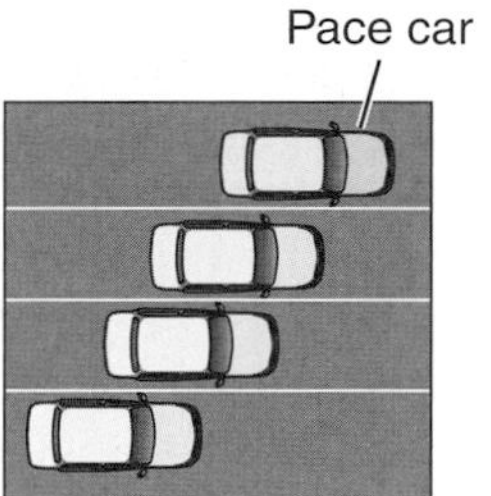

Do You Know...

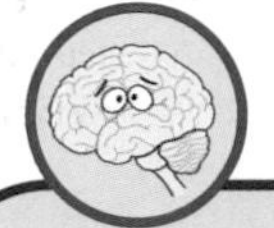

That there is the pacemaker and a bunch of slower pacemakers?

The SA node is *the* pacemaker of the heart because it normally sets the heart rate between 60 to 100 beats/min. There are many other pacemaker cells within the heart, but they fire at a slower rate. For instance, when the SA node fails to function as a pacemaker, the AV takes over and fires at a slower rate of 40 to 60 beats/min. Sometimes the ventricles assume the pacemaker role and fire at a much slower rate, 30 to 40 beats/min. Very slow heart rates cause a decrease in blood pressure and fainting. Impaired pacemaker activity often requires the insertion of an artificial pacemaker.

Atrial Conducting Fibers

The cardiac impulse spreads from the SA node through both atria along the **atrial conducting fibers.** The signal also spreads to the AV node.

Atrioventricular Node (AV Node)

The **atrioventricular (AV) node** is located in the floor of the right atrium, near the interatrial septum. (Note: Do not confuse the AV node with the AV valve.) The cardiac impulse slows as it moves through the AV node into the **bundle of His,** the specialized conduction tissue located in the interventricular septum. The slowing of the cardiac impulse as it moves through the AV node is important. The slow movement delays ventricular activation, thereby allowing the relaxed ventricle time to fill with blood after atrial contraction.

His-Purkinje System

The bundle of His divides into two branches, the right and left bundle branches. The right and left bundle branches send out numerous long fibers called **Purkinje** (PŬR-kĭn-jē) **fibers.** Purkinje fibers are distributed

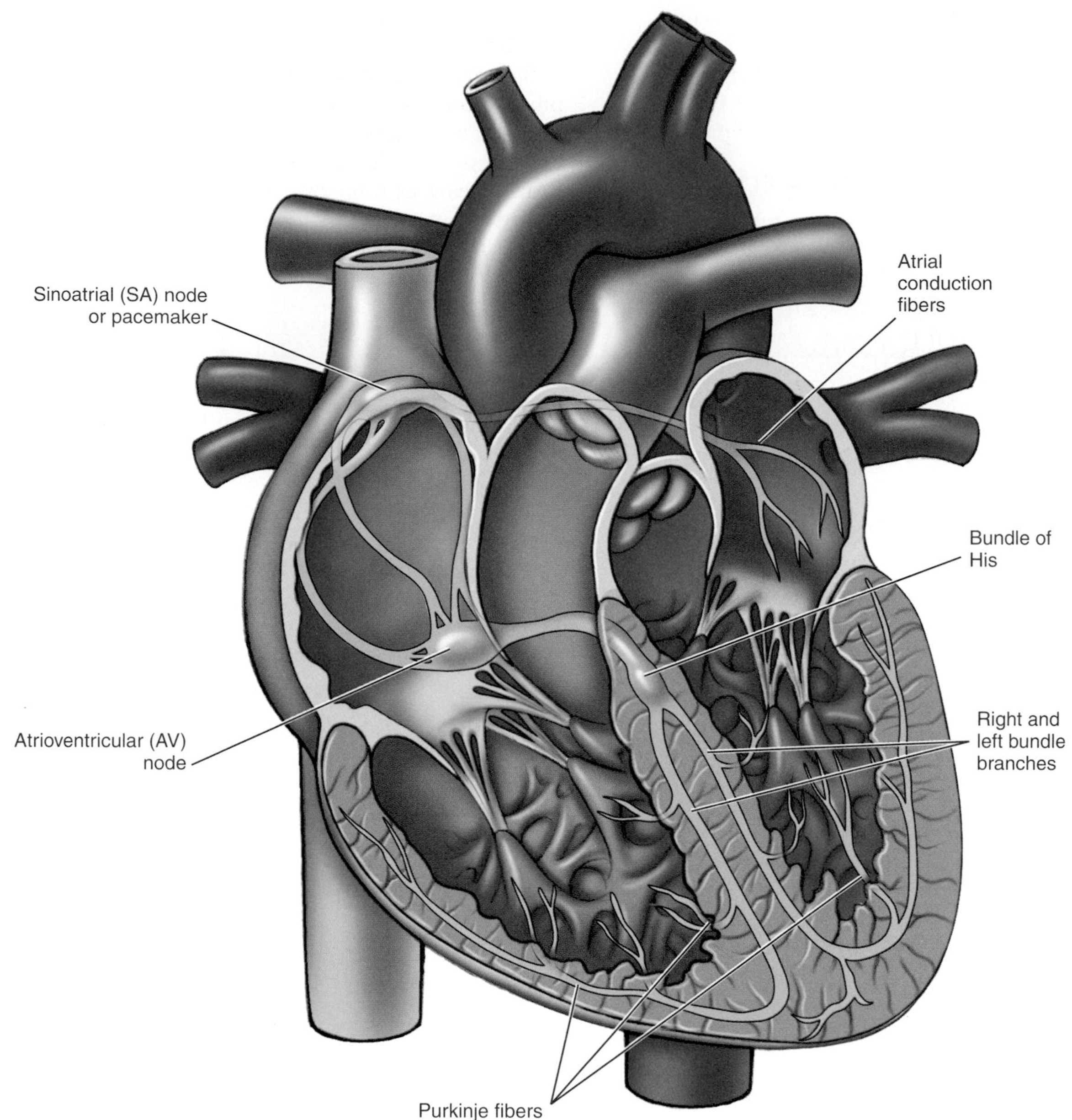

FIGURE 16-9 Conduction system of the heart.

throughout the ventricular myocardium. Purkinje fibers conduct the cardiac impulse very rapidly throughout the ventricles, thereby ensuring a coordinated contraction of both ventricles. The pathway followed by the cardiac impulse is summarized in Figure 16-10.

AUTOMATICITY AND RHYTHMICITY

Your heart beats automatically. The ability of cardiac tissue to create a cardiac impulse accounts for two characteristics of cardiac tissue: automaticity and rhythmicity. Because the cardiac impulse arises within cardiac tissue itself, cardiac tissue is said to have **automaticity.** (Note: a pacemaker cell creates the electrical signal with no help from extrinsic nerves.)

Your heart has rhythm. Because cardiac tissue fires a cardiac impulse regularly, the heart is said to have **rhythmicity.** The SA node, for instance, fires at a rate of 60 to 100 times per minute. At times, the rhythm of the heart is disturbed; the heart is then said to be dysrhythmic (difficulty with rhythm). Some dysrhythmias are relatively harmless. Others are life-threatening and demand immediate attention. For instance, ventricular fibrillation is a life-threatening dysrhythmia. Abnormal electrical activity causes the ventricular myocardium to fibrillate. A fibrillating muscle merely quivers and is unable to contract and pump blood. Dysrhythmias that are due to excess electrical activity are called tachydysrhythmias, while dysrhythmias characterized by diminished electrical activity are called bradydysrhythmias.

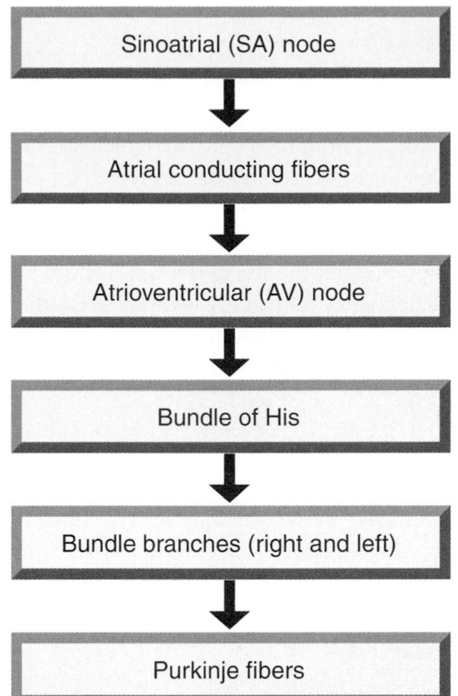

FIGURE 16-10 Pathway followed by a cardiac impulse.

"The pacemaker wanna-be." The SA node is normally the site where the cardiac impulse arises. At times, however, other areas of the heart take over the role of the pacemaker. For example, the area outside the SA node can produce a cardiac impulse. This impulse is called an ectopic focus. (Ectopic means that the beat originates in an area other than the normal site, the SA node.) The AV node can also assume the role of pacemaker (called nodal rhythm), as can other cells within the ventricular conduction system. Serious dysrhythmias occur when these other "wanna-be" sites act as pacemakers.

ELECTROCARDIOGRAM

The cardiac impulse that stimulates muscle contraction is an electrical signal. The electrical activity of the heart is measured by placing electrodes on the surface of the chest and attaching the electrodes to a recording device. The record of these electrical signals is called an **electrocardiogram,** or ECG (Figure 16-11).

The components of the ECG include a P wave, a QRS complex, and a T wave. The **P wave** reflects the electrical activity associated with atrial depolarization. Depolarization precedes and triggers contraction of the heart muscle. (See Chapter 10 for a review of polarization,

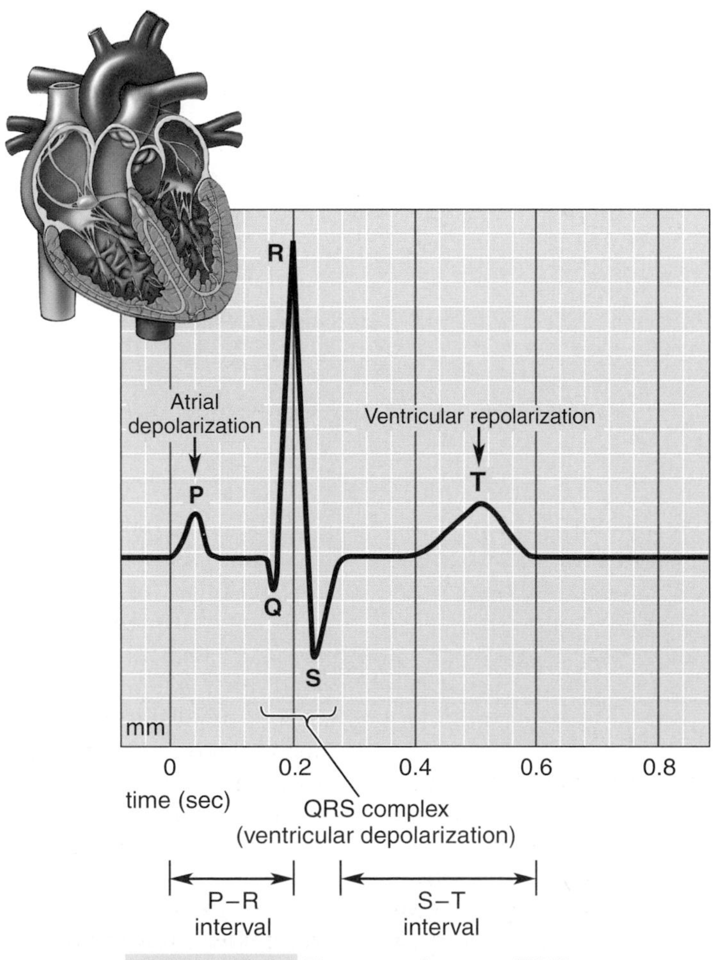

FIGURE 16-11 Electrocardiogram (ECG).

depolarization, and repolarization.) The **QRS complex** reflects the electrical activity associated with ventricular depolarization. The **T wave** reflects the electrical activity associated with ventricular repolarization.

In addition to identifying areas of depolarization and repolarization, the P, QRS, and T deflections (waves) of the ECG provide other useful information. For instance, the **P-R interval** represents the time it takes for the cardiac impulse to travel from the atria (P wave) to the ventricles (QRS complex). Other measurements include the width of the QRS complex and the length of the S-T interval. **Normal sinus rhythm (NSR)** means that the ECG appears normal and that the impulse originates in the SA node.

Note that the ECG is recorded on special graph paper that allows electrical events to be timed. The cardiologist can determine whether the electrical signals are moving too fast or are delayed.

Sum It Up!

Heart muscle contracts in response to an electrical signal called the cardiac impulse, which spreads throughout the heart, coordinating cardiac muscle contraction. The cardiac impulse normally arises within the SA node and spreads throughout both atria over specialized conduction tissue. The cardiac impulse then enters the AV node, where it is momentarily delayed before entering the His-Purkinje system in the ventricles. Cardiac conduction tissue displays automaticity and rhythmicity. The electrical events are recorded as the electrocardiogram (ECG).

SUMMARY OUTLINE

The heart is a four-chambered pump that delivers blood to the lungs and the systemic circulation.

I. Function, Location and Size of the Heart

A. The heart (size of a fist) is located in the mediastinum toward the left side.

B. The heart pumps blood throughout the body delivering nutrients and picking up waste.

II. The Heart's Layers and Covering

A. The heart has three layers: endocardium, myocardium, and epicardium.

B. The heart is supported by a slinglike pericardium.

C. Two layers of the pericardium form the pericardial space.

III. A Double Pump and Two Circulations

A. The right heart pumps blood to the lungs for oxygenation (called the pulmonary circulation).

B. The left heart pumps blood throughout the rest of the body (called the systemic circulation).

IV. The Heart's Chambers and Great Vessels

A. The heart has four chambers, two atria and two ventricles.

B. The atria receive the blood, and the ventricles pump the blood.

V. Heart Valves

A. The purpose of heart valves is to keep blood flowing in a forward direction.

B. Two atrioventricular (AV) valves are the tricuspid valve (right heart) and the bicuspid (mitral) valve (left heart).

C. The two semilunar valves are the pulmonic valve (right heart) and the aortic valve (left heart).

VI. Heart Sounds

A. The heart sounds ("lubb-dupp") are made by the vibrations caused by closure of the valves.

B. The "lubb" is due to the closure of the AV valves at the beginning of ventricular contraction. The "dupp" is due to the closure of the semilunar valves at the beginning of ventricular relaxation.

VII. Pathway: Blood Flow Through the Heart

A. The right heart receives blood from the venae cavae and pumps it to the lungs for oxygenation. The left heart receives oxygenated blood from the lungs and pumps it to the systemic circulation.

B. Blood flow through the heart is summarized in the flow chart (see Figure 16-7).

VIII. Blood Supply to the Myocardium

A. The left and right coronary arteries supply the myocardium with oxygen and nutrients.

B. The coronary veins drain the unoxygenated blood and empty it into the coronary sinus (which empties into the right atrium).

IX. Cardiac Conduction System

A. The heart generates an electrical signal (cardiac impulse) that moves throughout the heart in a coordinated way. The electrical signal causes the myocardium to contract.

B. The pathway followed by the cardiac impulse is summarized in Figure 16-10.

C. Cardiac muscle displays automaticity and rhythmicity.

D. The electrical activity of cardiac muscle is recorded as an electrocardiogram.

Review Your Knowledge

Matching: Structures of the Heart

Directions: Match the following words with their descriptions below. Some words may be used more than once.

a. left ventricle
b. coronary artery
c. right atrium
d. left atrium
e. right ventricle
f. myocardium
g. pericardium
h. precordium

1. ____ Slinglike structure that supports the heart
2. ____ Delivers oxygenated blood to the myocardium
3. ____ Layer of the heart that contains actin and myosin; arranged in sarcomeres
4. ____ Chamber that receives unoxygenated blood from the venae cavae
5. ____ Chamber that receives oxygenated blood from the four pulmonary veins
6. ____ Chamber that pumps blood into the aorta
7. ____ Chamber that has the thickest myocardium
8. ____ Chamber that pumps blood into the pulmonary artery
9. ____ The left ventricle receives oxygenated blood from this chamber
10. ____ Refers to the area of the chest that overlies the heart

Matching: Valves

Directions: Match the following words with their descriptions below. Some words may be used more than once.

a. aortic
b. tricuspid
c. bicuspid
d. pulmonic

1. ____ The semilunar valve through which blood exits the right ventricle
2. ____ The exit valve for the right ventricle
3. ____ The atrioventricular valve that "sees" unoxygenated blood
4. ____ The valve that is also called the mitral valve
5. ____ The semilunar valve through which blood exits the left ventricle
6. ____ The AV valve that "sees" oxygenated blood
7. ____ The AV valve located between the left atrium and left ventricle
8. ____ This leaky valve allows blood to flow backward from the pulmonary artery
9. ____ This valve is located in the right heart and does not have chordae tendineae
10. ____ This valve is located in the left heart and has chordae tendineae

Multiple Choice

1. Which of the following is not true of the heart?
   a. The heart is located within the mediastinum.
   b. The apex is located to the left of the sternal midline at the level of the fifth intercostal space.
   c. The base of the heart is located at the level of the second rib.
   d. The precordium is composed of cardiac muscle.
2. Which of the following is least descriptive of the myocardium?
   a. Composed of contractile proteins (actin and myosin)
   b. Thicker in the ventricles than the atria
   c. Thicker in the left ventricle than the right ventricle
   d. Oxygenated by oxygen that diffuses across the ventricular walls
3. Which of the following is the function of a valve?
   a. Regulates the direction of the flow of blood through the heart
   b. Regulates the amount of oxygen bound to hemoglobin
   c. Regulates heart rate
   d. Directs the progression of the cardiac impulse
4. Which of the following is true regarding the structures of the electrical conduction system?
   a. The AV node is the pacemaker.
   b. In normal sinus rhythm the electrical signal arises within the SA node.
   c. The His-Purkinje system spreads the electrical signal from the right atrium to the left atrium.
   d. The purpose of the AV node is to increase the speed at which the cardiac impulse moves from the atria to the ventricles.
5. Which of the following is least true of the aortic valve?
   a. "Sees" oxygenated blood
   b. Causes left ventricular hypertrophy if the valve is stenotic
   c. Allows blood to flow from the ventricle into the pulmonary artery
   d. Classified as a semilunar valve

CHAPTER 17

Function of the Heart

KEY TERMS

Afterload, p. 304
Cardiac cycle, p. 299
Cardiac reserve, p. 303
Chronotropic effect, p. 305
Diastole, p. 299
Dromotropic effect, p. 305
Heart failure, p. 306
Inotropic effect, p. 303
Preload, p. 303
Pulmonary edema, p. 306
Starling's law of the heart, p. 302
Stroke volume, p. 302
Systole, p. 299

OBJECTIVES

1. Define *cardiac cycle* with respect to systole and diastole.
2. Define *cardiac output* and explain how changes in heart rate and/or stroke volume change cardiac output.
3. Describe the autonomic innervation of the heart.
4. Describe the effect of Starling's law of the heart on myocardial contraction.
5. Describe the inotropic effect on myocardial contraction.
6. Define *preload* and explain how it affects cardiac output.
7. Define *afterload* and identify the major factors that determine afterload.
8. Define the special clinical vocabulary used to describe cardiac function.
9. Define *heart failure* and differentiate between right-sided and left-sided heart failure.

The heart functions as a pump supplying blood to every cell in the body. Moreover, the heart is an adaptable pump. For instance, the heart alters its pumping activity to meet the demands of day-to-day physiologic functions such as eating, exercise, and responding to changes in environmental temperature; it also adapts to disease. How does the heart know when to beat faster or slower, weaker or stronger? The coordinated and adaptable heart is the focus of Part A. Part B is called Heart Talk and defines terminology that is commonly used in clinical situations. Part C describes the failing heart.

PART A. THE COORDINATED AND ADAPTABLE PUMP

CARDIAC CYCLE

The **cardiac cycle** is the sequence of events that occurs during one heartbeat. A cardiac cycle is a coordinated contraction and relaxation of the chambers of the heart. Contraction of the heart muscle (myocardium) is called **systole** (SĬS-tō-lē). Contraction of the heart muscle during systole pumps blood out of a chamber. Relaxation of the myocardium is called **diastole** (dī-ĂS-tō-lē). Blood fills a chamber during diastole.

Atrial and ventricular muscle activity is closely coordinated. For example, during atrial systole, the ventricles are in diastole. In this way, when the atria contract, they pump blood into the relaxed ventricles.

The cardiac cycle has three stages (Figure 17-1).

- Atrial systole: The atria contract (systole) and pump blood into the ventricles. During atrial systole the AV valves are open and the ventricles are relaxed.
- Ventricular systole: At the end of atrial systole, the ventricles contract; this is called ventricular systole. As ventricular contractions begin, blood is forced against the AV valves, causing them to snap shut. The blood pushes the semilunar valves open, allowing blood to flow into the pulmonary artery and aorta. Note that the heart valves open and close in response to changing pressures within the chambers.
- Diastole: For a brief period during the cardiac cycle, both the atria and the ventricles are in diastole. As the chambers relax, blood flows into the atria. Because the AV valves are open at this time, much of this blood also flows passively into the ventricles. The period of diastole therefore is a period of filling (of blood); atrial systole follows. The cycle then repeats itself.

How long does the cardiac cycle last? With a heart rate of 70 beats per minute, the duration of the cardiac cycle is 0.8 seconds. All chambers rest for 0.4 seconds. As heart rate increases, the duration of the cardiac cycle shortens. With a dramatic increase in heart rate the period of rest (diastole) may shorten so much that cardiac function is compromised. Why? First, because of a decreased filling time, the amount of blood that enters the ventricles diminishes so that less blood is pumped. Second, because coronary blood flow to the myocardium occurs during diastole, the diminished period of diastole decreases coronary blood flow.

Sum It Up!

The cardiac cycle is the sequence of events that occurs during one heartbeat. The cardiac cycle has three stages: atrial systole, ventricular systole, and diastole. Cardiac muscle contraction is called systole; cardiac muscle relaxation is called diastole. The duration of the cardiac cycle (resting heart) is 0.8 sec.; duration changes with changes in heart rate.

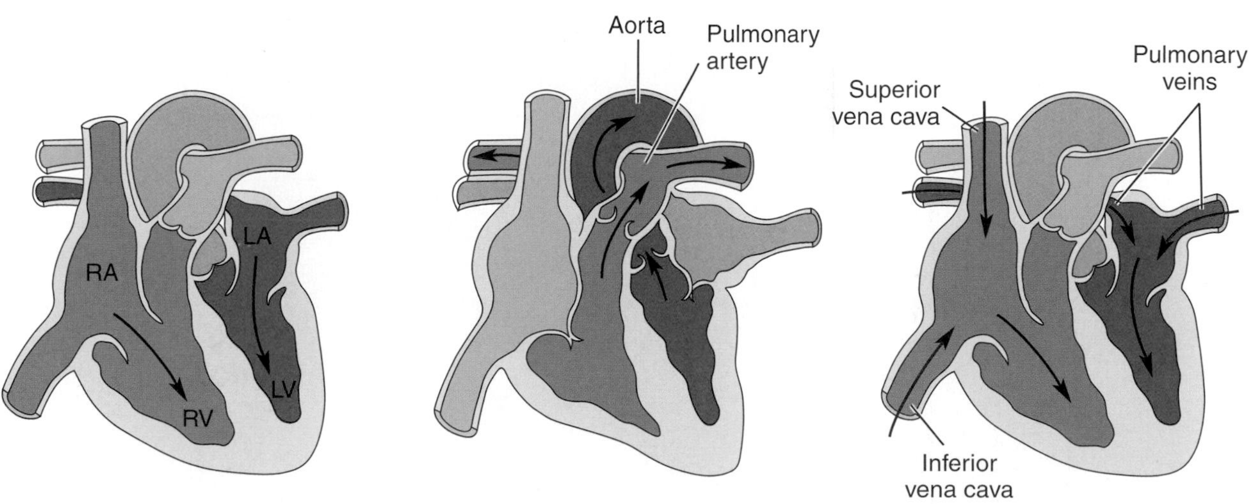

FIGURE 17-1 Stages of the cardiac cycle. **A,** Atrial systole. **B,** Ventricular systole. **C,** Diastole.

AUTONOMIC CONTROL OF THE HEART

The autonomic nervous system (ANS) plays an important role in coordinating and adapting cardiac function.

WHY THE AUTONOMIC NERVOUS SYSTEM?

In the previous chapter we learned that specialized cardiac tissue displays automaticity and rhythmicity. The electrical signal, the cardiac impulse, arises within the cardiac cells and then spreads throughout the heart, causing the heart muscle to contract. If the heart is capable of initiating its own cardiac impulse, then why are the autonomic nerves needed? Although the ANS does not cause the cardiac impulse, it can affect the rate at which the cardiac impulse is fired and the speed it travels throughout the heart. The ANS can also make the heart muscle contract more forcefully; thus the ANS can change the pumping activity of the heart. For instance, if a person suddenly sprints down the street, his or her heart autonomically responds to the increased need for more oxygenated blood; it beats faster and stronger.

AUTONOMIC WIRING

As described in Chapter 12, Autonomic Nervous System, the ANS has two branches, the sympathetic and parasympathetic branches. Refer to Figure 17-2 and note the autonomic wiring of the heart. Sympathetic nerves supply the SA node, AV node, and ventricular myocardium (the sarcomere represents heart muscle). Parasympathetic nerves, also called the vagus nerve, innervate the SA node and the AV node; there is no parasympathetic innervation of the ventricular myocardium.

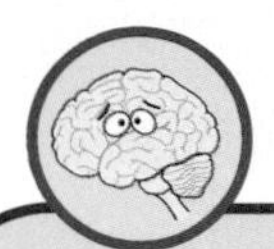

Do You Know...

Why a patient may "brady-down"?

Sometimes a patient may respond to fear or anxiety by an intense discharge of the parasympathetic (vagus) nerves. Vagal discharge to the heart causes a dangerous bradycardia and decline in cardiac output and blood pressure. The administration of a vagolytic drug, such as atropine, relieves the vagal effects and restores heart rate to normal.

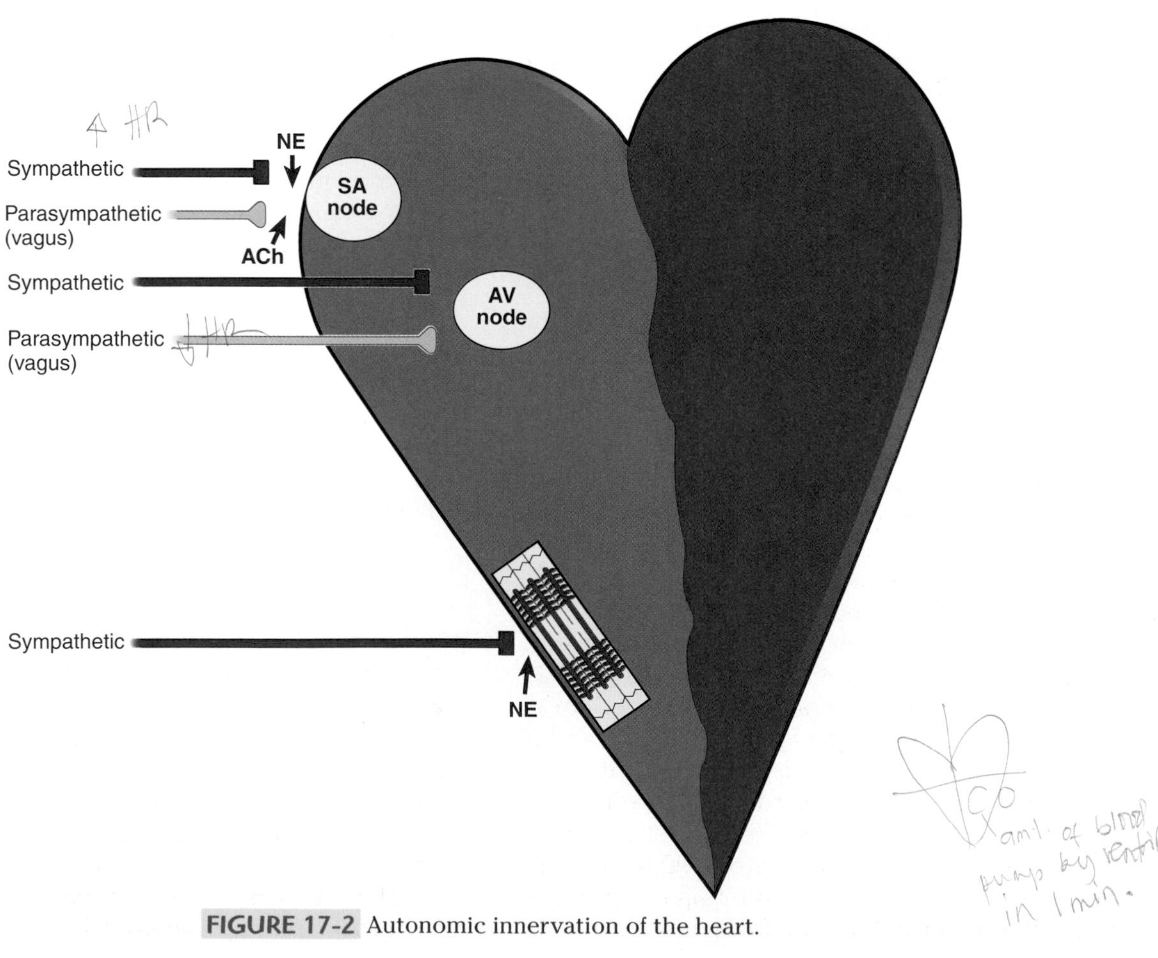

FIGURE 17-2 Autonomic innervation of the heart.

SNS
↑HR

AUTONOMIC FIRING

What happens when the ANS fires?

Sympathetic stimulation

- Increases SA node activity, thus increasing heart rate
- Increases the speed at which the cardiac impulse travels from the SA node throughout the His-Purkinje system
- Increases the force of myocardial contraction, thereby strengthening the force of myocardial contraction

There are four clinically important points regarding excess sympathetic activity on the heart and blood vessels:

- Excess sympathetic activity produces the "fight or flight" response. You will often observe these symptoms (racing and pounding heart) in people who are very anxious, such as during panic attacks. The symptoms are frightening, and the person is convinced of an impending heart attack. Many trips to the ER are panic related.
- Excess sympathetic activity plays a key role in some disease states. For instance, most of the signs and symptoms of circulatory shock are due to excess sympathetic firing. Likewise, the progressive deterioration of patients with heart failure is due in large measure to persistent sympathetic nerve stimulation. Some of the drugs used to treat heart failure are aimed at minimizing the sympathetic effects.
- Excess sympathetic activity often causes tachydysrhythmias.
- You will be giving drugs that resemble or block the effects of sympathetic activity. For instance, epinephrine (Adrenalin) and dopamine increase heart rate and myocardial contractile force. Because the effects mimic stimulation of the sympathetic nervous system (SNS), these drugs are called **sympathomimetic** drugs. Drugs that produce effects that are similar to an inhibition of the SNS are called **sympatholytic** drugs (*-lytic* refers to inhibition).

Parasympathetic (vagus nerve) stimulation

- Decreases SA node activity, thereby decreasing heart rate
- Decreases the speed at which the cardiac impulse travels from the SA node to the AV node
- Exerts no effect on the strength of myocardial contraction (since there are no parasympathetic fibers innervating the ventricular myocardium)

There are three clinically important points about parasympathetic (vagal) nervous system activity:

- In the resting heart, vagal tone is more intense than sympathetic activity. For instance, the SA node would like to fire at a rate of 90 beats/min. However, the "braking" or inhibiting effect of the vagus nerve slows SA node firing to a rate of 72 beats/min, the normal resting heart rate. If the vagus nerve were interrupted, the heart rate would increase to 90 beats/min.
- Certain conditions (heart attack) and drugs (digoxin) can cause excess vagal discharge. Excess vagal discharge causes **bradycardia** (<60 beats/min) and increases the tendency of the heart to develop life-threatening electrical rhythm disturbances. Excess vagal discharge also slows the conduction of the cardiac impulse through the heart causing heart block (a condition in which the signal has difficulty traveling from the atria to the ventricles). The abnormally slow rhythms are called bradydysrhythmias.
- You will be giving drugs that alter the effects of vagal activity. For instance, digoxin decreases heart rate and slows the speed at which the cardiac impulse travels from the atria to the ventricle. Because the effects of digoxin "mimic" vagal stimulation it is called a **vagomimetic** drug. A drug may also produce effects that are similar to an inhibition of vagal discharge. For instance, atropine is used to relieve bradycardia (following a heart attack), because it blocks the effects of vagal stimulation and increases heart rate. Because of its effects on the vagus nerve, atropine is called a **vagolytic** drug. Vagomimetic drugs are also called **parasympathomimetic** drugs and vagolytic drugs are also called **parasympatholytic** drugs.

CARDIAC OUTPUT

To understand how the heart alters its pumping activity, you must understand cardiac output. **Cardiac output** is the amount of blood pumped by each ventricle in 1 minute. The normal cardiac output is about 5 L per minute. Because the total blood volume is about 5 L (5000 ml), the entire blood volume passes through the heart every minute.

Two factors determine cardiac output: heart rate and stroke volume. The relationship is expressed as follows:

Cardiac Output = Heart Rate X Stroke Volume

HEART RATE

The **heart rate (HR)** is the number of times the heart beats each minute. The heart rate is due to the rhythmic firing of the SA node. The normal adult resting heart rate is between 60 and 100 beats per minute, with an average of 72 beats per minute. Resting heart rates differ for many reasons: size, gender, and age.

- Size: Size affects heart rate; generally, the larger the size, the slower the rate. Our feathered and furry friends dramatically illustrate this point.

The heart rate of a hummingbird, for instance, is greater than 200 beats per minute, whereas that of a grizzly is only about 30 beats per minute. Why do heart rates differ? The small hummingbird has a very high metabolism and therefore requires a large amount of oxygen. The metabolism of a grizzly is much slower, requiring less oxygen. Similarly, a tiny baby has a faster HR than a larger adult.

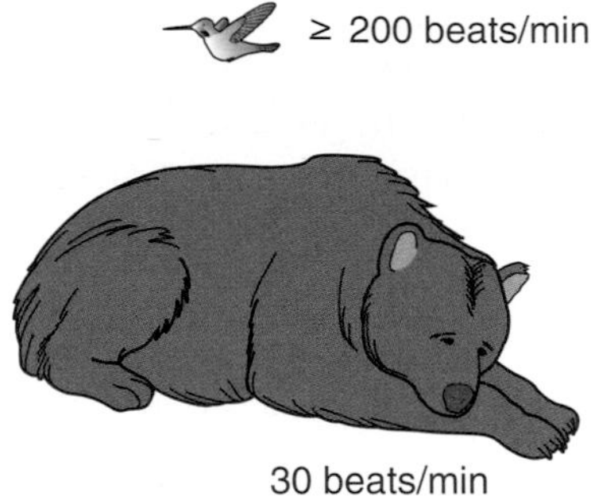

- Gender: Women have slightly faster heart rates than men.
- Age: Generally, the younger the person, the faster the rate. The normal adult heart rate, for example, is 70 to 80 beats per minute, whereas a normal child's heart rate is around 100 beats per minute. An infant's heart rate is about 120 beats per minute, and fetal heart rates are about 140 beats per minute.

In addition to the variation in heart rate according to size, age, and gender, a person's heart rate can change for a variety of other reasons, such as exercise, stimulation of the autonomic nerves, hormonal influence, pathology, and various medications.

- Exercise: Exercise increases heart rate. Check your pulse as you exercise and note the increase. Note also the decrease in pulse when you rest. At rest, the heart rate may be 65 but may increase well over 100 beats per minute with exercise.
- Stimulation of the autonomic nerves: Firing of the sympathetic nerve stimulates the SA node, causing an increase in heart rate. Stimulation of the parasympathetic (vagus) nerve slows the rate.
- Hormonal influence: Several hormones affect heart rate. Epinephrine and norepinephrine (adrenal gland) and thyroid hormone increase heart rate.
- Pathology: Certain disease states can affect heart rate. For instance, a sick SA node may fire too slowly, thereby slowing the heart too much. Vagal discharge following a heart attack (myocardial infarction) slows the rate, predisposing the heart to lethal rhythm disorders. A high fever can increase heart rate, overworking the heart and causing it to fail. Persistent sympathetic activity can also exhaust the heart, causing it to fail.
- Medications: Certain drugs can affect heart rate. Digoxin slows heart rate, whereas epinephrine and dopamine increase heart rate. Heavy coffee drinkers often experience palpitations (the heart feels "jumpy," as if it has extra beats) because of the stimulatory effect of caffeine on the heart. Because some drugs can profoundly alter heart rate, heart rate must be monitored when these drugs are used. For instance, digoxin should not be administered if the heart rate is less than 60 beats per minute.

STROKE VOLUME

Stroke volume is the second factor affecting cardiac output. **Stroke volume (SV)** is the amount of blood pumped by the ventricle per beat. An average resting stroke volume is 60 to 80 ml per beat (about 2 ounces). At rest the ventricles pump out only about 67% of the blood in the ventricles. Therefore if the ventricles can be made to contract more forcefully, a greater percentage of the blood can be pumped per beat. In other words, a greater force of contraction can increase stroke volume.

HOW TO CHANGE STROKE VOLUME

The stroke volume can be altered in two ways: through Starling's law of the heart and through an inotropic effect.

STARLING'S LAW OF THE HEART

Starling's law of the heart depends on the degree of stretch of the myocardial fibers. The greater the stretch, the stronger is the force of contraction. For instance, an increase in the amount of blood entering the ventricle causes the ventricle to stretch (Figure 17-3). Stretch increases the force of contraction, which, in turn, increases stroke volume. Conversely, a decrease in the amount of blood entering the ventricles causes less stretch. As a result, the force of contraction decreases, thereby decreasing stroke volume.

What is the purpose of Starling's law of the heart? It allows the heart to pump out the same amount of blood it receives. In other words, Starling's law allows the heart to match cardiac output with venous return (of blood).

INOTROPIC EFFECT

A second way to increase stroke volume is by strengthening the force of myocardial contraction without stretching the myocardial fibers. This is called a (+)

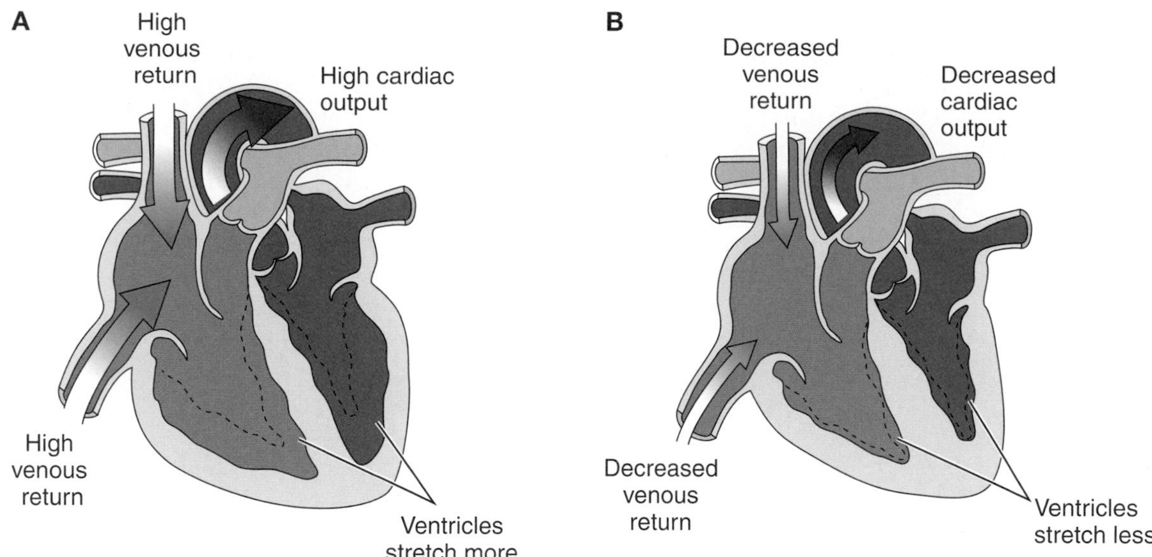

FIGURE 17-3 Starling's law of the heart: matching venous return with cardiac output. **A,** A large venous return. **B,** A smaller venous return.

inotropic (ĭn-ō-TRŌ-pĭk) **effect.** Stimulation of the heart muscle by sympathetic nerves causes a (+) inotropic effect. Certain hormones and drugs, such as epinephrine, also cause this effect. Digoxin is the most famous of the (+) inotropic drugs. Some medications cause a (–) inotropic effect. A (–) inotropic effect is a decrease in the force of contraction, resulting in a weaker myocardial contraction. Excessive dosing with a (–) inotropic agent can depress the myocardium to the point of failure.

CHANGING CARDIAC OUTPUT

Since cardiac output is determined by HR and SV, cardiac output can be altered by changing either or both. The healthy heart can increase cardiac output four to five times the resting cardiac output; an Olympic athlete can do even better! The capacity to increase cardiac output above the resting cardiac output is called the **cardiac reserve.** A person with a diseased heart may have little cardiac reserve and therefore becomes easily fatigued with mild exercise.

Sum It Up!

Cardiac output is determined by multiplying heart rate and stroke volume. The heart rate is the number of times the heart beats each minute. The normal adult resting heart rate is between 60 and 100 beats per minute (average: 72 beats/min). Heart rates differ for three reasons: size, gender, and age. A person's heart rate changes in response to exercise, stimulation of the ANS, hormonal influence, pathology, and various medications. Stroke volume is the amount of blood ejected by the ventricle in one beat. Stroke volume can be altered through Starling's law of the heart or an inotropic effect.

Parts B and C are clinically focused and may be omitted in nonmedical courses. Two topics are developed: Heart Talk (B, terms that are used clinically to describe cardiac function), and Heart Failure (C).

PART B. HEART TALK

HEART TALK: CLINICAL TERMS

Clinically, cardiac function is described using special vocabulary.

END-DIASTOLIC VOLUME

The end-diastolic volume (EDV) refers to the amount of blood in the ventricle at the end of its resting phase (diastole). Remember: The ventricle fills with blood during diastole. The EDV determines how much the ventricle is stretched and is the basis of Starling's law of the heart.

PRELOAD

The **preload** is the amount of blood in the ventricles at the end of diastole; it is the same as the EDV. Note Figure 17-4. The filling of the right heart by the funnel illustrates preload. An increased preload stretches the ventricles, causing a stronger force of contraction. The stronger contraction increases stroke volume and

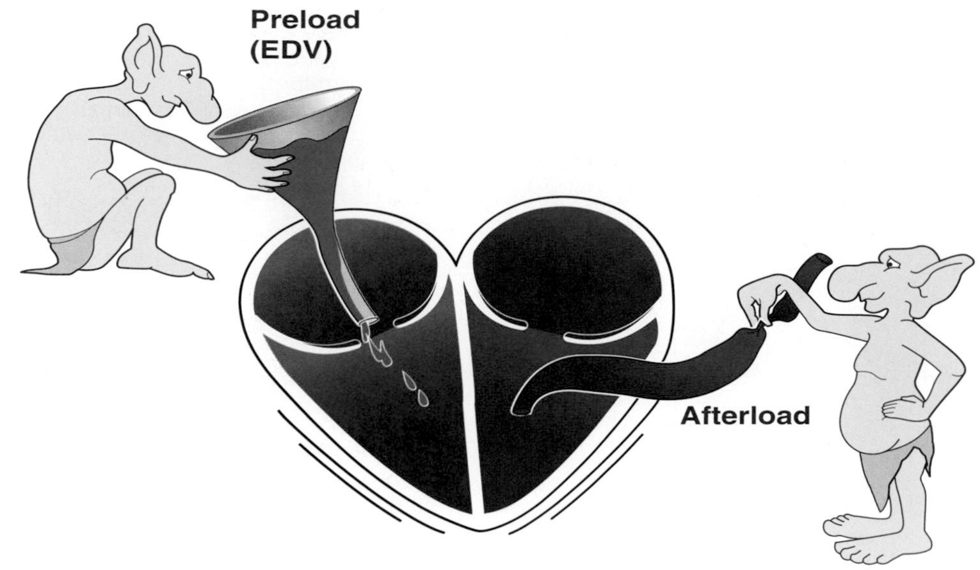

FIGURE 17-4 Preload and afterload.

cardiac output. Drugs can also affect preload. For instance, a drug may dilate the veins, causing blood to pool in the veins, decreasing the amount of blood returned to the heart; thus decreasing preload, stroke volume, and cardiac output. Another drug may constrict the veins; this increases blood flow to the ventricles thereby increasing preload, stroke volume, and cardiac output.

EJECTION FRACTION

When the ventricle contracts it pumps about 67% of its volume (EDV); therefore, some blood remains in the ventricle. The percentage of the EDV that is pumped is called the **ejection fraction.** The ejection fraction is an indication of cardiac health. For instance, a healthy heart can increase its ejection fraction to 90% with exercise. A weakened, failing heart is characterized by a decrease in ejection fraction, maybe as low as 30%.

AFTERLOAD

Afterload refers to resistance or opposition. For example, in order for the left ventricle to pump blood into the aorta, it must push against blood that is already in the aorta. The aortic blood pressure is the resistance or the afterload. Note Figure 17-4. The pinched aorta represents an increased afterload demanding that the left ventricle work harder to overcome the resistance. The pinched aorta can represent a number of clinical conditions such as aortic valve stenosis and hypertension. If the person develops high blood pressure, afterload increases and the ventricle must work harder to pump blood into the aorta. Like any other muscle that overworks, the left ventricular myocardium enlarges or hypertrophies. The enlarged left ventricle will eventually fail as a pump.

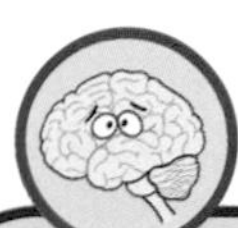

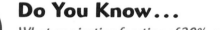

Do You Know...

What an ejection fraction of 30% means?

An ejection fraction of 30% means that the person's heart is failing. An ejection fraction refers to the percentage of blood that is pumped out of the ventricle with each beat. Normally the heart contracts and ejects or pumps out 67% of the blood that is in the ventricle. As the myocardial contraction weakens as the heart fails, the amount of blood ejected decreases. Thus the failing heart is associated with a low ejection fraction, such as 30%.

What about afterload and the right ventricle? Its afterload is determined by the pressure within the pulmonary artery. If pulmonary artery pressure rises (increased afterload) the right ventricle must work harder to pump blood and therefore hypertrophies. Right ventricular hypertrophy frequently occurs in response to chronic lung diseases such as emphysema and asthma. The elevation in pulmonary artery pressure and right ventricular hypertrophy is called cor pulmonale. Cor pulmonale often causes the right ventricle to fail as a pump.

Afterload can be altered by drugs. For instance, a drug that relaxes and dilates the blood vessels in the peripheral circulation can lower blood pressure and therefore decrease the afterload. The reduction in afterload reduces the work of the heart. Conversely, a drug that constricts blood vessels in the periphery increases afterload, thereby increasing the workload of the heart.

INOTROPIC EFFECT

An inotropic effect refers to a change in myocardial contraction that is not due to stretch. A (+) inotropic effect refers to an increase in contractile force, while a (−) inotropic effect refers to a decrease in contractile force. Sympathetic nerve stimulation causes a (+) inotropic effect.

CHRONOTROPIC EFFECT

A **chronotropic effect** refers to a change in heart rate. Anything that increases heart rate exerts a (+) chronotropic effect, while anything that decreases heart rate exerts a (−) chronotropic effect. Sympathetic nerve stimulation causes a (+) chronotropic effect while vagal (parasympathetic) stimulation causes a (−) chronotropic effect.

DROMOTROPIC EFFECT

A **dromotropic effect** refers to a change in the speed at which the cardiac impulse travels from the SA node through the AV node and the His-Purkinje system. If the speed of the cardiac impulse increases it is called a (+) dromotropic effect; a decrease in the speed causes a (−) dromotropic effect. Sympathetic nerve stimulation causes a (+) dromotropic effect, while vagal (parasympathetic) stimulation causes a (−) dromotropic effect. The (−) dromotropic effect may be so pronounced that the person develops a heart block.

HEART TALK: RECEPTOR LANGUAGE

Heart talk often involves the autonomic receptors of the heart and their responses to autonomic stimulation and to drugs. (Review Chapter 12, Autonomic Nervous System.)

BETA$_1$-ADRENERGIC RECEPTOR ACTIVATION

The sympathetic nerves innervate the SA node, AV node, His-Purkinje system, and the ventricular myocardium. The neurotransmitter for the adrenergic neuron is norepinephrine (NE). The cardiac adrenergic receptors for NE are called beta$_1$-adrenergic receptors. Activation of the beta$_1$ receptors causes a (+) chronotropic effect, a (+) dromotropic effect, and a (+) inotropic effect. The increase in heart rate and stroke volume increases cardiac output. A drug that activates beta$_1$-adrenergic receptors is called a beta$_1$-adrenergic agonist. Examples include dopamine and epinephrine. Note that beta$_1$-adrenergic receptor activation is the same as a sympathomimetic effect.

BETA$_1$-ADRENERGIC RECEPTOR BLOCKADE

Blockade of the beta$_1$-adrenergic receptors prevents cardiac beta$_1$-adrenergic receptor activation. People taking beta$_1$-adrenergic blockers, such as propranolol, will not increase their heart rate when their sympathetic nerves fire as in exercise or stress. If a person is **tachycardic** (heart rate>100 beats/min) from excessive sympathetic nervous stimulation, a beta$_1$-adrenergic blocker can decrease heart rate and force of myocardial contraction; this results in a decrease in cardiac output and blood pressure. Note that beta$_1$-adrenergic receptor blockade is the same as a sympatholytic effect.

MUSCARINIC (CHOLINERGIC) RECEPTOR ACTIVATION

The parasympathetic (vagus) nerves supply the SA and the AV nodes. The neurotransmitter for the cholinergic neuron is acetylcholine (ACh). The cardiac cholinergic receptors for ACh are called muscarinic receptors. Activation of the muscarinic receptors causes a (−) chronotropic effect and a (−) dromotropic effect. There is no effect on myocardial contractile force because there is no parasympathetic innervation to the ventricular myocardium. The administration of a cholinergic (muscarinic) agonist causes a (−) chronotropic effect and a (−) dromotropic effect. Note that muscarinic-receptor activation is the same as a parasympathomimetic effect.

MUSCARINIC (CHOLINERGIC) RECEPTOR BLOCKADE

The muscarinic receptors can also be blocked. Muscarinic-blocking drugs act by blocking the effects of ACh at the muscarinic receptors. Muscarinic blockade relieves the inhibiting effects of ACh at the receptors, thereby increasing heart rate and increasing the speed of the cardiac impulse from the atria to the ventricles. Atropine is an example of a muscarinic blocker that is often used to relieve bradycardia and heart block. Note that muscarinic-receptor blockade is the same as a parasympatholytic effect.

Note the duplication in terminology; your worst terminology nightmare! The muscarinic receptors are activated by ACh. Since ACh is secreted by a cholinergic fiber, a muscarinic agonist is also called a cholinergic agonist. A muscarinic blocker is also called an antimuscarinic agent, a cholinergic blocker, or an anticholinergic agent. Unfortunately this terminology is used frequently in pharmacology, so you need to start building your understanding now.

Sum It Up!

Cardiac function is often described using special vocabulary, such as end-diastolic volume (EDV), preload, ejection fraction, and afterload. Inotropic, chronotropic, and dromotropic effects describe changes in cardiac contractile force, heart rate, and conduction velocity (through the heart). Cardiac function is also described in receptor terminology, specifically the beta$_1$-adrenergic and muscarinic receptors.

PART C. THE FAILING HEART: WHEN THE HEART CAN'T PUMP

The heart functions as a double pump. The right ventricle pumps blood to the lungs for oxygenation, while the left ventricle pumps blood into the aorta for distribution to the systemic circulation. What happens when either or both pumps fail?

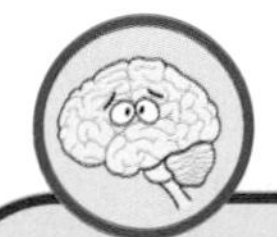

Do You Know...

Why BNP is used in the assessment of heart failure?

BNP, brain natriuretic peptide, is secreted by the walls of the ventricles in response to stretch. The failing heart is characterized by pooling of blood in the cardiac chambers (cardiac dilation), thereby increasing the secretion of BNP.

A new class of drugs that mimics BNP is also used to treat heart failure. The BNP-like drug increases the excretion of Na^+ in the urine, suppresses the renin-angiotensin system, and decreases sympathetic activity.

LEFT-HEART FAILURE

When the left ventricle fails to pump blood into the aorta, two things happen: blood backs up in the lungs, and the heart is unable to pump a sufficient amount of blood to the systemic circulation.

BACKWARD FAILURE

What happens when the blood backs up? (Figure 17-5) The blood backs up into the structures "behind" the left ventricle, namely the left atrium, pulmonary veins, and most importantly the pulmonary capillaries. The pooled blood increases the pressure within the pulmonary capillaries and forces fluid into the lungs. The presence of fluid in the lungs impairs oxygenation of blood. The accumulation of fluid within the lungs is called **pulmonary edema (PE).** The signs and symptoms (S&S) of PE are: exertional dyspnea (difficulty breathing upon exertion), cyanosis (bluish appearance), blood-tinged sputum and cough, orthopnea (inability to breathe while lying down), tachycardia, and restlessness. Since these symptoms are largely due to the backup of blood behind the failed ventricle, the condition is called backward failure. Note that the S&S of left-sided heart failure are predominantly respiratory! Treatment? In addition to a (+) inotropic agent, such as digoxin or dopamine, **NO MUD**!

N nitroglycerin (decrease the work of the heart)
O oxygen (relieve anxiety, oxygenate the myocardium)
M morphine (relieve anxiety, decrease work of the heart)
U upright position (ease breathing)
D diuretic (excrete excess fluid, relieve edema)

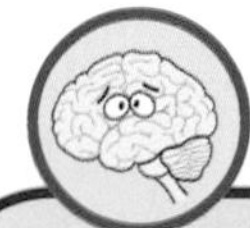

Do You Know...

About two- and three-pillow edema?

A patient with **heart failure** may develop pulmonary edema and dyspnea. There is a simple way to determine how severe the dyspnea is; ask patients how many pillows they sleep on at night. Patients with no pulmonary edema can lie flat and use a single pillow. As fluid collects in the alveoli, patients must sit up in order to breathe (orthopnea). Thus they tend to use two or three pillows, depending on the severity of the edema and dyspnea. Hence, the name two- or three-pillow edema.

FORWARD FAILURE

There is also a "forward" component to left-heart failure. For instance, if the damaged left ventricle cannot pump adequate blood to the systemic circulation, all of the organs of the body receive inadequate oxygen. The decreased cardiac output causes additional S&S to develop. For instance, the kidneys filter less water for excretion as urine. The kidneys also reabsorb excess salt and water, causing an increase in blood volume and edema formation. The decrease in cardiac output also stimulates the sympathetic nervous system. Sympathetic activity stimulates the heart and blood vessels in a way that temporarily improves cardiac output. Over time, however, the improvement diminishes and additional signs of heart failure develop. The heart begins to show the wear and tear of continuous and excessive sympathetic activity.

What usually causes the left heart to fail? Two common causes include myocardial infarction (MI) and chronic hypertension (increased blood pressure). If a person suffers an acute MI, a part of the left ventricular myocardium may be destroyed. The damaged myocardium is unable to contract and fails as a pump. More

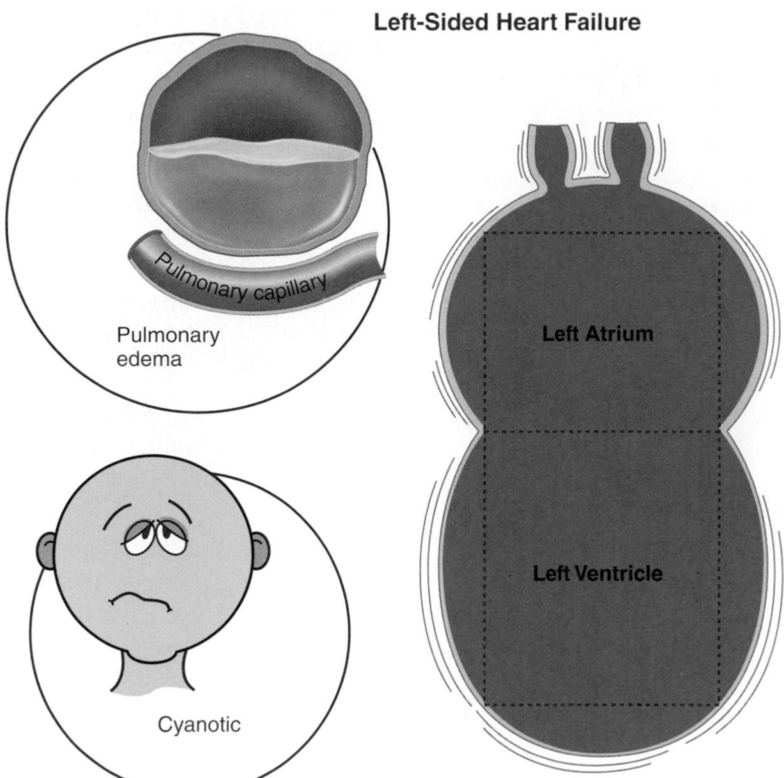

FIGURE 17-5 Left-sided heart failure.

commonly the left heart fails in response to chronic hypertension. Increased blood pressure overworks the heart, eventually causing the left ventricle to enlarge and then fail.

RIGHT-HEART FAILURE

When the right ventricle fails (Figure 17-6), blood backs up into the veins that return blood to the right heart. Blood backs up into the superior vena cava, thereby slowing venous drainage from the head via the jugular veins. The congestion of the jugular veins causes jugular vein distention (JVD), which is visible as the veins in the neck pulsate. Blood also backs up into the veins that drain the liver, spleen, and digestive organs, causing hepatomegaly (enlarged liver), splenomegaly (enlarged spleen), and digestive symptoms. Right-sided failure is also characterized by ankle, or pedal, edema; ankle edema can be so severe that the skin remains indented when you depress an area of skin with your thumb. This "indentation" response is called pitting edema.

The right heart most often fails as a consequence to left-sided failure; when one side of the heart fails, the other side will eventually fail. Another common cause is chronic lung disease, such as emphysema. The diseased lungs make it difficult for the right ventricle to pump blood into the pulmonary circulation. The overworked right ventricle becomes enlarged (right ventricular hypertrophy) and eventually fails.

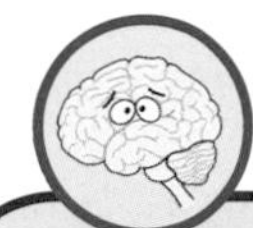

Do You Know...

Why CVP is elevated in heart failure?

Central venous pressure (CVP) is considered a direct measurement of the pressure in the right atrium and vena cava (the large vein that empties blood into the right atrium). The CVP reading is obtained by threading a catheter through the subclavian vein into the superior vena cava. When the heart fails, blood backs up in the vena cava thereby elevating venous pressure. Thus an elevated CVP is indicative of a failing heart.

GOALS OF TREATMENT OF HEART FAILURE

The treatment of heart failure is aimed at:

- Strengthening of myocardial contractile force
- Removal of excess water (edema)
- Decreasing the work of the heart
- Protection of the heart from excess sympathetic nerve activity.

Let's see if you can follow the rationale for the treatment in the following case studies:

Case #1. A patient in left-sided heart failure and pulmonary edema is given a (+) inotropic drug, a potent diuretic, oxygen, and morphine. Rationale: The failing heart muscle contracts weakly. A (+) inotropic drug such as digoxin or dopamine strengthens myocardial

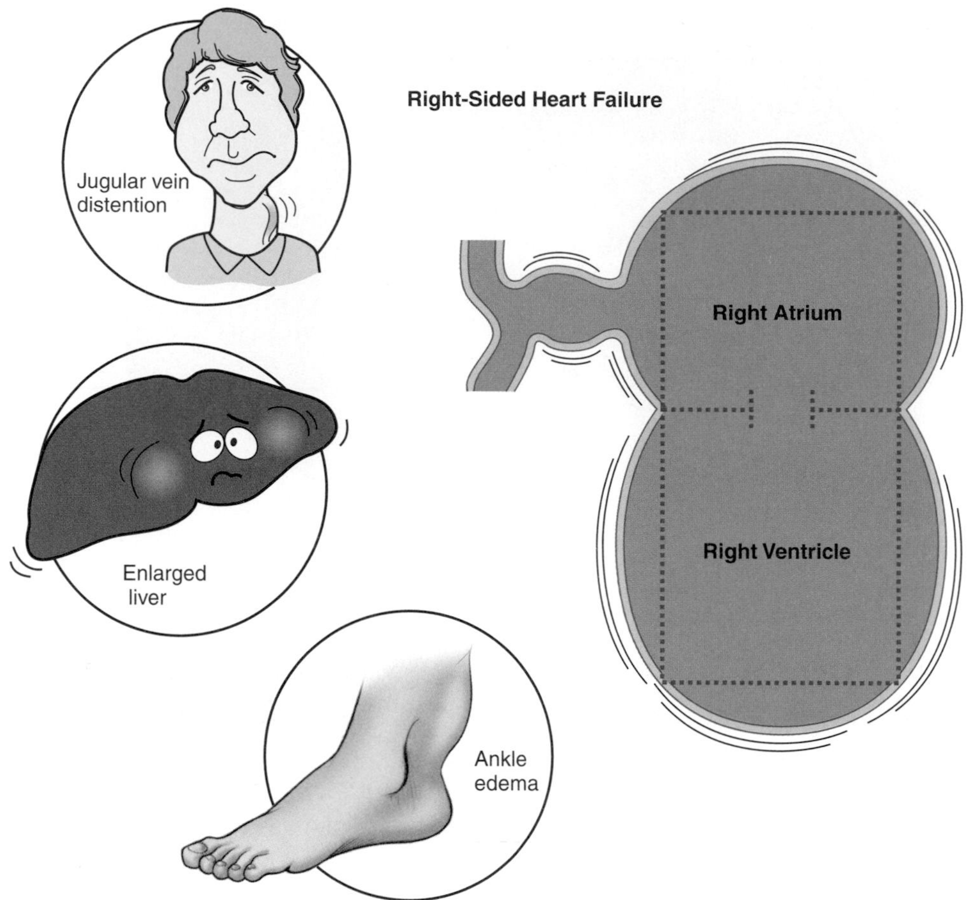

FIGURE 17-6 Right-sided heart failure.

contraction. The increased force of contraction results in an increased cardiac output, decreased pooling of blood in the pulmonary capillaries (decreases pulmonary edema), and increased blood flow to the kidney that results in greater excretion of urine. A potent diuretic, such as furosemide (Lasix), blocks the absorption of sodium and water by the kidney, thereby ridding the body of excess water and decreasing the edema. The oxygen and morphine improve oxygenation and relieve the anxiety caused by poor oxygenation.

Case #2. An elderly patient with symptoms of right-sided failure and fast heart rate is given a beta$_1$-adrenergic receptor blocker. Rationale: Heart failure is characterized by excess sympathetic nerve stimulation. Long-term sympathetic stimulation damages the heart causing the heart to eventually fail. The administration of a beta$_1$-adrenergic receptor blocker diminishes the response to sympathetic activity and protects the heart from further damage.

Case #3. An elderly patient has mild right-sided failure and is given an ACE inhibitor. An ACE inhibitor decreases afterload, acts like a diuretic, and decreases the secretion of aldosterone from the adrenal cortex. Rationale: The decreased afterload decreases the workload of the heart. The diuretic effect excretes water and relieves the edema. The decrease in the secretion of aldosterone has two effects: it causes diuresis and it prevents myocardial damage. (Chronic secretion of aldosterone causes structural damage, called remodeling, to the heart muscle.)

Clearly, the healthy heart is a magnificent, adaptable pump. Pump failure adversely affects the functioning of every organ system and is a common cause of disability and death.

Sum It Up!

The heart functions as a double pump. Either or both pumps can fail. When the left heart fails, fluid backs up into the lungs, causing pulmonary edema. The failing left heart is also unable to pump sufficient blood to the organs of the body; the result is poor tissue oxygenation. Right-sided failure causes JVD, ankle edema, and congestion of the abdominal organs. The treatment of heart failure is aimed at: strengthening of myocardial contractile force, removal of excess water, decreasing the work of the heart, and protection of the heart from excess sympathetic nerve activity.

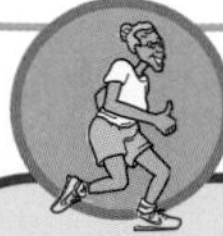

As You Age

1. Contrary to popular opinion, no significant age-related decline occurs in resting cardiac output. When cardiac output declines, it is secondary to age-related disease processes such as arteriosclerosis.
2. An age-related decline occurs in exercise cardiac output. The heart cannot respond as quickly or as forcefully to the increased workload of the exercised heart. Exertion, sudden movements, and changes in position may cause a decrease in cardiac output, resulting in dizziness, and loss of balance and falls.
3. Several structural changes in the heart contribute to the impaired response to exercise: heart muscle loses elasticity and becomes more rigid; heart valves become thicker and more rigid; the number of pacemaker cells decreases; and the aging heart cells have a decreased ability to use oxygen.
4. An age-related increase occurs in blood pressure, which increases the work the heart must do to pump blood into the systemic circulation.

Disorders of the Heart

Angina pectoris	From the Latin word meaning to strangle. The chest pain is due to inadequate oxygenation of the myocardium. The decreased oxygenation is generally caused by a decrease in coronary artery blood flow and is therefore called myocardial ischemia. Anginal pain is often triggered by exercise and emotional stress.
Cardiac dysrhythmias	Abnormal electrical conduction in the heart or abnormal changes in heart rate and rhythm. Fibrillation refers to an irregular, quivering, and ineffective type of myocardial contraction. Both the atria and the ventricles can fibrillate. Ventricular fibrillation causes a severe decrease in cardiac output and blood pressure with loss of consciousness; it is life threatening and demands immediate treatment. Flutter refers to a regular but rapid pace (200 to 300 beats per minute). An atrioventricular block occurs when the electrical signal cannot pass from the atria to the ventricles. Blocks are classified as first-, second-, and third-degree.
Congenital heart defects	A heart defect present at birth but not necessarily hereditary. Heart defects often involve the atrial and ventricular septa. An interatrial septal defect is an opening between the two atria. Blood flows through the hole and does not follow the correct path through the heart. A ventricular septal defect is a hole in the ventricular septum; it allows blood to flow back and forth between the ventricles. Other congenital heart defects include tetralogy of Fallot and a patent ductus arteriosus.
Coronary heart disease	A commonly used term for any disease affecting the heart.
Inflammation of the heart	Inflammation of the layers of the heart. Pericarditis is inflammation of the pericardium. Myocarditis is inflammation of the heart muscle, the myocardium. Endocarditis is inflammation of the endocardium, the heart valves, and the inner lining of the blood vessels attached to the heart. Bacterial endocarditis is the most common infectious disease of the heart.
Myocardial infarction (MI)	Also called a heart attack. An infarct is an area of tissue that has died. A myocardial infarction is an area of dead myocardium caused by a lack of oxygenated blood. Coronary artery blood supply may be decreased because of fatty plaque buildup inside the arteries (atherosclerosis), a blood clot (coronary thrombosis), spasm of the blood vessel wall, or low blood pressure.
Rheumatic fever	An infectious disease generally caused by a *Streptococcus* bacterium. The body develops antibodies to the streptococcal microorganism; then the antibodies attack the heart (particularly the valves) and joints, causing rheumatic heart disease.
Valvular heart disease	Dysfunction of any of the four valves. When blood flows through a diseased valve, it produces a characteristic sound called a murmur. Dysfunctional valves may produce regurgitation, or backflow of blood (e.g., mitral insufficiency). Valves may also be narrowed or stenosed (mitral stenosis).

SUMMARY OUTLINE

The heart pumps blood through the blood vessels, supplying the cells of the body with oxygen and nutrients, and carrying away the waste products of metabolism. The heart functions in a coordinated and adaptable manner to perform its tasks.

Part A. The Coordinated and Adaptable Pump

I. Cardiac Cycle

A. The cardiac cycle is a sequence of events that occurs during one heart beat.

B. The events of the cardiac cycle include atrial and ventricular systole (contraction) and diastole (relaxation).

II. Heart: Autonomic Control

A. The autonomic nervous system (ANS) allows the heart to respond to changing body needs.

B. Stimulation of the sympathetic nerves increases heart rate (SA node), conduction velocity (AV node), and contractile force (myocardium).

C. Stimulation of the parasympathetic nerves (vagus) decreases heart rate and conduction velocity.

III. Cardiac Output (CO)

A. CO is the amount of blood pumped by the ventricle in 1 minute.

B. CO is determined by heart rate and stroke volume.

C. There are many factors that change HR and or SV.

IV. How Stroke Volume (SV) Can Be Changed

A. SV can be changed by Starling's law of the heart (stretch).

B. SV can be changed by an inotropic effect (nonstretch).

Part B. Heart Talk

I. Heart Talk: Clinical Terms: Includes the definition and description of commonly used clinical terms such as preload, afterload, ejection fraction, and inotropic effect.

II. Heart Talk: Receptor Terminology: Includes the definitions of $beta_1$-adrenergic receptor activation, $beta_1$-adrenergic receptor blockade, muscarinic-receptor activation, and muscarinic-receptor blockade.

Part C. The Failing Heart: When the Heart Can't Pump

I. Left-Sided Heart Failure

A. The left heart can fail, producing symptoms due to a backup of blood into the pulmonic circulation (pulmonary edema).

B. The failing left heart is unable to pump adequate blood to the systemic circulation, producing S&S related to poor tissue oxygenation.

II. Right-Sided Heart Failure

A. Blood backs up behind the failed right ventricle, causing jugular vein distention, hepatomegaly, splenomegaly, digestive problems, and ankle edema.

III. Heart failure is also described as backward heart failure and forward heart failure.

Review Your Knowledge

Matching: Cardiac Function Terms

Directions: Match the following words with their descriptions below. Some words may be used more than once.

a. inotropic effect
b. cardiac output
c. stroke volume
d. diastole
e. systole
f. Starling's law of the heart

1. ____ 5000 ml/min
2. ____ 70 ml/beat
3. ____ Stroke volume times heart rate
4. ____ Phase of the cardiac cycle that refers to myocardial contraction
5. ____ Phase of the cardiac cycle when the ventricles fill with blood
6. ____ Phase of the cardiac cycle that refers to myocardial relaxation
7. ____ Change in myocardial contraction that is due to stretching of the heart muscle
8. ____ Change in myocardial contraction that is not due to stretching of the heart muscle
9. ____ Amount of blood pumped by the ventricle in one beat
10. ____ Amount of blood pumped by the ventricle in one minute

Matching: Loads and Effects

Directions: Match the following words with their descriptions below. Some words may be used more than once.

a. afterload
b. preload
c. ejection fraction
d. dromotropic effect
e. chronotropic effect

1. ____ Amount of blood in the ventricle at the end of its resting phase

2. ____ Percentage of the end-diastolic volume (EDV) pumped by the ventricle
3. ____ Arteriolar constriction and hypertension cause the ______ to increase
4. ____ Forms the basis of Starling's law of the heart
5. ____ The effect of a drug that changes heart rate
6. ____ Digoxin slows the speed of the cardiac impulse through the conduction system thereby causing a heart block
7. ____ Same as end-diastolic volume (EDV)
8. ____ May decline from 67% to 30% in the failing heart

Multiple Choice

1. Which of the following statements is correct about cardiac output?
   a. Cardiac output is determined by the heart rate and pulse.
   b. Stimulation of the sympathetic nerves decreases cardiac output.
   c. Vagal discharge increases cardiac output.
   d. Cardiac output is determined by heart rate and stroke volume.
2. What statement is true of ventricular diastole?
   a. Blood is ejected from the ventricles.
   b. The semilunar valves are open.
   c. The atrioventricular valves are closed.
   d. Blood fills the ventricles.
3. Increased return of blood to the heart stretches the heart muscle thereby
   a. stimulating the vagus nerve.
   b. increasing stroke volume.
   c. closing the atrioventricular valves.
   d. increasing coronary blood flow.
4. Ventricular systole refers to
   a. ventricular depolarization.
   b. the opening of the valves of the ventricles.
   c. ventricular filling.
   d. contraction of the ventricular myocardium.
5. Which of the following is least related to the vagus nerve?
   a. Parasympathetic
   b. Slows heart rate
   c. (+) Inotropic effect
   d. Autonomic nerve
6. Which of the following is least characteristic of sympathetic nerve stimulation?
   a. (−) Inotropic effect
   b. Increased heart rate
   c. Increased stroke volume
   d. Increased cardiac output
7. Which of the following is least related to bradycardia?
   a. <60 beats/min
   b. Vagal discharge
   c. (−) Chronotropic effect
   d. Beta$_1$-adrenergic receptor activation
8. Which of the following is least apt to increase cardiac output?
   a. Increased heart rate
   b. Increased stroke volume
   c. Increased venous return (Starling's law of the heart)
   d. Vagal discharge

CHAPTER 18

Anatomy of the Blood Vessels

KEY TERMS

Aorta, p. 316
Arteriole, p. 315
Artery, p. 315
Capacitance vessel, p. 316
Capillary, p. 315
Conductance vessel, p. 315
Exchange vessel, p. 316
Pulmonary circulation, p. 313
Resistance vessel, p. 315
Splanchnic circulation, p. 324
Systemic circulation, p. 313
Vein, p. 315
Vena cava, p. 319
Venule, p. 315

OBJECTIVES

1. Describe the pulmonary and systemic circulations.
2. Describe the structure and function of arteries, capillaries, and veins.
3. List the three layers of tissue found in arteries and veins.
4. Explain the functions of conductance, resistance, exchange, and capacitance vessels.
5. List those major arteries of the systemic circulation that are branches of the ascending aorta, aortic arch, and descending aorta.
6. List the major veins of the systemic circulation.
7. Describe the following special circulations: blood supply to the head and brain, hepatic circulation, and fetal circulation.

The circulatory system consists of the heart and blood vessels. The historical description of the heart and blood vessels is intriguing. The ancients knew that the heart played an important role in pumping blood through the body, but no one described the intricate role of the blood vessels. The ancient Greeks thought that blood moved throughout the body like an ocean tide. Blood was seen as washing out from the heart through a series of blood vessels and then ebbing back to it through those same blood vessels, with impurities removed from the blood as it washed through the lungs. Not until the seventeenth century did the English physician William Harvey, described as a crackpot by his fellow scientists, identify the system of blood vessels and thus provide the first accurate description of the circulation.

CIRCLES, CIRCUITS, AND CIRCULATIONS

The blood vessels are a series of connected, hollow tubes that begin and end in the heart. The blood vessels form a path through the body, much like the system of highways and roads that enables us to travel from place to place. Note the path of the delivery truck in Figure 18-1. Leaving the bakery, the truck travels a major highway and exits onto a smaller road. The truck then arrives at a grocery store where it makes a delivery. The empty truck returns to the bakery through a number of connecting roads. Note the circle, or circuit, from bakery to grocery store to bakery.

The heart and blood vessels also form a circuit. The heart pumps blood into the large artery. The blood flows through a series of blood vessels back to the heart. Moving from heart to blood vessels to heart, the blood forms a circuit, or circulation. This arrangement ensures a continuous one-way movement of blood. As Chapter 16 explained, the two main circulations are the pulmonary circulation and the systemic circulation.

The **pulmonary circulation** carries blood from the right ventricle of the heart to the lungs and back to the left atrium of the heart (see Figure 16-3). The pulmonary circulation transports unoxygenated blood to the lungs, where oxygen is loaded, and carbon dioxide is unloaded. Oxygenated blood then returns to the left side of the heart to be pumped into the systemic circulation.

The **systemic circulation** is the larger circulation; it provides the blood supply to the rest of the body. The systemic circulation carries oxygen and other nutrients to the cells and picks up carbon dioxide and other waste.

BLOOD VESSELS

NAMING THE BLOOD VESSELS

Note the different types of blood vessels (Figure 18-2), their relationship to the heart, and the color coding. The blood vessels are the body's highways and byways; they are classified as arteries, capillaries, and veins (Table 18-1).

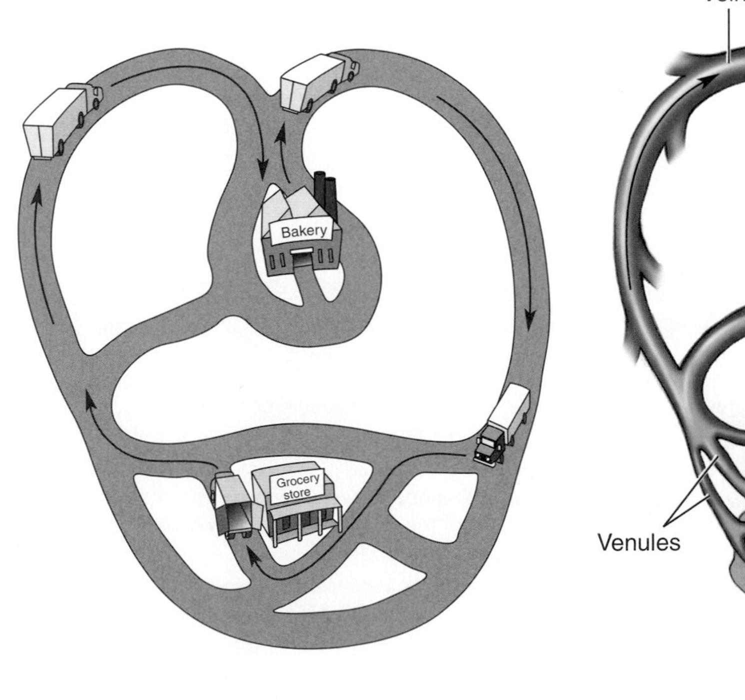

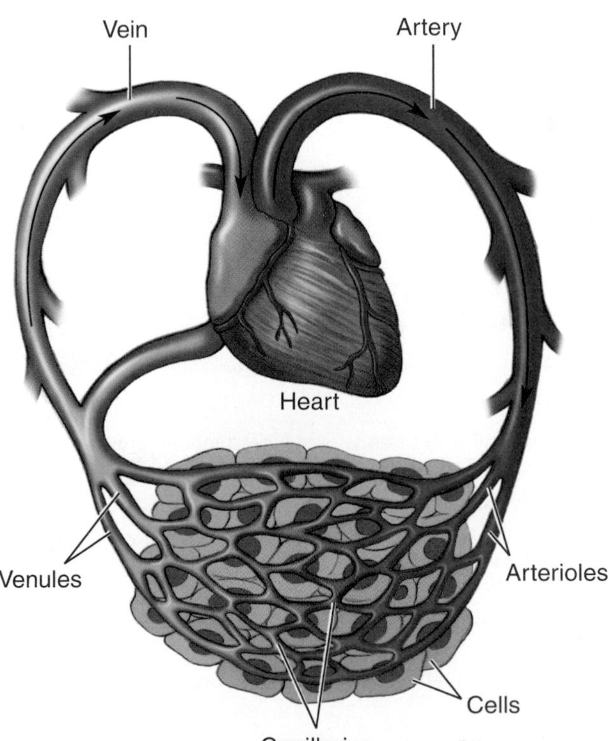

FIGURE 18-1 A circuit or route. The circulatory system.

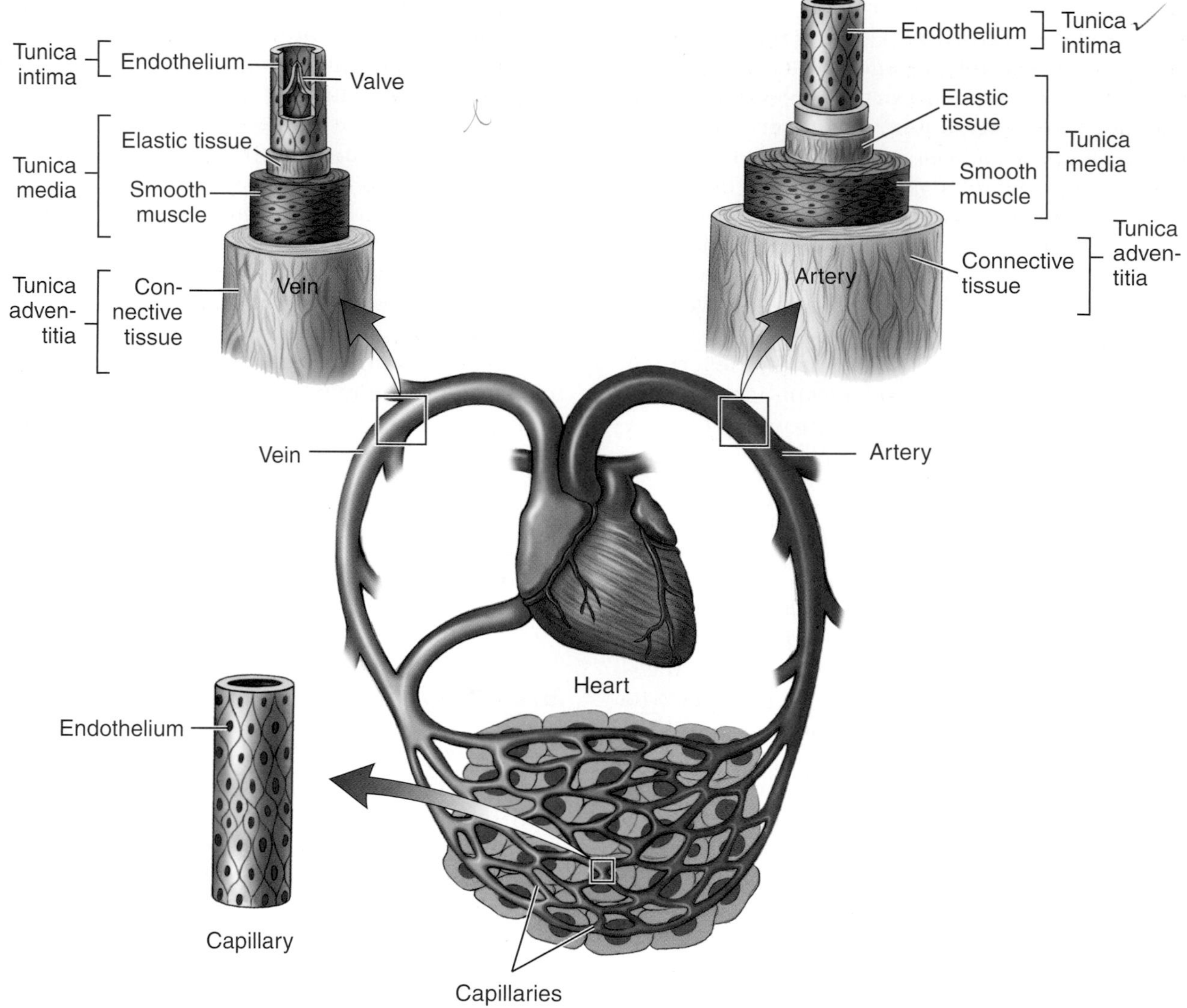

FIGURE 18-2 Blood vessel wall layers: tunica intima, tunica media, and tunica adventitia.

Table 18-1 Structure and Function of Blood Vessels

Vessel	Structure	Function
Artery	Thick wall with three layers: tunica intima (endothelial lining), tunica media (elastic tissue and smooth muscle), and tunica adventitia (connective tissue)	Called conductance vessels because they carry blood from the heart to the arterioles
Arteriole	Thinner than the wall of an artery but with three layers, mostly smooth muscle	Called resistance vessels because the contraction and relaxation of the muscle changes vessel diameter, which alters resistance to blood flow
Capillary	Layer of endothelium	Called exchange vessels because nutrients, gases, and wastes exchange between the blood and interstitial fluid
Venule	Thin wall with less smooth muscle and elastic tissue than an arteriole	Venules and veins collect and return blood from the tissues to the heart. They are called capacitance vessels because they hold or store blood (most of the blood is located in the venous side of the circulation).
Vein	Three layers (intima, media, and adventitia), but thinner and less elastic than an artery; veins contain valves	

Arteries

Arteries are blood vessels that carry blood away from the heart. The large arteries repeatedly branch into smaller and smaller arteries as they are distributed throughout the entire body. As they branch, the arteries become much more numerous but smaller in diameter. The smallest of the arteries are called **arterioles** (ăr-TĒ-rē-ōlz). The arteries are red in Figure 18-2 because they carry oxygenated blood.

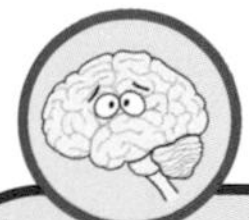

Do You Know...

What happens if an aneurysm "pops"?

An aneurysm is a weakening in the wall of an artery. The blood vessel is enlarged, and the aneurysm appears as an outpouching in the wall. This condition may "pop" or rupture, resulting in a massive hemorrhage. If the ruptured aneurysm involves a cerebral artery, a hemorrhage into the brain may cause severe neurologic damage and death.

Capillaries

Blood flows from the arterioles into the capillaries. The **capillaries** are the smallest and most numerous of all the blood vessels. They connect the arterioles with the venules. Because the body has so many of them, a capillary is close to every cell in the body. This arrangement provides every cell with a continuous supply of oxygen and other nutrients. The capillaries are colored from red to purple to blue. Why? Because, at the capillary level, the blood gives up its oxygen to the tissues; the unoxygenated blood leaving the tissues is therefore bluish.

Veins

Blood flows from the capillaries into the veins. **Veins** are blood vessels that carry blood back to the heart. The smallest of the veins are called **venules** (VĒN-ūlz). The small venules converge to form fewer but larger veins. The largest veins empty the blood into the right atrium of the heart. The veins are colored blue because they transport unoxygenated blood.

BLOOD VESSEL WALLS: THE LAYERED LOOK

With the exception of the capillaries, the blood vessels are composed of three layers (or tunics) of tissue (see Figure 18-2). The three layers are the tunica intima, tunica media, and tunica adventitia.

1. Tunica intima: The **tunica intima** is the innermost layer, an endothelium. The endothelial lining forms a slick, shiny surface continuous with the endocardium, the inner lining of the heart. Blood flows easily and smoothly along this surface.
2. Tunica media: The **tunica media** is the middle layer. It is the thickest layer and is composed primarily of elastic tissue and smooth muscle; the thickness and composition varies according to the function of the blood vessel. The large arteries, for instance, contain considerable elastic tissue so that they can stretch in response to the pumping of blood by the heart. The smallest of the arteries, the arterioles, are composed primarily of smooth muscle. The muscle allows the arterioles to contract and relax, thereby changing the diameter of the arteriole.
3. Tunica adventitia: The outer layer is called the **tunica adventitia.** Composed of tough connective tissue, its main function is to support and protect blood vessels.

BLOOD VESSELS: WHAT THEY DO

Note how the structure of the blood vessels changes from artery to capillary to vein (see Figure 18-2). As always, the structure is related to its function.

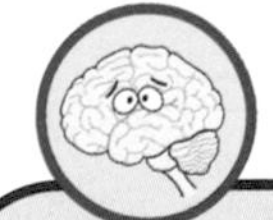

Do You Know...

What the consequences of poor ventilation are in a head-injured person?

The blood gases, oxygen (O_2) and carbon dioxide (CO_2), are vasoactive, meaning that they affect the lumen of the cerebral blood vessels. Poor ventilation (breathing) causes an accumulation of CO_2, which dilates the cerebral blood vessels, increases cerebral blood flow, increases cerebral edema, and increases intracranial pressure (ICP). The elevated ICP damages brain tissue and causes displacement of the brain structures. Particularly lethal is the downward herniation of the brain stem. Meticulous attention to respiratory function is especially important in the care of patients who have suffered brain trauma.

Arteries

The walls of the large arteries are thick, tough, and elastic because they must withstand the high pressure of the blood pumped from the ventricles. Because the primary function of the large arteries is to conduct blood from the heart to the arterioles, the large arteries are called **conductance vessels.**

Arterioles

The arterioles are the smallest of the arteries. They are composed primarily of smooth muscle and spend most of their time contracting and relaxing. By changing their diameter, the arterioles affect resistance to the flow of blood. A narrow (constricted) vessel offers an increased resistance to blood flow; a wider (dilated) vessel offers less resistance. Because of their effect on resistance, the arterioles are called **resistance vessels.**

Capillaries

The capillaries have the thinnest walls of any of the blood vessels. The capillary wall is made up of a single layer of endothelium lying on a delicate basement membrane. The thin capillary wall enables water and dissolved substances, including oxygen, to diffuse from the blood into the tissue spaces, where they become available for use by the cells. The capillary also allows waste from the metabolizing cell to diffuse from the tissue spaces into the capillaries for transport by the blood to the organs of excretion. The capillaries are called **exchange vessels** because they allow for an exchange of nutrients and waste.

Veins and Venules

As the capillaries begin to converge to form venules, the structure of the wall again changes. The venule wall is slightly thicker than the capillary wall. As the venules converge to form larger veins, the walls become even thicker. The tunica media of the vein, however, is much thinner than the tunica media of the artery. This difference is appropriate, because pressure within the veins is much less than the pressure in the arterial blood vessels.

Do You Know...

That an artery was named after air and not blood?

An artery is a blood vessel that carries blood. The word *artery,* however, comes from a Greek word meaning windpipe, because the early body dissectors thought that arteries carried air and not blood. When the ancients dissected corpses, blood was observed in the veins but not in the arteries. Why? At the time of death, the heart pumped the blood out of the arteries, and it accumulated in the veins. Now we are stuck with the word *artery* . . . anything but a wind bag!

In addition to thinner walls, the veins differ in another way: most veins contain one-way valves. These valves direct the flow of blood toward the heart. The valves are most numerous in the veins of the lower extremities, where they prevent backflow, helping move blood up and away from the ankles.

In addition to carrying blood back to the heart, the veins play another role. The veins store blood. In fact, about 70% of the total blood volume is found on the venous side of the circulation. Because the veins store blood, they are called **capacitance** (kă-PĂS-ĭ-tăns) **vessels.** (Capacitance refers to storage.) When this stored blood is needed the veins constrict (venoconstriction) and move blood to the heart for circulation.

Sum It Up!

The blood vessels are a series of connected, hollow tubes that form a circuit. There are two circulations: the pulmonary circulation and the systemic circulation. The three types of blood vessels are arteries (conductance), capillaries (exchange), and veins (capacitance). The arterioles are tiny arteries that are called resistance vessels.

MAJOR ARTERIES OF THE SYSTEMIC CIRCULATION

The major arteries of the systemic circulation include the aorta and the arteries arising from the aorta.

AORTA

The **aorta** (ā-ŎR-tă) is the mother of all arteries; its average diameter is that of a garden hose. The aorta originates in the heart's left ventricle (Figure 18-3), extends upward from the left ventricle, curves in an archlike fashion, and then descends through the thorax (chest) and abdomen. The aorta ends in the pelvic cavity where it splits into two common iliac arteries.

The aorta is divided into segments, each named according to two systems. One system is the path that the aorta follows as it courses through the body. In this system, the aorta is divided into the **ascending aorta,** the **arch of the aorta,** and the **descending aorta.** In the second naming system, the aorta is named according to its location within the body cavities. Thus we have the **thoracic aorta** and the **abdominal aorta.** Like most texts, we use both naming systems.

BRANCHES OF THE AORTA

All systemic arteries are either direct or indirect branches of the aorta. In other words, the arteries arise directly from the aorta, or they arise from vessels that are themselves branches of the aorta. For instance, the coronary arteries arise directly from the ascending aorta. The brachial artery in the right arm, however, arises from the axillary artery. The axillary artery has its origin in the brachiocephalic artery, which arises from the arch of the aorta. The brachial artery therefore arises indirectly from the aorta.

The systemic arteries are described in the order in which they arise from the aorta. Refer to Figure 18-4 as you read the text. You should be able to identify the arteries and the structures they supply.

Branches of the Ascending Aorta

The ascending aorta arises from the left ventricle. It begins at the aortic semilunar valve and extends to the aortic arch. The **right** and **left coronary arteries** branch

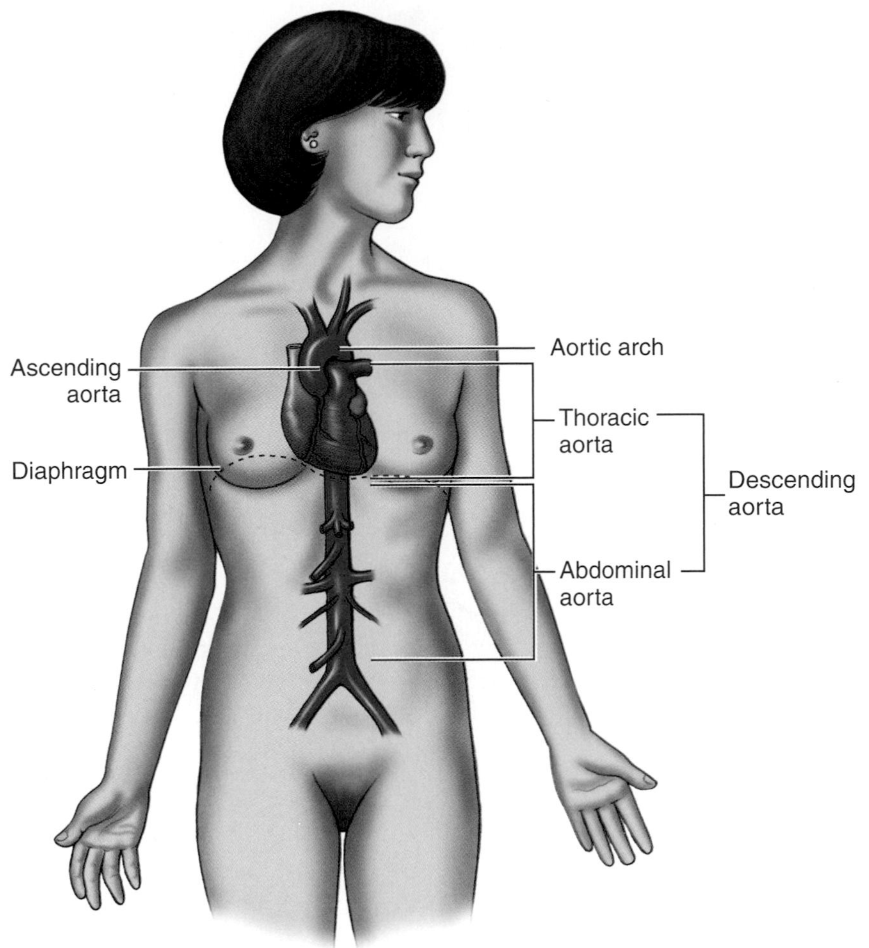

FIGURE 18-3 Naming the parts of the aorta.

from the ascending aorta. The coronary arteries are distributed throughout the heart and supply oxygenated blood to the myocardium.

Branches of the Aortic Arch

The aortic arch extends from the ascending aorta to the beginning of the descending aorta. The following three large arteries arise from the aortic arch:

- The **brachiocephalic artery** is a large artery on the right side of the body. It supplies blood to the right side of the head and neck, right shoulder, and right upper extremity. Refer to Figure 18-4 for the names of the arteries that extend from, or branch off the brachiocephalic artery. These arteries supply the right side of the head and neck and the arm and hand regions.
- The **left common carotid artery** extends upward from the highest part of the aortic arch and supplies the left side of the head and neck. Note that the left common carotid artery arises directly from the aorta, while the right common carotid arises from the brachiocephalic artery. (There is no left brachiocephalic artery.)

Do You Know...

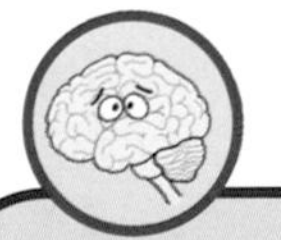

Which blood vessel refers to stupor or heavy sleep?

The name of the carotid arteries comes from the Greek word *karos,* meaning heavy sleep. The carotid arteries are blood vessels that supply blood to the brain. When pressure is exerted over the carotid artery, the vagus nerve is stimulated. Vagal stimulation results in a lowered blood pressure that can cause one to lose consciousness (the stupor or heavy sleep referred to earlier).

- The **left and right subclavian arteries** supply blood to the shoulders and upper arms.

Branches of the Descending Aorta (Thoracic Aorta)

The thoracic aorta is the upper portion of the descending aorta. It extends from the aortic arch to the diaphragm. **Intercostal arteries** arise from the aorta and supply the intercostal muscles between the ribs. Other small arteries supply the organs in the thorax.

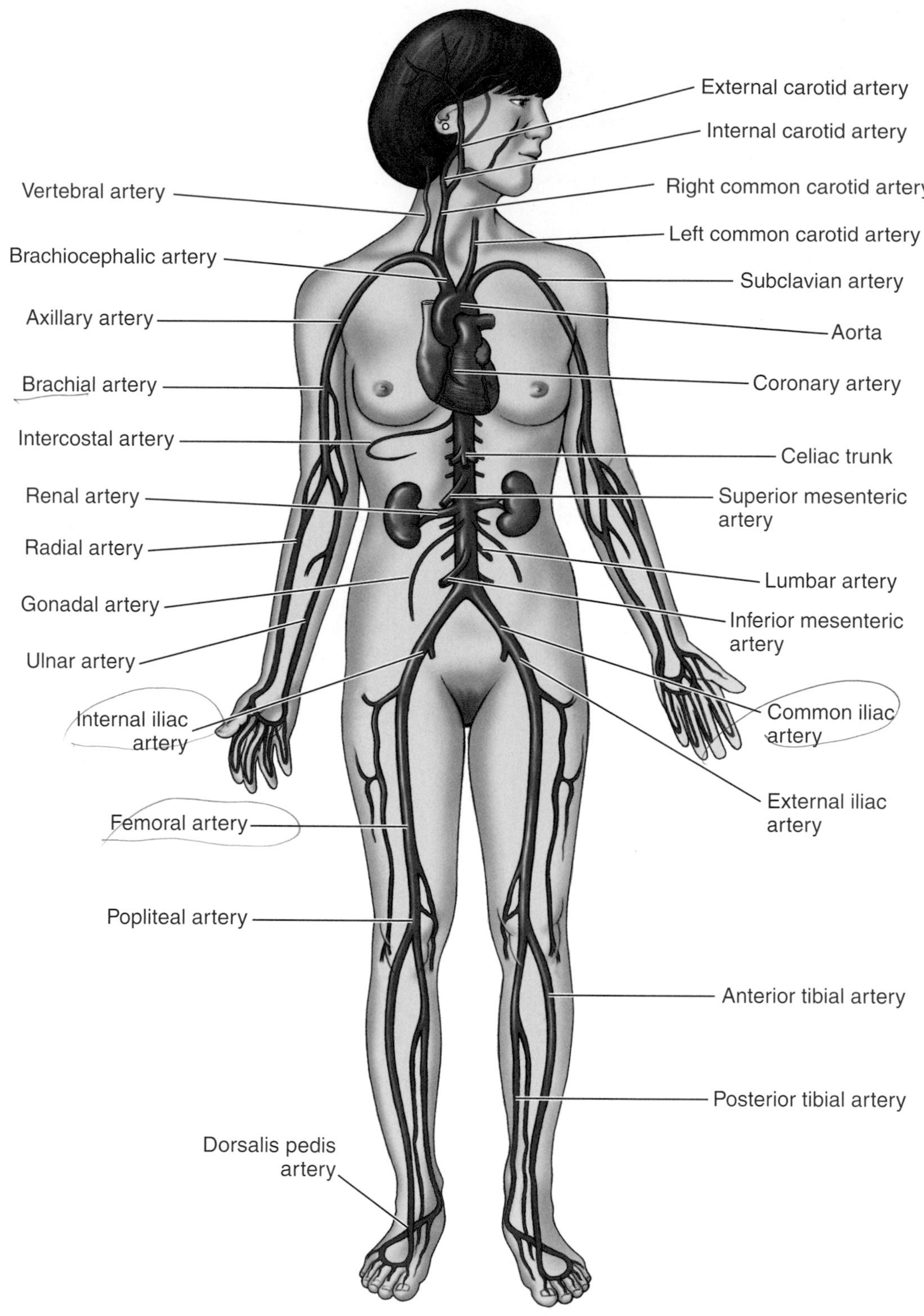

FIGURE 18-4 Major arteries.

Branches of the Descending Aorta (Abdominal Aorta)

The abdominal aorta extends from the thoracic aorta to the lower abdomen. Branches of the abdominal aorta include the following:

- The **celiac trunk** is a short artery that further divides into three smaller arteries. The **gastric artery** supplies the stomach; the **splenic artery** supplies the spleen; and the **hepatic artery** supplies the liver.
- Two **mesenteric arteries** are the superior and inferior segments. The **superior mesenteric artery** supplies blood to most of the small intestine and part of the large intestine. The other part of the

large intestine receives its blood supply from the **inferior mesenteric artery.**

- Two **renal arteries** supply blood to the right and left kidneys. Other branches of the abdominal aorta include the **gonadal arteries** and the **lumbar arteries.**

The distal abdominal aorta splits into the **right** and **left common iliac arteries** that supply the pelvic organs, thigh, and lower extremities. Identify the major arteries of the thigh and leg **(internal and external iliac arteries, femoral, popliteal, anterior,** and **posterior tibial arteries).** The anterior and posterior tibial arteries give rise to arteries that supply the foot. The anterior tibial artery becomes the **dorsalis pedis artery** in the foot.

MAJOR VEINS OF THE SYSTEMIC CIRCULATION

If you look at the back of your hand, you can see several veins but no arteries. Why? The arteries are usually located in deep and well-protected areas. Many of the veins, however, are located more superficially and can be seen. These are called **superficial veins. Deep veins** are located more deeply and usually run parallel to the arteries. With few exceptions, the names of the deep veins are the same as the names of the companion arteries. For instance, the femoral artery is accompanied by the femoral vein. In Figure 18-5, note the similarity in the names of many of the arteries and veins. Good news! If you learn the names of the arteries, you'll also know most of the names of the veins.

VENAE CAVAE

The veins carry blood from all parts of the body to the venae cavae for delivery to the heart.

The **vena cava** (VĒnă KĂ-vă) is the main vein. It is divided into the **superior vena cava (SVC)** and the **inferior vena cava (IVC).** Veins draining blood from the head, shoulders, and upper extremities empty into the SVC. Veins draining the lower part of the body empty into the IVC. The SVC and IVC empty into the right atrium.

VEINS THAT EMPTY INTO THE SUPERIOR VENA CAVA

The SVC receives blood from the head, shoulder, and upper extremities. Veins may drain directly or indirectly into the SVC. For instance, the brachiocephalic veins empty directly into the SVC. The **axillary vein,** however, drains into the **subclavian vein,** which drains into the brachiocephalic vein, which in turn drains into the SVC. Refer to Figure 18-5 so that you can trace the flow of venous blood from a distal site to the vena cava as follows:

- The **cephalic vein** is a superficial vein that drains the lateral arm region and carries blood to the axillary vein toward the SVC.
- The **basilic vein** is a superficial vein that drains the medial arm region. The cephalic and the basilic veins are joined by the **median cubital vein** (anterior aspect of the elbow). Blood samples are often drawn from the median cubital vein.
- The **subclavian veins** receive blood from the axillary veins and from the jugular veins. Blood is carried by these veins to the brachiocephalic veins that empty into the superior vena cava.
- The jugular veins drain blood from the head and drain into the subclavian veins. The **external jugular veins** drain blood from the face, scalp, and neck. The **internal jugular veins** drain blood from the brain. The internal jugular vein, in fact, is the main vein that drains the brain. Because the jugular veins are so close to the heart (right atrium), the pressure in the jugular veins reflects the pressure of blood in the right side of the heart. A person in right-sided heart failure has a higher than normal pressure in the right heart. This is observed clinically as pulsating jugular veins and is referred to as jugular vein distension (JVD). As a nurse, you will be observing, measuring, and recording JVD.
- The **brachiocephalic veins** are large veins that are formed by the union of the subclavian and internal jugular veins. The right and left brachiocephalic veins drain into the SVC.
- The **azygos vein** is a single vein that drains the thorax and empties directly into the SVC.

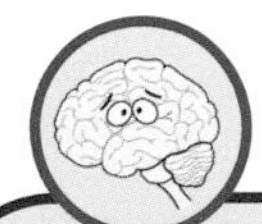

Do You Know...

What the subclavian stole?

Thou shalt not steal! Good advice! It even applies to blood. There is a condition called "subclavian steal syndrome." This is how the heist goes down. A person develops an occlusion in the subclavian artery proximal to the origin of the vertebral artery. (Remember the vertebral artery supplies blood to the posterior brain, while the subclavian artery supplies blood to the shoulder and arm.) When the affected arm is exercised the subclavian artery is unable to supply adequate blood. Blood pressure within the exercising shoulder and arm decreases, causing a retrograde (backward) flow of blood from the vertebral artery to the subclavian artery. The subclavian artery robs the posterior brain of blood, causing neurological symptoms such as impaired vision, dizziness, and syncope (fainting).

VEINS THAT EMPTY INTO THE INFERIOR VENA CAVA

The IVC returns blood to the heart from all regions of the body below the diaphragm. Follow the venous drainage in the lower leg in Figure 18-5.

- The **tibial veins** and the **peroneal veins** drain the calf and foot regions. The **posterior tibial vein** drains into the **popliteal vein** (behind the knee)

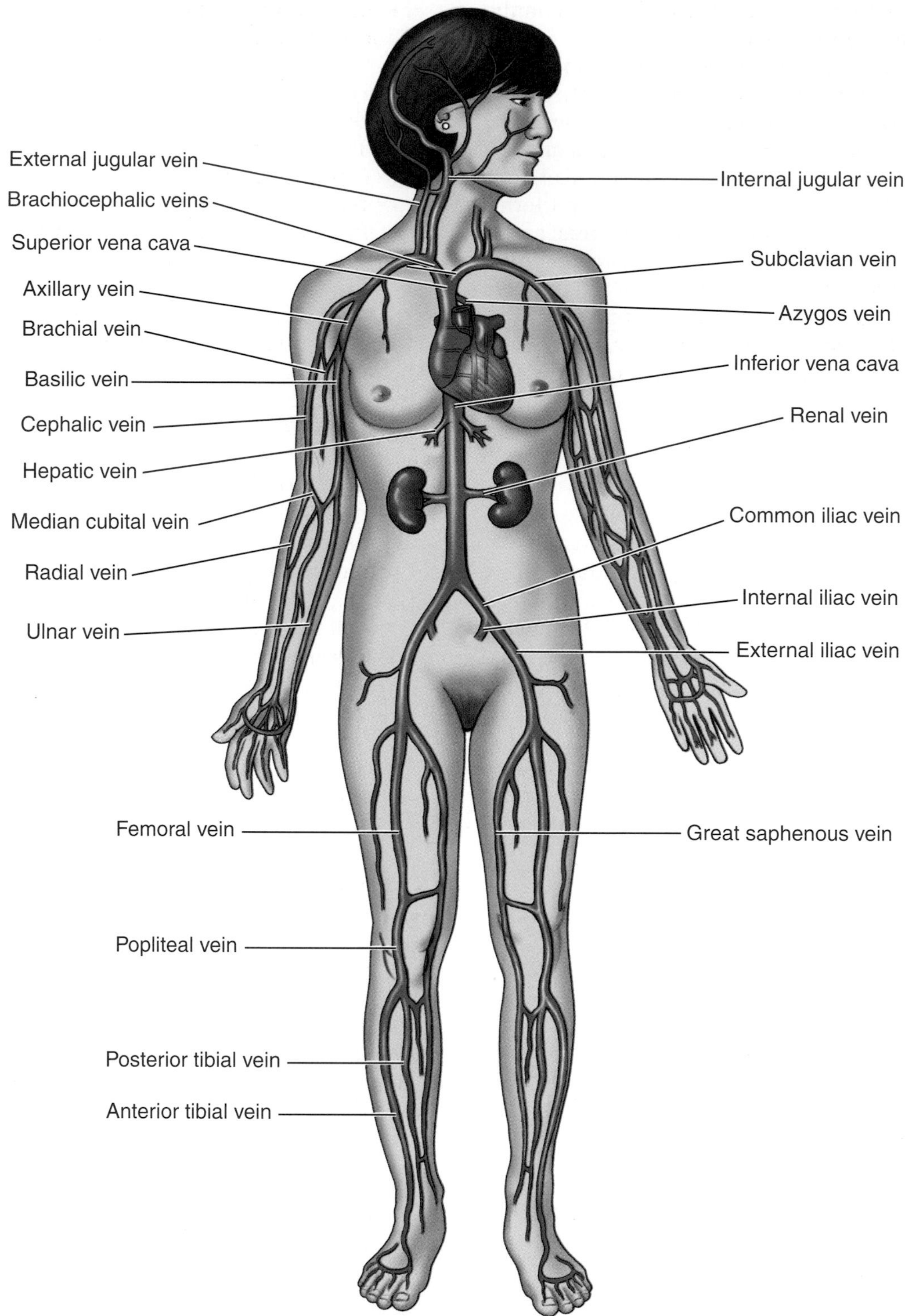

FIGURE 18-5 Major veins.

and then the **femoral vein** (in the thigh). The femoral vein enters the pelvis as the **external iliac vein** and empties into the **common iliac vein.** The common iliac vein continues as the IVC.

- The **great saphenous veins** are the longest veins in the body. They begin in the foot, ascend along the medial side, and merge with the femoral vein to become the external iliac vein. These veins receive drainage from the superficial veins of the leg and thigh region. The great saphenous veins also connect with the deep veins of the leg and thigh. Thus, blood can return from the lower extremities to the heart by several routes. The great saphenous veins are sometimes "borrowed" by surgeons. Portions of vein are surgically removed and transplanted into the heart in order to bypass clogged coronary arteries.

- The internal and external iliac veins unite to form the common iliac veins. The common iliac veins converge to form the inferior vena cava that ascends through the abdominal and thoracic regions to the right atrium of the heart.
- The **renal veins** drain the right and left kidneys, emptying blood directly into the IVC.
- The **hepatic veins** drain the liver, emptying blood directly into the upper IVC. Because the hepatic veins are so close to the heart, congestion of the right heart often causes congestion in the hepatic veins and liver.

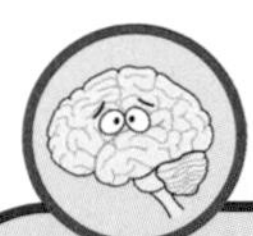

Do You Know...

What varicose veins look like?

Varicose veins are distended and twisted veins, usually involving the superficial veins in the legs. Varicosities can develop in other veins. Hemorrhoids, for instance, are varicose veins that affect the veins in the anal region. Persons who are alcoholic often develop varicose veins at the base of the esophagus. These are called esophageal varices. These varices are apt to rupture, causing a massive, life-threatening hemorrhage.

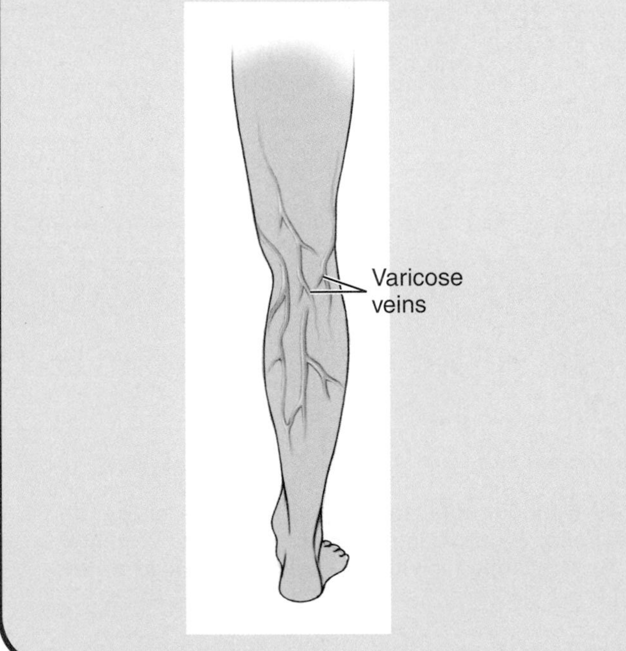

SPECIAL CIRCULATIONS

Most organs receive oxygen-rich blood from arteries, while oxygen-poor blood is drained by veins. Several organs have circulations that are arranged differently. They include the blood supply to the head and brain, the blood supply to the liver, and the arrangement of the blood vessels in the unborn child (fetal circulation).

BLOOD SUPPLY TO THE HEAD AND BRAIN

The brain requires a continuous supply of blood; even a few minutes without oxygen causes brain damage. To ensure a rich supply of blood, the head is supplied by two pairs of arteries, **carotid arteries** and **vertebral arteries** (Figure 18-6, *A*).

Arteries of the Head and Neck

The **right common carotid artery** arises from the brachiocephalic artery and the **left common carotid artery** arises directly from the aortic arch (see Figure 18-6, *B*). At about the level of the mandible, the common carotid arteries split to form the external and internal carotid arteries. The **external carotid arteries** supply the superficial areas of the neck, face, and scalp. The **internal carotid arteries** extend to the front part of the base of the brain. Once inside the cranium, each internal carotid artery divides, sending numerous branches to various parts of the brain. The internal carotid arteries supply most of the blood to the brain. Near the base of each internal carotid artery is an enlarged area called the carotid sinus. The carotid sinus contains special receptors called baroreceptors that help regulate blood pressure.

Vertebral arteries pass upward from the subclavian arteries toward the brain and back of the neck. As the vertebral arteries extend up into the cranium, they join to form a single **basilar artery** (see Figure 18-6, *B*). Numerous branches from the basilar artery supply areas of the brain around the brain stem and cerebellum. Other branches of the basilar artery connect with branches of the internal carotid arteries.

The branches from the internal carotid arteries and the basilar artery form a circle of arteries at the base of the brain. This circular arrangement of arteries is an **anastomosis** or connection, called the **circle of Willis** (see Figure 18-6, *B*). Arising from the circle of Willis are many arteries that penetrate the brain and maintain its rich supply of blood.

Most of the blood supply to the brain runs through the internal carotid arteries. What about knotted or clotted carotids? If the carotid arteries become blocked, the vertebral arteries cannot supply sufficient blood to the brain, which results in impaired brain function. Impaired brain function is most often observed as a cognitive (thinking) impairment and dizziness.

Venous Drainage of the Head and Brain

The **external** and **internal jugular veins** are the two major veins that drain blood from the head and neck (see Figure 18-6, *C*). The external jugular veins are more superficial and drain blood from the posterior head and neck region. They empty into the subclavian veins. The internal jugular veins drain

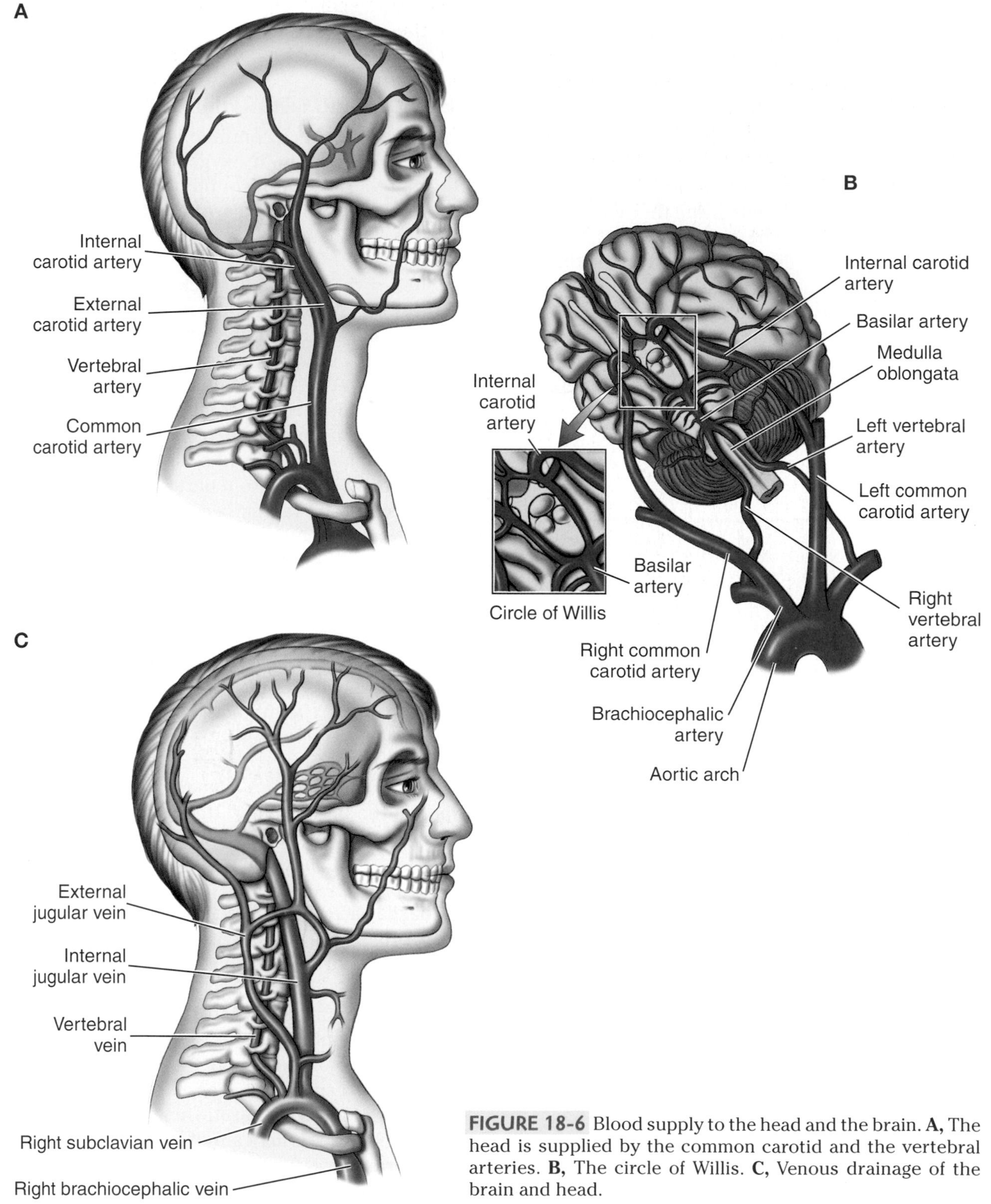

FIGURE 18-6 Blood supply to the head and the brain. **A,** The head is supplied by the common carotid and the vertebral arteries. **B,** The circle of Willis. **C,** Venous drainage of the brain and head.

the anterior head, face, and neck. The deep internal jugular veins drain most of the blood from the venous sinuses of the brain. The internal jugular veins on each side of the neck join with the subclavian veins to form the brachiocephalic veins. The brachiocephalic veins empty blood into the SVC.

BLOOD SUPPLY TO THE LIVER AND THE HEPATIC PORTAL CIRCULATION

The blood vessels of the liver have a unique arrangement. Three groups of blood vessels are associated with hepatic circulation; they are the portal vein, the hepatic veins, and the hepatic artery.

Hepatic Portal Circulation

The **portal vein** is a large vein that carries blood from the organs of digestion to the liver (Figure 18-7). It is formed by the union of two large veins: the **superior mesenteric vein** and the **splenic vein.** The superior mesenteric vein receives blood from the small intestine (where most digestion and absorption occur) and the first part of the large intestine. The splenic vein receives blood from the stomach, spleen, and pancreas. In addition, the splenic vein receives blood from the **inferior mesenteric vein,** which drains the last part of the large intestine.

The purpose of the hepatic portal circulation is to carry blood rich in digestive end products from the organs of digestion to the liver. Because it plays such a critical role in metabolism, the liver needs easy access to the digestive end products. As the blood flows through the liver, many of the nutrients are extracted from the blood and modified in some way. For instance, the liver prevents nitrogen from entering the general

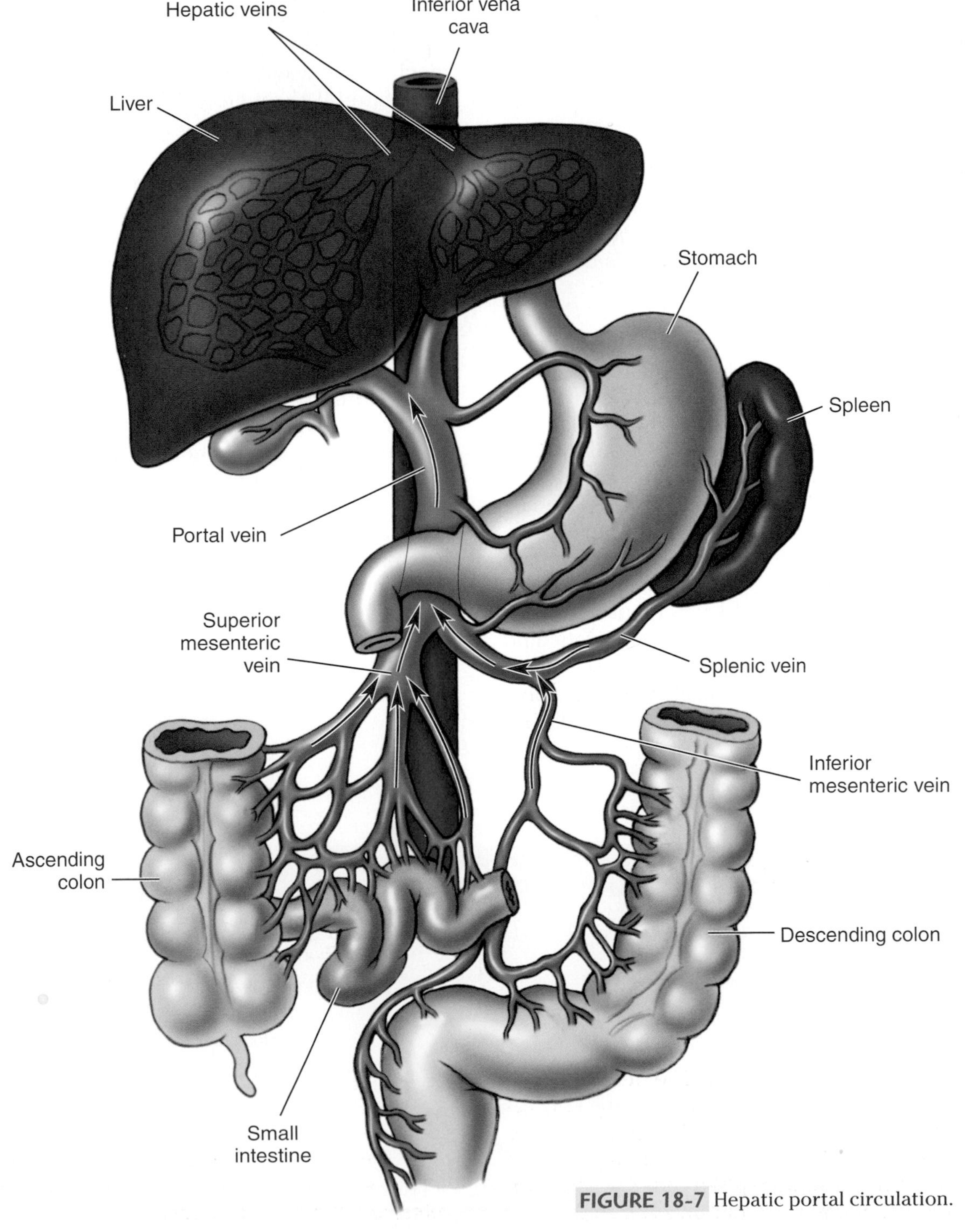

FIGURE 18-7 Hepatic portal circulation.

circulation as ammonia. Instead the nitrogen is excreted by the liver into the blood in the form of urea. Urea is less toxic than ammonia and is easily eliminated by the kidneys. In conditions such as cirrhosis, some of the blood bypasses the liver, allowing ammonia to enter the general circulation. Not good; ammonia severely impairs brain activity, causing disorientation and encephalopathy. Thus it is crucial that blood from the digestive organs first goes to the liver!

In addition to the portal vein, the liver has two other blood vessels: the **hepatic artery** and the **hepatic veins.** The hepatic artery is a branch of the celiac trunk, a large artery that branches off the abdominal aorta. The hepatic artery carries oxygen-rich blood to the liver. The hepatic veins drain blood from the liver and deliver it to the IVC.

Note that both the hepatic artery and the portal vein carry blood toward the liver. The hepatic artery carries oxygen-rich blood, and the portal vein carries blood rich in the products of digestion to the liver. One-third of the hepatic blood flow is delivered by the hepatic artery while 2/3 of the hepatic blood flow is delivered by the portal vein.

Another Way to Say It: The Splanchnic Circulation

The blood flow to the stomach, spleen, pancreas, intestines, and liver is referred to as the **splanchnic circulation.** The splanchnic circulation is very adjustable. Blood flow may increase up to eight times following a meal. When digestion is complete, the blood can then be diverted from the splanchnic blood vessels to other organs such as exercising skeletal muscles. Your mother was right! Do not go for a vigorous swim immediately after eating. Your splanchnic blood vessels are using the blood that your swimming skeletal muscles need. Cramping and drowning are possible. The splanchnic circulation also responds vigorously to a severe hemorrhage; the vessels constrict so intensely that they cause an ischemic or blood-deprived gut (intestines). The damaged gut is characterized by bloody diarrhea and absorption of toxins from the intestine into the blood, and it is potentially lethal.

FETAL CIRCULATION

Look at your "belly button," or **umbilicus.** At one time, you had a long **umbilical cord,** a lifeline that attached you to a structure called the **placenta** embedded in the wall of your mother's uterus. Why was this attachment necessary? As a fetus, you were submerged in amniotic fluid and were unable to eat or breathe. All your nutrients and oxygen had to be supplied by your mother. Your mother also absorbed much of the waste produced by your tiny body and eliminated it through her excretory organs. The exchange of all your nutrients, gases, and waste occurred at the placenta.

Because of these special needs, the fetal heart and circulation have several modifications that make them different from "life on the outside" (Figure 18-8). The following modifications are described and summarized in Table 18-2:

- *Umbilical blood vessels:* The umbilical cord contains three blood vessels: one large **umbilical vein** and two smaller **umbilical arteries.** The umbilical vein carries blood rich in oxygen and nutrients from the placenta to the fetus. The two umbilical arteries carry carbon dioxide and other waste from the fetus to the placenta. (Note: In the fetal circulation the umbilical vein is carrying oxygen-rich blood, whereas it is the umbilical arteries that are carrying oxygen-poor blood.)
- *Ductus venosus:* Blood flows through the umbilical vein into the fetus. Within the body of the fetus, the umbilical vein branches. Some blood flows through one branch to the fetal liver. Most of the blood, however, bypasses the liver and passes through the **ductus venosus** into the IVC. The ductus

Table 18-2 Special Features in the Fetal Circulation

Structure	Location	Function
Umbilical arteries (2)	Umbilical cord	Transport blood from fetus to the placenta
Umbilical vein (1)	Umbilical cord	Transports blood from the placenta to the fetus
Ductus venosus	Between the umbilical vein and the inferior vena cava	Carries blood from umbilical vein to inferior vena cava; allows some of the blood to bypass the liver
Foramen ovale	Septum between the right and left atria	Allows blood to go directly from the right atrium into the left atrium to bypass the pulmonary circulation
Ductus arteriosus	Between the pulmonary artery and the aorta	Allows blood in the pulmonary artery to go directly into the descending aorta and to bypass the pulmonary circulation

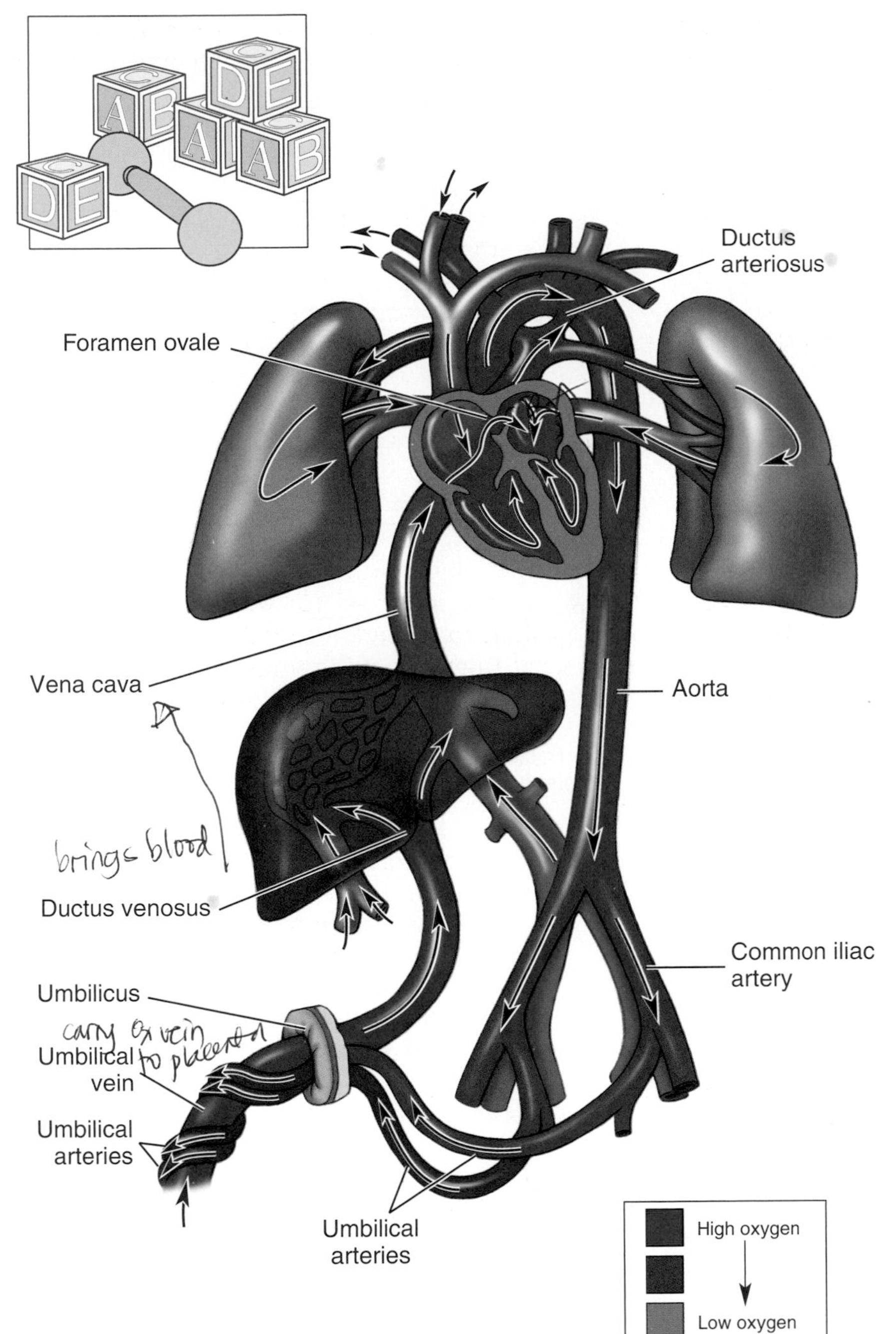

FIGURE 18-8 Fetal circulation.

venosus is a vessel that connects the umbilical vein with the IVC in the fetus, but after birth, the ductus venosus closes and serves no further purpose.

Because the deflated fetal lungs are not used for gas exchange, they have no need for blood pumped through the pulmonary circulation. Two modifications in the fetal heart and large vessels reroute most of the blood around the lungs. The two modifications are the **foramen ovale** and the **ductus arteriosus:**

- Foramen ovale: The foramen ovale is an opening in the interatrial septum of the heart. This opening allows most of the blood to flow from the right atrium directly into the left atrium.
- Ductus arteriosus: Although most blood flows through the foramen ovale into the left atrium, some blood enters the right ventricle and is pumped into the pulmonary artery. How does this blood bypass the lungs? The fetus has a short tube, or opening, called the ductus arteriosus, that connects the pulmonary artery with the aorta. Blood pumped into the pulmonary artery bypasses the lungs by flowing through the ductus arteriosus directly into the aorta. After birth, these fetal structures close. Why is it not a good idea for a pregnant woman to take aspirin or similar drugs such as indomethacin? Naturally secreted

prostaglandins help keep the ductus arteriosus open. Drugs such as aspirin and indomethacin block prostaglandin synthesis, thereby causing a premature closure of the ductus arteriosus. This can be lethal for the baby!

Occasionally, the fetal structures do not close and appear as congenital heart defects. For instance, the ductus arteriosus may fail to close, thereby allowing blood continuously to shunt from the aorta to the pulmonary artery. A patent ductus arteriosus (PDA) creates a left-to-right shunt. Fortunately, a PDA is easily corrected.

See Figure 18-8 for color coding of the fetal veins and arteries. Blood vessels carrying oxygenated blood are in red; these are usually the arteries. Vessels carrying unoxygenated blood are in blue; these are usually veins. Note, however, that the umbilical vein is red, indicating oxygenated blood. The umbilical arteries are blue, indicating unoxygenated blood.

Note the color of the upper portion of the vena cava. The adult vena cava is colored blue because it contains unoxygenated blood. The fetal vena cava, however, is violet, indicating that the blood is a mixture of unoxygenated blood (coming from the metabolizing fetal tissue) and oxygenated blood (coming from the umbilical vein). Note also the color of the blood in the fetal aorta; it is not the bright red that is characteristic of the adult aorta. The adult aorta carries only oxygenated blood, but the fetal aorta mixes oxygenated and unoxygenated blood.

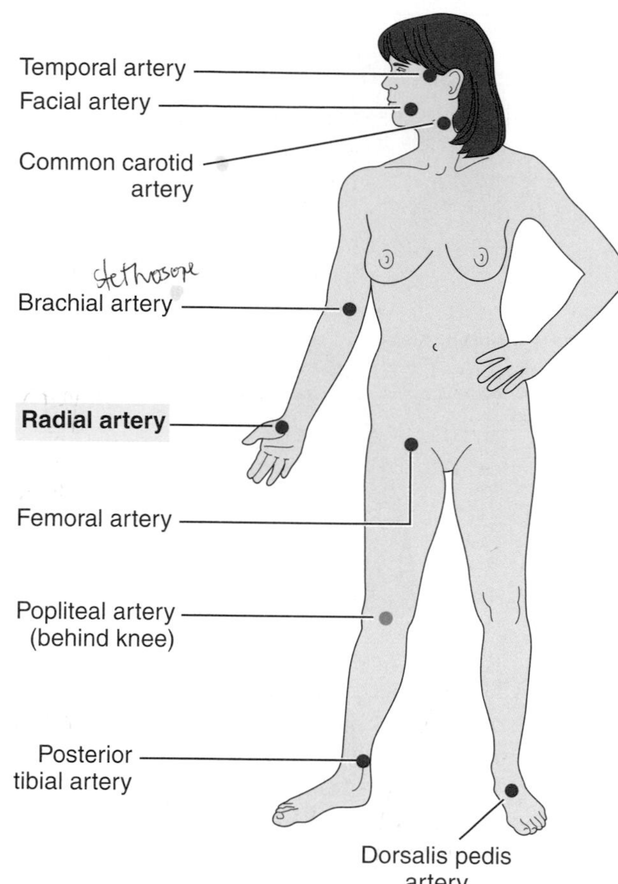

FIGURE 18-9 Pulse points.

PULSE

WHAT IS THE PULSE?

The ventricles pump blood into the arteries about 72 times per minute. The blood causes an alternating expansion and recoil of the arteries with each beat of the heart. This alternating expansion and recoil creates a pressure wave (similar to vibration), which travels through all the arteries. This wave is called the **pulse.**

Because it is due to the rhythmic contraction of the ventricles of the heart, the pulse is often described as a "heartbeat that can be felt at the wrist." Although a pulse can be felt in any artery lying close to the surface of the body, the site most often used to feel the pulse is the radial artery in the wrist area. Determine your own radial pulse and then try feeling a pulse at any of the nine "pulse points" identified in Figure 18-9.

WHAT CAN YOU LEARN ABOUT PATIENTS BY FEELING THEIR PULSE?

By feeling a person's pulse, you can determine the heart rate. A normal heart rate is about 72 beats per minute. You can also determine if the heart is beating regularly (rhythmically) or irregularly. By assessing the regularity of the pulse, you may detect a cardiac dysrhythmia (disturbance of rhythm).

You can also assess the pulse for its strength. Does the pulse feel strong or weak? At times the heart contracts so weakly that the heartbeat cannot be felt over the radial artery; this happens in a person who has lost a lot of blood and is in shock. It is also possible that you may not be able to detect a pulse in a particular artery. The pulse may be absent if the artery is blocked or occluded. For instance, if a person has poor arterial circulation to the feet, as occurs with many diabetic persons, the dorsalis pedis pulse may be undetectable. Thus a correct assessment of the pulse can provide much useful information about the patient's condition.

Sum It Up!

The arrangement and names of the major arteries and veins are summarized in Figures 18-4 and 18-5. There are three special circulations: circulation to the head and brain, the hepatic portal circulation, and the fetal circulation. The pulse is described as a "heartbeat that can be felt at the wrist." There are numerous pulse points that can be used to assess the pulse.

SUMMARY OUTLINE

The circulatory system is a series of blood vessels, or hollow tubes, that begin and end in the heart. The circulatory system delivers blood to all the body's cells and then returns the blood to the heart.

I. Circles, Circuits, and Circulations
- A. The heart and blood vessels form a circle.
- B. Two circulations: pulmonic and systemic.

II. Blood Vessels
- A. Naming the Blood Vessels
  1. Arteries carry blood away from the heart; the smallest arteries are the arterioles.
  2. Capillaries connect arteries and veins; a capillary is close to every cell in the body.
  3. Veins carry blood back to the heart; small veins are called venules.
- B. Layers of Blood Vessels
  1. The tunica intima is the smooth innermost layer.
  2. The tunica media is the middle layer that contains elastic tissue and smooth muscle.
  3. The tunica adventitia is the outermost layer of connective tissue.
- C. Blood Vessels: What They Do
  1. Arteries conduct blood from the heart to the organs and are called conductance vessels.
  2. The arterioles constrict and dilate, thereby determining resistance to the flow of blood. The arterioles are called resistance vessels.
  3. Capillaries are concerned with the exchange of water and dissolved substances between the blood and tissue fluid. Capillaries are called exchange vessels.
  4. Veins and venules return blood to the heart from the body. The veins also store blood and are therefore called capacitance vessels.

III. Major Arteries of the Systemic Circulation
- A. The major arteries include the aorta and the arteries arising from the aorta.
- B. See Figure 18-4 for the names and locations of the major arteries.

IV. Major Veins of the Systemic Circulation
- A. The major veins include the venae cavae and the veins that empty into them.
- B. See Figure 18-5 for the names and locations of the major veins.

V. Special Circulations
- A. The head and brain are supplied by two sets of arteries: the carotid arteries and the vertebral arteries. The internal carotid arteries and the basilar artery form the circle of Willis. Blood from the head and brain drains into the jugular veins.
- B. The blood supply of the liver is composed of the portal vein, hepatic artery, and hepatic veins. The hepatic artery brings oxygen-rich blood to the liver.
- C. The portal vein carries blood from the digestive tract to the liver. The hepatic veins carry blood from the liver to the inferior vena cava.
- D. The fetal circulation has several unique features. The fetus uses the placenta as lungs. The umbilical blood vessels carry blood between the placenta and the fetus. Three special structures are the ductus venosus, foramen ovale, and ductus arteriosus.

VI. The Pulse
- A. The pulse is due to the alternating expansion and recoil of the artery creating a pressure wave (similar to vibration).
- B. The pulse is often described as a "heartbeat that can be felt at the wrist."
- C. Figure 18-9 identifies the pulse points.

Review Your Knowledge

Matching: Blood Vessels: Structure and Function

Directions: Match the following words with their descriptions below. Some words may be used more than once.

a. large arteries
b. arterioles
c. capillaries
d. veins

1. ____ Exchange vessels
2. ____ Resistance vessels
3. ____ Composed of a single layer of epithelium sitting on a basement membrane
4. ____ The most numerous of the blood vessels
5. ____ Capacitance vessels
6. ____ Blood pressure is lowest in these blood vessels
7. ____ Generally colored blue and contain valves
8. ____ These are the strongest of the blood vessels
9. ____ Blood pressure is highest in these blood vessels
10. ____ Connect the arteries and veins

Matching: Names of Blood Vessels

Directions: Match the following words with their descriptions below. Some words may be used more than once.

a. aorta
b. vena cava
c. carotids
d. circle of Willis
e. portal vein
f. hepatic artery
g. jugular
h. brachial artery
i. renal artery
j. median cubital vein
k. saphenous
l. radial artery
m. coronaries

1. ____ Carries oxygen-rich blood to the liver
2. ____ Carries oxygen-rich blood to the kidneys
3. ____ Carries blood that is rich in digestive end-products to the liver
4. ____ Classified as ascending, arch, and descending
5. ____ The superior mesenteric and splenic veins merge to form this vein
6. ____ Classified as thoracic and abdominal
7. ____ Vein in the arm that is used to "draw" a sample of blood
8. ____ Main vein that drains the brain
9. ____ Arterial blood supply at the base of the brain
10. ____ Arteries that ascend along the anterior neck to the brain
11. ____ Longest superficial vein in the thigh and leg
12. ____ The iliac veins drain into this blood vessel
13. ____ Blood pressure is usually taken over this artery
14. ____ This artery is usually used in "taking a pulse"
15. ____ These arteries supply the myocardium

Matching: Fetal Circulation

Directions: Match the following words with their descriptions below.

a. umbilical arteries
b. umbilical vein
c. ductus arteriosus
d. ductus venosus
e. foramen ovale

1. ____ Carry blood from the fetus to the placenta
2. ____ Opening that connects the right and left atria in the fetal circulation
3. ____ Structure that connects the pulmonary artery and the aorta in the fetal circulation
4. ____ Structure that bypasses the fetal liver
5. ____ Carries oxygen-rich blood from the placenta to the fetus

Multiple Choice

1. Which of the following is not true about the capillaries?
   a. Are called the exchange vessels
   b. Capillary membranes have holes or pores
   c. Connect the arteries and the veins
   d. Have valves
2. The common carotid
   a. supplies oxygenated blood to the brain.
   b. is the main vein that drains the brain.
   c. is part of the hepatic portal system.
   d. ascends along the back part of the neck to the brain to form the basilar artery.
3. The purpose of the hepatic portal system is to
   a. provide the fetus with oxygenated blood.
   b. deliver blood that is rich in digestive end-products to the liver.
   c. drain unoxygenated blood from the brain.
   d. deliver oxygenated blood to the liver.
4. Which statement is true about the fetal circulation?
   a. The umbilical arteries deliver oxygenated blood to the fetus.
   b. The umbilical vein delivers oxygenated blood to the fetus.
   c. The ductus venosus connects the right and left fetal atria.
   d. The ductus arteriosus bypasses the fetal liver.
5. Which of the following is descriptive of the aorta?
   a. It is the largest and strongest of the arteries.
   b. It carries unoxygenated blood and so is colored blue.
   c. It is lined with large valves.
   d. Blood pressure in the aorta is lower than blood pressure within the veins.

CHAPTER 19

Functions of the Blood Vessels

KEY TERMS

Baroreceptor reflex, p. 336
Blood pressure, p. 330
Diastolic blood pressure, p. 331
Hypertension, p. 331
Hypotension, p. 335
Ischemia, p. 330
Oncotic pressure, p. 340
Pulse pressure, p. 331
Systolic blood pressure, p. 331
Vascular resistance, p. 335
Vasoconstriction, p. 335
Vasodilation, p. 335
Vasopressor, p. 336

OBJECTIVES

1. Explain how the blood vessels act as a delivery system.
2. Describe the factors that determine blood pressure.
3. Explain the baroreceptor reflex.
4. Describe the factors that determine capillary exchange.
5. Describe mechanisms of edema formation.
6. Explain how the blood vessels respond to changing body needs.
7. Describe the role of the blood vessels in the regulation of body temperature.

As mentioned earlier, it took seemingly forever for the ancients to "connect" the heart and the peripheral blood vessels. After that connection was made, scientists realized that blood was pumped out of the left heart, circulated around the body, and returned to the right side of the heart. But we still had no real understanding of the functions (physiology) of the peripheral blood vessels.

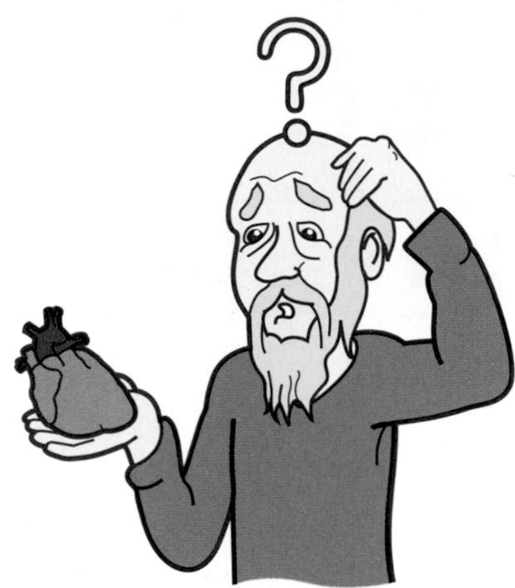

Today we know that the blood vessels do more than allow blood to run around in circles. The blood vessels perform five important functions:

1. Act as a delivery system
2. Regulate blood pressure
3. Engage in the exchange of nutrients and waste between the capillaries and cells
4. Redistribute blood in response to changing body needs
5. Help regulate body temperature

THE BLOOD VESSELS DELIVER

The primary purpose of the cardiovascular system is to deliver oxygen, hormones, and nutrients to the cells; the blood also collects cellular waste and delivers it to organs of excretion such as the kidney. The delivery of oxygen is especially critical. All cells need oxygen; without oxygen they die. Thus an adequate blood flow to an organ system is vital.

Clinically, you will spend a great deal of time assessing oxygen delivery to the tissues, since impaired blood flow (called **ischemia**) is a common cause of tissue damage and death. By analyzing the consequences of diminished cellular oxygenation, you can better appreciate the need for an adequate blood flow. As an example, a patient has an occlusion (blockage) in the large arteries in the lower left extremity. Why does he develop these "5 Cool Ps" of occlusive arterial disease?

1. **P**ain. Diminished oxygen stimulates pain receptors.
2. **P**ulselessness. The blocked artery decreases the flow of blood to the extremity; the pulse distal to the occlusion is diminished or absent.
3. **P**allor. Because of the lack of blood the extremity is pale, especially when elevated.
4. **P**aresthesia. Diminished blood flow decreases the supply of oxygen to the nerves of the leg, causing numbness and tingling.
5. **P**aralysis. Persistent oxygen deficit causes permanent nerve damage and paralysis (late sign).
6. **Cool**ness. Since blood carries heat, the decreased blood flow results in a decrease in the temperature of the affected extremity. Moreover, the damaged blood vessels cannot dilate and increase the flow of warm blood to the extremity.

BLOOD VESSELS REGULATE BLOOD PRESSURE

Why do you need a blood pressure? Blood pressure is needed to push blood through the blood vessels to an organ. No blood pressure—no organ perfusion! **Blood pressure** is the force blood exerts against the walls of the blood vessels. Blood pressure is determined by the pumping action of the heart and the size (lumen diameter) of the blood vessels, especially the arterioles.

MEASUREMENT OF BLOOD PRESSURE

120/80 mm Hg: What It Means

You just had a physical examination. The physician nodded approvingly that your blood pressure is normal at 120/80 mm Hg. Although you are thrilled to be normal, what exactly does 120/80 mm Hg mean?

The blood pressure in the large arteries is caused by the heart's pumping activity. When the ventricles contract, a volume of blood (stroke volume) is pumped out of the ventricle into the artery, thereby increasing pressure. The pressure in the arteries at the peak of

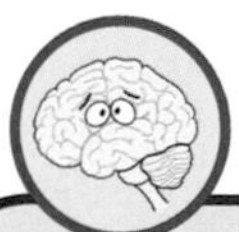

Do You Know...

About the MABP?

The normal blood pressure is expressed as 120/80 mm Hg. What is the mean arterial blood pressure (MABP)? MABP is calculated as follows:

$$\text{MABP} = 2/3 \text{ diastolic pressure} + 1/3 \text{ systolic pressure}$$

or

$$\text{MABP} = \text{diastolic pressure} + 1/3 \text{ pulse pressure}$$

For a blood pressure of 120/80 mm Hg, the MABP is 94 mm Hg. Why is the MABP important? Because the organs are perfused by or "feel" the MABP. Note that the MABP expresses more of the diastolic pressure than the systolic pressure. The dominance of the MABP by the diastolic pressure is the basis for the clinical concern for the diastolic reading.

ventricular contraction **(systole)** is called the **systolic pressure;** it is the top number—120 mm Hg. The **diastolic pressure** is the pressure in the large arteries when the ventricles of the heart are relaxing **(diastole).** The diastolic reading is the bottom number—80 mm Hg.

By measuring blood pressure, you can also calculate **pulse pressure.** The pulse pressure is the difference between the systolic and the diastolic pressure. For instance, your blood pressure is 120/80 mm Hg. Your pulse pressure is 40 mm Hg (120 minus 80).

Normal and Abnormal

A blood pressure range of 100 to 140 mm Hg (systolic) to 60 to 90 mm Hg (diastolic) is considered normal for adult males. Blood pressure readings vary according to age, gender, and size. For instance, the normal blood pressure of a 2-year-old child is 95/65 mm Hg. The maintenance of normal blood pressure is extremely important. If blood pressure becomes too low, blood flow to vital organs decreases, and the person is said to be in shock. Without immediate treatment, the person may die. If the blood pressure becomes elevated, the blood vessels may burst, or rupture. A ruptured blood vessel in the brain, for example, is a major cause of stroke, resulting in loss of speech, paralysis, and possible death. **Hypertension,** a long-term, or chronic, elevation of blood pressure, also causes serious problems. It puts added strain on the heart, damages the blood vessels in the kidneys, and damages the retina, causing loss of vision. Chronic hypertension is a major cause of heart failure. Because of the importance of maintaining a normal blood pressure, you will often be asked to assess blood pressure in your patients.

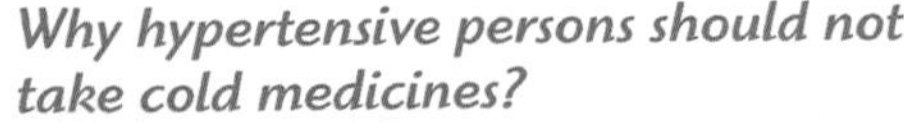

Do You Know...

Why hypertensive persons should not take cold medicines?

Hypertensive persons have high blood pressure that is often caused by increased systemic vascular resistance (SVR). Cold and cough medications usually include drugs (phenylephrine) that are alpha$_1$ agonists. Alpha$_1$ agonists cause arteriolar constriction, thereby further elevating SVR and blood pressure.

Measuring Blood Pressure

Measurement of blood pressure provides valuable information regarding a person's general health. Blood pressure is most commonly measured over the brachial artery in the upper arm. The pressures are expressed in mm Hg (millimeters of mercury). Unless otherwise stated, the term blood pressure refers to the blood pressure in the large arteries.

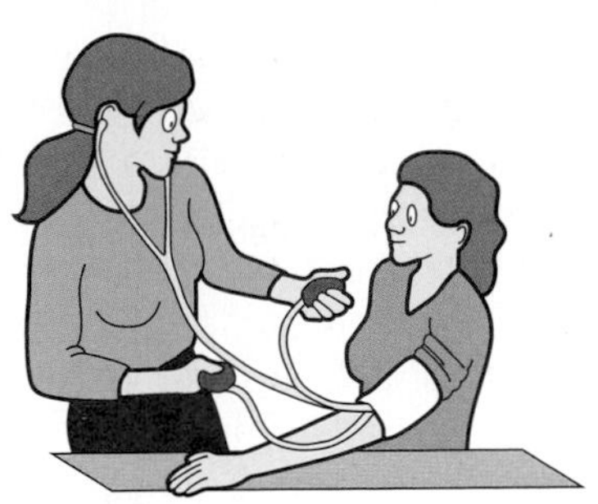

The instrument used to take a blood pressure recording is the sphygmomanometer. The sphygmomanometer is a device with two basic components, a dial indicating the pressure and an inflatable cuff. The cuff is wrapped around the patient's upper arm and inflated with air until the brachial artery is compressed, and the flow of blood through the artery is stopped. Then, with a stethoscope placed over the brachial artery distal to, or below, the cuff, the examiner listens for "tap tap tap" sounds. These sounds, called **Korotkoff sounds,** are caused by the flow of blood through the brachial artery. The measurement of blood pressure is explained in Figure 19-1.

BLOOD PRESSURE IN DIFFERENT BLOOD VESSELS

Blood pressures vary from one kind of blood vessel to the next (Figure 19-2). Note that the blood pressure is highest in the aorta because it is closest to the left ventricle; the left ventricle pumps blood with great force. The blood pressure gradually declines as the blood flows from the large arteries into the arterioles, into the capillaries, into the venules, and finally, into the veins. This difference in pressure causes blood to flow from the arterial side of the circulation to the venous side. Note that a blood pressure of 120/80 mm Hg is normal only for large blood vessels. Capillary pressure is generally much lower. Pressure within the large veins is around 0 mm Hg.

HOW VENOUS BLOOD FLOWS BACK TO THE HEART

Although blood pressure is very high in the arterial circulation, it decreases to almost 0 mm Hg in the veins. The blood pressure in the veins is so low, in fact, that it alone cannot return blood from the veins back to the heart. Three other mechanisms return venous blood to the heart: skeletal muscle action, respiratory movements, and constriction of the veins.

Skeletal Muscle Action

As Figure 19-3 shows, the large veins in the leg are surrounded by skeletal muscles. As the skeletal muscles

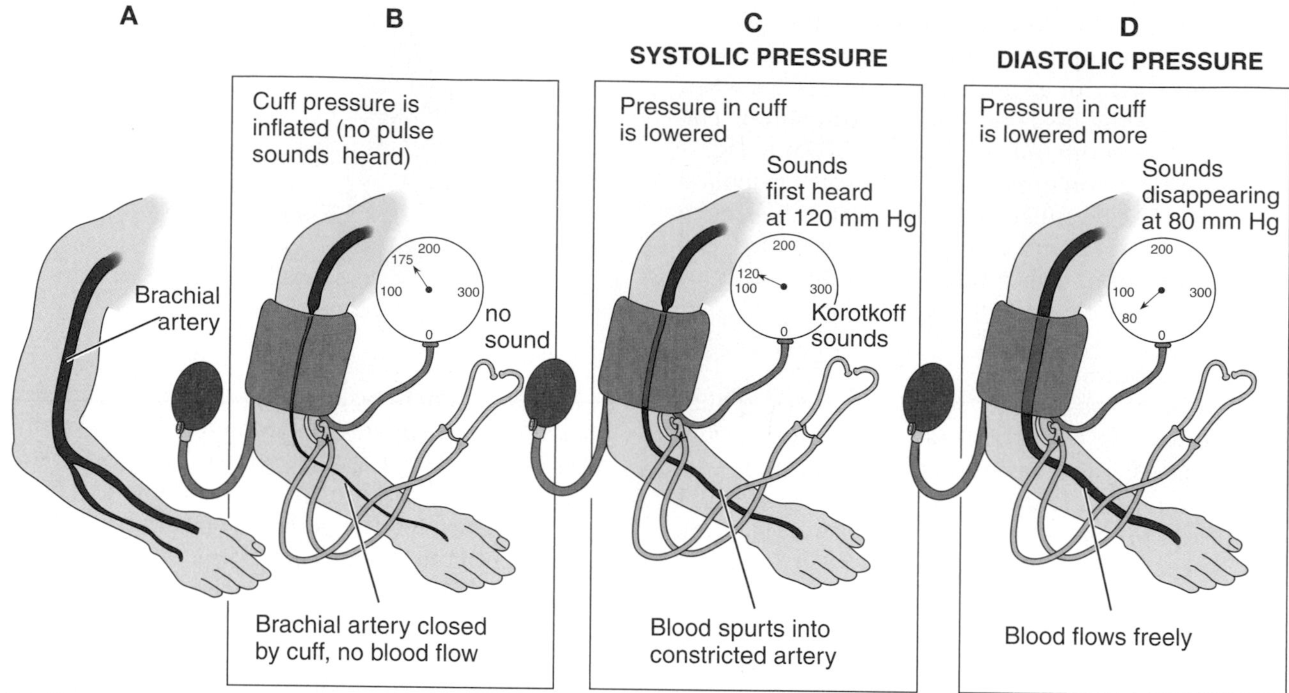

FIGURE 19-1 Taking a blood pressure. The measurement of blood pressure requires a sphygmomanometer and a stethoscope. Follow the panels for an explanation of the systolic (120 mm Hg) and diastolic (80 mm Hg) pressures. **A,** Identify the location of the brachial artery. **B,** Inflate the cuff, thereby squeezing the upper arm. At this point, the cuff pressure has become greater than the blood pressure within the brachial artery. The cuff pressure collapses the brachial artery, thereby stopping the flow of blood. No sound can be heard through the stethoscope. **C,** As the pressure within the cuff gradually diminishes, the artery opens slightly, and blood spurts through the blood vessel in response to the pressure within the brachial artery. You can hear the spurting effect of the blood as soft tapping sounds. The number on the sphygmomanometer that corresponds to the tapping sounds is recorded as the systolic blood pressure (120 mm Hg). With further reduction in cuff pressure, the brachial artery opens wider and allows blood flow through the artery to increase. The sound of the blood flowing through the partially opened artery sounds different from the tapping sounds of the spurting blood; it sounds louder and more distinct. **D,** As cuff pressure declines even further, the brachial artery opens completely, and normal blood flow through the artery resumes. At this point the sounds (heard through a stethoscope) disappear. The pressure at which the sounds disappear is read as the diastolic blood pressure (80 mm Hg).

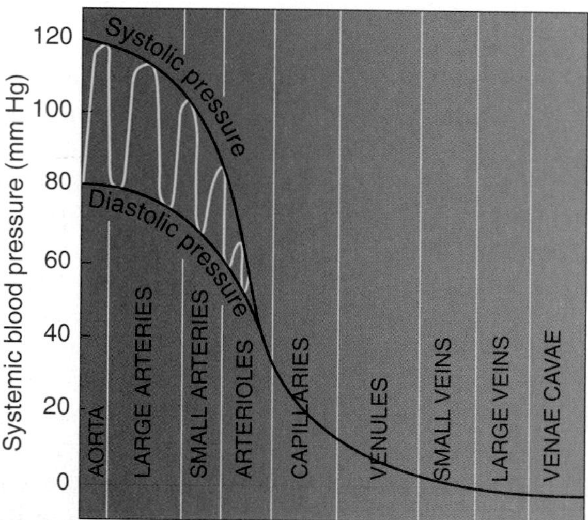

FIGURE 19-2 Blood pressure in the different blood vessels.

contract, they squeeze the large veins, thereby squirting blood toward the heart. Note that blood does not squirt backward because of the closed valves. Thus contraction of the skeletal muscles of the legs assists with the return of venous blood to the heart. This mechanism is called the **skeletal muscle pump.** The pump helps explain the beneficial effects of exercise for your patients. Exercise improves venous blood flow, thereby preventing stagnation of blood and blood clot formation.

Respiratory Movements

The act of breathing is performed by the contraction and relaxation of the skeletal muscles of the chest. These respiratory movements cause the pressures in the chest cavity to change. During inhalation, the diameter of the chest increases. The increase in thoracic size has two effects: it decreases pressure within the thorax and increases pressure within the abdominal cavity. The increased abdominal pressure, in turn, compresses or squeezes the vena cava, thereby pushing more blood toward the heart. The effect of respiratory activity on venous blood flow is called the **respiratory pump.** Encouraging your patient to "deep breathe" not only improves respiratory function, it also improves the circulation of blood.

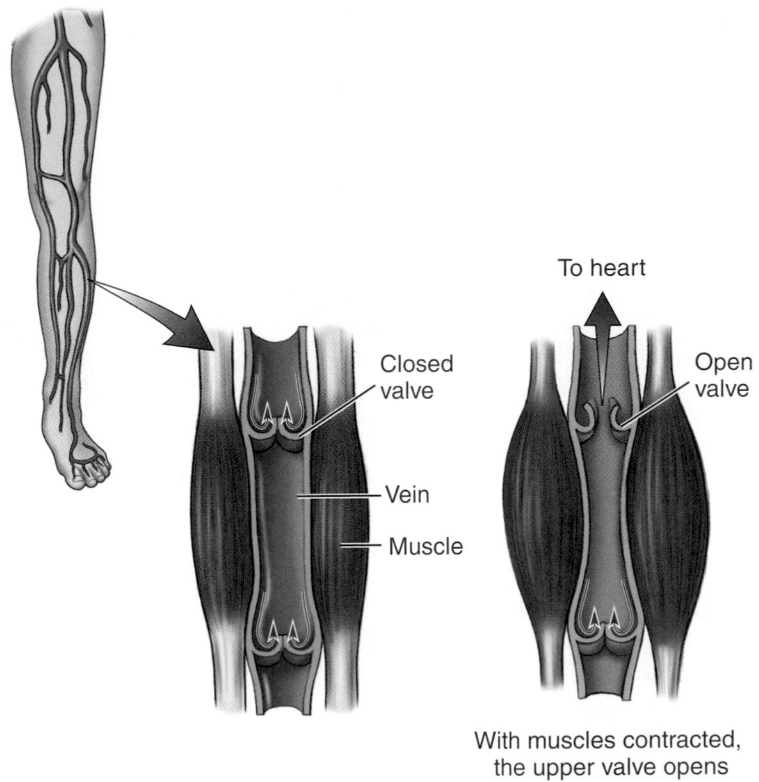

FIGURE 19-3 Skeletal muscle pump.

Constriction of the Veins

Because most of the blood is located in the venous side of the circulation (capacitance vessels), constriction of the veins pushes additional blood out of the veins toward the heart. Both sympathetic nervous system stimulation and some hormones cause **venoconstriction,** thereby increasing venous return.

HOW THE HEART AND BLOOD VESSELS DETERMINE BLOOD PRESSURE

Heart

How does myocardial function affect blood pressure? You have watched enough television to know that when the heart stops beating, the blood pressure drops to 0 mm Hg, and the person dies, indicating an obvious relationship between cardiac function and blood pressure. Figure 19-4 illustrates the relationship between pressure (blood pressure) and force (force of myocardial contraction). In Figure 19-4, *A,* the barrel of a syringe is filled with water. As you push on the plunger of the syringe, the pressure in the barrel increases, causing water to flow out of the syringe through the needle. Water flows from an area of high pressure (x) to an area of lower pressure (y). Figure 19-4, *B,* illustrates the similarity between the plunger-barrel model and the heart-blood vessel. The heart is similar to the plunger; when it contracts, it pushes the blood along the blood vessel. The blood vessel is similar to the barrel and needle of the syringe; the blood moves through the blood vessel from an area of high pressure to an area of lower pressure. Note: Blood pressure is caused by contraction of the heart muscle. It's simple: The stronger the force of contraction, the higher the blood pressure. No myocardial contraction, no blood pressure—dead!

Blood Vessels

How do the blood vessels affect blood pressure? A garden hose illustrates the blood vessels' effect on blood pressure. In Figure 19-5, *A,* the hose is hooked up to a faucet. When the faucet is turned on, water flows through the hose and falls to the ground in big droplets. In Figure 19-5, *B,* a nozzle has been attached to the end of the hose, thereby narrowing the end of the hose. The nozzle has increased the resistance to the flow of water. Because of the resistance of the nozzle, water does not fall out of the hose in big droplets, as Figure 19-5, *A;* instead, water squirts out of the end of the hose. Notice how much further the squirted water travels. What is the reason for this difference? If you were to measure the pressures at point X, you would record a higher pressure in the nozzled hose. The nozzle increases resistance to the flow of water and causes the pressure behind the nozzle to increase. The increased pressure in the nozzled hose simply pushes the water further.

How does the example of the hose apply to blood pressure? The large blood vessels are similar to the hose. The smaller vessels, especially the arterioles, act

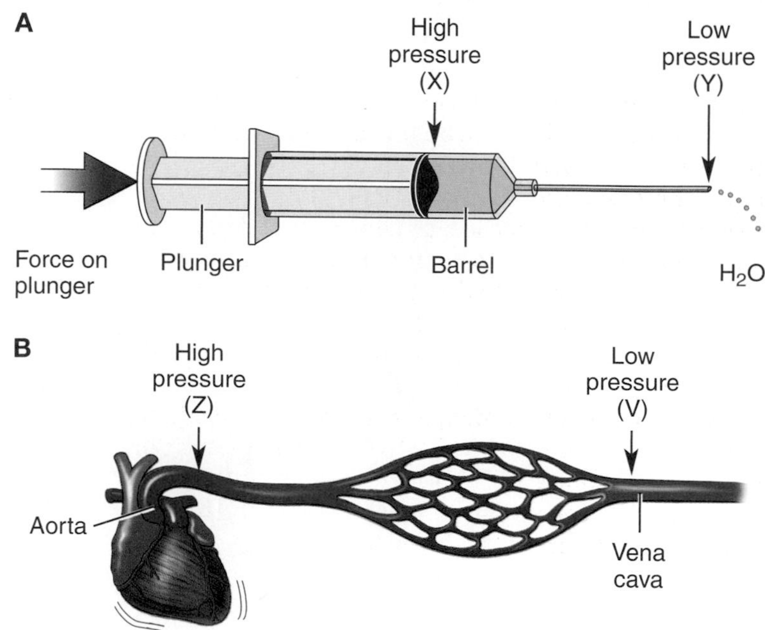

FIGURE 19-4 Relationship between pressure and force. **A,** The higher pressure within the barrel pushes water out through the needle, where pressure is lower. **B,** The contracting myocardium (force) pushes on the blood in the aorta. The higher arterial pressure pushes blood from the arterial side to the venous side of the circulation.

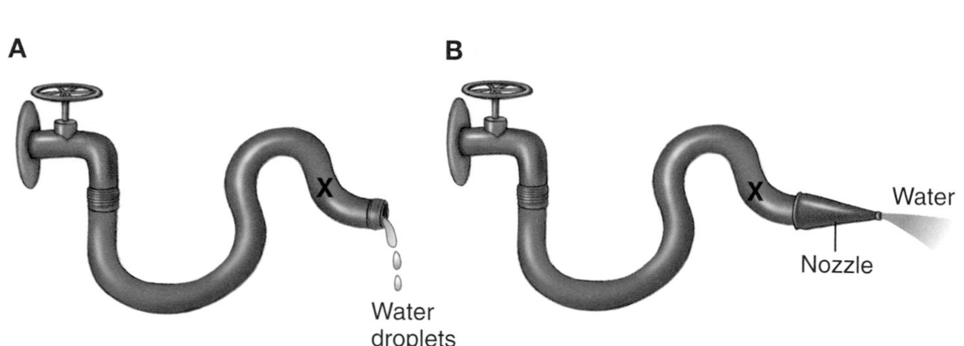

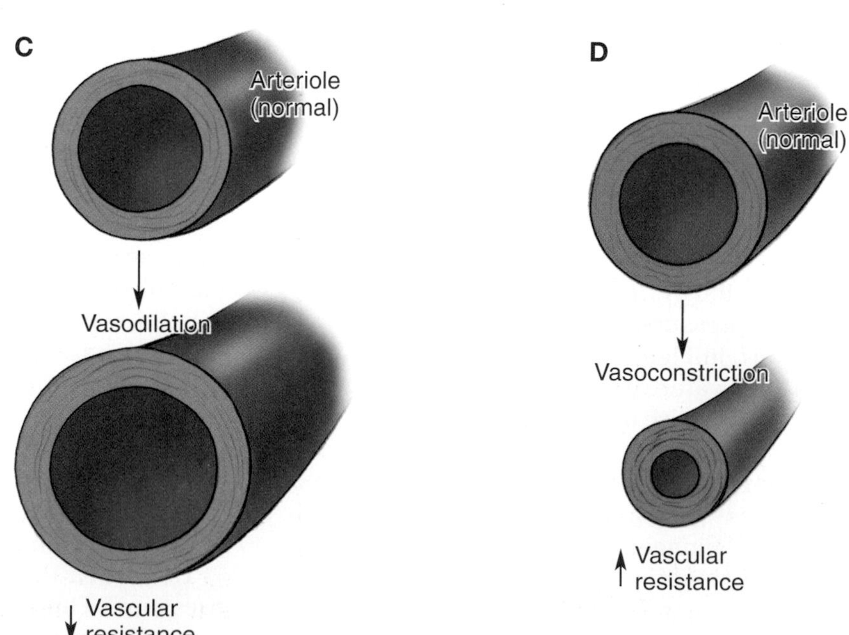

FIGURE 19-5 The effect of resistance on pressure. **A,** Low resistance and low pressure. **B,** High resistance and high pressure. **C,** Vasodilation, a low resistance, and low pressure. **D,** Vasoconstriction, a high resistance, and high pressure.

as nozzles. Because the arterioles are composed largely of smooth muscle, the contraction and relaxation of the muscle allow the arterioles to change their size (diameter). For instance, when the muscle relaxes, the opening of the arteriole increases, causing **vasodilation.** The process is comparable to removing the nozzle at the end of the hose (Figure 19-5, *C*). Vasodilation decreases resistance in the blood vessels.

When the smooth muscle contracts, the opening (diameter) of the arteriole becomes smaller. This process is known as **vasoconstriction;** it is comparable to adding a nozzle to the hose (Figure 19-5, *D*). Vasoconstriction increases resistance in the blood vessels. Note the effect of resistance on pressure. When vascular resistance decreases, blood pressure decreases. When resistance increases, pressure increases. Thus, the arterioles' ability to dilate and constrict affects blood pressure.

Do You Know...

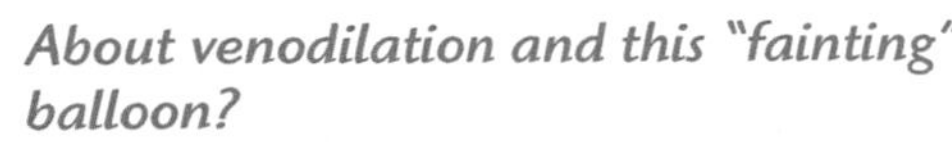

About venodilation and this "fainting" balloon?

If a patient takes a drug that causes venodilation, the following events occur: blood "pools" in the veins, less blood returns to the heart (decrease venous return), myocardial contraction decreases (Starling effect), cardiac output decreases, and blood pressure decreases **(hypotension).** If the patient attempts to change position quickly, as in rising from a supine (lying down) to a standing position, insufficient blood is pumped to the brain, causing dizziness, fainting, and falling. This series of events is called **postural hypotension,** since it usually occurs when the patient assumes an upright posture. The balloon illustrates venodilation and pooling when the position of the balloon changes from a lying down (horizontal) to a standing (vertical) position. Lesson? Advise your patients, especially the elderly, to get up slowly from lying, to sitting (dangling feet), to upright. Other common causes of postural hypotension are blood volume depletion (dehydration) and autonomic dysfunction.

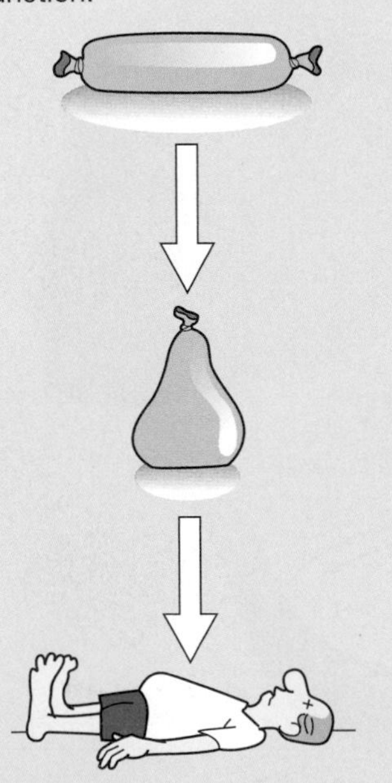

PUTTING IT TOGETHER: DETERMINING BLOOD PRESSURE

Now that you understand why blood pressure is affected by both the heart and the blood vessels, you can put it together as follows:

$$\text{Blood pressure} = \underset{\text{(heart)}}{\text{Cardiac output}} \times \underset{\text{(blood vessels)}}{\text{Vascular resistance}}$$

Heart: Cardiac Output

The amount of blood pumped by the heart each minute is the **cardiac output.** Recall from Chapter 17 that cardiac output is determined by heart rate and stroke volume (amount of blood pumped per beat). Thus an increase in heart rate or stroke volume, or both, can increase cardiac output and thus increase blood pressure. Conversely, a decrease in heart rate or stroke volume, or both, can decrease cardiac output and blood pressure. For instance, if a person hemorrhages severely, blood volume decreases. This decrease in blood volume, in turn, decreases stroke volume and cardiac output. The decreased cardiac output causes a decrease in blood pressure. A classic sign of hemorrhagic shock is a low blood pressure (less than 90 mm Hg systolic).

Do You Know...

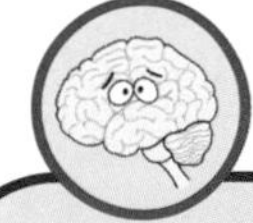

About obesity and the miles and miles of new blood vessels?

Blood pressure is determined by cardiac output and systemic vascular resistance (SVR). SVR is usually determined by changes in the diameter of the arterioles. Other resistance terms such as blood vessel length and blood viscosity are ignored. However, the accumulation of excess fat tissue not only adds pounds; it also contributes miles of additional new blood vessels, making blood vessel length a significant contributor to SVR. Fat tissue also secretes hormones that narrow or constrict blood vessels. Excess fat therefore elevates SVR making the person hypertensive. What to lower that BP? Lose weight!

Blood Vessels and Vascular Resistance

The relaxation and contraction of the arterioles cause changes in **vascular resistance** and therefore in blood pressure. Several factors affect the arterioles and therefore change vascular resistance; these factors include sympathetic nerve activity, various hormones, and numerous pharmacologic agents. What effect does sympathetic nerve activity exert on the arterioles? The arterioles are richly supplied by fibers of the sympathetic nervous system. When the sympathetic nerves fire, vascular smooth muscle contracts, causing vasoconstriction. Vasoconstriction increases vascular resistance and elevates blood pressure. Vasodilation is achieved when the sympathetic firing diminishes and the vascular smooth muscle relaxes.

Several hormones also affect vascular resistance. Epinephrine (Adrenalin) and angiotensin II cause vasoconstriction and elevate blood pressure. Because these substances elevate blood pressure, they are called **vasopressors.** Other hormones induce vasodilation, decreasing vascular resistance. Lastly, numerous pharmacologic agents affect vascular resistance. Drugs causing vasoconstriction elevate blood pressure and are often used in the treatment of shock. Antihypertensive agents induce vasodilation, lower vascular resistance, and therefore lower blood pressure.

HOW BLOOD PRESSURE STAYS WITHIN NORMAL LIMITS

Under normal conditions, blood pressure remains relatively constant, approximately 120/80 mm Hg. Regulation of blood pressure involves both rapidly acting and slowly acting mechanisms.

Rapidly Acting Mechanisms

The most important of the rapidly acting mechanisms is a nervous mechanism called the **baroreceptor reflex** (Figure 19-6). This reflex consists of the following structures: receptors, sensory nerves, medulla oblongata, and motor nerves.

- Receptors: The special receptors, called **baroreceptors,** or pressure receptors, are located in the walls of the aortic arch and carotid sinus. The baroreceptors sense any change in blood pressure.
- Sensory nerves: Once the baroreceptors have been activated, the sensory information travels along the nerves to the brain. The nerves that carry the sensory information are cranial nerves IX (glossopharyngeal) and X (vagus).
- Medulla oblongata: The medulla oblongata of the brain interprets sensory information. The medulla then decides what to do. If the blood pressure is low, the medulla tells the heart and blood vessels to increase blood pressure. If the medulla receives information that the blood pressure is high, the medulla tells the heart and blood vessels to decrease blood pressure.

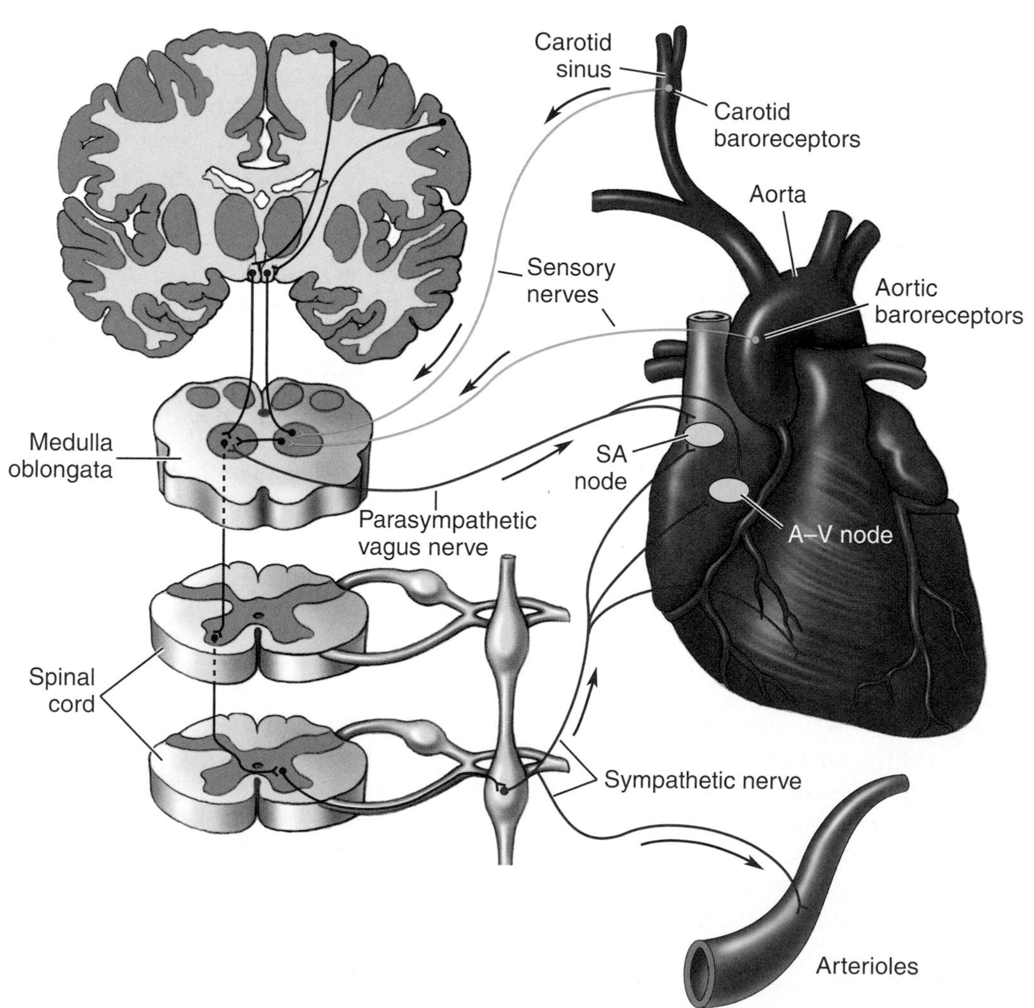

FIGURE 19-6 Baroreceptor reflex.

- Motor nerves: Once the medulla has identified adjustments needed to restore blood pressure to normal, the motor nerves carry information to the heart and blood vessels. The motor nerves involved are the nerves of the ANS (sympathetic and parasympathetic nervous system).

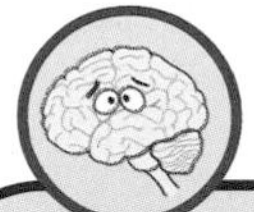

Do You Know...

About Val Salva's most embarrassing medical moment?

Val was constipated! Sounds like an insignificant problem, but in a person with a history of coronary artery disease (CAD), constipation can prove fatal. While "straining at stools," Val suffered a near-fatal heart attack. This is what happened. "Straining at stools" initiates the Valsalva maneuver. The Valsalva maneuver occurs when a person tries to force exhale with the mouth and nose closed (as in having a bowel movement). The forced exhalation increases pressure within the chest, which, in turn, increases blood pressure. The sudden increase in blood pressure activates the baroreceptor reflex, causing a sudden burst of parasympathetic activity that not only slows heart rate, but triggers a fatal electrical dysrhythmia leading to cardiac arrest. Unfortunately it is a rather common occurrence that a person with a history of CAD has a heart attack while "on the throne." How embarrassing—and to think it might have been prevented by a stool softener or laxative.

How does stimulation of the sympathetic nervous system increase blood pressure? Note the sympathetic nerve supply to the heart (see Figure 19-6). Sympathetic nerves supply the sinoatrial (SA) node, atrioventricular (AV) node, and ventricular myocardium. Stimulation of the sympathetic nerves causes the SA node to fire more quickly, thereby increasing heart rate. Sympathetic firing also causes the ventricular myocardium to contract more forcefully, increasing stroke volume. Both of these responses increase cardiac output and blood pressure. Firing of the sympathetic nerves also causes vasoconstriction of the peripheral blood vessels (arterioles), thereby increasing resistance and blood pressure.

How does stimulation of the parasympathetic nervous system decrease blood pressure? Note the parasympathetic innervation to the heart (see Figure 19-6). Parasympathetic nerves (vagus) supply the SA node and the AV node. (No parasympathetic nerves supply the ventricular myocardium or the peripheral blood vessels.) Parasympathetic stimulation decreases heart rate and therefore decreases cardiac output and blood pressure. Blood pressure also decreases because the blood vessels dilate, thereby decreasing resistance. If the blood vessels do not contain parasympathetic nerves, why do they dilate? The vasodilation is not due to parasympathetic activity; it occurs because the sympathetic nerves become less active when the parasympathetic nerves fire.

The Case of the Tight Collar. Some people have hypersensitive carotid sinuses. A tight collar exerts pressure on the carotid sinus baroreceptors. The baroreceptors falsely interpret this pressure as an elevation in blood pressure. Information sent from the brain to the heart and blood vessels lowers the BP. The BP may decrease so much that the person faints. This response is called carotid sinus syncope (fainting). Other stimuli for carotid sinus syncope include shaving over the neck region, showering with strong spurts of water, and the use of shoulder-strap seatbelts. The baroreceptor reflex has huge pharmacologic implications. For instance, if a drug such as nitroglycerin quickly lowers BP, the baroreceptors are activated, causing an increased heart rate (reflex tachycardia). The tachycardia can overburden a damaged heart, causing angina (chest pain) and further myocardial damage.

A second, but less important, rapidly acting mechanism is the secretion of epinephrine and norepinephrine from the medulla of the adrenal gland. These hormones increase cardiac output and cause vasoconstriction, thus increasing blood pressure.

Slower-Acting Mechanisms

Several mechanisms act slowly to control blood pressure. These mechanisms are more concerned with the long-term regulation of blood pressure. The most important of the slowly acting mechanisms is the renin-angiotensin-aldosterone mechanism. Activation of this mechanism increases blood volume and causes vasoconstriction. Both of these effects increase blood pressure (see Chapter 24). Other hormones that affect blood pressure include antidiuretic hormone (ADH). ADH is also called vasopressin because it exerts a vasopressor effect (increases blood pressure). Atrial natriuretic peptide (ANP) and brain natriuretic peptide (BNP), secreted by the distended walls of the heart, lower blood pressure by causing vasodilation and by decreasing blood volume through the renal (kidney) secretion of sodium (Na^+) and water.

Sum It Up!

The circulatory system maintains an adequate flow of blood to every cell in the body. Blood moves through the blood vessels because of a pressure difference between the arteries and veins. Blood pressure is determined by the activity of both the heart (cardiac output) and blood vessels (vascular resistance), especially the arterioles. Several mechanisms regulate blood pressure. The most important rapidly acting mechanism is the baroreceptor reflex. The secretion of epinephrine and norepinephrine contributes to the rapid-response system. More long-term mechanisms include the renin-angiotensin-aldosterone mechanism, ADH, and the natriuretic peptides.

BLOOD VESSELS ACT AS EXCHANGE VESSELS

The capillaries are the most numerous of the blood vessels. If all the capillaries in the body were lined up end-to-end they would encircle the earth 2.5 times. The capillaries function as exchange vessels.

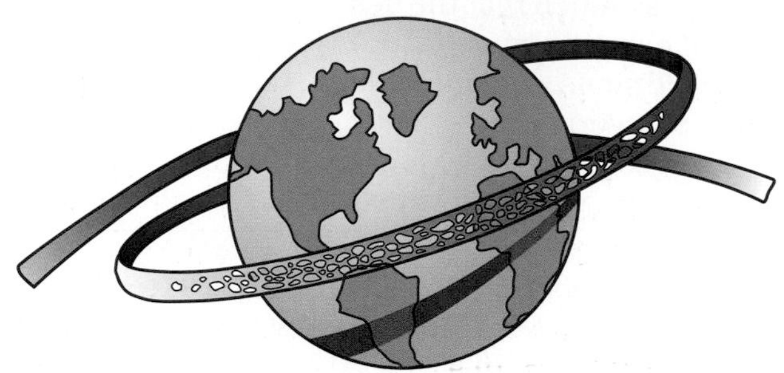

WHAT IS AN EXCHANGE VESSEL?

An exchange vessel exchanges or swaps substances, much like a waiter (Figure 19-7). For instance, a waiter delivers food to hungry guests. After a period has passed, the waiter picks up the waste—the empty trays, dirty dishes, and leftover food. Note the exchange part: food is dropped off and waste is picked up.

The capillaries work like the waiter (Figure 19-7, *B*). As blood flows through the capillaries, substances move out of the capillary into the surrounding tissue spaces (interstitium). These substances include oxygen, water, electrolytes, and various nutrients such as glucose; they are the substances the cell needs to live, work, and grow.

Oxygen and nutrients are taken up and used by the cells. As the cells carry on their work, they produce waste material such as carbon dioxide. The cellular waste diffuses out of the cell, into the interstitium, and then into the blood within the capillary. The blood carries the waste away from the capillary to the organs of excretion, such as the kidneys and the lungs.

WHY CAPILLARIES ARE GOOD EXCHANGE VESSELS

Three characteristics make the capillaries good exchange vessels: thin capillary walls, large numbers of capillaries, and slow blood flow through the capillaries.

Thin Capillary Walls

The capillary wall consists of a single layer of epithelium that sits on a delicate basement membrane. The epithelial layer has many holes or pores through which water and solute move.

Millions of Capillaries

The millions of capillaries provide a huge surface for exchange; the greater the capillary surface, the greater the rate of exchange.

A

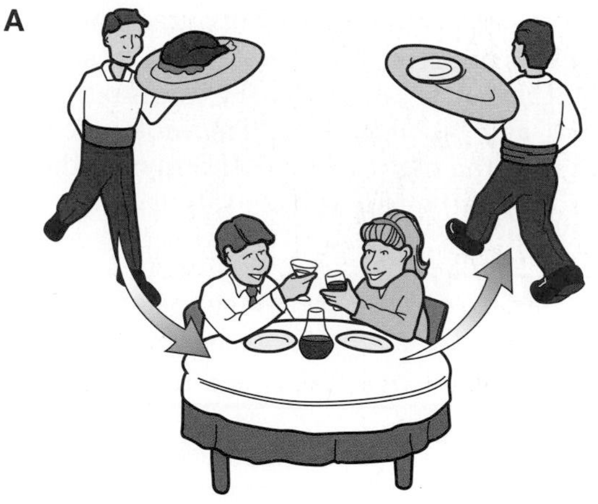

B

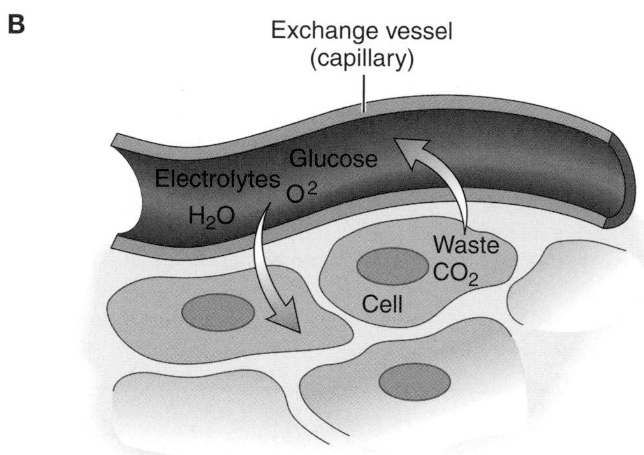

FIGURE 19-7 Capillary exchange: deliveries and pickup. **A,** A waiter. **B,** Capillary exchange.

Slow Velocity of Blood Flow

The large numbers of capillaries also affect the rate of blood flow. The more capillaries there are, the slower the flow of blood. The slow blood flow allows more time for exchange (Figure 19-8).

CAPILLARY FORCES: RUNNING DOWNHILL, PUSHING, AND PULLING

How do the nutrients and waste "know" where to go? There are forces that push and pull the nutrients and waste in and out of the capillaries. These forces are diffusion and exchange involving a filtration-osmosis balancing act.

Exchange Involving Diffusion

Diffusion is the primary process causing substances to move across the capillary wall. Diffusion means that a substance moves downhill from an area of high concentration to an area of low concentration. For instance, the concentration of oxygen is higher in the capillary than in the tissue fluid. Thus oxygen diffuses from the

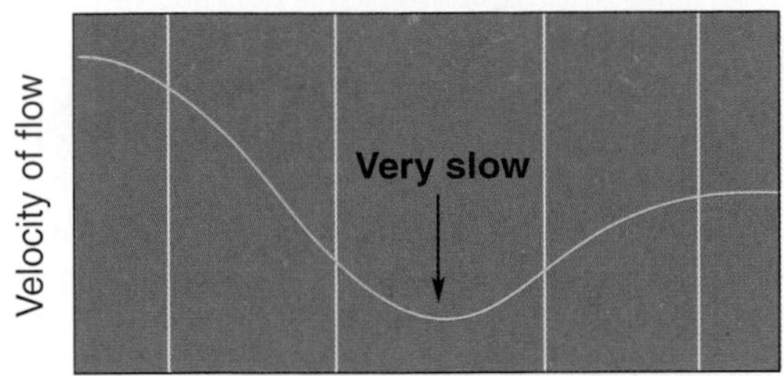

FIGURE 19-8 Blood flow in the capillaries is very slow.

capillary into the interstitium. On the other hand, carbon dioxide concentration is higher in the interstitium than in the capillaries. Thus carbon dioxide diffuses from the interstitium into the capillary.

Exchange Involving Filtration-Osmosis: The Push and Pull of Exchange

A secondary process of exchange involves filtration-osmosis. Filtration is illustrated in the syringe in Figure 19-9, *A*. A syringe is loaded with water. If you were to punch holes in the side of the syringe and push on the plunger, what would happen? Not only would water flow out of the needle-end, but it would also squirt out of the side of the syringe in response to the pressure.

The plunger and syringe are similar to the heart and capillaries (Figure 19-9, *B*). The heart pushes blood through the capillaries. Because of the blood pressure, blood moves forward from the arterial to the venous

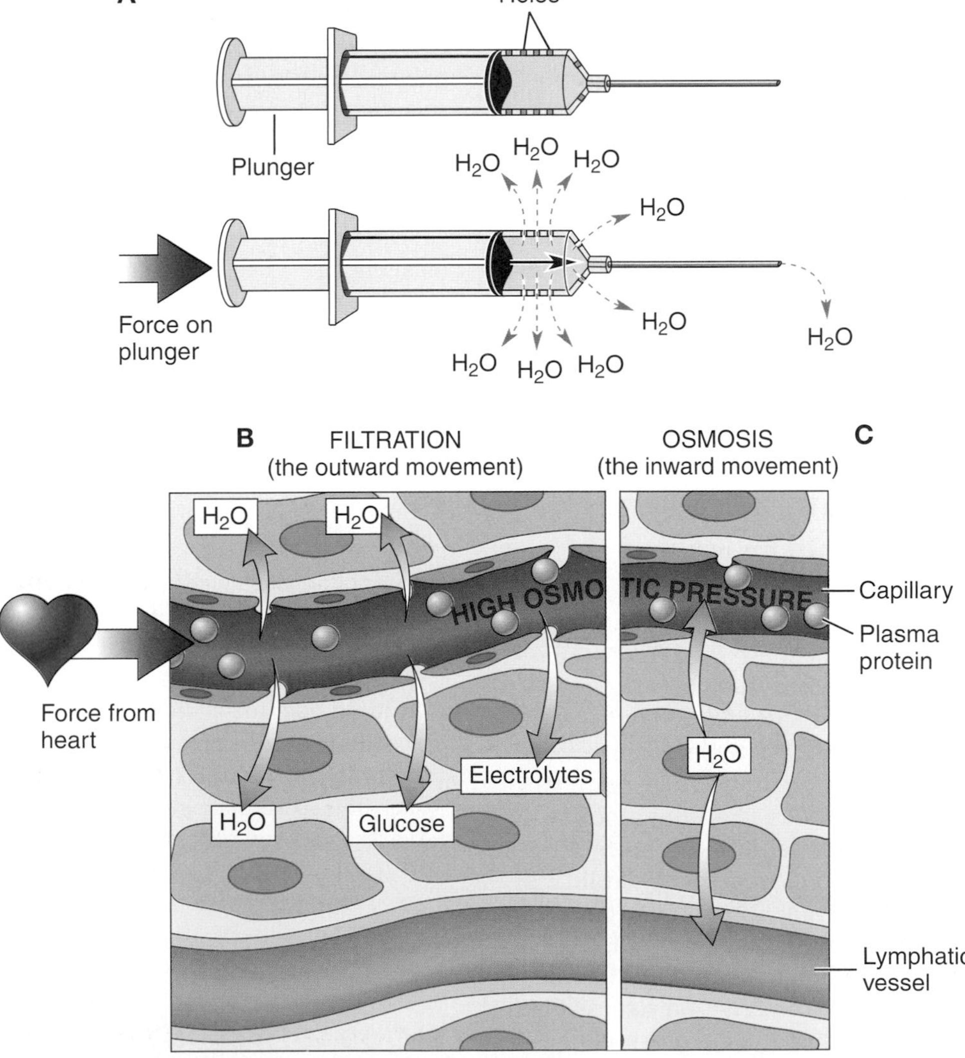

FIGURE 19-9 Filtration and osmosis. **A,** A syringe filled with water; the plunger pushes the water out of the syringe. **B,** Capillary filled with blood; the heart pushes blood out of the capillary. **C,** Movement of water back into the capillary because of the osmotic (oncotic) pressure within the capillary.

circulation. Because of the holes, or pores, in the capillary wall, however, water and the smaller substances (electrolytes, glucose) squirt into the interstitium.

The pushing of the water and dissolved substances through the pores is filtration. Note that the cause of filtration is blood pressure. Note also the direction. In response to the pressure in the capillary, water and the dissolved substances are pushed out of the capillary into the interstitium. What happens to all the material pushed into the interstitium? The nutrients are used by the cell while the water is reabsorbed by the capillary.

What about the water in the interstitial space? The water and dissolved waste must return to the capillaries. This effect involves osmosis. Figure 19-9, *C*, shows that the osmotic pressure in the capillary is higher than in the interstitium. The capillary oncotic pressure is higher because of the plasma proteins trapped within the capillaries. (Recall that the plasma proteins are too large to fit through the capillary pores.) The plasma proteins create a high **oncotic pressure** and pull the water from the interstitium into the capillary. Any excess water that the plasma proteins cannot pull back into the capillary is removed from the interstitium by the lymphatic vessels (see Chapter 20).

What is the balancing act? The exact amount of water filtered at one end of the capillary is reabsorbed at the other end. The balancing act is important. If the amount of water filtered out of the capillary exceeds the amount reabsorbed from the tissue space, fluid collects in the tissue space. Excess fluid collection in the interstitium is called **edema.** If more water is reabsorbed from the tissue space than was filtered, the tissue space becomes depleted and the patient appears dehydrated (the raisin-grape effect). Fluid imbalances occur in many clinical conditions.

Mechanisms of Edema Formation

The forces that push and pull water across the capillary walls are disrupted in many clinical conditions. Some of the more common conditions are described. Try to understand the case-study information in the light of Figure 19-9.

Heart Failure. A patient in heart failure retains water and develops excess blood volume (hypervolemia). The expanded blood volume, in turn, increases capillary filtration pressure, thereby increasing the amount of water filtered out of the capillaries into the interstitium. The excess filtration of water exceeds the ability of the capillaries to reabsorb water. Thus, the excess water remains in the interstitium, causing edema. Excess filtration of water into the lungs is called pulmonary edema and results in impaired oxygenation. Excess fluid accumulation in the feet is called pedal edema.

Severe Burn. A patient is admitted to the ER with severe burns on his lower extremities. In response to the thermal injury, the capillary pores dilate, thereby allowing the escape of excess water and plasma proteins into the interstitium. The "leaked" protein causes edema for two reasons. The decrease in plasma protein decreases the ability of the capillaries to osmotically "pull" water from the interstitium into the capillaries. Second, the protein in the interstitium osmotically "holds" the water in the interstitium, preventing it from returning to the capillaries.

Kidney Disease. A child is diagnosed with a kidney disease called nephrotic syndrome. The child's mother first noticed edema around his eyes (periorbital edema) and difficulty in fastening the waist of his pants. Nephrotic syndrome is characterized by the excretion of large amounts of the plasma protein, albumin, in the urine (albuminuria); this results in low plasma levels of albumin (hypoalbuminemia). The edema of nephrotic syndrome is due in part to the hypoalbuminemia, causing a decreased plasma oncotic pressure; there is not enough plasma protein in the blood to pull water from the interstitium into the capillaries.

Blocked Lymphatic Drainage. An adult female goes to a clinic complaining of a grossly swollen leg and is eventually diagnosed with a large tumor in the lower pelvis. The tumor has compressed the lymphatic vessels, thereby impairing the drainage of lymph; impaired lymph drainage causes the accumulation of fluid in the interstitium (edema). For this same reason (impaired lymphatic drainage), edema develops with the surgical removal of a breast (mastectomy) and lymph node dissection.

Thus, the pressures that are responsible for normal capillary exchange can cause serious problems with abnormal interstitial fluid accumulation as edema. An analysis of capillary pressures provides the clinical rationale for edema formation.

Sum It Up!

As blood flows through the capillaries, an exchange of nutrients and gases occurs between the capillary blood and the interstitium. Nourishing substances are continuously delivered to the cells, while waste products are removed from the interstitium for eventual elimination from the body. The processes of diffusion, filtration, and osmosis play key roles in the exchange and distribution of these substances. Diffusion accounts for most of the capillary exchange. The exchange forces can be disrupted and cause water accumulation in the interstitium (edema).

BLOOD VESSELS DISTRIBUTE BLOOD FLOW

In addition to regulating blood pressure, vasodilation and vasoconstriction also participate in the distribution of blood flow. As Figure 19-10 shows, blood flow to a

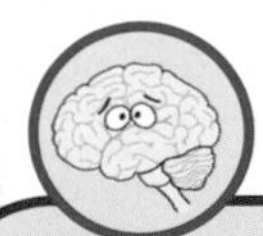

Do You Know...

The difference between osmotic pressure and oncotic pressure?

Osmotic pressure is normally determined by particles such as Na^+ and Cl^- ions. The greater the number of solute, the higher the osmotic pressure. Because the capillary membranes are permeable to these ions, the osmotic pressure within the vasculature (blood vessels) is determined by large particles that are trapped within the vasculature. The large, osmotically active particles are the plasma proteins such as albumin. The osmotic pressure created by the plasma proteins is called the oncotic (swelling) pressure. When the amount of plasma proteins diminishes, the oncotic pressure also decreases, and interstitial water cannot be drawn into the capillaries. The water remains in the interstitium, causing edema.

particular area of the body can change. For instance, in the resting state, the skeletal muscle receives 20% of the total blood flow, and the kidney and abdomen receive 19% and 24%, respectively. Note what happens during strenuous exercise. Blood flow is redirected; the percentage of blood flow pumped to skeletal muscle greatly increases (to 71% of total flow). Why? Exercising muscle needs more oxygen and nutrients. In addition, the increased blood flow carries heat and waste products away from the exercising muscles. At the same time, the percentage of blood that flows through the kidney and abdomen decreases (3.5% of total flow). In other words the blood is directed to sites where it is most needed, such as the skeletal muscle. Note also that the blood flow to the skin increases from 9% to 11% of total flow. The increased blood flow to the skin helps lose the excess heat, thereby helping to regulate body temperature. The change in blood vessel diameter is caused by the sympathetic nervous system firing and by the actions of various hormones that are released during exercise.

BLOOD VESSELS REGULATE BODY TEMPERATURE

The regulation of body temperature is described in Chapter 7. In essence, the blood vessels help to dissipate (get rid of) or conserve heat. For example, with exercise and temperature elevation, the blood vessels dilate, thereby allowing more blood to flow to the skin. This activity transfers heat from the deeper tissues to the surface of the body. The heat radiates from the flushed skin, thereby lowering body temperature. Conversely, heat is conserved when the blood vessels of the skin constrict, diverting the warm blood from surface blood vessels into deeper parts of the body.

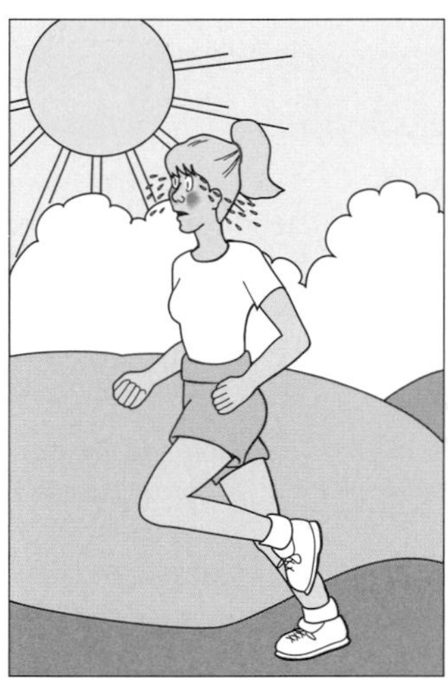

Sum It Up!

The circulatory system does more than run around in circles. It acts as a delivery system, regulates blood pressure, engages in the exchange of nutrients and waste with the cells, distributes blood in response to changing body needs, and helps in the regulation of body temperature.

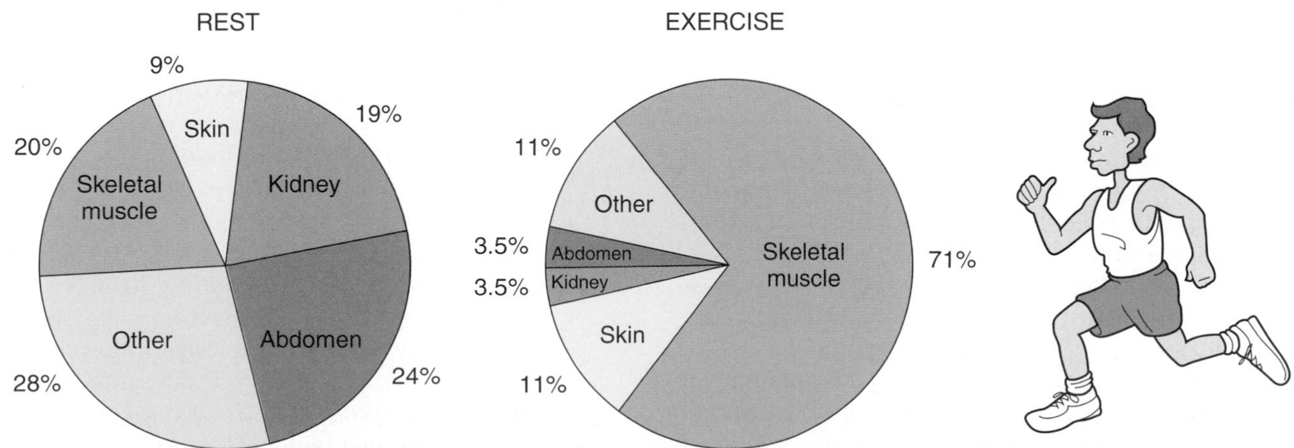

FIGURE 19-10 Distribution of blood flow at rest and during exercise.

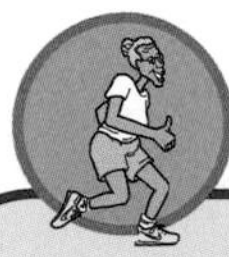

As You Age

1. The circulatory system is one of the body systems most affected by age. The walls of the arteries thicken and become less elastic and stiffer. Two major consequences occur: blood flow to vital organs (e.g., the brain) decreases and blood pressure increases.
2 Changes occur in both the walls and the valves of the veins. As a result, the elderly are more prone to the development of varicose veins.
3. The inner surface of the blood vessels becomes roughened because of age-related changes in the vessel wall and the development of fatty plaques. As a result, elderly persons are more prone to thrombus formation.
4. The baroreceptors become less sensitive. Cardiovascular adjustments to changes in position are slowed, and the person may become dizzy and tend to fall.
5. Permeability of the capillary membrane increases with age, thereby increasing edema formation in the elderly.

Disorders of Blood Vessels and Circulation

Aneurysm	A bulging of a weakened arterial wall most often affecting the aorta. The major concern is that the aneurysm will rupture, causing a massive hemorrhage. Rupture of a cerebral aneurysm causes a stroke.
Arterial occlusive disease	Narrowing of the arterial vessels, commonly affecting the lower extremities. The narrowing is due to changes in the arterial wall structure and the development of fatty plaques on the inner wall.
Arteriosclerosis	Hardening, or calcification, of arterial walls, often causing the blood pressure to increase.
Atherosclerosis	From the Greek meaning porridge and hardening. The arterial walls fibrose, harden, and accumulate lipids. Atherosclerosis is a major cause of myocardial infarction, stroke, and occlusive arterial disease of the lower extremities. The narrowing of the arteries decreases blood flow, deprives the cells of nutrients and oxygen, and causes gangrene. Persons with diabetes mellitus are particularly prone to arterial occlusive disease; it is a major cause of toe, foot, and leg amputations in the patient with diabetes.
Hypertension	A persistent, abnormally elevated blood pressure. By itself, hypertension causes no symptoms and is therefore called the silent killer. Hypertension is serious because it increases the risk of stroke, heart attack, and kidney failure.
Phlebitis	An inflammation of a vein, causing pain and swelling. Thrombophlebitis is caused by thrombotic (clot) occlusion of a vein. A serious consequence is the dislodging of the thrombus, which causes a fatal pulmonary embolus.
Shock	A condition characterized by inadequate blood flow to the tissues. Shock is often caused by hemorrhage and a severe decrease in blood pressure. The persistent low blood pressure impairs tissue oxygenation. Unless the hypotensive state is corrected, the patient develops irreversible shock and dies.

SUMMARY OUTLINE

The circulatory system performs five main functions.

I. Functions as a Delivery System

A. The circulatory system delivers oxygen and nutrients to the cells.

B. The circulatory system picks up waste from the cells and delivers it to the organs of excretion.

II. Regulates Blood Pressure

A. The circulatory system maintains a blood pressure to ensure an adequate flow of blood to the body.

B. The normal blood pressure is 120/80 mm Hg; 120 is the systolic reading, and 80 is the diastolic reading.

C. Blood pressure varies throughout the circulatory system; it is highest in the aorta and lowest in the venae cavae.

D. Blood pressure is determined by the action of the heart and blood vessels. The heart affects blood pressure by increasing or decreasing cardiac output. The blood vessels affect blood pressure by constricting or dilating the arterioles.

E. Blood pressure is regulated on a day-to-day basis by the baroreceptor reflex. Other mechanisms can correct blood pressure more slowly. The most important is the renin-angiotensin-aldosterone mechanism.

III. Acts as Exchange Vessels

A. The capillaries are the site of exchange of nutrients and waste between the blood and tissue fluid.

B. Factors that make the capillaries ideal exchange vessels are the thin capillary walls with many pores, millions of capillaries, and a slow rate of blood flow through the capillaries.

C. Water and dissolved substances move out of the capillary into the tissue spaces by diffusion and filtration. The capillary pressure pushes water out of the capillaries. Water and dissolved waste move from the tissue fluid into the capillaries by osmosis.

IV. Distributes Blood According to Need

V. Regulates Body Temperature

A. Vasodilation of the blood vessels of the skin encourages heat loss.

B. Vasoconstriction of the blood vessels of the skin decreases heat loss.

Review Your Knowledge

Matching: Blood Pressure Terms

Directions: Match the following words with their descriptions below. Some of the words may be used more than once.

a. systolic pressure
b. diastolic pressure
c. pulse pressure
d. MABP
e. reflex tachycardia
f. Korotkoff sounds
g. brachial artery
h. baroreceptors

1. ____ 2/3 diastolic pressure + 1/3 systolic pressure
2. ____ Silent . . . tap . . . tap . . . tap . . . tap . . . muffle
3. ____ Pressure reading that reflects myocardial contraction
4. ____ Areas in the carotid sinus and aortic arch that detect changes in blood pressure
5. ____ Usual site of blood pressure recording
6. ____ The top number of a blood pressure recording
7. ____ The bottom number of a blood pressure recording
8. ____ The difference between the systolic and diastolic pressure
9. ____ Pressure reading that reflects myocardial relaxation
10. ____ A consequence of a sudden drop in blood pressure

Matching: Blood Pressure Readings

Directions: Match the following blood pressure readings to their descriptions below.

a. 120/80 mm Hg
b. 70/45 mm Hg
c. 220/120 mm Hg

1. ____ Normal blood pressure recorded in the aorta
2. ____ Normal blood pressure recorded in the brachial artery
3. ____ A "shocky" blood pressure
4. ____ A hypertensive blood pressure
5. ____ A hypotensive blood pressure
6. ____ Normotensive reading
7. ____ A postoperative blood pressure that may require a vasopressor drug
8. ____ A blood pressure that requires immediate treatment with an antihypertensive drug
9. ____ Has a pulse pressure of 40
10. ____ Blood pressure that is most apt to cause a reflex tachycardia

Matching: Changes in Blood Pressure

Directions: Indicate if the following (a) increases blood pressure or (b) decreases blood pressure.

1. ____ Sympathetic nerve stimulation
2. ____ Vagal discharge
3. ____ Effects of a vasopressor agent
4. ____ Effects of epinephrine and angiotensin II
5. ____ Increased SVR
6. ____ Decreased cardiac output
7. ____ Arteriolar constriction
8. ____ Administration of an alpha$_1$-adrenergic blocker
9. ____ IV infusion of Levophed (norepinephrine)
10. ____ Administration of a beta$_1$-adrenergic agonist

Multiple Choice

1. The ability of the arterioles to contract and relax allows them to
   a. regulate heart rate.
   b. prevent the backflow of venous blood.
   c. function as resistance vessels.
   d. function as exchange vessels.
2. Which of the following is not a consequence of sympathetic nerve stimulation?
   a. Increased cardiac output
   b. Peripheral vasoconstriction
   c. Elevation of blood pressure
   d. Decreased peripheral resistance

3. A decrease in blood pressure is most apt to cause
   a. edema.
   b. reflex tachycardia.
   c. increase in the synthesis of albumin.
   d. arteriolar dilation.
4. Which of the following is an effect of the activation of the renin-angiotensin-aldosterone system?
   a. Secretion of a vasopressor hormone
   b. Vasodilation and decrease in vascular resistance
   c. Decreased blood pressure
   d. Sodium excretion and decreased blood volume
5. Pain, pallor, pulselessness, paresthesia, and paralysis are caused by
   a. hypertension.
   b. ischemia.
   c. decreased oncotic pressure.
   d. a failure of the renin-angiotensin-aldosterone system.
6. In the dehydrated state
   a. capillary oncotic pressure decreases; fluid accumulates in the tissue spaces.
   b. capillary filtration pressure decreases; tissue fluid is absorbed.
   c. capillary filtration rate increases thereby increasing lymph formation.
   d. plasma protein is filtered into the tissue spaces thereby causing edema.

CHAPTER 20

Lymphatic System

KEY TERMS

Lymph, p. 346
Lymph nodes, p. 348
Lymphatic duct, p. 347
Lymphatic vessels, p. 346
Spleen, p. 350
Thymus gland, p. 350
Tonsils, p. 348

OBJECTIVES

1. List three functions of the lymphatic system.
2. Describe the composition and flow of lymph.
3. Describe the four lymphoid organs: lymph nodes, tonsils, thymus gland, and spleen.
4. State the location of the following lymph nodes: cervical nodes, axillary nodes, and inguinal nodes.

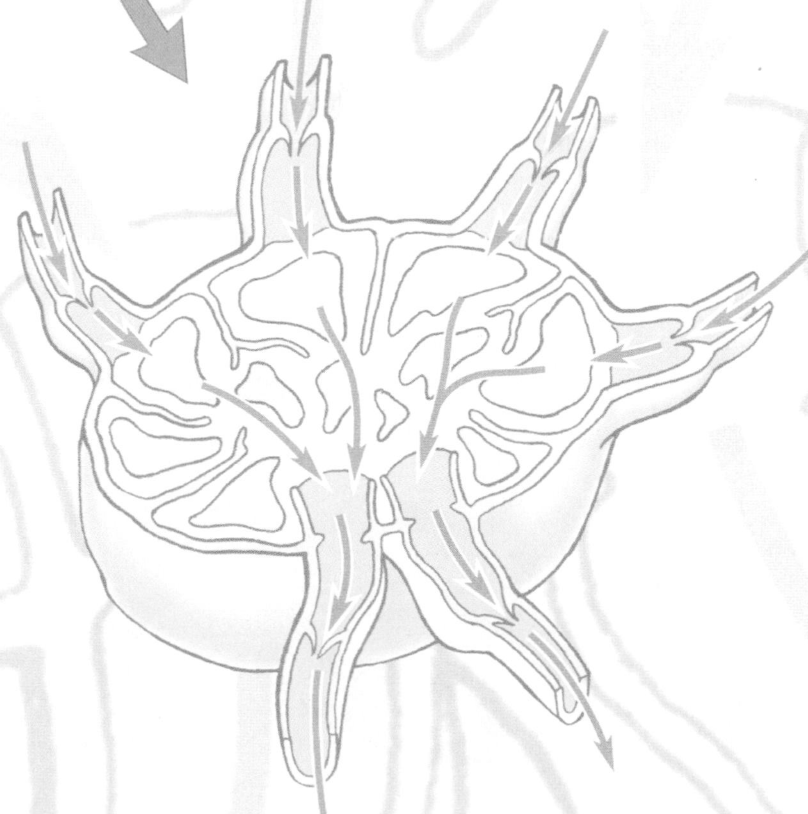

The woman in Figure 20-1 has a condition called elephantiasis. The name is an obvious reference to the size and shape of her leg. Elephantiasis is caused by the invasion and blockage of the lymphatic vessels by small worms called filariae. The amount of swelling illustrates the importance of the lymphatic system, which drains fluid from our tissue spaces.

The lymphatic system contains lymph, lymphatic vessels, lymphoid organs, and lymphoid tissue, which are widely scattered throughout the body. The three main functions of the lymphatic system are as follows:

- The lymphatic vessels return tissue fluid to the blood. Elephantiasis provides ample evidence for the importance of adequate drainage.
- Specialized lymphatic vessels play an important role in the intestinal absorption of fats and fat-soluble vitamins.
- Lymphoid tissue helps the body defend itself against disease.

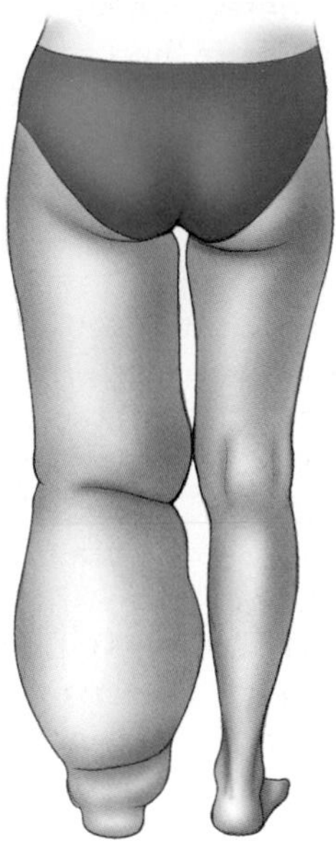

FIGURE 20-1 Elephantiasis, a form of lymphedema.

THE LYMPHATIC SYSTEM

LYMPH: WHAT IT IS, WHERE IT COMES FROM

Lymph (lĭmf) is a clear fluid that resembles plasma. Lymph is composed primarily of water, electrolytes, waste from metabolizing cells, and some protein that leaks out of the capillaries of the systemic circulation. Where does lymph come from? It is formed from the plasma during capillary exchange. About 20 L/day of lymph is filtered from the blood into the interstitium, or tissue spaces. It leaves the interstitium through the lymphatic vessels, which then carry the lymph toward the heart and eventually empty it into the blood.

Water and dissolved substances are continuously filtered out of the blood capillaries into the interstitium to form tissue fluid. Approximately 85% of this tissue fluid moves back into the blood capillaries and is carried away as part of the venous blood. What about the 15% of the tissue fluid that does not reenter the blood capillaries? This fluid is drained by the lymphatic capillaries that surround the blood capillaries (Figure 20-2). The tissue fluid entering the lymphatic vessels is the lymph.

LYMPHATIC VESSELS

The **lymphatic** (lĭm-FĂT-ĭk) **vessels** include lymphatic capillaries and several larger lymphatic vessels. Like the blood vessels, the lymphatic vessels form an extensive network. The distribution of lymphatic vessels is similar to the distribution of veins, and the vessels "run with" the veins. With the exception of the CNS, every

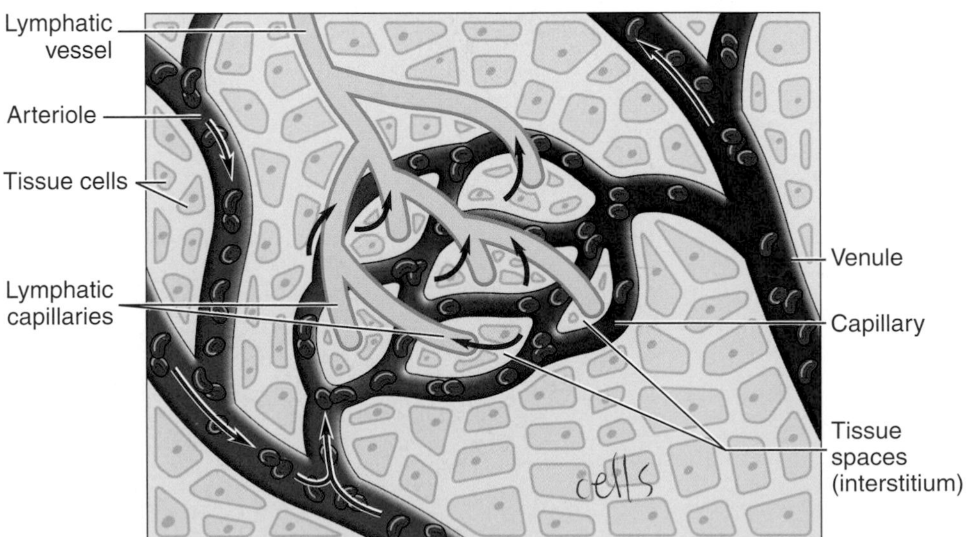

FIGURE 20-2 Lymph capillaries and blood capillaries.

organ in the body has a rich supply of lymphatic vessels. They pick up tissue fluid and transport it toward the heart. Figure 20-3 shows the relationship between the circulatory system and the lymphatic system.

The walls of the lymphatic capillaries are made up of a single layer of epithelium and have large pores. This large-pore structure allows the lymphatic capillaries to drain tissue fluid and proteins, thereby forming lymph. Once absorbed by the lymphatic capillaries, the lymph flows toward the heart through a series of larger and larger lymphatic vessels until it reaches the large **lymphatic ducts.**

For example, lymph from the right arm and the right side of the head and thorax drains into the right lymphatic duct. Lymph from the rest of the body drains into the **thoracic duct** (Figure 20-4). Both ducts empty the lymph into the subclavian veins. The right lymphatic duct drains lymph into the right subclavian vein; the thoracic duct drains lymph into the left.

MOVEMENT THROUGH THE LYMPHATIC VESSELS

Whereas blood moves because it is pumped by the heart, lymph depends on other means for movement. Lymph moves in response to the following:

- The "milking" action of the skeletal muscles. As the skeletal muscles contract, they squeeze the surrounding lymphatic vessels, thereby pushing lymph toward the heart.
- The movement of the chest during respiration. Contraction and relaxation of the chest muscles cause changes in the pressure within the thorax. The changes in intrathoracic pressure increase the flow of lymph.
- The rhythmic contraction of the smooth muscle in the lymphatic vessels. The alternating contraction and relaxation of the smooth muscle cause lymph to flow.

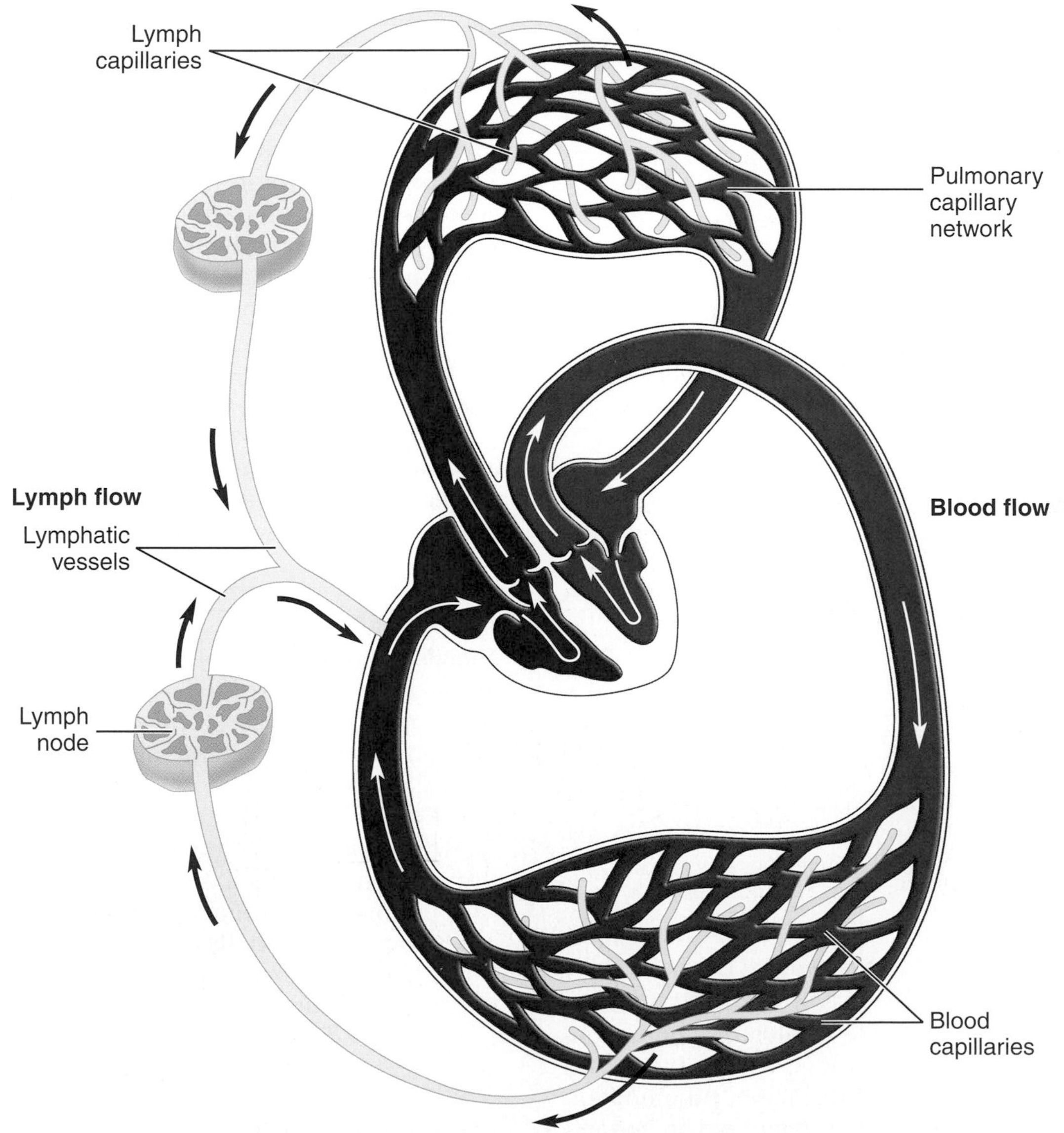

FIGURE 20-3 Lymphatic vessels "run with" the veins.

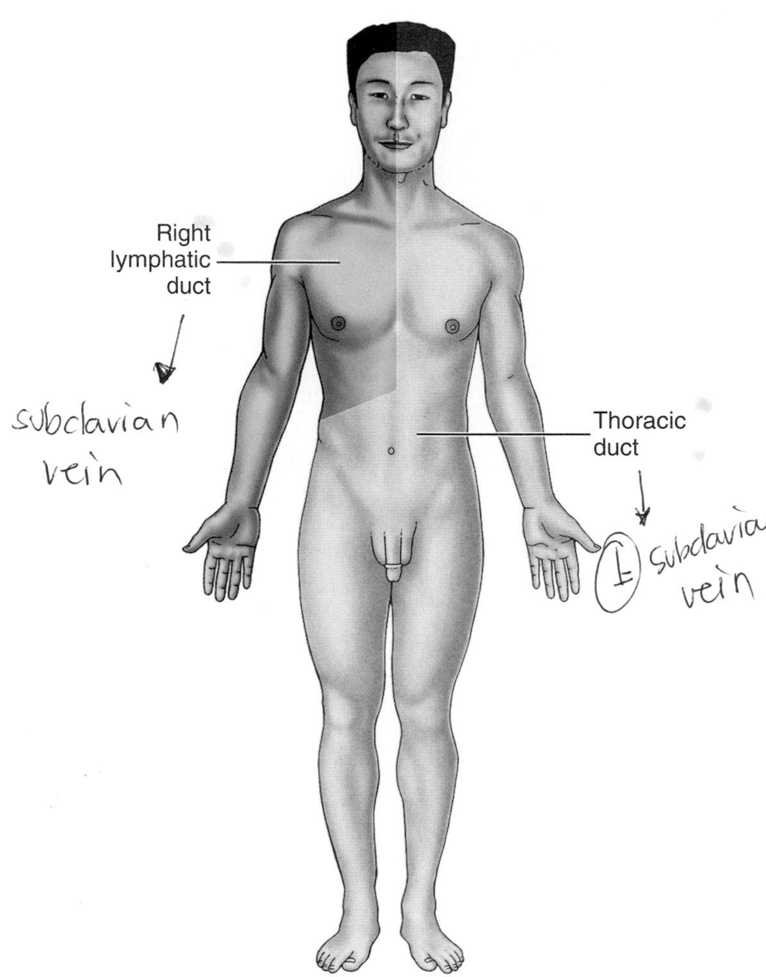

FIGURE 20-4 The main lymphatic ducts: right lymphatic duct and thoracic duct.

The lymphatic vessels form a one-way path, and lymph flows from the tissue spaces toward the heart. Why? Like the veins, the lymphatic vessels contain valves. Valves prevent any backflow of lymph; if lymph moves at all, it must move toward the heart.

Sum It Up!

Lymphatic vessels accompany venous blood vessels throughout the body. They drain fluid and protein from tissue spaces as lymph; the lymph eventually returns to venous blood by larger lymphatic vessels.

LYMPHOID ORGANS

The **lymphoid organs** include the lymph nodes, tonsils, thymus gland, and spleen (Figure 20-5). Lymphoid tissue is also found scattered throughout the body in many other organs. In general, the lymphoid organs and lymphoid tissue help defend the body against disease by filtering particles such as pathogens and cancer cells from the lymph, tissue fluid, and blood and by supporting the activities of the lymphocytes, which provide immunity against disease.

LYMPH NODES

Lymph nodes are small pea-shaped patches of lymphatic tissue strategically located so as to filter the lymph as it flows through the lymphatic vessels. Lymph nodes tend to appear in clusters (see Figure 20-5, *B*). The larger clusters include the following:

- **Cervical lymph nodes** drain and cleanse lymph coming from the head and neck areas. Enlarged, tender cervical lymph nodes often accompany upper respiratory infections.
- **Axillary lymph nodes** are located in the axillary area, or armpit. These nodes drain and cleanse lymph coming from the upper extremities, shoulders, and breast area. Cancer cells that escape from the breast are often found in the axillary lymph nodes.
- **Inguinal lymph nodes** are located in the groin region. These nodes drain and cleanse lymph from the lower extremities and external genitalia.

What does a lymph node look like? A lymph node contains several compartments, called **lymph nodules,** that are separated by **lymph sinuses** (Figure 20-6). The lymph nodules are masses of lymphocytes and macrophages. These cells are defensive cells; they are concerned with immunity and phagocytosis. They protect the body against disease. The lymph nodules are separated by lymph sinuses; these are lymph-filled spaces. Afferent lymphatic vessels carry lymph into the node for cleansing. The lymph leaves the node through the efferent lymphatic vessels as it continues its journey toward the heart.

TONSILS

Tonsils are partially encapsulated lymph nodes in the throat area (see Figure 20-5, *A* and *C*). They filter tissue fluid contaminated by pathogens that enter the body through the nose or mouth, or both. The three sets of tonsils are as follows:

- **Palatine tonsils** are small masses of lymphoid tissue located at the opening of the oral cavity into the pharynx. A tonsillectomy is most often performed on this particular set of tonsils.
- **Pharyngeal tonsils** are also called the **adenoids.** They are located near the opening of the nasal cavity in the upper pharynx. The adenoids atrophy during adolescence. Enlargement of the adenoids may interfere with breathing and require surgical removal called adenoidectomy.
- **Lingual tonsils** are located at the back of the tongue.

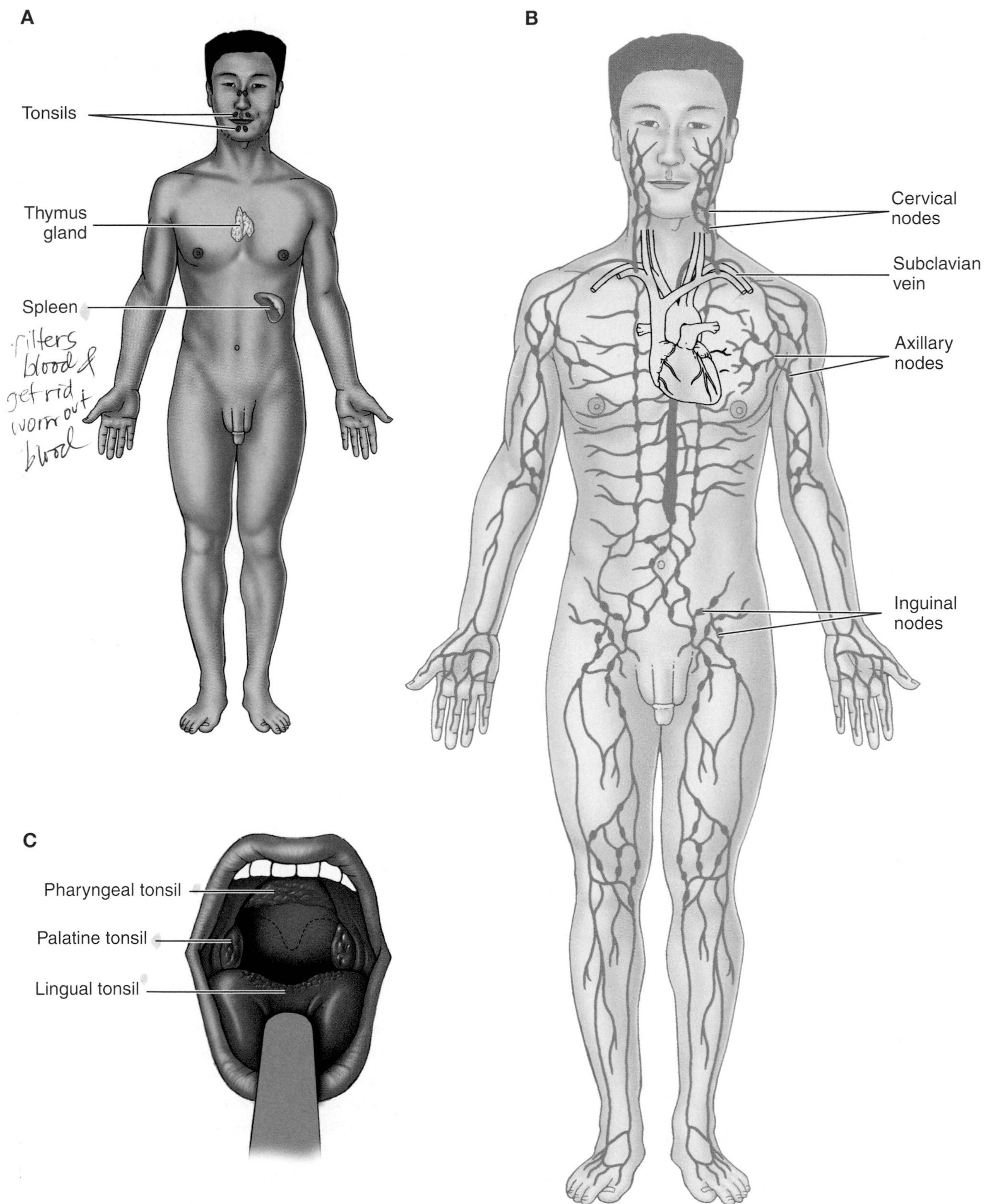

FIGURE 20-5 Location of lymphoid tissue. **A,** Lymphoid organs. **B,** Distribution of lymph nodes. **C,** Tonsils.

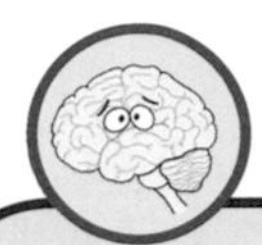

Do You Know...

Why the axillary lymph nodes are removed during a mastectomy (surgical breast removal)?

Many cancers metastasize or spread by way of the lymphatic vessels. Cancer of the breast commonly metastasizes to the axillary lymph nodes. In an attempt to rid the body of all cancer cells, the surgeon removes the breast and the associated axillary lymph nodes. Each lymph node is then biopsied; further treatment often depends on how many of the lymph nodes are positive (i.e., are cancerous, or malignant). Removal of the axillary lymph nodes frequently impairs lymphatic drainage. Consequently, the woman may develop edema of the affected arm and shoulder. Because the edema develops in response to impaired drainage of lymph, it is called lymphedema.

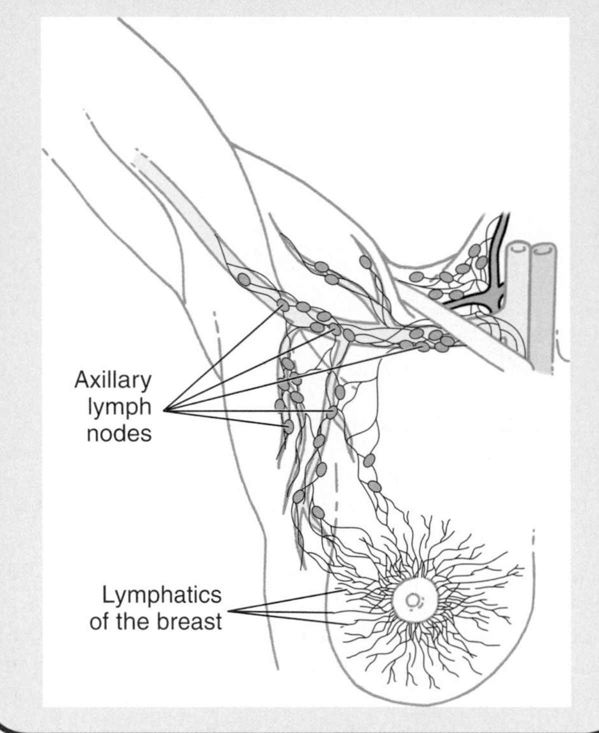

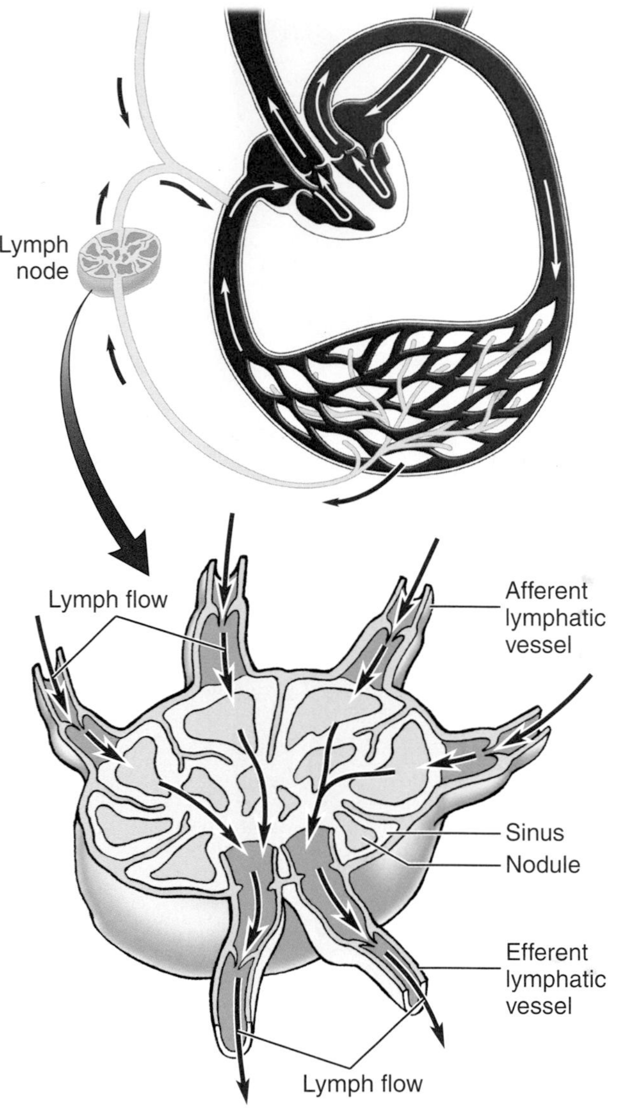

FIGURE 20-6 Cross section of a lymph node.

THYMUS GLAND

The **thymus** (THĪ-mŭs) **gland** is located in the upper mediastinum thoracic cavity (see Figure 20-5, *A*). The thymus gland plays a crucial role in the development of the immune system before birth and in the first few months after birth. After puberty, the gland shrinks (involutes), but remains active throughout life.

The thymus gland secretes hormones called thymosins. **Thymosins** promote the proliferation and maturation of special lymphocytes (T cells) in lymphoid tissue throughout the body (see Chapter 21).

SPLEEN

The **spleen** is the largest lymphoid organ in the body. It is located in the upper left quadrant of the abdominal cavity, just beneath the diaphragm and is normally protected by the lower rib cage (Figure 20-7). Although the spleen is much larger, it resembles a lymph node.

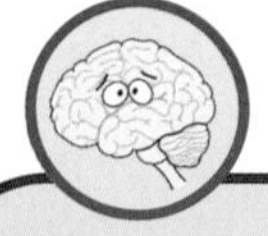

Do You Know...

Why you sometimes get swollen glands when you have a sore throat?

As the lymph drains from the throat, it flows through the closest lymph nodes, where it is cleansed by the resident phagocytes. The lymph nodes may become tender and enlarged as they work to kill the pathogens. This condition is called lymphadenitis. Calling the condition swollen glands is somewhat misleading. The swelling and tenderness are associated with the enlarged lymph nodes and not with glands.

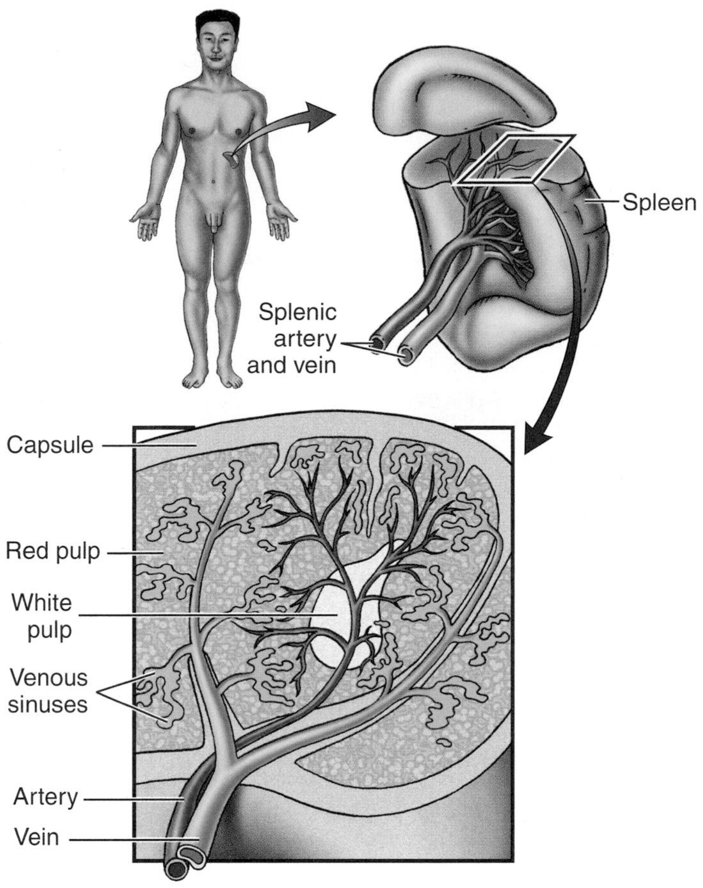

FIGURE 20-7 Spleen, composed of white pulp and red pulp.

The spleen filters blood rather than lymph. The spleen is composed of two types of tissue called white pulp and red pulp. The **white pulp** is lymphoid tissue consisting primarily of lymphocytes surrounding arteries. The **red pulp** contains venous sinuses filled with blood and disease-preventing cells such as lymphocytes and macrophages. Blood enters the spleen through the splenic artery. The blood is cleansed as it slowly flows through the spleen. Microorganisms trapped by the spleen are destroyed by the leukocytes within the spleen. The cleansed blood leaves the spleen through the splenic vein.

In addition to its cleansing role, the spleen has other functions. The spleen stores blood, especially platelets. (As much as 30% of the platelets are stored in the spleen.) The spleen also destroys and phagocytoses old, worn-out red blood cells. For this reason, the spleen is called the "graveyard" of the RBCs. Finally, the spleen plays a role in erythropoiesis, as a site of red blood cell production before birth. After birth the spleen stops producing RBCs but continues its lifelong production of lymphocytes.

Because of its location the spleen is commonly injured. Because it is difficult to repair and prone to bleed the spleen is often removed surgically. The splenectomized patient can live nicely without a spleen but may be more prone to infection.

Do You Know...

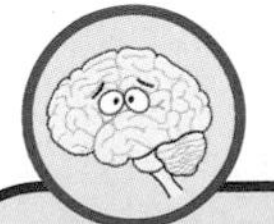

Why "lose that spleen" was a slogan for ancient Roman marathoners?

In ancient Roman times, the rumor in marathon circles was that removal of the spleen would make one a faster runner. The spleen was removed surgically or burnt out with a hot iron! Ugh! Trouble was, the rumor was based on a misreading of a biblical text. The biblical text does indeed say that the removal of the spleen made for a faster runner. The misreading? The shrinkage of the biblical spleen was achieved by an oral medicine concocted by the priests and not by surgery or a hot poker. Fortunately, the practice died out quickly.... Unfortunately, so did the victims of this "misreading."

Sum It Up!

Lymphocyte-containing organs, called lymphoid organs, include the lymph nodes, tonsils, thymus gland, and spleen. Lymphoid tissue, in general, plays a crucial role in the prevention of disease.

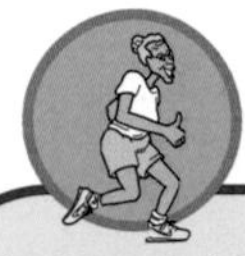

As You Age

1. Lymphoid tissue reaches its peak development at puberty and then progressively shrinks with age.
2 After puberty, the thymus gland involutes, or shrivels up, and is replaced by connective tissue. This process involves a decrease in the amount of thymosins produced. Because of these changes, the defensive mechanisms of the body diminish with age.

Disorders of the Lymphatic System

Cancer (lymphomas)	Several types of malignant tumors affect lymphatic tissue. Lymphosarcoma is a malignant tumor of lymphoid tissue (involving the connective tissue). Most lymphomas (tumors that occur in lymphoid tissue) are malignant. Hodgkin's disease and non-Hodgkin's disease are malignant lymphomas. Both are characterized by painless and progressive enlargement of lymphoid tissue.
Lymphadenitis	Inflammation of the lymph nodes. The nodes become swollen and tender as they fight an infection. With a sore throat a cervical lymphadenitis often occurs.
Lymphadenopathy	Disease of the lymph nodes. Lymphadenopathy often accompanies infection and cancer. HIV infection involves generalized lymphadenopathy.
Lymphangitis	Inflammation of the lymphatic vessels characterized by fine red streaks from the affected area to the groin or axilla. The condition is usually due to a staphylococcal or streptococcal infection.

HIV, Human immunodeficiency virus.

SUMMARY OUTLINE

The main functions of the lymphatic system are defense of the body against infection, return of fluid from the tissue spaces to the blood, and absorption of fat and fat-soluble vitamins from the digestive tract.

I. The Lymphatic System

A. Lymph
1. Lymph is a clear fluid containing water, electrolytes, waste, and some protein.
2. Water and electrolytes are filtered from the plasma into the tissue spaces. Tissue fluid leaves the interstitium by way of the lymphatic vessels (within the lymphatic vessels the fluid is known as lymph).

B. Lymphatic Vessels
1. Lymphatic vessels are similar to the blood capillaries and the veins. The large holes in the lymphatic capillaries absorb fluid and protein from the tissue spaces.
2. Lymph drains into the right lymphatic duct and the thoracic duct; both ducts drain into the subclavian veins.

C. Movement of Lymph
1. Lymph is not pumped like blood (by the heart).
2. Lymph moves in response to skeletal muscle contraction (through milking action), chest movement, and contraction of smooth muscle in the lymphatic vessels.

II. Lymphoid Organs

A. Lymph Nodes
1. The major clusters of lymph nodes are the cervical, axillary, and inguinal nodes.
2. Lymph nodes help protect the body against infection.

B. Tonsils
1. Tonsils are encapsulated lymph nodes.
2. The tonsils are the palatine, pharyngeal, and lingual tonsils.

C. Thymus Gland
1. The thymus gland produces and helps differentiate the lymphocytes.
2. The thymus gland secretes thymosins.

D. Spleen
   1. The spleen functions as a large lymph node.
   2. The spleen has resident WBCs that phagocytose microorganisms.
   3. The spleen stores blood and removes worn-out red blood cells and platelets.

Review Your Knowledge

Matching: Lymph Terms

Directions: Match the following words with their descriptions below.

a. lymph nodes
b. subclavians
c. thoracic duct
d. spleen
e. tonsils

1. __e__ Pharyngeal, lingual, palatine lymphoid organs
2. __c__ Most of the lymph drains into this large duct
3. __b__ The large lymphatic ducts empty lymph into these blood vessels
4. __d__ Contains red pulp and white pulp; it is the largest lymphoid organ in the body
5. __a__ Small, pea-shaped lymphoid structures that filter lymph as it flows through the lymphatic vessels

Multiple Choice

1. Which of the following is least characteristic of adenoids?
   a. Considered lymphoid organs
   b. Are tonsils
   c. Cannot be surgically removed
   d. Contain cells that fight infection
2. The spleen
   a. is located in the right upper quadrant.
   b. cannot be removed without causing death.
   c. removes worn-out RBCs and platelets from the circulation.
   d. is avascular.
3. An overly active spleen may prematurely remove platelets from the circulation thereby
   a. making the person hypertensive.
   b. predisposing the person to infection.
   c. predisposing the person to bleeding.
   d. causing hyperbilirubinemia and jaundice.
4. Which complication is most apt to develop in the patient who has had a breast removal (mastectomy) and lymph node dissection?
   a. Infectious mononucleosis
   b. Bleeding
   c. Lymphedema
   d. Jaundice
5. Which of the following is a tonsil-true statement?
   a. Tonsils are nonlymphoid tissue.
   b. The pharyngeal tonsils are called adenoids.
   c. The lingual tonsils are the tonsils most often removed surgically.
   d. The pharyngeal tonsils may enlarge but never get infected.

CHAPTER 21

Immune System

KEY TERMS

Active immunity, p. 363
Allergen, p. 365
Antibody, p. 360
Antibody-mediated immunity, p. 360
Antigen, p. 359
Artificially acquired immunity, p. 364
Autoimmunity, p. 366
B cell (B lymphocyte), p. 360
Cell-mediated immunity, p. 360
Clone, p. 361
Complement proteins, p. 358
Immunity, p. 355
Immunoglobulin, p. 362
Inflammation, p. 357
Interferons, p. 358
Macrophage, p. 357
Naturally acquired immunity, p. 363
Passive immunity, p. 363
Phagocytosis, p. 357
T cell (T lymphocyte), p. 360
Vaccine, p. 364

OBJECTIVES

1. Differentiate between specific and nonspecific immunity.
2. Describe the process of phagocytosis.
3. Explain the causes of the signs of inflammation.
4. Explain the role of fever in fighting infection.
5. Explain the role of T cells in cell-mediated immunity.
6. Explain the role of B cells in antibody-mediated immunity.
7. Differentiate between genetic immunity and acquired immunity.
8. Describe naturally and artificially acquired active and passive immunity.
9. Identify the steps in the development of anaphylaxis.

Joey was born with severe combined immunodeficiency disease; his immune system was not functioning well. This condition put Joey at high risk for life-threatening infections. As a result of this constant danger of infection, Joey spent most of his life in the sterile environment of a bubble. The bubble protected him from a world of microorganisms. For persons with healthy immune systems, most microorganisms are harmless, but for Joey, the same microorganisms became dangerous pathogens. Recently, the use of bone marrow transplants has eliminated the life-long use of bubbles and has offered new hope for children with immune deficiency diseases. Today we are more apt to encounter persons who are immunosuppressed because of HIV infection, or bone marrow depression caused by cancer chemotherapy.

Study of the immune system is called **immunology.**

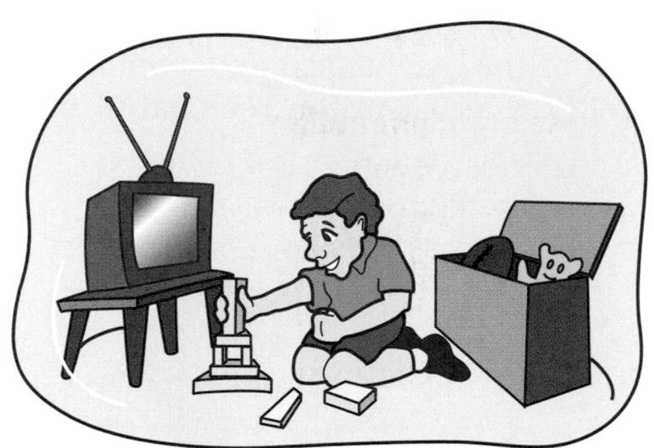

Do You Know...

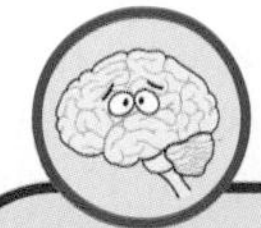

That you will probably get more "colds" if you are stressed out?

"Stressed-out" persons secrete excessive amounts of steroids, one of which is cortisol. Cortisol suppresses the immune response. This response explains, in part, why persons who are stressed out experience a higher rate of upper respiratory infections. Some scientists have suggested that high levels of stress might encourage the development of cancer.

The human body has an elaborate defense system called **immunity.** In addition to protecting the body from pathogens, the immune system protects the body from all other foreign agents, including pollens like ragweed, toxins like bee stings, and our own cells that have gone astray (cancer cells).

CLASSIFICATION OF THE IMMUNE SYSTEM

The defense mechanisms are classified as nonspecific and specific immunity. Table 21-1 lists the many types of cells involved in the immune response.

Table 21-1 Cells Involved in Immunity

Cell Type	Production Site	Function
Granular Leukocytes		
Neutrophils	Bone marrow	Phagocytosis
Basophils	Bone marrow	Secrete histamine and heparin
Eosinophils	Bone marrow	Destroy parasites
Nongranular Leukocytes		
Monocytes	Bone marrow	Phagocytosis; they enter tissues and are transformed into macrophages
Lymphocytes		
• B cells	Bone marrow	Antibody-mediated immunity: accounts for 20% to 30% of blood lymphocytes
—Plasma cells		Secrete antibodies
—Memory B cells		Remember the antigens
• T cells	Bone marrow	Cell-mediated immunity; accounts for 70% to 80% of blood lymphocytes
—Killer T cells		Kill cells
—Helper T cells		Secrete lymphokines, which activate B cells, and other cells
—Suppressor T cells		Inhibit B cell and T cell activity (help control immune response)
—Memory T cells		Remember the antigens
• Natural killer (NK) cells	Lymphoid tissue	Kill cells
Other Cells		
Macrophages	Almost all organs and tissues	Phagocytosis; present antigens to lymphocytes
Mast cells	Almost all organs and tissues, especially liver and lungs	Release histamine and other chemicals involved in inflammation

NONSPECIFIC IMMUNITY

Nonspecific immunity protects the body against many different types of foreign agents. With nonspecific immunity, the body need not recognize the specific foreign agent. A number of defense mechanisms are included in the category of nonspecific immunity (Figure 21-1). Nonspecific immunity can be divided into lines of defense. The first line of defense includes mechanical barriers, chemical barriers, and certain reflexes. The second line of defense includes phagocytosis, inflammation, fever, protective proteins (interferons and complement proteins), and natural killer (NK) cells. Remember: The nonspecific defense mechanisms work against all foreign agents; no recognition of a specific agent is necessary.

First Line of Defense

The first line of defense includes mechanical barriers, chemical barriers, and certain reflexes. Intact skin and mucous membranes serve as **mechanical barriers;** pathogens cannot cross these structures and enter the body. Destruction of mechanical barriers is an invitation to invasion and subsequent infection (see Figure 21-1). Assisting the skin and mucous membranes with their defensive functions are their secretions, called the **chemical barriers.**

For example, tears, saliva, and perspiration provide chemical barriers that wash away microorganisms. They also establish a hostile environment, thereby killing the potential pathogens. The acid and digestive enzymes secreted by the cells of the stomach kill most of the microorganisms swallowed. Tears secrete a substance called **lysozyme,** which discourages the growth of pathogens on the surface of the eye.

Other secretions make the environment sticky and so provide another kind of chemical barrier. The mucus secreted by the mucous membranes of the respiratory tract traps inhaled foreign material. Then the cilia, which line most of the respiratory structures, sweep the entrapped material toward the throat so that the material can eventually be coughed up or swallowed. In addition to the mechanical and chemical barriers, certain reflexes assist in the removal of pathogens.

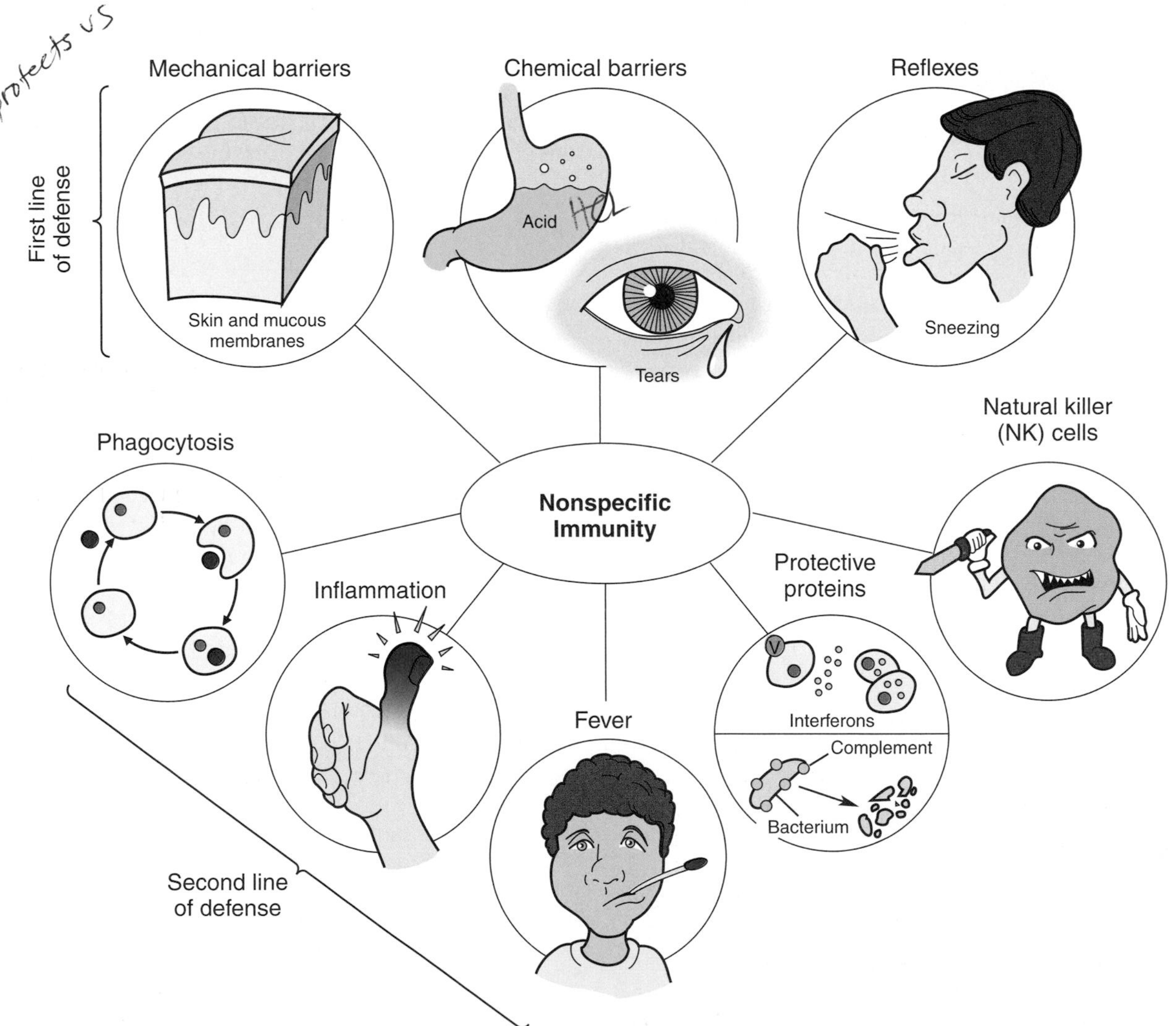

FIGURE 21-1 Nonspecific immunity. First line of defense: mechanical barriers, chemical barriers, and reflexes. Second line of defense: phagocytosis, inflammation, fever, protective proteins, and natural killer (NK) cells.

Sneezing and coughing help to remove pathogens from the respiratory tract, whereas vomiting and diarrhea help to remove pathogens from the digestive tract.

Mechanical barriers, chemical barriers, and reflexes are not an adequate defense against all pathogens, however. If a pathogen penetrates this first line of defense, it encounters processes that make up the second line of defense.

Second Line of Defense

The second line of defense includes phagocytosis, inflammation, fever, protective proteins (interferons and complement proteins), and natural killer (NK) cells.

Phagocytosis. Some of the white blood cells (leukocytes) can ingest and destroy pathogens and other foreign substances by phagocytosis. Some phagocytes, the neutrophils and monocytes, are motile; they wander around the body through the blood and tissue fluid, doing their job. Other phagocytes are confined within a particular tissue and are called fixed.

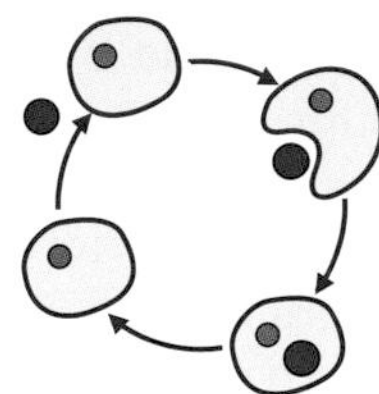

Traveling through the blood to the site of infection, the neutrophils and monocytes can squeeze through the tiny gaps between the endothelial cells of the capillary walls and enter the tissue spaces at the site of infection. The process of squeezing through the tiny gaps is called **diapedesis.** How do the neutrophils and monocytes know where to go? Chemicals released by injured cells attract them to the injured site. This signaling to attract phagocytes is called **chemotaxis.** This process is similar to a bloodhound tracking a scent. The hound picks up the signal (odor), which identifies its source.

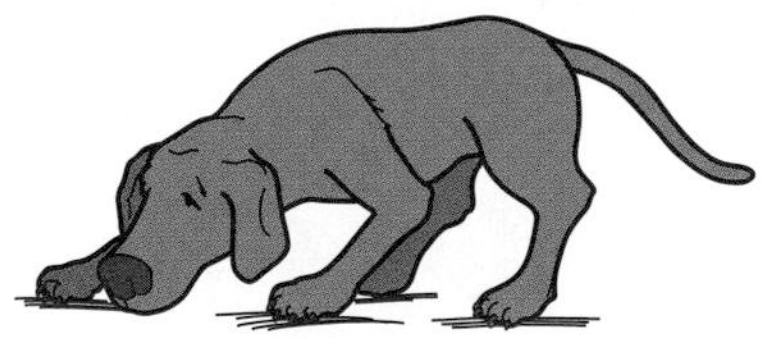

What Does a Phagocyte Do? A phagocyte engulfs, or eats, particles or pathogens much like an ameba does (see Figure 21-1). The phagocyte's plasma membrane sends out "false feet" (pseudopods) that surround the pathogen. The surfaces of the pseudopods then fuse, thereby capturing the pathogen within the phagocyte. The entrapped pathogen encounters a lysosome; the lysosomal membrane fuses with the pathogen, releasing potent enzymes that destroy the pathogen. The process of phagocytosis can be summarized as "ingested (eaten) and digested."

One group of phagocytic cells, the monocytes, deposit themselves in various organs and give rise to **macrophages** (MĂK-rō-făj-ĕs). As the name implies, the macrophages are big eaters. They become fixed within a particular organ and are thus nonmotile. They can, however, divide and produce new macrophages at their fixed site. The **Kupffer cells** in the liver, for instance, are fixed to the walls of the large capillaries called **sinusoids.** As blood flows through the sinusoids, pathogens and other foreign substances are removed from the blood and phagocytosed. The liver, spleen, lungs, and lymph nodes have a particularly rich supply of fixed phagocytes.

Inflammation. Inflammation refers to the responses the body makes when confronted by an irritant. The irritant can be almost anything; common irritants include pathogens, friction, excessive heat or cold, radiation, injuries, and chemicals. If the irritant is caused by a pathogen, the inflammation is called an **infection.**

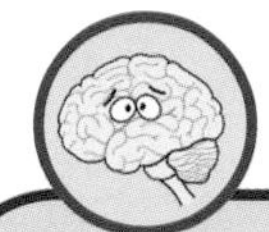

Do You Know...

Where you have seen rubor, calor, tumor, *and* dolor?

Enough with the Latin! These Latin words refer to the classic signs of inflammation: redness, heat, swelling, and pain. Note that the Latin word for swelling is tumor. When the ancients used the term tumor, it referred to any type of swelling—even the swelling of edema. When we use the word tumor today, we generally mean a solid mass, as in cancer.

Inflammation is characterized by redness, heat, swelling, and pain (see Figure 21-1). What are the causes of these symptoms? When the tissues are injured or irritated, injured cells release **histamine** and other substances. These substances cause the blood vessels in the injured tissue to dilate. The dilated blood vessels bring more blood to the area, and the increased blood flow causes redness and heat. The histamine causes the blood vessel walls to leak fluid and dissolved substances into the tissue spaces, causing swelling. Fluid and irritating chemicals accumulating at the injured site also stimulate pain receptors; therefore the person experiences pain. Redness, heat, swelling, and pain are the classic signs of inflammation.

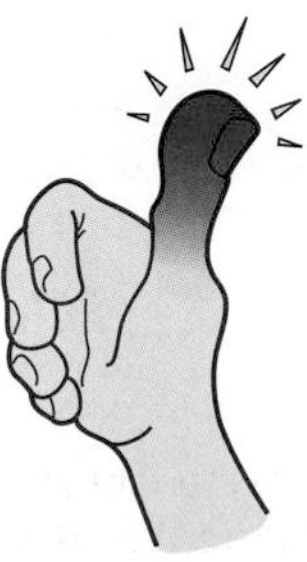

The increased blood flow also carries an increased number of phagocytes (neutrophils and monocytes) to the injured site. As the phagocytes do their job, many are killed in the process. In a severe infection, the area becomes filled with dead leukocytes, pathogens, injured cells, and tissue fluid. This thick, yellowish accumulation of dead material is called **pus.** The presence of pus indicates that the phagocytes are doing their job.

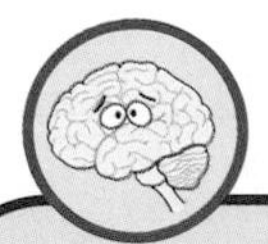

Do You Know...

How and why the body "walls off the pus"?

When an area becomes infected, the cells involved in the inflammatory response do two things. First, they kill the pathogens. As the war continues, dead cells (including phagocytes, injured cells, and pathogens) and secretions accumulate in the area as pus. Second, the cells build a wall of tissue around the infected debris. This walled-off area is an abscess. An abscess performs a beneficial role in that it restricts the spread of the infection throughout the body. A large abscess may require a surgical procedure in which the abscess is lanced and drained.

Because of the leaky blood vessels, fluid collects in the tissue spaces. This tissue fluid contains some blood-clotting factors, such as fibrinogen, a protein present in plasma. Fibrinogen creates fibrin threads within the tissue spaces. Later, fibroblasts, the cells that form connective tissue, may also invade the injured area. The connective tissue helps to contain, or restrict, the area of inflammation and thereby prevents the infection from spreading throughout the body. Fibroblastic activity is also involved in tissue repair.

Fever. Fever, also known as **pyrexia,** is an abnormal elevation in body temperature. As phagocytes perform their duty, they release fever-producing substances called **pyrogens** (from the Latin word for fire). The pyrogens stimulate the hypothalamus in the brain to reset the body's temperature, producing a fever. The elevation in temperature is thought to be beneficial in two ways: a fever both stimulates phagocytosis and decreases the ability of certain pathogens to multiply. In fact, the elimination of mild fevers may do more harm than good.

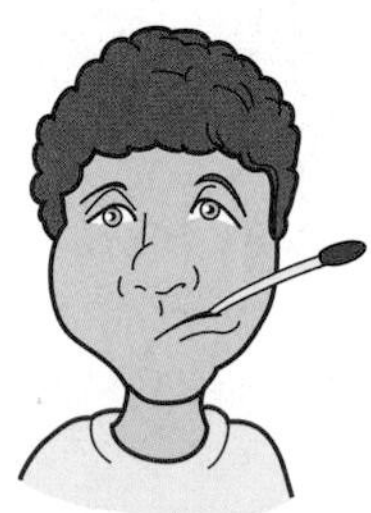

What happens when the hypothalamus resets the body temperature? First, the person shivers in an attempt to generate heat; the heat is conserved as the blood vessels of the skin constrict. The person may have chills and feel cold and clammy even though body temperature is rising. The elevated temperature hovers around the new set point while the pathogen is active, but when the infection is contained and the secretion of pyrogens diminishes, the hypothalamus resets its thermostat back to normal. Heat-losing mechanisms are activated, and the blood vessels of the skin dilate, thereby losing heat as the person sweats.

Evidence suggests that the reduction of fever prolongs an infection. Note, however, that a very high fever must be reduced because high body temperature may cause severe and irreversible brain damage. High fever, especially in children, is frequently accompanied by seizures. Seizures due to an elevated body temperature are called febrile (fever) seizures.

Protective Proteins. Two groups of protective proteins, the interferons and the complement proteins, act nonspecifically to protect the body (see Figure 21-1). **Interferons** (ĭn-tĕr-FĒR-ŏnz) are a group of proteins secreted by cells infected by a virus. The interferons diffuse to surrounding cells where they prevent viral replication. Researchers first found interferons in cells infected by the influenza virus. They called them interferons because they interfered with viral replication. Interferons also activate NK cells and macrophages, thus boosting the immune system.

A second group of proteins that protect the body are the complement proteins. **Complement proteins** circulate in the blood in their inactive form. When the complement proteins are activated against a bacterium, they swarm over it. The complement attaches to the bacterium's outer membrane and punches holes in it. The holes in the membrane allow fluid and electrolytes to flow into the bacterium, causing it to burst and die. The activated complements perform other functions that enhance phagocytosis and the inflammatory response.

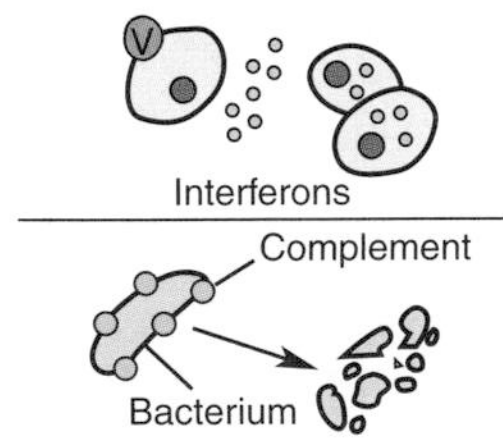

Natural Killer Cells. Natural killer (NK) cells are a special type of lymphocyte that acts nonspecifically to kill a variety of cells. NK cells are effective against many microbes and certain cancer cells. The NK cells cooperate with the specific defense mechanisms to mount the most effective defense possible.

FIGURE 21-2 The immune system wages its battle with three lines of defense. (Read from bottom to top.)

> **Sum It Up!**
> Figure 21-2 summarizes the functions of the nonspecific defense mechanisms. The wall of the fortress is the first line of defense. It protects the body from invaders such as bacteria, fungi, and viruses. Parts of this first line of defense are mechanical barriers, chemical barriers, and reflexes. Behind the wall of the fortress is the second line of defense: phagocytes, processes that cause inflammation and fever, protective proteins, and the NK cells.

SPECIFIC IMMUNITY: THIRD LINE OF DEFENSE

Specific immunity homes in on a foreign substance and provides protection against one specific substance but no others. They protect against a specific foreign agent such as the measles virus (a specific pathogen) or ragweed pollen. The two cells that play key roles in these specific immunity are the lymphocytes (B lymphocytes and T lymphocytes) and the macrophages. Understanding the function of lymphocytes requires an understanding of antigens.

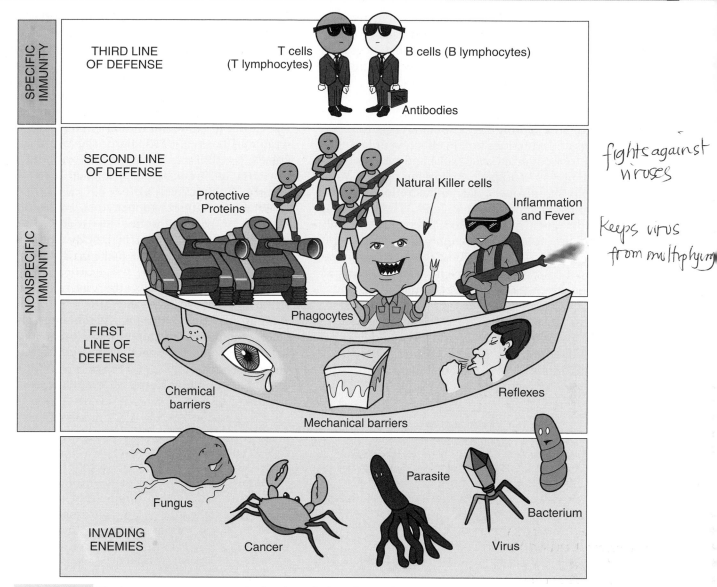

Antigens

An **antigen** is a substance that stimulates the formation of antibodies. Antigens are generally large molecules; most are proteins, but a few are polysaccharides and lipids. Antigens are found on the surface of many substances, such as pathogens, red blood cells, pollens, foods, toxins, and cancer cells. Foreign substances that display antigens are described as antigenic. Antigenic substances are attacked by lymphocytes.

Self and Nonself: Is That Me?

Before birth, your lymphocytes somehow get to know who belongs and who does not. In effect, your lymphocytes learn to recognize "you" (self) and take steps to eliminate "not you" (nonself, or foreign agent). Your body perceives your own cells and secretions as nonantigenic and other cells as antigenic. The antigenic cells are subsequently eliminated. Recognition of self is called **immunotolerance.** Sometimes a person's immune system fails to identify self and mounts an immune attack against its own cells. This attack is the basis of **autoimmune diseases,** such as rheumatoid arthritis.

Lymphocytes

The two types of lymphocytes are **T lymphocytes (T cells)** and **B lymphocytes (B cells).** Although they both come from the stem cells in the bone marrow, they differ in their development and functions (Table 21-1).

Why the Names T and B Cells? During fetal development, stem cells in the bone marrow produce lymphocytes. The blood carries lymphocytes throughout the body. About one half of the lymphocytes travel to the thymus gland, where they mature and differentiate. These cells are transformed and become T cells (thymus-derived lymphocytes). Eventually, the blood carries T cells away from the thymus gland to various lymphoid tissues, particularly the lymph nodes and spleen. T cells live and work in the lymphoid tissue and also circulate in the blood, making up 70% to 80% of the blood's lymphocytes.

What about the B lymphocytes? B cells differentiate in the fetal liver and bone marrow (the B is for bone marrow). Like the T cells, the B cells take up residence in lymphoid tissue. B cells make up 20% to 30% of the circulating lymphocytes.

Both T cells and B cells attack antigens, but they do so in different ways. T cells attack antigens directly, through cell-to-cell contact. This immune response is called **cell-mediated immunity.** B cells, on the other hand, interact with the antigen indirectly, through the secretion of **antibodies.** This response is called **antibody-mediated immunity.** Because the antibodies are carried

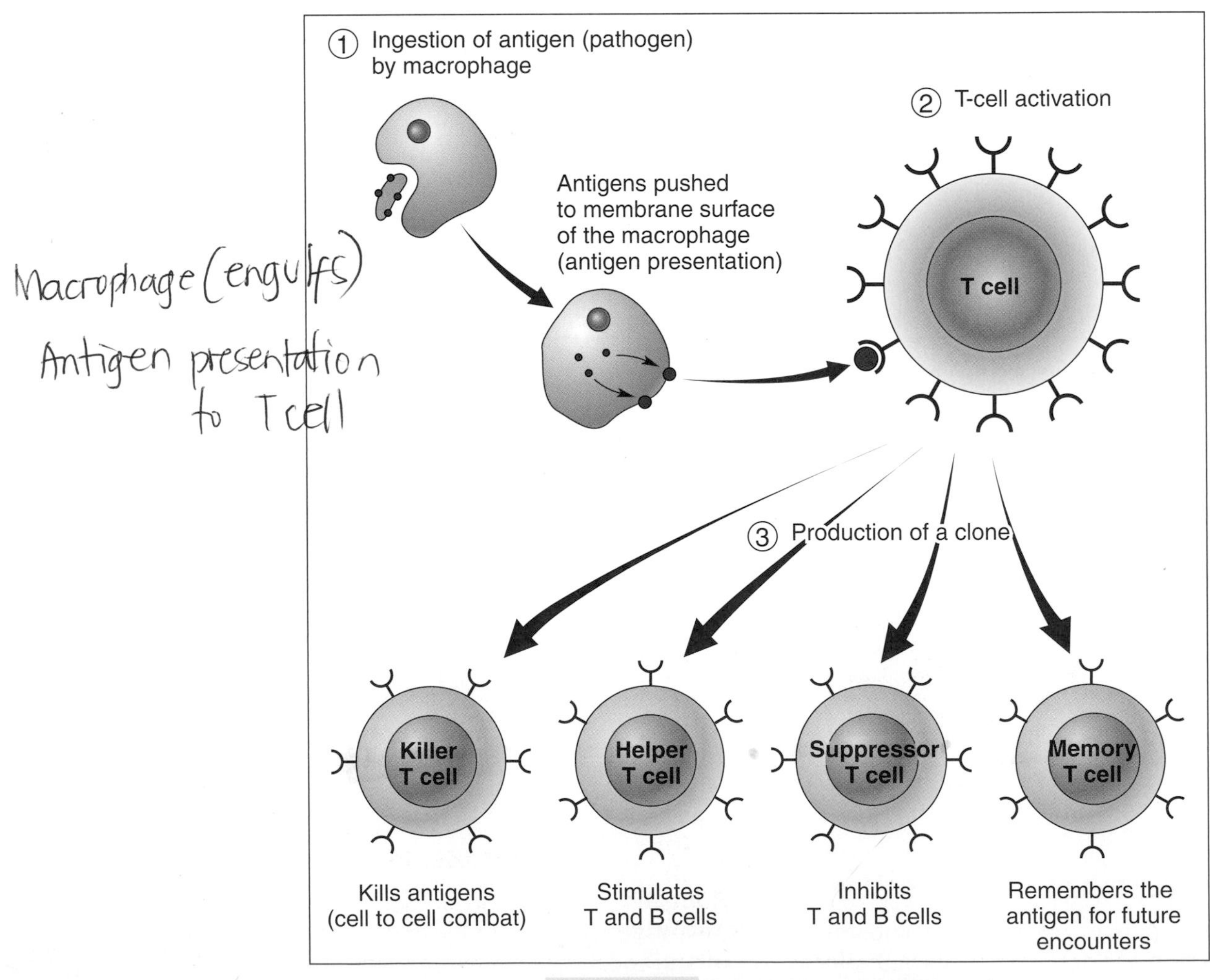

FIGURE 21-3 Cell-mediated immunity.

by the blood and other tissue fluid (the body "humors"), this type of immunity is also called **humoral immunity.**

Cell-Mediated Immunity: T Cell Function. Cell-mediated immunity is effective against many pathogens, tumor cells, and foreign tissue such as organ transplants. Refer to Figure 21-3 as you read about the following steps in cell-mediated immunity:

- Step 1: The antigen, on the surface of the pathogen is phagocytosed by a macrophage. The macrophage digests the antigen and pushes the antigen to its surface. The macrophage's ability to push the antigen to its surface is called **antigen presentation.**
- Step 2: T cells that have receptor sites bind to the antigen and become activated. This process is called **T-cell activation.** Activation of the T cell always requires an antigen-presenting cell, such as a macrophage.
- Step 3: The activated T cell divides repeatedly, resulting in large numbers of T cells. This group of T cells is called a **clone,** a group of identical cells formed from the same parent cell. Four subgroups are within the clone: killer T cells, helper T cells, suppressor T cells, and memory T cells.

The **killer T cells** destroy the antigen (pathogen) through the use of two mechanisms: punching holes in the pathogen's cell membrane and secreting substances called **lymphokines,** which enhance phagocytic activity. The killer T cells engage in cell-to-cell combat. The **helper T cells** also secrete a lymphokine that stimulates both T cells and B cells and, in general, enhances the immune response. The **suppressor T cells** inhibit the immune response when the antigen has been destroyed. The suppressor T cells control B and T cell activity.

The **memory T cells** do not participate in the destruction of the antigen. These cells "remember" the initial encounter with the antigen. If the antigen is presented at some future time, the memory cells quickly reproduce and thus allow a faster immune response to occur.

Antibody-Mediated Immunity: B Cell Function. B cells engage in antibody-mediated immunity. Activated B cells produce a clone of cells that secrete antibodies. The antibodies are carried by the blood and body fluids to the antigen-bearing pathogens. Individual B cells can produce over 10 million different antibodies, each of which reacts against a specific antigen. The large numbers of antibodies allow the body to develop immunity against many different diseases. Follow Figure 21-4 as

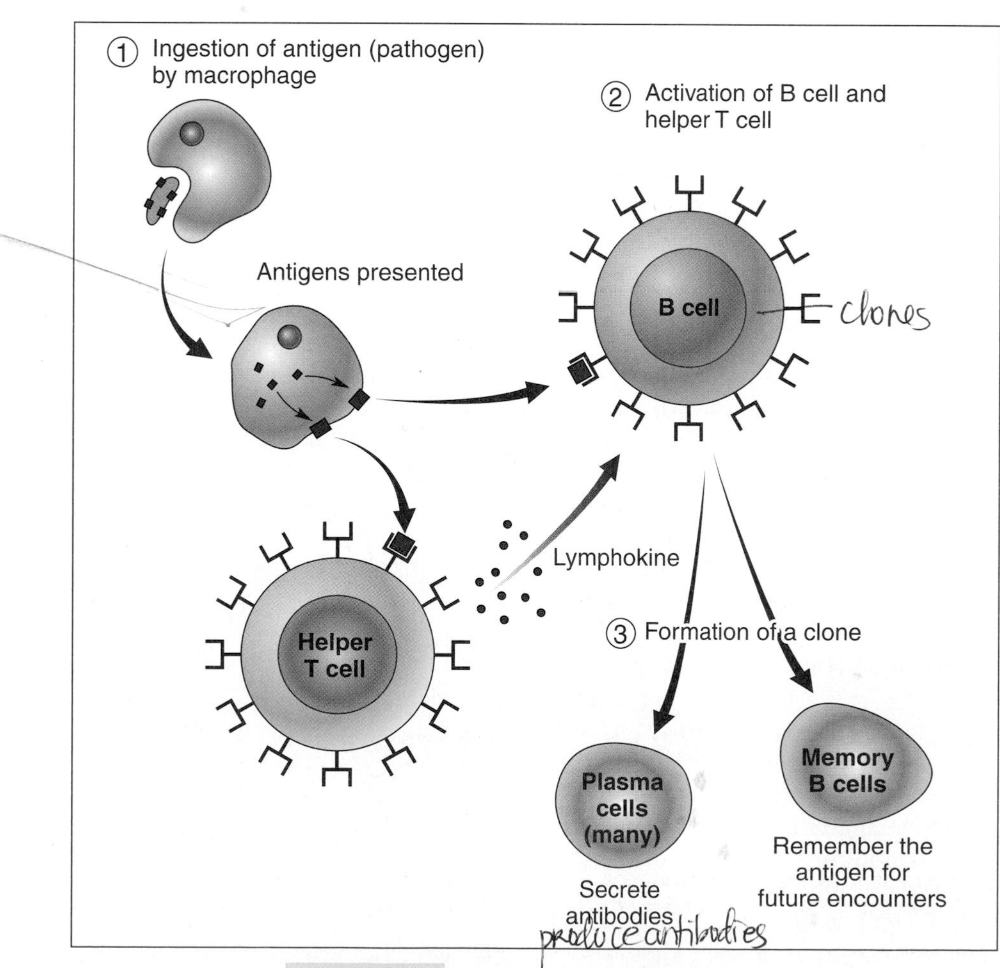

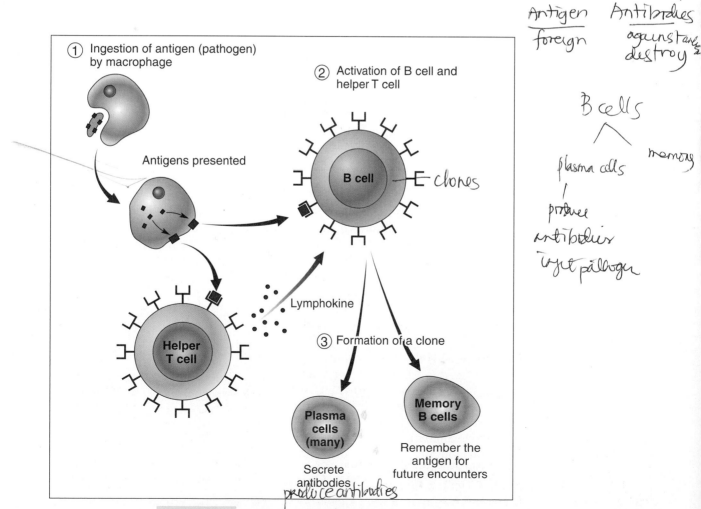

FIGURE 21-4 Antibody-mediated immunity.

body-mediated

processes an
the surface of
both the B cell

nd to both the
ting both cells.
cells with the

secrete a lym-
to reproduce,
ps of the clone
B cells. **Plasma cells** produce large quantities of antibodies that travel through the blood to the antigens (pathogens). The memory B cells do not participate in the attack; they remember the specific antigen during future encounters and allow a quicker response to the invading antigen.

Note that B and T cell activation both depend on helper T cell activity. Human immunodeficiency virus (HIV) attacks the helper T cells, thereby producing severe impairment of the immune system. This syndrome is called acquired immunodeficiency syndrome (AIDS). Because of the impairment of their immune system, persons with HIV infection and AIDS experience numerous bouts of infection.

The helper T cell is also called the $CD4^+$ T cell (because of a surface protein called CD4). The $CD4^+$ T cell is a marker for immune function and the progression of HIV infection is monitored by the $CD4^+$ T cell count. The $CD4^+$ T cell count usually decreases as the infection progresses.

Antibodies

What Antibodies Are. The antibodies secreted by the B cells are proteins called **immunoglobulins** (ĭm-ū-nō-GLŎB-ū-lĭnz). The immunoglobulins are found primarily in the plasma in the gamma globulin part of the plasma proteins. There are five major types of immunoglobulins. The three most abundant immunoglobulins are immunoglobulin G, immunoglobulin A, and immunoglobulin M. A fourth immunoglobulin, immunoglobulin E, is involved in hypersensitivity reactions and is described later.

- **Immunoglobulin G (IgG)** is an antibody found in plasma and body fluids. It is particularly effective against certain bacteria, viruses, and toxins.
- **Immunoglobulin A (IgA)** is an antibody found primarily in the secretions of exocrine glands. IgA in milk, tears, and gastric juice helps protect against infection. Breast milk contains IgA antibodies and helps the infant ward off infection.
- **Immunoglobulin M (IgM)** is an antibody found in blood plasma. The anti-A and anti-B antibodies associated with red blood cells are a type of IgM antibody.

What Antibodies Do. Antibodies destroy antigens. They accomplish this task directly by attacking the membrane and indirectly by activating complement proteins that, in turn, facilitate the attack on the antigens.

When antibodies react with antigens directly, the antibodies bind to antigens. This process is called an **antigen-antibody reaction.** By engaging in an antigen-antibody reaction, the antigen-antibody components clump together, or **agglutinate.** Agglutination makes it easier for the phagocytic cells to destroy the antigen. Under normal conditions, direct attack by the antibodies is not very helpful in protecting the body against invasion by pathogens.

A more effective way for antibodies to attack an antigen is through activation of the complement proteins. These activated complement proteins cause a variety of effects: they stimulate chemotaxis (attract more phagocytes), promote agglutination, make pathogens more susceptible to phagocytosis, and encourage lysis, or rupture of the pathogen's cell membrane. Direct and indirect attacks by antibodies provide an effective defense against foreign agents.

Remember Me? Primary and Secondary Responses. Activated when exposed to an antigen, B cells produce many plasma cells and memory cells. The plasma cells secrete antibodies. This initial response to antigen is called the **primary response** (Figure 21-5). The primary response is associated with a slow development and a relatively low plasma level of antibodies. Note what happens when the immune system is challenged for a second time by the same antigen. The immune system responds quickly and produces a larger number of antibodies. This second challenge is called the **secondary response.** Compare the plasma levels of antibodies in the primary and secondary responses.

Why is the secondary response so much greater? The initial exposure to the antigen has stimulated the formation of both antibody-secreting plasma cells and memory cells. The memory cells, which live for a long time in the plasma, are activated very quickly on

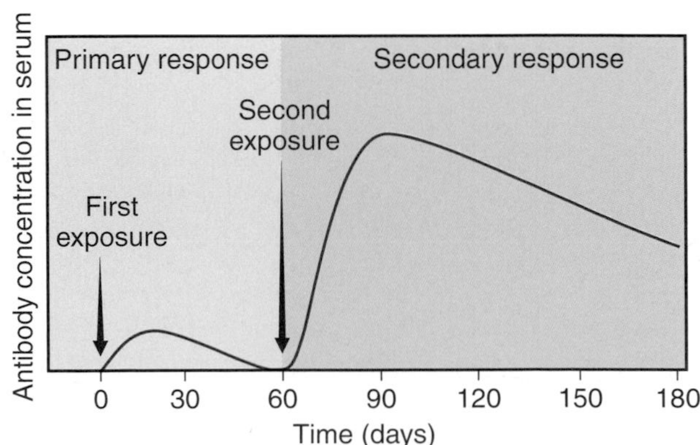

FIGURE 21-5 Primary and secondary responses to an antigen.

the second exposure. The activated memory cells, in turn, induce the formation of many antibody-secreting plasma cells. This fast reaction accounts for the larger number of antibodies associated with the secondary response.

What does the secondary response mean for you? It means that you won't get the disease a second time; you are **immune** to that disease. For example, if you had measles as a child, you developed measles antibodies and many memory cells. If you are then exposed to the measles virus later in life, the memory cells "remember" the first exposure and produce antibody-secreting plasma cells very quickly. The measles antibodies, in turn, attack the measles virus and prevent you from becoming ill.

The level of antibodies in your blood is called an **antibody titer.** If you have had measles, for instance, your measles antibody titer is higher than the titer of someone who has never had measles.

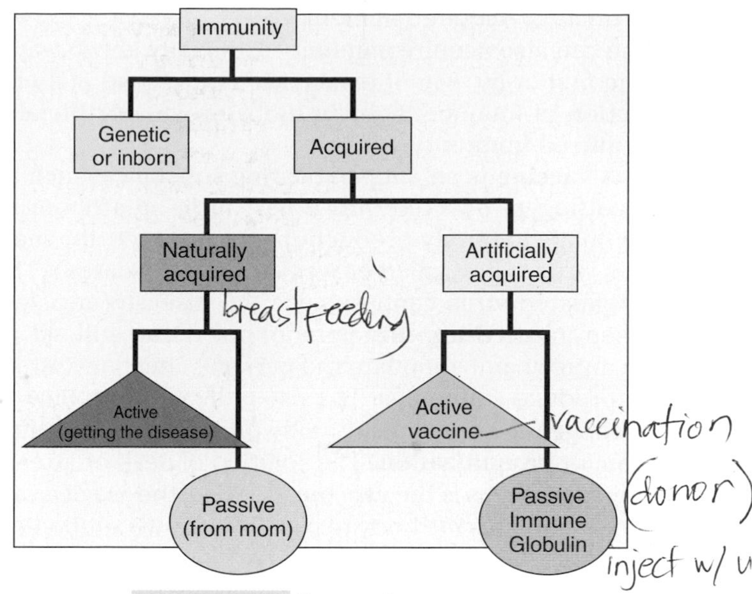

FIGURE 21-6 Types of immunity.

Sum It Up!

Specific immunity forms the third line of defense of the immune response. It allows the immune system to recognize and destroy specific substances called antigens. The lymphocytes (B and T cells) and the macrophages are the most important cells associated with specific immunity. T cells engage in cell-to-cell combat (cell-mediated immunity), whereas B cells fight at a distance through the mediation of antibodies. Macrophages not only engage in phagocytosis but also present the antigen to the lymphocytes.

TYPES OF IMMUNITY

The two main categories of immunity are genetic immunity and acquired immunity (Figure 21-6).

GENETIC IMMUNITY

Do you ever wonder why you have never gotten heartworms from your dog or why your dog did not pick up chickenpox from you? As a human, you have inherited immunity to certain diseases such as canine heartworm; you are immunologically protected from your pet. Likewise, your dog will never contract chickenpox; Rover is immunologically protected from you. Another comforting thought: neither you nor your dog is in danger of contracting Dutch elm disease from your tree. Each of you was born with genetic information that conveys immunity to certain diseases. **Genetic immunity** is also called inborn, innate, or species immunity. As you can see, your species protects you from many diseases that afflict other species.

ACQUIRED IMMUNITY

Unlike genetic immunity, **acquired immunity** is received during a person's lifetime. Acquired immunity comes either naturally or artificially.

Naturally Acquired Immunity

You can acquire immunity naturally in two ways. The first is by getting the disease. As a child you probably had one of the childhood diseases such as chickenpox. Your body responded to the specific pathogen by developing antibodies. After that first exposure, you never became ill with chickenpox again because your immune system had a ready supply of antibodies and memory cells with which to respond quickly to the second invasion of the chickenpox virus. Because your own body produced the antibodies, this type of **naturally acquired immunity** is called **active immunity.** Active immunity is generally long-lasting.

The second way to acquire immunity naturally is by receiving antibodies from your mother. Some antibodies (IgG) crossed the placenta from your mother into you as a fetus. Your mother developed these antibodies in response to the pathogens she encountered throughout her lifetime. Because your immune system did not produce these antibodies (you received them as a gift from your mother), this type of immunity is called **passive immunity.** Antibodies can also be transferred passively from mother to infant through breast milk. Breast milk contains IgA antibodies.

Unlike active immunity, which often lasts a lifetime, passive immunity is short-lived. The antibodies that are acquired passively are broken down and eliminated from the baby's body. The mother's antibodies afford protection to the infant for about the first 6 months after birth. Breastfeeding may extend the length of **immunoprotection.**

Artificially Acquired Immunity

You can also acquire immunity artificially in two ways. The first is by way of a vaccine. The second is by injection of immune globulin. Both provide **artificially acquired immunity.**

A **vaccine** is an antigen-bearing substance, such as a pathogen, injected into a person in an attempt to stimulate antibody production. For instance, the measles virus is first killed or **weakened (attenuated).** The attenuated virus cannot cause the disease (measles) when injected into the person, but it can still act as an antigen and stimulate the person's immune system to produce antibodies. The use of dead or attenuated pathogen to stimulate antibody production is **vaccination,** or **immunization.** The solution of dead or attenuated pathogens is the **vaccine.** Because the use of a vaccine stimulates the body to produce its own antibodies, vaccines induce active immunity.

A vaccine can also be made from the toxin secreted by the pathogen. The toxin is altered to reduce its harmfulness, but it can still act as an antigen to induce immunity. The altered toxin is called a **toxoid.** Because a toxoid stimulates the production of antibodies, it causes active immunity.

The purpose of vaccination is to provide an initial exposure and stimulate the formation of memory cells (the primary response). The purpose of a booster shot is to stimulate the secondary response by administering another dose of the vaccine.

Vaccines have almost eradicated certain diseases. For instance, infants routinely receive a series of DTP injections. DTP injections stimulate active immunity for diphtheria (diphtheria toxoid); tetanus (tetanus toxoid); and pertussis, or whooping cough (pertussis vaccine). MMR vaccine (measles-rubeola, mumps, and rubella) is also used preventively during early childhood.

Immune globulin differs from a vaccine. Immune globulin is obtained from a donor (human or animal) and contains antibodies (immune globulins). The antibodies are formed in the donor in response to a specific antigen. These preformed antibodies are taken from the donor and injected into a recipient, thereby conveying passive immunity.

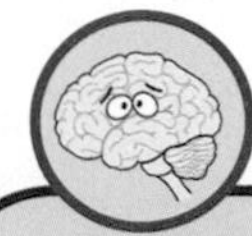

Do You Know...

Why Joey is mooing?

Here's the story. Vaccination against smallpox was originally accomplished by injecting the cowpox virus, a cousin to the smallpox virus. Although Edward Jenner (circa 1850) had demonstrated some success with vaccination, many doctors opposed the procedure. The doctors therefore spread a nasty rumor designed to scare the peasant population. The rumor claimed that the injection of the cowpox virus makes the child take on the characteristics of a cow ... moooooo! Pictures were widely distributed of Joey mooing, swatting flies with his tail, and clanging a cow bell hung around his neck.

Mooooooooooooooo!

Fortunately the peasants weren't duped because they knew that milkmaids never came down with smallpox. Most attributed the immunity of the milkmaids to the cowpox lesions that developed when the milkmaid milked the cows infected with the cowpox virus. Holy cow! This sounds like bull. Just remember, the Latin word for cow is *vacca,* the root word for vaccination.

Why might this procedure be done? Assume for the moment that you are not immune to hepatitis B and so do not have antibodies against the hepatitis B virus. You are then exposed to the virus. Because you have no immunity to the virus, you may receive immune globulin (antibodies) in an attempt to provide immediate protection against the virus. Because this is a form of passive immunity, the immunity is short-lived. Immune globulins are available for rubella (German measles); hepatitis A and B; rabies; and tetanus. A comparison of the different types of acquired immunity appears in Table 21-2.

Other forms of passive immunity are commonly used to prevent the disease or the development of severe symptoms of the disease. **Antitoxins** contain antibodies that neutralize the toxins secreted by the pathogens but have no effect on the pathogens themselves. Examples of antitoxins include tetanus antitoxin (TAT) and the antitoxins for diphtheria and botulism. **Antivenoms** contain antibodies that combat the effects of the poisonous venom of snakes.

Table 21-2 Types of Acquired Immunity

Type	Stimulus	Result
Naturally Acquired		
Active immunity	Exposed to live pathogens (e.g., get the disease)	Long-term immunity; makes antibodies
Passive immunity	Antibodies are passed from mother to infant (across placenta and/or by breastfeeding)	Short-term immunity (lasts approximately for the first 6 months and for duration of breast-feeding); does not stimulate the production of antibodies
Artificially Acquired		
Active immunity	Vaccination	Long-term immunity; makes antibodies
Passive immunity	Injection with gamma globulin (antibodies)	Short-term immunity; does not stimulate the production of antibodies

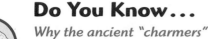

Do You Know...

Why the ancient "charmers" ate snake venom?

Long ago, Indian snake charmers squeezed the venom from their cobras and drank it. Why? They realized that by eating the venom, they developed resistance to the bite of the family pet. This practice was observed by a number of physicians. The concept eventually evolved into our modern-day immunology.

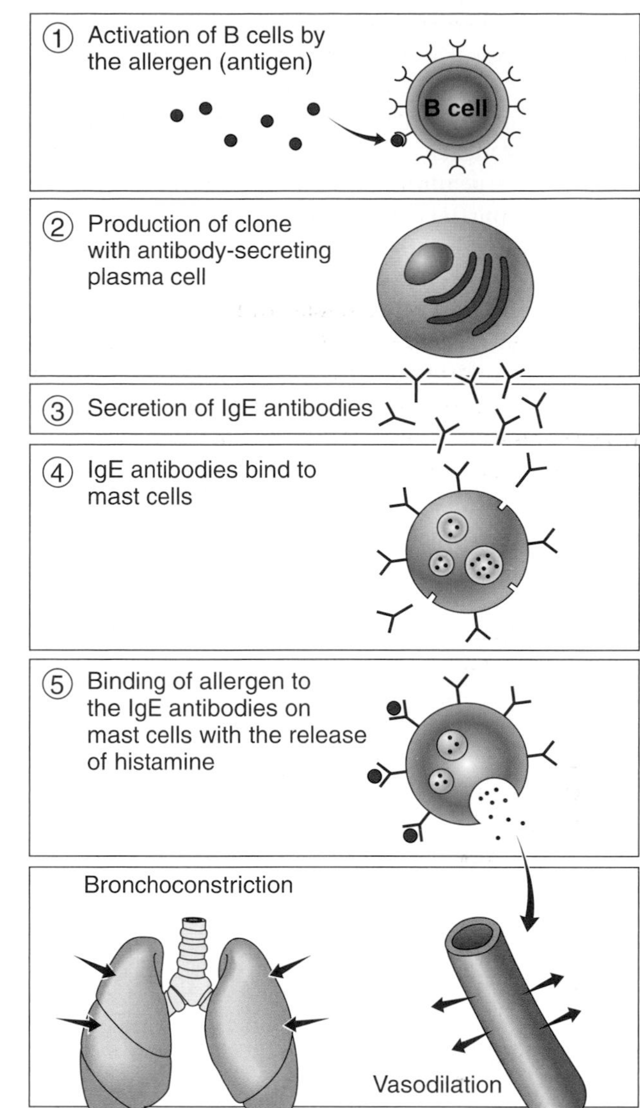

FIGURE 21-7 Immediate-reaction allergy (immediate hypersensitivity reaction).

OTHER IMMUNOLOGIC RESPONSES

Normally, the immune system protects the body from nonself; foreign agents are recognized and eliminated. Sometimes, however, the immune system goes awry: it attacks self, causing **autoimmune disease,** or it overreacts, causing **allergies.**

ALLERGIC REACTIONS

The immune system sometimes forms antibodies to substances not usually recognized as foreign. This response forms the basis of **allergic reactions.** The two common allergic reactions are the delayed-reaction allergy and the immediate-reaction allergy.

The **delayed-reaction allergy** is so named because it usually takes about 48 hours to occur; its onset is delayed. This type of allergic response can occur in anyone. It usually results from the repeated exposure of the skin to chemicals such as household detergents. Repeated exposure to the chemical activates T cells, which eventually accumulate in the skin. Local tissue response to T cell activity causes skin eruptions and other signs of inflammation. This skin response is called contact dermatitis. Other forms of contact dermatitis are associated with poison ivy, poison oak, certain cosmetics, and soaps.

The immediate-reaction allergy, as its name implies, occurs rapidly in response to its stimulus. It is more commonly called **immediate hypersensitivity reaction** and involves immunoglobulin E, the IgE antibodies. **Allergens** (antigens) are substances capable of inducing allergy. Allergens that are apt to be involved in this type of allergic response include pollens, such as ragweed, insect venom, drugs such as penicillin, and foods such as peanuts. Figure 21-7 illustrates the following steps involved in the development of an immediate hypersensitivity reaction:

- Step 1: An allergen activates a B cell.
- Step 2: The activated B cell forms a clone of antibody-secreting plasma cells.
- Step 3: The plasma cells secrete large amounts of IgE antibodies against the specific allergen.
- Step 4: The IgE antibodies bind to the mast cells in body tissues.
- Step 5: More of the allergen invades the body. The allergen binds with the IgE antibodies on the mast cells. The mast cells release large amounts of histamine, leukotrienes, and other chemicals that cause systemic effects. The systemic effects can be severe; they include a massive vasodilation, which causes a sharp drop in blood pressure and severe constriction of the respiratory passages (bronchoconstriction), making breathing extremely difficult and, in some cases, impossible. This severe form of the immediate hypersensitivity reaction is called **anaphylaxis** or **anaphylactic shock.** Persons allergic to penicillin are at risk for anaphylaxis. As a result, always ask a person about allergies to medications before administering any type of drug, particularly antibiotics.

AUTOIMMUNE DISEASE

Sometimes people's T cells attack their own body, causing extensive tissue damage and organ dysfunction. This process is **autoimmunity.** Diseases that develop in response to self attack are called **autoimmune diseases.** A surprisingly large number of diseases are considered autoimmune. A partial list includes thyroiditis, myasthenia gravis, systemic lupus erythematosis, rheumatic fever, rheumatoid arthritis, and some forms of diabetes mellitus.

Consider this. The immune system is affected by both your endocrine system and your nervous systems. Your endocrine and nervous systems are both affected by your emotional state (happy, sad, angry). What are the chances that your emotional state can affect your immune system and hence your physical well-being? In other words, does happiness promote health, while anger and depression cause disease? A new branch of science called **psychoneuroimmunology** seeks to explore this relationship. In the meantime, be happy!

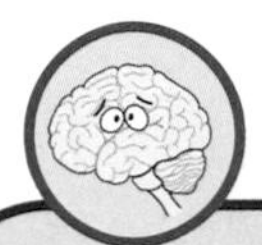

Do You Know...

Why might this bee kill Auntie Bea?

Auntie Bea has become sensitized to bee venom (antigen). IgE antibodies to the bee venom attached to the surface of her mast cells. If Auntie is stung again, the bee venom antigen will bind to the IgE antibodies on the mast cells, causing a massive release of histamine. The histamine causes an anaphylactic reaction. Unless treated immediately, she is apt to die in anaphylactic shock. Treatment is usually an injection of epinephrine (Adrenalin), which opens breathing passages and elevates blood pressure. Steroids (cortisol) are also given to suppress the immune response.

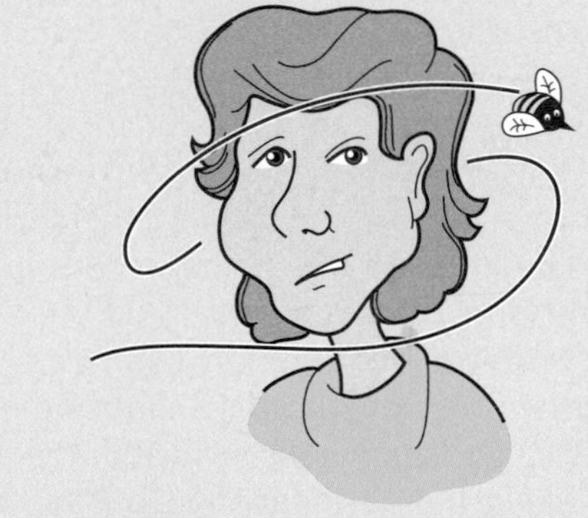

ORGAN REJECTION

Organ transplants have become common means of dealing with organ failure. A patient in kidney failure, for instance, may receive a kidney transplant. One of the greatest problems associated with this new surgical technology is the problem of organ rejection. The recipient's immune system recognizes the donated kidney as foreign and mounts an immune attack against it. When the immune attack is successful, the organ is destroyed and is said to be rejected.

There are several ways to prevent organ rejection. The physician first selects a donor organ that is immunologically similar to the recipient's tissues. The physician then administers drugs that suppress the recipient's immune system. Cyclosporine is a commonly used immunosuppressant that inhibits the secretion of certain lymphokines, which, in turn, diminishes the immune attack against the donated organ. Unfortunately, these measures are not always successful, and the recipient may ultimately reject the organ.

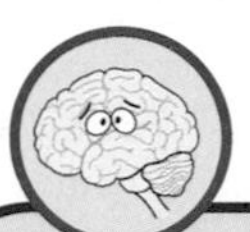

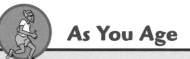

Do You Know...

About the ultimate rejection?

When dealing with transplant patients we watch closely for signs of organ rejection by the host (recipient). However, some patients experience the opposite—the transplanted organ (or blood) rejects the host. This response is called graft-versus-host (GVH) disease; GVH disease usually occurs in immunodeficient patients and is due in part to transplanted T cells. The target organs for rejection are the skin, digestive tract, and the liver. The biggest clinical problem is a variety of infections that gradually overwhelm the granulocytic patient. Imagine being rejected by an organ?

Sum It Up!

Immunity is classified as either genetic or acquired. Immunity may be acquired naturally or artificially. If a person makes antibodies within his or her own body, the immunity is active. If the person merely receives antibodies that were made by another person or animal, the immunity is passive. While the immune system normally works to protect the body, it can go awry, causing allergic reactions and autoimmune disease.

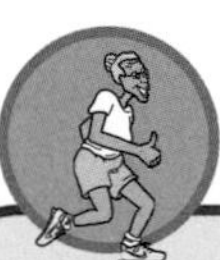

As You Age

1. T cell and B cell function are somewhat deficient in the elderly. Depressed lymphocyte function is accompanied by a decrease in macrophage activity. Consequently, the elderly are more prone to develop infections, and they recover more slowly. Depressed lymphocyte function might also explain the higher incidence of cancer in the elderly population.
2. The elderly often have a reduced fever-response to infection and may therefore have difficulty in combating infection.
3. The elderly have increased levels of circulating autoantibodies (antibodies directed against self). This increase explains, in part, why the elderly are more prone to the development of autoimmune disease.
4. The elderly often take drugs or have therapies that depress the immune system. For instance, the use of steroids in the treatment of arthritis and the use of drugs and radiation in the treatment of cancer all cause immunosuppression.

Disorders of the Immune System

Allergic responses	Delayed hypersensitivities and immediate hypersensitivities. These include contact dermatitis and anaphylaxis.
Autoimmune diseases	Immune system disorders in which the person's immune system produces antibodies against its own cells. There are many autoimmune diseases including rheumatoid arthritis; Hashimoto thyroiditis; diabetes mellitus (type 1); and rheumatic fever. Rheumatic fever is an immune disorder in which the antibodies produced in response to a streptococcal infection attack the heart muscle and its valves.
Immunodeficiency diseases	An incompetent or deficient immune system. Immunodeficiencies can be congenital or acquired. Severe combined immunodeficiency disease (SCID) is a congenital type of immunodeficiency. Children are defenseless against most pathogens and readily succumb to minor infections unless isolated from the environment of microorganisms. Immunodeficiency disease can also be acquired. The acquired immunodeficiency syndrome (AIDS) is an example of a virally induced immunodeficiency.

SUMMARY OUTLINE

The immune system is a defense system that protects the body from foreign agents such as pathogens, pollens, toxins, and cancer cells.

I. Nonspecific Immunity
- A. Nonspecific immune mechanisms protect the body against many different types of foreign agents and do not require recognition of the specific agent.
- B. Lines of Defense
  1. The first line of defense include mechanical barriers, chemical barriers, and reflexes.
  2. The second line of defense includes phagocytosis, inflammation, fever, protective proteins, and natural killer (NK) cells.

II. Specific Immunity
- A. Specific immunity protects the body against specific foreign agents and requires recognition of the specific agent involved.
- B. T Cells, or T Lymphocytes
  1. The T cells make up 70% to 80% of the blood's lymphocytes.
  2. T cells engage in cell-mediated immunity.
  3. Activated T cells produce a clone (killer T cells, helper T cells, suppressor T cells, and memory T cells).
- C. B Cells, or B Lymphocytes
  1. B cells make up 20% to 30% of the blood's lymphocytes.
  2. B cells engage in antibody-mediated immunity.
  3. Activated B cells produce a clone (memory cells and plasma cells). The plasma cells secrete antibodies that travel through the blood to the antigens.
  4. The antibodies are called immunoglobulins.

III. Types of Immunity
- A. Genetic or Acquired Immunity
  1. With genetic immunity, a person is genetically immune to an antigen.
  2. A person can acquire immunity naturally or artificially.
  3. A person can acquire immunity naturally in two ways: by getting the disease or by receiving antibodies from the mother across the placenta and/or through breast milk.
  4. Immunity can be acquired artificially in two ways: by the use of a vaccine or by injection of immune globulin made by another person or animal.
- B. Active or Passive Immunity
  1. Active immunity means that a person's body makes the antibodies.
  2. Passive immunity means that the antibodies are made by another animal and then injected into a patient's body.

IV. Other Immunologic Responses
- A. Allergic Reactions
  1. Allergic reactions are due to the formation of antibodies to substances usually not recognized as foreign.
  2. There are two types of allergic reactions: delayed-onset allergy and immediate-reaction allergy.

3. A delayed-onset allergy takes about 48 hours to develop. Contact dermatitis to a household chemical is a common example.
4. An immediate-reaction allergy (also called an immediate hypersensitivity reaction) is often due to exposure to pollens and drugs such as penicillin. The most severe form is anaphylaxis.

B. Autoimmunity and Tissue or Organ Rejection
1. Autoimmune disease develops when the immune system mounts an attack against self.
2. Tissue or organ rejection occurs when the immune system recognizes the transplanted organ as foreign and attacks it.

Review Your Knowledge

Matching: Nonspecific Immunity

Directions: Match the following words with their descriptions below. Some words may be used more than once.

a. protective proteins
b. phagocytosis
c. inflammation
d. fever

1. ____ Caused by pyrogens
2. ____ Eats debris and pathogens
3. ____ Redness, heat, swelling, and pain
4. ____ Neutrophils and monocytes
5. ____ Complement and interferons

Matching: Specific Immunity

Directions: Match the following words with their descriptions below.

a. immunotolerance
b. cell-mediated immunity
c. antibody-mediated immunity
d. macrophage
e. plasma cells

1. ____ A subgroup of the B cell clone that secretes antibodies
2. ____ Recognition of self
3. ____ The cell responsible for antigen presentation
4. ____ Also called humoral immunity
5. ____ T-cell immunity

Matching: Active and Passive Immunity

Directions: Indicate if the following conveys (a) active immunity or (b) passive immunity.

1. ____ Vaccine
2. ____ Antivenom
3. ____ Antitoxin
4. ____ Toxoid
5. ____ Gamma globulin
6. ____ Getting the disease

Multiple Choice

1. Complement and interferons are
   a. considered to be specific immunity.
   b. protective proteins engaged in nonspecific immunity.
   c. secreted by the B and T cells.
   d. vaccines.
2. Plasma cells
   a. refer to T cells.
   b. are the same as NK cells.
   c. secrete antibodies.
   d. secrete interferons.
3. What is the primary concern regarding the care of a person experiencing an anaphylactic reaction?
   a. Inability to breathe
   b. Development of hives
   c. Development of febrile seizures
   d. Intense itching and discomfort
4. Which of the following is least characteristic of a vaccine?
   a. Artificially acquired immunity
   b. Active immunity
   c. Conveys long-lasting immunity
   d. Passive, immediate-onset, and short-lived immunity
5. Inflammation is
   a. specific immunity.
   b. characterized by redness, heat, swelling, and pain.
   c. known as cell-mediated immunity.
   d. synonymous with infection.

CHAPTER 22

Respiratory System

KEY TERMS

Alveolus, p. 376
Bronchus, p. 374
Bronchioles, p. 376
Compliance, p. 381
Epiglottis, p. 372
Exhalation, p. 381
Glottis, p. 372
Hyperventilation, p. 390
Hypoventilation, p. 390
Inhalation, p. 381
Intrapleural pressure, p. 380
Larynx, p. 372
Partial pressure, p. 386
Pleura, p. 377
Surfactant, p. 379
Tidal volume, p. 387
Trachea, p. 374
Ventilation, p. 381
Vital capacity, p. 387

OBJECTIVES

1. Describe the structure and functions of the organs of the respiratory system.
2. Trace the movement of air from the nostrils to the alveoli.
3. Describe the role of pulmonary surfactants.
4. Describe the relationship of Boyle's law to ventilation.
5. Explain how respiratory muscles affect thoracic volume.
6. List three conditions that make the alveoli well-suited for the exchange of oxygen and carbon dioxide.
7. List lung volumes and capacities.
8. Describe common variations and abnormalities of breathing.
9. Explain the neural and chemical control of respiration.

Is he breathing? This is the first question asked about a person who has been seriously injured. The question indicates the importance of each breath. To breathe is to live; to not breathe is to die. Each breath is a breath of life.

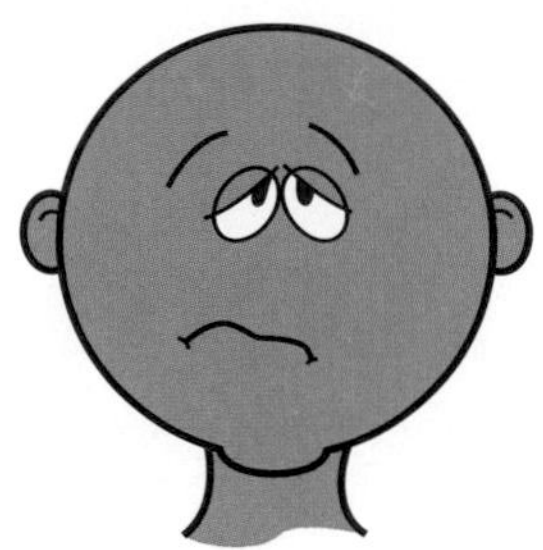

Because of its close connection with life, ancient peoples attributed the act of breathing to the divine. Even the phases of breathing are called inspiration and expiration, references to a divine spirit moving into and out of our lungs. The creation story in Genesis, in which God breathes life into the little clay figure Adam, vividly expresses an image of divine breath. Poetry also describes breathing as the life force. For example, the great Persian poet Sa'di echoed the sacredness of breath in a prayer: "Each respiration holds two blessings. Life is inhaled, and stale, foul air is exhaled. Therefore, thank God twice every breath you take."

STRUCTURE: ORGANS OF THE RESPIRATORY SYSTEM

UPPER AND LOWER RESPIRATORY TRACT

The respiratory system contains the upper and lower respiratory tracts (Figure 22-1). The **upper respiratory tract** contains the respiratory organs located outside the chest cavity: the nose and nasal cavities, pharynx, larynx, and upper trachea. The **lower respiratory tract** consists of organs located in the chest cavity: the lower trachea, bronchi, bronchioles, alveoli, and lungs. The lower parts of the bronchi, bronchioles, and alveoli are located in the lungs. The pleural membranes and the muscles that form the chest cavity are also part of the lower respiratory tract.

Most of the respiratory organs are concerned with conduction, or movement, of air through the respiratory passages. The alveoli are the tiny air sacs located at the end of the respiratory passages. They are concerned with the exchange of oxygen and carbon dioxide between the air and the blood.

NOSE AND NASAL CAVITIES

The **nose** includes an external portion that forms part of the face and an internal portion called the **nasal cavities.** The nasal cavities are separated into right and left halves by a partition called the **nasal septum.** The septum is made of bone and cartilage. Air enters the nasal cavities through two openings called the **nostrils,** or **nares.** Nasal hairs in the nostrils filter large particles of dust that might otherwise be inhaled. In addition to its respiratory function, the nasal cavity contains the receptor cells for the sense of smell. The olfactory organs cover the upper parts of the nasal cavity and a part of the nasal septum.

Three bony projections called **nasal conchae** appear on the lateral walls of the nasal cavities. The conchae increase the surface area of the nasal cavities and support the ciliated mucous membrane, which lines the nasal cavities. The mucous membrane contains many blood vessels and mucus-secreting cells. The rich supply of blood warms and moistens the air, and the sticky mucus traps dust, pollen, and other small particles, thereby cleansing the air as it is inhaled. Because the nose helps warm, moisten, and cleanse the air, breathing through the nose is better than mouth breathing.

Do You Know...

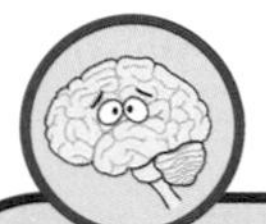

That your nose is more than just a smeller?

The nose does a few things real well; as you know, the nose knows smells. It also "nose" how to clean and humidify air. Equally important, the nose plays a big cosmetic role—it makes us look good and, if it doesn't, we simply rearrange it surgically until it is fashioned into a great-looking nose. Nose-related medical conditions or procedures are named after the rhino, who sports the mother of all noses. For instance, a rhinoplasty refers to the surgical reshaping, resizing, or realigning of the nose. Rhinorrhea refers to a runny nose, as in the common cold or the discharge of cerebrospinal fluid from the nose. Rhinokyphosis is a humpback nose and of course you can have a pain in the nose—rhinodynia. It is interesting that the rhino has captured the nose words, since the rhino's nose is merely hardened hair; it doesn't sniff or drip, and it certainly doesn't check itself in for a nose job.

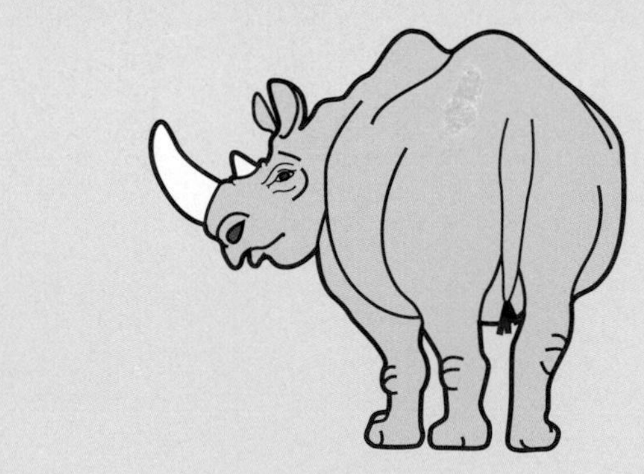

The nasal cavities contain several drainage openings. Mucus from the **paranasal sinuses** drains into the nasal cavity. The paranasal sinuses include the maxillary, frontal, ethmoidal, and sphenoidal sinuses. Tears from

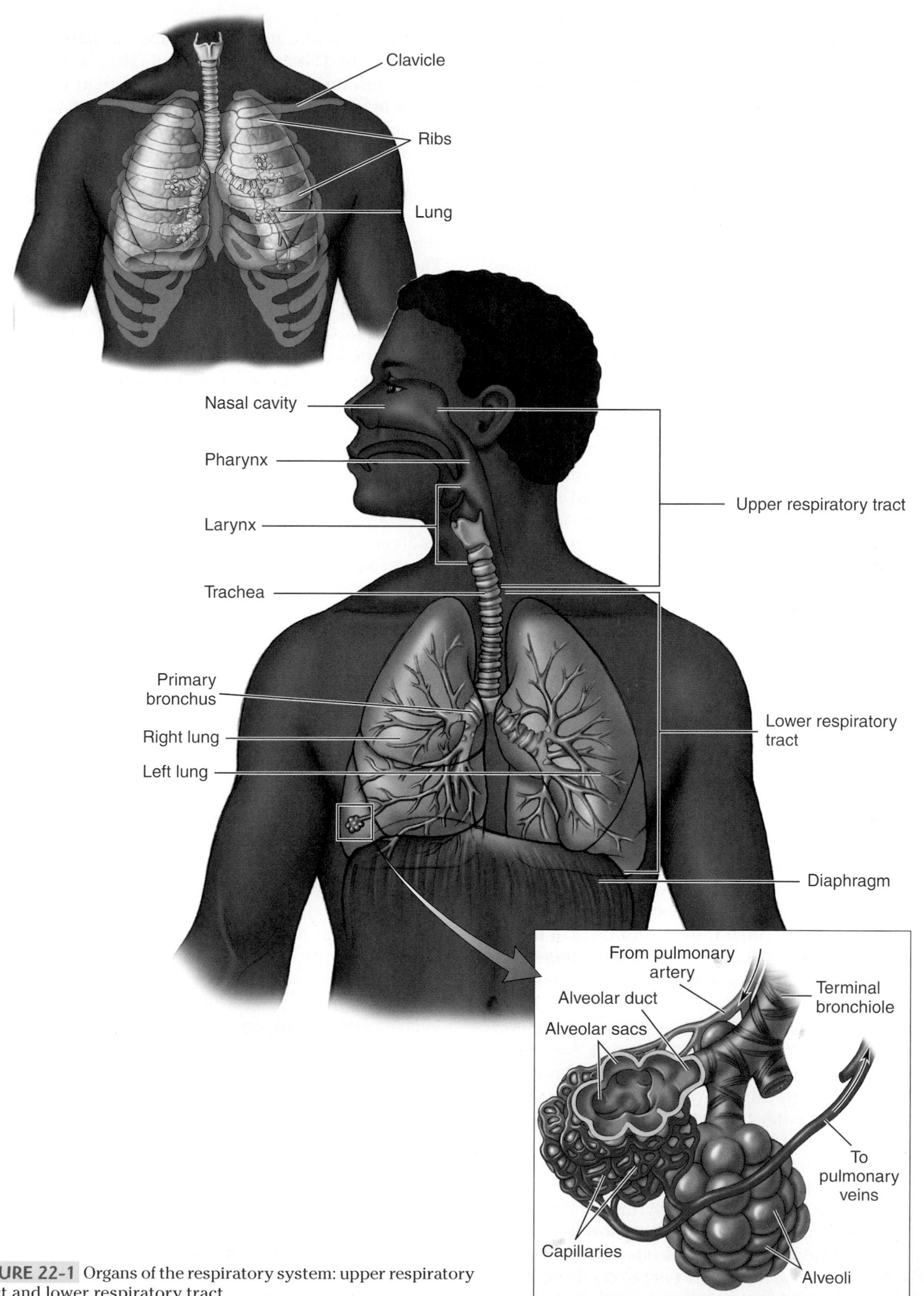

FIGURE 22-1 Organs of the respiratory system: upper respiratory tract and lower respiratory tract.

the nasolacrimal ducts also drain into the nasal cavities. As you know, crying means a runny nose.

In some persons, the nasal septum may bend toward one side or the other, thereby obstructing the flow of air and making breathing difficult. The abnormal positioning of the septum is called a deviated septum. Surgical repair of the deviated septum (septoplasty) corrects the problem.

PHARYNX

The **pharynx** (FĂR-ĭnks), or throat, is behind the oral cavity and between the nasal cavities and the larynx (Figure 22-2). The pharynx includes three parts: an upper section called the **nasopharynx,** a middle section called the **oropharynx,** and a lower section called the **laryngopharynx.** The oropharynx and the laryngopharynx are part of both the digestive and respiratory systems and function as a passageway for both food and air. The pharynx conducts food toward the esophagus (tube for food to enter the stomach). The pharynx also conducts air to the larynx as it moves toward the lungs.

The pharynx contains two other structures: the openings from the eustachian tubes (auditory tubes) and the tonsils. The eustachian tube connects the nasopharynx with the middle ear.

LARYNX

Where and What Is Your Voicebox?

The **larynx** (LĂR-ĭnks), also called the voicebox, is located between the pharynx and the trachea (see Figure 22-2, *A*). The larynx has three functions: it acts as a passageway for air during breathing; it produces sound, your voice (hence the name voicebox); and it prevents food and other foreign objects from entering the breathing structures (trachea). The larynx is a triangular structure made primarily of cartilage, muscles, and ligaments (see Figure 22-2, *C* and *D*).

The largest of the cartilaginous structures in the larynx is the **thyroid cartilage.** It is a tough hyaline cartilage and protrudes in the front of the neck. The thyroid cartilage is larger in men and is called the **Adam's apple.**

The **epiglottis** (ĕp-ĭ-GLŎT-ĭs) is another cartilaginous structure, located at the top of the larynx (see Figure 22-2, *A*). The epiglottis acts as a flap, a very important flap. It covers the opening of the trachea during eating so food does not enter the lungs.

Say, What?

The larynx is called the voicebox because it contains the **vocal cords** (see Figure 22-2, *A* and *C*). The vocal cords are folds of tissue composed of muscle and elastic ligaments and covered by mucous membrane. The cords stretch across the upper part of the larynx. The **glottis** is the space between the vocal cords.

True or False

The two types of vocal cords are the false and true vocal cords. The **false vocal cords** are called false because they do not produce sounds. Instead, the muscle fibers in this structure help to close the airway during swallowing. The **true vocal cords** produce sound. Air flowing from the lungs through the glottis during exhalation causes the true vocal cords to vibrate, thereby producing sound.

Shhhh!

The loudness of your voice depends on the force with which the air moves past the true vocal cords. The pitch of your voice depends on the tension exerted on the muscles of the true vocal cords. You form sound into words with your pharynx, oral cavity, tongue, and lip movement. The nasal cavities, sinuses, and pharynx act as resonating chambers, thereby altering the quality of your voice. Listen to the different voices of your friends. One voice may sound high and squeaky, while another may sound low and booming.

Down the Wrong Way

As Figure 22-2, *A*, shows, the pharynx acts as a passageway for food, water, and air. Food and water in the pharynx, however, should not enter the larynx. How is food and water normally kept out of the larynx? When you breathe in air, the glottis opens, and air moves through the glottis into tubes that carry it to the lungs.

When you swallow food, however, the epiglottis covers the glottis, thereby preventing food from entering the lower respiratory passages. Instead, the food enters the esophagus, the tube that empties into the stomach. How does this happen? During swallowing, the larynx moves upward and forward while the epiglottis moves downward. If you place your fingers on your larynx as you swallow, you can feel the larynx move upward and forward. In addition to the movement of the epiglottis, the glottis closes. Compare the size of the glottis in Figure 22-2, *C* and *D*.

Note that swallowing plays a key role in preventing the entrance of food or water into the respiratory tubes. Some patients develop difficulty in swallowing, particularly those patients who suffer neurological damage such as stroke. Any patient who experiences difficulty in swallowing is at risk for aspiration (entrance of food or water into the lungs)!

From Boy to Young Man

Why is Jack's voice lower than Jill's? At puberty, under the influence of testosterone, the male larynx enlarges and the vocal cords become longer and thicker. The larger vocal cords deepen the male voice. Changes in the larynx and vocal cords cause the boy's voice to "break" as he matures into a young man. In an earlier period in history, young choir boys with beautiful high voices were castrated. Castration, the surgical excision

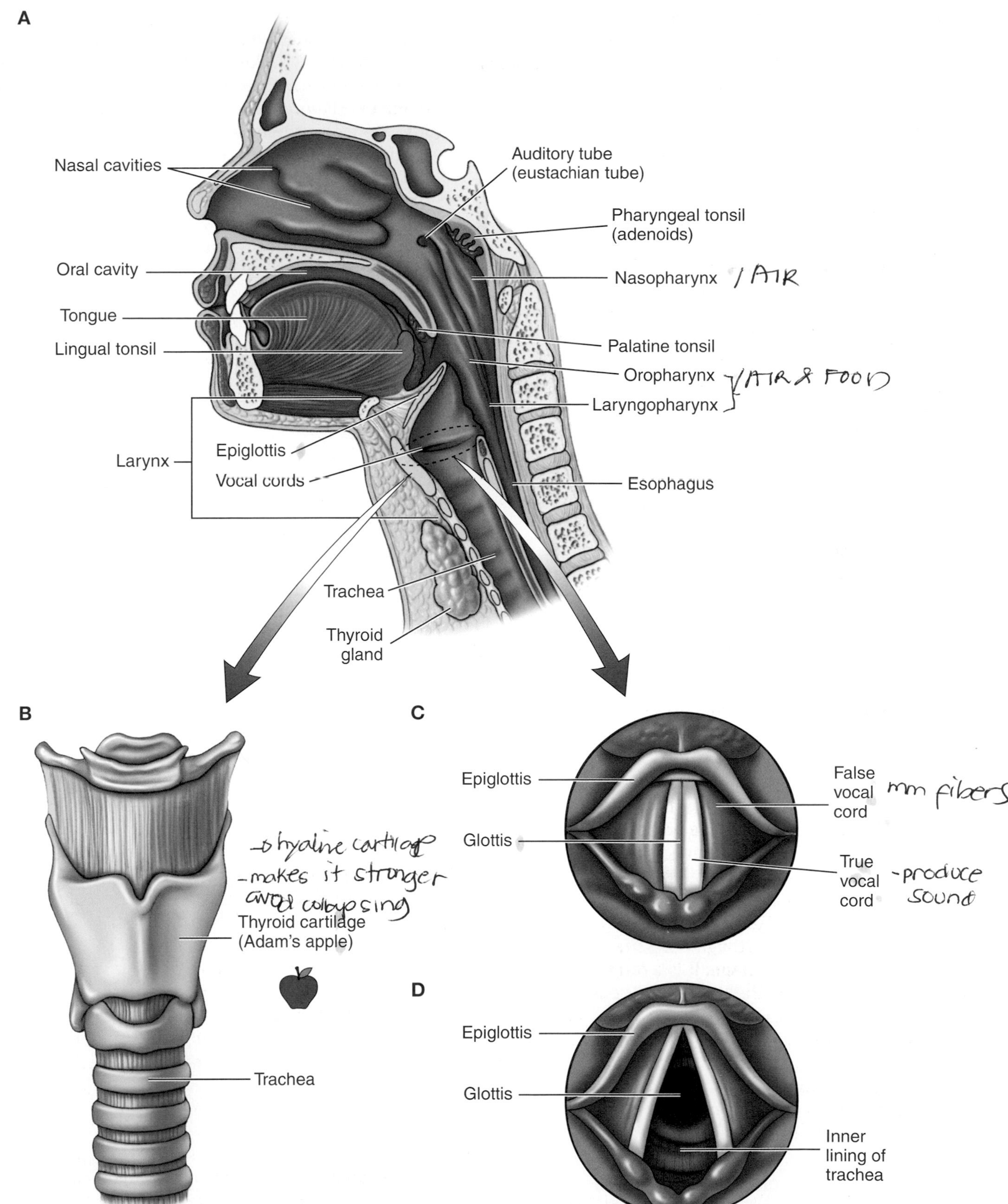

FIGURE 22-2 **A,** Organs of the upper respiratory tract. **B,** Larynx showing the thyroid cartilage (Adam's apple). **C,** Vocal cords and glottis (closed). **D,** Vocal cords and glottis (open).

Do You Know...

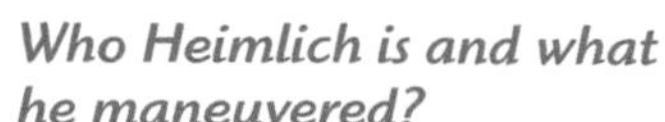

Who Heimlich is and what he maneuvered?

Dr. Heimlich is a physician who developed a procedure designed to dislodge the obstructing object in a choking person. The Heimlich maneuver, or abdominal thrust, is a simple technique. The "bear hug" procedure is demonstrated on an adult below. Here are the steps for the adult:

1. Stand behind the choking person and wrap your arms around the person's waist.
2. Position your hands (fist position) between the person's navel and the bottom of the rib cage.
3. Press your fist into the abdomen with a quick upward movement.
4. Repeat several times as necessary.

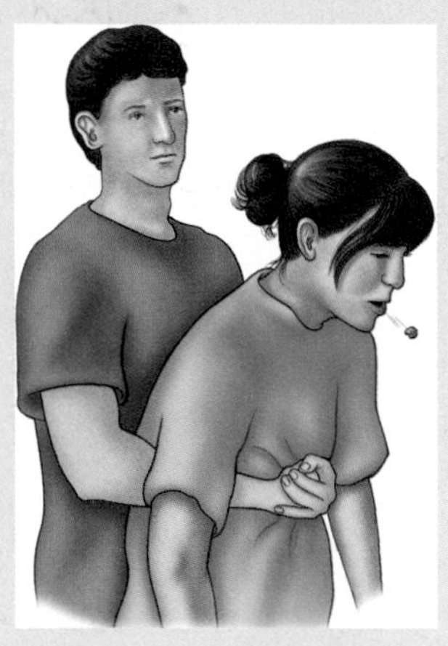

of the testes, removes the source of testosterone and prevents thickening of the vocal cords. These unfortunate, castrated boys continued to sing beautifully as members of the castrati choir. For obvious reasons, this practice eventually disappeared.

Do You Know...

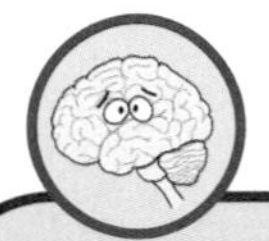

How "dumb plant" was used to control gossip (without, of course, killing the gossiper)?

A tea made from dieffenbachia ("dumb plant") was given to Roman slaves before they were sent to the market to shop. The tea caused the slave's tongue and mouth to swell and paralyzed the throat. The slave was therefore unable to speak and gossip about household affairs. It is still used by some African tribes as a punishment for gossip. An overdose of the poison causes excessive swelling, obstruction of the respiratory passageways, and death by suffocation.

TRACHEA

Where It Sits and Where It Splits

The **trachea** (TRĀ-kē-ă), or windpipe, is a tube 4 to 5 inches (10 to 12.5 cm) long and 1 inch (2.5 cm) in diameter (Figure 22-3). The trachea extends from the lower edge of the larynx downward into the thoracic cavity, where it splits into the right and left bronchi (singular: **bronchus** [BRŎNG-kŭs]). The trachea splits, or bifurcates, at a point called the **carina** at the manubriosternal junction (where the manubrium of the sternum meets the sternal body). Why is the carina so

Do You Know...

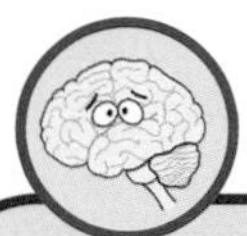

What a tracheostomy is?

Sometimes a part of the upper respiratory tract becomes blocked, thereby obstructing the flow of air into the lungs. To restore airflow, an emergency tracheostomy may be performed. This procedure is the insertion of a tube through a surgical incision into the trachea below the level of the obstruction. The tracheostomy bypasses the obstruction and allows air to flow through the tube into the lungs.

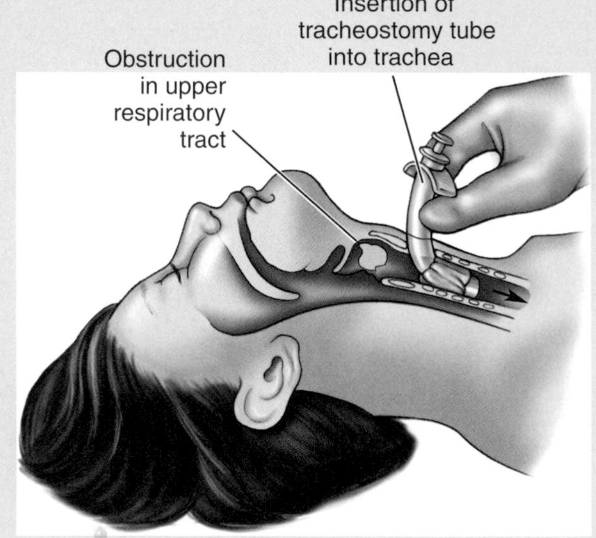

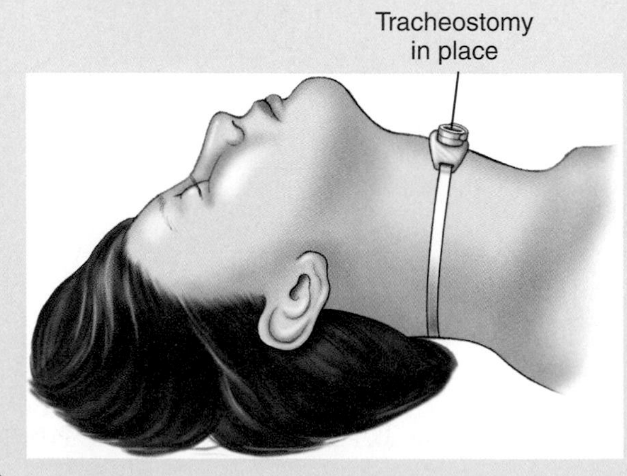

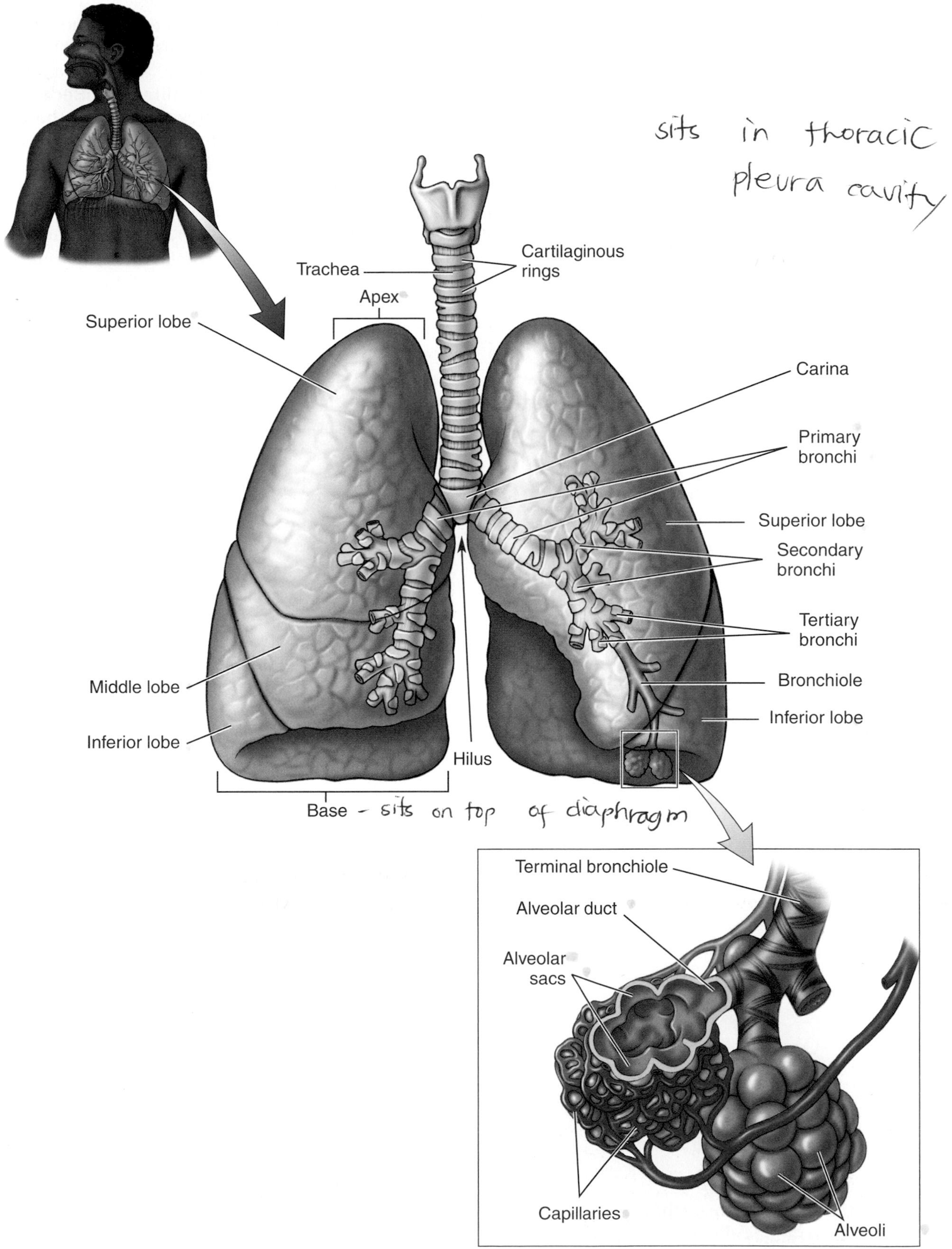

FIGURE 22-3 Trachea and bronchial tree (bronchi, bronchioles, and alveoli).

important clinically? The carina is very sensitive; touching it during suctioning causes vigorous coughing. The trachea conducts air to and from the lungs.

Keeping It Open

The trachea lies in front of the esophagus, the food tube. C-shaped rings of cartilage partially surround the trachea for its entire length and serve to keep it open. The rings are open on the back side of the trachea so that the esophagus can bulge forward as food moves along the esophagus to the stomach. You can feel the cartilaginous rings if you run your fingers along the front of your neck. Without this strong cartilaginous support, the trachea would collapse and shut off the flow of air through the respiratory passages. Because of the cartilaginous rings, a tight collar or necktie does not collapse the trachea. A severe blow to the anterior neck, however, can crush the trachea and cause an acute respiratory obstruction.

Keeping It Closed

What is a tracheoesophageal (TE) fistula? Occasionally, an infant is born with an opening between the trachea (respiratory passage) and the esophagus (digestive passage). This condition is a tracheoesophageal fistula (TE fistula). When the infant eats, food enters the trachea and lungs through this fistula. When this condition occurs, the infant experiences severe respiratory distress with violent coughing and cyanosis. Surgical correction is necessary for survival. The trachea must remain closed to food and water.

BRONCHIAL TREE: BRONCHI, BRONCHIOLES, AND ALVEOLI

The bronchial tree consists of the bronchi, the bronchioles, and the alveoli. It is called a tree because the bronchi and their many branches resemble an upside-down tree. Most of the bronchial tree is in the lungs.

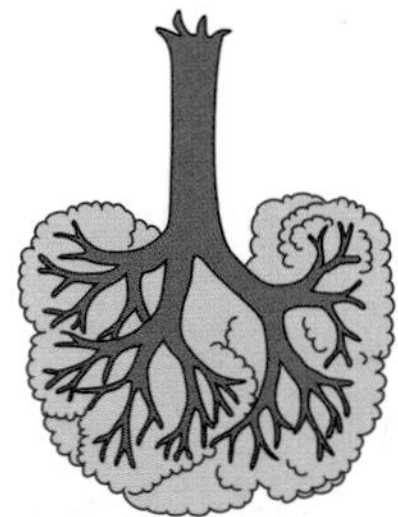

Bronchial tree

Bronchi

The right and left primary bronchi are formed as the lower part of the trachea divides into two tubes. The **primary bronchi** enter the lungs at a region called the **hilus.** The primary bronchi branch into **secondary bronchi,** which branch into smaller **tertiary bronchi.** Because the heart lies toward the left side of the chest, the left bronchus is narrower and positioned more horizontally than the right bronchus. The right bronchus is shorter and wider than the left bronchus and extends downward in a more vertical direction. Because of the differences in the size and positioning of the bronchi, food particles and small objects are more easily inhaled, or aspirated, into the right bronchus.

Why are tiny toys not good for tiny tots? Young children generally put toys in their mouths. The tiny toy may become lodged in the larynx or bronchus, causing an acute respiratory obstruction. Unless relieved immediately the obstruction can be fatal.

The upper segments of the bronchi have C-shaped cartilaginous rings, which help to keep the bronchi open. As the bronchi extend into the lungs, however, the amount of cartilage decreases and finally disappears. The finer and more distal branches of the bronchi contain no cartilage.

Bronchioles

The bronchi divide repeatedly into smaller tubes called **bronchioles.** The walls of the bronchioles contain smooth muscle and no cartilage. The bronchioles regulate the flow of air to the alveoli. Contraction of the bronchiolar smooth muscle causes the bronchioles to constrict, thereby decreasing the bronchiolar lumen (opening) and so decreasing the flow of air. Relaxation of the bronchioles causes the lumen to increase, thereby increasing the flow of air.

An asthma attack illustrates the effect of bronchiolar smooth muscle constriction. In a person with asthma, the bronchioles hyperrespond to a particular stimulus. The bronchiolar smooth muscle then constricts, decreasing the flow of air into the lungs. The person complains of a tight chest and expends much energy trying to force air through the constricted bronchioles into the lungs. Forced air causes a wheezing sound. Bronchiolar smooth muscle relaxants are medications that cause bronchodilation, thereby improving airflow and relieving the wheezing.

Translation into autonomic pharmacology. The bronchioles contain $beta_2$-adrenergic receptors. Stimulation of these receptors causes relaxation of the bronchiolar smooth muscle, thus inducing bronchodilation and improved airflow. Albuterol, a $beta_2$-adrenergic agonist, is a bronchodilator drug.

Alveoli

The bronchioles continue to divide and give rise to many tubes called **alveolar ducts** (see Figure 22-3). These ducts end in very small, grape-like structures called alveoli (singular: **alveolus** [ăl-VĒ-ō-lŭs]). The alveoli are tiny air sacs that form at the ends of the respiratory passages. A pulmonary capillary surrounds each alveolus. The alveoli function to exchange oxygen and carbon dioxide across the alveolar-pulmonary capillary membrane. The term atelectasis refers to collapsed and airless alveoli. Atelectasis occurs commonly as a postoperative complication and secondary to conditions such as pneumonia and cancer of the lung.

Do You Know...

Why you may diagnose cystic fibrosis by kissing your baby's face?

Cystic fibrosis (CF) is a hereditary disease that is characterized by thickened secretions of most exocrine glands. Consequently CF affects many organs including the liver, pancreas, and especially the lungs. The production of thick bronchial secretions is of particular concern because the secretions block narrow breathing passages, causing atelectasis and pulmonary infections. Eventually lung tissue is destroyed; for this reason the clinical picture of CF is dominated by lung dysfunction. In addition, sweat glands and salivary glands produce a very salty secretion; mothers often notice the salty taste of their infants upon kissing them.

Certain respiratory diseases may destroy alveoli or cause a thickening of the alveolar wall. As a result, the exchange of gases is slowed. Oxygenation of the blood may decrease, causing hypoxemia, and the blood may retain carbon dioxide, causing a disturbance in acid-base balance (acidosis).

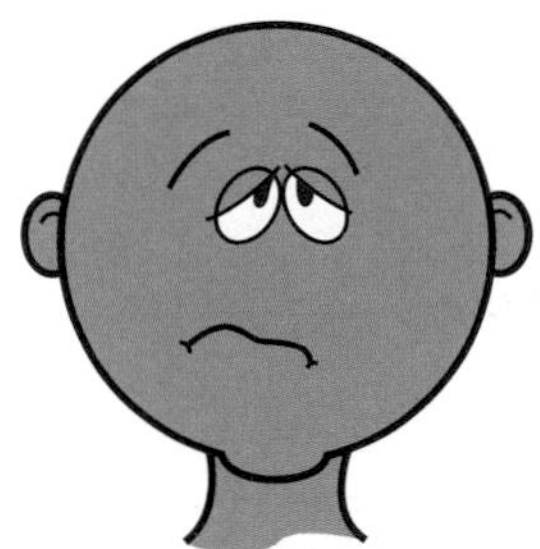

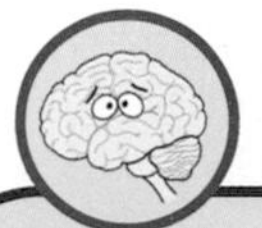

Do You Know...

Why your fingers go "clubbing"?

Patients who experience chronic hypoxemia, such as those with emphysema, often develop clubbing of the fingers and toes. Clubbing is characterized by enlarged fingertips and toes and changes in the thickness and shape of the nails. The enlargement is due to the formation of additional capillaries and tissue hypertrophy in an attempt to deliver oxygen to the O_2-deprived cells.

LUNGS

Right and Left

The two **lungs,** located in the pleural cavities, extend from an area just above the clavicles to the diaphragm. The lungs are soft, cone-shaped organs so large that they occupy most of the space in the thoracic cavity (see Figure 22-3). The lungs are subdivided into lobes. The right lung has three lobes: the superior, middle, and inferior lobes. Because of the location of the heart in the left side of the chest, the left lung has only two lobes: the superior lobe and the inferior lobe.

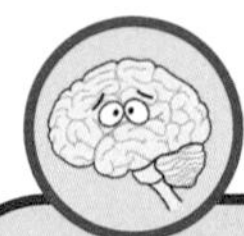

Do You Know...

About the lungs as giant fans?

According to Plato and Aristotle, the life force was contained in the heat of the body. The heat was thought to be produced by a fire that burned within the heart. The intracardiac fire was called the *flamma vitalis.* This fire, however, could burn too hot, go out of control, and cause disease. Enter the lungs! It was initially believed that the lungs acted as giant fans that cooled the flame and prevented excessive bubbling of the blood. Despite the genius of Plato and Aristotle, none of this fan stuff is true.

Top and Bottom

The upper, rounded part of the lung is called the **apex,** and the lower portion is called the **base.** The base of the lung rests on the diaphragm. The lungs contain the bronchial trees.

The amount of air the lungs can hold varies with a person's body build, age, and physical conditioning. For instance, a tall person has larger lungs than a short person. A swimmer generally has larger lungs than a "couch potato." And the trained singer has larger lungs than the singer whose talents are heard only in the shower.

PLEURAL MEMBRANES

Pleura

The outside of each lung and the inner chest wall are lined with a continuous serous membrane called the **pleura** (Figure 22-4). The pleura are named according to their location. The membrane on the outer surface of each lung is called the visceral pleura. The membrane lining the chest wall is called the parietal pleura. The visceral pleura and the parietal pleura are attracted to each other like two flat plates of glass whose surfaces are wet. The plates of glass can slide past one another but offer some resistance when you try to pull them apart.

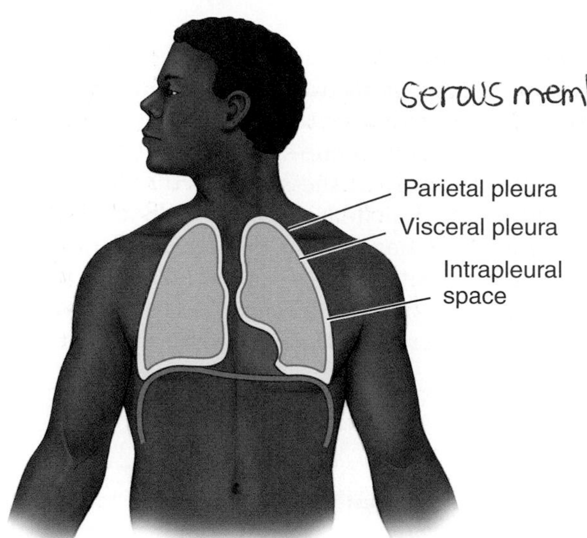

FIGURE 22-4 Lungs, pleural membranes, and the intrapleural space.

Pleural Cavity: A Potential Space

Between the visceral pleura and the parietal pleura is a space called the **intrapleural space,** or **pleural cavity.** The pleural membranes secrete a small amount of serous fluid (approximately 25 ml). The fluid lubricates the pleural membranes and allows them to slide past one another with little friction or discomfort. Under abnormal conditions, the intrapleural space has the potential to accumulate excess fluid, blood, and air. An excess secretion of pleural fluid is called pleural effusion. Purulent (pus) pleural effusion is called empyema.

> **Sum It Up!**
>
> Air moves through the following structures: from the nasal cavities, to the pharynx, to the larynx, to the trachea, to the bronchi, to the bronchioles, and to the alveoli. When the air reaches the alveoli, the tiny air sacs at the end of the bronchial tree, the respiratory gases, oxygen and carbon dioxide, diffuse across the alveolar-pulmonary capillary membrane. Most of the respiratory structures conduct air to and from the lungs. Only the alveoli function in the exchange of the respiratory gases between the outside air and the blood. The lungs contain the structures of the lower respiratory tract. Pleural membranes surround the lungs and line the thoracic cavity, creating the intrapleural space or pleural cavity.

COLLAPSED AND EXPANDED LUNGS

Figure 22-4 shows that the lungs occupy most of the thoracic cage, but this statement must be qualified: the *expanded* lungs occupy most of the thoracic cage. Under normal conditions, the lungs expand like inflated balloons. Under certain abnormal conditions, however, a lung may collapse. What determines whether or not the lungs collapse or expand?

WHY LUNGS COLLAPSE

If the thoracic cavity is entered surgically, the lungs collapse. There are two reasons that the lungs collapse: elastic recoil and surface tension.

Elastic Recoil

Consider a balloon and a lung (Figure 22-5, *A*). If you blow up a balloon but fail to tie off the open end, the

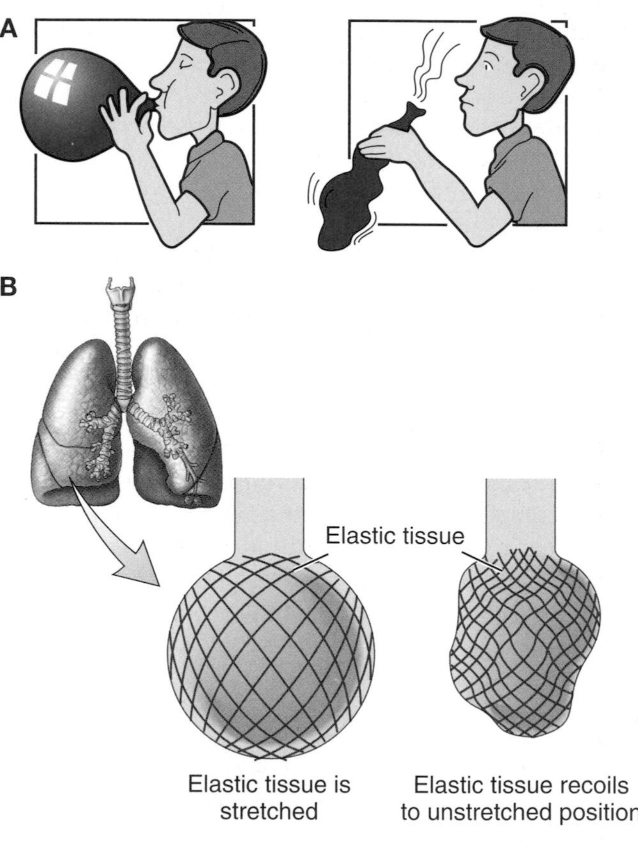

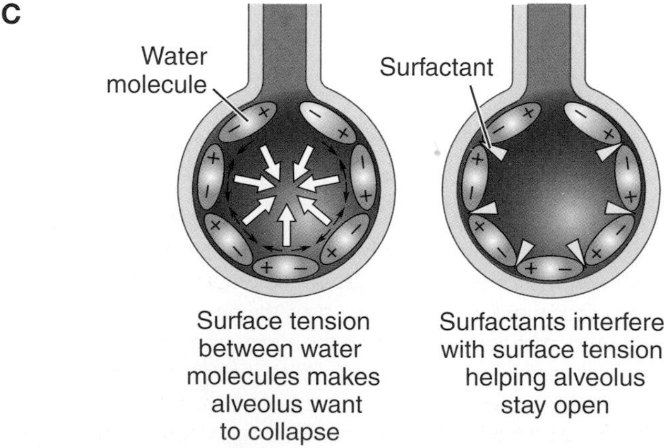

FIGURE 22-5 **A** and **B,** Elastic recoil. **C,** Surface tension: water and the effect of surfactants.

air rushes out, and the balloon collapses. It collapses because of the arrangement of its elastic fibers. When these fibers stretch, they remain stretched only when tension is applied (the air blown into the balloon stretches the balloon). If the end of the balloon is not tied off, the elastic fibers recoil, forcing air out and collapsing the balloon. The same can be said of the lung. The arrangement of the lung's elastic tissue is similar to the arrangement of the elastic fibers in the balloon. The elastic tissue of the lung can stretch, but it recoils and returns to its unstretched position if tension is released (see Figure 22-5, *B*). This is called elastic recoil.

Surface Tension

The lung can also collapse for a second reason, a force called **surface tension.** The single alveolus in Figure 22-5, *C*, illustrates surface tension. A thin layer of water lines the inside of the alveolus. Water is a polar molecule; one end of the water molecule has a positive (+) charge, while the other end of the molecule has a negative (–) charge. Note how the water molecules line up. The positive (+) end of one water molecule is attracted to the negative (–) charge on the second water molecule. Each water molecule pulls on the other. The electrical attraction of the water molecules is the surface tension. As the water molecules pull on one another, they tend to make the alveolus smaller; in other words, they collapse the alveoli.

NOTE: The surface tension of pure water is normally very high. In the mature, normal lung, certain cells secrete pulmonary surfactants. **Surfactants** (sŭr-FĂK-tănts) are lipoproteins secreted by special alveolar cells. Pulmonary surfactants are like detergents. They decrease surface tension by interfering with the electrical attraction between the water molecules on the inner surface of the alveolus (see Figure 22-5, *C*). The secretion of surfactant is stimulated by a sigh. After every 5-6 breaths, a person takes a larger-than-normal breath (a sigh); the sigh stretches the alveoli promoting the secretion of surfactant. Surfactants lower surface tension but do not eliminate it. Surface tension remains a force that acts to collapse the alveoli.

Do You Know...

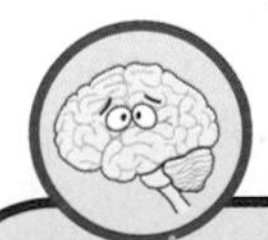

Why a premature infant is more apt than a full-term infant to develop respiratory distress syndrome?

Surfactant-secreting cells appear only during the later stages of fetal development. An infant born 2 to 3 months prematurely generally has insufficient surfactant-secreting cells. As a result, surface tension within the alveoli is excessively high, the alveoli collapse, and the infant experiences respiratory distress. The infant may die in respiratory failure. This condition is commonly called respiratory distress syndrome. Premature infants are given surfactants through inhalation in an attempt to prevent this life-threatening condition.

WHY LUNGS EXPAND

If elastic recoil and surface tension collapse the lungs, why do they remain expanded in the normal closed thorax? Lung expansion depends on pressure within the intrapleural space. A series of diagrams in Figure 22-6 illustrates this point. In Figure 22-6, *A,* the three pressures are labeled P1, P2, and P3. P1 is the pressure outside the chest (the pressure in the room), also called the atmospheric pressure. P2 is the pressure in the lung; it is called the **intrapulmonic pressure.** P3 is the pressure in the intrapleural space, also called the

Do You Know...

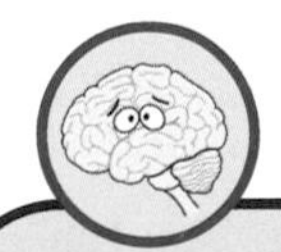

Why this person's chest looks like a barrel?

This person has emphysema, a condition characterized by damaged tissue in the lower respiratory structures and overinflated alveoli. As a result the lungs cannot exhale the proper amount of air, and the air remains trapped in the alveoli. (*Emphysema* means "puffed up" alveoli.) Consequently, the alveoli and lungs become overinflated and cause the chest to be shaped like a barrel. A person with severe emphysema is described as barrel-chested.

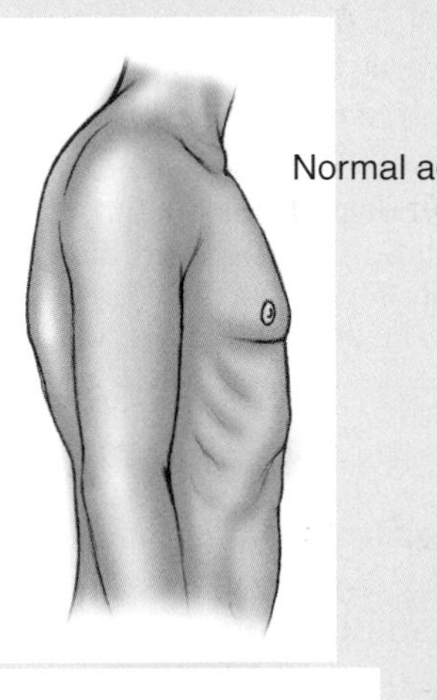

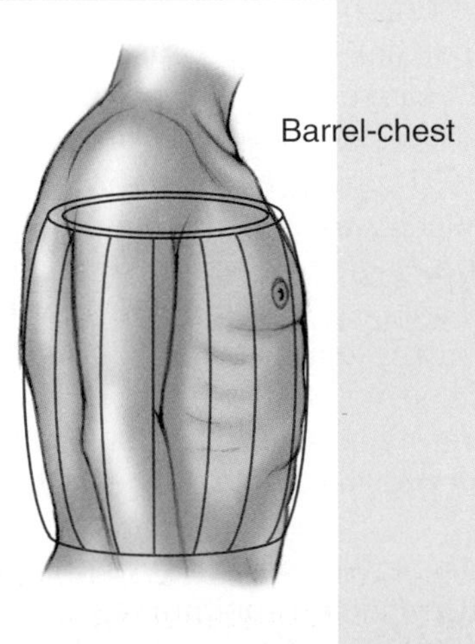

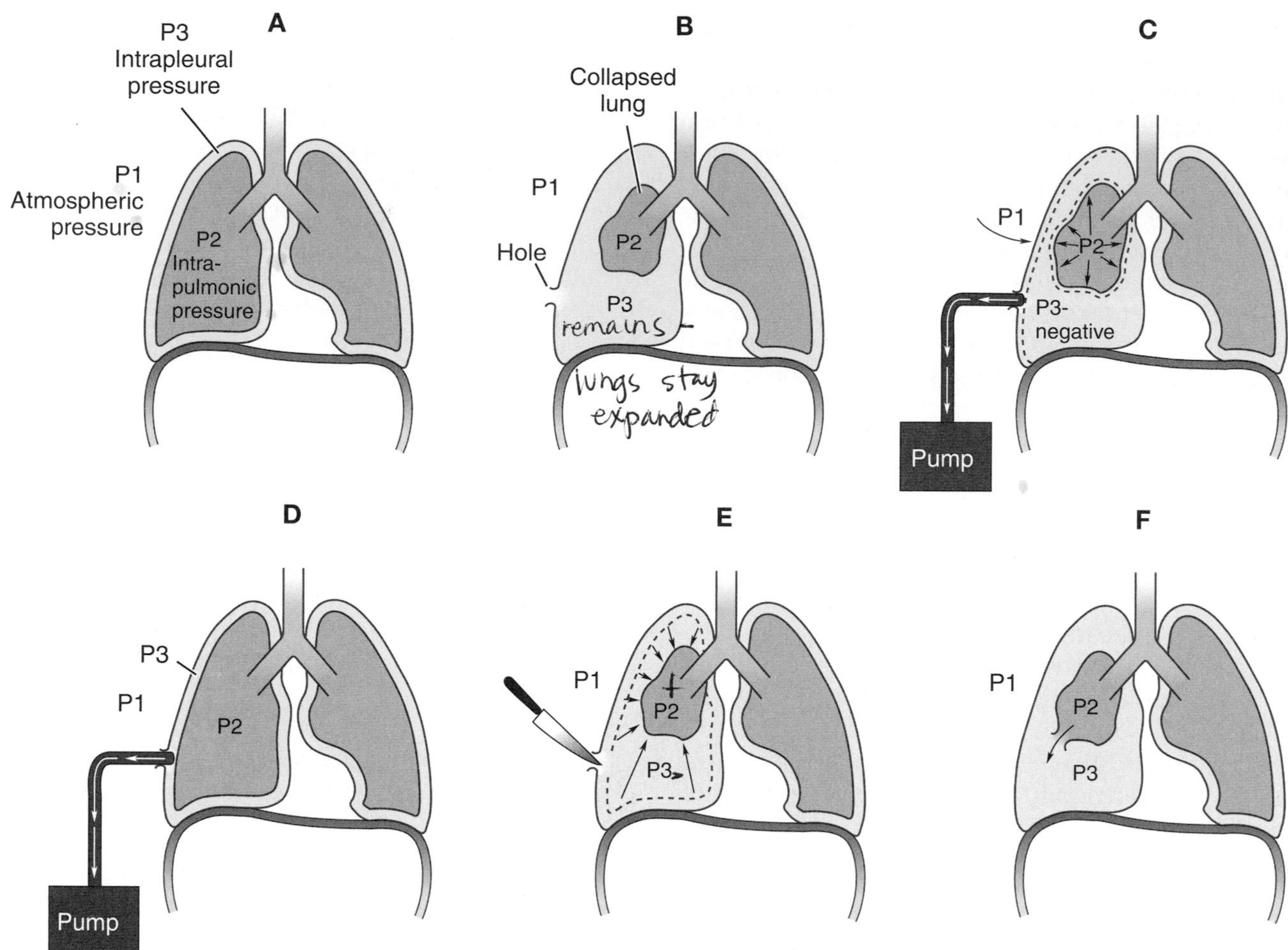

FIGURE 22-6 Lung expansion and collapse. **A,** The lungs expand. **B,** The right lung collapses because of the hole in the chest wall. **C,** Air is pumped out of the intrapleural space, creating a negative intrapleural pressure. **D,** The lung expands because of the negative intrapleural pressure. **E,** The lung collapses because of the hole (knife wound) in the chest wall. **F,** The lung collapses because of a hole in the lung.

intrapleural pressure. Note in Figure 22-6, *A,* that the lungs are normally expanded.

Figure 22-6, *B* and *C,* explain why the lungs expand. To illustrate this point, a hole is created in the right chest wall so that the right lung collapses. Note the pressures. Because of the hole in the chest wall, all the pressures are equal. In other words, P1 = P2 = P3. In Figure 22-6, *C,* a tube is inserted through the hole of the right chest wall into the intrapleural space. The tube is attached to a pump, which removes air from the intrapleural space. As air moves from the intrapleural space, the intrapleural pressure (P3) decreases and becomes negative. This negative intrapleural pressure (P3) merely means that it is less than either the atmospheric pressure (P1) or the intrapulmonic pressure (P2).

What is the effect of a negative intrapleural pressure? Because P2 (intrapulmonic pressure) is greater than P3 (intrapleural pressure), the lung is pushed toward the chest wall, causing the lung to expand. Also, because P1 (atmospheric pressure) is greater than P3, the chest wall is pushed inward toward the lung. When the chest wall and the lungs meet, the lung is expanded (see Figure 22-6, *C* and *D*). The important point is this: the lung expands and remains expanded because the intrapleural pressure is negative.

What happens if the pump is removed, thereby recreating the hole in the chest wall? Because P1 is greater than P3, air rushes into the intrapleural space through the hole and eliminates the negative intrapleural pressure. As a result, the lung collapses. Remember: the lung expands only when the intrapleural pressure is negative.

Figure 22-6, *E,* illustrates the effects of a stab wound to the chest. The hole created by the knife allows the air to rush into the intrapleural space and eliminate the negative intrapleural pressure. The introduction of air into the intrapleural space and subsequent collapse of the lung is called a pneumothorax (*pneumo* means air; *thorax* means chest). Air in the intrapleural space is also the reason that the lungs collapse when a surgical incision is made into the chest wall.

Figure 22-6, *F*, shows the effect of a hole in the lung. Because the intrapulmonic pressure (P2) is greater than the intrapleural pressure (P3), air rushes into the intrapleural space through the hole in the lung, thereby eliminating the negative intrapleural pressure and collapsing the lung. Sometimes people with emphysema develop blebs, or blisters, on the outer surface of their lungs. The blebs rupture and create a hole between the intrapulmonic and the intrapleural spaces, causing air to rush into the intrapleural space and collapsing the lung.

What can be done for a collapsed lung? The physician inserts a tube through the chest wall into the intrapleural space and pulls air out of the intrapleural space. As the air leaves the intrapleural space, negative pressure is reestablished, and the lung expands. Sometimes the physician inserts a large needle into the intrapleural space to aspirate, or withdraw, air, blood, and pus. This procedure is called a thoracentesis. It facilitates lung expansion. NOTE: The intrapleural pressure remains negative only when no hole exists in either the chest wall or the lungs.

SAYING IT ANOTHER WAY: COMPLIANCE

Compliance is the measure of elastic recoil and is illustrated by two balloons. One balloon has never been inflated and is stiff. A second balloon has been inflated many times and has lost some of its elasticity (elastic recoil); it appears baggy. Which balloon is easier to inflate? The baggy balloon is easier to inflate because it has lost some of its elasticity and is less stiff. Translation: the baggy balloon is more compliant (stretchy). The new balloon is less compliant (stiff) and is therefore more difficult to inflate. Which balloon expels air more efficiently? The new balloon expels air more efficiently because it has a greater elastic recoil.

Same with the lungs. When lung compliance decreases (stiff lungs) the lungs are more difficult to inflate. Some conditions that are associated with decreased lung compliance are pulmonary edema, respiratory distress syndrome, and pulmonary fibrosis. Decreased lung compliance is not good.

What about increased lung compliance? Lungs that are too stretchy also cause problems. For instance, the patient with emphysema has damaged lung structure and minimal elastic recoil. Lung compliance has increased too much; there is not enough elastic recoil to completely expel air on exhalation. The increased compliance also contributes to the formation of the barrel-chest appearance that characterizes a person with chronic lung disease.

Sum It Up!

The expanded lungs normally fill the thoracic cavity. Unless pressure conditions in the pleural cavity are correct, the lungs collapse. The tendency of the lungs to collapse is due to two factors: elastic recoil and the alveolar surface tension. The expansion of the lungs is due to a negative intrapleural pressure within the chest cavity. If the negative intrapleural pressure is eliminated, the lungs collapse.

RESPIRATORY FUNCTION

THREE STEPS IN RESPIRATION

Most of us equate breathing with respiration. Respiration includes breathing, but it is more than breathing; it involves the entire process of gas exchange between the atmosphere and the body cells. Respiration includes the following three steps:

- Ventilation, or breathing
- Exchange of oxygen and carbon dioxide
- Transport of oxygen and carbon dioxide by the blood

Ventilation or Breathing

What It Is. Movement of air into and out of the lungs is called **ventilation;** it is more commonly called breathing. Two phases of ventilation are **inhalation** and **exhalation.** Inhalation, also called inspiration, is the breathing-in phase. During inhalation, oxygen-rich air moves into tiny air sacs in the lungs. Exhalation, also called expiration, is the breathing-out phase. During exhalation, air rich in carbon dioxide is moved out of the lungs. One inhalation and one exhalation make up one **respiratory cycle.**

Boyle's Law: Pressure and Volume. To understand ventilation, you need some background information. You need to know the relationship between pressure and volume, a relationship called **Boyle's law.** Note the two tubes in Figure 22-7. Tube A is a small tube that fits into a bicycle tire. When filled, the tube can hold 1 liter (L) of air. Tube B is larger and fits into a truck tire. When filled, it can hold 10 L of air. Thus the volume of the truck tube (B) is 10 times greater than the volume of the bicycle tube (A).

In the upper panel of Figure 22-7, both tubes are empty. Let's add 1 L of air to each tube and measure the pressure in each tube. By touching the surfaces of the tubes, you can get a rough estimate of the pressures. Tube A feels firm, whereas tube B feels soft. In other words, the pressure in tube A is greater than the pressure in tube B. Both tubes received the same amount of air, so why are the pressures different? The different

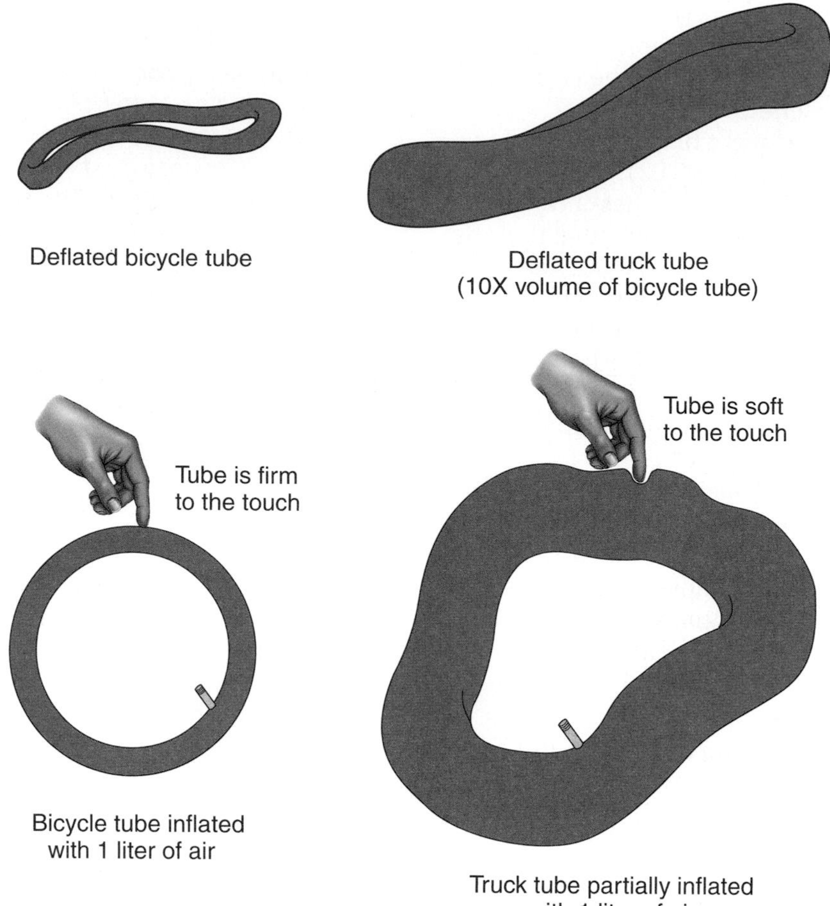

FIGURE 22-7 Boyle's law: relationship between pressure and volume.

volumes of the tubes cause the different pressures. The pressure is higher in tube A because the volume of tube A is small; 1 L of air completely fills the tube. The pressure in tube B is lower because its volume is large (10 L). One liter of air only partially fills the truck tube. The smaller the volume, the higher the pressure, or the greater the volume, the lower the pressure. If volume changes, the pressure changes. This is Boyle's law, the principle upon which ventilation is based.

Boyle's Law and Breathing. What does Boyle's law have to do with ventilation? On inhalation (breathing in), air flows into the lungs. What is the force that causes the air to flow in? Place your hands on your rib cage. Inhale. Notice that the thoracic cage moves up and out on inhalation (Figure 22-8, *A* and *C*). This movement increases the volume of the thoracic cavity and lungs. As the volume in the lung increases, the pressure in the lung (P2) decreases (satisfying Boyle's law). As a result, P2 becomes less than P1 (atmospheric pressure, the air you breathe). Air flows from high pressure to low pressure, through the nose into the lungs.

What happens on exhalation? Another change in lung volume. Place your hands on your rib cage and exhale. The thoracic and lung volumes decrease as the rib cage returns to its resting position (see Figure 22-8, *B* and *D*). The decreased lung volume causes the pressure within the lungs (P2) to increase. Now P2 is greater than P1, and air flows out of the lungs through the nose. Let us clarify the relationship between Boyle's law and ventilation.

Do You Know...

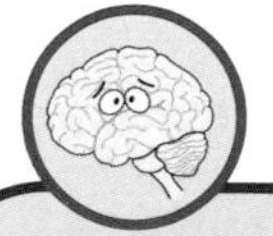

What a boa constrictor knows about ventilation?

Your friendly boa constrictor knows all about Boyle's law—that in order to inhale air, the victim must increase chest volume. Using this knowledge, Boa wraps itself around the victim's chest. During exhalation when chest diameter decreases, Boa further constricts, thereby preventing chest expansion and inhalation (Boyle's law). The victim soon suffocates, and our reptilian friend dines for days. "Get a grip" sums up the hunting technique of the boa. And if Boa can figure out Boyle's law, so can you!

- Air flows in response to changes in pressure. As the lung volume increases on inhalation, the intrapulmonic pressure (P2) decreases, and air flows into the lungs.

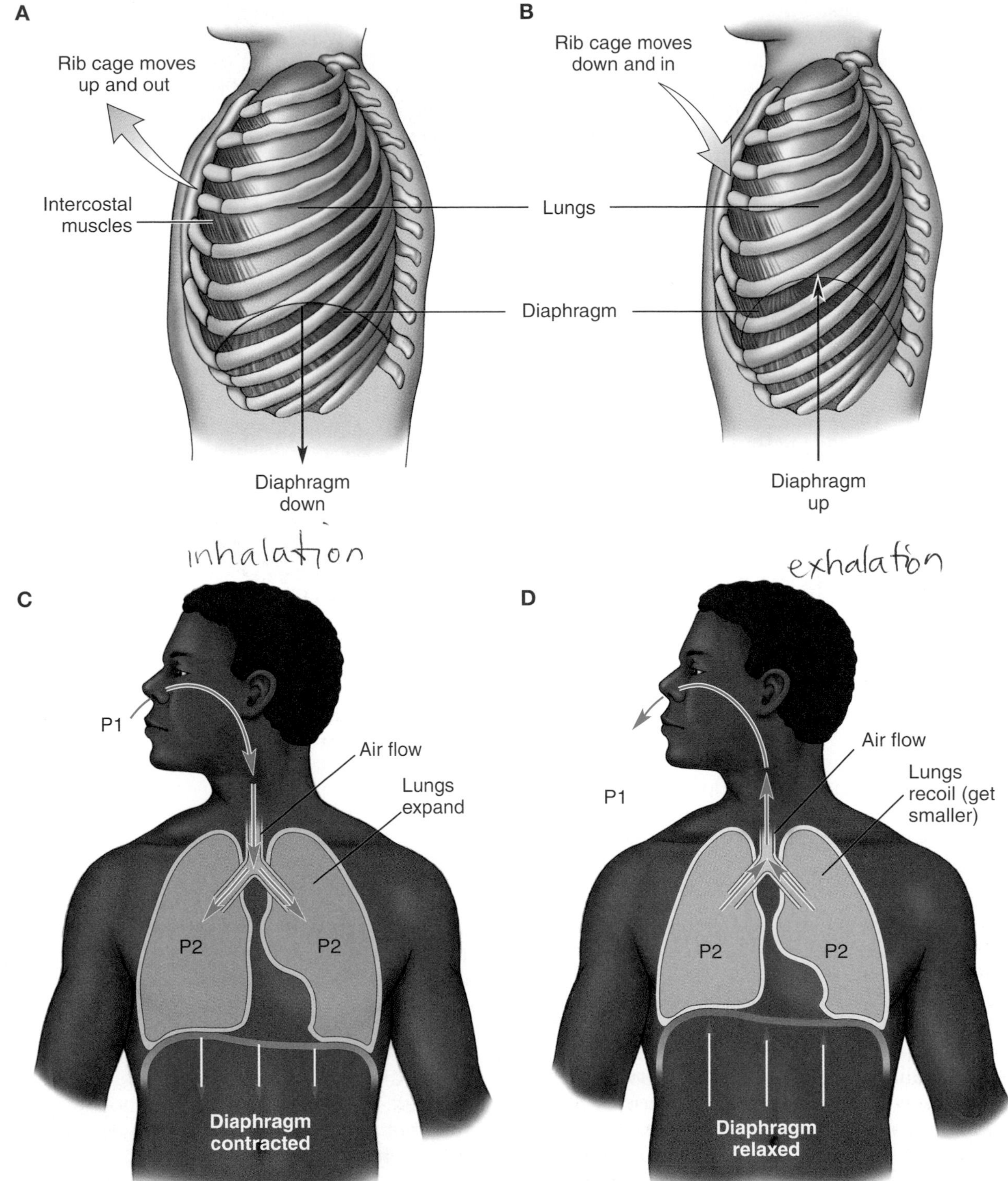

FIGURE 22-8 Inhalation and exhalation. The thoracic volume increases, and air rushes into the lungs (**A** and **C**). The thoracic volume decreases, and air rushes out of the lungs (**B** and **D**).

- On exhalation, lung volume decreases, intrapulmonic pressure (P2) increases, and air flows out of the lungs.
- Air flows in response to pressure changes. Pressure changes occur in response to changes in volume. Inhalation is associated with an increase in thoracic volume; exhalation is associated with a decrease in thoracic volume.

The Muscles of Respiration. What causes the thoracic volume to change? The change in thoracic volume is due to the contraction and relaxation of the respiratory muscles. On inhalation, the respiratory muscles,

diaphragm, and **intercostal muscles** contract (see Figure 22-8, *A* and *C*). The diaphragm is a dome-shaped muscle that forms the floor of the thoracic cavity and separates the thoracic cavity from the abdominal cavity. The diaphragm is the chief muscle of inspiration. Contraction of the diaphragm flattens the muscle and pulls it downward, toward the abdomen. This movement increases the length of the thoracic cavity. During quiet breathing, the diaphragm accounts for most of the increase in the thoracic volume.

The two intercostal muscles, the external and internal intercostals, are between the ribs. When the external intercostal muscles contract, the rib cage moves up and out, thereby increasing the width of the thoracic cavity. Note that the size of the thoracic cavity increases in three directions: from front to back, from side to side, and lengthwise. Why is this increase in thoracic volume so important? As the thoracic volume increases, so does the volume of the lungs. According to Boyle's law, the increase in volume decreases the pressure in the lungs, and as a result, air flows into the lungs. Some of the accessory muscles of respiration, located in the neck and chest, can move the rib cage even further during exertion.

On exhalation, the muscles of respiration relax and allow the ribs and the diaphragm to return to their original positions (see Figure 22-8, *B* and *D*). This movement decreases thoracic and lung volume and increases pressure in the lungs. Consequently, air flows out of the lungs. Elastic recoil of lung tissue and surface tension within the alveoli aid with exhalation. Forced exhalation uses the **accessory muscles of respiration.** These include the muscles of the abdominal wall and the internal intercostal muscles. Contraction of the accessory muscles of respiration pulls the bottom of the rib cage down and in, and it forces the abdominal viscera upward toward the relaxed diaphragm. These actions force additional air out of the lungs.

How much energy does it take to breathe? Inhalation is due to the contraction of the respiratory muscles. It is an active process. The muscles use up energy (ATP) as they contract. Exhalation associated with normal quiet breathing is passive. Exhalation is due to muscle relaxation; no energy is required for muscle relaxation. Thus in normal quiet breathing, we use up energy during half of the respiratory cycle, inhalation. We rest on exhalation. During forced exhalation (as in exercise), however, the accessory muscles of respiration must contract, and exhalation becomes energy-using, or active.

With certain lung diseases such as emphysema, exhalation can be achieved only when the accessory muscles of respiration are used. The patient with emphysema therefore uses energy during both inhalation and exhalation. This process is physically exhausting, and these patients usually complain of being very tired.

Nerves That Supply the Respiratory Muscles. Ventilation occurs in response to changes in the thoracic volume, and the changes in thoracic volume are due to muscle contraction and relaxation. The respiratory muscles, being skeletal muscles, must be stimulated by motor nerves in order to contract. The motor nerves supplying the respiratory muscles are the **phrenic nerve** and the **intercostal nerves.** The phrenic nerve exits from the spinal cord at the level of C4, travels within the cervical plexus, and is distributed to the diaphragm. Firing of the phrenic nerve stimulates the diaphragm to contract. The intercostal nerves supply the intercostal muscles. Thus inhalation is initiated by the firing of the phrenic and intercostal nerves.

Do You Know...

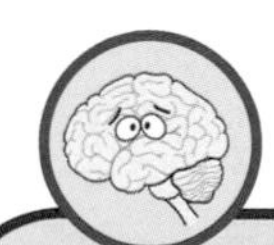

If a boa constrictor knows more about Boyle's law than the early corset makers?

The boa knows that by wrapping itself around an animal's chest, it can suffocate the victim by preventing chest expansion and inhalation (Boyle's law). The early corset makers, however, lacked or ignored this basic information. Corsets were designed to constrict the waist—the tighter the corset, the smaller the waist. A successfully corseted young lady might boast of a 12-inch-diameter waist! Problem was, the upper part of the corset included the lower part of the rib cage. What was the result of this constant binding? The corset prevented adequate ventilation and caused a permanent deformity of the rib cage—to say nothing of the displaced abdominal organs. The corseted young lovely couldn't breathe and often fainted. Herein lies the physiologic basis of the swoon and delicate weakness that characterized wealthy young women. They were not weak because of their female X chromosomes; they were merely hypoxic—no oxygen going to the brain. Fortunately, only the wealthiest could make this fashion statement.

You will be caring for patients whose nerve-muscle function is impaired. For instance, if the spinal cord is severed above C4, the phrenic nerve cannot fire. As a result, the skeletal muscles cannot contract. The person not only is quadriplegic but also can breathe only with the assistance of a ventilator. Other patients experience difficulty in breathing because of the effects of certain drugs. Curare, for instance, is a drug commonly used during surgery to cause muscle relaxation. It is a neuromuscular blocking agent that interferes with the transmission of the electrical signal from nerve to muscle. The block occurs within the neuromuscular junction. The patient is not only unable to move the body voluntarily but also is unable to breathe.

Translation into Receptor Terminology. The receptors located on the muscle membrane within the neuromuscular junction are nicotinic (N_M) receptors.

Activation of the N_M receptors stimulates skeletal muscle contraction. Blockade of the N_M receptors by a drug such as curare or succinylcholine (Anectine) inhibits skeletal muscle contraction, causing paralysis (including the muscles of respiration). NOTE: The N_M receptors are cholinergic but not autonomic. (Review Chapter 12.)

Sum It Up!

The three steps in respiration are ventilation, exchange of oxygen and carbon dioxide in the lungs and the cells, and transport of oxygen and carbon dioxide by the blood. Ventilation occurs in response to changes in thoracic volumes, which in turn cause changes in intrapulmonic pressures. Inhalation occurs when the respiratory muscles contract and enlarge the thoracic cage. Exhalation occurs when the respiratory muscles relax, allowing the thorax to return to its smaller, resting thoracic volume. The muscles of respiration contract in response to stimulation of the phrenic and intercostal nerves.

Exchange of Oxygen and Carbon Dioxide

Inhalation delivers fresh oxygen-rich air to the alveoli, and exhalation removes carbon dioxide–laden air from the alveoli. The second step of respiration is the exchange of the respiratory gases. Exchange occurs at two sites: in the lungs and at the cells (Figure 22-9).

Why the Lungs Are Good Gas Exchangers. Gas exchange occurs in the lungs, specifically across the membranes of the alveolus and the pulmonary capillary. There are three conditions that make the alveoli well suited for the exchange of oxygen and carbon dioxide: a large surface area, thin alveolar and pulmonary capillary walls, and a short distance between the alveoli and the pulmonary capillaries.

- Large surface area. Millions of alveoli, approximately 350 million per lung, create a total surface area about one half the size of a tennis court. The large surface increases the amount of oxygen and carbon dioxide exchanged across the alveolar membranes.

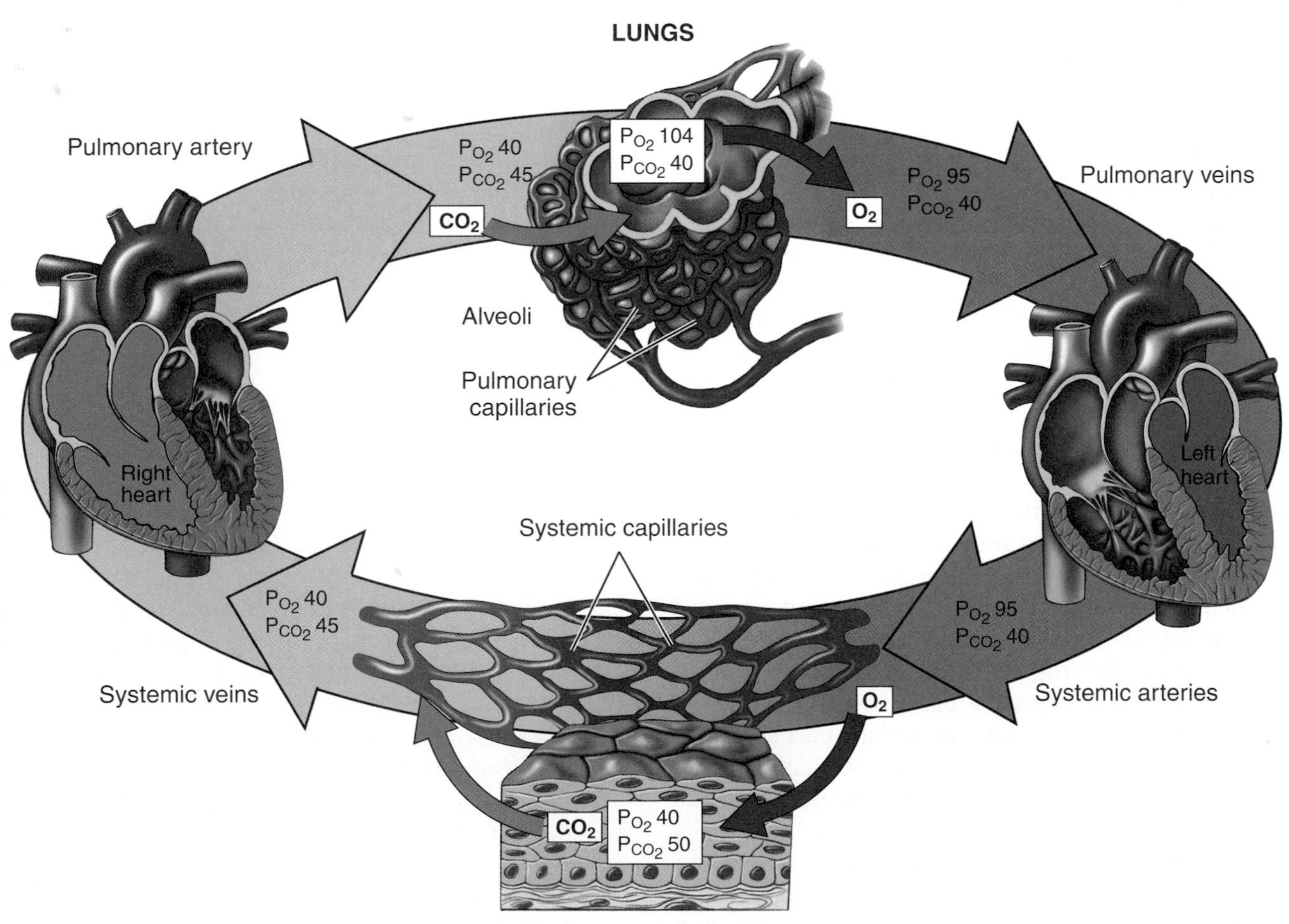

FIGURE 22-9 Partial pressures of oxygen and carbon dioxide within the lungs and at the cellular level.

- Thin alveolar and pulmonary capillary walls. The thin walls favor diffusion because they do not offer much resistance to the movement of oxygen and carbon dioxide across the membranes.
- Closeness of the alveoli to the pulmonary capillaries. Each alveolus is very close to a pulmonary capillary. For diffusion, closeness ensures a high rate of diffusion.

Partial Pressures and the Diffusion of Gases.

What Causes the Respiratory Gases to Diffuse? Chapter 3 describes how molecules diffuse from an area of greater concentration to an area of lesser concentration. For gases such as oxygen and carbon dioxide, however, concentration is related to pressure. When the molecules of a gas are highly concentrated, the gas creates a high pressure. Consequently, we can talk about diffusion from areas of high pressure to areas of low pressure.

Ordinary room air is a gas composed of 78% nitrogen, 21% oxygen, and 0.04% carbon dioxide. Each part of the gas contributes to the total pressure. The amount of pressure each gas contributes is called the **partial pressure.** The partial pressure of oxygen is symbolized as Po_2; the partial pressure of carbon dioxide is symbolized as Pco_2. (Because the body does not use nitrogen gas, we can ignore it.)

Partial Pressures Within the Lungs. Let us analyze the partial pressures of the respiratory gases in the alveoli and the pulmonary capillary (see Figure 22-9). The Po_2 of air in the alveoli is 104 mm Hg, whereas the Po_2 of venous blood (the blue end of the pulmonary capillary) is 40 mm Hg. Oxygen diffuses from the area of high pressure (the alveolus) to the area of low pressure (the pulmonary capillary). Note that the Po_2 in the blood goes from 40 mm Hg (blue) to 95 mm Hg (red). The partial pressure of oxygen increases because the blood has been oxygenated.

As for the waste, the carbon dioxide, the Pco_2 in the blood (blue capillary) is 45 mm Hg, while the Pco_2 in the alveolus is only 40 mm Hg. CO_2 diffuses from the capillary, the area of high pressure, to the alveolus, the area of low pressure. Because of the diffusion of CO_2 out of the blood, the Pco_2 of the blood goes from 45 mm Hg (the blue end of the capillary) to 40 mm Hg (the red end of the capillary). What has been accomplished? The blood coming from the right side of the heart (blue) has been oxygenated and the oxygenated blood (red) eventually returns to the left side of the heart so that it can be pumped throughout the body. As oxygenation occurs, CO_2 has been removed; it leaves the lungs during exhalation.

Partial Pressure at the Cells. What happens to the gases at the tissues, or body cells? Two events occur. First, oxygen leaves the blood and diffuses into the cells, where it can be used during cell metabolism. Second, carbon dioxide diffuses into the blood as metabolism occurs in the cell.

What partial pressures cause these events to happen? The Po_2 of the arterial blood is 95 mm Hg, whereas the cellular Po_2 is only 40 mm Hg. During gas exchange, oxygen diffuses from the blood into the space surrounding the cells. The Pco_2 of the cells is 50 mm Hg, and the arterial Pco_2 is only 40 mm Hg. CO_2 therefore diffuses from the cells into the blood. The blood then carries the CO_2 to the lungs for excretion. Thus oxygenated blood from the lungs carries the oxygen to the cells; the oxygen then diffuses from the blood into the cells. The CO_2, the waste produced by the metabolizing cells, diffuses into the blood, which carries it to the lungs for excretion. Note the venous blood leaving the cells. The Po_2 is 40 mm Hg because the O_2 has been used up by the cells. The Pco_2 is 45 mm Hg because the waste was removed from the cells.

Transport of Oxygen and Carbon Dioxide

The third step in respiration is the blood's mechanism for transporting oxygen and carbon dioxide between the lungs and body cells. Although the blood transports both oxygen and carbon dioxide, the way in which blood transports each gas differs.

Oxygen Transport. Almost all of the oxygen (98%) is transported by the hemoglobin in the red blood cells. The remaining 2% of the oxygen is dissolved in the plasma. As soon as oxygen enters the blood in the pulmonary capillaries, it immediately forms a loose bond with the iron portion of the hemoglobin molecule. This new molecule is **oxyhemoglobin.** As the oxygenated blood travels to the cells throughout the body, the oxygen unloads from the hemoglobin molecule and diffuses across the capillary walls to the cells. The oxygen is eventually used up by the metabolizing cells.

Carbon Dioxide Transport. Blood carries carbon dioxide from the metabolizing cells to the lungs, where it is exhaled. Blood carries carbon dioxide in the following three forms:

- Ten percent of the carbon dioxide is dissolved in plasma.
- Twenty percent of the carbon dioxide combines with hemoglobin to form **carbaminohemoglobin.** Note that the hemoglobin carries both oxygen and carbon dioxide but by different parts of the hemoglobin molecule. The oxygen forms a loose bond with the iron portion of the hemoglobin, whereas the carbon dioxide bonds with the globin, or protein portion, of the hemoglobin.
- Seventy percent of the carbon dioxide is converted to the bicarbonate ion (HCO_3^-). Note that the blood carries most of the carbon dioxide in the form of bicarbonate.

Sum It Up!

The exchange of the respiratory gases occurs at two sites: in the lungs and in the cells. Oxygen diffuses from the alveoli into the pulmonary capillaries. Carbon dioxide diffuses from the pulmonary capillaries into the alveoli. At the cellular sites, oxygen diffuses from the capillaries into the cells; carbon dioxide diffuses from the cells into the capillaries. Blood transports oxygen and carbon dioxide. Hemoglobin carries most of the oxygen as oxyhemoglobin. The blood carries most of the carbon dioxide in the form of a bicarbonate ion (HCO_3^-).

AMOUNTS OF AIR

Lung Volumes

Think about all the ways you can vary the amount of air you breathe. For instance, you can inhale a small amount of air, or you can take a deep breath. How are you breathing now? Probably slowly and effortlessly. With strenuous exercise, you would breathe more rapidly and deeply. If you become anxious, your breathing pattern becomes more rapid and shallow. With certain diseases, your respirations might increase or decrease. In other words, the amount, or volume, of air you breathe can vary significantly.

The different volumes of air you breathe have names. The four pulmonary volumes are tidal volume, inspiratory reserve volume, expiratory reserve volume, and residual volume. A spirometer measures pulmonary volumes. The patient blows into the spirometer, and it measures the amount of air and prints the results on graph paper. A recording of the volumes appears in Figure 22-10 and is summarized in Table 22-1:

- Tidal volume: Breathe in and out. The amount of air moved into or out of the lungs with each breath is called the **tidal volume.** The average tidal volume during normal quiet breathing is about 500 milliliters (ml).
- Inspiratory reserve volume: Inhale a normal volume of air. Now, in addition to this normal amount of air, inhale as much as you possibly can. The additional volume of air is called the **inspiratory reserve volume.** This extra volume is approximately 3000 ml.
- Expiratory reserve volume: Exhale a normal amount of air. Now in addition to this normal amount of air, exhale as much as you possibly can. The extra volume of exhaled air is called the **expiratory reserve volume.** It is about 1100 ml.
- Residual volume: Even after a forced exhalation, about 1100 ml of air remains in the lungs. This remaining air is the **residual volume.** Residual air remains in the lungs at all times, even between breaths. Note in Figure 22-10 that the four pulmonary volumes add up to the total lung capacity.

Lung Capacities

In addition to four pulmonary volumes, there are four pulmonary capacities. A **pulmonary capacity** is a combination of pulmonary volumes. For instance, **vital**

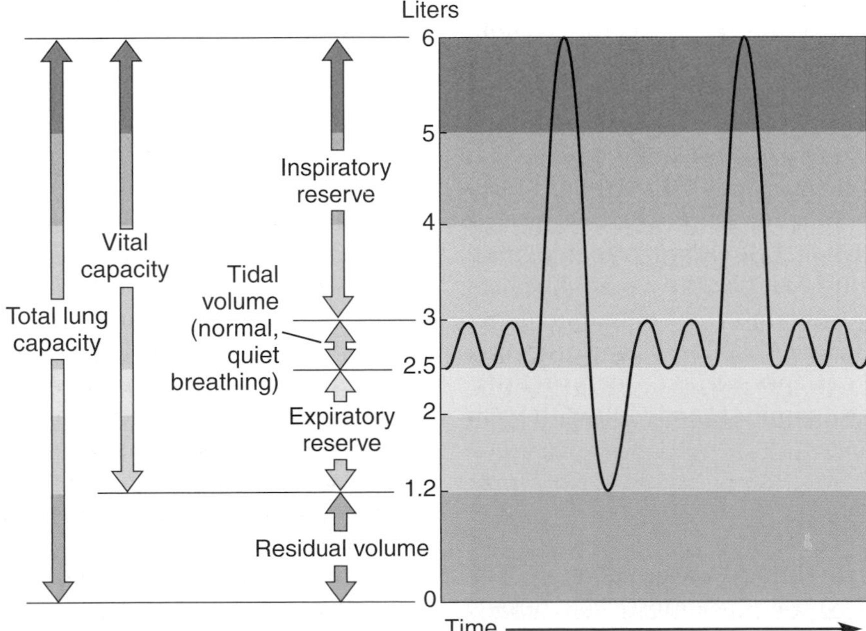

FIGURE 22-10 Pulmonary volumes and capacities.

Table 22-1 Lung Volumes and Capacities

Name	Description	Amount (ml)
Volumes		
Tidal volume	The volume of air moved into or out of the lungs during one respiratory cycle.	500
Residual volume	The volume of air that remains in the lungs after a forceful exhalation.	1200
Inspiratory reserve volume	The volume of air that can be forcefully inhaled after normal inhalation.	3000
Expiratory reserve volume	The volume of air that can be forcefully exhaled after normal exhalation.	1100
Capacities		
Vital capacity	The maximum volume of air that can be exhaled following maximal inhalation.	4600
Functional residual capacity	The amount of air remaining in the lungs following exhalation during quiet breathing.	2300
Total lung capacity	The total amount of air in the lung following a maximal inhalation.	5800

capacity (4600 ml) refers to the combination of tidal volume (500 ml), inspiratory reserve volume (3000 ml), and expiratory reserve volume (1100 ml). The measurement of vital capacity is a commonly used pulmonary function test.

You can measure vital capacity as follows. Take the deepest breath possible. Exhale all the air you possibly can into a spirometer. The spirometer measures the amount of air you exhale. The amount exhaled should be approximately 4600 ml. In other words, vital capacity is the maximal amount of air exhaled after a maximal inhalation. Vital capacity measures pulmonary function in patients with lung diseases such as emphysema and asthma. Other pulmonary capacities are listed in Table 22-1.

Dead Space

Some of the air you inhale never reaches the alveoli. It stays in the conducting passageways of the trachea, bronchi, and bronchioles. Because this air does not reach the alveoli, it is not available for gas exchange and is said to occupy **anatomical dead space.** The dead space holds about 150 ml of air. Breathing slowly and deeply increases the amount of well-oxygenated air that reaches the alveoli. Conversely, rapid panting delivers a poorer quality of air to the alveoli because a greater percentage of the inhaled volume of air remains in the anatomical dead space. Therefore when you encourage your patients to take deep breaths, you are also helping to supply the alveoli with well-oxygenated air.

CONTROL OF BREATHING

Normal breathing is rhythmic and involuntary. For instance, as you read, you are breathing effortlessly, about 16 times per minute. (The normal respiratory rate ranges from 12 to 20 breaths per minute in an adult and from 20 to 40 breaths per minute in a child, depending on the age and size of the child.) You do not have to remember to breathe in and out. Nor do you have to calculate how deeply to breathe. Fortunately, breathing occurs automatically.

You can voluntarily control breathing up to a point. Hold your breath for 5 seconds. Now hold your breath for 3 minutes. You can't do it; you must breathe. The need to breathe means that Sammy should not hold you hostage with his temper tantrums. No matter how good his performance and how long he holds his breath, he will eventually take a really deep breath and live.

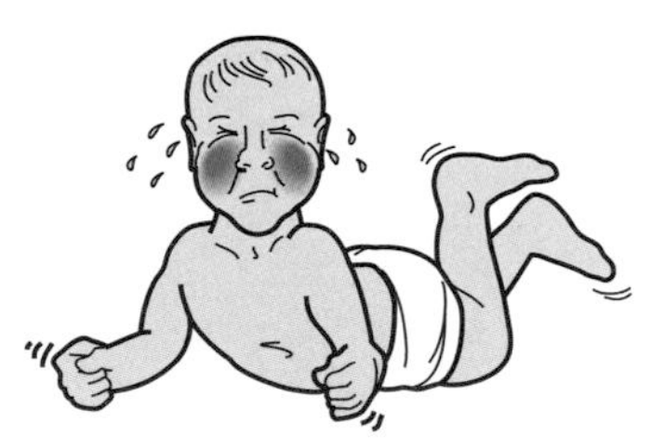

Neural Control of Respiration

How does the body control breathing? The two mechanisms that control breathing are nervous and chemical mechanisms. The nervous mechanism involves several areas of the brain, the most important being the brain stem. Special groups of neurons are widely scattered throughout the brain stem, particularly in the medulla oblongata and the pons (Figure 22-11). The main control center for breathing, in the medulla, is called the **medullary respiratory control center.** It sets the basic breathing rhythm.

Inhalation occurs when the inspiratory neurons in the medulla fire, giving rise to nerve impulses. The nerve impulses travel from the medulla along the phrenic and intercostal nerves to the muscles of respiration. Contraction of the respiratory muscles causes inhalation.

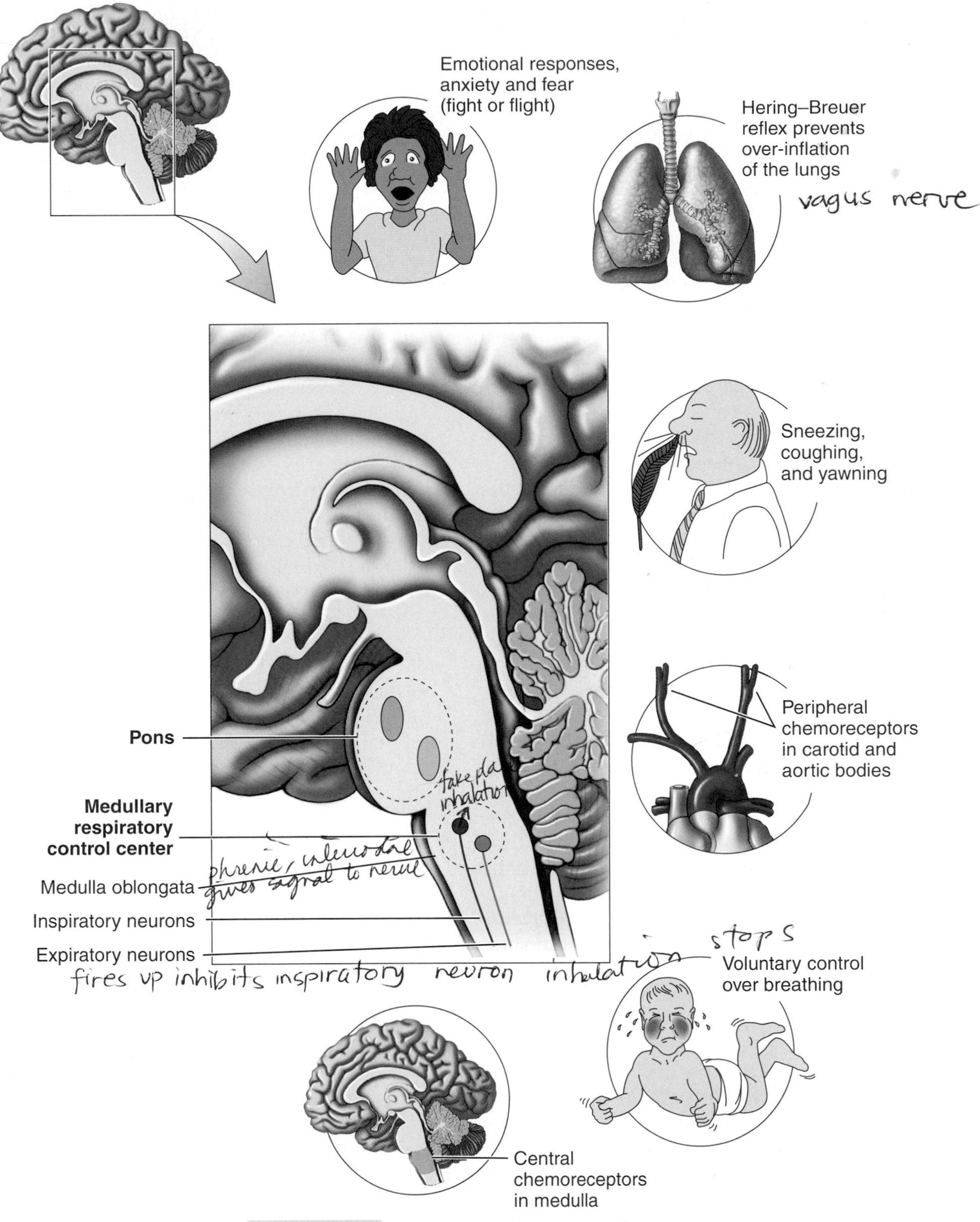

FIGURE 22-11 Factors that influence breathing.

Exhalation occurs when the expiratory neurons in the medulla oblongata fire and shut down the inspiratory neurons. This process inhibits the formation of nerve impulses and causes the respiratory muscles to relax. Thus breathing is due to the alternate firing of the inspiratory and expiratory neurons.

Although the medulla is the main control center for breathing, the pons also plays an important role. The pons contains the **pneumotaxic center** and the **apneustic center.** These areas in the pons modify and help to control breathing patterns.

The medullary respiratory center is very sensitive to the effects of narcotics. Narcotics (opioids), such as morphine, depress the medulla and slow respirations. If the narcotic overdose is large enough, respirations may even cease, causing respiratory arrest and death. Because of the profound effect of narcotics on respirations, you must check the patient's respiratory rate before administering narcotics.

Although the brain stem normally determines the basic rate and depth of breathing, other areas of the brain can also affect breathing patterns. These areas include the hypothalamus and the cerebral cortex. For instance, the hypothalamus processes our emotional responses such as anxiety and fear. The hypothalamus, in turn, stimulates the brain stem and changes the breathing pattern. Rapid breathing, a response to anxiety or fear, is part of the "fight or flight" response. The cerebral cortex can also affect respiration; cortical activity allows us voluntarily to control the depth and rate of breathing.

Several other nervous pathways affect the respiratory system. For instance, the vagus nerve carries nerve impulses from the lungs to the brain stem. When the lungs become inflated, nerve impulses travel to the brain stem, inhibiting the inspiratory neurons. This response is called the **Hering-Breuer reflex.** It prevents overinflation of the lungs. The nervous structures not only control breathing patterns but also affect several reflexes associated with the respiratory system. These include coughing, sneezing, and yawning.

Chemical Control of Respiration

Chemicals dissolved in the blood also affect breathing (see Figure 22-11). The chemicals include carbon dioxide, hydrogen ion (which determines the pH), and oxygen. These chemicals are detected by chemosensitive areas called **chemoreceptors.** When activated, the chemoreceptors stimulate the areas of the brain stem concerned with respiration. The two types of chemoreceptors are **central chemoreceptors,** located in the central nervous system (CNS), and **peripheral chemoreceptors,** located outside the CNS.

The central chemoreceptors in the medulla oblongata detect changes in the blood concentrations of carbon dioxide and hydrogen ions. If either carbon dioxide or hydrogen ion concentration increases, the central chemoreceptors signal the respiratory center to increase its activity. This response causes an increase in the rate and depth of breathing. As a result of the increase in breathing, carbon dioxide is exhaled, and the blood levels of carbon dioxide decrease. Conversely, if the blood levels of carbon dioxide and hydrogen ions decrease, breathing decreases, thereby allowing concentrations of both carbon dioxide and hydrogen ions to increase. Breathing is controlled primarily by blood concentrations of carbon dioxide and hydrogen ions, which trigger the central chemoreceptors.

The peripheral chemoreceptors are in the walls of the carotid arteries, and the walls of the aorta in the neck and chest region. They are called the **carotid** and **aortic bodies.** (Do not confuse the chemoreceptors with the baroreceptors, which are located in the same general area.) The peripheral chemoreceptors are sensitive primarily to low concentrations of oxygen and increased hydrogen ion concentration. Blood concentrations of oxygen, however, must be very low to trigger the peripheral chemoreceptors. Thus oxygen plays only a minor role in the regulation of breathing. **Remember: P_{CO_2} is the major regulator of respirations.**

VARIATIONS OF RESPIRATIONS

Respirations can vary considerably, depending on conditions in the body. For instance, a normal respiratory rate continues while the body is at rest. Respiratory depth and rate increase in association with exercise, anxiety, and conditions that increase metabolic rate (fever and hyperthyroidism). Respirations can also increase when the respiratory center in the brain is overstimulated (as in brain tumors or acidosis). Respirations decrease during relaxation, when the metabolic rate decreases (as in hypothermia and hypothyroidism) or when the respiratory center in the brain is depressed (as in overmedication with narcotics). A number of terms commonly describe some different types of respirations (Table 22-2):

Hyperventilation: an increase in the rate and depth of respirations. Hyperventilation causes excess exhaling of carbon dioxide, producing **hypocapnia** (diminished carbon dioxide in the blood). Hyperventilation occurs frequently during periods of anxiety and disease states, such as acidosis, pulmonary edema, and asthma.

Hypoventilation: a decrease in the amount of air entering the alveoli. Hypoventilation causes an insufficient amount of oxygen and an excessive amount of carbon dioxide in the blood. The many causes of hypoventilation include respiratory obstruction, lung diseases, and deformity of the chest wall. Other respiratory-related terms appear in Table 22-2.

Table 22-2 Common Respiratory Terms

Term	Description
Apnea	Temporary cessation of breathing
Dyspnea	Difficult or labored breathing
Tachypnea	Rapid breathing
Eupnea	Normal, quiet breathing
Orthopnea	Difficulty in breathing that is relieved by a sitting-up position. Orthopnea may be described in "pillow" terms; "two-pillow" orthopnea means that the dyspnea is relieved when lying in a bed supported by two pillows
Cheyne-Stokes respirations	An irregular breathing pattern characterized by a series of shallow breaths that gradually increase in depth and rate; the series of increased respirations is followed by breaths that gradually decrease in depth and rate. A period of apnea lasting 10 to 60 seconds follows; the cycle then repeats
Kussmaul breathing	An increase in rate and depth of respiration stimulated by acidosis
Cyanosis	A bluish color of the skin or mucous membrane due to a low concentration of oxygen in the blood
Hypoxia	An abnormally low concentration of oxygen in the tissues
Hypoxemia	An abnormally low concentration of oxygen in the blood
Hypercapnia	An abnormally high concentration of carbon dioxide in the blood
Hypocapnia	An abnormally low concentration of carbon dioxide in the blood

Sum It Up!

Normal breathing is rhythmic and involuntary. Nervous and chemical mechanisms control breathing. The nervous mechanism involves several areas of the brain, the most important of which is the brain stem. The inspiratory and expiratory neurons in the medulla oblongata determine the basic breathing pattern, which the apneustic center and the pneumotaxic center in the pons can modify. Chemicals in the blood help control respirations. The central chemoreceptors in the brain are sensitive to carbon dioxide and hydrogen ion, and the peripheral chemoreceptors are sensitive to low blood levels of oxygen and an increase in the hydrogen ion concentration. P_{CO_2} is the major regulator of respirations.

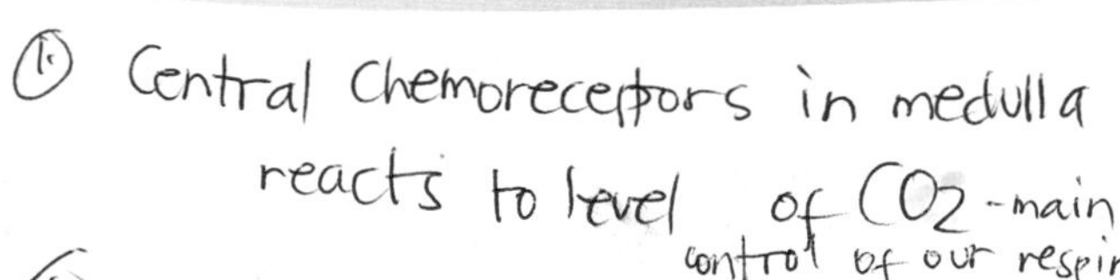

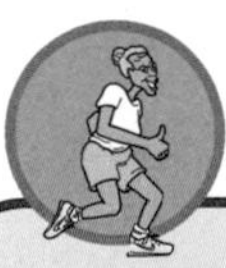

As You Age

1. As a person ages, lung capacity decreases. The decrease in lung capacity is due to the loss of elasticity of the lung tissue and diminished efficiency of the respiratory muscles. By the age of 70 years, vital capacity has decreased 33%.
2. With aging, many of the protective mechanisms of the respiratory system decline. The ciliary activity of the mucosa decreases, for example, and the phagocytes in the lungs become less effective. As a result, the elderly population is at greater risk for respiratory infections.
3. With age-related structural changes, the number of alveoli diminishes. The resulting decrease in oxygenation ultimately diminishes the capacity for physical activity.
4. Respiratory control is altered; consequently the P_{O_2} drops to a lower level while the P_{CO_2} increases to a higher level.
5. Having breathed a lifetime's worth of various harmful substances (e.g., cigarette smoke, pollutants, pollens, and pathogens), the lungs of an older person often show evidence of wear and tear.

Disorders of the Respiratory System

Asthma	A condition due to a hyperresponsiveness of the bronchiolar smooth muscle. Asthma causes difficulty with breathing, especially affecting the inhalation phase of respiration. Generally, the bronchiolar constriction is triggered by an allergen in the air but may be related to exercise or various pathogens.
Atelectasis	Incomplete expansion of the lung or a portion of the lung. The patient experiences varying degrees of dyspnea and hypoxia, depending on the extent of the atelectasis. Many respiratory diseases, such as cancer of the lung; mucous plugs (asthma); and pneumonia cause atelectasis.
Cancer of the lung	Bronchogenic carcinoma is a common form. As the tumor grows, it obstructs the air passages, causing them to collapse and eventually become infected. As the tumor grows and replaces normal lung tissue, less oxygen can be exchanged, and the person becomes dyspneic and hypoxic. Metastasis is common.
Chronic obstructive pulmonary disease (COPD)	Various combinations of asthma, chronic bronchitis, and emphysema. The most serious complications of COPD are heart and respiratory failure.
Common cold	Also called acute coryza. The common cold is the most common respiratory disease.
Emphysema	Means “puffed up” alveoli. As the lungs lose their elastic tissue, the airways collapse during exhalation, thereby obstructing the outflow of air. Overinflation of the lungs causes a permanently expanded “barrel chest.”
Inflammation of the respiratory tract	An inflamed part of the respiratory system. Most inflammations are caused by pathogens. Common inflammations include sinusitis (inflammation of the mucous membranes lining the paranasal sinuses); rhinitis (inflammation of the mucous membrane lining the nasal cavity); pharyngitis (sore throat); and laryngitis (hoarseness or lack of voice due to inflammation of the lining of the larynx).
Influenza	Also called flu. The flu is a contagious upper respiratory infection of viral origin. The flu may spread to the lungs, causing a severe form of pneumonia that is especially serious in the elderly population.
Pleurisy	Pleuritis. Occasionally, the pleural membranes become inflamed and dry out. As the inflamed pleural membranes slide past one another, friction arises between the two membranes, and the person experiences pain on breathing.
Pneumonia	Inflammation of the lungs in which the alveoli become filled with exudate. The exudate consists of serum and pus (products of infection). As the alveoli become filled with exudate, oxygenation decreases and the patient becomes hypoxemic.

SUMMARY OUTLINE

The respiratory system is primarily concerned with the delivery of oxygen to every cell in the body and the elimination of carbon dioxide.

I. Structures: Organs of the Respiratory System

A. The respiratory system consists of the upper and lower respiratory tracts.

B. Nose and Nasal Cavities

1. The nose and nasal cavities warm and humidify inhaled air.
2. Olfactory receptors are located in the nose.
3. The nasal cavities receive drainage from the paranasal sinuses and tear ducts.

C. Pharynx (throat)

1. The nasopharynx forms a passage for air only.
2. The oropharynx and laryngopharynx form passageways for both air and food.

D. Larynx (voicebox)

1. The larynx is a passage for air.
2. The epiglottis is the uppermost cartilage and covers the larynx during swallowing.

E. Trachea (windpipe)

1. Bifurcates into the right and left bronchi.
2. C-shaped rings of cartilage keeps the trachea open.

F. Bronchial Tree
   1. The bronchial tree contains the bronchi, bronchioles, and alveoli.
   2. The bronchioles determine the radius of the respiratory air passages and therefore affect the amount of air that can enter the alveoli.
   3. The alveoli are tiny, grapelike air sacs surrounded by pulmonary capillaries.
   4. Gas exchange occurs across the thin walls of the alveoli.

G. Lungs
   1. The right lung has three lobes, and the left lung has only two lobes.
   2. The lungs contain the structures of the lower respiratory tract.

H. Pleural Membranes
   1. The serous membranes in the chest cavity are the parietal pleura and the visceral pleura.
   2. Serous fluid between the pleural membranes prevents friction.
   3. For the lungs to remain expanded, pressure in the intrapleural space must be negative.

II. Respiratory Function

A. Respiration includes three steps: ventilation, exchange of respiratory gases, and transport of respiratory gases in the blood.
   1. Ventilation (Breathing)
      a. The two phases of ventilation are inhalation and exhalation.
      b. Ventilation occurs in response to changes in the thoracic volume (Boyle's law).
      c. Thoracic volume changes because of the contraction and relaxation of the respiratory muscles.
      d. The phrenic and intercostal nerves are motor nerves that supply the diaphragm and the intercostal muscles.
      e. Inhalation is an active process (ATP used is used during muscle contraction). Unforced exhalation is passive (no ATP used).
   2. Exchange of Gases
      a. Exchange of respiratory gases occurs by diffusion across the alveoli and pulmonary capillaries.
      b. Oxygen diffuses from the air in the alveoli into the blood while CO_2 diffuses from the blood into the alveoli.
      c. At the cellular layer, oxygen diffuses from the capillaries to the cells. Carbon dioxide diffuses from the cells into the capillaries where it is transported to the lungs for excretion.
   3. Transport of Gases in the Blood
      a. Most of the oxygen is transported by the red blood cell (oxyhemoglobin).
      b. The blood transports most carbon dioxide in the form of bicarbonate ion (HCO_3^-).

B. Amounts of Air
   1. Pulmonary Volumes
      a. Refers to the amounts of air moved into and out of the lungs.
      b. Pulmonary volumes are illustrated in Figure 22-10 and summarized in Table 22-1.
   2. Vital Capacity and Anatomic Dead Space
      a. Lung capacities are combinations of pulmonary volumes.
      b. Vital capacity is the amount of air that can be exhaled after a maximal inhalation.
      c. Anatomic dead space refers to air remaining in the large conducting passageways that is unavailable for gas exchange: ~150 ml of air.

C. Control of Breathing
   1. Neural control of breathing
      a. The respiratory center is located in the brain stem.
      b. The medullary respiratory center contains inspiratory and expiratory neurons. Nerve impulses travel along the phrenic and intercostal nerves to the muscles of respiration.
      c. The pneumotaxic center and the apneustic center are in the pons. These centers help control the medullary respiratory center to produce a normal breathing pattern.
      d. Two other areas of the brain can affect respirations: the hypothalamus and the cerebral cortex.
   2. Chemical control of respiration
      a. Central chemoreceptors are stimulated by carbon dioxide (P_{CO_2}) and [H^+].
      b. Peripheral chemoreceptors are sensitive to low concentrations of oxygen and increased hydrogen ion concentration in the blood.

Review Your Knowledge

Matching: Structures of the Respiratory Tract

Directions: Match the following words with their descriptions below. Some words may be used more than once.

a. pharynx
b. trachea
c. larynx
d. bronchus
e. paranasal sinuses
f. bronchioles
g. carina
h. alveoli

1. ___ The trachea branches into a right and left ___
2. ___ Called the voice box because it contains the vocal cords
3. ___ Mucus drains from these mucous membrane-lined structures into the nasal passages
4. ___ The respiratory structure that is connected to the middle ear by the eustachian tube
5. ___ Large tube supported by rings of cartilage; called the windpipe
6. ___ The respiratory structure(s) concerned with the exchange of the respiratory gases
7. ___ Structure that is closest to the pulmonary capillary
8. ___ Tiny respiratory passages that deliver air to the alveoli
9. ___ Respiratory passage that delivers air to the bronchioles
10. ___ The point at which the trachea splits; causes intense coughing when stimulated by a suction catheter

Matching: Thoracic Cavity and Ventilation

Directions: Match the following words with their descriptions below. Some words may be used more than once.

a. parietal pleura
b. thoracic cavity
c. intrapleural space
d. visceral pleura
e. phrenic
f. diaphragm

1. ___ Membrane on the outer surface of each lung
2. ___ Contains the pleural cavity, pericardial cavity, and mediastinum
3. ___ The lung collapses when air or fluid collects in this space
4. ___ The motor neuron that innervates the diaphragm
5. ___ Dome-shaped muscle is the chief muscle of inspiration
6. ___ Membrane that lines the walls of the chest cavity
7. ___ Must have a negative pressure here

Multiple Choice

1. Inhalation and exhalation are
   a. due to contraction of the diaphragm and intercostal muscles.
   b. caused by contraction and relaxation of the bronchiolar smooth muscle.
   c. referred to as ventilation.
   d. due to the relaxation of the diaphragm and intercostal muscles.
2. The bronchi, bronchioles, and alveoli are
   a. concerned with the exchange of respiratory gases.
   b. upper respiratory structures.
   c. collectively referred to as the bronchial tree.
   d. surrounded by rings of cartilage.
3. The diameter of the bronchioles determines the
   a. amount of mucus secreted by the respiratory membranes.
   b. rate of surfactant secretion.
   c. air flow to the alveoli.
   d. ventilatory rate.
4. Which of the following best describes the visceral and parietal pleura?
   a. Line the inner wall of the trachea and bronchi
   b. Line the mediastinum
   c. Are serous membranes
   d. Are surfactant-secreting membranes
5. If intrapleural pressure equals or exceeds intrapulmonic pressure
   a. surfactant secretion ceases.
   b. the lung collapses.
   c. the larynx can no longer generate sound.
   d. pulmonary edema develops.
6. Which of the following does not occur on inhalation?
   a. Air moves into the lungs.
   b. Thoracic volume increases.
   c. The diaphragm contracts.
   d. Pressure within the intrapleural space becomes positive.
7. Which of the following describes Boyle's law?
   a. An increase in thoracic volume causes an increase in intrapleural pressure.
   b. There is no relationship between intrapulmonic pressure and thoracic volume.
   c. An increase in thoracic volume decreases intrapulmonic pressure.
   d. An increase in thoracic volume forces air out of the lungs.

CHAPTER 23

Digestive System

KEY TERMS

Amylase, p. 414
Appendix, p. 405
Bile, p. 410
Biliary tree, p. 412
Cecum, p. 405
Chyle, p. 405
Chyme, p. 402
Colon, p. 405
Digestion, p. 396
Duodenum, p. 405
Esophagus, p. 400
Ileum, p. 405
Jejunum, p. 405
Lipase, p. 416
Mineral, p. 418
Peristalsis, p. 396
Protease, p. 415
Stomach, p. 401
Villus, p. 405
Vitamin, p. 418

OBJECTIVES

1. List four functions of the digestive system.
2. Describe the four layers of the digestive tract.
3. Describe the structure and functions of the organs of the digestive tract.
4. Describe the structure and functions of the accessory organs of the digestive tract.
5. Explain the physiology of digestion and absorption.
6. Describe the effects of amylases, proteases, and lipases.
7. Describe the role of bile in the digestion of fats.
8. Describe five categories of nutrients.

Most of us have no difficulty in eating our way through the Thanksgiving holiday turkey dinner, although the hours after the feeding frenzy can be a digestive challenge. Our digestive systems work very efficiently to digest and absorb as much of the food as possible. Before the holiday is over, the turkey dinner will be a part of every cell in your body.

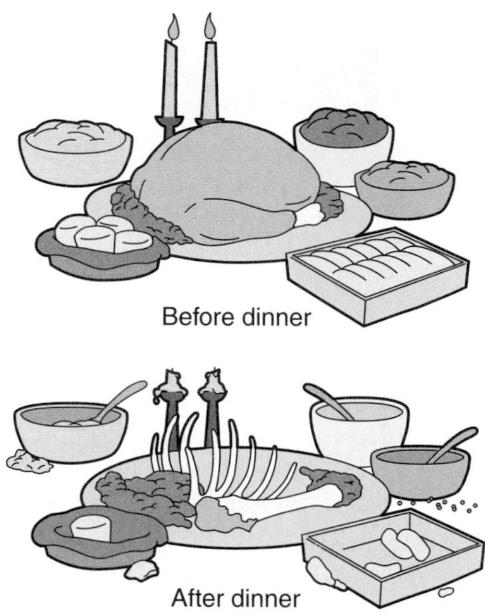

Cells require a constant supply of nutrients and energy. Food is their source. The purpose of the digestive system is to break down (digest) the food into particles that are small and simple enough to be absorbed. Thus, the digestive system ingests food, digests it, absorbs the end-products of digestion, and eliminates the waste. The study of the digestive tract is called **gastroenterology.**

OVERVIEW OF THE DIGESTIVE SYSTEM

The digestive tract and the accessory organs of digestion make up the **digestive system.** The digestive tract is a hollow tube extending from the mouth to the anus. It is also called the **alimentary canal** or the **gastrointestinal tract** (GI) tract (Figure 23-1). The structures of the digestive or GI tract include the mouth, pharynx, esophagus, stomach, small intestine, large intestine, rectum, and anus.

The accessory organs include the salivary glands, teeth, liver, gallbladder, and pancreas. The salivary glands empty their secretions into the mouth while the liver, gallbladder, and pancreas empty their secretions into the small intestine.

DIGESTION AND ABSORPTION

Digestion is the process by which food is broken down into smaller particles suitable for absorption. Digestion takes place within the digestive tract. **Absorption** is the process by which the end-products of digestion move across the walls of the digestive tract into the blood for distribution throughout the body.

The two forms of digestion are mechanical and chemical. **Mechanical digestion** is the breakdown of large food particles into smaller pieces by physical means. This process is usually achieved by chewing and by the mashing, or squishing, actions of the muscles in the digestive tract. **Chemical digestion** is the chemical alteration of food. For instance, a protein changes chemically into amino acids. Chemical substances such as digestive enzymes, acid, and bile accomplish chemical digestion.

The end products of digestion are absorbed by moving across the lining of the digestive tract into the blood. Digested nutrients eventually reach every cell in the body. The food that cannot be digested and absorbed is eliminated from the body as feces. Elimination of waste products is the last stage of the digestive process.

LAYERS OF THE DIGESTIVE TRACT

Although modified for specific functions in different organs, the wall of the digestive tract has a similar structure throughout its length (Figure 23-2). The wall of the digestive tract has four layers: the mucosa, the submucosa, the muscle layer, and the serosa.

Mucosa

The innermost layer of the digestive tract, the **mucosa,** is composed of mucous membrane. Glands secrete mucus, digestive enzymes, and hormones. Ducts from exocrine glands empty into the lumen of the digestive tract.

Submucosa

A thick layer of loose connective tissue, the **submucosa,** lies next to the mucosa. The submucosa contains blood vessels, nerves, glands, and lymphatic vessels.

Muscle Layer

The third layer of the digestive tract is the muscle layer. Two layers of smooth muscles are an inner circular layer and an outer longitudinal layer. Autonomic nerve fibers also lie between the two layers of muscles. The muscle layer is responsible for several types of movements in the digestive tract. Repeated contraction and relaxation of the stomach muscles mechanically digest the food and mix the particles with digestive juices.

A second type of muscle movement is **peristalsis** (pĕr-ĭ-STĂL-sĭs), a rhythmic alternating contraction and relaxation of the muscles. Peristalsis pushes the food through the digestive tract from one segment to the next. Peristalsis moves food in the same way that toothpaste squirts from a tube, as illustrated here by GI Joe. The toothpaste squirts in a forward direction because the bottom of the tube is squeezed. Peristaltic waves

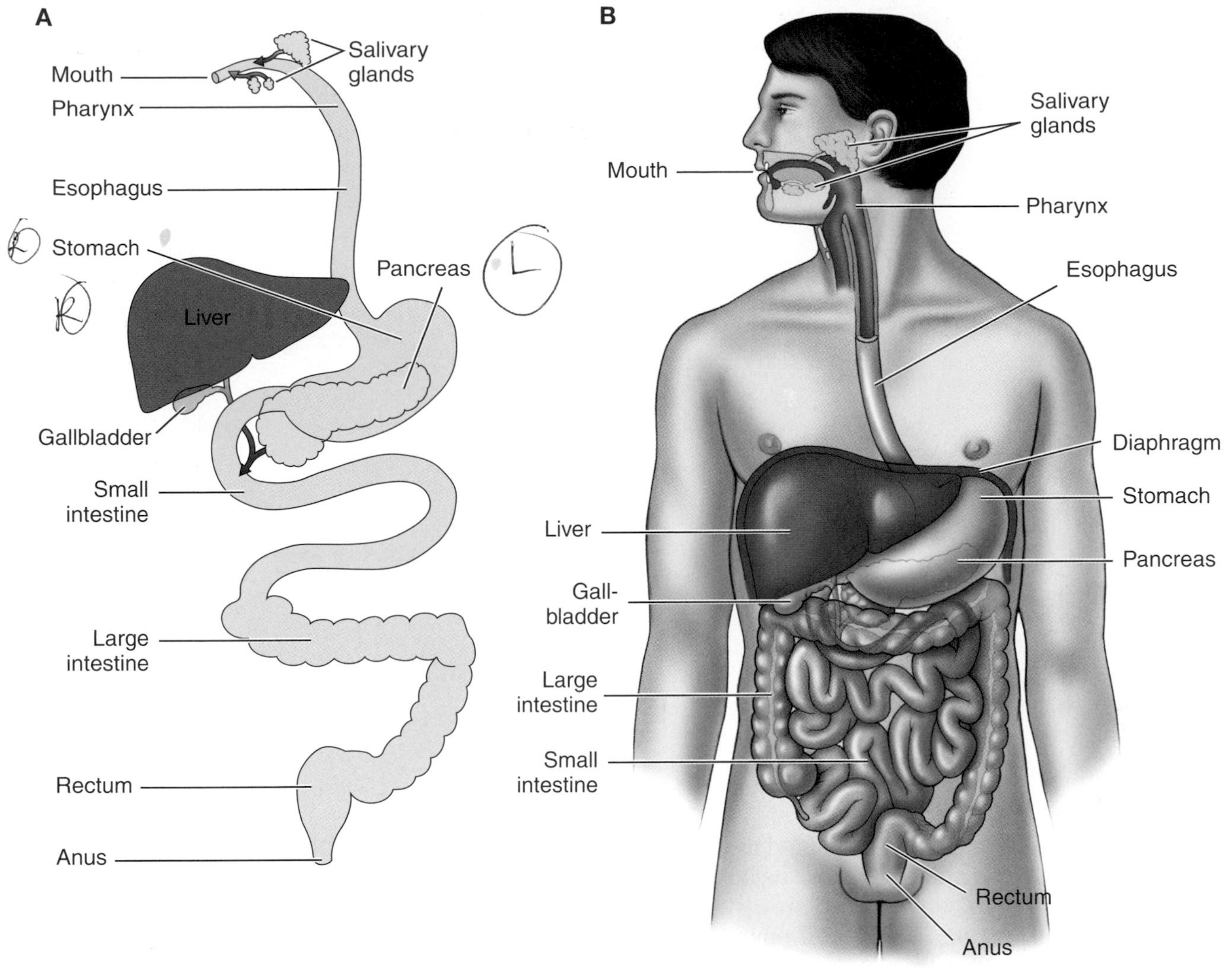

FIGURE 23-1 The digestive system. **A,** Hollow tube. **B,** Anatomical arrangement.

squeeze the food from behind and push it forward. Peristaltic waves are stimulated by the presence of food.

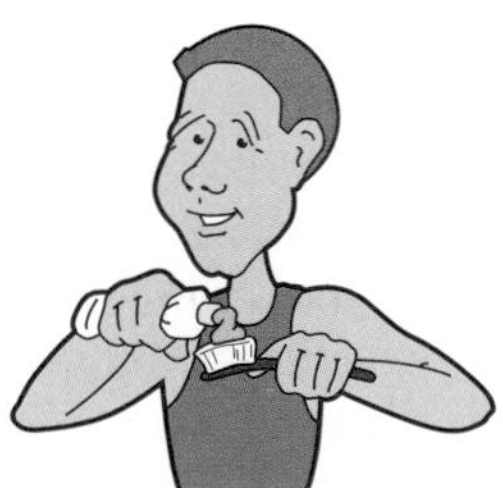

What happens if peristalsis stops? After surgery, intestinal peristalsis is often sluggish and may actually cease. This condition is called paralytic ileus. When this happens, food, gas, and liquid accumulate within the digestive tract, creating a life-threatening situation that demands immediate intervention.

Muscle activity is also responsible for other types of movement, such as swallowing and defecation (the elimination of waste from the digestive tract).

Serosa

The outermost lining of the digestive tract is the **serosa.** The serosa extends as peritoneal membranes.

INNERVATION

The digestive tract has a unique nervous network called the **enteral nervous system (ENS).** The ENS is part of the parasympathetic nervous system and responds to vagal nerve stimulation. The ENS regulates gut motility and secretion.

PERITONEAL MEMBRANES

The peritoneal membranes within the abdominal cavity are extensions of the serosa. These form large flat and folded structures that perform several important functions. They help anchor the digestive organs in place; carry blood vessels, lymph vessels, and nerves to the abdominal organs; and help restrict the spread of infection in the abdominal cavity.

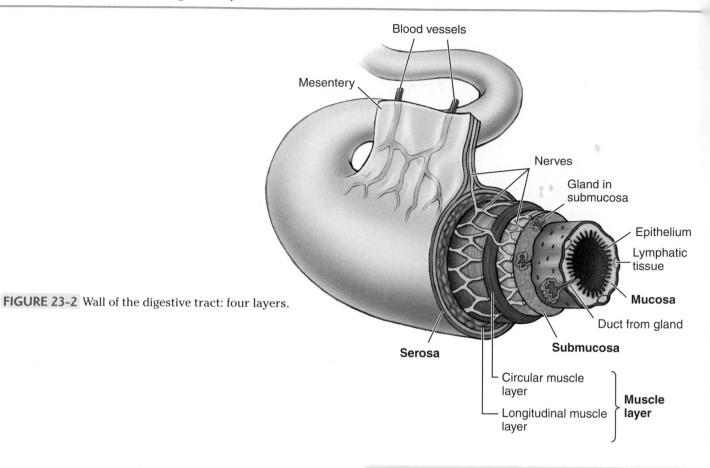

FIGURE 23-2 Wall of the digestive tract: four layers.

The peritoneal membranes, located behind the digestive organs, are called the **mesentery** and **mesocolon.** When located in front of the organs, they are called the **greater** and **lesser omentum.** The greater omentum is a double layer of peritoneum that contains a considerable amount of fat and resembles an apron draped over the abdominal organs.

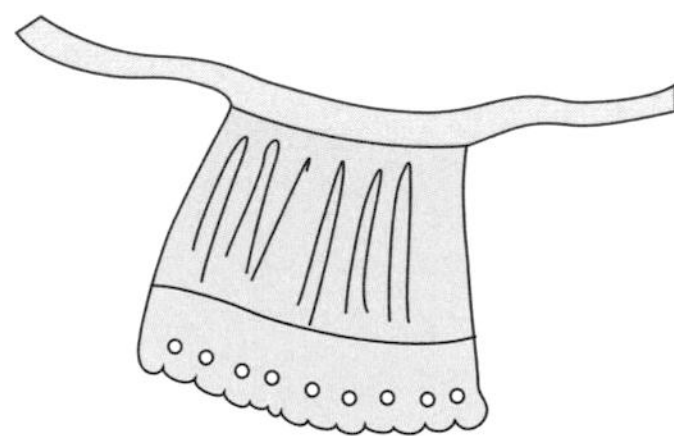

Sum It Up!

The digestive system is made up of a hollow tube that extends from the mouth to the anus and the accessory organs of digestion. The digestive system has four functions: ingestion, digestion, absorption, and elimination. The wall of the digestive tract has four layers: mucosa, submucosa, muscle layer, and serosa. The muscle layer enables the digestive tract to mix, mash, and move food through the tract; the forward movement of food is due to peristalsis. There are large, flat peritoneal membranes in the abdominal cavity that help anchor the digestive organs in place.

STRUCTURES AND ORGANS

MOUTH

The digestive tract begins with the mouth, also known as the **oral cavity.** The mouth contains structures that assist in the digestive process. These include the teeth, tongue, salivary glands, and several other structures. The **buccal cavity** is part of the oral cavity; it refers to the area between the gums and the cheek or lips.

Teeth

The purpose of the teeth is to chew food and to begin mechanical digestion. During the process of chewing, or **mastication,** the teeth break down large pieces of food into smaller fragments. Once moistened by the secretions in the mouth, the small pieces of food are easily swallowed.

During a lifetime, a person will have two sets of teeth, deciduous and permanent. The **deciduous teeth** are also called baby teeth or milk teeth. There are 20 deciduous teeth. They begin to appear at the age of 6 months and are generally in place by the age of 2½ years. Between the ages of 6 and 12 years, these teeth are pushed out and replaced by the **permanent teeth.** There are 32 permanent teeth (Figure 23-3, *A*).

Note the positions and names of the teeth: the incisors; cuspids (canines); premolars (bicuspids); and molars, including wisdom teeth. The shape and location of each tooth determines its function. For instance, the sharp, chisel-shaped incisors and cone-shaped cuspids are

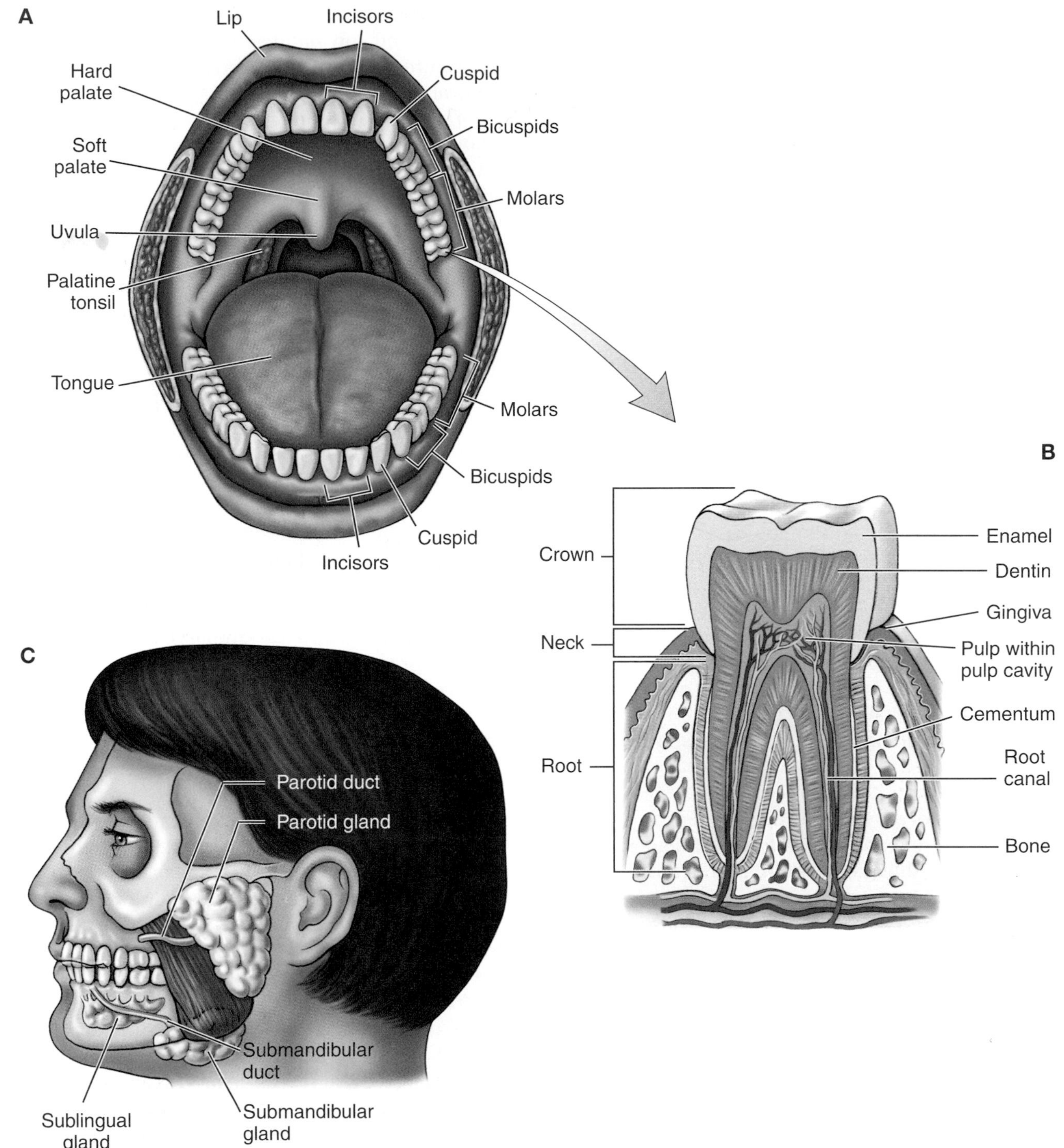

FIGURE 23-3 Oral cavity. **A,** Structures in the mouth. **B,** Longitudinal section of a tooth. **C,** Location of the salivary glands.

front teeth used to tear or grasp food. The larger, flatter molars, the back teeth, are more suited for grinding food.

A tooth has three parts: the crown, the neck, and the root (see Figure 23-3, *B*). The crown of the tooth is above the level of the gum, or gingiva, and is covered with hard, brittle enamel. The neck connects the crown with the root of the tooth. The root is that part of the tooth embedded in the jawbone. The outer surface of the root is anchored to the periodontal membrane by cementum. This holds the tooth in place. The bulk of the tooth consists of a bonelike material called dentin. Nerves, blood vessels, and connective tissue, called **pulp,** penetrate the dentin through the pulp cavity and supply the tooth with sensation and nutrients. As the pulp cavity extends into the root, it is called the root canal. Gingivitis and stomatitis are "mouth" conditions that are often drug-induced. Both cause considerable discomfort and interfere with nutrition. Gingivitis is inflammation of the gums. Stomatitis refers to inflammation or ulcers of the mouth area.

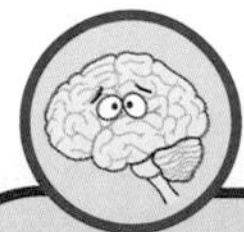

Do You Know...

What wisdom teeth are?

Four back molars can appear later in life (at 17-25 years of age when you have become wiser) and are therefore called wisdom teeth. In many individuals, the wisdom teeth remain imbedded in the jawbone and are said to be impacted. Because impacted teeth serve no function and are often a source of infection, they are frequently removed.

Tongue

The **tongue** is a muscular organ that occupies the floor of the mouth and serves two major roles in the digestive process. First, it facilitates chewing and swallowing by continuously repositioning the food in the mouth. As swallowing begins, the tongue pushes the food, which it has molded into a ball-like mass called a **bolus,** toward the pharynx. Second, the tongue contains the taste buds and allows us to taste food.

If you look under your tongue in the mirror, you will notice two structures. One is a small piece of mucous membrane called the **frenulum,** which anchors the tongue to the floor of the mouth and is the reason people cannot swallow their tongues. The second structure is an extensive capillary network that provides the sublingual (under the tongue) area with a rich supply of blood. Because the blood supply is so good, medications are absorbed rapidly when administered **sublingually.**

Salivary Glands

Three pairs of **salivary glands** secrete their contents into the mouth: the parotid glands, the submandibular glands, and the sublingual glands (see Figure 23-3, *C*). The **parotid glands** are the largest of the three glands and lie below and anterior to the ears. These are the glands infected by the mumps virus; the result is a chipmunk appearance. The **submandibular glands** are located on the floor of the mouth. The **sublingual glands** are located under the tongue and are the smallest of the salivary glands. Secretions from the salivary glands reach the mouth by way of tiny ducts. The salivary glands secrete **saliva,** a watery fluid that contains mucus and one digestive enzyme called salivary amylase, or ptyalin. Approximately 1 L of saliva is secreted per day. The most important function of saliva is to soften and moisten food and thereby facilitate swallowing.

What does one do with 1 L of saliva? Normally the saliva is swallowed. If someone is unable to swallow, however, the saliva must be suctioned so that it is not aspirated into the lungs. This problem occurs in patients who experience inflammation, tumors, or surgery of structures of the upper digestive tract.

Occasionally, one of the salivary ducts becomes obstructed by a stone. The condition is called sialolithiasis and is characterized by intense pain on eating when the salivary juices start to flow.

Other Structures Within the Mouth

The **hard** and **soft palates** form the roof of the mouth (see Figure 23-3, *A*). The anterior hard palate separates the oral cavity from the nasal passages, and the posterior soft palate separates the oral cavity from the nasopharynx. The soft palate extends toward the back of the oral cavity as the **uvula,** the V-shaped piece of soft tissue that hangs down from the upper back region of the mouth. The uvula plays a role in swallowing. The palatine tonsils are masses of lymphoid tissue located along the sides of the posterior oral cavity. These play a role in the body's defense against infection.

PHARYNX

The tongue pushes the food from the mouth into the **pharynx** (throat). The pharynx is involved in swallowing **(deglutition).** The three parts of the pharynx are the nasopharynx, the oropharynx, and the laryngopharynx (Figure 23-4). Only the oropharynx and laryngopharynx are part of the digestive system.

The pharynx communicates with nasal, respiratory, and digestive passages. The act of swallowing normally directs food from the throat into the esophagus, a long tube that empties into the stomach. Food does not normally enter the nasal or respiratory passages because swallowing temporarily closes off the openings to both. For instance, during swallowing, the soft palate moves toward the opening to the nasopharynx. Similarly, the laryngeal opening is closed when the trachea moves upward and allows the **epiglottis** to cover the entrance to the respiratory passages. You can see this process as the up-and-down movement of the Adam's apple, part of the larynx.

ESOPHAGUS

The **esophagus** (ĕ-SŎF-ă-gŭs) is the "food tube"; it carries food from the pharynx to the stomach (see Figure 23-1). The esophagus, which is approximately 10 inches (25 cm) in length, descends through the chest cavity and penetrates the diaphragm. The act of swallowing pushes the bolus of food into the esophagus. The presence of food within the esophagus stimulates peristaltic activity and causes the food to move into the stomach. Glands within the mucosa of the esophagus secrete mucus, which lubricates the bolus and facilitates its passage along the esophagus.

The two esophageal sphincters are the **pharyngoesophageal sphincter** located at the top of the esophagus, and the **gastroesophageal,** or **lower esophageal, sphincter (LES),** a thickening at the base of the esophagus (Figure 23-5). Swallowing pushes food past the pharyngoesophageal sphincter into the esophagus. Relaxation of the LES keeps the base of the esophagus open, thereby allowing the passage of food into the stomach. When contracted, however, the LES closes the base of

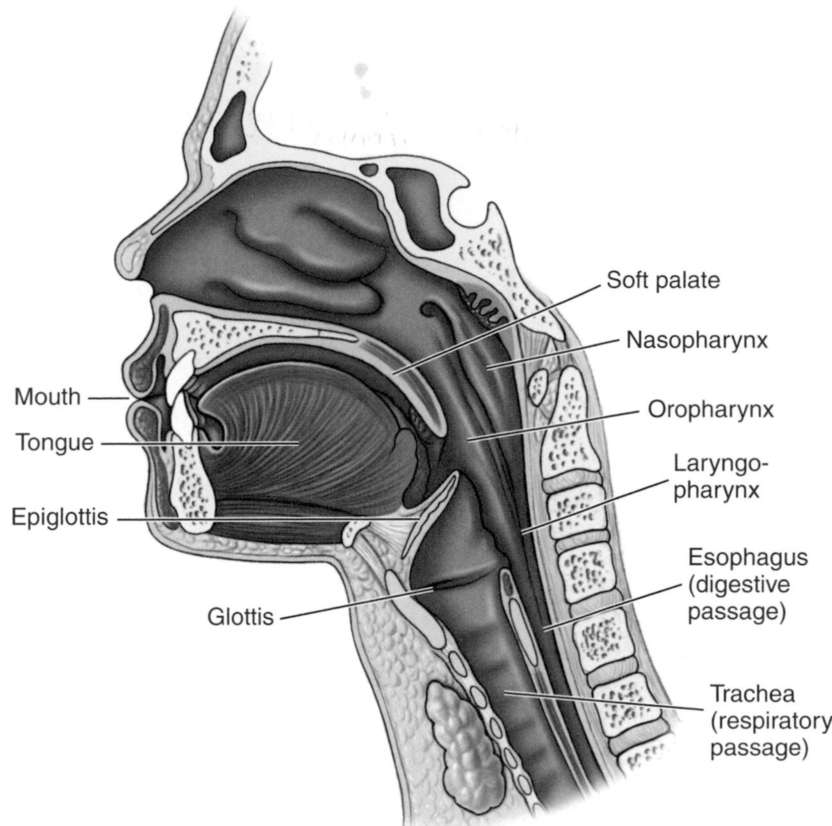

FIGURE 23-4 Eating and swallowing: from mouth to pharynx to esophagus.

the esophagus, thereby preventing reflux, or regurgitation, of stomach contents back into the esophagus.

In some persons a poorly functioning LES allows for reflux of stomach contents into the esophagus. The condition is called gastroesophageal reflux disease (GERD) and is characterized by a burning sensation called heartburn or pyrosis. The burning sensation is a result of the high acidity of stomach contents. (Note that the word pyrosis is related to the word pyromaniac, a person who loves to set fires, and to the word pyretic, referring to fever.)

STOMACH

What It Does

The **stomach** is a pouchlike organ that lies in the upper part of the abdominal cavity under the diaphragm (see Figure 23-1).

The stomach performs five important digestive functions:

- Secretion of gastric (stomach) juice, which includes digestive enzymes and hydrochloric acid as its most important substances.
- Secretion of gastric hormones and intrinsic factor.
- Regulation of the rate at which the partially digested food is delivered to the small intestine.
- Digestion of food. (Digestion within the stomach is limited.)
- Absorption of small quantities of water and dissolved substances. The stomach is not well suited for an absorptive role. It can, however, absorb alcohol efficiently. Therefore the consumption of alcoholic beverages on an empty stomach can quickly increase blood levels of alcohol.

Regions of the Stomach

The major regions of the stomach include the **fundus,** the **body,** and the **pylorus** (see Figure 23-5, *A*). The pylorus continues as the **pyloric canal.** A **pyloric sphincter** is located at the end of the pyloric canal and helps regulate the rate at which gastric contents are delivered to the small intestine. Other landmarks of the stomach include the **greater curvature** and the **lesser curvature.**

How big can your stomach get? The empty stomach lies in thick accordion-like folds called **rugae.** The rugae allow the stomach to expand. For instance, when the stomach is empty, it is the size and shape of a sausage. Following a large meal, however, the stomach may expand to approximately 1 L. Think of your turkey dinner sitting in your very expanded stomach—feels like you are going to pop! Sadly, the stomach can stretch in response to continued overeating.

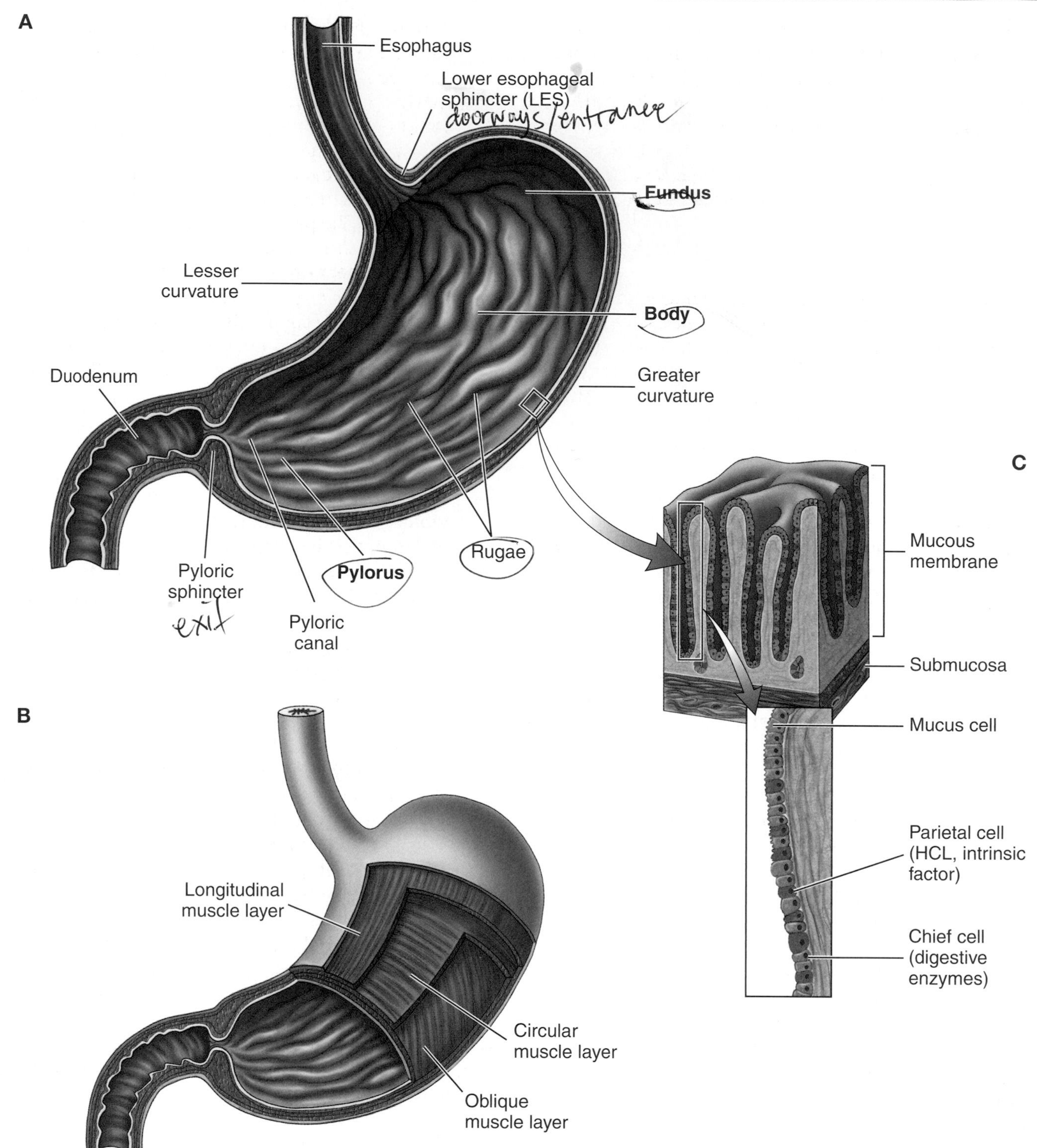

FIGURE 23-5 Stomach. **A,** Regions of the stomach: fundus, body, and pylorus. **B,** Three muscle layers of the stomach. **C,** Mucosa of the stomach showing the mucus, parietal, and chief cells.

Muscles of the Stomach

The stomach has three layers of muscles that lie in three directions: longitudinal, oblique, and circular (see Figure 23-5, *B*). This arrangement allows the stomach to churn and mix the food with gastric juice to create a thick, pastelike mixture called **chyme** (kīm). The muscles of the stomach also generate peristaltic waves that squeeze the food toward the pylorus.

Glands of the Stomach

The mucous membranes of the stomach contain gastric glands (see Figure 23-5, *C*). These glands contain three types of secretory cells: the **mucus cells,** which secrete mucus; the **chief cells,** which secrete digestive enzymes; and the **parietal cells,** which secrete hydrochloric acid (HCl) and intrinsic factor. The secretions of the gastric glands are called **gastric juice.** In addition to the gastric juice, other cells secrete thicker mucus that adheres closely to the stomach lining. This secretion forms a protective coating for the stomach lining and prevents the acidic gastric juices from digesting the stomach itself.

Vomiting

Vomiting, or emesis, is and is not a stomach event. It is a stomach event in that the stomach is emptied upon vomiting. However, vomiting is not a stomach event in terms of mechanism. Vomiting is part of the emetic reflex controlled by the medulla oblongata. In response to stimuli sent to the medullary vomiting center the LES relaxes and the diaphragm and the abdominal muscles contract, thereby squashing the stomach and ejecting its contents. You should become a keen observer of vomited stomach contents and its surrounding events. For instance, you will want to know if the vomiting was preceded by nausea or vertigo (dizziness), or related to food or drug intake. Record the frequency—is it an isolated event or more frequent? Record the amount and contents, including drugs; note the color and any evidence of blood (blood that is changed because of the stomach acid can have a bright red or coffee grounds–like appearance). A lot of clinically valuable information can be obtained through your observations. Don't rush to flush!

When the Stomach Is Not Working Right

The stomach gets a lot of attention clinically. Note the stomach collage (Figure 23-6):

- Ulcer (see Figure 23-6, *A*). A healthy digestive tract has an intact inner mucous membrane. The stomach lining may erode, or break down, thereby creating a lesion called an ulcer. Some ulcers are caused by the *Helicobacter pylori* (*H. pylori*) microorganism and are painful and prone to bleeding. An antiulcer drug plan for this type of ulcer includes an antibiotic in addition to drugs that decrease or neutralize acid.
- Hiatal hernia (see Figure 23-6, *B*). The stomach is located in the upper abdominal cavity immediately below the diaphragm. The esophagus enters the abdominal cavity through an opening in the diaphragm. If that opening is weakened or enlarged, the stomach may protrude, or herniate, from the abdominal cavity into the thoracic cavity. This condition is called a hiatal hernia.
- Nasogastric tube (see Figure 23-6, *C*). Many conditions require that a nasogastric (NG) tube be inserted through the nasal passages into the stomach. Most often the NG tube is used to empty the stomach to prevent vomiting. When a person cannot eat normally, a tube may be surgically inserted through the abdominal wall into the stomach. Food is introduced directly into the stomach through this tube. This procedure is called a gastrostomy.
- Gastric resection (see Figure 23-6, *D*). An important function of the stomach is to regulate the rate at which chyme is delivered to the duodenum. A person with cancer of the stomach may require a surgical procedure that removes the stomach or part of it. The procedure is called a gastric resection, or gastrectomy. A serious consequence of gastric resection is the inability to regulate the rate at which chyme is delivered to the duodenum. Because food (chyme) is literally dumped into the duodenum, since there is no stomach, a condition called dumping syndrome develops. The person experiencing dumping syndrome looks and acts "shocky" with severe nausea, perspiration, dizziness, and tachycardia.
- Pyloric stenosis (see Figure 23-6, *E*). The digestive tract is a hollow tube that must remain open. Occasionally during infancy, the pylorus is too narrow and impedes the movement of food out of the stomach. This condition is pyloric stenosis (narrowing). Pyloric stenosis is characterized by projectile vomiting immediately after feeding. Fortunately, a simple surgical procedure corrects the defect.
- Gastric hyperactivity (see Figure 23-6, *F*). Stimulation of the vagus nerve increases gastric secretion and motility. Certain drugs block the effects of the vagus nerve, thereby decreasing gastric secretion and motility. For instance, gastric hyperactivity, which occurs with some ulcers and a nervous stomach, may be treated with a drug that slows gastric motility and secretions. Atropine-like drugs are drugs that have a vagolytic effect and are used widely in the treatment of gastric hypermotility disorders. The administration of a vagolytic drug is like cutting the vagus nerve (vagotomy).

Autonomic translation. Stimulation of the vagus nerve activates muscarinic receptors. Drugs that activate muscarinic receptors stimulate gut motility and secretion. Anticholinergic or antimuscarinic (atropine) drugs block muscarinic receptors, thus slowing gut motility and decreasing gastric secretions.

Sum It Up!

The mouth begins the process of mechanical and chemical digestion. The bolus of food is swallowed and moves from the mouth, through the pharynx and esophagus, and into the stomach. The stomach continues the digestive process by mashing the food into chyme. Gastric juice helps to chemically break down food. The chyme is delivered to the duodenum by the stomach.

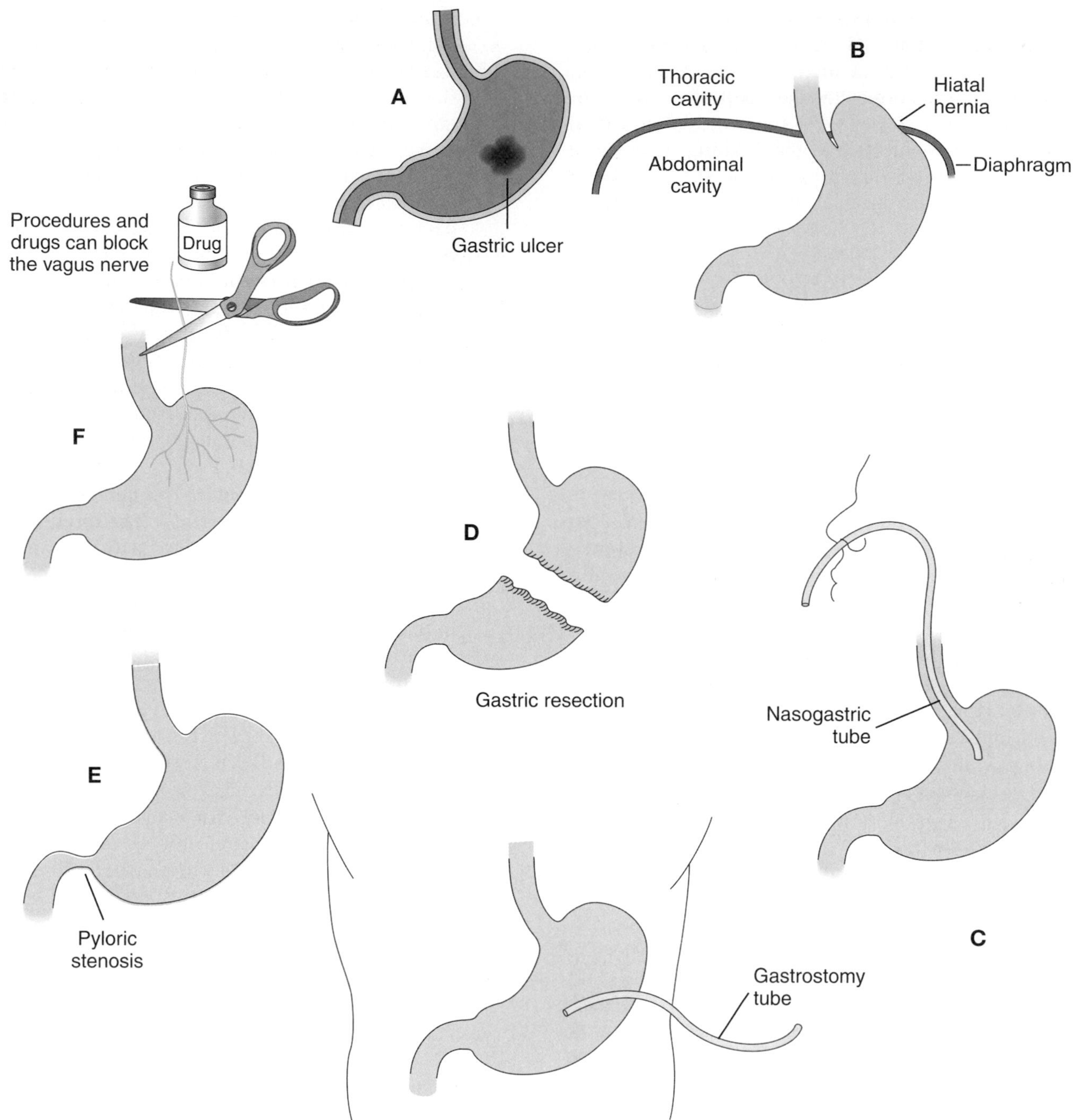

FIGURE 23-6 Stomach. Some clinical conditions that involve the stomach.

SMALL INTESTINE

Location and Parts

An acidic chyme is ejected by the stomach into the small intestine (see Figure 23-1). The small intestine is called small because its diameter is smaller than the diameter of the large intestine. The word small does not refer to its length; the small intestine is considerably longer than the large intestine. The small intestine is about 20 feet (6 m) long and the large intestine is about 5 feet (1.5 m) long. The small intestine is located in the central and lower abdominal cavity and is held in place by the mesentery. The small intestine is concerned primarily with chemical digestion and the absorption of food. The small intestine consists of three parts: the duodenum, the jejunum, and the ileum. While the stock market can make your guts churn, it can also help you remember the parts of the small intestine:

Dow	**D**uodenum
Jones	**J**ejunum
Industrials	**I**leum

Structures of the Small Intestine: What It Is

The **duodenum** (dŭ-ō-DĒ-nŭm) is the first segment of the small intestine. The word duodenum literally means twelve (duo means two, denum means ten). In this instance, the reference is to the width of 12 fingers. Thus the length of the duodenum is 12 fingerbreadths or approximately 10 inches (25 cm).

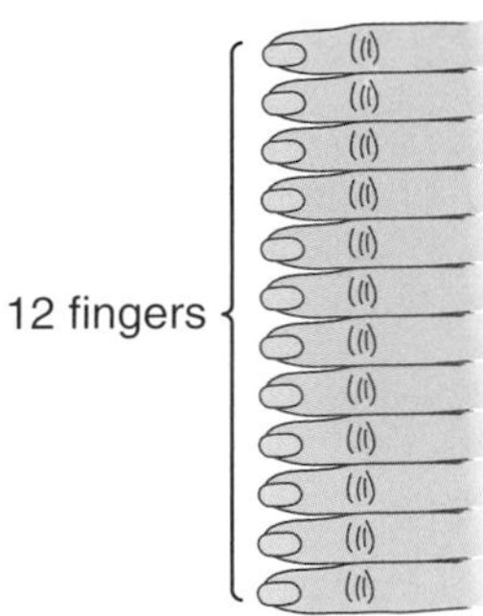

Why is the duodenum considered the meeting point for digestion? In addition to receiving chyme from the stomach, the duodenum also receives secretions from several accessory organs of digestion such as the liver, gallbladder, and pancreas (see Figure 23-1). These secretions, in addition to those from the mouth, stomach, and duodenum, are responsible for the digestion of all food. Most digestion and absorption occur in the duodenum. Repeat! Most digestion and absorption occur in the duodenum.

The **jejunum** (jĕ-JOO-nŭm) is the second segment of the small intestine. It is approximately 8 feet (2.4 m) in length. Some digestion and absorption of food occurs in the first part of the jejunum.

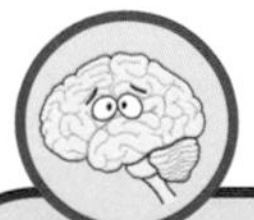

Do You Know...

What borborygmus is?

"Gurgle gurgle," growls your guts. How embarrassing is this as you look around the room! This gurgling sound that eminently emanates from your intestines is caused by the rapid movement of gas and liquid through the intestines. The sounds are louder and more noticeable when you are hungry because you tend to salivate more and swallow more air. "Gurgle, gurgle" is called **borborygmus** and comes from the Greek word meaning to rumble. Despite this long and ugly name, borborygmus is normal. Its only purpose? To embarrass you.

The **ileum** (ĬL-ē-ŭm) is the third segment of the small intestine and is approximately 12 feet (3.6 m) in length. It extends from the jejunum to the ileocecal valve. The **ileocecal** valve prevents the reflux of contents from the cecum (part of the large intestine) back into the ileum. The lining of the ileum contains numerous patches of lymphoid tissue called **Peyer's patches.** Peyer's patches diminish the bacterial content in the digestive system.

Functions of the Small Intestine: What It Does

What is so special about the wall of the small intestine? The wall of the small intestine forms circular folds with fingerlike projections called villi (VĬL-ī) (singular: **villus**) (Figure 23-7). The epithelial cells of each villus form extensions called **microvilli.** The large number of villi and microvilli increases the amount of digested food that can be absorbed.

What is a villus? Each villus consists of a layer of epithelial tissue that surrounds a network of blood capillaries and a lymphatic capillary called a **lacteal** (see Figure 23-7, *B*). The villus absorbs the end products of digestion from the duodenum into either the blood capillaries or the lacteal. The capillary blood within the villus drains into the hepatic portal vein and then into the liver. Thus the end products of carbohydrate and protein digestion first go to the liver for processing before being distributed throughout the body. The end products of fat digestion enter the lacteal, forming a milk-white lymph called **chyle** (kīl). The chyle empties directly into the lymphatic system. (Do not confuse the words chyle and chyme.)

In addition to forming a site for absorption, the cells of the intestinal wall also secrete several digestive enzymes and two important hormones, secretin and cholecystokinin (CCK). Table 23-1 lists the major intestinal enzymes and hormones.

LARGE INTESTINE

The **large intestine** is approximately 5 feet (1.5 m) long and extends from the ileocecal valve to the anus (Figure 23-8). The cecum, colon, rectum, and anal canal are parts of the large intestine.

Structure of the Large Intestine: What It Is

The first part of the large intestine is the **cecum** (SĒ-kŭm). The cecum is located in the lower right quadrant and ascends on the right side as the ascending **colon** (KŌ-lŏn). Attached to the cecum is the **appendix,** a wormlike structure that contains lymphocytes and is a source of immune cells.

Occasionally, the appendix becomes inflamed, causing appendicitis, and must be surgically removed through an appendectomy. Failure to remove an inflamed appendix causes it to rupture. The discharge of fecal material into the peritoneal cavity causes a life-threatening infection called peritonitis. RLQ pain? Think appendicitis and get thee to a doctor.

The ascending colon ascends on the right side and curves acutely near the liver at the hepatic flexure. As it crosses the upper abdomen, it is known as the **transverse colon.** The colon then bends near the spleen at the splenic flexure to become the descending colon. The **descending colon** descends on the left side of the abdomen into an S-shaped segment called

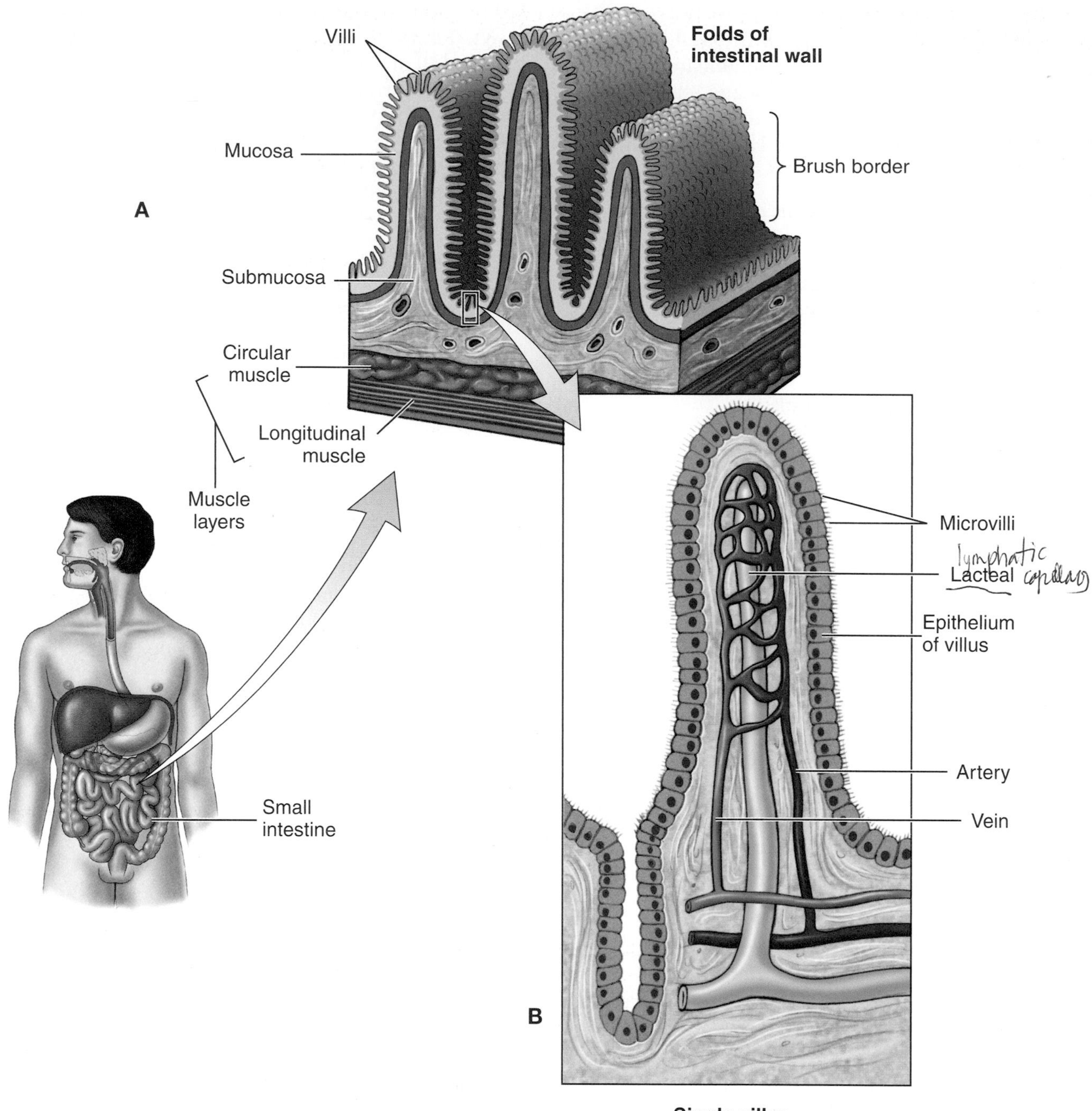

FIGURE 23-7 Small intestine. **A,** Folds of the intestinal wall. **B,** Single villus showing the blood capillaries and the lacteal.

the **sigmoid colon.** Structures distal to the sigmoid colon include the **rectum, anal canal,** and **anus.** The anal canal ends at the anus, a structure composed primarily of two sphincter muscles (an involuntary **internal sphincter** and a voluntary **external sphincter**). The sphincters are closed except during the expulsion of the feces. **Feces** is waste composed primarily of nondigestible food residue; it forms the stool, or bowel movement (BM). Expulsion of feces is called **defecation.**

Functions of the Large Intestine: What It Does

The four functions of the large intestine are:

- Absorption of water and certain electrolytes
- Synthesis of certain vitamins by the intestinal bacteria (especially vitamin K and some B vitamins)
- Temporary storage site of waste (feces)
- Elimination of waste from the body (defecation)

Peristalsis and Absorption. Intermittent and well-spaced peristaltic waves move the fecal material from the cecum through the colon. As the fecal material

Table 23-1 Major Secretions of the Digestive System

Name	Source	Digestive Function
Enzymes		
Salivary enzyme		
Amylase (ptyalin)	Salivary glands	Begins carbohydrate digestion to disaccharides
Gastric enzyme		
Pepsin	Gastric glands	Begins digestion of protein
Pancreatic enzymes		
Amylase	Pancreas	Digests polysaccharides to disaccharides
Lipase	Pancreas	Digests fats to fatty acids and glycerol
Proteases	Pancreas	Digest proteins to peptides and amino acids
Trypsin		
Chymotrypsin		
Intestinal enzymes		
Peptidases	Intestine	Digest peptides to amino acids
Disaccharidases	Intestine	Digest disaccharides to monosaccharides
Sucrase		
Lactase		
Maltase		
Lipase	Intestine	Digests fats to fatty acids and glycerol
Enterokinase	Intestine	Activates trypsinogen to trypsin
Digestive Aids		
Hydrochloric acid	Stomach	Helps to unravel proteins; kills microorganisms that are ingested in food
Intrinsic factor	Stomach	Assists in the absorption of vitamin B_{12}
Bile	Liver	Emulsifies fats; aids in the absorption of fatty acids and the fat-soluble vitamins (A, D, E, K)
Mucus	Entire digestive tract	Softens food; lubricates food and eases its passage through the digestive tract
Hormones		
Gastrin	Stomach	Stimulates gastric glands to secrete gastric juice
Cholecystokinin	Duodenum	Stimulates the gallbladder to contract and release bile; stimulates release of pancreatic digestive enzymes
Secretin	Duodenum	Stimulates the pancreas to secrete sodium bicarbonate

moves through the colon, water is continuously reabsorbed from the feces, across the intestinal wall, into the capillaries. Consequently, as the feces enter the rectum, it has changed from a watery consistency to a semisolid mass. Feces that remain in the large intestine for an extended period lose excess water, and the person experiences constipation. Rapid movement through the intestine allows insufficient time for water reabsorption, causing diarrhea.

Drugs may be administered to increase or decrease the motility of the large intestine. For instance, a person with diarrhea may take a drug that slows motility. Slower motility allows for more water reabsorption and the formation of a drier stool. In contrast, a person with constipation requires an increase in motility, so as to prevent additional water reabsorption. Thus a laxative, which increases motility, is often prescribed to relieve constipation.

Bacterial Action. What do bacteria do in the large intestine? The bacterial content within the feces is normally high, accounting for an impressive 30% of the fecal content. (The presence of bacteria in the intestinal tract is normal and is called the **normal flora.**) Some of these bacteria, *E. coli* for instance, synthesize vitamins. Although *E. coli* is normal and beneficial in the intestinal tract, it can cause serious medical conditions in urine and blood. Bacteria are also responsible for the formation of malodorous molecules that provide stools with their characteristic aroma.

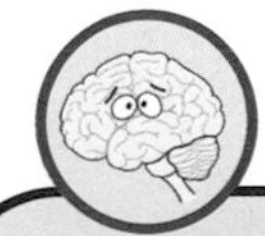

Do You Know...

Why Hirschsprung's disease is also called megacolon?

Hirschsprung's disease is a congenital disorder characterized by a lack of the enteral nerve network (no ganglia) in the distal colon (near the rectum). The aganglionic colon "feels" no urge to defecate and enlarges in response to accumulated feces (earning its alternative name, megacolon). When the megacolon finally produces a stool it is huge and noteworthy! Hirschsprung's disease, megacolon, congenital aganglionosis—all the same! This condition attests to the role of the enteral nerves in "moving things along."

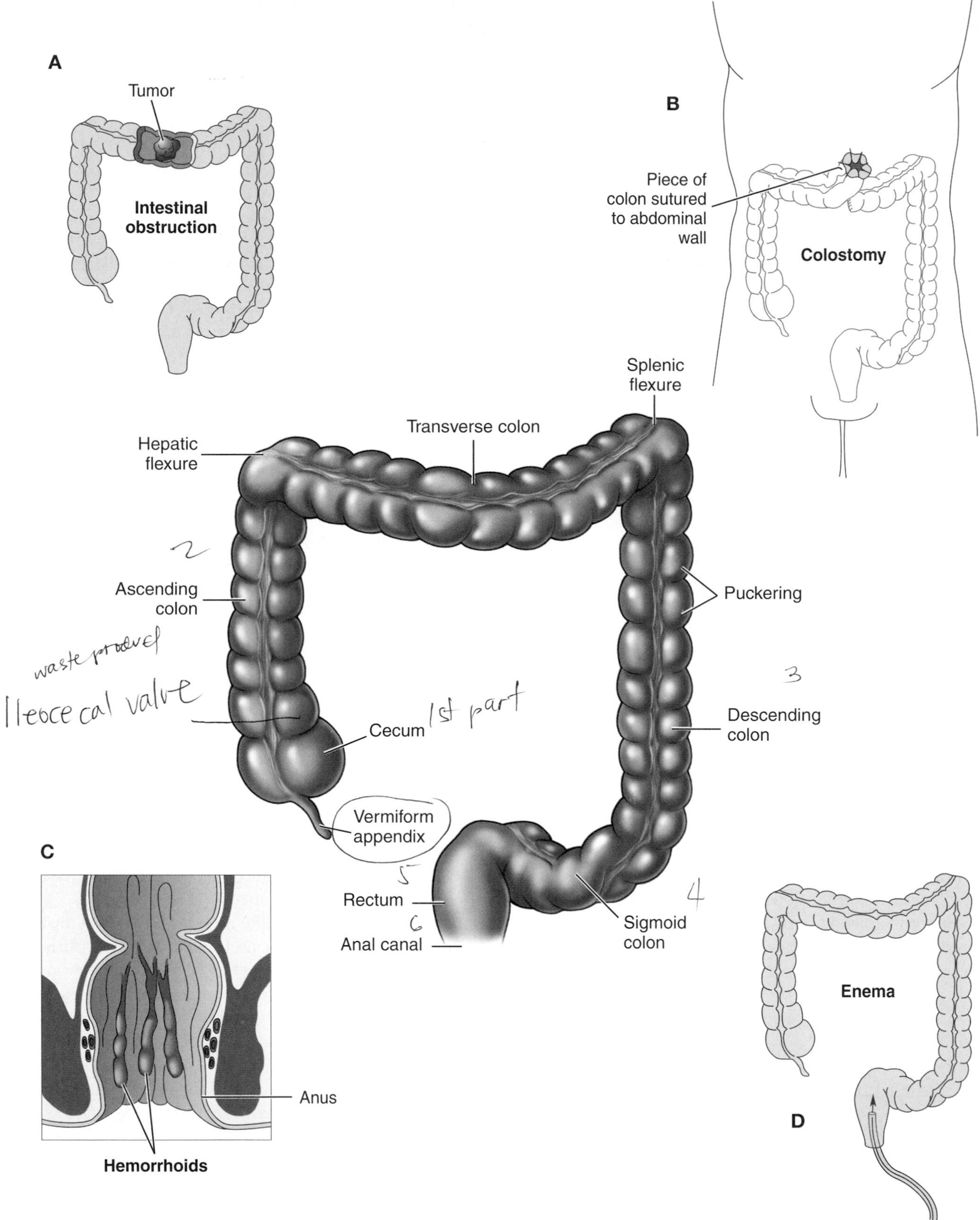

FIGURE 23-8 Large intestine (center), and some clinical conditions that affect the large intestine.

Do You Know...

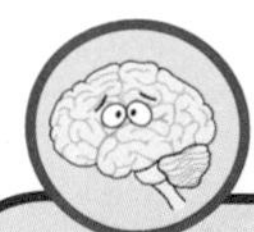

About the clinical concern for Clostridium difficile?

C. difficile, a Gram (+) bacillus, is a part of the intestinal normal flora; it normally causes no problems. If the intestinal flora is disrupted, as often occurs with antibiotic therapy, the number of *C. difficile* increases, causing a serious antibiotic-associated colitis. The combination of antibiotic therapy and severe diarrhea should red flag the possibility of superinfection with *C. difficile.* How did *C. difficile* get its name? From its uncooperative nature—it is difficult to grow in the lab.

Intestinal Gas. The average person expels about 500 ml gas/day (always a crowd pleaser). The expelled gas is called **flatus.** Gas is normally produced from air that is swallowed and as a byproduct of digestion. Conditions such as lactose intolerance produce excess gas causing severe cramping and discomfort. You will often hear surgeons ask patients if they have been "passing gas." A barely audible and embarrassed "yes" indicates that peristaltic activity, which often diminishes during surgery, has resumed. Passing gas post-surgically—very good. The intestinal gases include methane and hydrogen gas, both of which are flammable. This is a concern in the operating room where the use of electrical equipment (cautery) can cause the intestinal gas to explode. Not good.

When the Large Intestine Is Not Working Right

The large intestine is a common site of clinical disorders and discomfort. Note the collage (see Figure 23-8) that illustrates some clinical conditions and procedures involving the large intestine.

Because the digestive tract is a hollow tube that extends from the mouth to the anus, it occasionally becomes blocked, or occluded (see Figure 23-8, *A*). For instance, a tumor may grow large enough to block a segment of the large intestine completely. Or the bowel may become twisted on itself, causing a volvulus, and may occlude the lumen of the bowel. Both conditions result in intestinal obstruction, whereby the movement of feces is impaired.

In the event of an intestinal obstruction, a surgical procedure may be performed to relieve the obstruction (see Figure 23-8, *B*). An incision into the colon and the rerouting of the colon onto the surface of the abdomen (colostomy) allows the feces to bypass the obstruction. Because of insufficient water reabsorption, a colostomy performed on the ascending colon is characterized by drainage of liquid feces. Because of adequate water reabsorption along the length of the large intestine, however, a colostomy performed on the sigmoid colon is characterized by a well-formed stool.

All organs receive a supply of oxygen-rich blood from the arteries and are drained by veins. The walls of the veins are thin and may become damaged by excessive pressure. Sometimes the veins that drain the anal region become stretched and distorted (causing varicosities). These varicosities are called hemorrhoids (see Figure 23-8, *C*).

For several reasons (constipation, preparation for x-ray examination) cleansing of the rectum or colon may be necessary. This procedure is accomplished by infusing water through a tube inserted into the rectum (enema) (see Figure 23-8, *D*). The water stimulates the contraction of the muscle of the bowel, causing evacuation of its contents. Once the bowel is cleansed of fecal material, barium may be infused into the lower bowel (a procedure called a barium enema). The white, translucent barium appears on x-ray and outlines any tumor or other abnormality.

Do You Know...

That the "shepherd of the anus" was a high-profile ca—rear

Ancient Egyptian medicine was divided into many specialties. Each area of the body had its own physician or shepherd. The physician of the rectal area, comparable to today's proctologist, was called the "shepherd of the anus." Given the ancients' preoccupation with bowel irregularity and the popularity of emetics and purges, this shepherd was a very busy person—not too different from today if you note the staggering numbers of over-the-counter gastrointestinal drugs.

Do You Know...

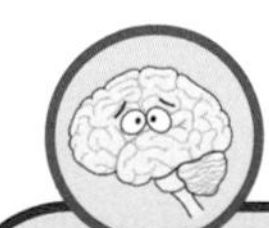

About Witch Hazel ... the rectal shrink?

Witch hazel lurks in many of our medicine cabinets. Check yours. As an astringent, it's busy shrinking those swollen hemorrhoids. Yes, witch hazel is a rectal shrink! Our shrink is called Hazel because the witch's broom was reputedly made from hazel-tree wood. Hazel survived the hunts at Salem and has served us as well. Which astringent? Witch Hazel!

Sum It Up!

Chyme is discharged from the stomach into the duodenum, the first segment of the small intestine, where most digestion and absorption occur. The end products of digestion are absorbed across the duodenal wall into the intestinal villi. Glucose and amino acids are absorbed into the capillaries of the villi. The fats and the fat-soluble vitamins are absorbed into the lacteals. Water and electrolytes are absorbed as the contents move through the small and large intestines. Digestive waste is eliminated as feces.

ACCESSORY DIGESTIVE ORGANS

Three important organs—the liver, the gallbladder, and the pancreas—empty their secretions into the duodenum (Figure 23-9). These secretions are necessary for the digestion of food.

LIVER

The liver is a large, reddish-brown organ located in the mid and right upper abdominal cavity (see Figure 23-9, *A*). It lies immediately below the diaphragm; much of the liver is tucked up under the right rib cage. The liver is the largest gland in the body and has two main lobes, a larger right lobe and a smaller left lobe separated by a ligament. This ligament secures the liver to surrounding structures. The liver is surrounded by a fibrous membrane called a capsule. The word hepatic refers to liver.

Functions of the Liver: What It Does

The liver is essential for life and performs many vital functions:

- Synthesis of bile salts and secretion of bile. Bile salts play an important role in fat digestion and in the absorption of fat-soluble vitamins. Bile secretion is the main digestive function of the liver.
- Synthesis of plasma proteins. The plasma proteins play an important role in maintaining blood volume and controlling blood coagulation.
- Storage. The liver stores many substances: glucose in the form of glycogen, the fat-soluble vitamins (A, D, E, and K), and vitamin B_{12}.
- Detoxification. The liver plays an important role in the detoxification of drugs and other harmful substances. The liver changes these toxic substances into substances that can be more easily eliminated from the body by the kidneys.
- Excretion. The liver excretes many substances, including bilirubin, cholesterol, and drugs.
- Metabolism of carbohydrates. The liver plays an important role in the regulation of blood glucose levels. If blood glucose levels rise above normal, the liver takes the glucose out of the blood, converts it to glycogen, and then stores it for future use. If the blood glucose levels decline below normal, the liver makes glucose from glycogen and nonglucose substances (gluconeogenesis) and releases it into the blood.
- Metabolism of protein. The liver can make a variety of different amino acids. Also, because only the liver contains the urea cycle enzymes, nitrogen (from ammonia) is converted to urea in the liver for eventual excretion by the kidneys. Free ammonia is toxic to humans.
- Metabolism of fats. The liver can break down fatty acids, synthesize cholesterol and phospholipids, and convert excess dietary protein and carbohydrates to fat.
- Phagocytosis. The Kupffer cells are hepatic macrophages and can phagocytose bacteria and other substances.

Blood Supply to the Liver

Blood Supply and the Hepatic Portal System. The liver has a unique arrangement of blood vessels called the hepatic portal system (see Figure 18-7). The liver receives a lot of blood, approximately 1.5 L/min, from two sources: the portal vein (which provides most of the blood) and the hepatic artery. The portal vein drains blood from all of the organs of digestion, and the hepatic artery delivers oxygen-rich blood from the aorta to the liver. Thus the portal vein brings blood rich in digestive end products to the liver. Blood leaves the liver through the hepatic veins and empties into the vena cava, where it is returned to the heart for recirculation. (Review the hepatic portal system in Chapter 18 so that you can understand absorption.)

Liver Lobules

The liver contains thousands of liver lobules, the functional unit of the liver (see Figure 23-9, *B*). The liver lobules consist of a special arrangement of blood vessels and hepatic cells. Note the central vein and the rows of hepatic cells that radiate away from the central vein. These cells are bathed by blood that enters the lobule from both the hepatic artery and the portal vein.

Blood from these two blood vessels mixes in the liver in spaces called **sinusoids.** The hepatic cells extract water and dissolved substances from the sinusoidal blood. Hepatic cells then secrete a greenish yellow substance called bile into tiny canals called **canaliculi.** These tiny bile canals merge with canals from other lobules to form larger hepatic bile ducts. Bile exits from the liver through the **hepatic bile ducts.**

Bile

Bile is a greenish yellow secretion produced by the liver and stored in the gallbladder. Bile is composed primarily of water, electrolytes, cholesterol, bile pigments, and bile salts. The bile pigments **bilirubin** and **biliverdin** are formed from the hemoglobin of worn-out red blood cells. The bile salts are the most abundant constituents of the bile. Only the bile salts have a digestive function; they play an important role in fat digestion and in the absorption of fat-soluble vitamins. Between 800 and 1000 ml of bile is secreted per day.

Bile pigments, especially urobilinogen (a breakdown product of bilirubin), also give the stool a brownish color. With gallbladder disease, a gallstone sometimes becomes lodged in the common bile duct, blocks the flow of bile into the duodenum, and deprives the stools of brown pigments. Common bile duct obstruction is therefore characterized by colorless, gray, or clay-colored stools.

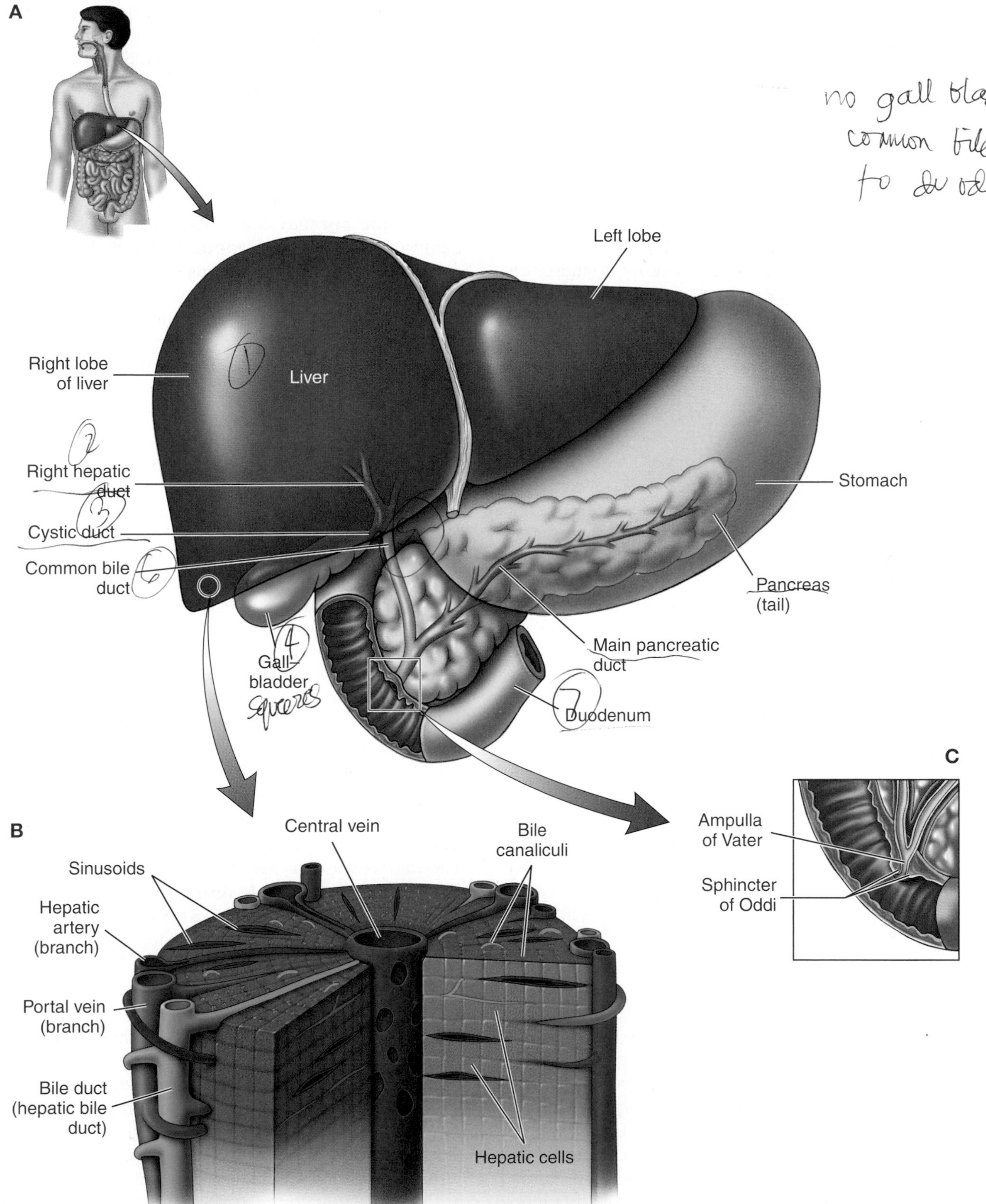

FIGURE 23-9 **A,** The relationship of the liver, gallbladder, and pancreas to the duodenum. **B,** Liver lobule. **C,** The entrance of the common bile duct into the duodenum.

Bile salts are made from cholesterol by the liver. If the liver is stimulated to make additional bile salts, more cholesterol is used up, thereby lowering the amount of cholesterol in the blood. The "statins," popular cholesterol-lowering drugs, stimulate the hepatic synthesis of bile salts and are therefore useful in the prevention of coronary artery disease.

Biliary Tree

The ducts that connect the liver, gallbladder, and duodenum are called the **biliary** (BĬL-ē-ăr-ē) **tree** (see Figure 23-9, *A*). This network of ducts, the bile aisle, includes the hepatic bile ducts, the cystic duct, and the common bile duct. The **hepatic bile ducts** receive bile from the canaliculi within the liver lobules. The hepatic ducts merge with the **cystic duct** to form the **common bile duct,** which carries bile from both the hepatic ducts (liver) and the cystic duct (gallbladder) to the duodenum.

The base of the common bile duct swells to form the **hepatopancreatic ampulla (ampulla of Vater)** (see Figure 23-9, *C*). The main pancreatic duct joins the common bile duct at this point. The **hepatopancreatic sphincter (sphincter of Oddi)** encircles the base of the ampulla, where it enters the duodenum. This sphincter helps regulate the delivery of bile to the duodenum and is sensitive to nervous, hormonal, and pharmacologic control.

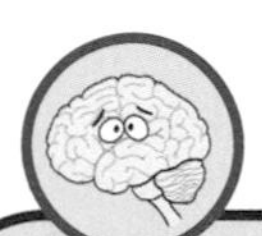

Do You Know...

With no hepatic cells—everything swells?

The liver is a very busy organ. One of its functions is to make plasma proteins such as albumin. Plasma proteins help to hold water in the blood vessels. In severe liver disease, insufficient protein is made, causing water to leak out of the blood vessels into the surrounding tissue. The waterlogged tissue is called edema. "Take care of that liver," says Sir Osis, who has cirrhosis, "And remember—too many drinks, liver shrinks. No hepatic cells—everything swells."

GALLBLADDER

The **gallbladder** is a pear-shaped sac attached to the underside of the liver (see Figure 23-9, *A*). The cystic duct connects the gallbladder with the common bile duct. Bile, produced in the liver, flows through the hepatic ducts and into the cystic duct and gallbladder. The gallbladder concentrates about 1200 ml of bile per day.

The fat in the duodenum stimulates the release of a hormone, **cholecystokinin (CCK).** This hormone enters the bloodstream and circulates back to the gallbladder, where it causes the smooth muscle of the gallbladder to contract. When the gallbladder contracts, the bile is ejected into the cystic duct and then into the common bile duct and duodenum.

Stones and groans. For unknown reasons bile components often form stones. The larger stones remain in the gallbladder. However, the smaller stones can be pushed out of the gallbladder when bile is ejected. The stones then lodge in the common bile duct. Bile that backs up behind the stones causes jaundice and impairs hepatic function. The stagnant bile can also be forced into the main pancreatic duct causing a life-threatening pancreatitis. Presence of stones in the gallbladder often causes an inflammation called cholecystitis. Presence of stones in the common bile duct is called choledocholithiasis. Both conditions may cause biliary colic (midepigastric pain that often radiates to the right subscapular area) and other digestive symptoms such as nausea, vomiting, and pain.

How can a fatty meal trigger biliary colic in a person with cholecystitis? When the fat enters the duodenum it causes the release of CCK. The CCK travels via the blood to the gallbladder and stimulates the inflamed gallbladder to contract. Ouch!

PANCREAS

The **pancreas** is an accessory organ of digestion located just below the stomach (see Figure 23-9, *A*). The head of the pancreas rests in the curve of the duodenum, and the tail lies near the spleen in the upper left quadrant of the abdominal cavity. The **main pancreatic duct,** which travels the length of the pancreas, joins with the common bile duct at the ampulla of Vater. The pancreatic duct carries digestive enzymes from the pancreas to the duodenum, the meeting point for digestion.

The pancreas secretes both endocrine and exocrine substances. The exocrine secretions include the digestive enzymes and an alkaline secretion. These secretions form the pancreatic juice: the pancreas secretes about 1400 ml/day. The pancreatic enzymes are the most important of all the digestive enzymes. Repeat! The pancreatic enzymes are the most important of all the digestive enzymes. **Acinar cells** secrete the pancreatic enzymes in their inactive form. The enzymes travel through the main pancreatic duct to the duodenum and are activated in the duodenum.

In addition to the digestive enzymes, the pancreas also secretes an alkaline juice rich in bicarbonate. The bicarbonate neutralizes the highly acidic chyme coming from the stomach into the duodenum. This neutralization is important because the digestive enzymes in the duodenum work best in an alkaline environment.

Control of Secretion

The secretion of the digestive enzymes and bicarbonate is under nervous (vagus) and hormonal control. The presence of food in the stomach and duodenum is the stimulus for the nervous and hormonal responses. For instance, the presence of chyme in the duodenum stimulates the release of the hormone CCK from the duodenal walls. CCK travels by way of the blood to the pancreas, stimulating the release of pancreatic digestive enzymes. Note that CCK affects both the gallbladder and the pancreas (see Table 23-1). The acid in the duodenum stimulates the release of a second hormone, **secretin,** from the duodenal walls. Secretin travels by way of the blood to the pancreas, stimulating release of the bicarbonate-rich juice.

WHEN ACCESSORY DIGESTIVE ORGANS ARE NOT WORKING RIGHT

Disorders involving the liver, gallbladder, biliary tree, and pancreas are common. Note the collage (Figure 23-10, *A-E*) for some clinical conditions.

- Jaundice (see Figure 23-10, *A*). The liver secretes bile, which is stored in the gallbladder for future use in the duodenum. When needed, bile travels through bile ducts to the duodenum. If the common bile duct become blocked with stones the flow of bile stops. The bile backs up into the liver. The bile pigments, especially bilirubin, accumulate in the blood and are eventually carried throughout the body, where they are deposited in the skin. The skin turns yellow, and the person is described as being jaundiced. Because the jaundice is due to an obstruction, it is called obstructive jaundice (in contrast to hemolytic jaundice, which is caused by the rapid breakdown of red blood cells; see Chapter 15). Jaundice can also occur in response to liver disease (hepatitis). A person with hepatitis may become jaundiced because the inflamed

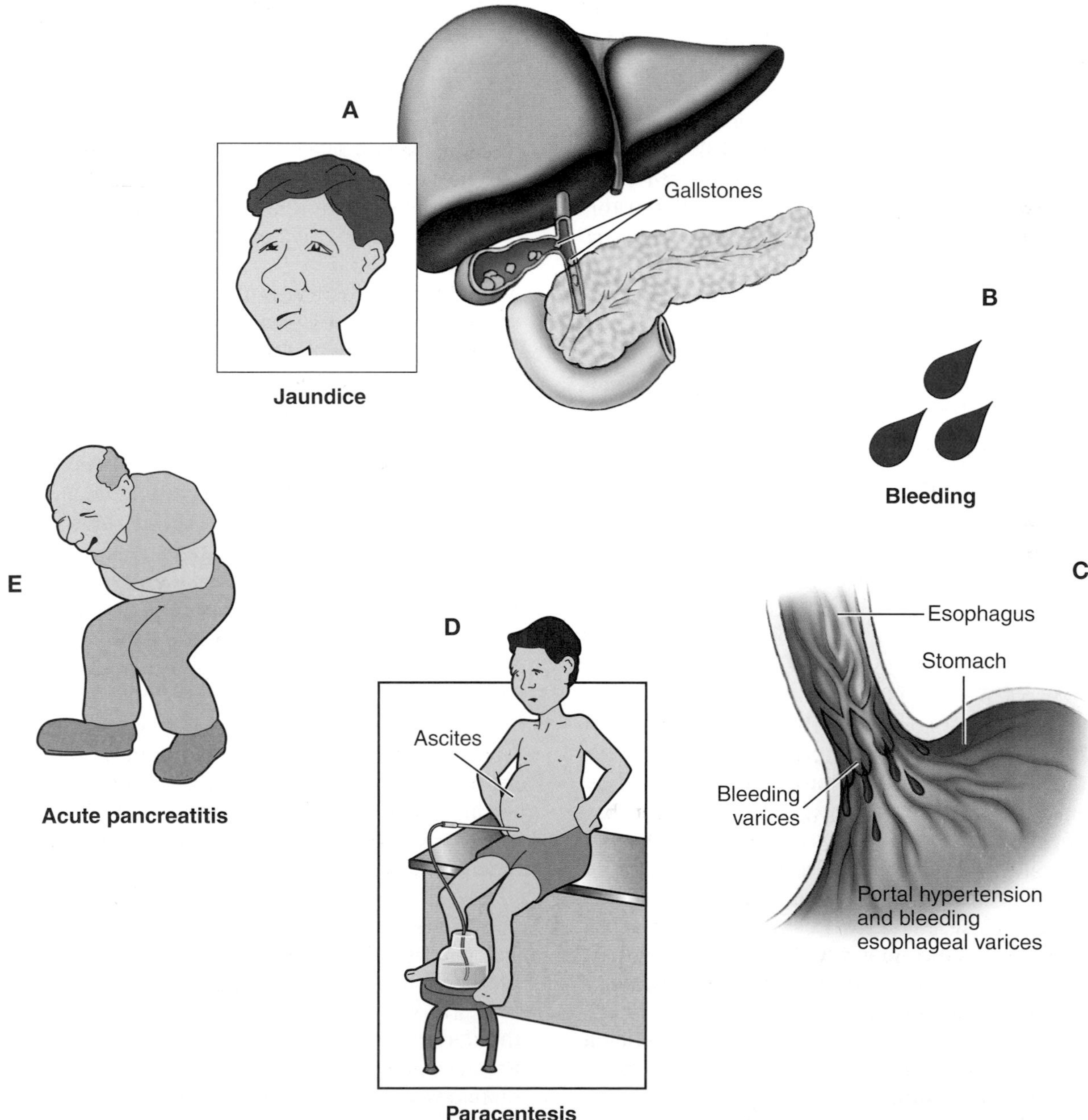

FIGURE 23-10 Some clinical conditions that affect the liver, gallbladder, and pancreas.

hepatic tissue causes the bile canaliculi to swell and close. This closure diminishes the excretion of bile from the liver and causes backup of bilirubin in the blood.

- Bleeding (see Figure 23-10, *B*). The liver synthesizes clotting factors such as prothrombin. What can make a person hypoprothrombinemic (a diminished amount of prothrombin in the blood)? A gallstone lodged in the common bile duct may cause hypoprothrombinemia. Because bile is necessary for the absorption of fat-soluble vitamins, bile duct obstruction causes diminished absorption of vitamin K. Vitamin K is necessary for the hepatic synthesis of a number of clotting factors, including prothrombin. Thus common bile duct obstruction diminishes the hepatic synthesis of prothrombin, causing hypoprothrombinemia, a prolonged prothrombin time, and bleeding.
- Portal hypertension and hemorrhage (see Figure 23-10, *C*). The liver receives a large flow of blood from the portal vein. Normally, the blood passes through the liver quickly and easily with very little resistance to the flow of blood. In alcoholic cirrhosis, however, the liver is so damaged that the flow of portal blood through the liver is greatly impeded. The blood backs up in the portal vein, elevating the pressure in the vein and causing portal hypertension. The increased portal pressure is felt not only by the portal vein but also by all the veins that drain into the portal vein, including the small veins at the base of the esophagus. Over time the small veins become stretched and damaged (varicose veins). If the portal pressure becomes too great, the weak varicose veins (esophageal varices) at the base of the esophagus may rupture, causing a massive hemorrhage.
- Portal hypertension and ascites (see Figure 23-10, *D*). In alcoholic cirrhosis, the portal hypertension may also cause fluid to seep across the blood vessels into the peritoneal cavity. The collection of fluid in the peritoneal cavity is called ascites. The ascites may be so severe that the accumulated fluid pushes up on the diaphragm and interferes with breathing. The fluid may be siphoned off by the insertion of a tube into the peritoneal cavity. This procedure is called paracentesis.
- Pancreatitis (see Figure 23-10, *E*). The pancreas secretes potent digestive enzymes in their inactive forms. These inactive enzymes normally flow through the main pancreatic duct into the duodenum, where the enzymes are activated. Sometimes, the enzymes become activated within the pancreas and digest the pancreatic tissue, causing severe inflammation in the form of acute pancreatitis. This condition is very painful and dangerous, demanding immediate intervention.

Sum It Up!

The accessory digestive organs include the liver, gallbladder, and pancreas. These organs secrete substances that are eventually emptied into the duodenum, the meeting place for digestion. The liver performs many functions. The liver's primary digestive role is the secretion of bile. Bile is stored in the gallbladder and is released in response to cholecystokinin. The pancreas secretes the most potent digestive enzymes. The pancreatic enzymes empty into the duodenum. In addition to the digestive enzymes, bicarbonate-rich pancreatic secretions assist the digestive process.

DIGESTION AND ABSORPTION

The primary purpose of the digestive system is to break down large pieces of food into small particles suitable for absorption. Food is digested mechanically and chemically. Mechanical digestion is the physical breakdown of food into small fragments. It is achieved by the chewing activity of the mouth and by the mixing and churning activities of the muscles of the digestive organs.

Chemical digestion is the chemical change occurring primarily in response to the digestive enzymes. Whereas mechanical digestion refers to a breakdown in the size of the piece of food, chemical digestion refers to a change in the chemical composition of the food molecule.

Food is made of carbohydrates, proteins, and fats. Digestive enzymes and several digestive aids (mucus, hydrochloric acid, and bile) play key roles in chemical digestion. Specific enzymes digest each type of food (see Table 23-1). (Review the structures of carbohydrates, protein, and fat in Chapter 4.)

CARBOHYDRATES AND CARBOHYDRATE-SPLITTING ENZYMES

Carbohydrates are organic compounds composed of carbon, hydrogen, and oxygen; they are classified according to size (see Figure 4-2). **Monosaccharides** are single (mono) sugars (saccharides). The three monosaccharides are glucose, fructose, and galactose. Glucose is the most important of the three monosaccharides. **Disaccharides** are double (di) sugars. The three disaccharides are sucrose (table sugar), lactose, and maltose. **Polysaccharides** are many (poly) glucose molecules linked together. The shorter monosaccharides and disaccharides are called **sugars.** The longer-chain polysaccharides are **starches.**

A polysaccharide is digested in two stages (Figure 23-11, *A*). First, enzymes called **amylases** (ĂM-ĭ-lās-ĕs)

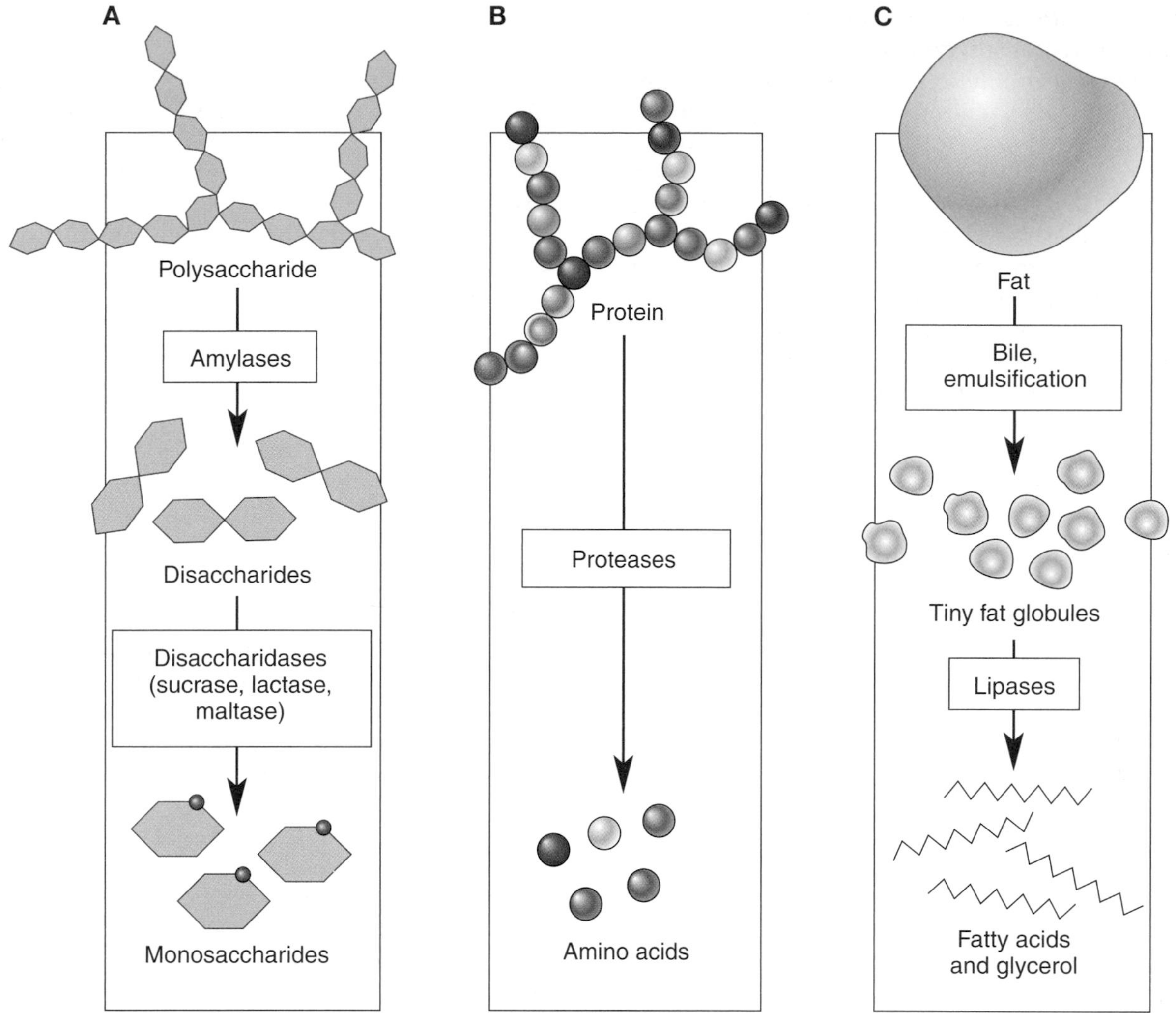

FIGURE 23-11 Chemical digestion. **A,** Carbohydrate digestion. **B,** Protein digestion. **C,** Fat emulsification and digestion.

break the polysaccharide into disaccharides. The two amylases are salivary amylase (ptyalin) and pancreatic amylase. Second, disaccharidases break disaccharides into monosaccharides. The three disaccharidases are sucrase, lactase, and maltase. (The ending *-ase* indicates an enzyme.) The cells of the intestinal villi secrete disaccharidases. Disaccharides therefore are split into monosaccharides in the duodenum at the surface of the villus. They are immediately absorbed across the villus into the blood capillaries.

Certain carbohydrates **(cellulose)** cannot be digested and therefore remain within the lumen of the digestive system. While providing no direct nourishment, dietary cellulose is beneficial in that it provides fiber and bulk to the stool.

Many persons suffer from a deficiency of the enzyme lactase. They are unable to digest the sugar found in milk (lactose) and are said to be lactose intolerant. This enzyme deficiency prevents lactose-intolerant people from ingesting milk and many milk products.

PROTEINS AND PROTEIN-SPLITTING ENZYMES

The building blocks of proteins are amino acids. Several amino acids linked together form a peptide. Many amino acids linked together form a polypeptide. **Proteins** are very long polypeptide chains; some proteins contain more than one polypeptide chain (see Figure 23-11, *B*). To be absorbed across the wall of the digestive tract, these chains must be uncoiled and broken down into small peptides and amino acids.

Enzymes called **proteases** (PRŌ-tē-ās-ĕs) or proteolytic enzymes, digest proteins. Proteases are secreted by three organs: the stomach secretes pepsin; the intestinal cells secrete enterokinase; and the pancreas secretes trypsin and chymotrypsin. The pancreatic proteases are the most potent proteases. Proteins are broken down into small peptides and amino acids and are absorbed across the intestinal villi into the blood capillaries.

Although not an enzyme, gastric hydrochloric acid (HCl) aids protein digestion. First, the HCl unravels the strands of protein, making the protein fragments more sensitive to the proteases. Second, the HCl activates a gastric proteolytic enzyme, pepsinogen, into pepsin. Pepsin then facilitates breaking protein into small peptides.

FATS, BILE, AND FAT-SPLITTING ENZYMES

Fats are long-chain molecules composed of carbon, hydrogen, and oxygen. Enzymes called **lipases** (LĪ-pās-ĕs) digest fats. The most important is pancreatic lipase (see Figure 23-11, *C*). The end products of fat digestion are fatty acids and glycerol; fat is absorbed into the lacteals of the villus.

Why is bile necessary for fat digestion (see Figure 23-11, *C*)? Fats, unlike carbohydrates or proteins, are not soluble in water; they tend to clump together into large fat globules when added to water. If, for instance, oil and water are placed in a test tube, the oil and water separate; the oil rises to the surface, and the water settles at the bottom. Oil and water simply do not mix. The same separation occurs in the digestive tract. Dietary fat tends to form large fat globules. The lipase cannot readily digest the fat. It can attack only the outside surface of the fat globule.

Bile solves the large fat globule problem. Bile can split the large fat globule into thousands of tiny fat globules. This process is **emulsification.** Because of emulsification, the lipases can work on the surfaces of all the tiny fat globules, thereby digesting more fat. Bile performs two other important roles. Bile salts prevent the fatty acids (end products of fat digestion) from reforming large fat globules in the intestine before they can be absorbed across the intestinal villi. Bile salts also help the absorption of the fat-soluble vitamins A, D, E, and K.

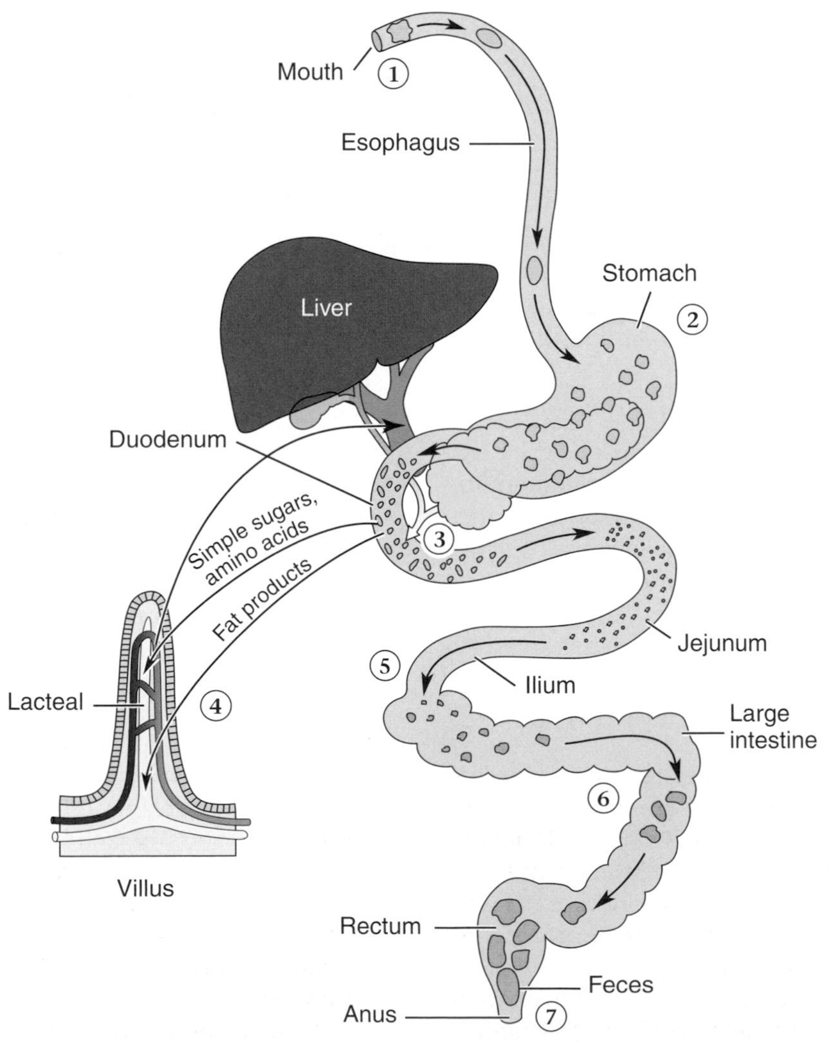

FIGURE 23-12 The digestion and absorption of the turkey meal.

Sum It Up!

How is a turkey dinner digested and absorbed (Figure 23-12)?

1. In the mouth, food is chewed into tiny pieces, and mixed with saliva.
2. The smaller pieces of food are transported through the esophagus to the stomach, where they are mixed, mashed, and churned into chyme.
3. The partially digested food (chyme) squirts into the duodenum, where it mixes with bile and the pancreatic and intestinal enzymes. Pancreatic amylase and the disaccharidases digest the polysaccharides to monosaccharides. The pancreatic proteases (trypsin and chymotrypsin) and the intestinal proteases digest the proteins to amino acids. A pendulum-like peristaltic motion washes the digested food across each villus, thereby enhancing absorption.
4. The simple sugars and the amino acids are absorbed into the blood capillaries of the villi. These capillaries eventually empty into the portal vein for transport to the liver.

   Bile emulsifies the fats, and the pancreatic and intestinal lipases digest them. The end products of fat digestion are fatty acids and glycerol. The fat products are absorbed into the lacteals of the villi. Most of the digestion and absorption occurs in the duodenum, the meeting point for digestion.
5. The unabsorbed food material moves along the jejunum and ileum and into the large intestine.
6. A large volume of water and certain electrolytes are absorbed along this route, and a semisolid stool is formed.
7. The presence of the fecal material in the rectum gives rise to an urge to defecate.

NUTRITION: CONCEPTS TO KNOW

Nutrition is the science that studies the relationship of food to the functioning of the body. Food consists of nutrients, substances the body uses to promote normal growth, maintenance, and repair. The five categories of nutrients are carbohydrates, proteins, lipids, vitamins, and minerals.

CARBOHYDRATES

Dietary carbohydrates are classified as simple sugars and complex carbohydrates. A **simple sugar** is composed of monosaccharides and disaccharides. Glucose, the simplest carbohydrate, is the major fuel used to make ATP in most body cells. Most of the carbohydrates come from plants. The sugars are derived primarily from fruit, sugar cane, and milk.

The **complex carbohydrates** are larger sugar molecules (polysaccharides) and consist primarily of starch and fiber. Starch is found in cereal grains (wheat, oats, corn, barley); legumes (peas, beans); and root vegetables such as potatoes. Fiber, or cellulose, is found primarily in vegetables. Cellulose cannot be digested by humans, but it is beneficial nutritionally because it provides bulk in the stool and aids in defecation.

Most carbohydrate ingestion should be in the form of complex carbohydrates for two reasons. First, complex carbohydrates usually provide other nutrients, whereas simple sugars provide "empty calories" (nothing but calories). Second, complex carbohydrates are absorbed at a slower rate than sugars thereby preventing a sudden spike in blood glucose. The spiking of blood glucose has been linked to an oversecretion of insulin, impaired cellular uptake of glucose, and hypertension. (The hypertension is due to the effect of insulin on the reabsorption of Na^+ and water by the kidney.) Our excessive intake of corn syrup is fattening us up. Is it also creating a nation of diabetics?

PROTEINS

Dietary proteins supply the body with amino acids. Because the body cannot store amino acids, a daily supply is necessary. Amino acids are classified as essential and nonessential. An **essential amino acid** cannot be synthesized by the body and must therefore be consumed in the diet. A **nonessential amino acid** can be synthesized by the body. It is not essential that these amino acids be consumed in the diet. Of the 20 amino acids, 9 are essential.

Proteins are classified as complete or incomplete. A **complete protein** contains all essential amino acids. Complete proteins are found in animal sources; meat, eggs, and dairy products are complete proteins. **Incomplete proteins** do not contain all of the essential amino acids. Vegetable proteins are incomplete proteins. These include nuts, grains, and legumes. Vegetable proteins, if eaten in combinations, can supply a complete complement of amino acids. For instance, a favorite Mexican dish containing rice and beans is complete in that it supplies all the essential amino acids, even though both the rice and the beans are incomplete proteins.

FATS (LIPIDS)

Most dietary lipids are **triglycerides,** molecules that contain glycerol and fatty acids. Fatty acids are classified as saturated or unsaturated. A **saturated fatty acid** (butter, lard) is solid at room temperature. Also included in this group are artificially hardened, or hydrogenated, fats such as vegetable shortening and margarine. Saturated fats come primarily from animal sources. An **unsaturated fat** is liquid at room temperature and is called an oil.

The body can synthesize all fatty acids, with one exception—linoleic acid, an important component of cell membranes. Because the body cannot synthesize it, linoleic acid is an **essential fatty acid** and must therefore be included in the diet.

Foods high in fat come from both animal and plant sources. Animal sources, however, tend to contain more saturated fat. They include meat, eggs, butter, and whole-milk products such as cheese. Plant sources include coconut oil and palm oil. Hydrogenated vegetable oils in shortening and margarine are also high in saturated fat. In addition to the fat content, these foods also tend to be high in cholesterol.

VITAMINS

Vitamins are small organic molecules that help regulate cell metabolism (Table 23-2). Vitamins are parts of enzymes or other organic substances essential for normal cell function and are classified as fat soluble or water soluble. The **fat-soluble vitamins** include vitamins A, D, E, and K. Because the body stores fat-soluble vitamins, excess intake (hypervitaminosis) may result in symptoms of toxicity.

The **water-soluble vitamins** include vitamins B and C. These vitamins, for the most part, are not stored by the body. Excess water-soluble vitamins are generally excreted in the urine. Excretion, however, does not rule out the possibility of toxicity in response to megadosing with water-soluble vitamins.

You can best appreciate the roles vitamins play by observing the effects of specific vitamin deficiencies. For instance, vitamin A is necessary for healthy skin. It also plays a vital role in night vision. Vitamin A deficiency is characterized by various skin lesions and by night blindness, the inability to see in a darkened room. Vitamin D is necessary for the absorption of calcium and the development and formation of strong bones. Vitamin D deficiency causes rickets in children, a condition in which the bones are soft and often bow in response to weight bearing. Because the skin can synthesize vitamin D in response to exposure to ultraviolet radiation, the incidence of rickets is higher in places with little sunlight. Vitamin D deficiency in adults results in a bone-softening condition called osteomalacia.

Vitamin K plays a crucial role in hemostasis. It is necessary for the synthesis of prothrombin and several other clotting factors. A deficiency of vitamin K causes hypoprothrombinemia (diminished amount of prothrombin in the blood) and a tendency to bleed excessively.

Finally, vitamin C is necessary for the integrity of the skin and mucous membranes. A deficiency of vitamin C causes scurvy, a condition involving skin lesions and inability of the tissues to heal. Historically, scurvy was common on ships that were at sea for months at a time. Having determined that limes prevented scurvy, the British sailors traveled around the world sipping lime juice. In response to this habit, they were dubbed limeys. Other vitamin deficiencies are included in Table 23-2.

MINERALS

Minerals are inorganic substances necessary for normal body function (Table 23-3). Minerals have numerous functions, ranging from regulation of plasma

Table 23-2 Selected Vitamins

Vitamin	Function	Deficiency
Fat Soluble		
Vitamin A	Necessary for skin, mucous membranes, and night vision	Night blindness; dry, scaly skin; disorders of mucous membranes
Vitamin D (calciferol)	Necessary for the absorption of calcium and phosphorus	Rickets in children; osteomalacia in adults
Vitamin E	Necessary for health of cell membrane	None defined
Vitamin K	Needed for the synthesis of prothrombin and other clotting factors	Bleeding
Water Soluble		
Thiamine (Vitamin B_1)	Helps release energy from carbohydrates and amino acids; needed for growth	Beriberi; alcohol-induced Wernicke's syndrome
Riboflavin (Vitamin B_2)	Essential for growth	Skin and tongue disorders; dermatitis
Niacin (Vitamin B_3)	Helps release energy from nutrients	Pellagra with dermatitis, diarrhea, mental disorders
Pyridoxine (Vitamin B_6)	Participates in the metabolism of amino acids and proteins	Nervous system and skin disorders
Vitamin B_{12}	Helps form red blood cells and deoxyribonucleic acid (DNA)	Anemias, particularly pernicious anemia
Folic acid	Participates in the formation of hemoglobin and DNA	Anemia; neural tube defects in embryo
Ascorbic acid (Vitamin C)	Necessary for synthesis of collagen; helps maintain capillaries; aids in the absorption of iron	Scurvy; poor bone and wound healing

Table 23-3 Selected Minerals

Mineral	Function	Deficiency
Potassium (K)	Nerve and muscle activity	Nerve and muscle disorders
Sodium (Na)	Water balance; nerve impulse conduction	Weakness, cramps, diarrhea, dehydration, confusion
Calcium (Ca)	Component of bones and teeth, nerve conduction, muscle contraction, blood clotting	Rickets, tetany, bone softening
Phosphorus (P)	Component of bones and teeth, component of adenosine triphosphate, nucleic acids, and cell membranes	Bone demineralization
Iron (Fe)	Component of hemoglobin (red blood cells)	Anemia, dry skin
Iodine (I)	Necessary for synthesis of thyroid hormones	Hypothyroidism; iodine-deficient goiter
Magnesium (Mg)	Component of some enzymes; important in carbohydrate metabolism	Muscle spasm, dysrhythmias, vasodilation
Fluorine (F)	Component of bones and teeth	Dental caries
Trace minerals	Small amounts required for certain specific functions	Nerve and muscle disorders
Zinc (Zn)	Nerve and muscle activity	Weakness, cramps, diarrhea, dehydration, confusion
Copper (Cu)	Water balance; nerve impulse conduction	Rickets, tetany, bone softening
Manganese (Mn)	Component of bones and teeth, nerve conduction, muscle contraction, blood clotting	Bone demineralization
Selenium (Se)	Component of bones and teeth, component of adenosine triphosphate, nucleic acids, and cell membranes	Anemia, dry skin

volume (sodium, chloride) to bone growth (calcium) to oxygen transport (iron) to the regulation of metabolic rate (iodine).

Mineral deficiencies can cause serious health problems. For instance, because iodine is necessary for the synthesis of the thyroid hormone thyroxine, iodine deficiency can cause an enlarged thyroid gland (goiter) and hypothyroidism. Because iron is necessary for the synthesis of hemoglobin, iron deficiency can cause anemia. This anemic state is characterized by fatigue and, depending on its severity, a diminished ability to transport oxygen around the body.

HEALTH AND A BALANCED DIET

A Balanced Diet

A balanced diet contains all the essential nutrients and includes a variety of foods. The balanced diet is often displayed in the form of a food pyramid. The newest food pyramid "personalizes" food intake since it also considers body build and level of activity. Exercise is a crucial part of the newest pyramid.

Poorly Balanced Diet and Disease

Many health problems are thought to originate in poor dietary choices. For instance, a diet high in cholesterol or fats, or both, has been implicated in coronary artery disease. Fatty plaques develop along the inside walls of the blood vessels and eventually occlude the flow of blood to the heart, causing a heart attack. Fatty plaques can also form within the blood vessels that supply the brain, causing a stroke and paralysis. A diet high in saturated fat has also been implicated in diabetes and cancer.

Although overeating has been linked with health problems, a number of health problems are also related to a deficiency of certain foods. For instance, infants who are fed fat-poor diets (skim milk) may become deficient in fats essential for the development of nervous tissue. Fat deficiency may cause nerve damage and developmental delay. In poverty-stricken areas of the world, protein-deficiency diseases are common. Kwashiorkor, for example, is a protein-deficient state in which protein intake is inadequate to synthesize plasma proteins, muscle protein, and the protein necessary for healthy skin. The condition is characterized by edema formation, particularly ascites, muscle wasting, and dermatitis. The ascites appears as the distended abdomen of a starving child.

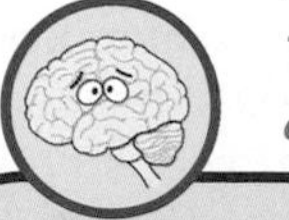

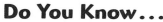

Do You Know...

That kwashiorkor refers to a "displaced" child?

Kwashiorkor is a condition of severe protein deficiency resulting in emaciation, edema formation, and ascites. The African word *kwashiorkor* (displaced or deposed) indicates the cause of the condition. A breast-fed infant is prematurely weaned from breast milk and placed on a protein-poor cereal diet. Why the premature weaning? To make room for baby brother. The 9-month-old infant is displaced or deposed by the newborn.

Malnutrition usually refers to starvation or a profound weight loss due to a caloric deficiency. Although malnutrition certainly takes this form in countries with limited food supplies, in the United States malnutrition appears most often in the overfed. The American diet and sedentary lifestyle have contributed to obesity, a national health problem. The magnitude of the problem is evident in the numbers of weight-reduction diets. The problem is so common that we now have a routine phrase, couch potato, to describe a sedentary person, one who may well be obese.

One form of extreme wasting that is common in the United States is called cachexia. It is most often seen in patients who are terminally ill with cancer and other chronic diseases. The severe anorexia and altered metabolism causes depletion of fat and protein stores, resulting in dramatic weight loss and starvation.

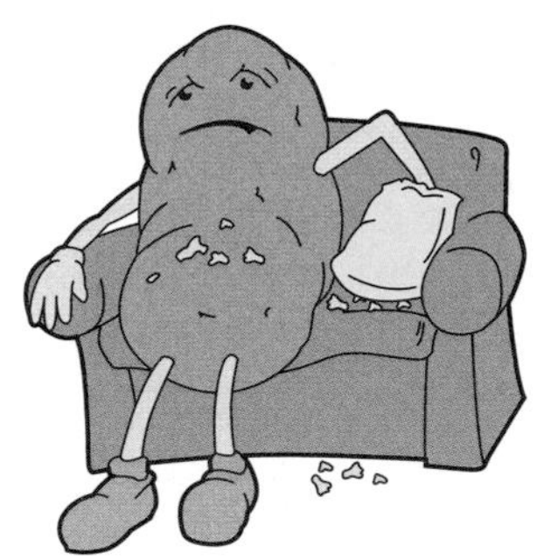

Appetite Control and the Couch Potato

What makes us eat and stop eating? Don't know! We know that the hypothalamus plays an important role. There is an area of the lateral hypothalamus called the **feeding center.** When destroyed it leads to anorexia and starvation. Another hypothalamic area is called the **satiety center;** damage to it causes overeating and morbid obesity. There are numerous theories about what satisfies (satiety) and therefore suppresses appetite. The **glucostat hypothesis** states that the satiety center contains neurons called glucostats that absorb glucose and send inhibitory information to the feeding center. In response, appetite diminishes. The **lipostat hypothesis** states that adipocytes (fat cells) secrete a hormone called leptin. Leptin is an appetite suppressant. Other appetite suppressants have been identified. CCK secreted by the duodenum suppresses the feeding center in the brain. Alas! Couch Potato keeps eating, apparently ignoring the "stop eating" signals from his bombarded hypothalamus.

BODY ENERGY

Energy is essential for two reasons: (1) it provides the body with the power to do its work, and (2) it maintains body temperature.

Measurement of Energy

Energy is measured in units called kilocalories (kcal) meaning the "large calorie." (A capital C means a "large calorie.") One **Calorie** is the amount of energy required to raise the temperature of 1 kilogram (kg) of water by 1° Celsius (C). The energy yield of the three food groups, carbohydrates, proteins, and fats, is expressed in calories.

Carbohydrate yields 4 Cal/g
Protein yields 4 Cal/g
Fat yields 9 Cal/g

NOTE: The metabolism of 1 g of fat yields twice as many calories as the metabolism of 1 g of carbohydrate or protein.

Energy Balance

Energy balance occurs when the input of energy (food) equals the output of energy (energy expenditure). Energy balance is not always achieved. If food intake exceeds energy expenditure, the excess energy is converted to and stored as fat, causing weight gain. Conversely, if food intake is less than the energy expended, weight loss occurs. Weight management programs therefore encourage both dietary restriction and exercise regimens.

Energy Expenditure

Energy expenditure differs depending on whether the body is in a resting or nonresting state. The amount of energy the body requires per unit time to perform essential activities at rest is the **basal metabolic rate (BMR).** These activities include breathing, kidney function, cardiac muscle contraction—whatever minimal functions the body must perform to remain alive.

Several factors affect BMR (Figure 23-13). These include gender, age, body surface area, emotional state, overall health status, and several hormones. Men have a higher BMR than women. An adolescent has a higher BMR than an elderly person. A tiny bird has a higher BMR than an elephant. A person livid with rage has a higher metabolism than a peaceful person. A patient with an infection has a higher BMR than an infection-free person. The thyroid hormone thyroxine exerts the most profound effect on BMR. The hyperthyroid patient has a higher BMR than a euthyroid (normal thyroid) person. The metabolism of a hyperthyroid patient can be so high that the patient can consume in excess of 6000 Cal/day and still lose weight. In contrast, the hypothyroid patient has a lower-than-normal BMR and often consults a physician because of loss of energy and weight gain.

The body needs a certain amount of energy to maintain minimal function but requires additional energy when the person engages in activity above and beyond the resting state. In general, the more active the person is, the higher the metabolic rate and the greater the expenditure of energy.

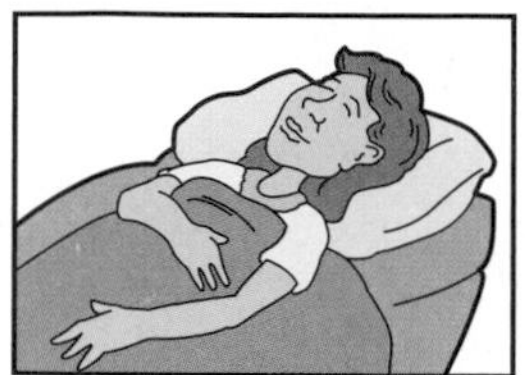

Basal metabolic rate (BMR)

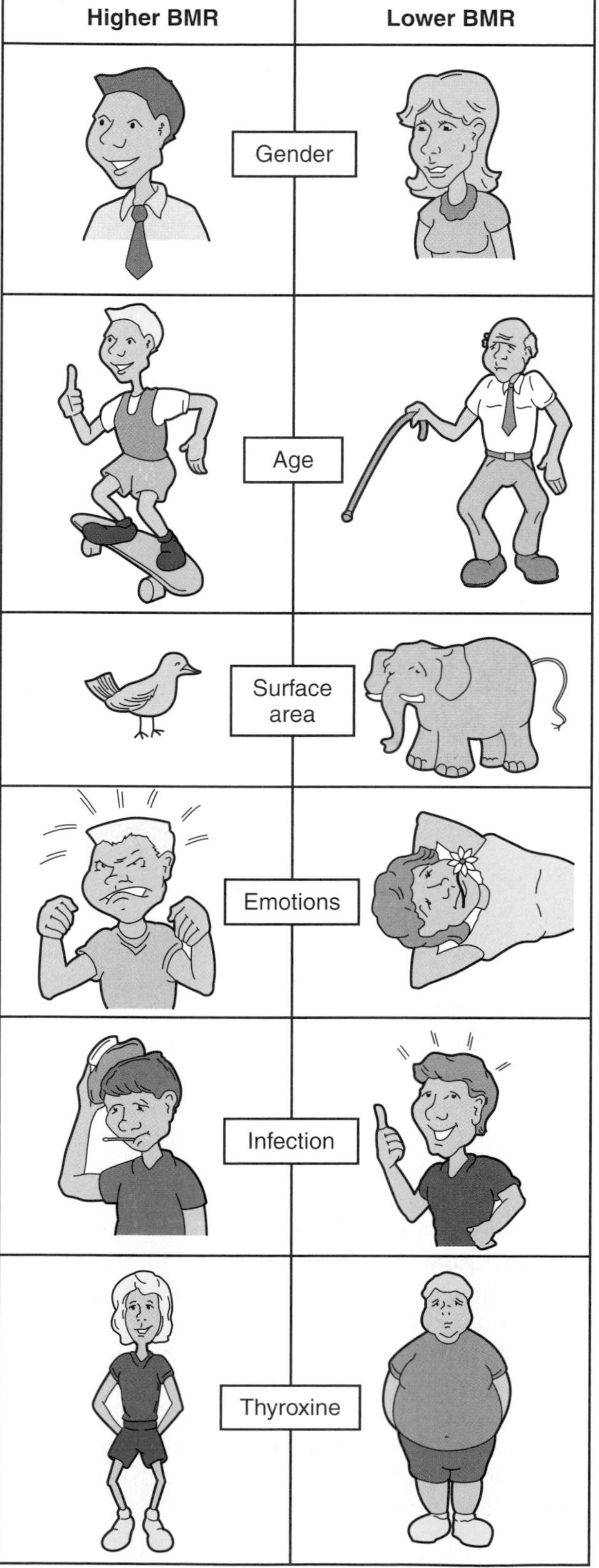

Sum It Up!

The body uses food for energy, repair, and maintenance. A balanced diet contains specific amounts and types of nutrients: carbohydrates, proteins, fats, vitamins, and minerals. Failure to ingest certain nutrients causes malnutrition, deficiency states, and illness.

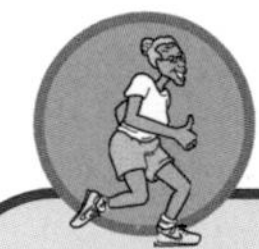

As You Age

1. The muscular wall of the digestive tract loses tone, causing constipation due to a slowing of peristalsis.
2. Secretion of saliva and digestive enzymes decreases, thereby decreasing digestion. The decrease in secretions also impairs the absorption of vitamins (vitamin B_{12}) and minerals (iron and calcium).
3. The sensations of taste and smell diminish with age. Consequently, food tastes different, and appetite may be affected.
4. The loss of teeth and an inability to chew food effectively makes eating difficult. The loss of teeth may also affect the choice of food, causing the elderly person to select a less nutritious diet such as tea and toast.
5. Peristalsis in the esophagus is no longer triggered with each swallow, and the lower esophageal sphincter relaxes more slowly. These changes hamper swallowing and cause an early feeling of fullness.
6. A weakened gag reflex increases the risk of aspiration.
7. The liver shrinks and receives a smaller supply of blood. The rate of drug detoxification by the liver declines, thereby prolonging the effects of drugs and predisposing the person to a drug overdose. (Remember: the liver is the chief organ of drug inactivation.)

FIGURE 23-13 Factors that affect basal metabolic rate.

Disorders of the Digestive System

Anorexia	Loss of appetite due to many causes, ranging from simple emotional upset to serious diseases and adverse drug reactions. Anorexia nervosa is a severe psychological disorder characterized by a fear of becoming obese. A significant loss of weight is achieved through starvation and a binge-purge routine called bulimia, another eating disorder.
Cirrhosis	A chronic disease of the liver in which the liver cells are replaced by scar tissue. Cirrhosis is often caused by chronic alcoholism or hepatitis. Cirrhosis leads to progressive loss of liver function, a life-threatening increase in portal pressure, ascites, esophageal varices, and massive hemorrhage.
Diverticulitis	An inflammation of the pouches (diverticula) in the lining of the intestinal wall.
Hepatitis	An inflammation of the liver commonly caused by a virus. The many types of hepatitis are designated as A, B, C, D, and E. All cause hepatic cell damage; some increase the risk of cirrhosis and cancer of the liver. All forms of hepatitis are serious.
Inflammation of the lining of the gastrointestinal (GI) tract	Inflamed lining of the GI tract has many causes. Gastritis, an inflammation of the stomach lining, is commonly caused by an infection (food poisoning); ingestion of ulcer-causing drugs (such as steroids, aspirin, nonsteroidal antiinflammatory drugs [NSAIDs]); and smoking of tobacco. Enteritis is an inflammation of the intestinal lining commonly caused by infection. Gastroenteritis refers to an inflammation of the stomach and intestinal lining.
Inflammatory bowel disease	An umbrella term that includes ulcerative colitis and Crohn's disease. Both conditions are characterized by severe cramping, diarrhea, bleeding, and fever.
Pancreatitis	An inflammation of the pancreas. Pancreatitis causes severe pain and signs and symptoms that may end in death.

SUMMARY OUTLINE

I. Overview of the Digestive System

A. Functions of the Digestive System
1. Ingestion (eating).
2. Digestion.
3. Absorption.
4. Elimination.

B. The Wall of the Digestive Tract and Membranes
1. There are four layers: mucosal, submucosa, muscle, serosa.
2. Peritoneal membranes: mesentery, mesocolon, greater and lesser omentum.

II. Structures and Organs of the Digestive System

A. Mouth
1. Teeth and tongue.
2. Salivary glands: parotid, submandibular, and sublingual.

B. Pharynx (Throat)

C. Esophagus
1. The esophagus is a long tube that connects the pharynx to the stomach.
2. There are two sphincters.

D. Stomach
1. The three parts of the stomach are the fundus, body, and pylorus.
2. The stomach functions in digestion; its most important role is regulate the rate at which chyme is delivered to the small intestine.

E. Small Intestine
1. The three parts of the small intestine are the duodenum, jejunum, and ileum.
2. Most of the digestion and absorption occurs within the duodenum.
3. The end products of digestion are absorbed into villi.

F. Large Intestine
1. The large intestine consists of the cecum, ascending colon, transverse colon, descending colon, sigmoid colon, rectum, and anus.
2. The large intestine functions in absorption of water and electrolytes.

III. Accessory Digestive Organs

A. Liver
1. The liver has many functions; its most important digestive function is the secretion of bile.
2. The liver receives blood from the portal vein; portal blood is rich in digestive end products.

B. Biliary Tree
   1. The biliary tree is composed of the bile ducts that connect the liver, gallbladder, and duodenum.
   2. The common bile duct empties into the duodenum.

C. Gallbladder
   1. The gallbladder functions to store and concentrate bile.
   2. The gallbladder contracts and releases bile in response to the hormone cholecystokinin (CCK).

D. Pancreas
   1. The pancreas secretes the most important digestive enzymes.
   2. The pancreatic enzymes empty into the duodenum.

IV. Digestion and Absorption

A. Carbohydrate Digestion
   1. To be absorbed, carbohydrates must be broken down into glucose.
   2. Carbohydrates are digested by enzymes called amylases and disaccharidases.

B. Protein Digestion
   1. To be absorbed, proteins must be broken down into amino acids.
   2. Proteins are broken down by proteolytic enzymes or proteases.

C. Fat Digestion
   1. To be absorbed, fats must be broken down into fatty acids and glycerol.
   2. Fats are digested by enzymes called lipases. Fats are first emulsified by bile.

V. Nutrition and Body Energy

A. Carbohydrates
   1. Carbohydrates are either simple or complex.
   2. Glucose, the simplest carbohydrate, is the major fuel used by the body for energy.

B. Protein
   1. The body needs essential amino acids, which it cannot synthesize, and nonessential amino acids, which it can synthesize.
   2. Dietary proteins are complete or incomplete.

C. Fats (Lipids)
   1. Most dietary lipids are triglycerides.
   2. Fats are either saturated fats (like butter) or unsaturated fats (like oils).

D. Vitamins
   1. Vitamins are small organic molecules that help regulate cell metabolism. Dietary vitamin deficiencies give rise to many diseases (see Table 23-2).
   2. Vitamins are either water soluble (vitamins B and C) or fat soluble (vitamins A, D, E, and K).

E. Minerals
   1. Minerals are inorganic substances necessary for normal body function.
   2. Mineral deficiencies can cause serious health problems.

F. Body Energy
   1. The body needs energy to do its work and maintain body temperature.
   2. The basal metabolic rate (BMR) is the amount of energy the body requires per unit time to perform essential activities at rest.
   3. Metabolism is determined by many factors, including age; gender; surface area; emotional state; overall health status; and hormones (especially thyroxine).

Review Your Knowledge

Matching: Structures: Making the Connections

Directions: Match the following words with their description below.

a. ileum
b. sigmoid
c. jejunum
d. common bile duct
e. transverse colon
f. duodenum
g. esophagus
h. stomach

1. ____ Connects the duodenum to the ileum
2. ____ Connects the cystic and hepatic ducts to the duodenum
3. ____ Connects the rectum to the descending colon
4. ____ Connects the ascending colon to the descending colon
5. ____ Connects the esophagus to the duodenum
6. ____ Connects the pharynx to the stomach
7. ____ Connects the stomach to the jejunum
8. ____ Connects the jejunum to the cecum

Matching: Enzymes, Hormones, and Digestive Aids

Directions: Match the following words with their description below. Some words may be used more than once

a. amylases
b. hydrochloric acid
c. disaccharidases
d. secretin
e. bile
f. proteases
g. cholecystokinin
h. intrinsic factor
i. lipase

1. ____ Classification of trypsin and chymotrypsin
2. ____ Secreted by the parietal cells of the stomach; lowers gastric pH
3. ____ Digests sucrose, maltose, and lactose
4. ____ An emulsifying agent
5. ____ Digests fats to fatty acids and glycerol
6. ____ Hormone secreted by the duodenum in response to the presence of fat
7. ____ Digests starch and polysaccharides to disaccharides
8. ____ Hormone that stimulates the pancreas to secrete a bicarbonate-rich secretion
9. ____ Hormone that stimulates the gallbladder to contract
10. ____ Digests protein to small peptides and amino acids
11. ____ Secreted by the liver and stored in the gallbladder
12. ____ Necessary for the absorption of vitamin B_{12}
13. ____ Classification of sucrase, maltase, and lactase

Multiple Choice

1. The esophagus
   a. secretes potent proteolytic enzymes.
   b. secretes intrinsic factor that is necessary for the absorption of vitamin B_{12}.
   c. is a hollow tube that carries food from the pharynx to the stomach.
   d. is the primary site of digestion and absorption.
2. Which of the following is true regarding the stomach?
   a. Its most important function is the digestion of fat.
   b. It is lined with microvilli so as to maximize absorption.
   c. It is attached distally to the jejunum and proximally to the esophagus.
   d. Its most important function is to deliver chyme to the duodenum at the proper rate.
3. Which of the following is not descriptive of bile?
   a. Aids in fat digestion
   b. Is an emulsifying agent
   c. Is classified as a lipase
   d. Is stored by the gallbladder
4. Lipases, proteases, and amylases are
   a. gastric hormones.
   b. synthesized by the liver and stored in the gallbladder.
   c. digestive enzymes.
   d. digestive enzymes that split carbohydrates to disaccharides.
5. Which of the following is not a function of the liver?
   a. Makes blood clotting factors such as prothrombin
   b. Makes bile
   c. Secretes cholecystokinin and secretin
   d. Stores fat soluble vitamins
6. Which of the following best describes emulsification?
   a. A fat is chemically digested to fatty acids and glycerol.
   b. The fatty acids are absorbed into the lacteal becoming chyle.
   c. A large fat globule is mechanically broken into smaller fat globules.
   d. A large protein forms ammonia.
7. The pancreas
   a. secretes the most potent digestive enzymes.
   b. secretes CCK and secretin.
   c. is only important because of its endocrine (insulin) function.
   d. empties its digestive enzymes into the appendix.
8. The duodenum is most concerned with
   a. the secretion of intrinsic factor and the absorption of vitamin B_{12}.
   b. digestion and absorption.
   c. the synthesis of clotting factors and plasma proteins.
   d. the synthesis of bile and emulsification.

CHAPTER 24

Urinary System

KEY TERMS

Aldosterone, p. 431
Angiotensin, p. 431
Antidiuretic hormone (ADH), p. 431
Collecting duct, p. 428
Creatinine, p. 430
Detrusor muscle, p. 438
Dialysis, p. 435
Diuresis, p. 430
Glomerulus, p. 428
Kidney, p. 426
Loop of Henle, p. 428
Micturition, p. 438
Nephron, p. 428
Renal tubule, p. 428
Renin, p. 431
Specific gravity, p. 433
Ureter, p. 426
Urethra, p. 426
Urinary bladder, p. 426

OBJECTIVES

1. List four organs of excretion.
2. Describe the major organs of the urinary system.
3. Describe the location, structure, blood supply, nerve supply, and functions of the kidneys.
4. Explain the role of the nephron unit in the formation of urine.
5. Explain the three processes involved in the formation of urine: filtration, reabsorption, and secretion.
6. Describe the hormonal control of water and electrolytes by the kidneys.
7. List the normal constituents of urine.
8. Describe the structure and function of the ureters, urinary bladder, and urethra.

Sammy with his soggy diaper is a friendly reminder of our hard-working urinary system. Indeed, Sammy may be a bundle of joy, but he is generally a wet bundle. What makes Sammy wet? Like a round-the-clock factory, Sammy's body burns fuel and produces waste products. To remain healthy, his kidneys must remove the waste and constantly adjust the amount of water and the concentration of electrolytes in his body. The kidneys work hard to do this; a wet Sammy is a healthy Sammy.

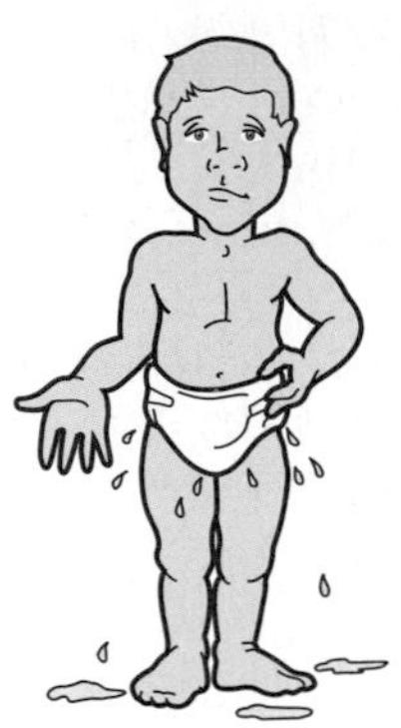

EXCRETION

ORGANS OF EXCRETION

The kidneys are the most important excretory organs. They eliminate nitrogenous waste, water, electrolytes, toxins, and drugs. Other organs perform excretory functions. The sweat glands secrete small amounts of nitrogen compounds, water, and electrolytes. The lungs eliminate carbon dioxide and water, and the intestines excrete digestive wastes, bile pigments, and other minerals (Table 24-1). While the skin, lungs, and intestines eliminate waste, only the kidneys can fine-tune the excretion of water and electrolytes to maintain the normal volume and composition of body fluids.

URINARY SYSTEM ORGANS

The urinary system, shown in Figure 24-1, makes urine, temporarily stores it, and finally eliminates it from the body. The major organs of the urinary system include the following:

- Two kidneys. The **kidneys** form urine from the blood.
- Two ureters. The **ureters** (ū-RĒ-tĕrz) are tubes that conduct urine from the kidneys to the urinary bladder.
- One **urinary bladder.** The bladder acts as a temporary reservoir; it receives urine from the ureters and stores the urine until it can be eliminated.
- One **urethra** (ū-RĒ-thră). The urethra is a tube that conducts urine from the bladder to the outside for elimination. (Do not confuse the ureters with the urethra.)

Table 24-1 Organs of Excretion

Organ	Substance Excreted
Kidneys	Water Electrolytes Nitrogenous waste
Skin (sweat glands)	Water Electrolytes Nitrogenous waste
Lungs	Carbon dioxide Water
Intestines	Digestive waste (feces) Bile pigments

URINARY SYSTEM TERMS

There are several words that refer to the urinary system and specifically to the kidneys. The word **renal** refers to the kidney. Thus renal physiology refers to the study of kidney function. **Nephrology** also refers to the study of kidney function. The term comes from the nephron unit, the unit in the kidney that makes urine. **Urology** is the study of the urinary system.

KIDNEYS

LOCATION

The kidneys are located high on the posterior wall of the abdominal cavity, behind the parietal peritoneum (retroperitoneal) (see Figure 24-1, *A*). The kidneys are cushioned and protected by the renal fascia, adipose tissue pads, and the lower rib cage.

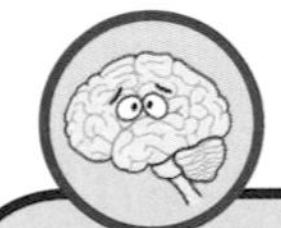

Do You Know...

What a floating kidney is?

The kidney is normally held in position by connective and adipose tissue. A very thin person has little adipose tissue. The kidney is more loosely attached to surrounding structures and may move about, or float. As you might expect, the floating kidney has a fancy medical name: nephroptosis. The downward displacement of the kidney causes the ureters to kink and the flow of urine to be restricted.

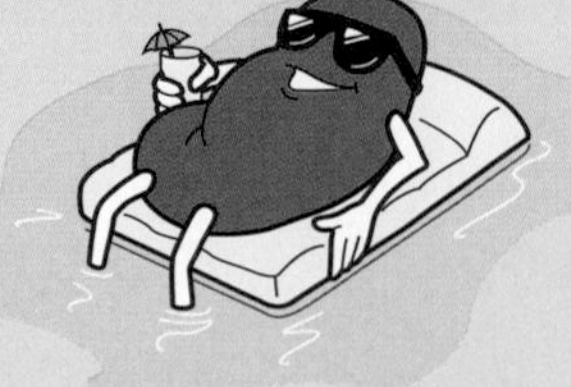

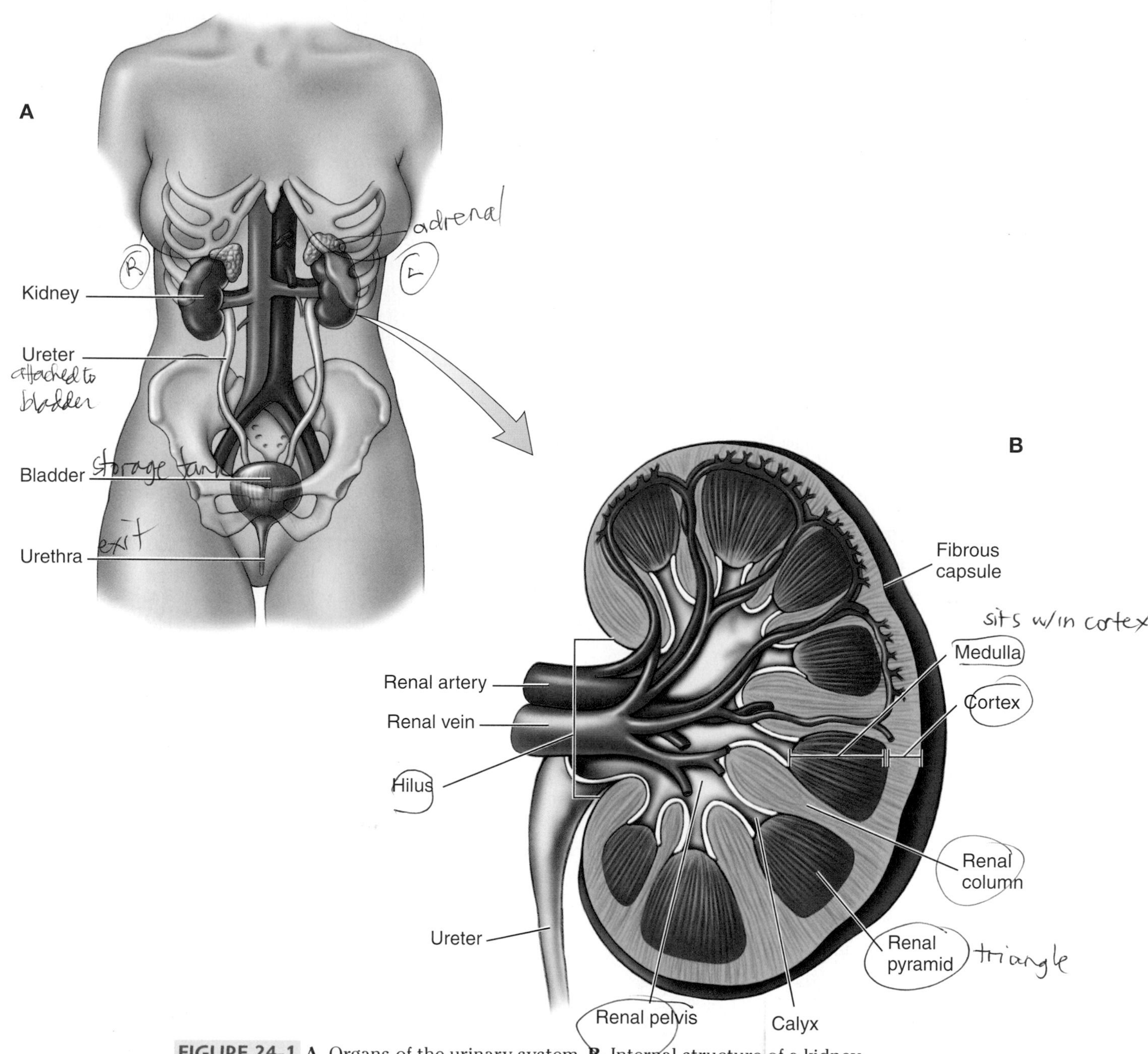

FIGURE 24-1 **A,** Organs of the urinary system. **B,** Internal structure of a kidney.

STRUCTURE

The kidney is a reddish-brown, beanlike structure enclosed in a tough fibrous capsule. Each kidney is about 4 inches (10 cm) long, 2 inches (5 cm) wide, and 1 inch (2.5 cm) thick. The indentation of the bean-shaped kidney is called the **hilus.** It is the point where the blood vessels, ureter, and nerves enter and exit the kidney.

What do you see when you cut open a kidney? As Figure 24-1, *B,* shows, a kidney has three distinct regions: the renal cortex, the renal medulla, and the renal pelvis. The lighter, outer region is the **renal cortex.** The darker triangular structure, the **renal medulla,** is located deeper within the kidney. The renal medulla forms striped, cone-shaped regions called **renal pyramids.** Each pyramid is separated by a **renal column.** These are extensions of the outer renal cortex. The lower ends of the pyramids point toward the **renal pelvis,** a basin that collects the urine made by the kidney and helps form the upper end of the ureter. The cuplike edges of the renal pelvis, closest to the pyramids, are calyces. **Calyces** (KĀ-lĭ-sēz) (singular: **calyx**) collect the urine formed in the kidney.

BLOOD SUPPLY

Blood is brought to the kidney by the renal artery, which arises from the abdominal aorta (see Figure 24-1, *B*). The renal arteries deliver a large amount of blood (about 20% to 25% of the cardiac output) to the kidneys. After entering the kidney, the renal artery branches into a series of smaller and smaller arteries, which make contact with the nephron units, the urine-making structures of the kidney. Blood leaves the kidneys through a series of veins that finally merge to form the renal vein. The renal vein empties into the inferior vena cava.

NERVE SUPPLY

The renal nerves travel with the renal blood vessels to the kidney. The nerves are primarily sympathetic nerves that help control blood flow to the kidney and regulate the release of renin (a blood pressure–controlling substance).

FUNCTIONS OF THE KIDNEYS

In general, the kidneys cleanse the blood of waste products, help regulate the volume and composition of body fluids, and help regulate the pH of body fluids. Specifically, the kidneys perform the following tasks:

- Excrete nitrogenous waste such as urea, uric acid, ammonia, and creatinine
- Regulate blood volume by determining the amount of water excreted
- Help regulate the electrolyte content of the blood
- Play a major role in the regulation of acid-base balance (blood pH) by controlling the excretion of hydrogen ions (H^+) (See Chapter 25 for the renal regulation of acid-base balance.)
- Play a role in the regulation of blood pressure through the secretion of renin
- Play a role in the regulation of red blood cell production through the secretion of a hormone called erythropoietin

URINE MAKING: THE NEPHRON UNIT

STRUCTURES

The **nephron** is the functional unit, or urine-making unit, of the kidney. Each kidney contains about 1 million nephron units. The number of nephron units does not increase after birth, and they cannot be replaced if damaged. Each nephron unit has two parts: a tubular component (renal tubule) and a vascular component (blood vessels).

Renal Tubules

The **renal tubules** consist of a number of tubular structures. The glomerular capsule, called **Bowman's capsule,** is a C-shaped structure that partially surrounds a cluster of capillaries called a **glomerulus** (glō-MĔR-ū-lŭs). Note that Figure 24-2 shows two views of a nephron unit: a realistic one and a schematic one. You should become familiar with both views.

Bowman's capsule extends from the glomerulus as a highly coiled tubule called the **proximal convoluted tubule.** The proximal convoluted tubule dips toward the renal pelvis to form a hairpin-shaped structure called the loop of Henle. The **loop of Henle** contains a descending and ascending limb. The ascending limb becomes the **distal convoluted tubule.** The distal convoluted tubules of several nephron units merge to form a **collecting duct.** The collecting ducts run through the renal medulla to the calyx of the renal pelvis. Urine is formed within these tubules.

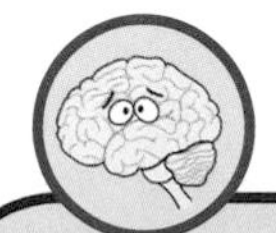

Do You Know...

Why the desert kangaroo rat has a loop of Henle that "just won't quit"?

The desert 'roo rat has a very long loop of Henle—much longer than yours. Why is that, you say? The 'roo rodent eats only seeds, other dry foods, and drinks no water (as in, it's a desert). But the water that is formed from the metabolism of its food is sufficient because the very long loops of Henle reabsorb almost all of the water that is filtered across its glomeruli. K Rat excretes urine that is about 15 times more concentrated than its plasma. You excrete urine that is 4 times as concentrated as your plasma.

Renal Blood Vessels (Vascular Structures)

The kidney receives blood from the renal artery. The renal artery branches into smaller blood vessels that form the afferent arteriole. The **afferent arteriole** branches into a cluster, or tuft, of capillaries called a glomerulus. The glomerulus sits in Bowman's capsule and exits from Bowman's capsule as the efferent arteriole. The **efferent arteriole** then forms a second capillary network called the peritubular capillaries. The **peritubular capillaries** empty into the venules, larger veins, and, finally, into the renal vein. The peritubular capillaries surround the renal tubule. (You need to understand the relationships of the vascular structures to the tubular structures. Become thoroughly familiar with Figure 24-2.)

URINE FORMATION

Urine is formed in the nephron units as water and dissolved substances move between the vascular and tubular structures. Three processes are involved in the formation of urine: glomerular filtration, tubular reabsorption, and tubular secretion.

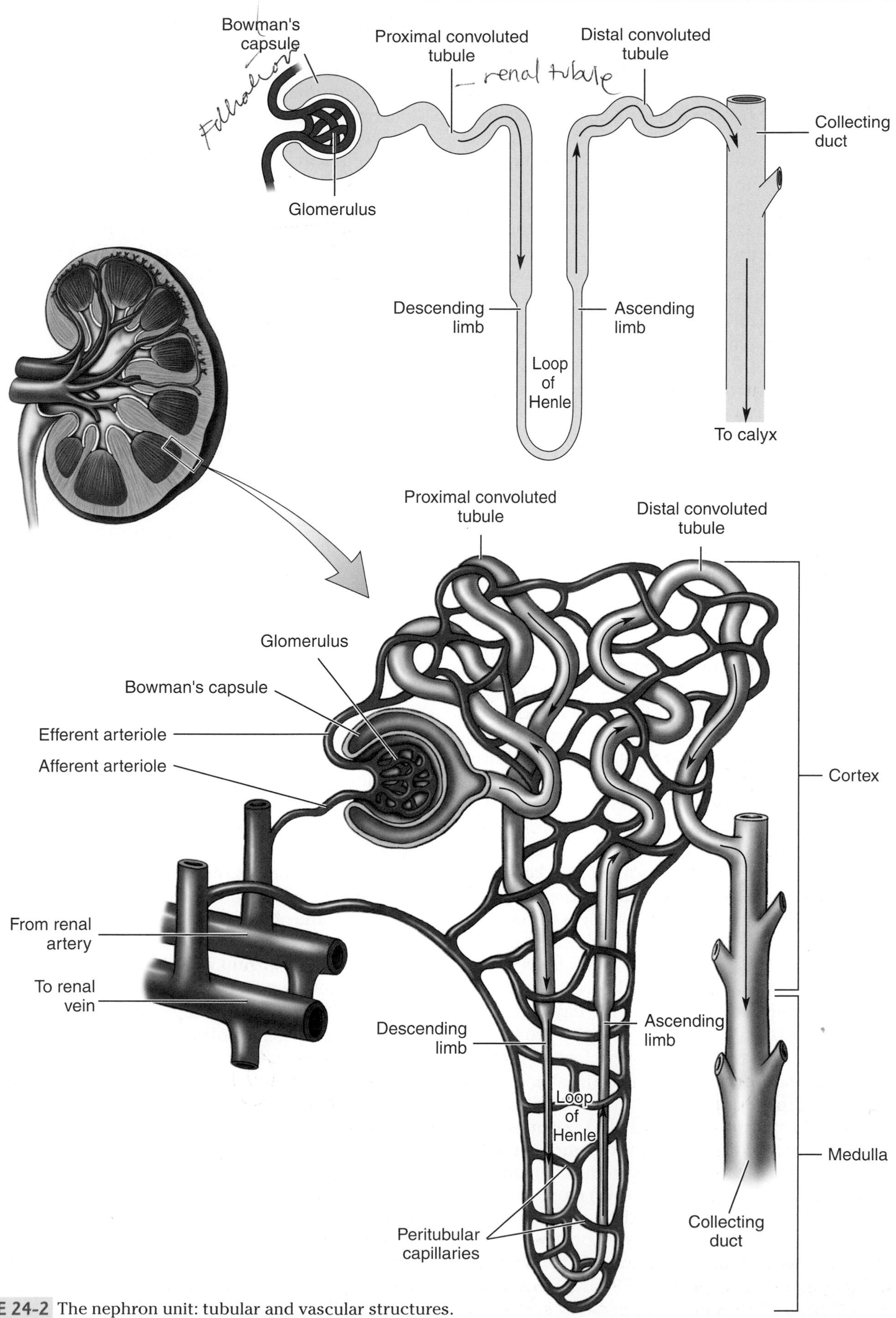

FIGURE 24-2 The nephron unit: tubular and vascular structures.

Glomerular Filtration

Urine formation begins in the glomerulus and Bowman's capsule. **Glomerular filtration** causes water and dissolved substances to move from the glomerulus into Bowman's capsule. Understanding filtration means answering two questions: why does filtration occur and what substances are filtered across the glomerular membrane?

Why Filtration Occurs. Filtration occurs when the pressure on one side of a membrane is greater than the pressure on the opposite side. Blood pressure in the glomerulus is higher than the pressure within Bowman's capsule. It is this pressure difference that provides the driving force for filtration. This pressure difference is called the glomerular filtration pressure.

What Substances Are Filtered. The wall of the glomerulus contains pores and acts like a sieve or a strainer. The size of the pores determines which substances can move across the wall from the glomerulus into Bowman's capsule. Small substances such as water, sodium, potassium, chloride, glucose, uric acid, and creatinine move through the pores very easily. These substances are filtered in proportion to their plasma concentration. In other words, if the concentration of a particular substance in the plasma is high, much of that substance is filtered. Large molecules such as red blood cells and large proteins cannot fit through the pores and therefore remain within the glomerulus. The water and the dissolved substances filtered into Bowman's capsule are called the **glomerular filtrate.** Note that the glomerular filtrate is protein-free; the presence of protein in the urine indicates abnormal nephron function (abnormally large holes in the glomerulus).

The rate at which glomerular filtration occurs is called the **glomerular filtration rate,** or **GFR.** Here is the amazing thing about GFR: the amount of filtrate formed is 125 ml/min, or 180 L (45 gal) in 24 hours. Picture in your mind 180 1-L bottles of cola. This is the amount of filtrate formed by your kidneys in one day. Obviously, you do not excrete 180 L of urine per day. Otherwise, you would do little more than drink and urinate, and you would literally wash away within a few hours. You excrete only about 1.5 L per day; so the big question is what happens to the 178.5 L that are filtered but not excreted?

Tubular Reabsorption

Most of the filtrate, approximately 178.5 L, is reabsorbed in the kidney and returned to the circulation. **Tubular reabsorption** is the process by which water and dissolved substances (glomerular filtrate) move from the tubules into the blood of the peritubular capillaries. Although reabsorption occurs throughout the entire length of the renal tubule, most occurs in the proximal convoluted tubule.

What is reabsorbed, and what is excreted? The kidney chooses the type and quantity of substances it reabsorbs. Some substances, such as glucose, are completely reabsorbed. For example, the amount of glucose filtered is the same as the amount reabsorbed, so glucose normally does not appear in the urine. Some substances are incompletely reabsorbed. For instance, over 99% of water and sodium is reabsorbed, whereas only 50% of urea is reabsorbed. Some waste products such as creatinine are not reabsorbed at all. Those substances not reabsorbed remain in the tubules, becoming part of the urine.

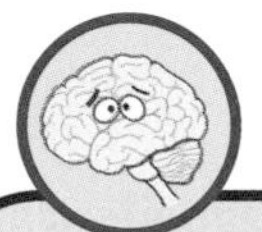

Do You Know...

Why serum creatinine is a measure of kidney function?

Creatinine (krē-ĂT-ĭ-nēn) is a waste product removed from the blood by the kidneys and eliminated in the urine. If kidney function declines, creatinine accumulates in the plasma. Thus serum creatinine levels are used to monitor kidney function.

The reabsorption of substances by the kidney also varies with the mechanism of reabsorption. Absorption occurs through either active or passive transport. For instance, sodium is actively transported from the tubules into the peritubular capillaries. Water and chloride passively follow the movement of sodium. In general, when sodium is pumped from one location to another, water follows passively. This sequence is the basis for the action of most **diuretics,** drugs that increase the production of urine. The excess secretion of urine is **diuresis** (dī-ūr-RĒ-sĭs). Most diuretics block the tubular reabsorption of sodium and therefore also block the reabsorption of water. The excess sodium and water remain in the tubules and are eliminated as urine. Hormones regulate the reabsorption of some substances. These hormones are described later in the chapter.

Tubular Secretion

Although most of the water and dissolved substances enter the tubules because of filtration across the glomerulus, a second process moves very small amounts of substances from the blood into the tubules. This is **tubular secretion.** It involves the active secretion of substances such as potassium ions (K^+), hydrogen ions (H^+), uric acid, ammonium ions, and drugs from the peritubular capillaries into the tubules.

Sum It Up!

The urinary system is composed of the urine-making kidneys and the structures that transport, store, and eliminate urine from the body. The urine is made by the nephron units, the functional units of the kidney. Urine is formed by three processes: filtration, reabsorption, and secretion. Filtration causes water and dissolved substances to move from the glomeruli into the tubules. Reabsorption causes water and selected substances to move from the tubules into the peritubular capillaries. Secretion causes small amounts of specific substances to move from the peritubular capillaries into the tubules.

HORMONES THAT WORK ON THE KIDNEYS

Several hormones act on the kidney to regulate water and electrolyte excretion. Thus these hormones play an important role in the regulation of blood volume, blood pressure, and electrolyte composition of body fluids (Table 24-2).

ALDOSTERONE

Aldosterone is a hormone secreted by the adrenal cortex. Aldosterone acts primarily on the distal tubule of the kidney. It stimulates the reabsorption of sodium and water and the excretion of potassium. Because of its effect on salt (NaCl), aldosterone is called the "salt-retaining" hormone. Aldosterone expands or increases blood volume. Because aldosterone increases blood volume, it also increases blood pressure. A deficiency of aldosterone causes severely diminished blood volume, decline in blood pressure, and shock.

What causes the release of aldosterone? One of the most important stimuli for the release of aldosterone is renin. **Renin** (RĒ-nĭn) is an enzyme that stimulates the **renin-angiotensin-aldosterone system.** Renin is secreted by a specialized collection of cells called the **juxtaglomerular apparatus,** located in the afferent arterioles. The renin-secreting cells are stimulated when either blood pressure or blood volume declines. As Figure 24-3 shows, renin sets off the following series of events:

- Renin activates **angiotensinogen** to form **angiotensin I** (ăn-jē-ō-TĔN-sĭn). Angiotensinogen is secreted by the liver and circulates within the blood; angiotensinogen is inactive.
- An enzyme called **converting enzyme** acts to change angiotensin I to **angiotensin II.** (Converting enzyme is found in the blood but is particularly high in the lungs.)
- Angiotensin II stimulates the adrenal cortex to release aldosterone. The aldosterone, in turn, stimulates the distal tubule to reabsorb sodium and water and to excrete potassium.

In addition to stimulating the release of aldosterone, angiotensin II is also a potent **vasopressor.** Angiotensin II causes vasoconstriction and an elevation in blood pressure. Thus the activation of the renin-angiotensin-aldosterone system regulates blood volume and blood pressure. A class of drugs called ACE inhibitors is used to lower blood pressure. (ACE stands for angiotensin-converting enzyme.) ACE inhibitors prevent the production of angiotensin II and aldosterone, both of which increase blood pressure. The ACE inhibitors include the *-pril* drugs, such as lisinopril and captopril.

ANTIDIURETIC HORMONE

A second hormone affecting water reabsorption is **antidiuretic hormone (ADH).** The action of ADH allows the kidneys to concentrate urine. (Think of the name antidiuretic hormone. It literally means against diuresis, or urine production.) The posterior pituitary gland (neurohypophysis) secretes ADH.

Antidiuretic hormone works primarily on the collecting duct by determining its permeability to water. In the presence of ADH, the collecting duct becomes permeable to water. Water is reabsorbed from the collecting duct into the peritubular capillaries. In other words,

Table 24-2 Effects of Hormones on the Kidney

Hormone	Secreted by	Function
Aldosterone	Adrenal cortex	Stimulates the reabsorption of sodium and water; stimulates the excretion of potassium; acts primarily on the distal tubule
Atrial natriuretic peptide (ANP)	Atria of the heart	Decreases the reabsorption of sodium; causes greater excretion of sodium and water by the kidney
Brain natriuretic peptide (BNP)	Ventricles of the heart	Decreases the reabsorption of sodium; causes greater excretion of sodium and water by the kidney
Antidiuretic hormone (ADH)	Neurohypophysis (posterior pituitary)	Stimulates the reabsorption of water primarily by the collecting ducts
Parathyroid hormone (PTH)	Parathyroid gland	Stimulates the reabsorption of calcium and excretion of phosphate

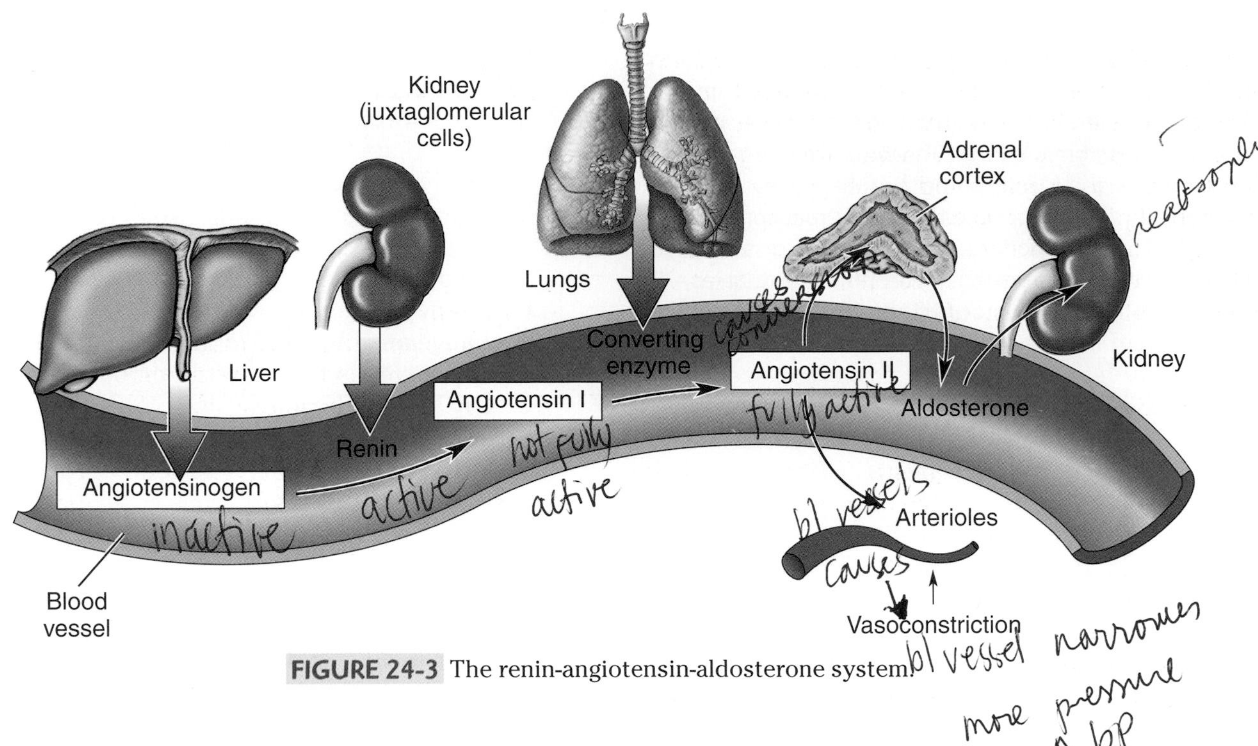

FIGURE 24-3 The renin-angiotensin-aldosterone system.

Do You Know...

Why both diabetes mellitus and diabetes insipidus cause polyuria?

Diabetes mellitus is a disease of insulin deficiency that results in hyperglycemia. The hyperglycemia, in turn, leads to excess filtration of glucose by the kidneys. Because all of the filtered glucose cannot be reabsorbed, glycosuria develops. The excess glucose in the tubules requires the excretion of large amounts of water. Thus the person with diabetes mellitus experiences polyuria (*poly* means much; *uria* means urine). Diabetes insipidus is a disease of ADH deficiency. ADH is necessary for the reabsorption of water from the collecting duct. In the absence of ADH, the person may excrete up to 10 L of a pale dilute urine. Note that both diabetes mellitus and diabetes insipidus are characterized by polyuria. The word diabetes refers to diuresis.

ADH decreases the excretion of water and causes excretion of a highly concentrated urine. In the absence of ADH, the membrane permeability of the collecting duct decreases, and water cannot be reabsorbed; the result is excretion of a very dilute urine. Because ADH affects the amount of water excreted by the kidneys, it plays an important role in the determination of blood volume and blood pressure. Excess ADH expands blood volume, while a deficiency of ADH diminishes blood volume.

What is the stimulus for the release of ADH? The two stimuli are a decrease in blood volume and an increase in the concentration of solutes in the plasma. Consider a person who becomes dehydrated by vomiting. The person loses large amounts of water and electrolytes. When the volume of blood decreases and the concentration of the blood increases, ADH is released. The ADH increases the reabsorption of water by the kidneys, expanding blood volume and diluting the blood. The increased blood volume eventually stops the stimulus for the release of ADH.

The hypersecretion of ADH is associated with many clinical conditions. Head injuries are a common cause of the syndrome of inappropriate ADH release. Excess ADH increases the reabsorption of water (not salt) and an expansion of a dilute blood volume. A dilute blood can cause serious CNS effects such as seizures. Hyposecretion of ADH causes diabetes insipidus, a condition characterized by the excretion of a large volume of pale dilute urine.

NATRIURETIC PEPTIDES

Atrial natriuretic peptide (ANP) and **brain natriuretic peptide (BNP)** cause excretion of sodium (Na^+), a process called **natriuresis.** ANP is secreted by the walls of the atria of the heart in response to an increase in the volume of blood. BNP is secreted by the walls of the ventricles in response to elevated ventricular pressure. (BNP is used diagnostically in the assessment of heart failure.) ANP and BNP decrease the secretion of aldosterone by the adrenal cortex. The effect is decreased sodium and water reabsorption. The effects of the natriuretic peptides are opposite to the effects of aldosterone and ADH.

PARATHYROID HORMONE

Parathyroid hormone (PTH) is secreted by the parathyroid glands. It does not affect water balance but plays an important role in the regulation of two electrolytes, calcium and phosphate. PTH stimulates the renal tubules to reabsorb calcium and excrete phosphate. The excretion of phosphate is called the "phosphaturic effect" of PTH. The primary stimulus for the release of PTH is a low plasma level of calcium (see Chapter 14 for a detailed description of PTH).

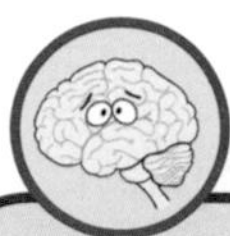

Do You Know...

What happens when Griz doesn't whiz?

As you know, Griz hibernates during the long winter months. Ever think about why he doesn't have to get up to whiz (urinate)? Griz has the ability to metabolically recycle his nitrogenous waste, such as urea. In other words, the waste is converted into metabolic fuel and reused all winter until Mr. Lazy awakens. If Griz would give up his biochemical secret to scientists, perhaps persons with impaired renal function could do the recycle thing. "No Whiz Griz" is just fine. He awakens in the spring . . . to have his fling . . . then off to sleep, without a peep. Ol' Griz . . . no whiz.

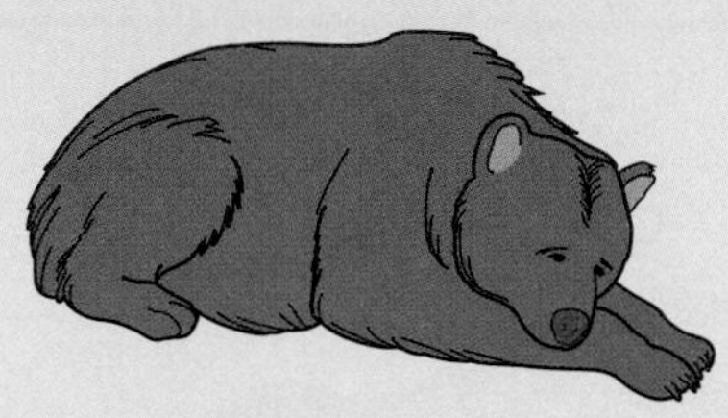

COMPOSITION OF URINE

Finally, we can answer this question: What is in urine? Urine is a sterile fluid composed mostly of water (95%), nitrogen-containing waste, and electrolytes. Important nitrogenous waste includes urea, uric acid, ammonia, and creatinine. The light yellow color of urine is due to a pigment called urochrome, formed from the breakdown of hemoglobin in the liver. The average output of urine is 1500 ml/24 hrs. The term oliguria (*oligo* means "scanty") refers to a urine output of <400 ml/24 hrs. Table 24-3 summarizes the composition of urine along with the significance of some abnormal constituents.

What is meant by the specific gravity of urine? **Specific gravity** is the ratio of the amount of solute to volume (solute/volume). The specific gravity of urine ranges from 1.001 to 1.035, depending on the amount of solute (substances such as Na^+ and creatinine) in the urine. The more solute, the higher is the specific gravity. If a patient is dehydrated, the kidneys filter less water; as a result, the volume of urine decreases. The ratio of solute to volume in the urine therefore increases. Thus dehydration is characterized by an increase in urinary specific gravity. Very dilute urine has a low specific gravity.

Odor? Not too bad if fresh. However, over time bacteria degrades the urea to ammonia. That explains the diaper-pail odor. Whoa! Similarly, a bladder infection can often be detected by the rotten odor of the urine. Your sense of smell can help you in your medical sleuthing. Use it.

Table 24-3 Characteristics of Urine

Characteristic	Description
Amount (volume)	Average 1500 ml/24 hrs
pH	Average 6.0
Specific gravity	Slightly heavier than water (1.001-1.035)
Color	Yellow (amber, straw colored, deep yellow in dehydration, pale yellow with overhydration)
Some Abnormal Constituents of Urine	
Albumin (protein)	Albuminuria: indicates an increased permeability of the glomerulus (e.g., nephrotic syndrome, glomerulonephritis, hypertension); sometimes exercise or pregnancy will result in albuminuria
Glucose	Glycosuria (glucosuria): usually indicates diabetes mellitus
Red blood cells	Hematuria: bleeding in the urinary tract; indicates inflammation, trauma, or disease
Hemoglobin	Hemoglobinuria: indicates hemolysis (transfusion reactions, hemolytic anemia)
White blood cells	Pyuria (pus): indicates infection within the kidney or urinary tract
Ketone bodies	Ketonuria: usually indicates uncontrolled diabetes mellitus (fats are rapidly and incompletely metabolized)
Bilirubin	Bilirubinuria: usually indicates disease involving the liver and/or biliary tree

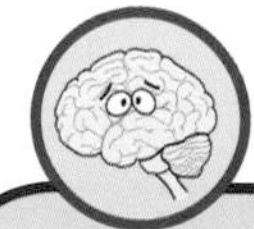

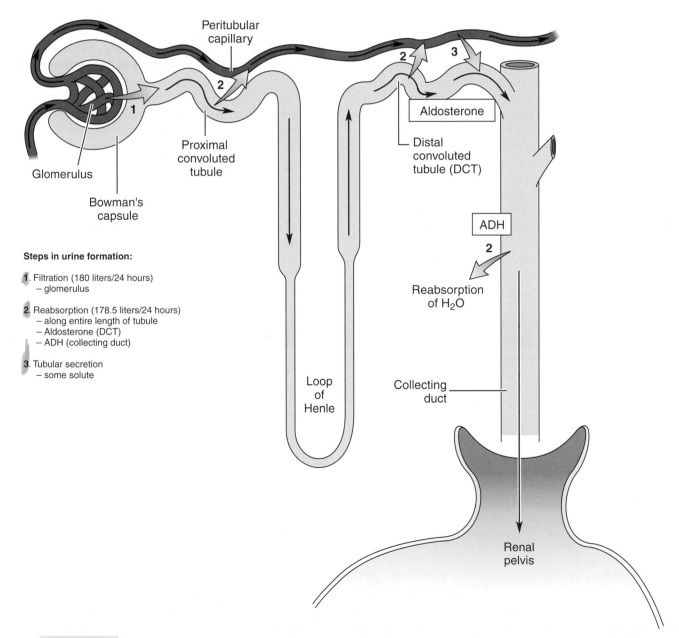

Do You Know...

About urine as a first aid wash?

A scene from the old war stories journal! A soldier is seriously wounded in battle. He is propped up against a charred tree stump as the battle rages on. As his fellow soldiers pass by, they note a large gaping wound in his thigh. Each soldier stops and urinates on the wounded area. Seems like a rather disgusting thing to do! However, urine is sterile and acidic. Given the unsanitary wartime conditions, the "cleansing" of the wounded area with urine helped to prevent wound infection. A urine wash? Not recommended today, but better than nothing in the good ol' days.

Sum It Up!

Figure 24-4 summarizes the steps in urine formation. Water and dissolved solute (180 L/24 hrs) are filtered across the glomerulus into Bowman's capsule. While reabsorption occurs throughout the entire length of the tubule, most occurs in the proximal tubule. Approximately 1.5 L of urine is excreted from the body in 24 hours. Water (178.5 L/24 hrs) moves from the tubules into the blood (peritubular capillaries). The kidney responds to several hormones in regulating the composition of blood: aldosterone ("salt-retaining" hormone), ADH, ANP, BNP, and PTH.

Peritubular capillary

2

3

2

1

Aldosterone

Glomerulus

Bowman's capsule

Proximal convoluted tubule

Distal convoluted tubule (DCT)

ADH

2

Reabsorption of H_2O

Steps in urine formation:

1. Filtration (180 liters/24 hours)
   - glomerulus
2. Reabsorption (178.5 liters/24 hours)
   - along entire length of tubule
   - Aldosterone (DCT)
   - ADH (collecting duct)
3. Tubular secretion
   - some solute

Loop of Henle

Collecting duct

Renal pelvis

FIGURE 24-4 Steps in urine formation: filtration, reabsorption, and secretion. Effects of aldosterone and ADH.

WHEN THE PARTS DON'T WORK

What happens when parts of the nephron don't work correctly?

NEPHROTIC SYNDROME

Nephrotic syndrome provides an excellent example of what happens when the pores in the glomerular membrane become too large. Remember: the size of the glomerular pores determines what gets filtered; proteins such as albumin are normally too large to pass through the pores. Nephrotic syndrome is characterized by the excretion of large amounts of protein in the urine (albuminuria). The loss of protein from the blood results in hypoalbuminemia. Since albumin helps keep water in the blood vessels, a decrease of plasma albumin results in a shift of water from the blood into the tissue spaces, causing generalized edema and ascites. Nephrotic syndrome can develop in response to different insults: trauma, drugs, infection, chronic diseases such as diabetes mellitus, and collagen diseases. Nephrotic syndrome often responds favorably to steroid (prednisone) therapy; the prednisone decreases the size of the glomerular pores thereby decreasing the glomerular filtration of albumin.

GLOMERULONEPHRITIS

The glomeruli can be injured in response to an autoimmune reaction to a pathogen, usually the group A beta hemolytic streptococcus. This is what happens. A person develops a streptococcal throat infection. The person's immune system responds to the streptococcus in a way that the glomeruli are damaged. The damaged glomeruli cannot function normally and the person experiences hematuria (blood in the urine), albuminuria, edema, and hypertension. As glomerular function declines, GFR decreases and serum creatinine rises (an indication of renal failure). The person develops azotemia, the accumulation of nitrogenous waste such as urea and creatinine. The autoimmune reaction to streptococcus is called glomerulonephritis; it may be acute or chronic. Note! Glomerulonephritis is not an infection and therefore cannot be treated with an antibiotic. What is treatable is the initial streptococcal throat infection. An antibiotic can cure the throat infection and prevent glomerulonephritis. Poststreptococcal glomerulonephritis is preventable!

ACUTE TUBULAR NECROSIS (ATN)

ATN is an example of the consequences of renal tubular damage. A common cause of ATN is a prolonged period of hypotension (as in shock) in which the tubules are deprived of blood and the tubular cells die. The injured tubular cells cannot reabsorb tubular fluids and electrolytes properly. Initially the damaged cells cause excessive but nonselective reabsorption and the person becomes oliguric and azotemic (requiring dialysis). As the tubular cells heal, reabsorption improves.

There are many reasons that the kidneys fail. Nephrotoxic drugs, such as the aminoglycosides, and poisons such as antifreeze (ethylene glycol) destroy the kidneys. Infections, such as *E. coli* found in contaminated beef, can destroy the kidneys and is capable of causing a lethal hemolytic uremic syndrome (HUS). Lastly, chronic diseases such as hypertension, diabetes mellitus, and gout are capable of destroying the kidneys.

Do You Know...

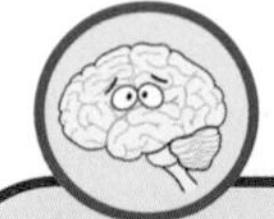

Why a patient in renal failure may have to take the drug epoetin?

The kidneys normally produce erythropoietin, a hormone that stimulates the bone marrow to make red blood cells. A patient in renal failure does not produce erythropoietin and therefore develops anemia ("the anemia of chronic renal failure"). The drug epoetin is erythropoietin; it stimulates the bone marrow to produce RBCs.

UREMIA AND DIALYSIS

Kidney failure is called **renal suppression.** The kidneys no longer make urine. The blood is not cleansed of its waste, and substances that should have been excreted in the urine remain in the blood. This condition is called **uremia,** which literally means urine in the blood. Uremia may be prevented with an **artificial kidney,** a form of **dialysis** (Figure 24-5). The artificial kidney consists of a cylinder filled with a plasmalike solution called the **dialysate.** The patient's blood is passed through a series of tiny tubes immersed in the dialysate. Waste products in the blood, such as potassium, creatinine, uric acid, and excess water, diffuse out of the tubules into the dialysate. The blood is thus cleansed of these waste products and returned to the patient. Because this procedure cleanses blood like a kidney, it is called an artificial kidney.

Do You Know...

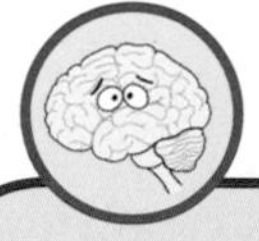

Why a sharp drop in blood pressure causes oliguria?

In a state of circulatory shock, blood pressure is severely decreased. The low blood pressure decreases glomerular filtration, thereby reducing urinary output. A low urinary output is called **oliguria** (ŏl-ĭ-GŪ-rē-ă) (*oligo* means scanty; *uria* means urine). Oliguria is a urinary output of less than 400 ml/24 hrs.

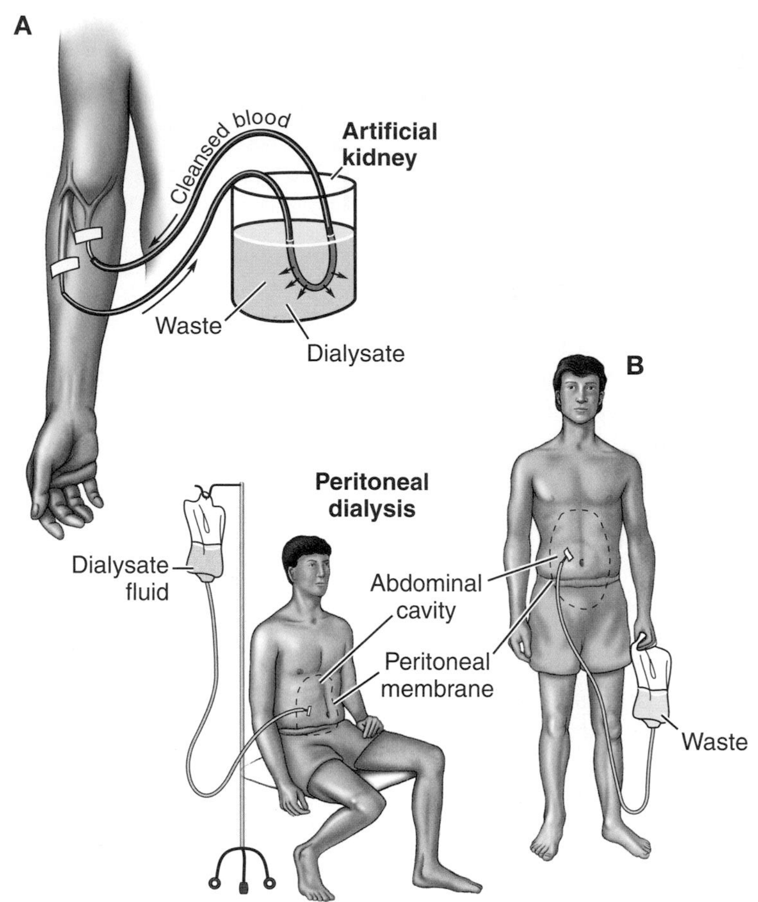

FIGURE 24-5 Types of dialysis: **A,** artificial kidney and **B,** peritoneal dialysis.

A second form of dialysis is peritoneal dialysis. With this procedure, the peritoneal cavity of the patient is used as the cylinder of an artificial kidney, and dialysate is infused into the peritoneal cavity. Waste products diffuse from the blood into the dialysate. The dialysate eventually drains out of the peritoneal cavity and is discarded.

YOUR PLUMBING

While the kidneys form urine, the remaining structures of the urinary system (ureters, bladder, and urethra) function as plumbing and form the **urinary tract** (Figure 24-6). They do not alter the urine in any way; instead, they store and conduct urine from the kidney to the outside of the body. The urinary tract has an outer layer of connective tissue and a middle layer of smooth muscle. The tract is lined with mucous membrane.

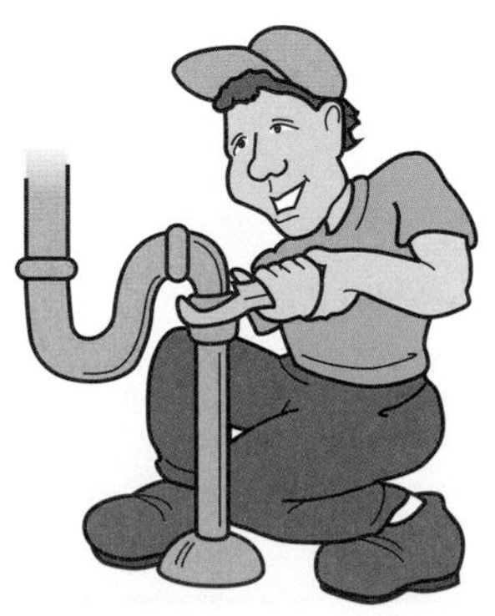

URETERS

Two ureters connect the kidneys with the bladder. The ureters originate in the pelvis of the kidneys and terminate in the bladder. The ureters are long (10 to 13 inches or 25 to 33 cm), slender, muscular tubes capable of peristalsis. Urine moves along the ureters from the kidneys to the bladder in response to gravity and peristalsis.

Sometimes a kidney stone (renal calculus, nephrolithiasis) lodges in the slender ureter, and the urine backs up behind the stone, increasing pressure within the renal pelvis (hydronephrosis). The increased pressure causes severe pain (renal colic) and can adversely affect the kidney, causing a severe decline in GFR and irreversible kidney damage. The stone must be removed. Most stones simply wash out with the urine. Some must be extracted with an instrument inserted into the ureters via the bladder. Other methods include lithotripsy (crushing by ultrasound) and surgical removal.

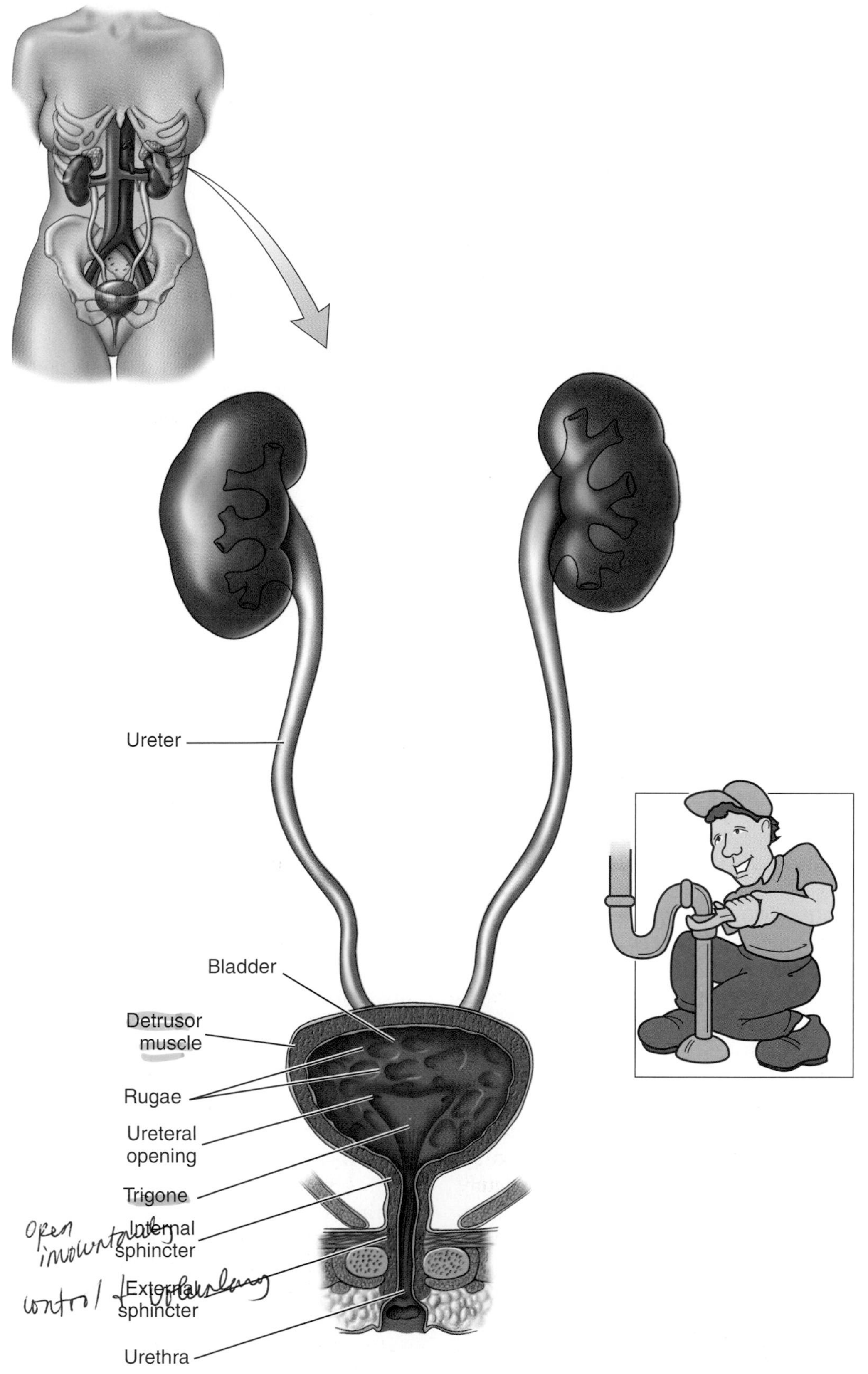

FIGURE 24-6 Organs of the urinary tract: ureters, bladder, and urethra ... "your plumbing."

Do You Know . . .

What Ka-plunk . . . and Gush have to do with the lithotomy position?

"Ka-plunk!" echoed the giant stone as it flew out of the bladder into a bucket. So went the very first lithotomy, a crude and desperate surgical procedure used to extract stones (from the Greek word *lithos*) from the urinary bladder. A stone in the bladder acted like a plug, preventing the outflow of urine and causing the urine to accumulate in the bladder. Imagine the discomfort of not being able to urinate for days on end. Generally, the patient was in such excruciating pain that he agreed to have a sharp and dirty instrument pushed through the perineum into the bladder. Out popped the stones, followed by a major gush of urine and blessed relief of pressure. Because this position was used to perform the surgical procedure (removal of lithos, that is, stones), the position itself was named the lithotomy position, a term (and position) that is still in use today in gynecologic practice.

URINARY BLADDER

The urinary bladder functions as a temporary reservoir for the storage of urine. When empty, the bladder is located below the peritoneal membrane and behind the symphysis pubis. When full, the bladder rises into the abdominal cavity. You can feel a distended bladder if you place your hand over the lower abdomen.

Four layers make up the wall of the bladder. The innermost layer is mucous membrane and contains several thicknesses of transitional epithelium. The mucous membrane is continuous with the mucous membrane of the ureters and urethra. The second layer is called the submucosa and consists of connective tissue and contains many elastic fibers. The third layer is composed of muscle. This involuntary smooth muscle is the **detrusor** (dē-TROO-sěr) **muscle.** The outermost layer of the upper part of the bladder is the serosa.

How much can you hold? The bladder wall is arranged in folds called rugae that allow the bladder to stretch as it fills. The urge to urinate usually begins when it has accumulated about 200 ml of urine. As the volume of urine increases to 300 ml, the urge to urinate becomes more uncomfortable. A moderately full bladder contains about 500 ml, or 1 pt of urine. An overdistended bladder may contain more than 1 L of urine. With overdistention, the urge to urinate may be lost.

One specific area of the floor of the bladder is the **trigone.** It is a triangular area formed by three points: the entrance points of the two ureters and the exit point of the urethra. The trigone is important clinically because infections tend to persist in this area. The exit of the urinary bladder contains a sphincter muscle, called the **internal sphincter.** The internal sphincter is composed of smooth muscle that contracts involuntarily to prevent emptying. Below the internal sphincter, surrounding the upper region of the urethra, is the **external sphincter.** This sphincter is composed of skeletal muscle and is voluntarily controlled. Contraction of the external sphincter allows you to resist the urge to urinate.

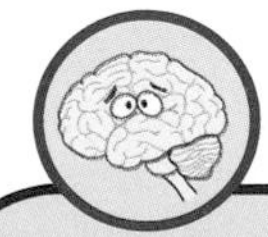

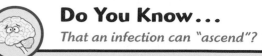

Do You Know . . .

That an infection can "ascend"?

The urinary bladder, especially in the female, is a frequent site of infection. An infection of the urinary bladder is called cystitis. If cystitis is not treated promptly, pathogens can travel from the bladder up the ureter into the kidney, causing a kidney infection (pyelonephritis). Because the pathogens travel to the kidney from the bladder, a kidney infection is often called an ascending infection. In the female the offending pathogen is usually *E. coli,* a resident of the lower digestive tract. Because the female urethra is short, *E. coli* has a short journey from the meatus to the bladder.

URINATION

Urination, also called **micturition** or **voiding,** is the process of expelling urine from the bladder. What causes micturition? As the bladder fills with urine, stimulated stretch receptors send nerve impulses along sensory nerves to the spinal cord. The spinal cord reflexively sends motor nerve impulses back to the bladder, causing the bladder wall to contract rhythmically and the internal sphincter muscle to relax. This response is called the micturition reflex.

The **micturition reflex** gives rise to a sense of urgency. Contraction of the external sphincter prevents involuntary urination. In an infant, the micturition reflex causes the bladder to empty involuntarily. This is what caused baby Sammy to be a wet bundle of joy. As baby Sammy matures, he will learn to override this reflex by voluntarily controlling the external sphincter. Only then can Sammy move from diapers to training pants.

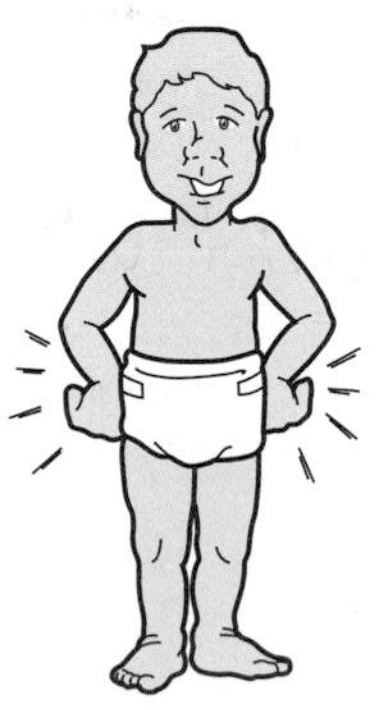

A patient may experience urinary retention, the inability to void or to empty the bladder. Urinary retention is usually due to the effects of drugs used during surgery. Note the difference between renal suppression and urinary retention. Renal suppression means that the kidneys do not make urine. Urinary retention means that the bladder does not expel urine.

Many patients experience urinary incontinence, the involuntary leakage of urine from the bladder. There are many causes of incontinence: an incompetent bladder sphincter, bladder infection, excess external pressure as occurs during pregnancy. A chronically full bladder (from an obstruction) may cause an overflow incontinence. The patient does not urinate and empty his bladder; the excess dribbles out in small amounts. Lastly, a sudden rise in bladder pressure as occurs in coughing or laughing causes incontinence; this is called stress incontinence and is the source of much embarrassment.

URETHRA

The urethra is a tube that carries urine from the bladder to the outside. It is lined with mucous membrane that contains numerous mucus-secreting glands. The muscular layer of the urethra contracts and helps expel urine during micturition.

The male and female urethras differ in several ways. In the female, the urethra is short (1.5 inches [3.8 cm]) and is part of the urinary system. The urethra opens to the outside at the **urethral meatus.** The female urethral meatus is located in front of the vagina and between the labia minora.

In the male, the urethra is part of both the urinary and the reproductive systems. The male urethra (8 inches [20 cm]) is much longer than the female urethra. As the male urethra leaves the bladder, it passes through the prostate gland and extends the length of the penis. Thus the male urethra performs a dual purpose; it carries urine (its urinary function) and sperm (its reproductive function).

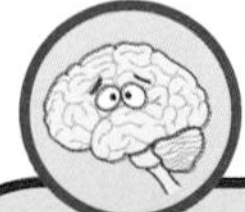

Do You Know...

Why an enlarged prostate gland "slows the stream" ... or even worse?

The male urethra is surrounded by the donut-shaped prostate gland. When the prostate gland enlarges, pressure is exerted on the outside of the urethra, closing the lumen of the urethra and impeding the flow or "stream" of urine from the bladder. Urination becomes difficult (dysuria), and the incomplete emptying of the bladder sets the stage for repeated bladder infections. The incomplete emptying also causes nocturia (needing to urinate at night, thereby interfering with sleep), a bothersome symptom that may cause men to seek medical help.

AN AUTONOMIC MOMENT

The detrusor muscle of the urinary bladder and the internal sphincter have muscarinic receptors. Activation of the muscarinic receptors causes the detrusor muscle to contract and the sphincter to relax; this action causes the bladder to expel the urine (urination). There are two pharmacology issues. First, if a patient is experiencing urinary retention, he may be given a muscarinic agonist such as Urecholine (bethanechol). The muscarinic agonist causes urination. Second, if a person has been taking medications that have antimuscarinic side effects, he may experience difficulty in urinating. This often happens to persons who take preoperative drugs such as atropine and persons who take anticholinergic antidepressants.

Sum It Up!

The kidneys make urine. The urine is stored and transported by the structures that make up the urinary tract: ureters, bladder, and urethra. The accumulation of urine in the bladder is the stimulus for the micturition reflex and creates the urge to void. Voluntary control of the external sphincter allows you to void at a particular time. Urine exits the body through the urethral meatus.

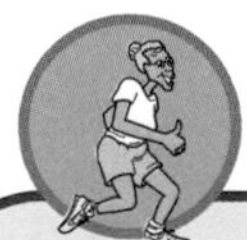

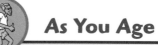

As You Age

1. The number of nephron units progressively decreases so that, by the age of 70 to 80 years, there has been a 50% reduction. Clinically, this decrease in nephron function causes a diminished ability to concentrate urine.
2. Glomerular filtration rate (GFR) declines with age. As a result, the elderly person excretes drugs more slowly and is at risk for drug overdose. The decrease in GFR also makes it difficult for the elderly person to excrete excess blood volume, so any intravenous fluids must be administered slowly and carefully. Overhydration is a common cause of heart failure in the elderly.
3. The aging urinary bladder shrinks and becomes less able to contract and relax. As a result, the elderly person must void more frequently. Because of less effective bladder contraction and residual urine, the incidence of bladder infection increases. The weakening of the external sphincter and a decreased ability to sense a distended bladder increase the incidence of bladder incontinence. Frequent urination in men may be caused by an enlarged prostate gland, a common age-related disorder.

Disorders of the Urinary System

Glomerulonephritis	Inflammation (antigen-antibody reaction) of the glomeruli that develops in response to streptococcal infection. The glomeruli are damaged in such a way that large amounts of albumin and other proteins are lost in the urine.
Inflammation of the lining of the urinary tract	Inflammation of the urinary tract, commonly caused by infection with *Escherichia coli.* Both urethritis and cystitis are lower urinary tract infections. Urethritis is an inflammation of the urethra. Cystitis is inflammation of the urinary bladder. Pyelitis is a form of upper urinary tract infection and refers to inflammation of the renal pelvis and calyces.
Polycystic kidney	A genetic disease characterized by the development of multiple fluid-filled sacs in the kidney. The sacs gradually cause destruction of kidney tissue and loss of kidney function.
Pyelonephritis	A bacterial infection of the pelvis of the kidney. Pyelonephritis is frequently caused by a neglected bladder infection that ascends through the ureters to the kidneys.
Renal calculi	Also called nephrolithiasis or kidney stones. Sharp stones (like those that form in the patient with gout) can damage the nephron units and cause gradual loss of renal function. Kidney stones typically get lodged in the ureter, blocking the flow of urine and causing accumulation of urine in the renal pelvis (hydronephrosis). The urine backs up in the kidney and may cause serious kidney damage and pain (renal colic).
Renal failure	Rapid kidney failure (acute renal failure) or gradual kidney failure (chronic renal failure). Renal failure has many causes: infections, acute hypotensive episodes, exposure to toxins, complications of diseases such as diabetes, genetic disorders such as polycystic kidney disease, and congenital defects. Unless dialyzed the blood of a patient in renal failure accumulates waste products (uremia) and makes the person toxic.

SUMMARY OUTLINE

The urinary system consists of organs that make urine, temporarily store it, and then eliminate it from the body. The kidneys contain the nephron units that make urine, thereby eliminating waste from the body and regulating water and electrolyte balance.

I. Excretion

A. There are several organs of excretion: kidney, skin, lungs, intestines.

B. The urinary system organs include the kidneys, ureters, urinary bladder, and urethra.

II. Kidneys

A. The kidney has three distinct regions: cortex, medulla, pelvis.

B. The kidneys have many functions: excrete nitrogenous waste, regulate blood volume, regulate electrolyte concentration, regulate pH and blood pressure, and stimulate red blood cell production.

III. Urine Making: Nephron Unit

A. The nephron unit is the functional (urine-making) unit of the kidney.

B. The nephron unit is composed of tubular structures and vascular structures.

C. There are three processes in urine formation.

1. Glomerular filtration filters 180 L of filtrate in 24 hours.
2. Tubular reabsorption causes the reabsorption of 178.5 L of filtrate.
   a. A substance is either completely or incompletely reabsorbed.
   b. A substance is either reabsorbed actively or passively.
3. Tubular secretion causes the secretion of small amounts of specific substances from the peritubular capillaries into the tubules.

IV. Hormones That Work on the Kidneys

A. Aldosterone

1. Aldosterone stimulates the distal tubule to reabsorb Na^+ and water and to excrete K^+.

2. The secretion of aldosterone is regulated by the renin-angiotensin-aldosterone system.

B. Antidiuretic Hormone (ADH)

1. ADH stimulates the collecting duct to reabsorb water.
2. ADH is released from the posterior pituitary gland in response to low blood volume and increased concentration of solute in the plasma.

C. Natriuretic peptides (ANP, BNP) inhibit the reabsorption of Na^+ and water, thereby causing natriuresis and the excretion of water.

D. Parathyroid hormone (PTH) stimulates the renal reabsorption of calcium and the excretion of phosphate.

V. Composition of Urine. (The characteristics of urine are summarized in Table 24-3.)

A. Amount
B. pH
C. Specific gravity
D. Color
E. Abnormal constituents

VI. When the Kidneys Don't Work

A. The parts of the kidney can be damaged or diseased.
B. Kidney failure causes a syndrome called uremia.
C. Dialysis can prevent uremia.

VII. Your Plumbing

A. Ureters: The two ureters are long, slender tubes that carry urine from the renal pelvis to the bladder.

B. Urinary Bladder

1. The urinary bladder is a temporary reservoir that holds the urine.
2. The detrusor muscle is a smooth muscle responsible for bladder contraction and the elimination of urine.
3. There are two sphincters: internal (involuntary) and external (voluntary).
4. The voluntary elimination of urine is called urination (micturition).

C. The urethra is a tube that carries urine from the bladder to the outside of the body.

Review Your Knowledge

Matching: Plumbing ... More or Less

Directions: Match the following words with their descriptions below. Some words may be used more than once.

a. urethra
b. kidneys
c. ureters
d. urinary bladder

1. ____ These two long tubes empty urine into the urinary bladder
2. ____ The urine-making organs
3. ____ Urine leaves the bladder through this structure
4. ____ The external urinary sphincter is located at the distal end of this structure
5. ____ Its walls contains the detrusor muscle
6. ____ Tubes that receive urine from the renal pelvis
7. ____ An enlarged prostate gland prevents the emptying of this structure
8. ____ Cystitis is an inflammation of this urinary structure
9. ____ Renal suppression is most associated with these structures
10. ____ Urinary retention is most associated with this structure

Matching: Nephron Unit

Directions: Match the following words with their descriptions below. Some words may be used more than once.

a. loop of Henle
b. glomerulus
c. afferent arterioles
d. collecting duct
e. proximal convoluted tubule
f. calyx
g. peritubular capillaries

1. ____ This structure receives urine from the distal convoluted tubule
2. ____ The tuft of capillaries that sits within Bowman's capsule
3. ____ Urine flows from the proximal tubule into this structure
4. ____ These capillaries surround the tubules and reabsorb huge amounts of water and solute
5. ____ Filtration occurs across the membrane of this vascular structure
6. ____ Most reabsorption occurs across this tubular structure
7. ____ These tiny blood vessels deliver blood to the glomeruli
8. ____ Hairpin tubular structure between the proximal and distal tubules

9. ______ A cuplike structure that receives urine from the collecting duct
10. ______ The tubular site that is most responsive to ADH

Matching: Hormones and Enzymes

Directions: Match the following words with their descriptions below. Some words may be used more than once.

a. aldosterone
b. renin
c. parathyroid hormone (PTH)
d. converting enzyme
e. antidiuretic hormone (ADH)
f. brain natriuretic peptide (BNP)
g. angiotensin II

1. ______ Secreted by the JGA cells; activates angiotensinogen
2. ______ Stimulates the distal tubule to reabsorb Na^+ and excrete K^+
3. ______ Determines the membrane permeability of the collecting duct to water
4. ______ Mineralocorticoid secreted by the adrenal cortex
5. ______ Secreted by the walls of the heart; it causes the renal excretion of Na^+ and water
6. ______ Called the "salt-retaining" hormone
7. ______ A deficiency of this hormone causes diabetes insipidus
8. ______ Stimulates the tubules to reabsorb calcium and excrete phosphate
9. ______ Secreted by the lungs; changes angiotensin I to angiotensin II
10. ______ A potent vasopressor that is generated by the action of converting enzyme

Multiple Choice

1. Micturition
   a. occurs within Bowman's capsule.
   b. refers to the filtration of 180 L water.
   c. refers to the storage of urine by the bladder.
   d. refers to urination.
2. Which of the following is least true of aldosterone?
   a. Is a mineralocorticoid
   b. Is the "salt-retaining hormone"
   c. Determines the membrane permeability of the collecting duct to water
   d. Causes the tubular reabsorption of sodium and water
3. ADH
   a. is released in response to excess blood volume and a dilute plasma.
   b. determines the membrane permeability of the collecting duct to water.
   c. makes the collecting duct impermeable to water.
   d. determines the pore size of the glomeruli.
4. A drug that blocks the renal reabsorption of Na^+ causes
   a. defecation.
   b. diuresis.
   c. oliguria.
   d. hypernatremia.
5. Why is glucose normally not excreted in the urine?
   a. No glucose is filtered.
   b. All filtered glucose is reabsorbed.
   c. Glucose is used up by the metabolizing nephron units.
   d. Glucose is converted to ammonia in the distal tubule and excreted as urea.
6. A drug that blocks the effects of aldosterone
   a. increases the reabsorption of Na^+ and water.
   b. is kaliuretic.
   c. may cause an increase in plasma K^+.
   d. causes oliguria.
7. Oliguria
   a. refers to a lowered serum potassium.
   b. most often develops in response to declining renal blood flow.
   c. is a sign of good renal function.
   d. most often accompanies a decline in serum creatinine.

CHAPTER 25

Water, Electrolyte, and Acid-Base Balance

KEY TERMS

Buffer, p. 449
Electrolyte balance, p. 446
Extracellular fluid, p. 444
Hyperkalemia, p. 448
Hyperventilation, p. 451
Hypokalemia, p. 448
Hypoventilation, p. 451
Intake, p. 445
Interstitial fluid, p. 444
Intracellular fluid, p. 444
Kussmaul respirations, p. 451
Metabolic acidosis, p. 451
Metabolic alkalosis, p. 452
Output, p. 445
Respiratory acidosis, p. 450
Respiratory alkalosis, p. 451
Skin turgor, p. 446
Transcellular fluid, p. 444

OBJECTIVES

1. Describe the two main fluid compartments.
2. Define *intake* and *output.*
3. List factors that affect electrolyte balance.
4. Describe the most common ions found in the intracellular and extracellular compartments.
5. List three mechanisms that regulate pH in the body.
6. Discuss acid-base imbalances: acidosis and alkalosis.

The old saying "you're all wet" has some truth to it. Between 50% and 70% of a person's weight is water. In the average adult male, the water makes up 60% of the weight (about 40 L); in the female, water makes up about 50%. An infant is composed of even more water, up to 75%. Because adipose tissue contains less water than muscle tissue, obese persons have less water than thin persons.

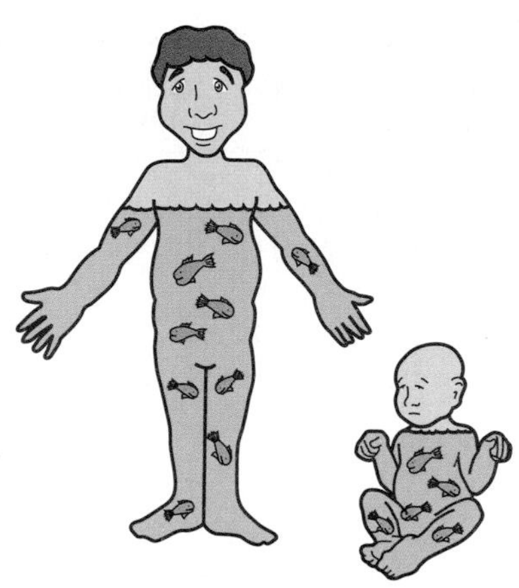

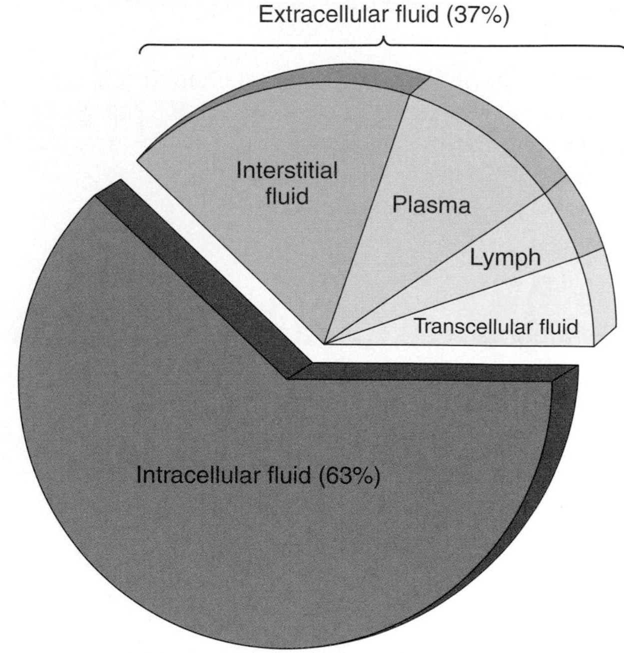

FIGURE 25-1 Fluid compartments: extracellular and intracellular.

BODY FLUIDS: DISTRIBUTION AND COMPOSITION

FLUID COMPARTMENTS

Water and its dissolved electrolytes are distributed into two major compartments: an intracellular compartment and an extracellular compartment (Figure 25-1). The intracellular compartment includes the water located in all the cells of the body. Most water, about 63%, is located in the intracellular compartment.

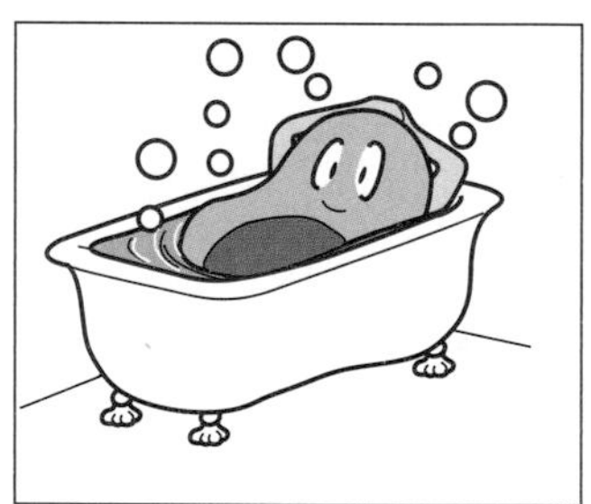

The extracellular compartment includes the fluid located outside all the cells and represents about 37% of the total body water. The extracellular compartment includes the water located between cells, called **interstitial** (ĭn-tĕr-STĬSH-ăl) **fluid;** water within blood vessels (plasma); and water within lymphatic vessels (lymph). **Transcellular fluid** is extracellular fluid and includes cerebrospinal fluid (CSF), the aqueous and vitreous humors in the eyes, the synovial fluids of joints, the serous fluids in body cavities, and the glandular secretions. Interstitial fluid and plasma are the largest extracellular compartments.

COMPOSITION OF BODY FLUIDS

Intracellular and extracellular fluids vary in their concentrations of various electrolytes. **Extracellular fluids** contain high concentrations of sodium (Na^+), chloride (Cl^-), and bicarbonate (HCO_3^-) ions. The plasma portion (extracellular) contains more protein than other extracellular fluids do. **Intracellular fluid** contains high concentrations of potassium (K^+); phosphate (PO_4^{3-}); and magnesium (Mg^{2+}) ions.

Smaller concentrations of other ions are present in both intracellular and extracellular fluids. Although distributed across the fluid compartments, water and electrolytes can move from one compartment to another. The movement of fluid and electrolytes between compartments is well regulated.

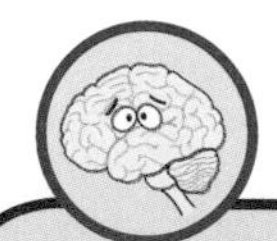

Do You Know...

What is so "normal" about normal saline and why it is normally given?

Some patients become deficient in body fluids. These may be surgical patients who are not permitted to drink, patients who have been vomiting, or those who are unconscious and unable to eat or drink. These patients often receive intravenous infusions of solutions that resemble plasma in ionic composition. Normal saline, for instance, contains 0.9% sodium chloride, a concentration equal to that of plasma. Because the concentration of "salt" in normal saline resembles that of plasma, it is called normal.

WATER BALANCE

Normally, the quantity of water taken in, **intake,** equals the amount of water eliminated from the body, which is **output.** Water balance exists when intake equals output (Figure 25-2). As part of your clinical responsibilities, you will be measuring intake and output.

WATER INTAKE

Although water intake can vary considerably, the average adult takes in about 2500 ml every 24 hours. About 60% comes from drinking liquids, and an additional 30% comes from water in foods. Ten percent comes from the breakdown of foods. This portion is called the **water of metabolism.**

Thirst is the primary regulator of water intake. The thirst center is in the hypothalamus of the brain. As the body loses water, the thirst center in the hypothalamus is stimulated, thus causing you to drink. Drinking restores the water content of the body. Both your thirst and your hypothalamus are satisfied. The elderly have a diminished thirst mechanism and are therefore prone to dehydration.

WATER OUTPUT

In a healthy person, 24-hour intake and output are approximately equal. The individual who takes in 2500 ml of water should therefore eliminate 2500 ml. Water can leave the body through several routes: kidneys, skin, lungs, and digestive tract. The kidneys eliminate about 60% of the water as urine. About 28% is lost from the skin and lungs. Six percent is eliminated in the feces, and another 6% is lost as sweat. The amount lost by sweat can vary considerably, depending on the level of exercise

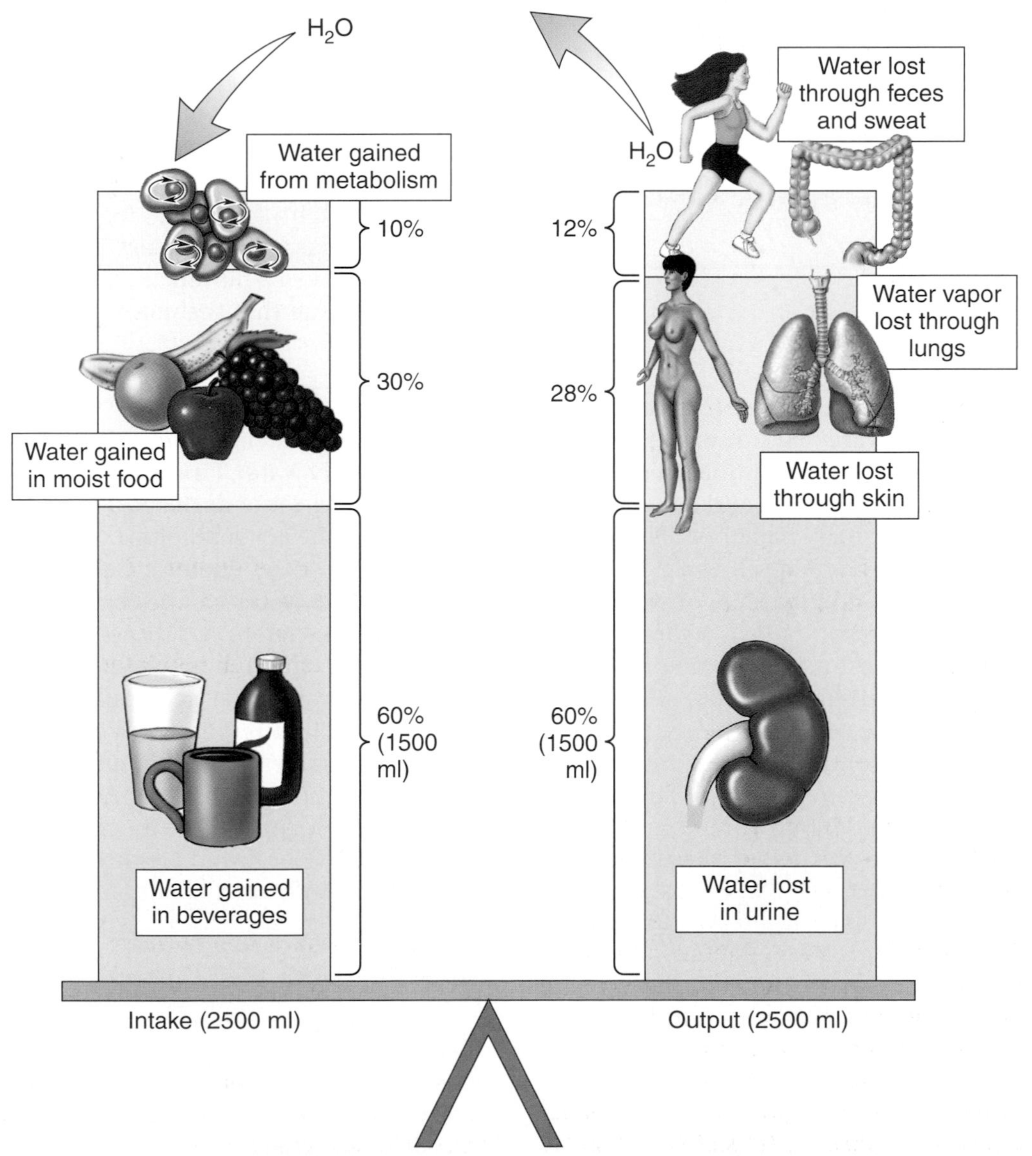

FIGURE 25-2 Water balance: intake equals output.

and environmental temperatures. Water loss through the skin and lungs increases in a hot, dry environment.

The kidneys are the primary regulator of water output. Water regulation occurs mainly through the action of antidiuretic hormone (ADH) on the collecting duct. When body water content is low, the posterior pituitary gland releases ADH. It stimulates the collecting duct to reabsorb water, thereby decreasing water in the urine and increasing blood volume. When body water content is high, the secretion of ADH decreases. As a result, less water is reabsorbed from the collecting duct, and the excess water is eliminated in the urine. Water balance is also regulated by aldosterone discussed later in the chapter.

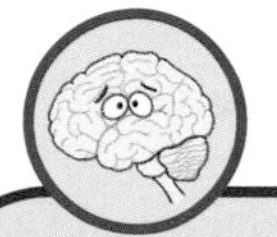

Do You Know...

What a prune and a dehydrated person have in common?

A prune is a dehydrated plum. As water is removed from the plum, the skin assumes a shriveled appearance. The same process occurs in a person who is dehydrated. As fluid is lost from the body, water moves from the interstitium (tissue spaces), into the blood vessels in an attempt to maintain adequate blood volume and blood pressure. As water is lost from the interstitium, the overlying skin appears shriveled, much like a prune. The dehydrated patient is said to have poor skin turgor.

WATER IMBALANCES

Dehydration

A deficiency of body water is called **dehydration.** Dehydration develops when water output exceeds water intake and commonly occurs in conditions such as excessive sweating, vomiting, diarrhea, and use of diuretics. A dehydrated person usually has poor skin turgor. **Skin turgor** is assessed by pinching the skin and then observing how quickly the skin flattens, or returns to its normal position. If a person is well hydrated, the pinched skin quickly flattens out. The skin of a dehydrated person, however, flattens out more slowly, giving the skin the appearance of a tent, hence the term **tenting** for the appearance of the skin of a dehydrated person. Tenting is due to the depletion of fluid in the interstitial space. If untreated blood volume and blood pressure continue to decline, the person develops a low volume (hypovolemic) shock.

Edema

The body can retain excess water and deposit it in various compartments, especially the interstitial space. Fluid retention is called **edema.** Edema can be intracellular or extracellular. Generally we are concerned with interstitial edema. Excess body water can accumulate in various parts of the body. For instance, water accumulation in the lungs is called pulmonary edema; it causes hypoxemia and cyanosis. Cerebral edema is the accumulation in the brain; it causes a life-threatening increase in intracranial pressure and evidence of neurological dysfunction. Water accumulation in the ankle region is called pedal edema. As you can see, the consequences can be mild (pedal edema) or life-threatening (pulmonary edema and cerebral edema). The goal of therapy is to remove excess fluid, relieve the symptoms, and to treat the underlying cause of the edema.

Why Does Fluid Shift?

The fluid shifts because of a change in the "pushing and pulling" forces of the capillaries. (See Chapter 19, capillary exchange and mechanisms of edema formation.) The forces include: the capillary filtration force, the plasma oncotic pressure, the effect of lymphatic drainage, and the effects of plasma protein that is trapped in the tissue space. Alteration of any of these factors affects water movement.

Daily Weights and Fluid Balance

The daily measurement of body weight provides a reliable estimate of fluid balance. For instance, if a person with heart failure suddenly gains 4.4 lbs, you should suspect fluid retention. How is the amount estimated? One liter of water weighs 2.2 lbs (1 kg). If a person has a sudden weight gain of 4.4 lbs, you can assume that that person has retained 2 L of fluid. Another example: A patient is given a diuretic and loses 2.2 lbs overnight. You can assume that the patient excreted 1 L of fluid.

FLUID SPACING—IN OTHER WORDS

Fluid spacing is a clinical term that refers to the distribution of body water. **First spacing** refers to the normal distribution of water as described earlier. **Second spacing** refers to the accumulation of water in the interstitial spaces (interstitial edema). Generally, with adequate treatment this water can be reabsorbed and excreted. **Third spacing** refers to the accumulation of water in spaces from which it is not easily absorbed. For instance, the water that accumulates in the abdominal cavity as ascites is not easily reabsorbed. Similarly, the excess water that accumulates within the digestive tract secondary to a paralytic ileus is unavailable for easy reabsorption. The amount of water that "third spaces" can be large and life-threatening. Monitoring of water distribution is a common clinical concern.

ELECTROLYTE BALANCE

Electrolyte balance exists when the amounts of the various electrolytes gained by the body equal the amounts lost. **Electrolyte imbalances** are common, serious clinical challenges. Electrolytes are important components of the body fluids. The kidneys control the composition

Table 25-1 Major Ions and Functions

Electrolyte	Plasma Levels	Function
Sodium (Na^+)	136-145 mEq/L	Chief extracellular cation Regulates extracellular volume Participates in nerve-muscle function
Potassium (K^+)	3.5-5.0 mEq/L	Chief intracellular cation Participates in nerve-muscle function
Calcium (Ca^{2+})	4.5-5.8 mEq/L	Strengthens bone and teeth Participates in muscle contraction Helps in blood clotting
Magnesium (Mg^{2+})	1.5-2.5 mEq/L	Strengthens bone Participates in nerve-muscle function
Chloride (Cl^-)	95-108 mEq/L	Chief extracellular anion Involved in extracellular volume control
Bicarbonate (HCO_3^-)	22-26 mEq/L	Part of bicarbonate buffer system Participates in acid-base balance
Phosphate (PO_4^{3-})	2.5-4.5 mEq/L	Strengthens bone Participates in acid-base balance

mEq/L, Milliequivalents per liter.

of body fluids by regulating the renal excretion of electrolytes. Table 25-1 includes the major electrolytes and their normal levels and functions.

QUICK REFERENCE

Chapter 2 describes the chemical characteristics of electrolytes. You will want to review several of the terms listed here for quick reference:

- **Ion:** An element or compound that carries an electrical charge. Common ions are Na^+, Cl^-, K^+, Ca^{2+}, and Mg^{2+}
- **Cation:** A positively charged ion, such as Na^+, K^+, and Ca^{2+}
- **Anion:** A negatively charged ion, such as Cl^- and HCO_3^- (bicarbonate). Most proteins (such as albumin) carry a negative charge
- **Electrolyte:** Substances that form ions when they dissolve in water, such as NaCl (salt):

$$NaCl \rightarrow Na^+ \text{ (cation)} + Cl^- \text{ (anion)}$$

- **Ionization:** The chemical reaction caused when an electrolyte splits into two ions

MOST IMPORTANT IONS

Sodium (Na^+)

Sodium is the chief extracellular cation, accounting for nearly 90% of the positively charged ions in the extracellular fluid. Sodium is necessary for nerve impulse conduction, and it also helps maintain body fluid balance. The primary mechanism regulating sodium concentration is aldosterone. Aldosterone stimulates the distal tubule of the nephron unit to reabsorb sodium. Usually, when "sodium moves, water moves"; this means that aldosterone causes the reabsorption of both Na^+ and water. **Hypernatremia** refers to excess Na^+ in the blood and is the result of excess water loss or increased Na^+ intake. Note the kinds of patients who develop hypernatremia:

- Elderly persons following surgery or fever. They are apt to have a low blood volume and diminished thirst mechanism.
- Patients who have been on prolonged diuretic therapy because of the loss of excessive water as urine.
- Uncontrolled diabetic patients with hyperglycemia. The glucosuria requires the excretion of large amounts of water (polyuria) leading to dehydration and hypernatremia.

Hyponatremia refers to a decrease in the concentration of plasma Na^+. Normal plasma Na^+ levels are essential for normal brain function. Often a patient becomes hyponatremic because of excess water in the blood. The blood literally is diluted out with water, causing a dilutional hyponatremia. For instance, a person with heart failure often has an expanded blood volume and a dilutional hyponatremia. Sometimes runners drink too much water during a marathon causing a dilutional hyponatremia, a condition that is serious because it can cause delirium and seizures. Psychiatric patients sometimes "water binge"; they too are at risk for dilutional hyponatremia and seizures.

Potassium (K^+)

Potassium is the chief intracellular cation. The primary hormone regulating potassium concentration is aldosterone. Aldosterone stimulates the distal tubule of the kidney to excrete potassium into the urine. The kidney is the primary organ responsible for the excretion of excess K^+. The monitoring of serum potassium levels is an important clinical responsibility. While only 2% of the K^+ is located in the extracellular space, plasma K^+ is important for normal muscle function, especially cardiac function. Changes in plasma levels of K^+ cause serious cardiac dysrhythmias.

Hyperkalemia refers to excess K^+ (>5.5 mEq/L) in the blood. The primary cause of hyperkalemia is kidney disease, since the kidneys play a major role in the elimination of K^+. Hyperkalemia is an emergency situation and is treated in several ways: dialysis or the IV administration of an insulin-glucose solution. Dialysis removes K^+ from the blood. The IV insulin drives the glucose and K^+ into the cells, lowering plasma levels of K^+.

Hypokalemia refers to a lower-than-normal amount of K^+ (<3.5 mEq/L) in the blood. Hypokalemia usually presents as muscle fatigue, leg cramps, abdominal distention, and cardiac rhythm disturbances. The most common cause of hypokalemia is the prolonged use of potassium-losing diuretics (kaliuretics). Some diuretics such as spironolactone are not kaliuretic and cause the kidney to reabsorb potassium. These diuretics are called "potassium sparers"; they can cause hyperkalemia. Maintaining normal potassium levels in a patient who requires diuretic therapy is a major clinical concern. You must know which diuretics waste potassium and which diuretics spare potassium. Large amounts of K^+ can also be lost through vomiting (or nasogastric tubes) and diarrhea. Hypokalemia is a serious condition and is treated by the administration of K^+.

Calcium (Ca^{2+})

Calcium is necessary for bone and teeth formation, muscle contraction, nerve impulse transmission, and blood clotting. Ninety-nine percent of the body's calcium is in the bones and teeth. Parathyroid hormone is the primary regulator of plasma levels of calcium. Hyper- and hypocalcemia are described in Chapter 14.

Magnesium (Mg^{2+})

Next to potassium, magnesium is the most abundant cation in the intracellular fluid. Magnesium is important in the function of the heart, muscles, and nerves. Kidney disease is the major cause of hypermagnesemia. Other causes include overuse of magnesium-containing antacids. (Thought the over-the-counter drugs couldn't kill you?) Hypomagnesemia is often seen in critically ill persons. It can be caused by aggressive diuretic therapy and is also seen in patients with chronic alcoholism, as well as in pregnant women with preeclampsia (high blood pressure of pregnancy).

Chloride (Cl^-)

Chloride is the chief extracellular anion. Chloride usually follows sodium. That is, when sodium is actively pumped from the tubules into the peritubular capillaries, chloride follows the sodium passively. Changes in the plasma levels of chloride affect acid-base balance through its effect on bicarbonate (discussed in the next section). For instance, when plasma chloride decreases (hypochloremia), plasma bicarbonate increases and causes alkalosis. Hyperchloremia, on the other hand, causes a decrease in plasma bicarbonate and a state of acidosis. Like Na^+, Cl^- is greatly affected by diuretic therapy.

Bicarbonate (HCO_3^-)

Bicarbonate is an important anion in acid-base balance. Bicarbonate is an alkaline (basic) substance that helps remove excess acid from the body. It is also the form in which carbon dioxide (CO_2) is transported in the blood. Bicarbonate excretion is controlled by the kidneys. Bicarbonate can be either reabsorbed or excreted, depending on the body's needs.

Other Ions

The plasma contains other ions, such as sulfate (SO_4^{2-}) and phosphate (PO_4^{3-}). The normal laboratory values for the major ions are summarized in Table 25-1.

> **Sum It Up!**
>
> The volume and composition of body fluids are closely regulated. Body fluids are found in two main compartments. Most body fluid (63%) is in the intracellular compartment. The remaining 37% is in the extracellular compartment. The extracellular compartment contains interstitial fluid, plasma, lymph, and transcellular fluid. The electrolyte composition of the body fluids is important. The chief extracellular cation is sodium; the chief intracellular cation is potassium. Excesses and deficiencies of water and electrolytes cause serious problems.

ACID-BASE BALANCE

A normally functioning body requires a balance between acids and bases. Acid-base balance is described according to its regulation of pH. Why is the regulation of pH so important? All chemical reactions in the body occur at a particular pH level; any alteration in pH interferes with these reactions. Chemical reactions that take place within extracellular fluids occur only when the pH is above 7. Changes in pH profoundly affect cardiac and neurologic function.

QUICK REFERENCE

Chapter 2 describes acids, bases, and pH. You will want to review several terms of the listed here for quick reference:

- **Acid:** A substance that dissociates (splits) into H^+ and an anion like Cl^- (e.g., $HCl \rightarrow H^+ + Cl^-$).

An acid donates a hydrogen ion (H^+) during a chemical reaction.

- **Base:** A substance that combines with H^+ during a chemical reaction and removes H^+ from solution (e.g., $OH^- + H^+ \rightarrow H_2O$). A base is an H^+ acceptor. The hydroxyl ion (OH^-), for example, combines with H^+ to form water (H_2O).
- **pH:** A unit of measurement that indicates the number of H^+ in solution. Remember: as the number of H^+ increases, the pH decreases. As the number of H^+ decreases, the pH increases. The normal plasma pH ranges from 7.35 to 7.45, with an average of 7.4. A plasma pH of less than 7.35 is called **acidosis.** A plasma pH of more than 7.45 is called **alkalosis** (Figure 25-3).

WHERE THE ACID (H^+) COMES FROM

Remember! H^+ is acid. Most H^+ comes from the body's chemical reactions during metabolism. For instance, when glucose is metabolized in the presence of oxygen, it produces carbon dioxide (CO_2), water, and energy. The CO_2 combines with water and forms an acid (carbonic acid). When glucose is metabolized in the absence of oxygen, it forms lactic acid (H^+). When fatty acids are metabolized very quickly, they yield ketoacids (H^+). Finally, when proteins are metabolized, some of them yield sulfuric acid (H^+). All these acids are produced by metabolizing cells. To maintain acid-base balance, the body must eliminate the acids.

HOW THE BODY REGULATES pH

Three mechanisms work together to regulate pH: buffers, respirations, and kidney function (see Figure 25-3, *B*).

Buffers

The buffer system is the first line of defense in the regulation of pH. A **buffer** is a chemical substance that prevents large changes in pH. There are two parts to a buffer, called a **buffer pair.** The buffer pair consists of a "taker" and a "giver" and works like this. If H^+ concentration in the blood increases, the "taker" part of the buffer removes

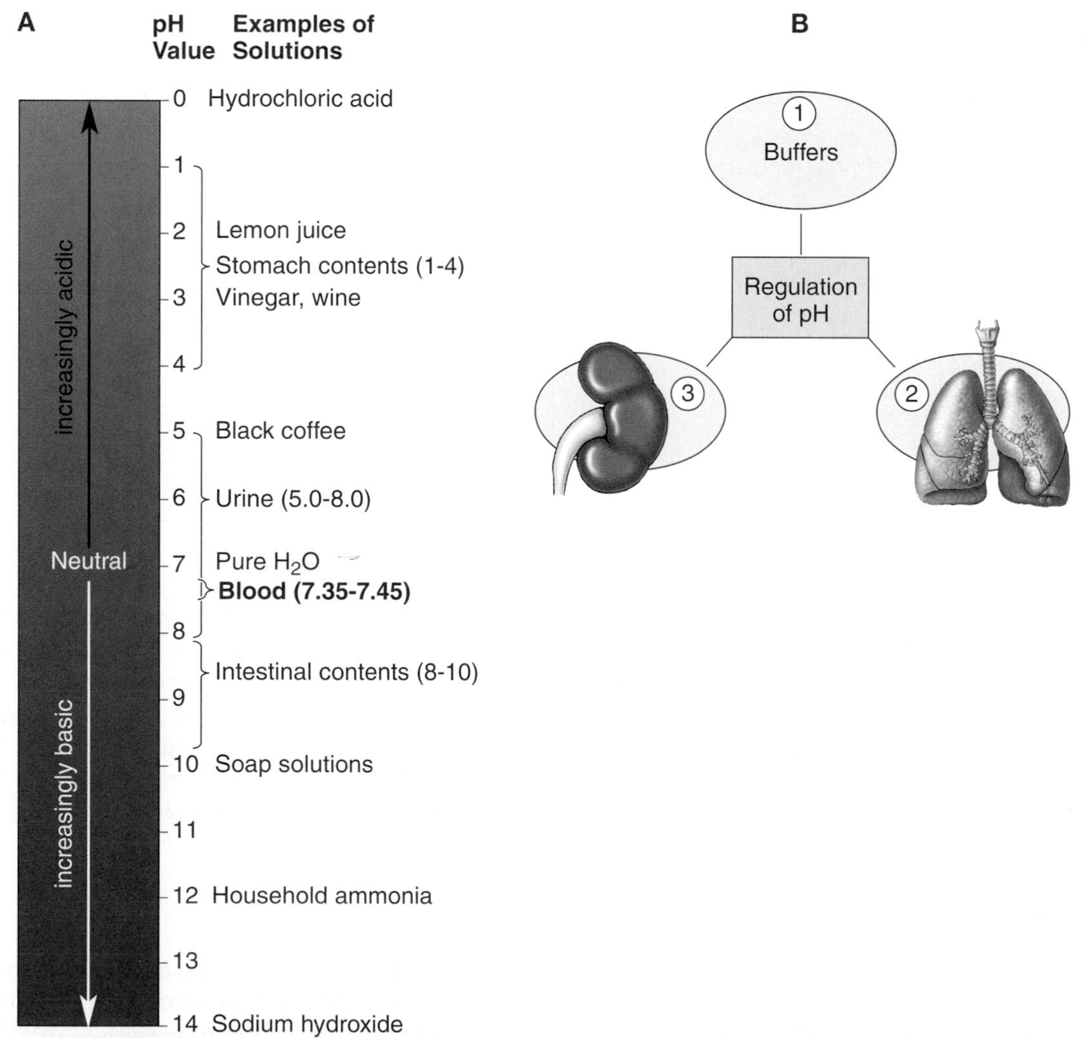

FIGURE 25-3 **A,** pH scale. **B,** Regulation of pH by buffers, lungs, and kidneys.

H^+ from the blood. If the H^+ concentration decreases, the "giver" part of the buffer donates H^+ to the blood. By removing or adding H^+, the buffer pair can maintain a normal blood pH. The body has numerous buffer systems. The most important are the bicarbonate buffers, phosphate buffers, hemoglobin, and plasma proteins.

Lungs

The respiratory system is the second line of defense in the regulation of pH. What does breathing have to do with pH? Carbon dioxide (CO_2) can combine with water to form an acid (H^+). Since breathing controls CO_2 levels, it also affects H^+ concentration or blood pH (Figure 25-4, *A*).

How Decreasing the Respiratory Rate Decreases pH. By decreasing the respiratory rate, the body retains or accumulates CO_2. The CO_2 combines with H_2O to form H^+. The increase in H^+ causes the pH to decrease. Note that CO_2 retention causes the formation of (H^+) and a decrease in pH; this is the basis for the development of respiratory acidosis (see Figure 25-4, *B*).

How Increasing the Respiratory Rate Increases pH. By increasing respiratory rate, the body exhales, or blows off, CO_2. The decrease in CO_2 causes a decrease in H^+ concentration and an increase in pH; this is the basis of respiratory alkalosis (see Figure 25-4, *C*).

How the Respiratory System Knows. How does the respiratory system know that it should increase or decrease the respiratory rate? The medulla oblongata, the respiratory center in the brain, senses changes in H^+ concentration. As plasma H^+ concentration increases, the respiratory center is stimulated. The respiratory center then increases the rate and depth of breathing, thereby increasing the excretion of CO_2 by the lungs. As plasma H^+ concentration decreases, the medullary respiratory center sends a slow-down signal, thereby decreasing the rate of breathing and the excretion of CO_2 by the lungs. As CO_2 accumulates in the plasma, it forms H^+ and decreases pH.

A

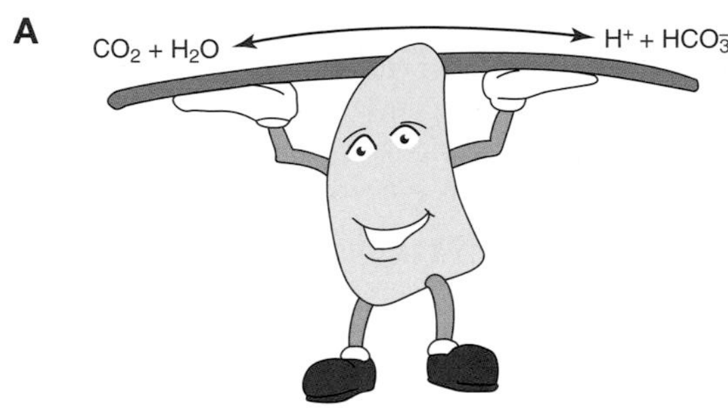
$CO_2 + H_2O$
$H^+ + HCO_3^-$
Normal lung maintains healthy acid-base balance.

B

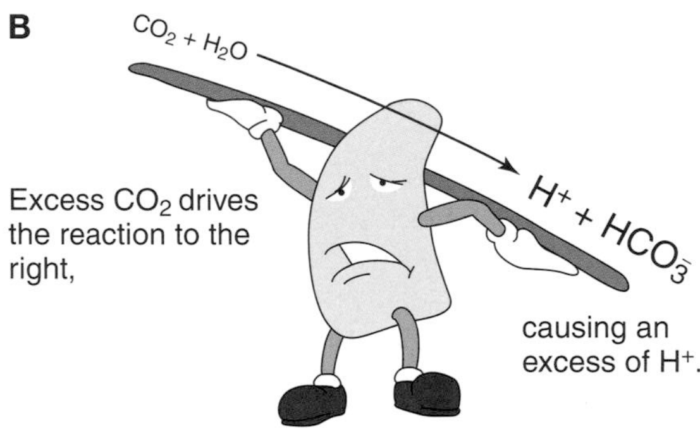
$CO_2 + H_2O$
$H^+ + HCO_3^-$
Excess CO_2 drives the reaction to the right,
causing an excess of H^+.
A lung that hypoventilates can cause respiratory acidosis.

C

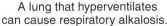

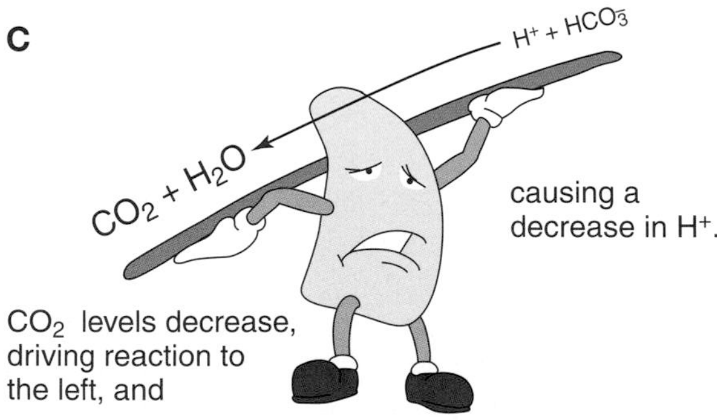
$H^+ + HCO_3^-$
$CO_2 + H_2O$
causing a decrease in H^+.
CO_2 levels decrease, driving reaction to the left, and
A lung that hyperventilates can cause respiratory alkalosis.

FIGURE 25-4 Respiratory control of acid-base balance. **A,** Normal respiratory rate. **B,** Hypoventilation causes respiratory acidosis. **C,** Hyperventilation causes respiratory alkalosis.

Kidneys

The kidneys are the third line of defense in the regulation of pH. The kidneys help regulate pH by reabsorbing or excreting H^+ as needed. The kidneys also help regulate bicarbonate (HCO_3^-), a major buffer. The kidneys can reabsorb bicarbonate when it is needed and can eliminate bicarbonate in the urine. Because the kidneys are major H^+ eliminators, patients in kidney failure are generally acidotic.

ACID-BASE IMBALANCES

When the body is unable to regulate pH, acid-base imbalances develop. The acid-base imbalances in the blood are called acidosis and alkalosis. These imbalances are common, exert generalized effects, and are often life-threatening (Table 25-2).

ACIDOSIS

A decrease in plasma pH below 7.35 is acidosis. (Remember: an increase in the plasma H^+ concentration results in a decrease in pH.) The two types of acidosis are respiratory acidosis and metabolic acidosis. **Respiratory**

Table 25-2 pH Imbalances

Imbalance	Causes	Compensations
Acidosis (pH <7.35)		
Respiratory acidosis	Any condition that causes hypoventilation (chronic lung disease such as emphysema, asthma, splinting of the chest, high doses of narcotic drugs, myasthenia gravis)	Kidneys excrete H^+ and reabsorb HCO_3^- (renal compensation for respiratory acidosis)
Metabolic acidosis	Kidney disease, diarrhea, diabetic ketoacidosis, lactic acidosis, and vomiting of intestinal contents	Increased respiratory rate to blow off CO_2; Kussmaul respirations (respiratory compensation for metabolic acidosis)
Alkalosis (pH >7.45)		
Respiratory alkalosis	Any condition that causes hyperventilation (anxiety)	Kidneys retain H^+ and excrete HCO_3^- (renal compensation for respiratory alkalosis)
Metabolic alkalosis	Persistent vomiting of stomach contents (loss of HCl), gastric suctioning, overingestion of antacids and bicarbonate-containing drugs	Decreased respiratory activity to retain CO_2 (respiratory compensation for metabolic alkalosis)

acidosis is caused by any condition that decreases the effectiveness of the respiratory system or causes prolonged **hypoventilation.** For example, chronic lung disease (emphysema); high doses of narcotics; splinting of the chest; and injury to the medulla oblongata may all cause a decrease in respiratory activity. The hypoventilation, in turn, increases the plasma levels of CO_2. The excess CO_2 forms H^+, decreases pH and causes acidosis (see Figure 25-4, *B*). Because the acidosis is caused by a respiratory dysfunction (hypoventilation), it is classified as a respiratory acidosis.

How does the body try to correct respiratory acidosis? First, the buffer systems remove some of the excess H^+. Then the kidneys excrete the excess H^+. The ability of the kidneys to correct respiratory acidosis is called the renal compensation of respiratory acidosis. The respiratory system, however, cannot correct this pH imbalance, because it is the dysfunctional respiratory system that is causing the acidosis.

Metabolic acidosis is a decrease in pH due to nonrespiratory conditions. For instance, kidney disease, uncontrolled diabetes mellitus, prolonged vomiting of intestinal contents (with loss of bicarbonate), and severe diarrhea (with loss of bicarbonate) are common causes of metabolic acidosis. A patient with poor kidney function is unable to excrete H^+ and becomes acidotic. A patient with uncontrolled diabetes mellitus produces excess ketoacids that overwhelm the buffer systems, accumulate in the plasma, and cause ketoacidosis.

How does the body try to correct metabolic acidosis? First, the buffer system removes some of the excess H^+. Second, the respiratory system helps remove excess H^+ through **hyperventilation** or **Kussmaul** (KOOS-mŭl) **respirations.** Hyperventilation decreases plasma CO_2 and therefore decreases H^+ concentration (increasing pH). The increased respiratory activity is called the respiratory compensation for metabolic acidosis.

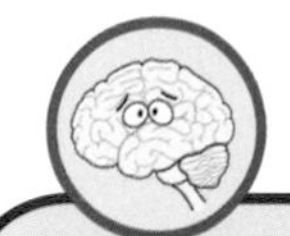

Do You Know...

Why you can hyperventilate yourself into a hypocalcemic tetany?

An anxious person often hyperventilates, causing a respiratory alkalosis. Calcium is less soluble in alkalotic blood. Consequently, the plasma levels of calcium decrease. Because calcium is necessary for normal nerve conduction, nerve function is impaired, and the person experiences numbness and tingling. If the person continues to hyperventilate, the plasma levels of calcium may decline so much that an episode of hypocalcemic tetany may occur. Chill!

ALKALOSIS

An increase in plasma pH above 7.45 is alkalosis. The two types of alkalosis are respiratory alkalosis and metabolic alkalosis. Respiratory alkalosis develops from hyperventilation and the resulting decrease in plasma CO_2. Common causes of respiratory alkalosis include anxiety and aspirin (salicylate) poisoning. Any condition that causes hyperventilation causes **respiratory alkalosis** (see Figure 25-4, *C*).

The body tries to correct respiratory alkalosis by the buffers and the kidneys. The buffers donate H^+ to the plasma, thereby decreasing pH. The kidneys decrease the excretion of H^+; H^+ retention decreases pH.

The kidneys also increase the excretion of bicarbonate. The ability of the kidneys to correct respiratory alkalosis is called the renal compensation of respiratory alkalosis. The respiratory system cannot correct this pH disturbance because it is the overactivity, or hyperventilation, of the respiratory system that is causing the alkalosis.

Metabolic alkalosis is an increase in pH caused by nonrespiratory disorders. Metabolic alkalosis can be caused by overuse of antacid and bicarbonate-containing drugs; persistent vomiting of stomach contents (loss of HCl); and frequent nasogastric suctioning (loss of HCl). The body tries to correct metabolic alkalosis through buffers, the kidneys, and the respiratory system. The buffers donate H^+, thereby decreasing pH. The kidneys decrease their excretion of H^+. Finally, the respiratory system corrects the pH by hypoventilation. Hypoventilation increases plasma CO_2 and H^+ and decreases pH.

Note that the respiratory system can both cause a pH imbalance and help correct a nonrespiratory pH imbalance. Similarly, the kidneys can both cause and correct pH imbalances. The ability of the lungs and the kidneys to correct a pH imbalance is called a **compensatory function.**

Sum It Up!

Plasma H^+ concentration is expressed as pH. The normal plasma pH is 7.4 (the range is 7.35 to 7.45). It is precisely regulated by three mechanisms: buffers, respirations, and kidney function. Acid-base balance is essential for the proper functioning of millions of chemical reactions in the body. Thus acid-base imbalances pose a serious threat to health. The imbalances are classified as either acidosis, a plasma pH less than 7.35 (respiratory and metabolic), or alkalosis, a plasma pH greater than 7.45 (respiratory and metabolic).

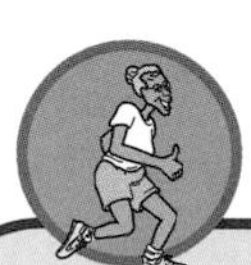

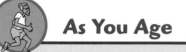

As You Age

1. As the kidneys age, the tubules become less responsive to antidiuretic hormone (ADH) and tend to lose too much water. The excess water loss is accompanied by a decrease in the thirst mechanism. As a result, the elderly person is prone to dehydration.
2. The ability to reabsorb glucose and sodium is also diminished. The presence of excess solute (sodium and glucose) in the urine contributes to excess urination and water loss. In addition, impaired reabsorption of glucose interferes with blood glucose monitoring in diabetes.
3. The kidney tubules are less efficient in the secretion of ions, including the hydrogen ion (H^+). As a result the elderly person experiences difficulty in correcting acid-base imbalances.
4. With immobility and diminished exercise, calcium moves from the bones into the renal tubules. There the calcium precipitates, causing kidney stones.

Disorders Resulting from Fluid and Electrolyte Imbalance

Dehydration	A condition in which the water content of the body is decreased below normal. Dehydration develops when water output exceeds water intake and commonly occurs in conditions such as excessive sweating, vomiting, diarrhea, and overuse of diuretics.
Potassium imbalances	Common and often life-threatening imbalances. Hypokalemia is a decrease in the amount of potassium in the blood and is usually due to prolonged diarrhea and the overuse of diuretics. Hyperkalemia is an increase in the amount of potassium in the blood. Common causes include impaired renal function, tissue injury, and the use of drugs such as potassium-sparing diuretics.
Sodium imbalances	Increased or decreased plasma levels of sodium. Hypernatremia is an increase in plasma sodium. It is most often seen in patients with high fever and excessive water loss through evaporation. Hypernatremia also accompanies sustained decreased secretion of ADH. Hyponatremia is a decrease in plasma sodium and is commonly seen with excess sweating, vomiting, diarrhea, and some forms of renal disease. Excess ingestion of water can dilute the plasma, thereby decreasing tonicity (hyponatremia) and causing water intoxication.

SUMMARY OUTLINE

Water, electrolytes, acids, and bases are tightly regulated. Fluids and electrolytes must be distributed in the body compartments in the correct volumes and concentrations.

I. Body Fluids: Distribution and Composition

A. Major Fluid Compartments
1. The two major fluid compartments are the intracellular compartment (63% of the water) and the extracellular compartment (37% of the water).
2. The extracellular compartment includes interstitial fluid, intravascular fluid (plasma), lymph, and transcellular fluid.

B. Composition of Body Fluids
1. Intracellular fluid contains high concentrations of potassium (K^+), phosphate (PO_4^{3-}), and magnesium (Mg^{2+}).
2. Extracellular fluid contains a high concentration of sodium (Na^+), chloride (Cl^-), and bicarbonate (HCO_3^-).

II. Water Balance: Intake Equals Output

A. Intake
1. The average intake of water is 2500 ml/24 hrs.
2. The primary regulator of fluid intake is thirst.

B. Output
1. The average output of water is 2500 ml/24 hrs.
2. Water is excreted by the kidneys (60%); skin and lungs (28%); digestive tract (6%); and sweat (6%).

C. Water: Deficiency and Excess
1. A deficiency of body water is called dehydration.
2. An excess of body water expands blood volume and causes edema.

III. Electrolyte Balance

A. Sodium (Na^+)
1. The chief extracellular cation.
2. Necessary for nerve-muscle conduction and helps maintain fluid balance.
3. Primarily regulated by aldosterone.

B. Potassium (K^+)
1. The chief intracellular cation.
2. Necessary for nerve-muscle conduction.
3. Primarily regulated by aldosterone.

C. Calcium (Ca^{2+})
1. Strengthens bones and teeth and is necessary for muscle contraction, nerve-muscle conduction, and blood clotting.
2. Is primarily regulated by parathyroid hormone.

D. Magnesium (Mg^{2+}) and Chloride (Cl^-)
1. Magnesium performs important functions in heart, muscles, and nerves.
2. Chloride is the chief extracellular anion and follows Na^+.

E. Bicarbonate (HCO_3^-)
1. A major extracellular anion.
2. Plays three important roles: it is the major form in which CO_2 is transported, it acts as a base (alkaline substance), and it plays an important role in acid-base balance.

IV. Acid-Base Balance

A. pH
1. The pH refers to the concentration of H^+.
2. The normal blood pH is 7.35 to 7.45. If blood pH is less than 7.35, the person is in acidosis. If blood pH is greater than 7.45, the person is in alkalosis.

B. Regulation of Blood pH
1. Blood pH is regulated by three mechanisms: buffers, the respiratory system, and the kidneys.
2. Buffers (the buffer pair) can donate or remove H^+.
3. The respiratory system affects pH by regulating CO_2.
4. The kidneys can vary their excretion of H^+.

V. Acid-Base Imbalances

A. Acidosis
1. Acidosis means that the blood pH is less than 7.35.
2. Respiratory acidosis is caused by hypoventilation.
3. Metabolic acidosis is due to nonrespiratory causes, including kidney disease, uncontrolled diabetes mellitus, diarrhea, and lactic acid production.

B. Alkalosis
1. Alkalosis means that the blood pH is greater than 7.45.
2. Respiratory alkalosis is caused by hyperventilation.
3. Metabolic alkalosis is caused by nonrespiratory conditions, including overingestion of antacids and loss of gastric contents.

Review Your Knowledge

Matching: Water Compartments

Directions: Match the following words with their description below. Some words may be used more than once.

a. interstitial
b. intracellular
c. plasma
d. transcellular

1. ____ Most body water is located within this compartment
2. ____ Water located within the vascular compartment (blood vessels)
3. ____ Water located between the cells
4. ____ Includes water within the eye, glandular secretions, and the cerebrospinal fluid
5. ____ Also called tissue fluid

Matching: Ions

Directions: Match the following words with their description below. Some words may be used more than once.

a. Na^+
b. K^+
c. H^+
d. Ca^{2+}

1. ____ Plasma concentration of this ion determines pH
2. ____ The chief extracellular cation
3. ____ The chief intracellular cation
4. ____ The ion that is elevated in hyperkalemia
5. ____ Aldosterone stimulates the distal tubule to reabsorb this cation
6. ____ Hypoventilation causes the accumulation of CO_2 and this cation
7. ____ Many diuretics are kaliuretic and therefore cause a loss of this cation
8. ____ Most diuretics work by blocking the renal reabsorption of this cation
9. ____ An increase in this ion causes acidosis
10. ____ This ion is regulated primarily by parathyroid hormone

Multiple Choice

1. Hyperkalemia
   a. refers to an elevated serum potassium.
   b. is never serious.
   c. develops in response to kaliuresis.
   d. refers to dangerously high levels of plasma sodium.
2. Which of the following best indicates the role of albumin in water balance?
   a. Blocks the renal reabsorption of Na^+
   b. Enhances the renal excretion of K^+
   c. Maintains plasma oncotic pressure
   d. "Plugs up" capillary pores keeping water within the plasma
3. Which of the following is not true of Na^+?
   a. Na^+ is the chief extracellular cation.
   b. Na^+ helps regulate extracellular volume.
   c. Na^+ is affected by aldosterone.
   d. Na^+ retention causes diuresis.
4. Which of the following is most apt to happen when fatty acids are broken down rapidly and incompletely?
   a. Plasma pH increases.
   b. The patient hypoventilates in an attempt to correct the pH disturbance.
   c. Ketoacids are produced causing metabolic acidosis.
   d. Plasma $[H^+]$ decreases.
5. Hypocalcemia is most apt to
   a. cause blood volume expansion (hypervolemia).
   b. be treated with IV potassium.
   c. cause tetany.
   d. be caused by excess parathyroid hormone activity.

CHAPTER 26

Reproductive Systems

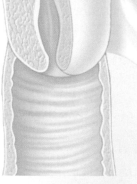

KEY TERMS

Cervix, p. 464
Endometrium, p. 464
Epididymis, p. 459
Estrogen, p. 463
Fallopian tube, p. 463
Gonad, p. 456
Gonadotropin, p. 461
Graafian follicle, p. 463
Menopause, p. 469
Menses, p. 466
Myometrium, p. 464
Ovarian follicle, p. 461
Ovulation, p. 463
Progesterone, p. 463
Prostate gland, p. 459
Scrotum, p. 456
Semen, p. 460
Spermatogenesis, p. 458
Testes, p. 456
Testosterone, p. 456
Uterus, p. 464
Vas deferens, p. 459

OBJECTIVES

1. List the structures and functions of the male and female reproductive systems.
2. Describe the structure and function of the testes.
3. Describe the structure and function of the male genital ducts.
4. Describe the accessory glands that add secretions to the semen.
5. Describe the hormonal control of male reproduction, including the effects of testosterone.
6. Describe the structure and function of the ovaries.
7. Describe the structure and function of the female genital tract.
8. Explain the hormonal control of the female reproductive cycle.

Few biologic drives are as strong as the urge to reproduce. As everyone knows and appreciates, human reproduction is sexual, meaning that both a female and a male partner are required. In contrast, reproduction in single-cell organisms is asexual, meaning that no partner is required. They simply divide by themselves. Think of how different your life would be in an asexual environment!

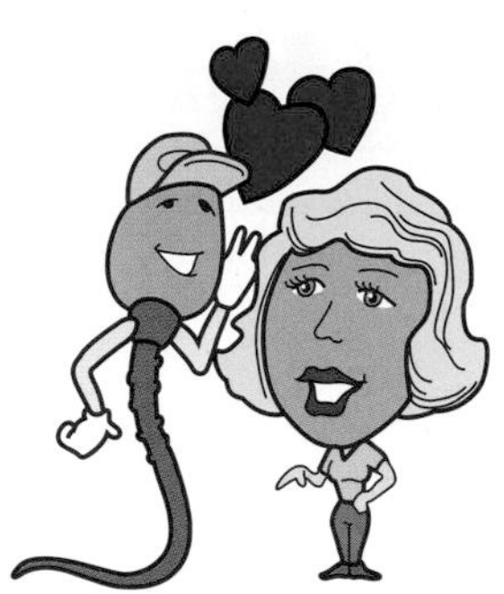

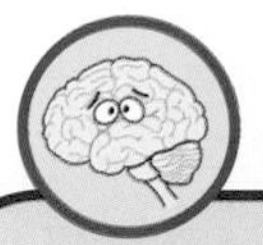

Do You Know...

Why Aristotle called the testicle the orchis?

The root of the orchid plant is olive shaped; in Greek the shape is called an *orchis.* Noticing the similarity between the shape of the orchid root and the testicles, Aristotle dubbed the testicle *orchis.* The word *orchis* is still used in medical terms. For example, orchitis refers to inflammation of the testicles, and orchiectomy refers to the surgical removal of the testicles. The word *testis* comes from the Latin and means to bear witness to. The word *testes* shares the same Latin root with the word *testify.* In ancient Rome, only men could bear witness, or testify, in a public forum. To show the importance of their testimony, they held their testicles as they spoke.

To carry out its role, the reproductive system performs two functions. It produces, nurtures, and transports ova and sperm, and it secretes hormones. The reproductive organs include the primary reproductive organs and the secondary reproductive organs. The primary reproductive organs are the **gonads.** The female gonads are the ovaries. The male gonads are the testes.

The gonads perform two functions: they secrete hormones, and they produce the gametes. The **gametes** are the ova (eggs) and the sperm. All other organs, ducts, and glands in the reproductive system are secondary, or accessory, reproductive organs. The secondary reproductive structures nourish and transport the eggs and sperm. They also provide a safe and nourishing environment for the fertilized eggs.

MALE REPRODUCTIVE SYSTEM

The male reproductive system performs three roles. It produces, nourishes, and transports sperm. It deposits the sperm within the female reproductive tract, and it secretes hormones. Figure 26-1, *A,* shows the organs of the male reproductive tract.

TESTES

The **testes** (TĔS-tēz), or **testicles,** are the male gonads. They perform two functions: the production of sperm and the secretion of the male hormone, **testosterone** (see Figure 26-1, *A*). The two oval testes are located outside the abdominal cavity and are suspended in a sac between the thighs called the **scrotum.**

The testes begin their development within the abdominal cavity but normally descend into the scrotum during the last 2 months of fetal development. Failure of the testes to descend into the scrotum is called cryptorchidism, a condition that can result in sterility if it is left untreated.

Location, Location, Location

Why are undescended testicles associated with infertility? It's a temperature thing. Sperm cannot live at body temperature; instead, they prefer the cooler temperature of the scrotum. To avoid infertility, a surgeon will pull the undescended testicles into the scrotum. Wearing tight underwear and jeans can also elevate the temperature in the testes, thereby lowering sperm count. What happens when the outside, environmental temperature becomes excessively cold during the winter months? The scrotum, with the assistance of the cremaster muscle, pulls the testes close to the body, thereby keeping the sperm toasty.

Lobules

The testis is divided into about 250 smaller units called **lobules** (Figure 26-2, *A*). Each lobule contains seminiferous tubules and interstitial cells. The tightly coiled **seminiferous tubules** form sperm. The **interstitial cells** lie between the seminiferous tubules and produce the male hormones called **androgens.** The most important androgen is testosterone. Thus the testes produce both sperm and testosterone.

Sperm Cells

Each day a man makes millions of sperm. Sperm are formed by the epithelium of the seminiferous tubules. The seminiferous tubules contain two types of cells, spermatogenic cells and supporting cells. The spermatogenic cells are sperm-producing cells. The supporting cells are also called sustentacular cells or Sertoli cells. They support, nourish, and regulate the spermatogenic cells.

A

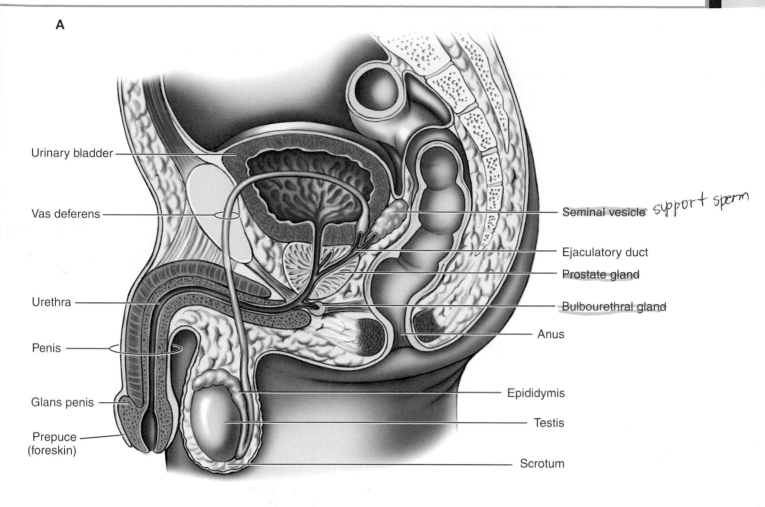

Urinary bladder
Vas deferens
Urethra
Penis
Glans penis
Prepuce (foreskin)
Seminal vesicle
Ejaculatory duct
Prostate gland
Bulbourethral gland
Anus
Epididymis
Testis
Scrotum

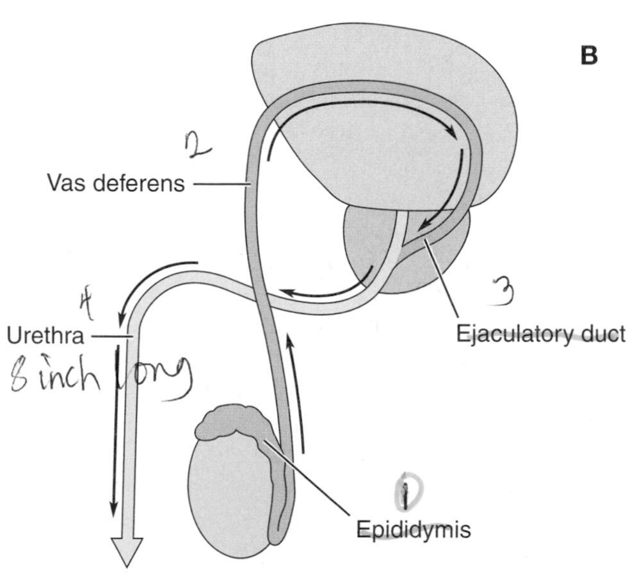

FIGURE 26-1 **A,** Male reproductive organs. **B,** The pathway for semen.

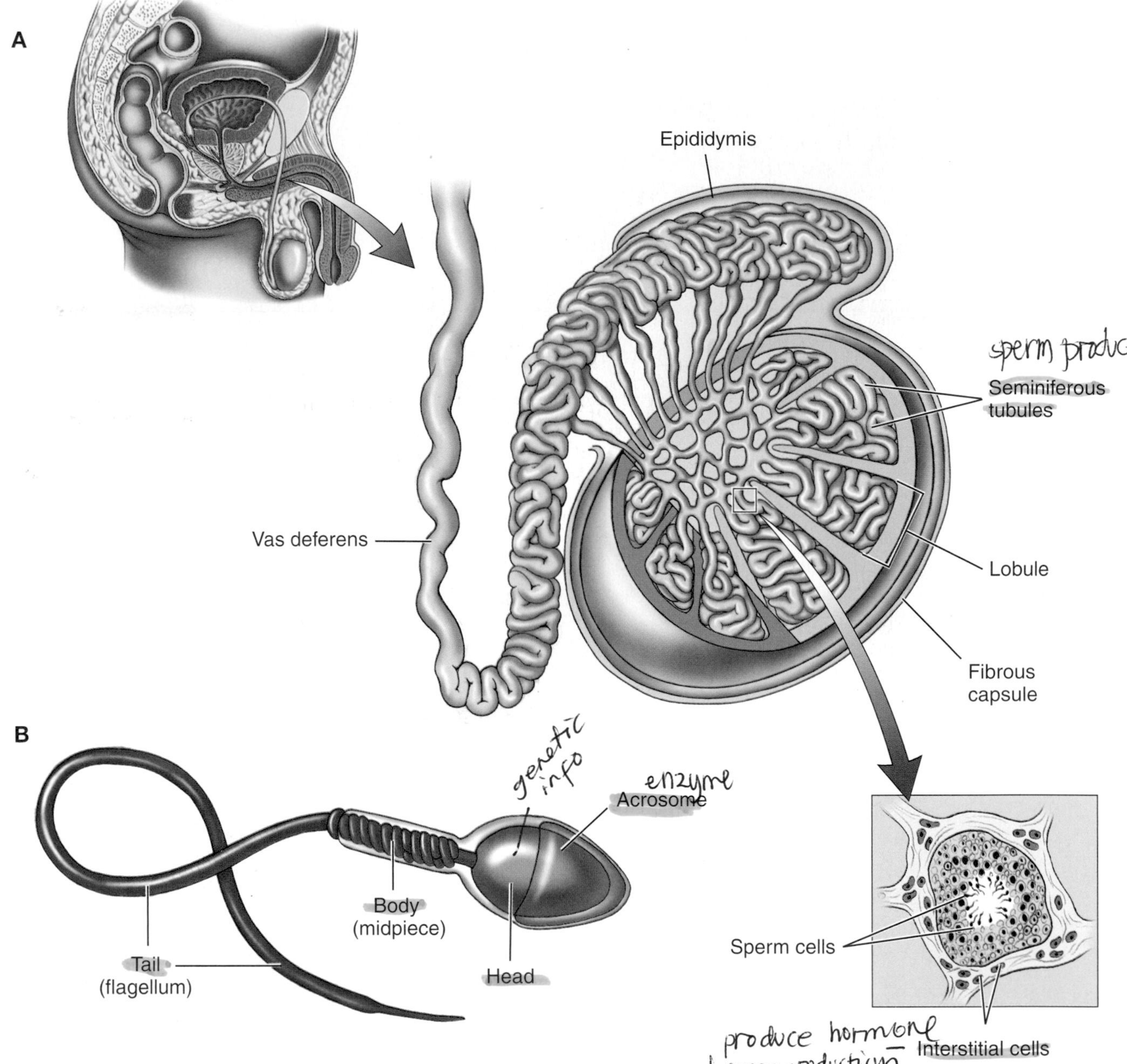

FIGURE 26-2 **A,** Male gonad. The testis consists of lobules containing seminiferous tubules surrounded by interstitial cells. **B,** Sperm.

Spermatogenesis

Spermatogenesis (spĕr-mă-tō-JĔN-ĕ-sĭs) is the formation of sperm. The undifferentiated spermatogenic cells are called **spermatogonia.** Each spermatogonium contains 46 chromosomes, the normal number of chromosomes for human body cells. Under the influence of testosterone, the spermatogonia enlarge to become primary spermatocytes. The **primary spermatocytes** divide by a special type of cell division called **meiosis.** The important point about meiosis is this: meiosis reduces the number of chromosomes by one half, from 46 to 23. Thus a sperm has only 23 chromosomes. When the sperm unites with an egg, which also has only 23 chromosomes (by meiosis), the fertilized egg contains 46 chromosomes, the normal number for human body cells. Newly formed sperm are not functional and must undergo several maturational changes.

A sperm looks like a tadpole (see Figure 26-2, *B*). The mature sperm has three parts: a head, a body, and a tail. The **head** is primarily a nucleus. The nucleus is important because it contains the genetic information. The front part of the head has a specialized structure called the **acrosome,** which contains enzymes that help the sperm penetrate the egg at the time of fertilization. The **body,** or **midpiece,** of the sperm is spiral-shaped structure that contains many mitochondria and supplies the sperm with the energy needed for the "big swim." The **tail** of the sperm is a flagellum. Its whiplike movements enable the sperm to swim. Most sperm live only hours after being deposited in the female reproductive tract, but the hardier ones may survive for up to 3 days.

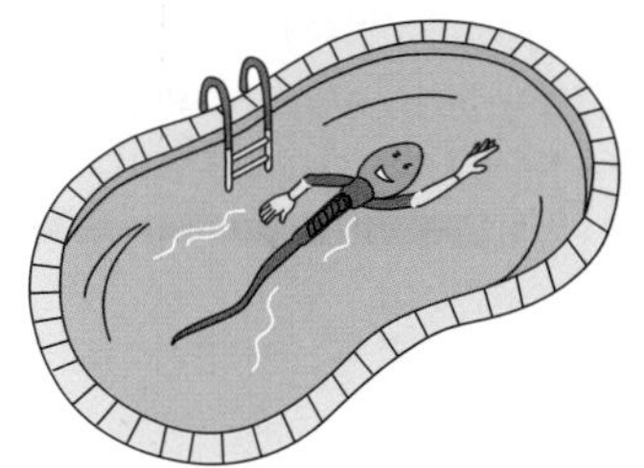

Sum It Up!

The purpose of the reproductive system is to produce offspring. Human reproduction is achieved sexually through the union of an egg and a sperm. The primary reproductive organs are the gonads: the ovaries in the female, and the testes in the male. The gonads produce the gametes. The ovaries produce the female gametes (eggs). The testes produce the male gametes (sperm). The mature egg and sperm each contain 23 chromosomes. On union, the fertilized egg contains 46 chromosomes, the number of chromosomes that human cells contain.

GENITAL DUCTS

As the sperm form, they gather in the seminiferous tubules and then move into a series of genital ducts, where they mature. They are then transported from the testes to the outside of the body. The ducts include two epididymides, two vas (ductus) deferens, two ejaculatory ducts, and one urethra.

Epididymis

The **epididymis** (ĕp-ĭ-DĬD-ĭ-mĭs) is the first part of the duct system. It is about 20 feet (6 m) in length, is tightly coiled, and sits along the top and posterior side of the testis (see Figure 26-1). While in the epididymis, the sperm mature, becoming motile and fertile. The walls of the epididymis contract and push the sperm into the next structure, the vas deferens.

Vas Deferens and Ejaculatory Ducts

The **vas deferens** (văs DĔF-ĕr-ĕnz) is continuous with the epididymis. It ascends as part of the **spermatic cord** through the inguinal canal in the groin region into the pelvic cavity. (There are two spermatic cords, one coming from the right and one from the left groin region.) In addition to the vas deferens, the spermatic cord includes blood vessels, lymphatic vessels, nerves, muscles, and connective tissue.

As the vas deferens courses through the pelvic cavity, it curves over the urinary bladder and joins with the duct of the seminal vesicle to form the **ejaculatory duct** (see Figure 26-1). The two ejaculatory ducts, from the right and left sides, pass through the prostate gland and join with the single urethra. Trouble remembering the directions? Let swimmer STEVE help!

ST Seminiferous Tubules
E Epididymis
V Vas deferens
E Ejaculatory duct

Urethra

The **urethra** extends from the base of the urinary bladder to the tip of the penis. The male urethra serves two organ systems, the reproductive and urinary systems. The urethra carries urine from the urinary bladder to the outside. It also carries semen from the ejaculatory ducts to the outside. However, the urethra can only do one thing at a time. It passes either urine or semen but never both simultaneously.

ACCESSORY GLANDS

Various secretions are added to the sperm as they travel through the genital ducts. The secretions come from three glands: the seminal vesicles, the prostate gland, and the bulbourethral glands (see Figure 26-1, *A*).

Seminal Vesicles

The **seminal vesicles** are located at the base of the bladder and secrete a thick, yellowish material rich in substances such as fructose (sugar), vitamin C, and prostaglandins. These substances nourish and activate the sperm as they pass through the ducts.

Prostate Gland

The single, donutlike **prostate gland** encircles the upper urethra just below the bladder. The prostate gland secretes a milky, alkaline substance that plays a role in increasing sperm motility. It also counteracts the acidic environment of the vagina and so helps protect the sperm as they enter the woman's body. During ejaculation, the smooth muscle of the prostate gland contracts and forces the secretions into the urethra.

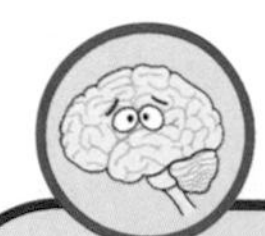

Do You Know...

If it is a prostrate or a prostate gland?

The donut-shaped gland of the male surrounds the urethra as it leaves the bladder. The word *prostate* means "one who stands before"; the prostate gland stands before the exit from the bladder. It sort of has a noble ring to it. However, sometimes the gland is mistakenly called the "prostrate" gland. A prostrate position is flat and helpless. Definitely not a flattering name for such equipment. So, it's *prostate,* not prostrate.

Bulbourethral Glands

The **bulbourethral glands,** or **Cowper's glands,** are tiny glands that secrete thick mucus into the urethra. The mucus serves as a lubricant during sexual intercourse.

SEMEN

The mixture of sperm and the secretions of the accessory glands is called **semen** (SĒ-mĕn). About 60% of the volume of semen comes from the seminal vesicles. Most of the remainder of the volume comes from the prostate gland. Semen is a milky white liquid with an alkaline pH. The alkaline pH is important because sperm are sluggish in an acidic pH. Because the pH of the female vagina is acidic, the alkaline pH of semen neutralizes the acid in the vagina and therefore protects the sperm from the destructive effects of acid.

The secretions of the accessory glands perform several other functions: they nourish the sperm, aid in the transport of sperm, and lubricate the reproductive tract. The amount of semen per ejaculation is small, about 2 to 6 ml, or 1 teaspoon. The number of sperm per ejaculation, however, is impressive (50 to 100 million).

EXTERNAL GENITALS

The **external genitals (genitalia)** of the male consist of the scrotum and the penis (see Figure 26-1). The scrotum is a sac, or pouch of skin, that hangs loosely between the legs and contains the testes.

The **penis** has two functions: it carries urine through the urethra to the outside of the body, and it acts as the organ of **sexual intercourse (copulation).** The penis deposits sperm in the female reproductive tract. The shaft, or body, of the penis contains three columns of erectile tissue and an enlarged tip called the **glans penis.** The opening of the urethra penetrates the glans penis.

The loose skin covering the penis extends downward and forms a cuff of skin around the glans and is called the **foreskin** or **prepuce.** Around puberty, small glands located in the foreskin and the glans secrete an oily substance. This secretion and the surrounding dead skin cells form a cheesy substance called **smegma.** As part of daily hygiene, a man should pull back the foreskin to remove the smegma. Occasionally, the foreskin is too tight and cannot be retracted. This condition is called phimosis. The foreskin is often surgically removed after birth in a process called circumcision. Although parents often have their sons circumcised to promote cleanliness, circumcision is also a common religious ritual.

MALE SEXUAL RESPONSE: ERECTION, EMISSION, EJACULATION, AND ORGASM

The urethra extends the length of the penis and is surrounded by three columns of spongy erectile tissue. When a man is sexually stimulated, the parasympathetic nerves fire, the penile arteries dilate, and the erectile tissue fills with blood. The accumulation of blood in the erectile tissue causes the penis to enlarge and become rigid. This process is an **erection.** It enables the penis to penetrate the reproductive tract of the female. For a number of reasons, a man may be unable to achieve an erection and is said to have erectile dysfunction. (The older term is impotence.)

Orgasm refers to the pleasurable sensations that occur at the height of sexual stimulation. Orgasm in the male is accompanied by emission and ejaculation. **Emission** is the movement of sperm and glandular secretions from the testes and genital ducts into the proximal urethra, where they mix to form semen. Emission is caused by the influence of the sympathetic nervous system on the ducts, causing rhythmic, peristaltic-type contractions. Remember the autonomics—Up and Out!

Up: Erection — Parasympathetic
Out: Emission — Sympathetic

Ejaculation is the expulsion of semen from the urethra to the outside. Ejaculation begins when the urethra fills with semen. Motor nerve impulses from the spinal cord stimulate the skeletal muscles at the base of the erectile columns in the penis to contract rhythmically. The rhythmic contraction provides the force necessary to expel the semen. The flow of semen during ejaculation is illustrated in Figure 26-1, *B.* Immediately after ejaculation, sympathetic nerve impulses cause the penile arteries to constrict, thereby reducing blood flow into the penis. This process is accompanied by increased venous drainage of blood from the penis. As a consequence, the penis becomes flaccid and returns to its unstimulated size. Remember the autonomics—Up and Down!

Up: Erect — Parasympathetic
Down: Flaccid — Sympathetic

MALE SEX HORMONES

Effects of Testosterone

The male sex hormones are called androgens, the most important being testosterone. Most of the testosterone is secreted by the interstitial cells of the testes. A small amount is secreted by the adrenal cortex.

Secretion of testosterone begins during fetal development and continues at a very low level throughout childhood. When a boy reaches age 10 to 13, testosterone secretion increases rapidly, transforming the boy into a man. This phase in reproductive development is called **puberty.** After puberty, testosterone is secreted continuously throughout the life of the male.

Testosterone is necessary for the production of sperm and is responsible for the development of the male sex characteristics. The **primary sex characteristics** include the enlargement and development of the testes and the various accessory organs such as the penis. Secondary sex characteristics refer to special features of the male body and include the following:

- Increased growth of hair, particularly on the face, chest, axillary region, and pubic region
- Deepening of the voice due to enlargement of the vocal cords
- Thickening of the skin and increased activity of the oil and sweat glands; at puberty, the adolescent is faced with new challenges such as acne and body odor
- Increased musculoskeletal growth and development of the male physique (broad shoulders and narrow waist)

Hormonal Control of Male Reproduction

The male reproductive system is controlled primarily by the hormones secreted by the hypothalamus, the anterior pituitary gland, and the testes. The hypothalamus secretes a releasing hormone, which then stimulates the anterior pituitary gland to secrete two **gonadotropins: follicle-stimulating hormone (FSH)** and **luteinizing hormone (LH)** (Figure 26-3). FSH promotes spermatogenesis by stimulating the spermatogenic cells to respond to testosterone. Note that spermatogenesis comes about through the combined action of FSH and testosterone. LH, also known as **interstitial cell–stimulating hormone (ICSH)** in the male, promotes the development of the interstitial cells of the testes and the secretion of testosterone.

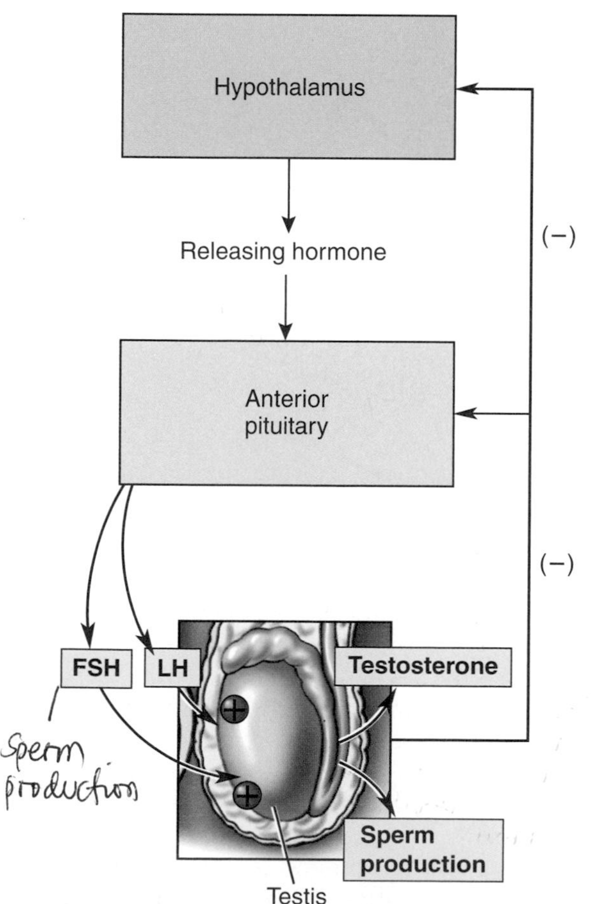

FIGURE 26-3 Hormonal control of sperm production and testosterone secretion.

After puberty, a negative feedback loop regulates testosterone production. When the level of testosterone in the blood increases, it causes the hypothalamus and the anterior pituitary gland to decrease their hormonal secretions, thereby decreasing the production of testosterone. As blood levels of testosterone decrease, the anterior pituitary gland increases its secretion of LH (ICSH), thereby stimulating the interstitial cells to secrete testosterone once again. The negative feedback mechanism maintains constant blood levels of testosterone.

> **Sum It Up!**
>
> Four hormones—releasing hormone, FSH, LH, and testosterone—control the male reproductive system. The releasing hormone (hypothalamus) stimulates the anterior pituitary gland to secrete FSH and LH (ICSH). FSH and testosterone stimulate spermatogenesis. LH stimulates the secretion of testosterone. Finally, testosterone stimulates the development of the male secondary sex characteristics. A male looks male because of testosterone.

FEMALE REPRODUCTIVE SYSTEM

The female reproductive system produces eggs, secretes hormones, and nurtures and protects a developing baby during the 9 months of pregnancy. Figure 26-4, *A,* shows the organs of the female reproductive system.

OVARIES

The **ovaries** are the female gonads. Two almond-shaped ovaries, located on either side of the uterus in the pelvic cavity, are anchored in place by several ligaments, including the ovarian and the broad ligaments. The ovaries, although not attached directly to the fallopian tubes, are close to them.

Egg Development: The Ovarian Follicle

Within the ovary are many tiny, saclike structures called **ovarian follicles.** A female is born with two million follicles. This number steadily declines with age, however, so that at puberty only about 400,000 follicles remain. Of these, only about 400 follicles ever fully mature, because a female usually produces only one egg per month throughout her reproductive years. The production of eggs begins at puberty and continues until menopause,

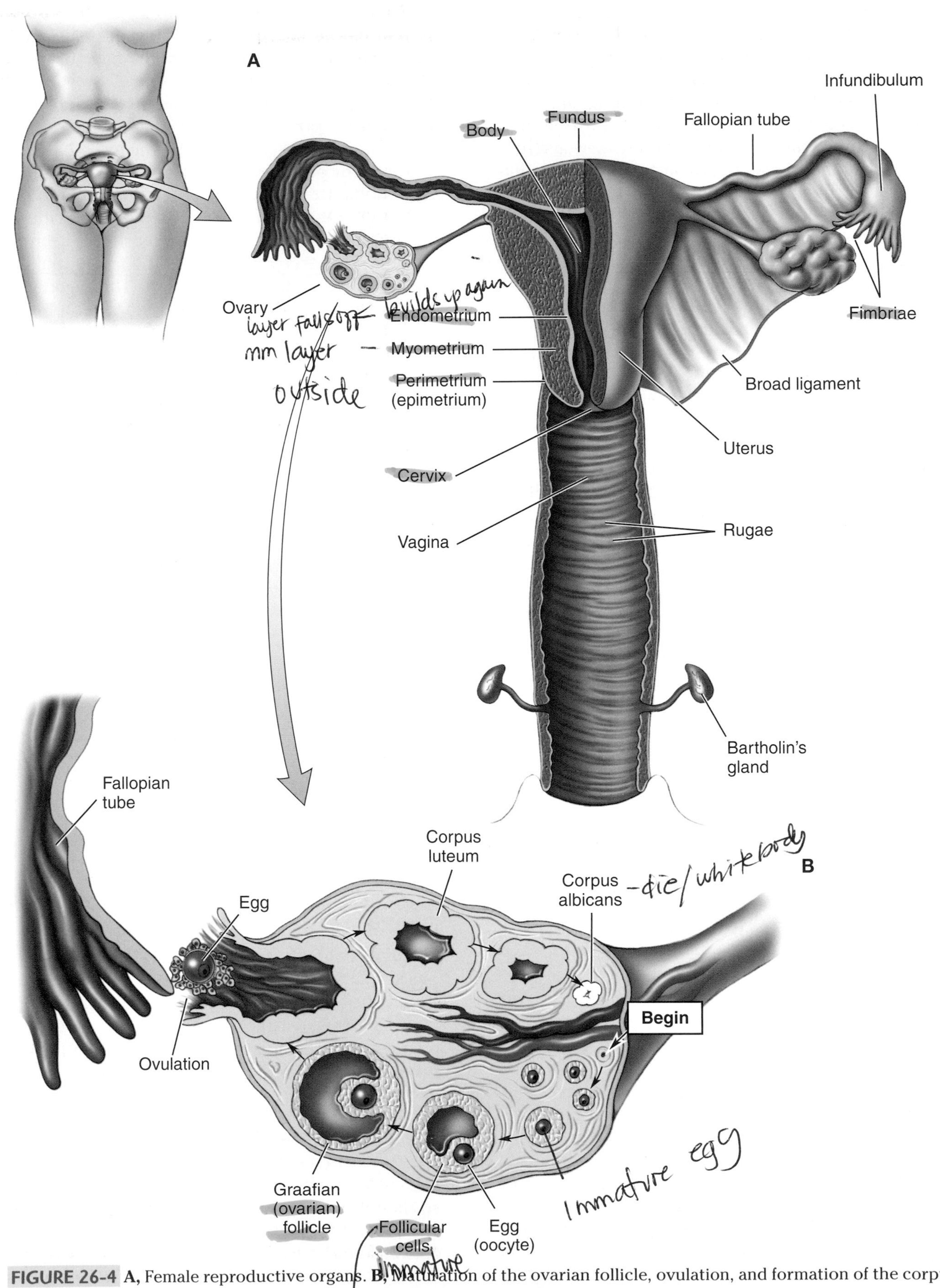

FIGURE 26-4 **A,** Female reproductive organs. **B,** Maturation of the ovarian follicle, ovulation, and formation of the corpus luteum.

at about 45 to 55 years of age. As with sperm, the supply of eggs far exceeds the actual need. This is Mother Nature's way of ensuring future generations.

Each ovarian follicle consists of an immature egg, called an **oocyte,** and cells surrounding the oocyte, called **follicular cells** (see Figure 26-4, *B*). Beginning at puberty, several follicles mature every month, although usually only one fully matures. As the egg matures, it begins to undergo meiotic cell division, which will reduce the number of chromosomes by one half, from 46 to 23.

At the same time, the follicle enlarges, a fluid-filled center is formed, and the follicular cells begin to secrete estrogen. The mature ovarian follicle is known as the **graafian follicle.** The graafian follicle looks like a blister on the surface of the ovary.

Ovulation

Once a month the ovarian follicle bursts. The ovary ejects a mature egg (ovum) with a surrounding layer of cells. This ejection phase is called **ovulation.** The egg travels from the surface of the ovary into the peritoneal cavity, where it is immediately swept into the fallopian tubes by the swishing motion of the **fimbriae** (fingerlike projections at the end of the fallopian tubes). The egg travels through the fallopian tubes to the uterus. If the egg is fertilized, it implants itself in the uterine lining and grows into a baby. If the egg is not fertilized, the egg dies and is eliminated in the menstrual blood. Some women feel twinges of pain at the time of ovulation; the pain is called mittelschmerz (from the German meaning middle pain).

Once ovulation has occurred, the follicular cells that remain in the ovary develop into a glandular structure called the **corpus luteum** ("yellow body"). The corpus luteum secretes two hormones, large amounts of progesterone (prō-JĔS-tĕ-rōn) and smaller amounts of estrogen. If fertilization does not occur, the corpus luteum deteriorates in about 10 days and becomes known as the **corpus albicans** ("white body"). The dead corpus albicans is not capable of secreting hormones. If fertilization occurs, however, the corpus luteum does not deteriorate. It stays alive and continues to secrete its hormones until this role can be taken over by the placenta, a structure you will read about in Chapter 27.

Sometimes the corpus luteum fills with fluid and forms an ovarian cyst. A blood-filled cyst is called a chocolate cyst. These cysts can resolve on their own but may require surgery.

Ovarian Hormones

At puberty, the ovaries begin to secrete the sex hormones estrogen and progesterone. The follicular cells of the maturing follicles secrete estrogen, and the corpus luteum secretes large amounts of progesterone and smaller amounts of estrogen. These hormones transform the girl into a woman.

Estrogen. Estrogen exerts two important effects: it promotes the maturation of the egg, and it helps develop the female secondary sex characteristics. Just as the male looks male because of testosterone, the female looks female because of estrogen. The feminizing effects of estrogen include the following:

- Enlargement and development of the organs of the female reproductive system
- Enlargement and development of the breasts
- Deposition of fat beneath the skin, especially in the thighs, buttocks, and breasts
- Widening of the pelvis
- Onset of the menstrual cycle
- Closure of the epiphyseal discs in long bones, thereby stopping further growth in height

Progesterone. The corpus luteum secretes **progesterone.** Progesterone has three important effects: it works with estrogen in establishing the menstrual cycle, helps maintain pregnancy, and prepares the breasts for milk production after pregnancy, increasing their secretory capacity. Although the corpus luteum secretes enough progesterone to maintain pregnancy in the early months, the woman's body needs larger amounts of both estrogen and progesterone during the later stages of pregnancy. This role is performed by the placenta.

Sum It Up!

The female gonad is the ovary. Once a month, an ovarian follicle matures, forming a graafian follicle. The follicle contains an egg and estrogen-secreting follicular cells. Under the influence of LH, the egg is expelled from the mature follicle; this event is ovulation. Following ovulation, the corpus luteum begins to secrete large amounts of progesterone. Estrogen helps the egg mature and is primarily responsible for the secondary sex characteristics of the female. Progesterone plays an important role in preparing the reproductive system for pregnancy.

GENITAL TRACT

The female genital tract includes the fallopian tubes, the uterus, and the vagina (see Figure 26-4, *A*).

Fallopian Tubes

The **fallopian tubes** are also called the **uterine tubes** or the **oviducts.** Each of the two fallopian tubes is about 4 inches (10 cm) long and extends from either side of the uterus to the ovaries. The funnel-shaped end of the fallopian tube nearest the ovary is called the **infundibulum** and has fingerlike projections called **fimbriae.** The fallopian tube does not attach directly to the ovary; the fimbriae hang over the ovary.

At ovulation, the fimbriae sweep the egg from the surface of the ovary into the fallopian tube. Once in the fallopian tube, the egg moves slowly toward the uterus. Because the egg cannot swim like sperm, the peristaltic activity of the fallopian tubes moves it forward.

The fallopian tubes have two functions. First, the tube transports the egg from the ovary to the uterus. Second, the tube is the usual site of fertilization of the egg by the sperm. The fertilized egg moves through the fallopian tube into the uterus, where it implants and grows into a baby. The journey through the fallopian tubes takes about 4 to 5 days.

Tube Troubles

- Occasionally, the fertilized egg implants in the fallopian tube rather than in the uterus. This condition is an ectopic pregnancy. The word *ectopic* means in an abnormal site; a tubal pregnancy is therefore an ectopic pregnancy. An ectopic pregnancy usually results in a miscarriage. It causes maternal bleeding, possible hemorrhage, and even death.
- What happens if the tubes scar and close? Scarring and closing, as occurs with repeated gonorrheal infections, blocks the movement of the egg through the tubes. This can cause sterility.
- PID. The fallopian tubes open directly into the pelvic cavity. An infection of the female reproductive tract can spread through the tubes into the pelvic cavity, causing pelvic inflammatory disease (PID). PID is most frequently associated with sexually transmitted diseases.

Uterus

The **uterus,** or **womb,** is shaped like an upside-down pear and is located between the urinary bladder and the rectum. The **broad ligament** holds the uterus in place. The primary function of the uterus is to provide a safe and nurturing environment for the growing baby. It is the baby's cradle for 9 comfortable months. During pregnancy, the size of the uterus increases considerably to hold the growing baby and the placenta.

The uterus has three parts. The **fundus** is the upper, dome-shaped region above the entrance of the fallopian tubes. The **body** is the central region. The **cervix** is the lower narrow region that opens into the vagina.

The uterus has three layers: an outer serosal layer called the **epimetrium,** or **perimetrium;** a middle, smooth muscular layer called the **myometrium;** and an inner layer called the **endometrium.** The endometrial uterine lining has two layers: the basilar layer and the functional layer. The basilar layer is thin and vascular and lies next to the myometrium. The functional layer responds to the ovarian hormones and thickens in preparation for the fertilized egg. It is also the layer that sloughs off during menstruation, when fertilization has not occurred.

The cervix is often associated with the Pap smear. The Pap smear is a diagnostic procedure used for detecting cancer of the cervix. The technique involves scraping cells from around the cervix and examining them for evidence of cancer. This simple and painless procedure has been used successfully to diagnose cancer in its early stages, when the cure rates are high. The technique is named for its developer, Dr. George Papanicolaou.

Do You Know...

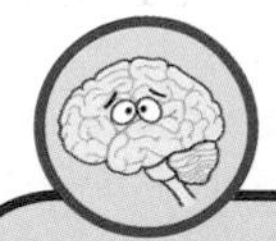

What Plato, hysteria, and the concept of the wandering womb have in common?

Plato believed that the womb (uterus), if unused for a long period, became "indignant." This indignant womb then wandered around the body, inhibiting the body's spirit and causing disease. According to the male thinkers of the day, a woman was so thoroughly controlled by her wandering womb that she was considered irrational and prone to emotional outbursts and fits of hysteria. This belief was the reason that the womb was named the *hystera.* The term has persisted in medical terminology. For example, a hysterectomy refers to the surgical removal of the uterus.

Do You Know...

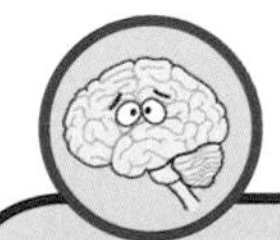

What the spots are on the outer surfaces of these organs?

These spots represent endometrial tissue adhering to the outer surface of the ovary, fallopian tube, rectum, and urinary bladder. How did the endometrial tissue get there? In some women, a portion of the menstrual discharge flows backward, into the fallopian tubes, and then into the pelvic cavity. The endometrial tissue adheres to the outer surface of the organs in the pelvic cavity. This condition is called **endometriosis.** The endometrial tissue acts as though it were still in uterus. It responds to the ovarian hormones by thickening, becoming secretory, and then sloughing. A woman then feels the discomfort of menstruation throughout the pelvic cavity. In addition to causing severe pain, endometriosis causes scarring and the formation of adhesions.

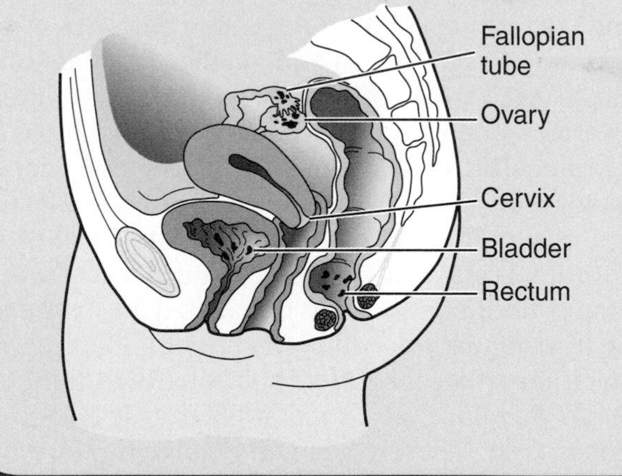

Vagina

The **vagina** is a 4-inch muscular tube that extends from the cervix to the vaginal opening in the perineum. The vaginal opening is usually covered by a thin membrane called the **hymen.** The hymen may be torn in a number of ways such as the first intercourse, use of tampons, or strenuous exercise. Much has been written about the hymen and whether or not it is intact. The upper portion of the vagina receives the cervix of the uterus. The cervix dips into the vagina so that pockets, or spaces, form around the cervix. The pockets are called **fornices.** The deepest is the posterior fornix, located behind the cervix.

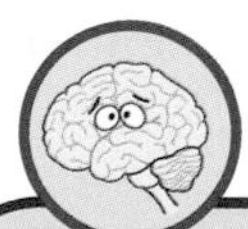

Do You Know...

Who rented the veil?

Anatomically, the veil refers to the **hymen,** a delicate membrane that partially closes the lower end of the vagina. The definition of hymen comes from the image of the vagina as a sanctuary of the virgin love goddess Aphrodite. The veil is rent, or torn, at marriage, the first intercourse. As you can imagine, there is much folklore (and many, many rules) concerning the hymen and who "rents" it. For instance, there was an ancient law that required a young girl to wear bells on the hem of her dress. If the bells rang while she was walking, she had to slow down, lest the vigorous walking movement tear the hymen. Female athletes, beware!

The mucosal lining of the vagina lies in folds (rugae) that are capable of expanding. The folding is important for childbearing because it permits the vagina to stretch and accommodate the baby during birth. In addition to forming a part of the birth canal, the vagina is also the organ that receives the penis during intercourse and serves as an exit for menstrual blood. The bacterial population (normal flora) in the vagina creates an acidic environment that discourages the growth of pathogens.

Sum It Up!

The genital tract consists of the fallopian tubes, the uterus, and the vagina. The fallopian tube, the usual site of fertilization, transports the egg from the ovary to the uterus. The uterus is the site where the fetus lives and grows for 9 months. The vagina receives the penis during intercourse and serves as part of the birth canal. A baby makes its entrance into the world through the vagina.

EXTERNAL GENITALS

The female external genitals (genitalia) are together called the **vulva** (Figure 26-5). The vulva includes the labia majora and labia minora, the clitoris, and the vestibular glands. (The external genitalia of the female are also called the pudendum, from a word meaning shameful. Go figure!)

The two **labia majora** are folds of hair-covered skin that lie external to the two smaller **labia minora.** The labia (the word means lips) are separated by a cleft containing the urethral and vaginal openings. The labia prevent drying of the mucous membranes. The labia majora merge anteriorly (in front) to form the rounded, hair-covered region over the symphysis called the **mons pubis.**

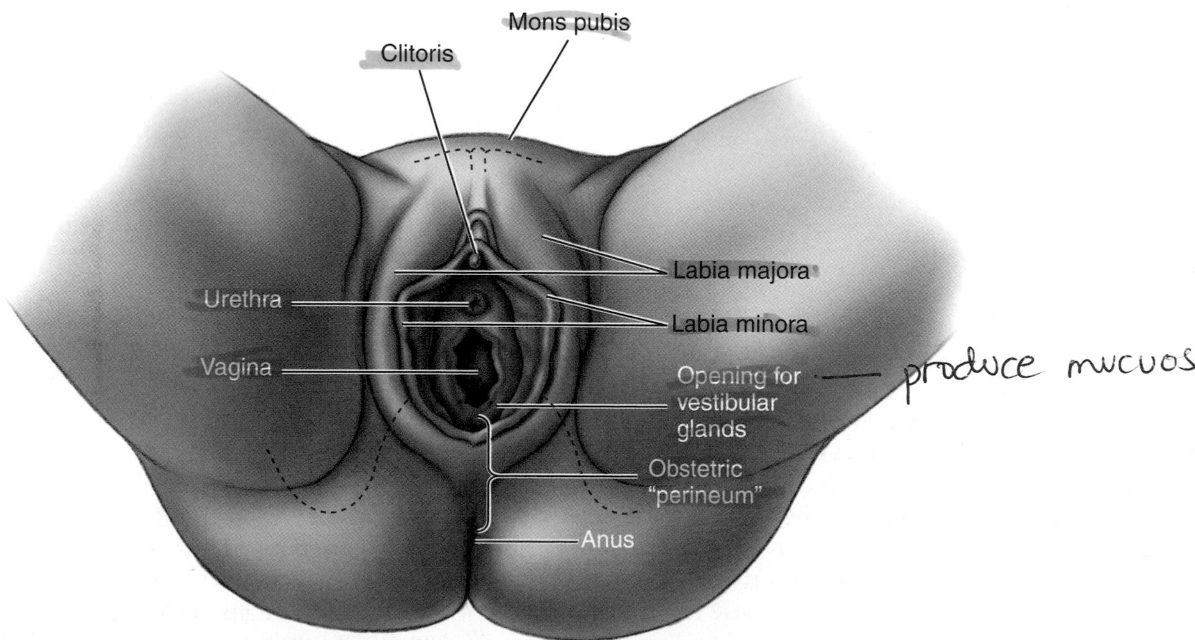

FIGURE 26-5 External genitals of the female.

The **clitoris** is the structure that resembles the penis. Although small, the clitoris contains erectile tissue and is capped by a thin membrane called the glans. The labia minora extend forward and partially surround the clitoris to form a foreskin. Like the penis, the clitoris contains sensory receptors that allow the female to experience pleasurable sexual sensations.

The **vestibule** is a cleft between the labia minora. It contains the openings of the urethra and the vagina. A pair of **vestibular glands (Bartholin's glands)** lie on either side of the vaginal opening and secrete a mucus-containing substance that moistens and lubricates the vestibule. Note that the female urinary system and the reproductive system are entirely separate. The female urethra carries only urine, whereas the male urethra carries both urine and semen.

The **perineum** refers to the entire pelvic floor. The common use of the word, however, is more limited. Most clinicians use the word *perineum* to mean the area between the vaginal opening and the anus (called the "obstetric perineum").

FEMALE SEXUAL RESPONSE

The female responds to sexual stimulation with erection and orgasm. Erectile tissue in the clitoris and the tissue surrounding the vaginal opening swell with blood in response to parasympathetically induced dilation of the arteries. Erectile tissue in the vaginal mucosa, breasts, and nipples also swell. Other responses include an engorgement of the vagina and secretion by the vestibular glands. At the height of sexual stimulation, a woman experiences orgasm.

The orgasm also stimulates a number of reflexes. These reflexes cause muscle contractions in the perineum, uterine walls, and uterine tubes; the muscular activity is thought to aid in directing and transporting the sperm through the genital tract.

HORMONAL CONTROL OF THE REPRODUCTIVE CYCLES

Let us review the female reproductive cycle. Each month, an egg is produced by the ovary in anticipation of producing a baby. As the egg develops in the ovary, the uterus prepares to receive the fertilized egg. Its preparation consists of the building up of a thick, lush endometrial lining. If the egg is not fertilized, the endometrial lining is no longer needed to nourish the fetus, and so it is shed in the menstrual flow. Then the process begins again. A second egg ripens in the ovary, and the uterine lining starts the rebuilding process. This process repeats itself throughout the female reproductive years, all for the purpose of reproducing.

A number of hormones control the female reproductive cycle. Unlike male hormones, female hormonal secretion occurs in a monthly cycle with a regular pattern of increases and decreases in hormone levels. In fact, the word **menses** (MĔN-sēz) comes from the Greek word for month or moon. The hypothalamus, anterior pituitary gland, and ovaries secrete most of the hormones involved in the menstrual cycle. The hypothalamus secretes a releasing hormone that then stimulates the anterior pituitary gland to secrete the two gonadotropins, FSH and LH. FSH and LH then stimulate the ovaries, causing them to secrete estrogen and progesterone. The hormones that regulate the female reproductive cycle are summarized in Table 26-1.

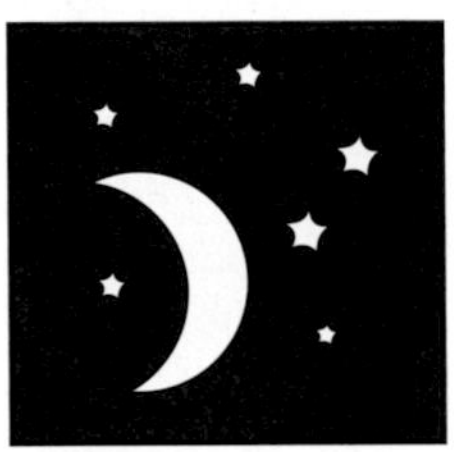

TWO REPRODUCTIVE CYCLES

There are two components of the female reproductive cycle; the ovarian cycle and the uterine cycle. These cycles begin at puberty and last about 40 years. Refer to Figure 26-6 as you read about the cyclic changes. Figure 26-6, *A*, illustrates the secretions of the anterior pituitary gland, FSH, and LH, over a 28-day monthly cycle. (The 28-day cycle is an average length; a normal cycle may be shorter or longer than 28 days.) The hypothalamic-releasing hormones are not shown, but they are responsible for stimulating the anterior pituitary secretion of the gonadotropins.

For each day of the period, you should be able to identify the secretions of the anterior pituitary gland, the maturation of the ovarian follicle, the changes in the blood levels of ovarian hormones, and the growth of the endometrial lining of the uterus. Figure 26-6, *B*, illustrates the growth and maturation of the ovarian follicle, which results in ovulation and the development of the corpus luteum. Figure 26-6, *C*, shows the blood levels of the ovarian hormones estrogen and progesterone. Figure 26-6, *D*, illustrates the monthly changes in the uterine lining. Together, the parts of Figure 26-6 describe events that occur over a 28-day period.

Ovarian Cycle

The **ovarian cycle** consists of two phases: the follicular phase and the luteal phase.

Follicular Phase. The **follicular phase** begins with the hypothalamic secretion of releasing hormones. These hormones, in turn, stimulate the release of

Table 26-1 Female Hormones

Hormone	Gland	Target Organ	Effects
Releasing hormone	Hypothalamus	Anterior pituitary	Stimulates the secretion of the gonadotropins (FSH and LH)
Follicle-stimulating hormone (FSH)	Anterior pituitary	Ovary	Initiates development of the ovarian follicle Stimulates the secretion of estrogen by the follicular cells
Luteinizing hormone (LH)	Anterior pituitary	Ovary	Causes ovulation Stimulates the corpus luteum to secrete progesterone
Estrogen	Ovary (follicle)	Locally (ovary) Uterus (endometrium)	Stimulates maturation of the ovarian follicle Stimulates the proliferative phase of endometrial development
		Other tissues and organs	Causes the development of the secondary sex characteristics
Progesterone	Ovary (corpus luteum)	Uterus (endometrium)	Stimulates the secretory phase of endometrial development
Human chorionic gonadotropin (hCG)	Trophoblastic cells of the embryo	Corpus luteum	Maintains the corpus luteum during early pregnancy

gonadotropins by the anterior pituitary gland. The FSH and small amounts of LH stimulate the growth and maturation of the ovarian follicle. The maturing ovarian follicle secretes large amounts of estrogen, causing the blood levels of estrogen to increase (see Figure 26-6, *C*).

Estrogen dominates the follicular phase. Estrogen affects both the ovary and the uterus and helps the ovarian follicle to mature. The blood also carries the estrogen to the uterus, where it helps build up the uterine lining in the first half of the uterine cycle (days 1 to 14) (see Figure 26-6, *D*).

The follicular phase ends when a sharp rise (midcycle surge) of LH on day 14 causes ovulation. (See Figure 26-6, *A,* for the midcycle surge of LH and Figure 26-6, *B,* for ovulation.)

Luteal Phase. The **luteal phase** immediately follows ovulation. Follicular cells of the ruptured follicle on the surface of the ovary form the corpus luteum. LH then stimulates the corpus luteum to secrete progesterone and small amounts of estrogen. The progesterone and estrogen exert a negative feedback effect on the anterior pituitary gland, thereby inhibiting further secretion of FSH and LH. Progesterone also supports the endometrial lining of the uterus during the second half of the cycle (days 14 to 28). Progesterone dominates the luteal phase.

When the corpus luteum dies, secretion of progesterone and estrogen declines. As a result of the decrease in estrogen and progesterone, FSH and small amounts of LH are once again secreted, and the cycle is repeated.

Uterine Cycle

The **uterine cycle,** also called the **menstrual cycle,** consists of the changes that occur in the endometrium over a 28-day period (see Figure 26-6, *D*). Estrogen and progesterone secreted by the ovaries cause the endometrial changes; thus the ovarian cycle controls the uterine cycle. The uterine cycle has three phases: the menstrual phase, the proliferative phase, and the secretory phase.

Menstrual Phase. Bleeding characterizes the menstrual phase. It begins on the first day and continues for 3 to 5 days, varying from person to person. During the menstrual phase, the functional layer of the endometrial lining and blood leave the uterus through the vagina as menstrual flow. This process is also called "having your period."

Proliferative Phase. The proliferative phase begins with the end of the menstrual phase. Repair and growth of the inner endometrial lining characterize the proliferative phase. The lining grows primarily because of estrogen secreted by the ovaries (see Figure 26-6, *B* and *C*). The proliferative phase is so named because the cells proliferate and thus repair the endometrial lining. Note in Figure 26-6, *D,* that the endometrial lining becomes thicker and acquires additional blood vessels during the proliferative phase.

Secretory Phase. The secretory phase is due to the secretion of progesterone by the corpus luteum of the ovary (see Figure 26-6, *C* and *D*). Progesterone causes the endometrial lining to thicken, thereby forming a nutritious environment awaiting the arrival of a fertilized ovum.

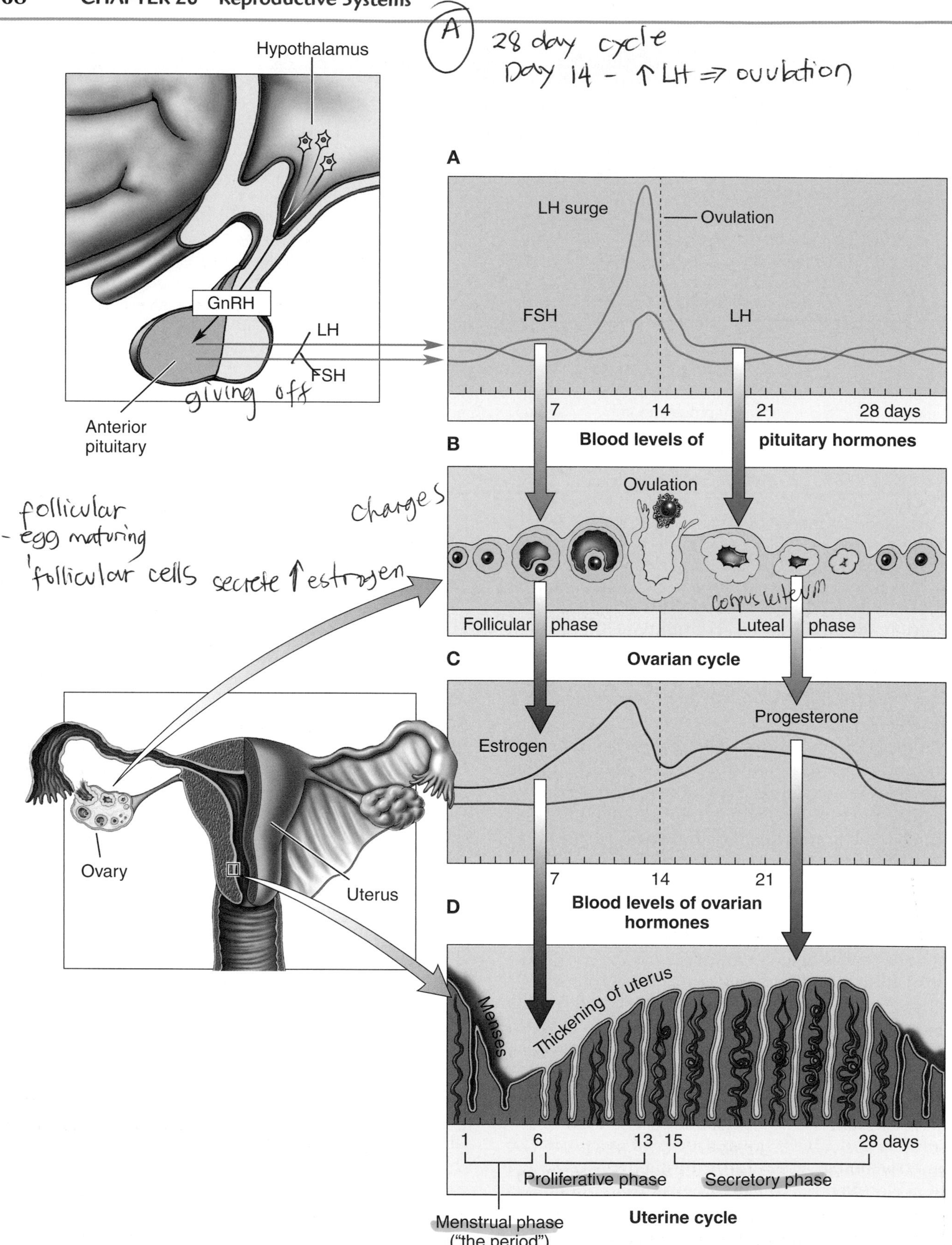

FIGURE 26-6 Hormonal control of the female reproductive cycle (28-day cycle). **A,** The anterior pituitary gland secretes the gonadotropins FSH and LH. **B,** Ovarian events. **C,** Blood levels of the ovarian hormones estrogen and progesterone. **D,** The uterine cycle.

Sum It Up!

Let us highlight the events of the ovarian and uterine cycles. Refer again to Figure 26-6:

- The development of the ovarian follicle, during the follicular phase of the ovarian cycle, is due primarily to FSH. FSH stimulates the follicle to secrete estrogen. The estrogen performs two functions: It stimulates the growth of the follicle, and it is responsible for the proliferative phase of the uterine cycle.
- Ovulation is the expulsion of the egg at midcycle (day 14) and is due to a surge of LH from the anterior pituitary gland.
- The follicular cells that remain on the surface of the ovary form the corpus luteum. The corpus luteum secretes progesterone and some estrogen. Blood carries the hormones to the uterus.
- Progesterone stimulates the uterine lining to become thick and lush, thereby forming a rich lining for the fertilized egg.
- When blood levels of estrogen and progesterone decline, the endometrial lining sloughs off and causes bleeding (menstruation).
- The ovarian hormones (estrogen and progesterone) exert a negative feedback effect on the anterior pituitary gland.

When blood levels of the ovarian hormones rise, secretions of FSH and LH are low. When the corpus luteum degenerates into the corpus albicans, however, the blood levels of estrogen and progesterone decrease. The decrease in the ovarian hormones in turn allows the anterior pituitary gland to secrete FSH and LH. The stimulated ovary then develops another follicle.

Implantation: Keeping the Corpus Luteum Alive

NOTE: The endometrial lining does not slough if blood levels of estrogen and progesterone are adequate. These levels are adequate if the corpus luteum does not deteriorate. How does the body prevent the deterioration of the corpus luteum?

If fertilization occurs, preserving the uterine lining is crucial. Menstruation must be prevented. How? Soon after fertilization, the egg implants in the uterine lining. Some of the cells at the site of implantation in the uterus secrete a hormone called **human chorionic gonadotropin (hCG).** Blood carries hCG from the uterus to the ovary where it stimulates the corpus luteum. hCG prevents the deterioration of the corpus luteum, thereby ensuring the continued secretion of estrogen and progesterone. hCG prolongs the life of the corpus luteum for 11 to 12 weeks, until the placenta can take over as the major estrogen- and progesterone-secreting gland. (Chapter 27 takes the story from here.)

Do You Know...

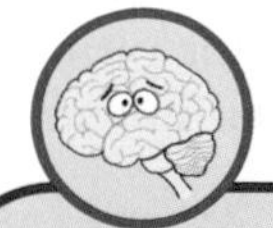

What the missing words in this "scientific" observation are?

According to the ancient scientist Pliny, "When a ________ ________ approaches, fermenting wine will be soured, seeds she touches become infertile, grass withers, garden plants shrivel, and fruit falls from the trees."

The missing words are "menstruating woman." Menstruating women were often feared, and a great lore grew up around menstrual blood. Casual observation might have suggested that the above charges were false. Pliny pondering periods! Not too observant for a scientist.

Menarche, Menses, and Menopause

In the female, puberty is marked by the first period of menstrual bleeding. This event is called **menarche.** Thereafter, the menstrual periods (menses) occur regularly until the woman reaches her late 40s or early 50s. At this time, the periods gradually become more irregular until they cease completely. This phase is called **menopause.** Menopause is also called the change of life, or the climacteric. Female reproductive function lasts from menarche to menopause.

The effects of menopause are due to a decrease in the ovarian secretion of estrogen and progesterone. Without ovarian hormones, the uterine cycle ceases, and the woman stops menstruating. Other symptoms associated with menopause include hot flashes, sweating, depression, irritability, and insomnia. The symptoms are highly variable. Some women experience severe disturbances; others hardly notice any systemic effects.

METHODS OF BIRTH CONTROL

Birth control is the voluntary regulation of reproduction. Birth control can limit the number of offspring produced and help determine the timing of conception. Methods of contraception are forms of birth control that prevent the union of egg and sperm.

BARRIER METHODS OF BIRTH CONTROL

Barriers prevent the sperm from entering the female: no union means no baby. Barrier methods are mechanical or chemical. The female and male condoms and the diaphragm are mechanical barriers. Spermicidal creams, foams, and jellies are chemical barriers. The effectiveness of the chemical barriers is improved considerably when they are used with a mechanical barrier.

HORMONAL CONTRACEPTIVES

The birth control pill is a pharmacologic agent that contains estrogen and progesterone. As the blood levels of estrogen and progesterone increase, negative feedback inhibits the secretion of FSH by the anterior pituitary gland. This process, in turn, prevents ovulation: no egg means no baby.

Implants containing progesterone act in much the same way. Progesterone-containing capsules, or rods, can be surgically implanted under the skin of a woman's upper arm or scapular region. The progesterone is slowly but continuously released from the implant. As with the birth control pill, the elevated blood levels of progesterone prevent ovulation. The same effect can be achieved by the injection of Depo-Provera (synthetic progesterone) 2 to 4 times per year.

SURGICAL METHODS OF BIRTH CONTROL

Surgical methods of contraception include a vasectomy in the male and a tubal ligation in the female (Figure 26-7). A vasectomy involves removing a small section of each vas deferens and tying the cut ends. A vasectomy is contraceptive because the sperm cannot leave the epididymis: no sperm means no baby.

In the female, a tubal ligation involves removing a small section of each fallopian tube and tying the cut ends. After a tubal ligation, the egg cannot be transported from the ovary through the fallopian tubes, where fertilization normally takes place: no egg means no baby.

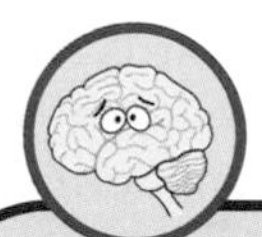

Do You Know...

If contraception is a new idea?

The practice of contraception has been around for centuries—and the methods are quite intriguing. For instance, one concoction used by Egyptian women included crocodile dung. The dung and herbal paste was inserted into the upper vagina. Croc dung is highly acidic and acted as a spermicidal agent. Others ate wild yam; this veggie contains large amounts of progesterone and acted physiologically like the pill, preventing ovulation. Condoms also made an early appearance. Men used the stomach of sheep as their preferred barrier type of contraception. Those ancients were very resourceful!

INTRAUTERINE DEVICES

An intrauterine device (IUD) is a small solid object placed in the uterine cavity. The IUD prevents pregnancy because it stimulates the uterus to prevent implantation of the fertilized egg. Note that the IUD is not technically contraceptive. In other words, it does not prevent conception; instead, it prevents implantation.

BEHAVIORAL METHODS OF BIRTH CONTROL

Sexual partners can behave in ways to prevent pregnancy. Behavioral methods include abstinence, the rhythm method, and coitus interruptus. Abstinence, or the avoidance of sexual intercourse, is the most effective method of birth control.

The rhythm method, also called natural family planning or timed coitus, requires avoiding sexual intercourse at a time when the female is ovulating, generally at midcycle. Because the menstrual cycle (and ovulation) are not always regular, the rhythm method is associated with a high pregnancy rate. Coitus interruptus involves the withdrawal of the penis from the vagina before ejaculation. It too is associated with a high pregnancy rate.

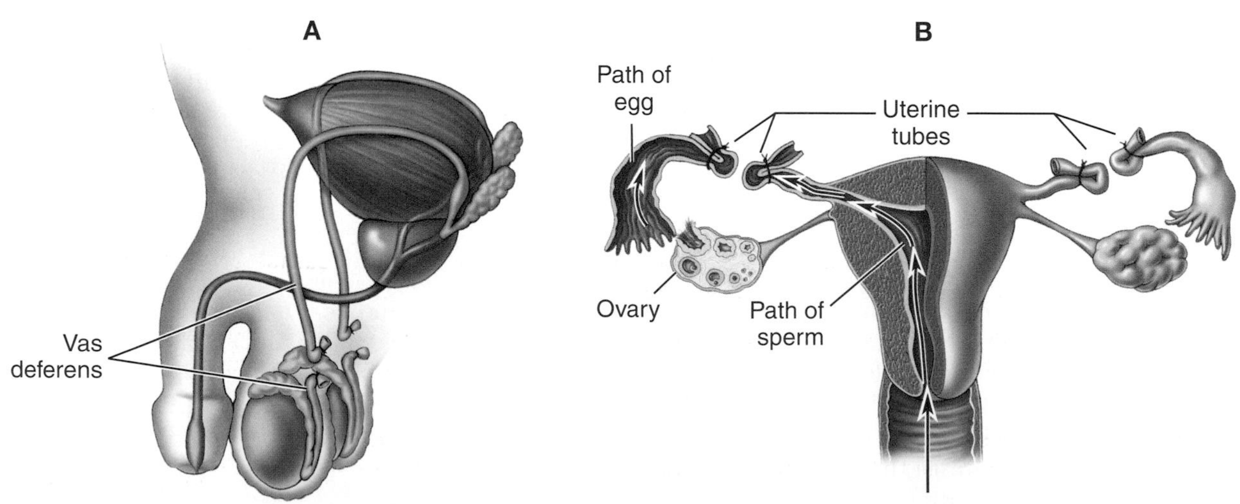

FIGURE 26-7 Surgical methods of birth control. **A,** Vasectomy. **B,** Tubal ligation.

EMERGENCY CONTRACEPTION

Emergeny contraception refers to contraception that is implemented after intercourse. It is accomplished by two types of drugs. Preven is an example of one group of drugs; it contains both estrogen and progesterone and works like "the pill" by preventing ovulation. It is also thought to inhibit implantation in the event that fertilization occurs. A second drug, mifepristone, or RU-486, causes the loss of the implanted embryo by blocking progesterone receptors in the endometrium. The loss of progesterone receptors causes the endometrium to slough, carrying the implanted embryo with it.

Sum It Up!

In the female, puberty is marked by the first period of menstrual bleeding. This event is called menarche. Thereafter, monthly menstrual periods (menses) occur regularly until menopause. Menopause, also called the climacteric or change of life, generally occurs when a woman is in her late 40s or early 50s. Menopause is caused by the decreased ovarian secretion of estrogen and progesterone. Birth control is the voluntary regulation of reproduction. There are numerous methods of contraception.

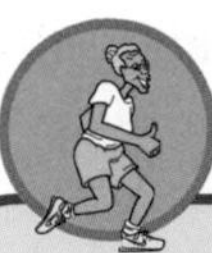

As You Age

1. As a woman ages, her ovaries begin to atrophy, or shrink. Between the ages of 40 and 50, estrogen secretion decreases and symptoms of menopause appear; menstrual periods cease, signaling the end of her reproductive years.
2. The decrease in estrogen secretion causes a change in the accessory organs of reproduction. Tissues become thinner, with a decrease in secretions. The changes in these structures make the woman more prone to vaginal infections. Also, a decrease in vaginal secretions can make intercourse uncomfortable. The decrease in estrogen is also thought to cause weakening of bone, causing osteoporosis, and an increase in the incidence of cardiovascular diseases.
3. By the age of 50, the size of the uterus has decreased by 50%. The ligaments that anchor the uterus, urinary bladder, and rectum weaken, allowing these organs to drop down. Surgical correction is sometimes needed.
4. Breast tissue changes; the supporting ligaments weaken; fibrous cells replace glandular cells; and the amount of fat tissue decreases. These changes cause breast tissue to sag.
5. Around the age of 40, testicular function declines. This decline is accompanied by a decrease in the secretion of testosterone and a decreased sperm count (up to 50%). Despite these changes, a man continues to produce sperm and is capable of fathering children throughout most of his life span.

Disorders of the Reproductive Systems

Benign prostatic hyperplasia (BPH)	A noncancerous enlargement of the prostate gland. The enlarged prostate gland compresses the urethra, impeding urination and making the person prone to bladder infections.
Cancer of the reproductive organs	A number of cancers in both men and women. Cancer of the breast is a leading cause of death in women. Cervical cancer is a common form of cancer that is about 90% curable if diagnosed early. The routine use of the Pap smear as a screening test plays an important role in the high cure rate. Ovarian cancer is a particularly deadly form of cancer. Symptoms of ovarian cancer develop late in the course of the disease, thereby delaying diagnosis and treatment. Cancer of the prostate gland is a common cancer in men. A digital rectal examination is done routinely to detect any enlargement or changes in the prostate. The incidence of testicular cancer is increasing, particularly in athletes.
Dysmenorrhea	Painful or difficult menstruation.
Ovarian cyst	Fluid-filled bubbles of tissue that generally occur in the follicles or in the corpus luteum. Most cysts disappear spontaneously and require no treatment. Some cysts are painful; others may burst and require surgical intervention. All cysts must be evaluated to rule out cancer.
Pelvic inflammatory disease (PID)	A general term that includes inflammation of the uterus; uterine tubes (salpingitis); pelvic peritonitis; and abscess formation. PID is a serious complication of infection by *Neisseria gonorrhoeae (N. gonorrhoeae)* and *Chlamydia trachomatis (C. trachomatis).*
Premenstrual tension	Also called premenstrual syndrome (PMS). Premenstrual tension is a syndrome characterized by abdominal bloating, fluid retention, and hyperirritability about 2 weeks before a menstrual period.

Continued

Disorders of the Reproductive Systems—cont'd

Sexually transmitted diseases (STDs)	Called venereal diseases, after Venus, the Roman goddess of love and beauty. STDs are infectious diseases transmitted from person to person mainly by sexual contact. Left untreated, most STDs cause sterility; some cause permanent disability and death. The most common STD is chlamydia, a nongonococcal urethritis, caused by a bacterium *(Chlamydia trachomatis).* Genital herpes is caused by the herpes simplex virus and is characterized by painful, blisterlike sores on the external genitalia. A woman who harbors the virus may infect the fetus on delivery. Pregnant women with genital herpes are encouraged to deliver their babies by cesarean section to prevent transmission of the virus to the baby. Other STDs include gonorrhea *(N. gonorrhoeae);* syphilis *(Treponema pallidum),* and trichomoniasis *(Trichomonas vaginalis).*

SUMMARY OUTLINE

The reproductive system produces the cells and hormones necessary for reproduction.

I. Male Reproductive System

A. Testes
1. The testes, or testicles, are the male gonads.
2. The testis is composed of lobules with two types of cells: the seminiferous tubules, which produce sperm, and the interstitial cells, which secrete testosterone.

B. Genital Ducts and Glands
1. The sperm move through a series of genital ducts: the epididymis, the vas deferens, the ejaculatory ducts, and the urethra.
2. Three glands—the seminal vesicles, the prostate gland, and the bulbourethral glands—secrete into the genital ducts. The mixture of sperm and glandular secretions is called semen.

C. External Genitals
1. The male genitals consist of the scrotum and the penis.
2. The penis performs two functions: it is the organ of copulation (sexual intercourse), and it carries urine.

D. Male Sexual Response
1. Erection
2. Emission
3. Ejaculation
4. Orgasm

E. Male Sex Hormones
1. The most important is testosterone.
2. Testosterone determines the primary and secondary sex characteristics.
3. The male reproductive system is controlled by hormones from the hypothalamus and from the anterior pituitary gland.

II. Female Reproductive System

A. Ovaries
1. The ovaries are the female gonads.
2. Each ovarian follicle consists of an oocyte and follicular cells.
3. On day 14 (of a 28-day cycle), ovulation occurs.
4. The ovarian follicular cells become the corpus luteum.
5. The ovaries secrete two hormones, estrogen and progesterone.

B. Genital Tract
1. The genital tract includes the fallopian tubes, the uterus, and the vagina.
2. The fallopian tubes transport the egg from the ovaries to the uterus, and are the site of fertilization.
3. The uterus is the baby's cradle during pregnancy.
4. The uterus has three layers: epimetrium, myometrium, and endometrium.

C. External Genitals: called the vulva (labia majora, labia minora, clitoris, and the vestibular glands.

D. Female Sexual Response
1. Erection
2. Orgasm

E. Hormonal Control of the Female Reproductive Cycles
1. Two cycles are the ovarian cycle and the uterine cycle.
2. The ovarian cycle is divided into the follicular phase and the luteal phase.
3. During the follicular phase the ovarian follicle matures and secretes estrogen.
4. The luteal phase of the ovarian cycle begins immediately after ovulation and is

dominated by the secretion of progesterone by the corpus luteum.

5. In the nonpregnant state the corpus luteum deteriorates. In the pregnant state the corpus luteum stays alive because of human chorionic gonadotropin (hCG).
6. The uterine cycle is divided into the menstrual phase, the proliferative phase, and the secretory phase. The menstrual phase refers to the loss of a part of the endometrial lining and blood ("having your period"). During the proliferative phase, the inner endometrial lining thickens and becomes vascular, primarily in response to estrogen. During the secretory phase, the endometrial lining is becoming lush and moist from increased secretory activity; the secretory phase is dominated by progesterone.
7. See Figure 26-6 for a summary of the day-to-day hormonal relationships between the anterior pituitary gland, the ovaries, and the uterus.

III. Methods of Birth Control. The regulation of childbearing can be achieved with the use of barrier methods, hormonal contraceptives, surgical methods, intrauterine devices, behavioral methods, and drugs used for emergency contraception.

Review Your Knowledge

Matching: Structures: Female

Directions: Match the following words with their description below. Some words may be used more than once.

a. fallopian tubes
b. uterus
c. ovaries
d. vagina

1. A Fertilization occurs here FALLOPIAN TUBES
2. C Female gonads OVARIES
3. B Contains the fundus, body, and cervix UTERUS
4. B Contains the endometrium, myometrium, and epimetrium UTERUS
5. C Home of the corpus luteum OVARIES
6. B Where implantation occurs UTERUS
7. C Home of the graafian follicle OVARIES
8. B Menstrual phase, proliferative phase, and secretory phase UTERUS
9. C Follicular phase and luteal phase OVARIES
10. D Birth canal; distal to the cervix VAGINA

Matching: Structures: Male

Directions: Match the following words with their description below. Some words may be used more than once.

a. interstitial cells
b. seminiferous tubules
c. urethra
d. epididymis
e. scrotum

1. B Structure that forms sperm SEMINIFEROUS
2. A Testosterone-secreting cells INTERSTI
3. D Tightly coiled ducts that sit on top of the testes EPIDIDYMIS
4. C Structure that is shared by both the reproductive and urinary tracts URETHRA
5. E Pouch that contains the testes SCROTUM

Matching: Hormones

Directions: Match the following words with their descriptions below. Some words may be used more than once.

a. estrogen
b. progesterone
c. hCG
d. gonadotropins
e. testosterone

1. E Primary androgen secreted by the testes TESTOS
2. D FSH and LH are called GONAD
3. A The proliferative phase (uterus) is dominated by this ovarian hormone ESTROGEN
4. B The secretory phase (uterus) is dominated by this ovarian hormone PROGESTERON
5. C Secreted by trophoblastic cells; preserves the secretion of the corpus luteum HCG
6. D The ovaries are the targets of this anterior pituitary secretion GONADO
7. E Its secretion is a response to interstitial cell-stimulating hormone (ICSH) TEST
8. A This hormone makes a female look like a woman ESTROGE
9. E This hormone makes a male look like a man TE
10. B The corpus luteum secretes large amounts of this hormone; makes the endometrium juicy or lush PROGESTERON

Multiple Choice

1. The gonadotropins
   a. are aimed at the testes.
   b. include FSH and LH (ICSH).
   c. stimulate sperm development and the secretion of androgen.
   d. all of the above.

2. Luteinizing hormone
   a. is also called ICSH and stimulates the interstitial cells to secrete testosterone.
   b. stimulates sperm production.
   c. causes emission.
   d. causes orgasm.
3. Estrogen and progesterone
   a. are gonadotropins.
   b. are secreted by the trophoblastic cells as they implant in the uterine wall.
   c. are secreted by the ovaries.
   d. exert their effects only on reproductive structures.
4. In the nonpregnant state
   a. the corpus albicans becomes hormonally active, secreting estrogen and progesterone.
   b. the endometrium secretes hCG.
   c. hormonal secretion of the corpus luteum gradually declines.
   d. the zygote becomes hormonally active.
5. Human chorionic gonadotropin (hCG)
   a. promotes the maturation of the egg.
   b. is responsible for female characteristics.
   c. maintains the corpus luteum.
   d. promotes the transformation of the corpus luteum into the corpus albicans.
6. The luteal phase of the ovarian cycle
   a. is responsible for menstruation.
   b. is responsible for the uterine secretory phase.
   c. elevates plasma levels of estrogen, progesterone, and hCG.
   d. precedes the LH surge.
7. Menstruation occurs in response to
   a. an LH surge.
   b. diminished plasma levels of estrogen and progesterone.
   c. elevated plasma levels of hCG.
   d. elevation of plasma levels of FSH and LH.

CHAPTER 27

Human Development and Heredity

KEY TERMS

Amnion, p. 478
Blastocyst, p. 478
Chorion, p. 480
Chromosome, p. 489
Embryo, p. 478
Fertilization, p. 476
Fetus, p. 483
Gene, p. 489
Human chorionic gonadotropin (hCG), p. 478
Karyotype, p. 490
Mammary gland, p. 486
Placenta, p. 480
Sex-linked trait, p. 492
Teratogen, p. 481
Umbilical cord, p. 480
Zygote, p. 476

OBJECTIVES

1. Describe the process of fertilization: when, where, and how it occurs.
2. Describe the process of development: cleavage, growth, morphogenesis, and differentiation.
3. Explain the three periods of prenatal development: early embryonic, embryonic, and fetal periods.
4. State two functions of the placenta.
5. Explain hormonal changes during pregnancy.
6. Describe the hormonal changes and stages of labor.
7. Describe the structure of the breast and lactation.
8. Describe the relationships among deoxyribonucleic acid (DNA), chromosomes, and genes.
9. Explain how the sex of the child is determined.
10. State the difference between congenital and hereditary diseases.
11. Define *karyotype*.

Nine months after conception, the reproductive process produces a baby. "Bundle of Joy" has arrived on the scene. Note that this term of endearment does not suggest "up, awake, and playing at 2 AM," gallons of the pink stuff (amoxicillin), and diapers, diapers, and more diapers. Nonetheless, Baby is cute, and the urge to reproduce is very strong. Let us follow Baby's start from fertilization through development and birth. Finally, we'll see what is meant by statements like "He's got his father's nose and his mother's smile." This is the genetic story.

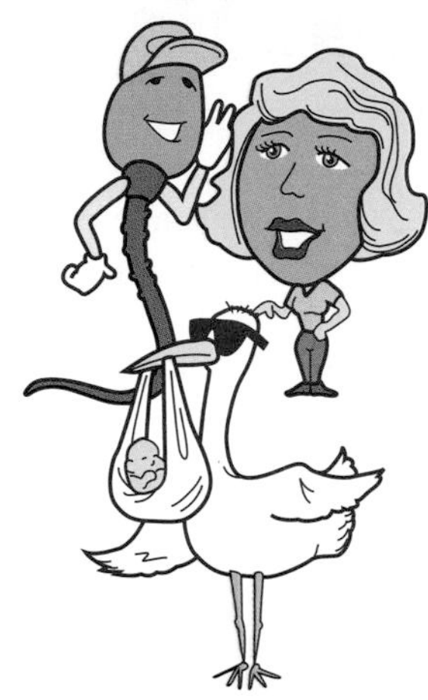

FERTILIZATION

Fertilization, also called **conception,** refers to the union of the nuclei of the egg and the sperm. When, where, and how does this union take place?

WHEN FERTILIZATION OCCURS

Timing is everything. In the female, ovulation occurs at midcycle, around day 14 (see Chapter 26). The egg lives for about 24 hours after ovulation. Sperm usually live between 12 and 48 hours, with some surviving up to 72 hours. For fertilization to occur, sexual intercourse must take place around the time of ovulation, generally no earlier than 72 hours (3 days) before ovulation and no later than 24 hours (1 day) after ovulation. Alert: Evidence suggests that some women are reflex ovulators. These women ovulate in response to having intercourse. Think about it: the chance of pregnancy goes waaaay up. Remember that rabbits are reflex ovulators, and we all know about the rabbit population.

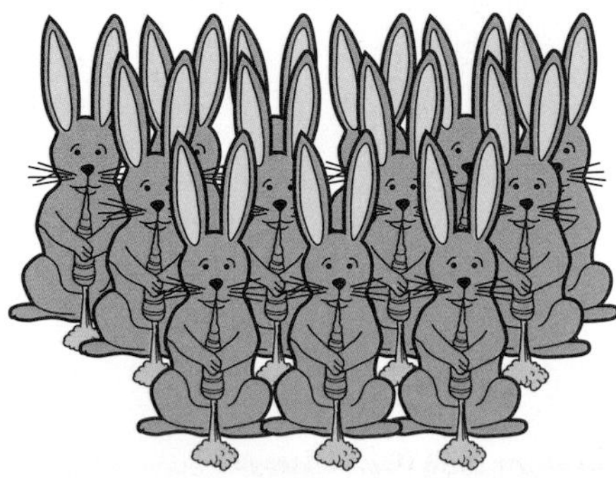

WHERE FERTILIZATION OCCURS

After ovulation, the egg enters the fallopian tube. Fertilization normally occurs in the first third of the fallopian tube.

HOW FERTILIZATION OCCURS

During intercourse, about 200 to 600 million sperm are deposited in the vagina, near the cervix of the uterus. Although many of the sperm are killed by the acidic environment of the vagina, about 100,000 survive and swim through the uterus and into the fallopian tube toward the egg. Within 1 to 2 hours after intercourse, thousands of sperm are gathered around the egg in the fallopian tube.

The acrosomes on the heads of the sperm rupture and release enzymes. The enzymes digest the linings of cells that surround the egg. Then, one (and only one) sperm penetrates the membrane of the egg. Upon penetration of the egg, the nuclei of the egg and sperm unite, thereby completing fertilization. The fertilized egg is called a **zygote** (ZĪ-gōt). The zygote is the first cell of a new individual. For swimmer STEVE, it's been a successful night of "zygoting"!

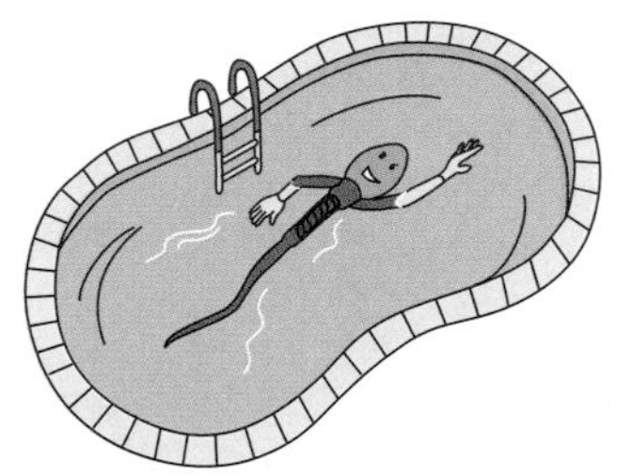

The single-cell zygote has 46 chromosomes, 23 from the egg and 23 from the sperm. The zygote begins to divide, forming a cluster of cells that slowly makes its way through the fallopian tube toward the uterus. When this cluster of cells reaches the uterus, it implants itself into the plush endometrial lining, where it grows and develops into a human being with billions of cells.

HUMAN DEVELOPMENT

Development is a process that begins with fertilization and ends with death. Human development is divided into two phases: prenatal development and postnatal development. **Prenatal development** begins with fertilization and is terminated at birth. The time of prenatal development is called **pregnancy,** or **gestation.** The normal gestation period lasts 38 weeks, or about 9 months. Pregnancy is divided into **trimesters** (3-month periods). The first trimester is the first 3 months of pregnancy. The second trimester is months 4, 5, and 6, and the third, or last, trimester is months 7, 8, and 9. Postnatal development begins with birth and terminates with death; it is what we are all doing now—it is called *life.*

PRENATAL DEVELOPMENT

What does prenatal development include? Prenatal development includes cleavage, growth, morphogenesis, and differentiation. **Cleavage** is cell division by mitosis. Mitosis produces two identical cells from a single cell. Thus one cell splits into two cells. The two cells split into four cells, four cells split into eight cells, and so on. Each new cell is identical to the parent cell. Mitotic cell division increases the numbers of cells but not their actual size. The size of the cell increases through **growth.** Thus as development progresses, both the number and the size of the cells increase.

Morphogenesis is the shaping of the cell cluster. Certain cells migrate to specific areas in the cell cluster. This process changes the shape of the cell mass. For instance, cells migrate to the side of the cell mass and take the appearance of tiny buds. These buds eventually become legs. Through morphogenesis, the round cluster of cells develops into an intricately and wonderously formed infant. Baby is shaping up!

Differentiation is the process whereby a cell becomes specialized. A cell differentiates to become a nerve cell, muscle cell, blood cell, or some other cell.

What are the periods of prenatal development? There are three periods: early embryonic, embryonic, and fetal periods.

EARLY EMBRYONIC PERIOD

From Zygote to Blastocyst

The **early embryonic period** lasts for 2 weeks after fertilization. During this period, the zygote undergoes mitosis and travels from the fallopian tube into the uterus. After fertilization (Figure 27-1, *A*) the zygote undergoes cleavage. Cleavage is accomplished by mitosis,

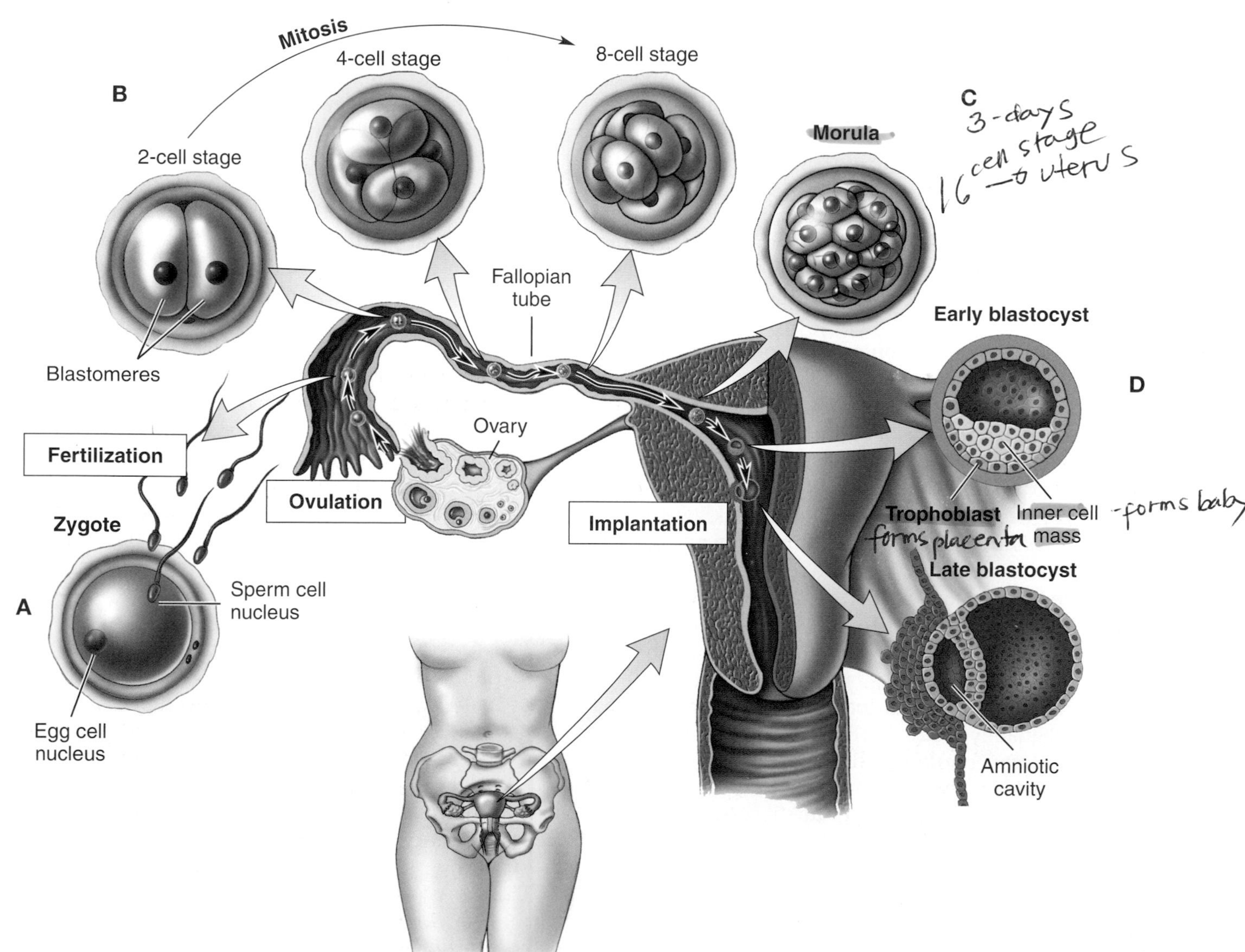

FIGURE 27-1 Stages of early embryonic development: from zygote to blastocyst.

cell division that increases the numbers of cells. The cells formed by mitotic cell division are **blastomeres** (see Figure 27-1, *B*). Note the two-cell cluster, four-cell cluster, and eight-cell cluster.

When the number of cells increases to 16, the collection of cells is called a **morula** (see Figure 27-1, *C*). The morula looks like a raspberry, so tiny that it is visible only through a microscope. Transformation from the zygote to a morula takes about 3 days. The morula enters the uterine cavity, where it floats around for 3 to 4 days and continues to undergo mitosis. By the end of the fifth day, the morula develops into a **blastocyst.**

Note the structure of the early blastocyst (see Figure 27-1, *D*). The **early blastocyst** contains a hollow cavity surrounded by a single layer of flattened cells and a cluster of cells at one side. The single layer of flattened cells surrounding the cavity is called the **trophoblast.** These cells will help form the placenta and also secrete an important hormone. The cluster of cells within the blastocyst is called the **inner cell mass.** These cells will eventually form a baby.

The **late blastocyst** develops by day 7. This stage shows the beginnings of the amniotic cavity. The late blastocyst burrows into the endometrial lining of the uterus, where it is gradually covered over by cells of the endometrial lining. The burrowing process is called **implantation.**

During implantation, the blastocyst also functions as a gland. The trophoblast, the flattened layer of cells that surrounds the cavity, secretes a hormone called **human chorionic gonadotropin (hCG),** which travels through the blood to the ovary, where it prevents the deterioration of the corpus luteum. In response to hCG, the corpus luteum continues to secrete estrogen and progesterone. The estrogen and progesterone stimulate the growth of the uterine wall and prevent menstruation.

The secretion of hCG continues at a high level for about 2 months, then steadily declines as the placenta develops. The placenta eventually takes over the role of the corpus luteum by secreting large amounts of estrogen and progesterone. The blastocyst thus helps preserve its own survival through its secretion of hCG. With the implantation of the blastocyst and the organization of the inner cell mass, the early embryonic period comes to a close.

Human chorionic gonadotropin (hCG) forms the basis of pregnancy tests. hCG is secreted in early pregnancy and can be detected in the mother's urine or blood. A pregnancy test may indicate positive results within about 8 to 10 days after fertilization.

Seeing Double: Twins

Each cell within the morula or blastocyst can become a complete individual. Sometimes these cells split, and two embryos begin developing at the same time, thereby producing two offspring (twins) rather than one. These are **identical,** or **monozygotic, twins** because they develop from the same zygote and have identical genetic information. For monozygotic twins to develop, one sperm fertilizes one egg, and the zygote then splits.

Sometimes a woman ovulates two eggs, which are then fertilized by two different sperm. Because two babies are produced, they are called twins. These twins, however, are not identical. They do not develop from the same egg and do not have the same genetic information. They are called **fraternal,** or **dizygotic, twins** (meaning that they come from two different zygotes). Triplets, quadruplets, and other multiple births can develop in the same two ways.

EMBRYONIC PERIOD

Embryonic development lasts for 6 weeks, from week 3 through week 8. During this period, the baby-to-be is called an **embryo.** The **embryonic period** involves the formation of extraembryonic membranes, the placenta, and all of the organ systems in the body.

Extraembryonic Membranes

The **extraembryonic membranes** form outside the embryo; hence the term *extra*embryonic. The membranes help to protect and nourish the embryo; they are also involved in the embryonic excretion of waste. At birth the membranes are expelled along with the placenta as the **afterbirth.** The four extraembryonic membranes are the amnion, the chorion, the yolk sac, and the allantois.

The **amnion** (ĂM-nē-ŏn) enlarges and forms a sac around the embryo (Figure 27-2). The sac is called the **amniotic sac** and is filled with a fluid called the **amniotic fluid.** The amniotic fluid forms a protective cushion around the embryo and helps protect it from bumps and changes in temperature. The amniotic fluid also nourishes embryos as they drink and digest it. About 1 L of amniotic fluid occupies the amniotic sac at full term.

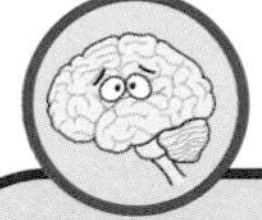

Do You Know...

About the new drink for low birth weight infants?

In utero Baby drinks and digests amniotic fluid. Seems that the amniotic fluid is rich in nutrients and growth factors necessary for fetal growth and development. When born prematurely, an infant is unable to digest milk and is usually fed intravenously. IV feedings, however, bypass the digestive tract and cause the intestines to deteriorate. A solution resembling amniotic fluid has been developed; it is fed to very low birth weight infants. The results so far are very promising—faster weight gain and less intestinal damage.

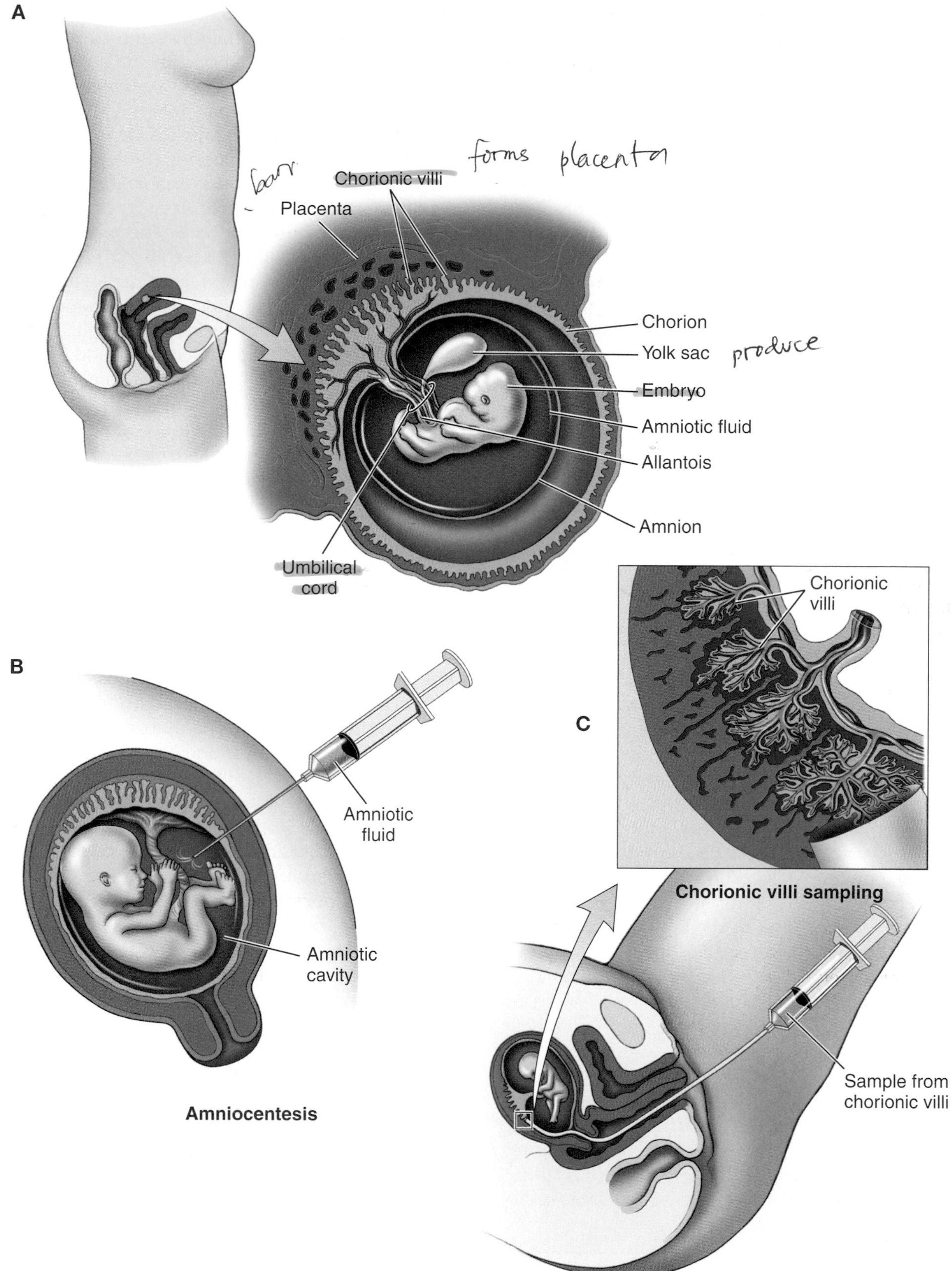

FIGURE 27-2 Extraembryonic membranes and the formation of the placenta. **A,** The embryo is surrounded by the amnion and the amniotic fluid in the amniotic cavity. **B,** Amniocentesis. **C,** Chorionic villi sampling.

The embryo secretes waste and sheds cells into the amniotic fluid. This process is the basis for a diagnostic test called an amniocentesis, in which a sample of amniotic fluid is aspirated from the amniotic cavity and examined for evidence of fetal abnormalities (see Figure 27-2, *B*). The amniotic sac is often called the bag of waters. It breaks before delivery and generally signals the onset of labor.

A second extraembryonic membrane is the chorion. The **chorion** (KŎR-ē-ŏn) is the outer extraembyronic membrane. It develops many fingerlike projections called **chorionic villi.** The chorionic villi penetrate the uterine wall and interact with the tissues of the mother's uterus to form the placenta. Sampling of the cells of the chorionic villi is another way to detect genetic defects (see Figure 27-2, *C;* Figure 27-3).

A third extraembryonic membrane is the **yolk sac.** The yolk sac in birds and reptiles helps nourish the offspring, but the yolk sac in humans serves different functions: it produces red blood cells and immature sex cells. After the sixth week, the yolk sac ceases to function. The embryonic liver then produces red blood cells, and by the seventh month the bone marrow has assumed this function. By then the yolk sac has become part of the umbilical cord.

The **allantois** is the fourth extraembryonic membrane. The allantois contributes to the formation of several structures, including the urinary bladder. The blood vessels of the allantois also help form the umbilical blood vessels, which transport blood to and from the placenta. After the second month, the allantois deteriorates and becomes part of the umbilical cord.

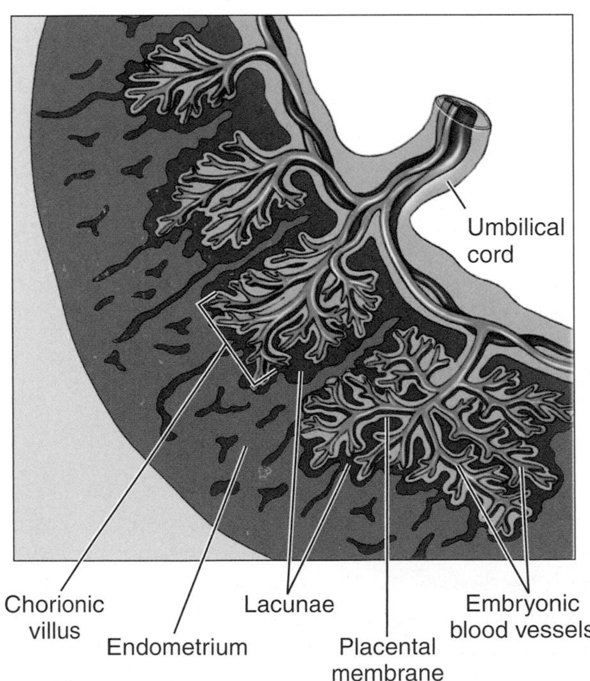

FIGURE 27-3 A cross section of the chorionic villi.

Placenta

The **placenta** is a disc-shaped structure about 7 inches (15 to 20 cm) in diameter and 1 inch (2.5 cm) thick. Normally, the placenta develops in the upper portion of the uterus. The placenta is a highly vascular structure formed from both embryonic and maternal tissue. By the end of the embryonic period (8 weeks), the placenta is functional. After the birth of the baby, the placenta is expelled as part of the afterbirth.

Formation of the Placenta. The placenta develops as the chorionic villi of the embryo burrow into the endometrial lining of the uterus (see Figure 27-3). The chorionic villi contain blood vessels that are continuous with the umbilical arteries and umbilical vein of the embryo. The chorionic villi sit in blood-filled spaces **(lacunae)** in the mother's endometrium.

Pay special attention to the arrangement of the embryonic and maternal blood vessels. The chorionic villi contain blood that comes from the embryo. The endometrial spaces (lacunae) contain blood from the mother. The embryonic and maternal blood supplies, although intimately close, are separated by the placental membrane. The placental membrane thus maintains two separate circulations: the embryonic and maternal circulations. The two circulations do not mix!

Functions of the Placenta. The placenta plays two important roles. First, it is the site across which nutrients and waste are exchanged between mother and baby. Oxygen, food, and other nutrients diffuse from the mother's blood into the blood of the embryo. Carbon dioxide and other waste diffuse from the embryo's blood into the mother's blood are then excreted. Baby-to-be "breathes," "eats," and excretes at the placenta. If the placenta is injured in any way, the oxygen supply to the embryo may be cut off, causing irreversible brain damage and possibly death.

Secondly, the placenta acts as a gland. It secretes hormones that help to maintain the pregnancy, prepare the body for the birthing process, and promote postnatal events such as breast-feeding. The placental hormones are listed and described in Table 27-1.

Hook Up: The Umbilical Cord

How does the embryo connect with the mother? The **umbilical cord** is the structure that connects embryo and mother at the placenta (see Figure 27-2). The umbilical cord contains two umbilical arteries and one umbilical vein (see Figure 18-8). Because the umbilical cord carries oxygen-rich blood to the developing infant, it is literally the baby's lifeline. Compression or injury to the umbilical cord can cause severe distress and possibly the death of the baby.

When the baby is delivered, the umbilical cord is cut, severing the placenta. The stump of the cord shrivels up, drops off, and leaves the navel, or belly button. The

Table 27-1 Hormones of Pregnancy

Hormone	Secreted by	Effects
Human chorionic gonadotropin (hCG)	Embryonic cells (trophoblasts) during implantation	Maintains the function of the corpus luteum; forms the basis of the pregnancy test.
Estrogen and progesterone	Corpus luteum during the first 2 months; placenta after 2 months	Both estrogen and progesterone stimulate the development of the uterine lining and mammary glands. Progesterone inhibits uterine contractions during pregnancy. Estrogen causes relaxation of the pelvic joints. At the beginning of labor, estrogen opposes the quieting effects of progesterone on uterine contractions and sensitizes the myometrium to oxytocin.
Prolactin	Anterior pituitary gland	Prolactin stimulates the breast to secrete milk.
Oxytocin	Posterior pituitary gland	Oxytocin causes the release of milk from the breast (part of the milk let-down reflex initiated by suckling). Causes uterine contraction (participates in labor and postpartum uterine contractions to decrease bleeding).
Prostaglandins	Placenta	Prostaglandins stimulate uterine contractions.
Aldosterone	Adrenal cortex	Aldosterone expands blood volume.

baby's organs such as the lungs, kidneys, and digestive system must then take over the functions previously performed by the placenta.

Organogenesis

The embryonic period is a time of **organogenesis,** the formation of body organs and organ systems. The inner cell mass of the blastocyst forms a flattened structure called the **embryonic disc.** The embryonic disc, in turn, gives rise to three primary germ layers, the ectoderm, the mesoderm, and the endoderm.

All of the tissues and organs of the body develop from these germ layers. For instance, the **ectoderm** gives rise to the nervous system, portions of the special senses, and the skin. The skin is one of the earliest organs to develop and forms during the third week. The **mesoderm** gives rise to muscle, bone, blood, and many of the structures of the cardiovascular system. The **endoderm** gives rise to the epithelial lining of the digestive tract, respiratory tract, and parts of the urinary tract. By the end of the embryonic period (week 8) the main internal organs are established. The embryo weighs about 1 g, is about 1 inch (2.5 cm) in length, and has a human appearance (Figure 27-4).

Be Careful: Teratogens

Because the organs of the body are being formed at this time, the embryonic period is most critical for development. Toxic substances such as alcohol, drugs, and certain pathogens can cross the placental membrane and interfere with embryonic development, causing severe birth defects. These toxic substances are called **teratogens** (TĔR-ă-tō-jĕn), a word that means monster-producing and attests to the severity of teratogenic birth defects. Hazardous conditions such as exposure to radiation can also act as teratogens (Figure 27-5).

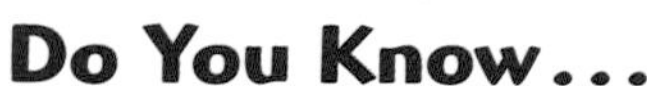
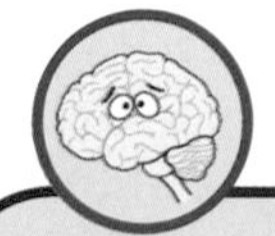

Do You Know...

How you get that extra inch OR "slackus the urachus"?

Following delivery of a baby, the umbilical cord is tied off or clamped. Traditionally, the cord of a girl baby was tied close to the abdominal wall. The cord of a male baby, however, was tied farther away from the abdominal wall. Why the difference in cord length?

In the baby there is a cordlike structure called the urachus, that extends from the top of the urinary bladder to the navel. It was thought that the urachus would be pulled up tight if the cord were tied too close to the abdominal wall. The tight urachus in turn would pull up on the penis, thereby stunting its growth. Conversely, by leaving the umbilical cord long, the urachus would relax, and the penis would grow longer. This obsession with penile length gave rise to the motto "slackus the urachus." Today the umbilical cord in both male and female babies is clamped about 1 to 2 cm from the abdominal wall. No penile shortening has been recorded.

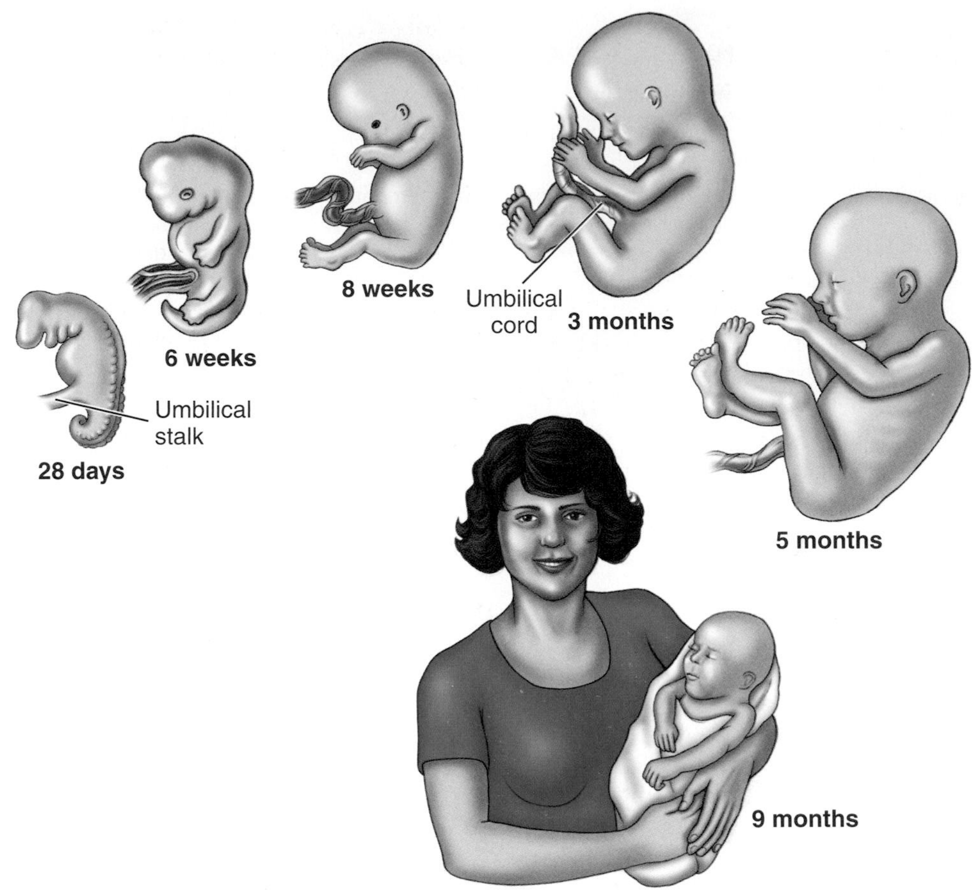

FIGURE 27-4 From embryo to fetus to baby.

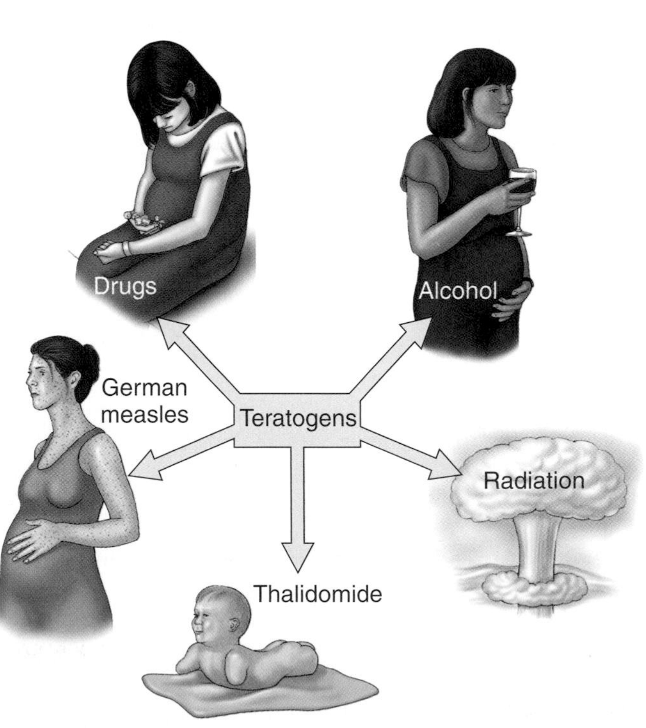

FIGURE 27-5 Teratogens: "monster-producing agents."

Alcohol is a potent teratogen. It can cause a cluster of birth defects known as fetal alcohol syndrome. In addition to causing facial deformities, alcohol interferes with neurologic and mental development. The tranquilizer thalidomide is another drug that produces teratogenic effects. The development of finlike appendages instead of arms and legs has been correlated with the ingestion of thalidomide during pregnancy. Because of the sensitivity of the embryo to teratogenic agents, the mother must be extremely careful to protect her unborn child from toxic substances and hazardous conditions. Many drugs are teratogenic!

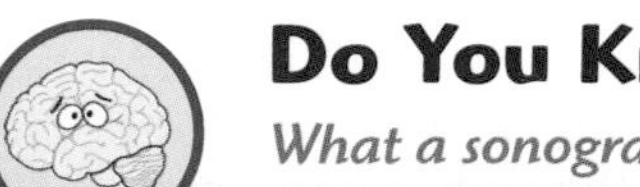

Do You Know...

What a sonogram is?

A sonogram is an image produced by sound waves as they encounter different tissues and organs. During the procedure, sound waves are directed through the mother's abdomen. As the sound waves "hit" the fetus, an image appears on the scope showing an outline of the fetus. The sex of the fetus can be determined by sonography, as can certain fetal abnormalities.

FETAL PERIOD

The **fetal period** extends from week 9 to birth. At this time, the developing offspring is called a **fetus** (FĒ-tŭs). The fetal period is primarily a time of growth and maturation; only a few new parts appear. Body proportions, however, continue to change. For instance, at 8 weeks the head is nearly as large as the body. At birth, the head is proportionately much smaller than the body. Note the change in body size and proportion in Figure 27-4.

Table 27-2 summarizes prenatal development. Note that a primitive nervous system begins to form in the third week. The heart and blood vessels originate during the second week. The heart is pumping blood to all the organs of the embryo by the second month, and a heartbeat can be detected during the third month, when the sex of the fetus can also be determined. Once the testes differentiate, they produce the male sex hormone testosterone. Testosterone stimulates the growth of the male external genitals. In the absence of testosterone, female genitals form.

The mother first feels the fetus move during the fifth month; this experience is called **quickening.** As the fetus grows, its skin becomes covered by a fine, downy hair called **lanugo** (during the fifth month). The lanugo is covered by a white, cheeselike substance called the **vernix caseosa.** The vernix is thought to protect the delicate fetal skin from the amniotic fluid. By the fifth month the fetus is in crowded quarters and is flexed in fetal position. During the last 2 months the baby is gaining weight rapidly as fat is deposited in the subcutaneous tissue. As the time for birth approaches, the fetus rotates so that the head is pointed toward the cervix. At the end of 38 weeks, the fetus is full term. During this period the fetal weight has increased from less than 0.5 oz (14 g) to 7.5 lbs (3.4 kg) (average weight of a full-term infant). The fetus has grown in length from about 1 inch (2.5 cm) to 21 inches (53 cm). Baby is ready to face the world!

Sometimes, the embryo or fetus is born too early, before the 9-month gestation period is completed. A number of terms are used to describe early birth. An **abortion** is the loss of an embryo or fetus any time during the gestational period; most commonly, abortion refers to the termination of the pregnancy before the twentieth week of development. (A fetus that is less than twenty weeks is considered to be nonviable.) A **spontaneous abortion** occurs naturally with no artificial interference. Usually, a spontaneous abortion is caused by some fetal abnormality. A **miscarriage** is the layperson's term for a spontaneous abortion. An **induced abortion** is an abortion deliberately caused by some artificial or mechanical means. An unwanted pregnancy is a common cause of an induced abortion. A **therapeutic abortion** is performed by a physician as a form of treatment for the mother. For instance, a pregnancy that threatens the life of the mother may be terminated to save her life or improve her medical condition.

Table 27-2 Human Development

Time	Developmental Event
Embryonic	
Second week	Implantation occurs. The inner cell mass is giving rise to the primary germ layers. Beginning of placental development.
Third week	Beginning of the nervous system.
Fourth week	Appearance of limb buds. Heart is beating. Embryo has tail. Other organ systems begin.
Fifth week	Enlarged head; nose, eyes, and ears are noticeable.
Sixth week	Fingers and toes are present; appearance of cartilage skeleton.
Second month	All organ systems are developing. Cartilaginous skeleton is being replaced by bone (ossification). Embryo is about 1.5 inches (3.8 cm) long.
Fetal	
Third month	Facial features present in crude form. Can determine gender (the external reproductive organs are distinguishable as male or female).
Fourth month	Sensory organs are present: eyes and ears attain shape and position. Eyes blink and the baby begins sucking movements. Skeleton is visible.
Fifth month	Vernix caseosa and a fine downy hair (lanugo) cover the skin. The proud parents first hear Baby's heartbeat during a prenatal visit. Quickening.
Sixth month	Continues to grow. Myelination of the spinal cord begins.
Seventh month	Eyes are open. Testes descend into scrotum. Weighs about 3 lbs (135 g). Bone marrow becomes the only site of blood cell formation.
Eighth month	Body is lean and well proportioned. Subcutaneous fat begins to be deposited.
Ninth month	Full term and ready to be delivered. Average weight is 7.5 lbs (338 g). Average length is 21 inches (53.3 cm).

A baby born before 38 weeks but capable of living outside the womb is a **premature** or **preterm infant.** A 20-week-old fetus is considered viable, that is, able to live outside the womb. A premature baby is small, but more importantly, it is immature and may require medical support. In particular, the hypothalamus is too immature to regulate body temperature well, and the surfactant produced by the fetal lungs is inadequate to maintain breathing. Generally, the more premature the birth, the greater is the need for medical support.

Sum It Up!

Fertilization takes place in the fallopian tube, when the nuclei of a sperm and egg unite, producing a zygote. The zygote gradually moves through the fallopian tube into the uterus, where it develops into an infant over a 9-month period. Prenatal development includes the processes of cleavage (mitosis), growth, morphogenesis, and differentiation. Prenatal development is divided into three periods: the early embryonic period (2 weeks), the embryonic period (6 weeks), and the fetal period (7 weeks to birth at 38 weeks). The zygote undergoes mitosis and develops into a blastocyst; trophoblastic cells help the blastocyst to implant. The major accomplishments of the embryonic period include the formation of extraembryonic membranes and the development of the placenta and umbilical cord. The embryonic period is also the period of organogenesis. The fetal period is primarily a period of rapid growth and maturation. Baby shapes up, fattens up, and moves about.

CHANGES IN THE MOTHER'S BODY DURING PREGNANCY

Throughout pregnancy the mother supplies all the food and oxygen for the fetus and eliminates all the waste. This added burden requires many changes in the mother's physiology:

- The rate of metabolism increases. For instance, the mother secretes greater amounts of the thyroid hormones triiodothyronine (T_3) and thyroxine (T_4).
- The mother's blood volume expands by as much as 40% to 50%. The increase in blood volume is due to an increase in the secretion of aldosterone by the adrenal cortex. To pump the additional blood and meet the demands of an increased metabolism, the activity of the cardiovascular system increases. For instance, heart rate, stroke volume, and cardiac output increase.
- Respiratory activity increases to provide additional oxygen and to eliminate excess carbon dioxide.
- The kidneys work harder and produce more urine because they must eliminate waste for both the mother and the fetus.
- Under the influence of estrogen and progesterone the size and weight of the uterus increase dramatically as the fetus grows to full term. To accommodate the growth of the uterus, the pelvic cavity expands as the sacroiliac joints and the symphysis pubis become more flexible. With growth, the uterus pushes the abdominal organs upward. In the later months of pregnancy especially, the upward displacement of abdominal organs exerts pressure on the diaphragm and hampers the mother's breathing.
- The mother's nutritional needs increase as the maternal organs (uterus and breasts) grow and she provides for the growing fetus. In particular the need for calcium increases, since an increase in parathyroid hormone (PTH) extracts calcium from the mother's bone, making it available to the growing fetus.

Pregnancy brings some discomforts for some women. Nausea and vomiting, generally referred to as morning sickness, commonly occur in the first 3 months. Morning sickness may be due to hormonal changes, especially to the elevated levels of hCG. During the later months of pregnancy, the woman gains approximately 2 to 3 pounds per month. The added weight causes a shift in the mother's center of gravity, thereby affecting her balance and forcing her to adjust her walking style (eventually, many women appear to be waddling).

The added weight may also cause discomfort in the lower back and a multitude of other aches as the uterine ligaments and other supporting structures stretch. The expanding uterus stretches the abdominal skin, causing stretch marks, or striae. It also displaces the stomach upward, causing heartburn. Frequent urination results from increased urine formation and compression of the urinary bladder by the uterus. Lastly, the expanded uterus hampers the return of blood through the veins of the lower body region. This inhibited blood flow, in turn, may cause varicose veins and hemorrhoids. No wonder the mother-to-be looks forward to giving birth!

Although these discomforts of pregnancy are normal, several pregnancy-related conditions are not normal and are instead dangerous to both the mother and the child. For instance, the mother may develop a toxemia of pregnancy. This condition is characterized by an elevated blood pressure and progresses in severe cases to generalized seizures. The early stage is called preeclampsia, and the later seizure stage is called eclampsia.

Sum It Up!

Pregnancy causes many changes in the mother. Hormonal changes are numerous and complex. Secretion of hCG, estrogen, and progesterone help maintain the pregnancy and prepare the organs of reproduction for 9 months of pregnancy. Other hormones, such as aldosterone, thyroid hormones, and parathyroid hormone, prepare the mother's body to nourish and sustain the growing unborn child. Almost every maternal organ responds to the presence of the fetus. The heart pumps more blood; the kidneys excrete more waste; and the increased metabolic rate indicates that every cell is working harder.

BIRTH OF BABY

Finally, Baby is ready to face the world. The birth process is called **parturition. Labor** is the process whereby forceful contractions expel the fetus from the uterus. Once labor starts, forceful and rhythmic contractions begin at the top of the uterus and travel down its length, forcing the fetus through the birth canal.

LABOR

Hormonal Basis of Labor

The precise mechanism that starts labor is unknown. A number of hormonal stimuli do, however, play a role. For example, progesterone, which normally quiets uterine contractions during pregnancy, is secreted in decreasing amounts after the seventh month. This decrease coincides with an increase in the secretion of estrogen. Estrogen has two effects on the uterus: it opposes the quieting effect of progesterone on uterine contractions, and it sensitizes the myometrium (uterine muscle) to the stimulatory effects of oxytocin.

The secretion of prostaglandins by the placenta also plays a role in initiating labor. Prostaglandins stimulate uterine contractions. Finally, the stretching of the uterine and vaginal tissue in the late stage of pregnancy stimulates nerves that send signals to the hypothalamus. The hypothalamus, in turn, stimulates the release of oxytocin from the posterior pituitary gland. Oxytocin exerts a powerful stimulating effect on the myometrium and is thought to play an important role in labor.

Labor can, however, have a false start. Sometimes, a very pregnant and embarrassed mother is admitted to the hospital in false labor. What has happened? She has indeed felt uterine contractions. These contractions, however, are weak, irregular, and ineffectual. They are called **Braxton Hicks contractions,** and they normally occur during late pregnancy. These contractions are due to the increased responsiveness of the uterus to various hormones, particularly changing concentrations of estrogen and progesterone. The mother returns home to await the onset of true labor.

Stages of Labor

The three stages of true labor are the dilation stage, the expulsion stage, and the placental stage (Figure 27-6). The **dilation stage** begins with the onset of labor and ends with full dilation of the cervix (10 cm). This stage is characterized by rhythmic and forceful contractions, rupture of the amniotic sac (the bag of waters), and cervical dilation. It is the longest stage of labor and generally lasts between 6 and 12 hours. The **expulsion stage** extends from complete cervical dilation to the expulsion of the fetus through the vagina (birth canal). This stage generally lasts less than 1 hour. During this stage the mother has the urge to push with abdominal muscles.

In a normal delivery, the head is delivered first. A head-first delivery allows the baby to be suctioned free of mucus and to breathe even before the baby's body has fully exited from the birth canal. Because the vaginal orifice may not expand enough to deliver the baby, however, an episiotomy may be performed. An **episiotomy** is a surgical incision into the perineum, the tissue between the vaginal opening and the anus. The incision enlarges the vaginal opening and facilitates the delivery of the baby.

The third stage is the **placental stage** and occurs 10 to 15 minutes after the birth of the baby. It involves the separation of the placenta from the uterine wall and expulsion of the placenta and attached membranes by forceful uterine contractions. The placenta and the attached membranes are collectively called the afterbirth. In addition to expelling the fetus and the placenta, the uterine contractions also cause vasoconstriction of the uterine blood vessels, thereby minimizing blood loss. Uterine contractions also help the uterus to return to its nonpregnant size and shape. About 500 ml of blood is lost during delivery.

Sometimes, the fetus does not come out head first. Instead, another part of the body, such as the buttocks, is delivered first. This presentation is called a **breech**

Do You Know...

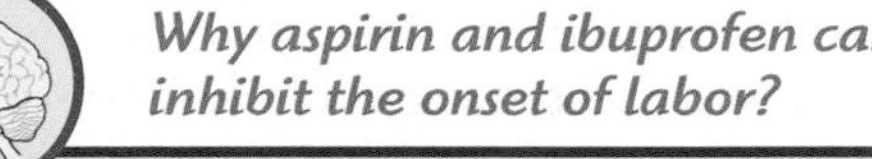

Why aspirin and ibuprofen can inhibit the onset of labor?

Aspirin and ibuprofen are antiprostaglandin drugs. Because prostaglandins stimulate uterine contractions, suppression of prostaglandin secretion by these drugs may inhibit uterine contractions, thereby inhibiting labor.

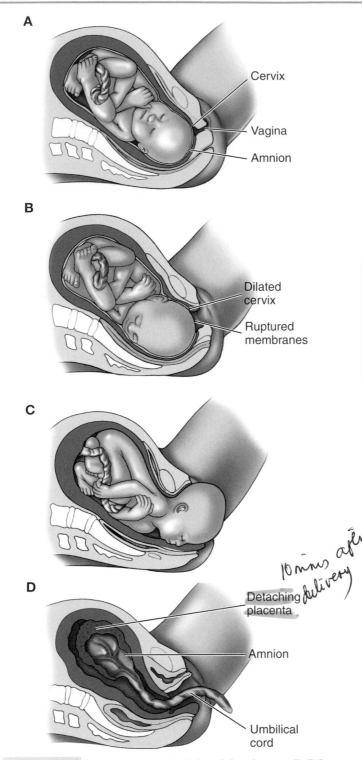

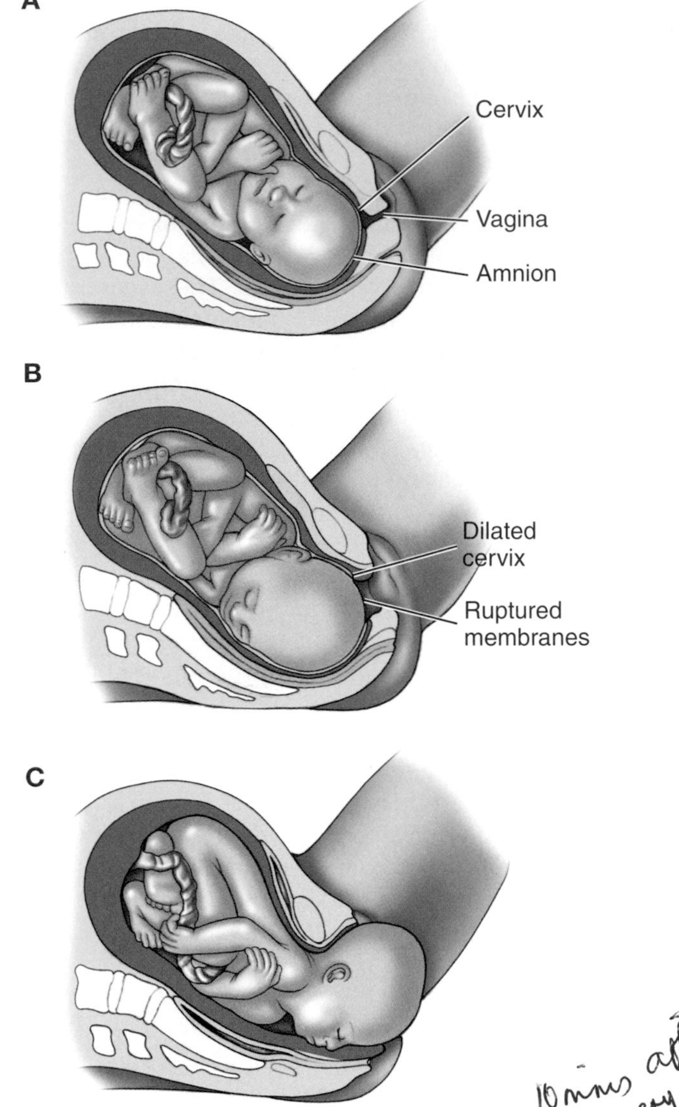

FIGURE 27-6 Stages of labor. **A,** Before labor begins. **B,** Dilation stage. **C,** Expulsion stage. **D,** Placental stage.

birth. A breech presentation makes delivery more difficult for both the mother and the infant.

There are a number of conditions that prevent a safe vaginal delivery, thereby requiring surgery. A C-section, or cesarean section, refers to the delivery of the infant through a surgical incision in the abdominal and uterine walls.

Sum It Up!

The birth process is called parturition. Labor is the forceful contractions that expel the baby and afterbirth from the uterus, through the birth canal. Labor begins in response to various hormones, particularly oxytocin. The three stages of labor are the dilation stage, the expulsion stage, and the placental stage.

Do You Know...

What placenta previa and abruptio placentae are?

Sometimes the placenta forms too low in the uterus, near the cervix. When the cervix dilates during the later stages of pregnancy, the placenta detaches from the uterine wall, causing bleeding in the mother and depriving the fetus of an adequate supply of oxygen and nutrients. This condition is called placenta previa. Abruptio placentae refers to the premature separation of an implanted placenta at about 20 or more weeks of pregnancy. Without immediate treatment, abruptio placentae results in severe hemorrhage in the mother and death for the fetus.

FEMALE BREAST AND LACTATION

STRUCTURE OF A BREAST: THE MAMMARY GLANDS

The anterior chest contains two elevations called **breasts** (Figure 27-7, *A*). The breasts are located anterior to the pectoralis major muscles and contain adipose tissue and mammary glands. **Mammary glands** are accessory organs of the female reproductive system. They secrete milk following the delivery of the baby. At the tip of each breast is a nipple surrounded by a circular area of pigmented skin called the **areola.** Each mammary gland contains 15 to 20 lobes. Each lobe contains many alveolar glands and a lactiferous duct. The **alveolar glands** secrete milk, which is carried toward the nipple by the **lactiferous duct.** Connective tissue, including the suspensory ligaments, helps support the breast.

Until a child reaches puberty, the mammary glands of male and female children are similar. At puberty, however, the female mammary glands are stimulated by estrogen and progesterone. The alveolar glands and ducts enlarge, and adipose tissue is deposited around these structures. The male breast does not develop because there is no hormonal stimulus to do so. If a male is given female hormones, however, he too develops breasts.

GOT MILK?

Hormones of Lactation. During pregnancy, the increased secretion of estrogen and progesterone have a profound effect on the breasts. The breasts may double

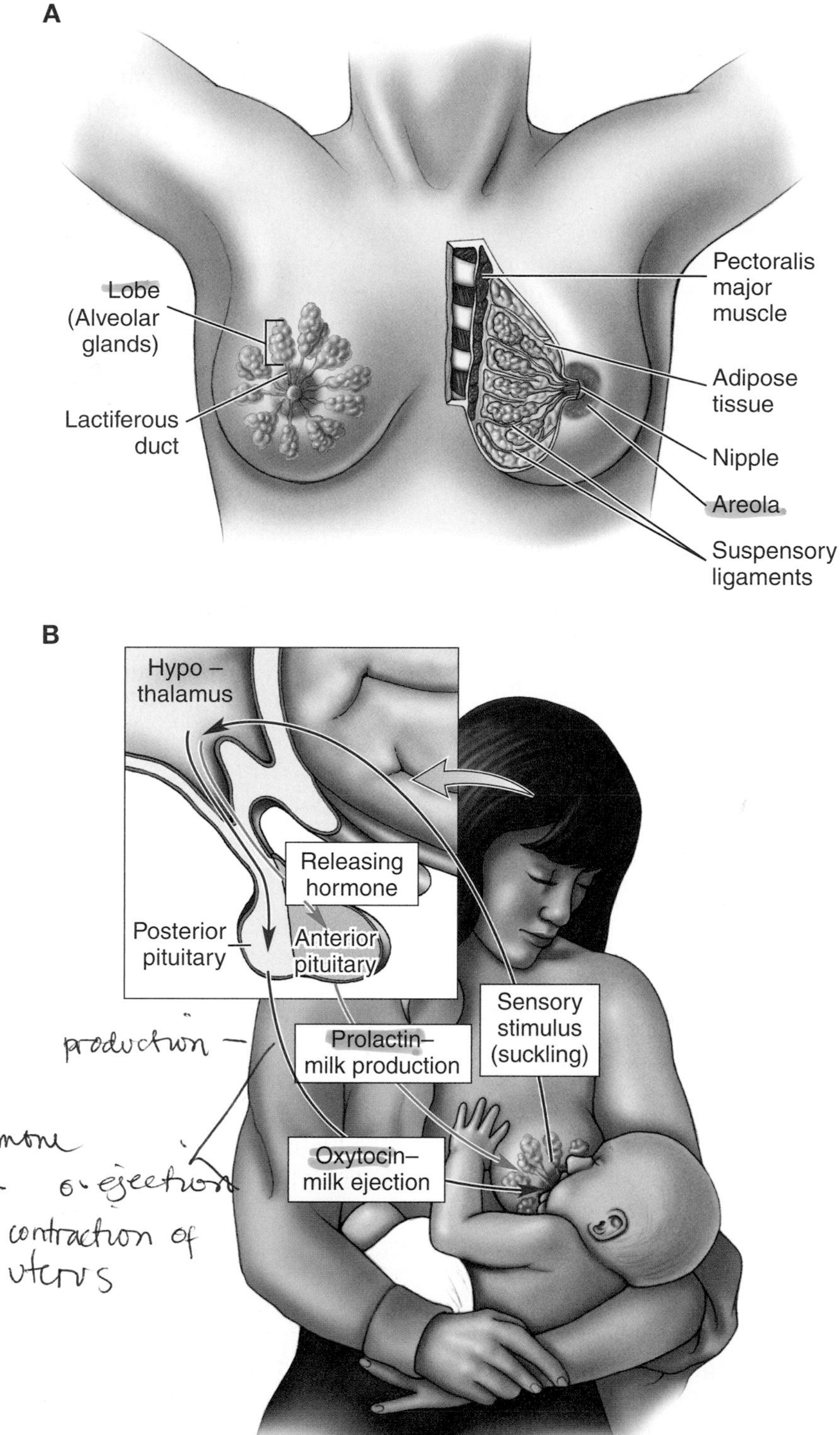

FIGURE 27-7 **A,** Breast and mammary glands. **B,** Hormones involved in breast-feeding; the milk let-down reflex.

in size in preparation for **lactation** (milk production) following birth. Usually there is no milk production during pregnancy because lactation requires prolactin, a hormone secreted by the anterior pituitary gland (see Figure 27-7, *B*). High plasma levels of estrogen and progesterone inhibit prolactin secretion during pregnancy. After delivery, however, plasma levels of estrogen and progesterone decrease, allowing the anterior pituitary gland to secrete prolactin. Milk production takes 2 to 3 days to begin. In the meantime, the mammary glands produce **colostrum,** a yellowish, watery fluid rich in protein and antibodies.

Prolactin is necessary for milk production, but a second hormone, **oxytocin,** is necessary for the *release* of milk from the breast. How does milk-release happen? When the baby suckles, or nurses, at the breast, nerve impulses in the areola are stimulated. Nerve impulses then travel from the breast to the hypothalamus; the hypothalamus, in turn, stimulates the posterior pituitary gland to release oxytocin. The oxytocin travels through the blood to the breast, causing contraction of the lobules. This process squeezes milk into the ducts, where it can be sucked out of the nipple by the nursing infant.

The effect of suckling and oxytocin release is called the **milk let-down reflex.** Note that the stimulus for the milk let-down reflex is suckling at the breast. Thus nursing mothers are encouraged to suckle their infants often. Breast-feeding encourages a good flow of milk. Note the distinction between the effects of prolactin and oxytocin. Prolactin stimulates milk production, or lactation. Oxytocin stimulates the milk let-down reflex and stimulates the flow of milk.

In addition to its effect on the flow of milk, oxytocin causes the uterus to contract. Uterine contraction helps minimize blood loss and more quickly returns the uterus to its nonpregnant state. A classification of drugs called oxytocic agents are sometimes administered to the mother after childbirth. Like oxytocin, these drugs, such as ergot preparations, cause uterine contractions and minimize postpartum bleeding.

POSTNATAL CHANGES AND DEVELOPMENTAL STAGES

IMMEDIATE ADJUSTMENTS

Immediately after birth, the baby must make many important adjustments to survive. Most importantly, the baby must begin breathing. The first deep breaths, drawn as the baby cries, expand the lungs and provide the infant with life-giving oxygen. The cardiovascular system also makes major adjustments, the most important being the establishment of blood flow to the lungs. Pulmonary blood flow occurs when the fetal heart structures, such as the foramen ovale and ductus arteriosus, close. (Review fetal circulation in Chapter 18.)

Just after birth, other organ systems also begin to function. For instance, the kidneys begin to make urine, and the digestive system begins a lifelong career of eating, digesting, and excreting. The first stool produced by the newborn is soft and dark green; it is called **meconium.** (During a long, difficult labor the baby may become stressed and excrete meconium into the amniotic fluid.)

One minute after birth, the infant's physical condition may be rated according to the Apgar scale. A score of 0, 1, 2, and so on, with a maximum score of 10, is given for the following signs: heart rate, respirations, color, muscle tone, and response to stimuli. An Apgar evaluation is also made at 5 minutes. Infants with low Apgar scores require prompt medical treatment.

DEVELOPMENT AS A LIFELONG PROCESS

After the newborn makes the immediate adjustments, the infant continues to grow and develop. Throughout life, the person will pass through the following developmental stages:

- *Neonatal period.* The **neonatal period** begins at birth and lasts for 4 weeks. During this time, the baby is called a neonate, or newborn.
- *Infancy.* The **period of infancy** lasts from the end of the first month to the end of the first year. Baby's first birthday marks the end of this stage.
- *Childhood.* The **period of childhood** lasts from the beginning of the second year to puberty.
- *Adolescence.* The **period of adolescence** lasts from puberty to adulthood. One word characterizes this stage: hormones. The period of adolescence is a period of tremendous growth and upheaval. Adolescents are physically capable of reproduction. The teen moves toward adulthood, leaving behind childish ways and coming to grips with becoming an adult.
- *Adulthood.* **Adulthood** is the period from adolescence to old age. During this period, the person is usually concerned with family matters and career goals. Most of us are still trying to give up childish ways.
- *Senescence.* **Senescence** is the period of old age, ending in death. It is not only a time to reflect on a life well lived but also a time to pursue other goals and to pass on the collected wisdom of a lifetime.

Sum It Up!

After the birth of the baby, both baby and mother make many physiologic adjustments. The mother's body returns to its nonpregnant state. For instance, cardiac output and blood volume decrease. She is physiologically prepared to breast-feed. Through the actions of prolactin and oxytocin, her mammary glands are producing milk and making it readily available to the suckling infant. The baby has made an initial adjustment to life on the outside and is breathing, urinating, and eating. The newborn continues postnatal development as a neonate. From there, it is on to infancy, childhood, adolescence, adulthood, and senescence.

HEREDITY

"He has his father's nose and his mother's smile." How often have we made that kind of statement when we recognize the traits of a parent in a child? The transmission of characteristics from parent to child is called **heredity,** and the science that studies heredity is called **genetics.** It was the work of an Austrian monk, Gregor Mendel, in the early nineteenth century that paved the way for the modern science of genetics. Using garden peas, Mendel demonstrated a pattern of specific traits passed on from parent to child.

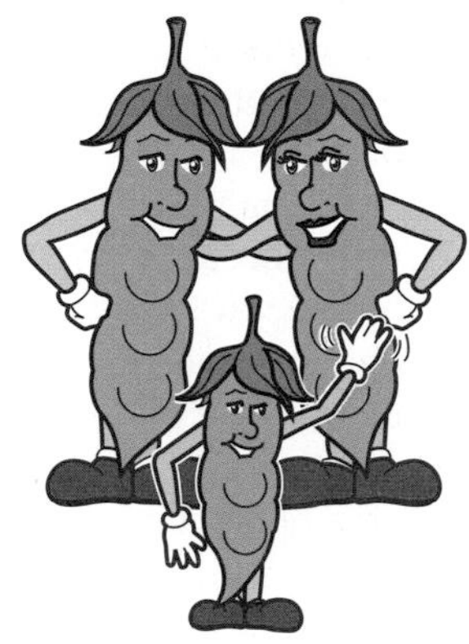

DNA, GENES, AND CHROMOSOMES

How are genetic structures related? Genetic information is located in the deoxyribonucleic acid (DNA) molecule and more specifically, in the DNA base-sequencing (Figure 27-8; see Chapter 4). DNA is tightly wound into threadlike structures called **chromosomes** found in the nucleus of most cells in the body. **Genes** are segments of the DNA strand and carry information for a specific **trait** such as skin color, freckles, and blood type. See Table 27-3 for other genetically determined characteristics. Some traits are determined by a single pair of genes, whereas other traits, such as height, require input from several genes. Each chromosome may carry thousands of genes, and each gene occupies a specific position on a chromosome.

Table 27-3 Examples of Genetic Traits

Trait	Dominant	Recessive
Hairline	Widow's peak	Continuous hairline
Hair color	Dark	Light
Hair texture	Curly	Straight
Hair on back of hand	Present	Absent
Freckles	Present	Absent to few
Dimples	Present	Absent
Eye color	Dark	Light
Color vision	Normal	Color-blind
Ear lobes	Unattached	Attached
Cleft chin	Present	Absent
Rh factor	Present	Absent

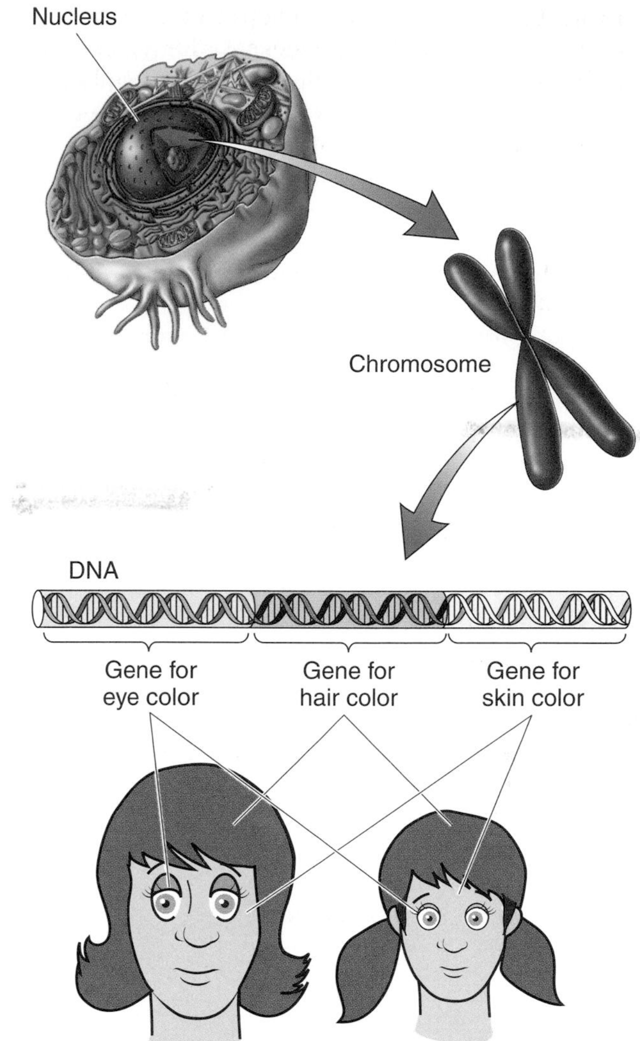

FIGURE 27-8 Chromosomes and genes.

Chromosomes exist in pairs. With the exception of the sex cells (egg and sperm), there are 23 pairs, or 46 chromosomes, in almost all human cells (red blood cells are the other exception). During fertilization, the egg and sperm each contribute 23 chromosomes to the zygote for a total of 23 pairs, or 46 chromosomes. One member of each pair comes from the egg; the other comes from the sperm. Thus for each trait, genetic instructions come from both the mother and the father. Forty-four chromosomes (22 pairs) are called **autosomes.** The autosomal gene pairs are numbered from 1 to 22. Two (one pair) of the 46 chromosomes are sex chromosomes; each is either an X or a Y chromosome.

Genetic Art: The Karyotype

It is possible to photograph the chromosomes in the cell. The photograph of the chromosomes is then cut apart, and the chromosomes are arranged in pairs by size and shape. The resulting display of the paired chromosomes is called a **karyotype** (KĂR-ē-ō-tīp) (Figure 27-9). This genetic artwork displays 22 pairs of autosomes and one pair of sex chromosomes. The karyotype is a diagnostic tool. It can reveal structural abnormalities and errors in the numbers of chromosomes.

Dominant, Recessive, and Codominant Genes

Remember: Each cell inherits two genes for each trait—tall or short, straight nose or curved nose, stubby fingers or long fingers, dark eyes or light eyes. Hence the choice: Will it be long or short, curved or straight? Genes can be dominant, recessive, or codominant. A **dominant gene** expresses itself; it gets noticed. The dominant gene overshadows the recessive gene, keeping it unnoticed, or unexpressed. Thus a **recessive gene** is not expressed if it is paired with a dominant gene. For instance, the genes for dark eyes are dominant, whereas the genes for light eyes are recessive. If the dominant genes (dark) and the recessive (light) genes are paired, the genes for dark eyes will be expressed (Figure 27-10). The genes for light eyes will not be expressed. **Codominant genes** express a trait equally. AB blood type is an example of codominance.

If recessive genes carry light eye coloring, how can an offspring develop blue eyes? Although blue eye coloring is recessive, a baby develops blue eyes because both the mother and the father are carrying the genes for blue eyes, a recessive trait (see Figure 27-10). If either the mother or the father had passed on a dominant gene for dark eyes, the child would have brown eyes.

The question put another way: If I have brown eyes, can any of my children have blue eyes? Yes! If I am carrying both a dominant (brown) and recessive (blue) gene for eye color, my child has a chance of having blue eyes. My recessive gene might pair with a recessive gene from my mate. If so, the pairing of two recessive genes produces a blue-eyed offspring. Brown-eyed-me is a carrier, one who shows no evidence of a trait (like blue eyes) but carries a recessive gene for that trait.

Too Many or Too Few Chromosomes

A person normally inherits 22 pairs of autosomal chromosomes. Sometimes, however, a person inherits too

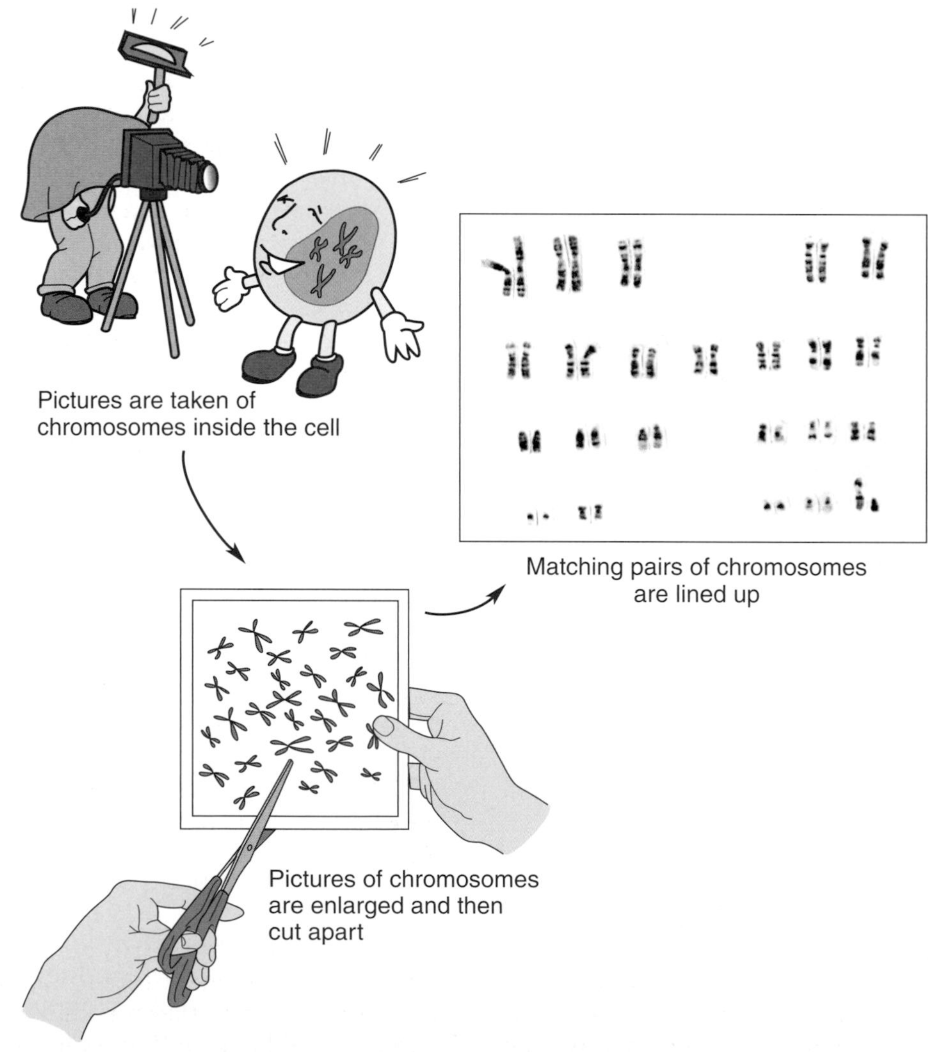
Pictures are taken of chromosomes inside the cell
Matching pairs of chromosomes are lined up
Pictures of chromosomes are enlarged and then cut apart

FIGURE 27-9 Genetic art: the karyotype.

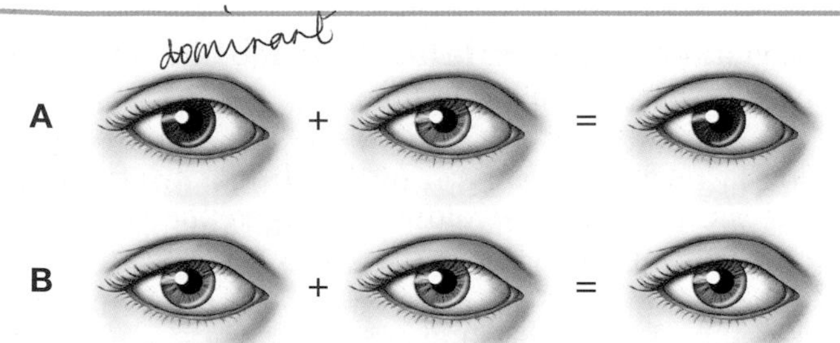

FIGURE 27-10 Eye color: dominant and recessive genes. **A,** The dominant brown-eye gene is expressed over the recessive blue-eye gene. **B,** Two recessive blue-eye genes produce a blue-eyed offspring.

many or too few autosomal chromosomes. The most common autosomal abnormality is called trisomy 21, or Down syndrome. A child with trisomy 21 has three copies of chromosome 21 instead of two copies. Other types of trisomy occur very infrequently in live births. Trisomy 18, called Edwards' syndrome, is due to three copies of chromosome 18, while trisomy 13, called Patau's syndrome, is due to three copies of chromosome 13. Autosomal abnormalities are usually due to nondisjunction.

Nondisjunction is the failure of the chromosomes to separate during meiosis, thereby causing the formation of eggs or sperm with too many or too few chromosomes. If these eggs and sperm lead to pregnancy, the embryo may have one too many or too few chromosomes. Most pregnancies with an unbalanced number of chromosomes miscarry in the first trimester. Down syndrome is the most common chromosomal abnormality because the condition is least likely to cause the pregnancy to miscarry. Even so, an estimated 70% of pregnancies with Down syndrome spontaneously miscarry, usually in the first trimester.

Genetic Expression

Genetic expression determines what the offspring looks like. A person's genetic makeup, in turn, determines genetic expression. A person's genetic expression can be influenced by a number of factors, including the person's sex, the influence of other genes, and environmental conditions. For instance, certain types of baldness and color blindness may be inherited by both males and females, but these traits are more apt to appear in the male. A child may also have the genetic capability of growing very tall. If the child is deprived of adequate nutrition and exercise, however, that child may not grow as tall as genetic makeup predicted.

Genetic Mutations

Normally, DNA replicates all information with few mistakes. Because of this precision, information is passed along reliably and efficiently to the next generation. Sometimes, however, a change occurs in a gene, or a chromosome breaks in some unexpected way. The result may be a unique feature or a birth defect. This change in the genetic code is called a **mutation.** Some mutations occur spontaneously. Others are caused by mutagenic agents. Certain chemicals, drugs, and radiation are mutagenic. Mutations can be beneficial or harmful and may even cause the death of the offspring. For instance, a mutation in the cells of the immune system may render a child resistant to a particular disease, thereby enhancing health. Another mutation, however, may weaken the immune system, making it more susceptible to pathogens.

IT'S A BOY, IT'S A GIRL: HOW THE SEX OF THE CHILD IS DETERMINED

Xs and Ys

Each human cell has 22 pairs of autosomal chromosomes and one pair of sex chromosomes (X and Y chromosomes). The female has two X chromosomes in her cells, a pair designated XX. A male has both an X and a Y chromosome in his cells, a pair designated XY (Figure 27-11).

Sex Determination: A Male Thing

The sex cells, the egg and the sperm, divide by a special type of cell division called **meiosis** (mī-Ō-sĭs). The important step in meiosis is the reduction (by one half) of the chromosomes. In other words, meiosis reduces the numbers of chromosomes from 46 to 23. The meiotic cell reduction also reduces the numbers of sex chromosomes by half. Consequently, each egg contains one X chromosome, and the sperm contains either an X chromosome or a Y chromosome. If a sperm containing an X chromosome fertilizes an egg, the child has an XX sex chromosome pair and is therefore female. If a sperm containing a Y chromosome fertilizes an egg, the child has an XY chromosome pair and is therefore male. Thus the sperm (male) determines the sex of the child.

Sometimes a person inherits an abnormal number of sex chromosomes. For instance, a female with Turner syndrome inherits only one sex chromosome, an X chromosome. Turner syndrome is designated as XO. The X signifies the female chromosome; the O signifies the absence of the second sex chromosome. A child with Turner syndrome does not develop secondary sex characteristics, is shorter than average, and has a webbed neck. People with Turner syndrome have normal intelligence.

Other genetic disorders involving extra sex chromosomes include Klinefelter syndrome (XXY) and the XYY male.

Sex-Linked Traits

The X and Y chromosomes differ structurally. The female X chromosome is larger than the Y chromosome and carries many genes for traits in addition to determining sex. The male Y chromosome is much smaller than the X chromosome and does not carry as much

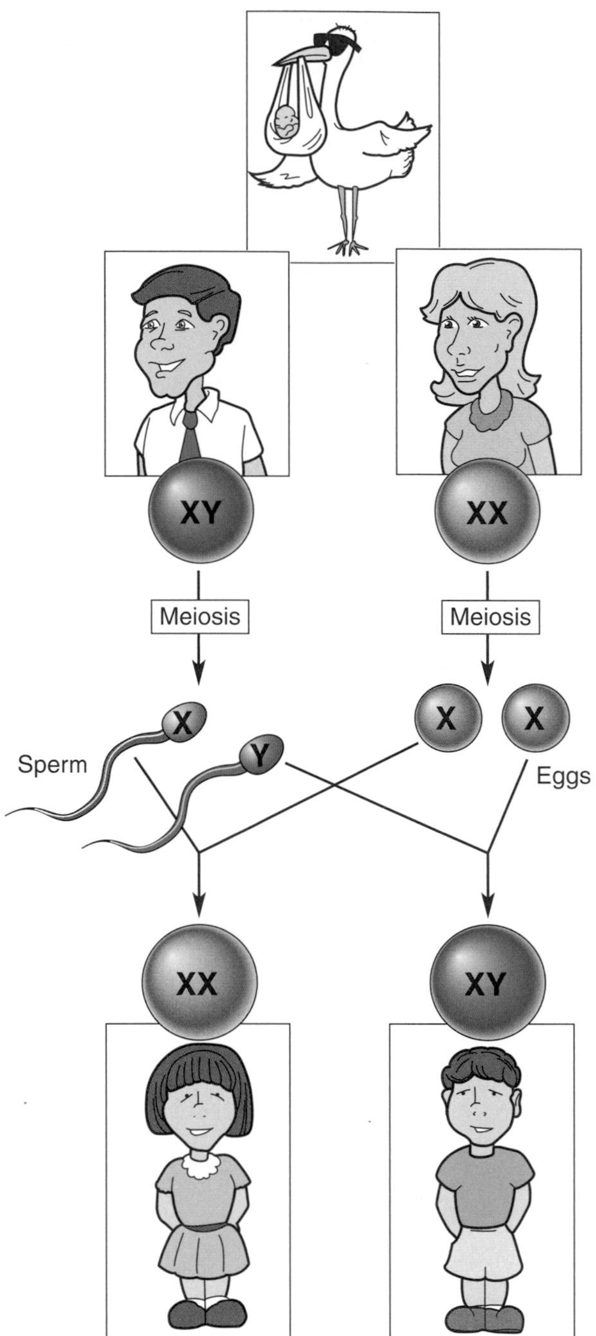

FIGURE 27-11 Determination of sex: Xs and Ys.

genetic information as the X chromosome does. Any trait that is carried on a sex chromosome is called a **sex-linked trait.** Because the X chromosome has more genetic information than the Y chromosome, most sex-linked traits are carried on the female X chromosome. Sex-linked traits carried on the X chromosomes are also called **X-linked traits.**

Although most sex-linked traits are carried on the X chromosome, they are expressed, or appear, in the male. Sex-linked diseases include hemophilia, Duchenne muscular dystrophy, and fragile X syndrome. Less serious sex-linked traits include baldness and red-green color-blindness.

CONGENITAL AND HEREDITARY DISEASE

You need to distinguish between hereditary diseases and congenital diseases and defects. **Hereditary diseases** are genetically transmitted. **Congenital** conditions are present at the time of birth. Any disease or defect present at birth is called congenital and includes both conditions that are inherited and those that are not. For instance, hemophilia is genetically transmitted and is therefore inherited. Because hemophilia is present at birth, it is also congenital.

A disease can, however, be congenital but not inherited. For instance, a mother may give birth to an infant who was exposed to the rubella virus (German measles) during her first trimester of pregnancy. This child may be born with cardiovascular defects, ocular defects, neural tube defects, and learning disabilities. These defects were not transmitted genetically from the parents to the child and are therefore not hereditary. The defects are congenital, however, because they were present at birth. Only 15% of congenital defects have a known genetic cause. Far fewer have a known environmental cause; for 70% of congenital birth defects, the cause is unknown.

Gene therapy offers hope for the treatment and eventual cure of genetic disorders. **Gene therapy** refers to the insertion of normal genes into cells that have abnormal genes. For instance, a person with congenitally high cholesterol levels might be successfully treated with genes that code for normal cholesterol production. Although in its early experimental stages, gene therapy provides hope for those with such genetic conditions as sickle cell disease, cystic fibrosis, and muscular dystrophy.

Sum It Up!

A child resembles the parents because he or she inherits genetic information from each parent. Genetic information is stored in the DNA molecules, which are arranged in strands called chromosomes. Almost every human cell contains 22 pairs of autosomal chromosomes and one pair of sex chromosomes. Genes are segments of DNA that contain codes for specific traits such as eye color or blood type. The child receives two genes for each inherited trait, one from the mother and one from the father.

Genes are dominant, recessive, or codominant. The sex chromosomes are designated X and Y. At fertilization, an XX combination produces a female child, while an XY combination produces a male. The father, with his Y chromosome, determines the sex of the child. Genetic information is passed along efficiently and reliably. Occasionally, incorrect or unhealthy information is passed along, thereby producing genetic diseases.

Disorders of Human Development

Cystic fibrosis	A disorder that results in the secretion of thick mucus. The mucus obstructs the respiratory passages and the ducts of the pancreas. The child's main problem concerns inadequate respiratory function. Cystic fibrosis is the most common genetic disease within the white population.
Duchenne muscular dystrophy	A disorder caused by a defective protein and characterized by the replacement of muscle tissue with fat and scar tissue. There is a progressive decline in muscle function so that the child is eventually confined to a wheelchair and dies because of poor muscle functioning of the heart and respiratory system.
Hemophilia	A disorder characterized by a deficiency of the antihemophilic factor (factor VIII). Hemophilia causes bleeding and immobility of the joints.
Huntington's disease	A neurologic disorder characterized by uncontrollable muscle contractions and deterioration of the memory and personality. The onset of symptoms is delayed until 30 to 50 years of age, making genetic counseling difficult.
Neurofibromatosis	Also called elephant man disease. Neurofibromatosis is a disorder characterized by the growth of multiple masses along nerves throughout the body. The growths result in severe deformities. Many persons with this disorder become socially isolated and suffer more emotionally than physically.
Osteogenesis imperfecta	Known as brittle bone disease and characterized by multiple fractures. Some bones may break in response to a simple change in posture.
Sickle cell disease	A genetic condition in which defective hemoglobin is synthesized (a single amino acid is out of place in the globin chain, causing a distortion of the hemoglobin molecule). The defective hemoglobin causes the red blood cells to sickle and then lyse, producing hemolytic anemia. The sickling also causes tissue hypoxia and severe pain.
Tay-Sachs disease	A disorder characterized by degeneration of the nervous system, resulting in death before the age of 2 years. Tay-Sachs disease is the most common genetic disease in persons of Jewish ancestry.

SUMMARY OUTLINE

The purpose of the reproductive system is to produce offspring whose genetic information is faithfully transmitted from generation to generation.

I. Fertilization to Birth

A. Fertilization
1. Fertilization (conception); refers to the union of an egg and a sperm.
2. Fertilization takes place around the time of ovulation.
3. Fertilization normally occurs within the fallopian tube.
4. The fertilized egg is called a zygote.

B. Human Development
1. Development is a process that begins with fertilization and ends with death.
2. The two phases are prenatal development and postnatal development.

C. Prenatal Development
1. Prenatal development includes four processes: cleavage, growth, morphogenesis, and differentiation.
2. The prenatal period consists of the early embryonic, embryonic, and fetal periods.
   a. The early embryonic period lasts for 2 weeks after fertilization. The zygote develops and implants into the uterine endometrial lining; its trophoblastic cells secrete hCG (maintains the corpus luteum).
   b. The two types of twins: monozygotic (identical) twins and dizygotic or fraternal (nonidentical) twins.
   c. The embryonic period lasts for 6 weeks and involves the formation of the extraembryonic membranes, the placenta, and all of the organ systems.
   d. The four extraembryonic membranes are the amnion, the chorion, the yolk sac, and the allantois.
   e. The placenta develops as the chorionic villi of the embryo burrow into the endometrial lining of the uterus. The mother and embryo form two separate circulations.
   f. The placenta has two functions: a. the site of "exchange" of nutrients and waste,

b. glandular function (estrogen and progesterone) throughout the pregnancy.

g. The embryo is hooked up to the placenta by the umbilical cord.

h. The embryonic period is a period of organogenesis. The organs arise from the primary germ layers: the ectoderm, the mesoderm, and the endoderm.

i. The fetal period extends from week 9 to birth; it is a time of growth and maturation.

j. Hormonal changes during pregnancy are summarized in Table 27-1.

D. Birth (Parturition)

1. Labor is the forceful contractions that expel the fetus from the uterus.
2. Labor is caused by hormones.
3. The three stages of labor are the dilation stage, the expulsion stage, and the placental stage.

E. Breasts and Lactation

1. The breasts contain mammary (milk-secreting) glands and adipose tissue.
2. The mammary glands and surrounding structures are affected by two hormones, prolactin and oxytocin. Prolactin stimulates the mammary glands to increase the production of milk. Oxytocin stimulates the smooth muscle in the breast to release the milk (part of the milk let-down reflex).

II. Postnatal Development

A. Immediate Postnatal Changes

1. The baby takes a first breath and the cardiovascular system makes some major adjustments.
2. The baby's transition to "life on the outside" is monitored by the Apgar scale.

B. Developmental Periods: Neonatal period, Infancy, Childhood, Adolescence, Adulthood, and Senescence

III. Heredity

A. DNA, Genes, and Chromosomes

1. Genetic information is stored in the DNA of genes, which are arranged into chromosomes.
2. Chromosomes exist in pairs. With the exception of sex cells, most human cells have 23 pairs of chromosomes, or 46 chromosomes.
3. Genes are dominant, recessive, or codominant.
4. A genetic mutation is due to a change in the genetic code.
5. The sex chromosomes are designated X and Y. A female has two X chromosomes, and a male has one X chromosome and one Y chromosome. Because only the male has the Y chromosome, the father determines the sex of the child.
6. Sex-linked traits are carried on the sex chromosomes. Most are carried on the X chromosome and are therefore also called X-linked traits.

B. Congenital and Hereditary Diseases

1. A congenital disorder is a condition present at birth.
2. Congenital disorders include inherited and noninherited birth defects and diseases. A hereditary disease is transmitted genetically from parent to child.

Review Your Knowledge

Matching: Fertilization and Development

Directions: Match the following words with their descriptions below.

a. primary germ layers
b. fetus
c. zygote
d. fertilization
e. embryo
f. parturition
g. trophoblasts
h. placenta
i. implantation
j. umbilical cord

1. ____ The fertilized ovum
2. ____ Cells that secrete hCG
3. ____ A zygote-making event
4. ____ The site where Baby breathes, eats, and excretes
5. ____ Baby's lifeline; contains the umbilical blood vessels
6. ____ Baby's name at age 3 to 8 weeks
7. ____ Process whereby the blastocyst baby-to-be burrows into the endometrium
8. ____ The birth process
9. ____ Endoderm, mesoderm, and ectoderm
10. ____ Baby's name from 9 weeks to birth

Matching: Hormones

Directions: Match the following words with their descriptions below. Some words may be used more than once.

a. hCG
b. prolactin
c. oxytocin
d. aldosterone

1. ____ Hormone that stimulates the mammary glands to make milk
2. ____ Posterior pituitary hormone involved in the milk let-down reflex
3. ____ Hormone that sustains the corpus luteum
4. ____ Hormone that stimulates the contraction of the myometrium
5. ____ Secretion of this hormone continues at a high level for about 2 months, then steadily declines as the placenta takes over
6. ____ Hormone that stimulates Na^+ reabsorption and expands blood volume during pregnancy

Matching: Heredity

Directions: Match the following words with their descriptions below.

a. sex-linked trait
b. mutation
c. autosomes
d. sex chromosomes
e. genes

1. ____ Segments of a DNA strand that carry the code for a specific trait such as eye color
2. ____ Twenty-two pairs (numbered 1-22) of chromosomes
3. ____ X and Y chromosomes
4. ____ Any trait that is carried on an X or Y chromosome
5. ____ A change in the genetic code that may express itself as a change in a particular trait

Multiple Choice

1. Implantation
   a. normally occurs within the fallopian tubes.
   b. is achieved by the morula.
   c. is a uterine event achieved by the blastocyst.
   d. occurs within the ovaries.
2. Human chorionic gonadotropin (hCG)
   a. promotes the maturation of the egg.
   b. is responsible for female characteristics.
   c. maintains the corpus luteum.
   d. promotes the transformation of the corpus luteum into the corpus albicans.
3. Trophoblastic cells
   a. secrete oxytocin.
   b. are responsible for the milk let-down reflex.
   c. assist with implantation.
   d. are incorporated within the graafian follicle.
4. The morula
   a. only occurs if there is an ectopic pregnancy.
   b. is the unfertilized ovum that gets discharged with the menstrual blood.
   c. refers to the adorable preembryonic cluster of cells.
   d. spends its life embedded within the endometrium.
5. Which of the following is least true of or associated with the placenta?
   a. Is the site at which Baby-to-be breathes
   b. Is very vascular
   c. Replaces the glandular secretion of the corpus luteum
   d. Nourishes the zygote as it matures into the morula

APPENDIX A

Medical Terminology and Eponymous Terms

MEDICAL TERMINOLOGY

Anatomy and physiology has its own vocabulary. You must learn this vocabulary to understand the scientific concepts and to communicate effectively with other medical professionals. This special vocabulary consists of prefixes, word roots, and suffixes arranged in various combinations. By recognizing the meanings of the various prefixes, word roots, and suffixes, you can understand most words.

The **word root** is the main part of the word; it provides the central meaning of the word. For instance, *cardi-* refers to heart, while *cerebr-* refers to brain. Sometimes, two word roots are combined. For instance, *cardio-* (heart) and *pulmon-* (lungs) are combined in *cardiopulmonary,* a reference to both the heart and the lungs. Refer to the list in Table A-1 for other common word roots.

The **prefix** is the part of the word placed before the word root. The prefix alters the meaning of the word root. For example, the prefix *mal-,* when placed before nutrition (*malnutrition*), modifies or alters the meaning of nutrition; it means bad or poor nutrition. The prefix *hyper-,* as in *hypersecretion,* means that there is excessive secretion, whereas the prefix *hypo-,* as in *hyposecretion,* means that secretion is insufficient. Refer to the list in Table A-1 for commonly used prefixes.

The **suffix** is the part of the word that follows the word root; it is a word ending that may modify or alter the meaning of the word root. For instance, the suffix *-cide,* as in *germicide,* refers to a substance that kills germs. Refer to the list in Table A-1 for commonly used suffixes.

EPONYMOUS TERMS

As you study anatomy and physiology, you will notice that some terms incorporate the name of a person. For instance, the Krebs cycle is named after Hans Krebs, the famous biochemist who worked out and described the chemical reactions of this cycle. The person for whom something is named is an **eponym;** the descriptive term is an **eponymous term.**

Because eponymous terms do not provide much useful information, they are being replaced with more informative terms. For instance, the Krebs cycle has been renamed the citric acid cycle, because citric acid plays an important role in the cycle.

The following list provides some of the commonly used eponymous terms and the newer, more descriptive terms.

Eponymous Term	Newer Term
Achilles tendon	calcaneal tendon
Adam's apple	thyroid cartilage
ampulla of Vater	hepatopancreatic ampulla
Bowman's capsule	glomerular capsule
bundle of His	atrioventricular bundle
canal of Schlemm	scleral venous sinus
cells of Leydig	interstitial cells
circle of Willis	cerebral arterial circle
Cowper's glands	bulbourethral glands
eustachian tube	auditory tube
fallopian tube	uterine tube, oviduct
fissure of Rolando	central sulcus
graafian follicle	vesicular ovarian follicle
haversian canal	central canal
haversian system	osteon
islets of Langerhans	pancreatic islet cells
Krebs cycle	citric acid cycle
loop of Henle	nephron loop
Sertoli cells	sustentacular cells
sphincter of Oddi	sphincter of the hepatopancreatic ampulla
Wernicke's area	posterior speech area

Table A-1 Prefixes, Suffixes, and Word Roots

Word Part	Meaning	Example
Prefixes		
a-, an-	lack of, without	anoxia (without oxygen)
ab-	away from	abduction (movement away from the midline)
ad- (af-)	to, toward	adduction (movement toward the midline), afferent (toward a center)
ante-	forward, before	antenatal (before birth)
anti-	against	antibiotic (against life), anticoagulant (against blood clotting)
bi-	two	biceps (two heads of a muscle)
bio-	life	biology (study of life)
brady-	slow	bradycardia (abnormally slow heart rate)
co-, com-, con-	with, together	congenital (born with)
contra-	against, opposite	contralateral (opposite side), contraception (against conception)
cyan-	blue	cyanotic (having a blue coloring)
de-	away from	dehydration (loss of water)
dextro-	right	dextrocardia (heart abnormally shifted to the right)
di-	two	disaccharide (double sugar)
dys-	difficult	dysphagia (difficulty swallowing)
ect-, exo-, extra-	outside	extracellular (outside the cell)
epi-	on, upon	epidermis (upon the dermis)
erythr-	red	erythrocyte (red blood cell)
eu-	good, well	euphoria (sense of well-being), eupnea (normal breathing)
hemi-, semi-	one half	hemiplegia (paralysis of one half or one side of the body), semilunar valve (valve that resembles a half-moon)
hyper-	over, above normal	hypersecretion (excessive secretion)
hypo-	under, below normal	hyposecretion (insufficient secretion)
inter-	between	intercellular (between the cells)
intra-	within	intracellular (within the cells)
leuk(o)-	white	leukocyte (white blood cell)
macro-	large	macrophage (large phagocytic cell)
mal-	bad	malnutrition (bad or inadequate nutrition), malfunction (bad or inadequate function)
micro-	small	microbiology (study of small life such as bacteria)
melan-, mele-	black	melena (darkening of the stool by blood pigments)
necr-	dead	necrosis (death, as of tissue)
neo-	new	neonate (newborn infant), neoplasm (new growth)
noct-	night	nocturia (excessive urination at night)
olig-	scanty	oliguria (scanty urine)
orth-	straight	orthopnea (ability to breathe easily only in an upright, or straight, position)
peri-	around	pericardium (membrane surrounding the heart)
pleur-	rib, side	pleural membranes (membranes that enclose the lungs)
poly-	much, many	polyuria (much urine); polysaccharide (many sugars)
post-	after	postnatal (after birth)
pre-	before	prenatal (before birth)
presby-	elder, old	presbyopia (diminished vision due to aging)
pseudo-	false	pseudopod (false foot)
retro-	behind, backward	retroperitoneal (behind the peritoneum)
sten-	narrow	mitral valve stenosis (narrowing of the mitral valve)
sub-	underneath	subcutaneous (underneath the skin)
super-, supra-	above	suprarenal glands (glands located above the kidneys)
syn-	with, together	synergistic muscle (a muscle that works with another muscle)
tachy-	rapid	tachycardia (abnormally rapid heart rate)
trans-	across	transcapillary exchange (movement across the capillary membrane)

Table A-1 Prefixes, Suffixes, and Word Roots—cont'd

Word Part	Meaning	Example
Suffixes		
-algia	pain	neuralgia (nerve pain)
-cele	hernia	omphalocele (umbilical hernia)
-centesis	puncture to remove fluid	thoracentesis (aspiration of fluid from the chest)
-cide	to kill	germicide (kills germs)
-cyte	cell	leukocyte (white blood cell)
-ectomy	removal of	hysterectomy (removal of the uterus)
-emia	blood	hypoglycemia (decreased glucose in the blood)
-gram	record	mammogram (x-ray or record of the breasts)
-iasis	condition of	cholelithiasis (condition of having gallstones)
-itis	inflammation of	appendicitis (inflammation of the appendix)
-logy	study of	physiology (study of the function of the body)
-lysis, lytic	breakdown	hemolysis (breakdown of blood)
-malacia	softening	osteomalacia (softening of the bones)
-megaly	enlargement	hepatomegaly (enlarged liver)
-oma	tumor	adenoma (tumor containing glandular tissue)
-osis	abnormal condition	leukocytosis (abnormal condition of white blood cells)
-ostomy	to create an abnormal opening	colostomy (an opening into the colon)
-pathy	disease	nephropathy (disease of the kidney)
-penia	deficiency, poor	thrombocytopenia (a deficiency of platelets)
-plasty	to shape	pyloroplasty (to surgically shape the pylorus)
-rrhaphy	to suture or sew	herniorrhaphy (to repair or sew a hernia)
-rrhea	discharge from	rhinorrhea (discharge from the nose, a runny nose)
-scopy	visualization	colonoscopy (insertion of a scope to see the inside of the colon)
-stasis	to stand still, stop	hemostasis (stop the flow of blood)
-uria	urine	glucosuria (glucose in the urine)
Word Roots		
aden	gland	adenoma (tumor of glandular tissue)
angi	vessel	angioma (tumor of a vessel)
arthr	joint	arthritis (inflammation of the joints)
blast	immature cell	osteoblast (immature bone cell)
brachi	arm	brachialgia (pain in the arm)
cardi	heart	cardioactive (having an effect on the heart)
cephal	head	cephalad (toward the head)
cervic	neck	cervicodynia (pain in the neck)
chondr	cartilage	chondroma (tumor of the cartilage)
crani	skull	craniometry (measurement of the skull)
derm(at)	skin	dermatitis (inflammation of the skin)
gastr	stomach	gastritis (inflammation of the lining of the stomach)
gingiv	gums	gingivitis (inflammation of the gums)
gloss	tongue	glossitis (inflammation of the tongue)
glyc(y), gluc	sugar, glucose	hyperglycemia (high blood sugar)
hem(at)	blood	hematuria (blood in the urine)
hepat	liver	hepatitis (inflammation of the liver)
hyster	uterus	hysterectomy (removal of the uterus)
lact, galact	milk	lactogenic hormone (milk-producing hormone)
lith	stone	cholelithiasis (condition of gallstones)
mast, mamm	breast	mastitis (inflammation of the breast)
myo	muscle	myocardium (heart muscle)
myel	marrow, spinal cord	myelosuppression (depression of the bone marrow)

Continued

Table A-1 Prefixes, Suffixes, and Word Roots—cont'd

Word Part	Meaning	Example
Word Roots—cont'd		
nephr	kidney	nephritis (inflammation of the kidney)
neur	nerve	neuritis (inflammation of a nerve)
oo	egg	oocyte (egg cell)
oophor	ovary	oophorectomy (removal of the ovary)
ophthalm	eye	ophthalmoscope (an instrument used to view the eye)
path	disease	pathology (study of disease)
ped, pedia	child	pediatrics (branch of medicine dealing with the child)
phag	eat, swallow	dysphagia (difficulty swallowing)
pharyng	throat	pharyngitis (sore throat)
phleb	vein	phlebitis (inflammation of the vein)
pneum	air, breath	pneumothorax (air in the chest)
pneumon, pulmo(n)	lung	pneumonectomy (removal of the lung)
psych	mind	psychology (study of the mind)
rhin	nose	rhinorrhea (discharge from the nose; runny nose)
therm	heat	hyperthermia (higher than normal temperature)
thorac	chest	thoracotomy (incision into the chest)
thromb	clot	thrombolytic (an agent that dissolves a clot)
trache	windpipe	tracheostomy (incision into the trachea)

APPENDIX B

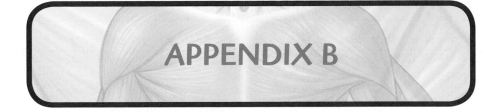

Laboratory Values

Test	Normal Values*	Clinical Significance
Blood Tests		
Blood Counts (Formed Elements)		
Platelet count	150,000-450,000/mm^3	Increases in heart disease, cirrhosis, and cancer; decreases in myelosuppression
Red blood cell count	Men: 4.5-6.0 million/mm^3 Women: 4.2-5.4 million/mm^3	Decreases in anemia; increases in polycythemia, dehydration
Reticulocyte count	0.5%-1.5% of RBCs/mm^3	Increases in anemia following hemorrhage, decreases in myelosuppression
White blood cell count	5000-10,000/mm^3	Increases in infection, inflammation, and dehydration; decreases in myelosuppression
White blood cell count (differential)		See Table 15-1
Other Counts		
Clotting time	5-10 min	Increases in severe liver disease and deficiencies of coagulation factors
Hematocrit	Men: 40%-50% Women: 37%-47%	Increases in dehydration and polycythemia; decreases in anemia and hemorrhage
Hemoglobin	Men: 13.5-17.5 g/100 ml Women: 12-16 g/100 ml	Increases in polycythemia and dehydration; decreases in anemia, bleeding, and hemolysis
Prothrombin time	11-15 sec	Increases in liver disease, vitamin K deficiency, and oral anticoagulation
Blood Electrolytes and Metabolites		
Albumin	3.5-5.5 g/100 ml	Decreases in kidney disease, liver disease, and burns
Bicarbonate	22-26 mEq/L	Increases in chronic lung disease; decreases in metabolic acidosis (uncontrolled diabetes mellitus) and diarrhea
Bilirubin (total)	0.3-1.4 mg/100 ml	Increases in hepatobiliary disease and hemolytic reactions
Calcium	9.0-11 mg/100 ml	Increases in hyperparathyroidism and cancer; decreases in alkalosis and hyperphosphatemia
Chloride	95-108 mEq/L	Increases in dehydration and heart failure; decreases when body fluids are lost, as in vomiting, diarrhea, and diuresis
Cholesterol	$<$200 mg/dl	Increases in coronary artery disease
Creatinine	0.6-1.5 mg/100 ml	Increases in kidney disease
Glucose	70-110 mg/100 ml (affected by meals)	Increases in diabetes mellitus, severe illness, pregnancy; decreases in insulin overdose
pH	7.35-7.45	Increases in hyperventilation and metabolic alkalosis; decreases in metabolic acidosis and hypoventilation
Potassium	3.5-5.0 mEq/L	Increases in kidney failure, cell destruction, and acidosis; decreases in loss of body fluid (vomiting, diarrhea, diuretic-induced polyuria)
Sodium	136-145 mEq/L	Increases in dehydration; decreases when body fluids are lost (burns, diuresis, vomiting, diarrhea)
Blood urea nitrogen (BUN)	8-25 mg/100 ml	Increases in kidney disease and high protein diet
Uric acid	3-7 mg/100 ml	Increases in gout, leukemia, and kidney disease

*Values vary from laboratory to laboratory. Most common values are given.

Continued

Test	Normal Values*	Clinical Significance
Urinalysis		
General Characteristics		
Color	Amber, straw	Affected by hydration; dehydration causes a deeper yellow color, overhydration causes a pale color; hepatobiliary disease causes a deeper yellow color; color changes in response to drugs
Clarity	Clear, slightly hazy	Becomes cloudy on refrigeration or in the presence of urinary tract infection (bacteria clouds urine)
Odor	Aromatic	Foul-smelling with a urinary tract infection; fruity odor in ketoacidosis (diabetes mellitus)
Specific gravity (SG)	1.003-1.035	Affected by hydration. In dehydration, the SG increases; in overhydration the SG decreases. Polyuria (as with diabetes) causes a low specific gravity; also decreases in kidney damage
pH	4.6-8.0	Decreases in acidosis and high protein diet; increases in alkalosis and vegetarian diet
Metabolites		
Ammonia	20-70 mEq/L	Increases in diabetes mellitus and liver disease
Bilirubin	Negative	Increases in liver disease and biliary obstruction
Creatinine	1.0-2.5 mg/24 hrs	Increases in infection; decreases in kidney disease
Glucose	Negative	Increases in diabetes mellitus
Ketone bodies	Negative	Increases in ketoacidosis (diabetes mellitus and starvation)
Protein	Negative	Increases in kidney disease
Uric acid	0.4-1.0 g/24 hrs	Increases in gout and liver disease; decreases in kidney disease
Urobilinogen	0-4 mg/24 hrs	Increases in liver disease and hemolytic anemia
Formed Elements, Other Large Substances		
Red blood cells	Few	Increases in inflammation and trauma to the urinary tract
White blood cells	Few	Increases in urinary tract infection
Bacteria	Few	Increases in urinary tract infection

APPENDIX C

Answers to Review Your Knowledge Questions

Chapter 1: Introduction to the Human Body

Matching: Directions of the Body

1. c 4. f 5. d
2. e 3. b

Matching: Regional Terms

1. d 5. g 9. a
2. f 6. b 10. j
3. i 7. c
4. h 8. e

Multiple Choice

1. c 3. c 5. b
2. d 4. d

Chapter 2: Basic Chemistry

Matching: Atoms and Elements

1. a 3. d 5. e
2. b 4. c

Matching: Structure of the Atom

1. f 3. b 5. d
2. a 4. d

Matching: Ions and Electrolytes

1. c 3. a 5. e
2. b 4. d

Matching: Acids and Bases

1. e 3. b 5. f
2. c 4. f

Multiple Choice

1. c 4. d 7. c
2. a 5. b 8. c
3. d 6. c

Chapter 3: Cells

Matching: Cell Structure

1. f 4. b 7. g
2. d 5. c
3. a 6. e

Matching: Transport and Tonicity

1. g 5. f 9. b
2. h 6. e 10. d
3. i 7. a
4. c 8. d

Multiple Choice

1. b 3. c 5. c
2. d 4. c

Chapter 4: Cell Metabolism

Matching: Carbohydrates, Proteins, and Fats

1. d 5. f 8. a
2. b 6. b 9. e
3. c 7. h 10. a
4. g

Matching: Biochemistry Terms

1. b 3. c 5. a
2. a 4. d 6. e

Matching: Genetic Code and Protein Synthesis

1. d 3. c 5. b
2. e 4. a

Multiple Choice

1. a 3. c 5. a
2. d 4. c 6. a

Chapter 5: Microbiology Basics

Matching: Microorganisms and Other Pathogens

1. b 5. d 9. c
2. a 6. c 10. b
3. e 7. e 11. f
4. d 8. b

Multiple Choice

1. a 3. c 5. d
2. b 4. c

Chapter 6: Tissues and Membranes

Matching: Tissues

1. a 5. b 9. b
2. b 6. c 10. d
3. a 7. b
4. a 8. b

Matching: Membranes

1. d 3. b 5. c
2. e 4. a

Multiple Choice

1. c 3. d 5. a
2. a 4. a

Chapter 7: Integumentary System and Body Temperature

Matching: Skin

1. d 3. a 5. d
2. b 4. c

Matching: Glands

1. b 3. a 5. d
2. b 4. c

Matching: Colors

1. c 3. a 5. e
2. b 4. d

Multiple Choice

1. b 3. c 5. c
2. b 4. c 6. a

Chapter 8: Skeletal System

Matching: Long Bone

1. d 5. j 9. h
2. c 6. a 10. e
3. g 7. b
4. i 8. f

Matching: Names of Bones

1. e 5. g 9. c
2. f 6. h 10. i
3. b 7. j
4. d 8. a

Matching: Joints and Joint Movement

1. c 5. c 9. d
2. j 6. a 10. g
3. i 7. f
4. h 8. b

Multiple Choice

1. b 3. c 5. b
2. c 4. d 6. a

Chapter 9: Muscular System

Matching: Muscle Terms

1. l 5. k 9. h
2. j 6. b 10. i
3. j 7. f
4. d 8. g

Matching: Names of Muscles

1. c 5. j 9. b
2. k 6. a 10. b
3. g 7. d
4. f 8. i

Multiple Choice

1. a 3. b 5. d
2. c 4. b 6. b

Chapter 10: Nervous System: Nervous Tissue and Brain

Matching: Nerve Cells

1. e 5. c 9. h
2. d 6. b 10. i
3. f 7. j
4. a 8. g

Matching: Brain

1. b 3. d 5. e
2. a 4. c

Multiple Choice

1. b 4. d 7. c
2. d 5. a 8. b
3. c 6. b 9. b

Chapter 11: Nervous System: Spinal Cord and Peripheral Nerves

Matching: Reflexes

1. f 3. e 5. a
2. b 4. c 6. d

Matching: Nerves

1. a 5. e 9. h
2. b 6. c 10. a
3. h 7. f
4. g 8. d

Multiple Choice

1. c 3. a 5. d
2. d 4. a

Chapter 12: Autonomic Nervous System

Matching: Sympathetic or Parasympathetic

1. S 5. S 9. P
2. P 6. S 10. S
3. S 7. P
4. S 8. P

Matching: Norepinephrine or Acetylcholine

1. NE 5. ACh 9. NE
2. NE 6. NE 10. ACh
3. ACh 7. NE
4. ACh 8. ACh

Multiple Choice

1. c
2. b
3. a
4. c
5. b

Chapter 13: Sensory System

Matching: Senses

1. a 4. e 7. d
2. d 5. b
3. c 6. a

Matching: Structures of the Eye

1. h 5. f 9. h
2. e 6. b 10. g
3. c 7. e
4. a 8. d

Matching: Structures of the Ear

1. b 5. c 9. b
2. b 6. c 10. c
3. a 7. a
4. c 8. b

Multiple Choice

1. b 3. b 5. a
2. c 4. c 6. b

Chapter 14: Endocrine System

Matching: Glands

1. a 5. h 9. d
2. b 6. c 10. g
3. b 7. f
4. e 8. a

Matching: Hormones

1. e 5. c 9. d
2. g 6. f 10. a
3. b 7. j
4. i 8. i

Multiple Choice

1. b 3. c 5. d
2. a 4. d 6. a

Chapter 15: Blood

Matching: Blood Cells

1. c 5. a 9. b
2. c 6. a 10. c
3. c 7. b
4. b 8. c

Matching: Blood Clots

1. e
2. d
3. a
4. b
5. c

Matching: Blood Types

1. d 3. c 5. d
2. d 4. a

Multiple Choice

1. b 3. a 5. d
2. b 4. c 6. d

Chapter 16: Anatomy of the Heart

Matching: Structures of the Heart

1. g 5. d 9. d
2. b 6. a 10. h
3. f 7. a
4. c 8. e

Matching: Valves

1. d 5. a 9. d
2. d 6. c 10. c
3. b 7. c
4. c 8. d

Multiple Choice

1. d 3. a 5. c
2. d 4. b

Chapter 17: Function of the Heart

Matching: Cardiac Function Terms

1. b 5. d 9. c
2. c 6. d 10. b
3. b 7. f
4. e 8. a

Matching: Loads and Effects

1. b 4. b 7. b
2. c 5. e 8. c
3. a 6. d

Multiple Choice

1. d 4. d 7. d
2. d 5. c 8. d
3. b 6. a

Chapter 18: Anatomy of the Blood Vessels

Matching: Blood Vessels: Structure and Function

1. c 5. d 9. a
2. b 6. d 10. c
3. c 7. d
4. c 8. a

Matching: Names of Blood Vessels

1. f 6. a 11. k
2. i 7. j 12. b
3. e 8. g 13. h
4. a 9. d 14. l
5. e 10. c 15. m

Matching: Fetal Circulation

1. a 3. c 5. b
2. e 4. d

Multiple Choice

1. d 3. b 5. a
2. a 4. b

Chapter 19: Functions of the Blood Vessels

Matching: Blood Pressure Terms

1. d 5. g 9. b
2. f 6. a 10. e
3. a 7. b
4. h 8. c

Matching: Blood Pressure Readings

1. a 5. b 9. a
2. a 6. a 10. b
3. b 7. b
4. c 8. c

Matching: Changes in Blood Pressure

1. a 5. a 9. a
2. b 6. b 10. a
3. a 7. a
4. a 8. b

Multiple Choice

1. c 3. b 5. b
2. d 4. a 6. b

Chapter 20: Lymphatic System

Matching: Lymph Terms

1. e 3. b 5. a
2. c 4. d

Multiple Choice

1. c 3. c 5. b
2. c 4. c

Chapter 21: Immune System

Matching: Nonspecific Immunity

1. d 3. c 5. a
2. b 4. b

Matching: Specific Immunity

1. e 3. d 5. b
2. a 4. c

Matching: Active and Passive Immunity

1. a 3. b 5. b
2. b 4. a 6. a

Multiple Choice

1. b 3. a 5. b
2. c 4. d

Chapter 22: Respiratory System

Matching: Structures of the Respiratory Tract

1. d 5. b 9. d
2. c 6. h 10. g
3. e 7. h
4. a 8. f

Matching: Thoracic Cavity and Ventilation

1. d 4. e 7. c
2. b 5. f
3. c 6. a

Multiple Choice

1. c 4. c 7. c
2. c 5. b
3. c 6. d

Chapter 23: Digestive System

Matching: Structures: Making the Connections

1. c 4. e 7. f
2. d 5. h 8. a
3. b 6. g

Matching: Enzymes, Hormones, and Digestive Aids

1. f 6. g 11. e
2. b 7. a 12. h
3. c 8. d 13. c
4. e 9. g
5. i 10. f

Multiple Choice

1. c 4. c 7. a
2. d 5. c 8. b
3. c 6. c

Chapter 24: Urinary System

Matching: Plumbing...More or Less

1. c 5. d 9. b
2. b 6. c 10. d
3. a 7. d
4. d 8. d

Matching: Nephron Unit

1. d 5. b 9. f
2. b 6. e 10. d
3. a 7. c
4. g 8. a

Matching: Hormones and Enzymes

1. b 5. f 9. d
2. a 6. a 10. g
3. e 7. e
4. a 8. c

Multiple Choice

1. d 4. b 7. b
2. c 5. b
3. b 6. c

Chapter 25: Water, Electrolyte, and Acid-Base Balance

Matching: Water Compartments

1. b
2. c
3. a
4. d
5. a

Matching: Ions

1. c 6. c
2. a 7. b
3. b 8. a
4. b 9. c
5. a 10. d

Multiple Choice

1. a
2. c
3. d
4. c
5. c

Chapter 26: Reproductive Systems

Matching: Structures (Female)

1. a 6. b
2. c 7. c
3. b 8. b
4. b 9. c
5. c 10. d

Matching: Structures (Male)

1. b
2. a
3. d
4. c
5. e

Matching: Hormones

1. e 6. d
2. d 7. e
3. a 8. a
4. b 9. e
5. c 10. b

Multiple Choice

1. d
2. a
3. c
4. c
5. c
6. b
7. b

Chapter 27: Human Development and Heredity

Matching: Fertilization and Development

1. c 6. e
2. g 7. i
3. d 8. f
4. h 9. a
5. j 10. b

Matching: Hormones

1. b
2. c
3. a
4. c
5. a
6. d

Matching: Heredity

1. e
2. c
3. d
4. a
5. b

Multiple Choice

1. c
2. c
3. c
4. c
5. d

GLOSSARY

PRONUNCIATION OF TERMS

The markings ¯ and ˘ above the vowels (a, e, i, o, and u) indicate the proper sounds of the vowels. When ¯ is above a vowel its sound is long, that is, exactly like its name; for example:

ā as in āpe
ē as in ēven
ī as in īce
ō as in ōpen
ū as in ūnit

The ˘ marking indicates a short vowel sound, as in the following examples:

ă as in ăpple
ĕ as in ĕvery
ĭ as in ĭnterest
ŏ as in pŏt
ŭ as in ŭnder

Abdominopelvic cavity (ăb-Dŏm-ĭ-nō-PĔL-vĭk KĂ-vĭ-tē) - Part of the ventral cavity that lies inferior to the diaphragm; includes upper abdominal cavity and lower pelvic cavity.

Abduction (ăb-DŬK-shŭn) - Movement of a body part away from the midline.

Absorption - Taking in of substances by cells or membranes; more specifically, referring to the movement of digested food from the digestive tract into the blood.

Accommodation - Adjustment of the lens for near vision.

Acetylcholine (ăs-Ē-tĭl-KŌ-lēn) - Neurotransmitter that is secreted from the nerve terminals of cholinergic fibers.

Acid (ĂS-ĭd) - Substance that donates or releases hydrogen ions when it ionizes in water.

Acidosis (ăs-ĭ-DŌ-sĭs) - Imbalance caused by excess H^+, causing the blood pH to decrease below 7.35; there is respiratory acidosis and metabolic acidosis.

Actin (Ăk-tĭn) - One of the contractile proteins in muscle; also called thin filaments.

Action potential - Sequence of changes in the membrane potential that occurs when a cell is stimulated to threshold; it includes depolarization and repolarization; also called the nerve impulse and the cardiac impulse.

Active immunity - Immunity achieved when the body makes antibodies against an antigen.

Active transport - Transport process that requires an input of energy (ATP) to move a substance from an area of low concentration to an area of high concentration.

Adaptation - Adjustment to a stimulus, such as the adaptation to odor.

Adduction (ăd-DŬK-shŭn) - Movement of a body part toward the midline of the body.

Adenohypophysis (ăd-ĕ-nō-hī-PŎF-ĭ-sĭs) - Anterior pituitary gland.

Adenosine triphosphate (ATP) - Energy-storing and energy-transferring molecule found in all cells.

Adipose (Ă-dĭ-pōs) tissue - Type of connective tissue that stores fat.

Adrenal gland - Endocrine gland that consists of an outer cortex and inner medulla. The cortex secretes steroids and the medulla secretes catecholamines.

Adrenergic fiber - A neuron that secretes norepinephrine (noradrenalin) as its neurotransmitter

Aerobic catabolism (ăr-Ō-bĭk kă-TĂB-ŏ-lĭzm) - Chemical reactions that break down complex substances into simpler substances in the presence of oxygen.

Aerobic metabolism - Chemical reactions that require oxygen; includes aerobic anabolism and catabolism.

Afferent (ĂF-ĕr-ĕnt) neuron - Carrying toward a center, such as afferent nerves carrying information toward the central nervous system.

Afterload - The force against which the heart contracts, such as the aortic blood pressure.

Agglutination (ă-gloo-tĭ-NĀ-shŭn) - Clumping of cells in response to an antigen-antibody reaction.

Albumin (ăl-BŪ-mĭn) - Plasma protein that helps regulate plasma osmotic pressure, thereby "holding" water within the blood vessels; responsible for the oncotic pressure.

Aldosterone (ăl-DŎS-tĕ-rōn) - Mineralocorticoid (steroid) secreted by the adrenal cortex; stimulates the kidney to reabsorb sodium and water and to excrete potassium.

Alkalosis (ăl-kă-LŌ-sĭs) - Imbalance associated with a decrease in H^+ concentration and an increase in blood pH greater than 7.45; there is a respiratory alkalosis and metabolic alkalosis.

Allergen (ĂL-ĕr-jĕn) - Foreign substance or antigen that stimulates an allergic reaction.

Alveolus (ăl-VĒ-ō-lŭs) (*pl.* alveoli) - Tiny, grapelike sac in the lungs; the site of gas exchange (oxygen and carbon dioxide) between the air and the blood.

Amino acids - Small nitrogen-containing organic compounds; the building blocks of protein.

Amnion (ĂM-nē-ŏn) - Extraembryonic membrane that surrounds the fetus and contains amniotic fluid.

Amylase (ĂM-ĭ-lās) - Enzyme that digests carbohydrates.

Anabolism (ă-NĂB-ŏ-lĭzm) - Metabolic reactions that build complex substances from simpler substances.

Anaerobic catabolism (ăn-ăr-Ō-bĭk kă-TĂB-ŏ-lĭzm) - Chemical reactions that break down complex substances into simpler substances, without the presence of oxygen.

Anaerobic (ăn-ăr-Ō-bĭk) metabolism - Chemical reactions that do not require oxygen.

Anastomosis (ă-năs-tō-MŌ-sĭs) - A connection between two tubular structures.

Anatomical position - Position of the body; the body is standing erect with the face forward and the arms at the side (palms and toes face in a forward direction).

Anatomy - Study of the structure of the body.

Anemia - Condition characterized by abnormally low amounts of hemoglobin or low numbers of red blood cells.

Angiotensin (ăn-jē-ō-TĔN-sĭn) - Blood pressure–elevating hormone produced by the action of renin on angiotensinogen.

Anion (ĂN-ī-ŏn) - Negatively charged ion.

Antagonist - A muscle that opposes another muscle.

Antibody - Substance that reacts with a specific antigen.

Antibody-mediated immunity - A type of immunity engaged in by the B lymphocyte. The B cell secretes antibodies that attack the antigen; also called humoral immunity.

Antidiuretic hormone (ADH) - Posterior pituitary hormone that stimulates the collecting duct in the kidney to reabsorb water and decrease urinary output.

Antigen (ĂN-tĭ-jĕn) - Foreign substance that stimulates the production of antibodies.

Aorta (ā-ŌR-tă) - Large artery that conducts blood from the left ventricle of the heart.

Apocrine (ĂP-ŏ-krĭn) gland - One of the sudoriferous (sweat) glands.

Aponeurosis (ăp-ō-nū-RŌ-sĭs) - Broad, flat sheet of fibrous connective tissue that connects muscle to another structure.

Appendicular skeleton - Part of the skeleton that includes the bones of the upper extremities, the lower extremities, the pelvic girdle, and the pectoral girdle.

Appendix - Worm-shaped outpouching of the wall of the cecum.

Areolar (ă-RĒ-ō-lăr) tissue - Loose connective tissue.

Arteriole (ăr-TĒ-rē-ōl) - Small artery that is composed largely of smooth muscle and is found between the larger artery and the capillaries; also called resistance vessel.

Artery - Blood vessel that carries blood away from the heart.

Articulation - Joining of structures at a joint.

Artificially acquired immunity - Immunity that is acquired through the use of such agents as vaccines, toxoids, and immunoglobulins.

Atom - Fundamental unit of an element; the smallest part of the element that has the characteristics of that element.

ATP - See *Adenosine triphosphate.*

Atrium (*pl.* atria) - Upper chamber of the heart that receives blood from veins.

Atrophy (ĂT-rŏ-fē) - A wasting or a decrease in the size of an organ or tissue, usually referring to a muscle.

Autoimmunity (ăw-tō-ĭ-MŪN-ĭ-tē) - Immunity against one's own tissue.

Autonomic nervous system - Involuntary or automatic nervous system that controls the organs, glands, cardiac muscle, and smooth muscle; two divisions, the sympathetic and parasympathetic nervous systems.

Axial skeleton - The part of the skeleton that includes the skull, vertebral column, ribs, and sternum.

Axon (ĂKs-ŏn) - Elongated part of the neuron that conducts nerve impulses away from the cell body.

Bacteria - Single-cell organisms that are classified as cocci, bacilli, and curved rods.

Baroreceptor (BĂR-ō-rĕ-SĔP-tŏr) - Receptor that detects or senses changes in blood pressure; located in the carotid sinus and aortic arch.

Baroreceptor (BĂR-ō-rĕ-SĔP-tŏr) reflex - An autonomic reflex that responds to a sudden change in blood pressure.

Basal metabolic rate (BMR) - The rate at which cells metabolize (use oxygen) in a resting state.

Base - Substance such as the hydroxyl ion (OH^-) that combines with hydrogen ion (H^+).

Base-pairing - Pairing of the bases of the nucleotides; adenine and thymine (DNA), guanine and cytosine (DNA and RNA), and adenine and uracil (RNA).

Base-sequencing - Sequence or arrangement of the bases in a strand of DNA or RNA.

Basophil (BĀ-sō-fĭl) - Type of granular leukocyte; stains blue.

B cell - B lymphocyte; secretes antibodies.

Belly - The thick part of a skeletal muscle between its origin and insertion.

Beta-adrenergic receptor - A type of receptor that is activated by norepinephrine.

Bicuspid (bī-KŬS-pĭd) valve - The atrioventricular valve between the left atrium and the left ventricle; also called the mitral valve.

Bile - A digestive aid secreted by the liver; it emulsifies fats.

Biliary (BĬL-ē-ăr-ē) tree - Arrangement of ducts that transports bile from the liver to the gallbladder and duodenum; includes hepatic ducts, cystic duct, and common bile duct.

Bilirubin (bĭl-ĭ-ROO-bĭn) - Pigment produced from the breakdown of hemoglobin and secreted into the bile; an accumulation of bilirubin in the skin causes jaundice.

Blastocyst - Early preembryonic cluster of cells with a hollow interior.

Blood pressure - The force that the blood exerts against the vessel wall.

Bowman's capsule - C-shaped tubular structure that partially surrounds the glomerulus. Water and dissolved substances are filtered from the glomerulus into the Bowman's capsule.

Brain stem - Lower part of the brain that connects the brain with the spinal cord; consists of the midbrain, pons, and medulla oblongata.

Breast - Elevation on the anterior chest that contains mammary glands.

Bronchioles (BRŎNG-kē-ōlz) - Small airway tubes in the respiratory tract; composed largely of smooth muscle.

Bronchus (*pl.* bronchi) - Large airway in the lungs that connects the trachea and the bronchioles; there is a right and left bronchus.

Buffer - Substance that resists changes in pH. A buffer can remove or add H^+, thereby adjusting pH.

Calyces (KĀ-lĭ-sēz) - Cuplike structures that collect urine from the collecting ducts of the nephron units.

Capacitance (kă-PĂS-ĭ-tăns) vessels - Storage vessels for blood; refers to veins.

Capillary - Smallest and most numerous of the blood vessels; site of exchange of nutrients and waste between the blood and tissue fluid.

Carbaminohemoglobin (căr-BAM-ē-nō-HĒ-mō-glō-bĭn) - Hemoglobin that has combined with carbon dioxide.

Carbohydrates - Types of organic compounds including simple sugars, starch, and glycogen; primary source of energy.

Carbon dioxide (CO_2) - The waste product of cellular metabolism.

Cardiac conduction system - Cardiac cells that have specialized to create and conduct the cardiac action potential; includes the SA node, AV node, and the His-Purkinje system.

Cardiac cycle - Events that occur in the heart during one heartbeat.

Cardiac muscle - Type of muscle found in the heart; the myocardium.

Cardiac output - Amount of blood pumped by the heart in one minute; about 5000 ml per minute.

Cardiac reserve - The potential increase in cardiac output above resting cardiac output.

Cardiology - The study of the heart.

Carrier - A living organism that harbors a pathogen and acts as a source of infection.

Catabolism (kă-TĂB-ŏ-lĭzm) - Metabolic breakdown of complex molecules into simpler molecules; the breakdown is accompanied by the release of energy.

Catalyst (KĂT-ă-lĭst) - Any substance that speeds up the rate of a chemical reaction; see *Enzyme*.

Catecholamine (kăt-ĕ-KŌL-ă-mēn) - Classification of hormones that is secreted by the adrenal medulla; includes epinephrine (adrenalin) and norepinephrine.

Cation (KĂT-ī-ŏn) - Positively charged ion.

Cecum (SĒ-kŭm) - Part of the large intestine that connects the ileum of the small intestine and the ascending colon of the large intestine.

Cell - Basic unit of life; the structural and functional unit of a living organism.

Cell cycle - The phases that a cell goes through as it divides.

Cell-mediated immunity - Type of immunity engaged in by the T cell; cell-to-cell combat.

Cell membrane - Membrane that surrounds the cell and regulates what enters and leaves the cell; also called the plasma membrane.

Cerebellum (sĕr-ĕ-BĔL-ŭm) - Part of the brain that is located under the cerebrum; it coordinates skeletal muscle activity.

Cerebrospinal fluid - Cushioning fluid that circulates within the subarachnoid space around the brain and the spinal cord.

Cerebrum (sĕ-RĒ-brŭm) - Largest and uppermost part of the brain, it is divided into two cerebral hemispheres. There are four lobes: frontal, parietal, temporal, and occipital.

Ceruminous (sĭ-RŪ-mĭ-nŭs) gland - Modified sweat gland found in the external ear canal; it secretes cerumen, or earwax.

Cervix - Constricted portion of an organ, usually referring to the lower portion of the uterus.

Chemoreceptor (KĒ-mō-rē-SĔP-tŏr) - Receptor that detects changes in the chemical composition of a substance.

Cholinergic (kō-lə-NŬR-jĭk) fiber - A neuron that secretes acetylcholine (ACh) as its neurotransmitter.

Chondrocyte (KŎN-drō-sīt) - A cartilage-forming cell.

Chordae tendineae (KŎR-dē tĕn-DĬN-ē-ē) - Tough fibrous bands of connective tissue that attach the cuspid valves to the walls of the ventricles of the heart.

Chorion (KŎR-ē-ŏn) - The outermost extraembryonic membrane surrounding the fetus; it helps form the placenta.

Chromosome - Coiled, threadlike structures that contain segments of DNA called genes.

Chronotropic (KRŎN-ə-trōp-ik) effect - A change in heart rate (HR). A (+) chronotropic effect is an increase HR, while a (−) chronotropic effect is a decrease in HR.

Chyle (kīl) - Milky fluid found in the lacteals of the villi; consists of emulsified fats and lymph.

Chyme (kīm) - Pastelike mixture of partially digested food, water, and digestive enzymes that is formed in the stomach.

Cilia (SĬL-ē-ă) (*s.* cilium) - Hairlike processes on the surface of many cells.

Clone - A group of cells that come from a single cell and are therefore genetically identical.

Coagulation - Clotting of blood.

Cochlea (KŎK-lē-ă) - Part of the inner ear that contains the organ of Corti, the receptors for hearing.

Collecting duct - The nephron structure that receives urine from the distal tubule and delivers it to the renal pelvis.

Colon (KŌ-lŏn) - Major portion of the large intestine that extends from the cecum to the rectum.

Columnar epithelium - Type of epithelium that has column-shaped cells.

Communicable disease - A disease that can be spread from one host to another.

Complement (KŎM-plĕ-mĕnt) proteins - Group of proteins in the blood that are concerned with phagocytosis.

Compound - Substance composed of two or more chemical elements, such as water (H_2O).

Conductance (kŏn-DŬK-tăns) vessels - Blood vessels that are primarily concerned with carrying blood to smaller blood vessels; functional name for arteries.

Conduction - Loss of heat energy as it is transferred from the warm body to a cooler object such as a cooling blanket.

Congenital (kŏn-JĔN-ĭ-tăl) - Present at birth.

Connective tissue - One of the four basic types of tissues that generally holds and supports body structures.

Contracture (kŏn-TRĂK-shŭr) - An abnormal formation of fibrous tissue within a muscle, causing it to freeze in a flexed position.

Convection - Loss of heat energy to the surrounding cooler air. The layer of heated air next to the body is constantly being removed by a fan (or breeze) and replaced by cooler air.

Cornea - Clear portion of the sclera that covers the anterior portion of the eye.

Corpus luteum (KŎR-pŭs LŪ-tē-ŭm) - Yellow body formed from the ovarian follicle after ovulation; it secretes large amounts of progesterone and smaller amounts of estrogen.

Covalent (Kō-VĀ-lĕnt) bond - Bond or attraction formed by the sharing of electrons between atoms.

Cranial cavity - Part of the dorsal cavity that contains the brain.

Cranial nerves - The 12 pairs of nerves that emerge from the brain.

Craniosacral (krā-nē-ō-SĀ-krəl) outflow - Parasympathetic activity.

Creatinine (krē-ĂT-ĭ-nēn) - A waste product that is excreted by the kidney.

Cuboidal epithelium (kyū-BOID-ăl ĕp-ĭ-THĒL-ē-ŭm) - Type of epithelium that has cells shaped like cubes.

Cutaneous (kū-TĀN-ē-ŭs) membrane - Skin.

Cytoplasm (CĪ-tō-plăzm) - Gel-like substance surrounded by the cell membrane but outside of the nucleus.

Dehydration - State in which there is a deficiency in body water.

Dendrite (DĔN-drīt) - Treelike process of the neuron that receives the stimulus and carries it toward the cell body.

Deoxyribonucleic (dē-ŎK-sē-rī-bō-nū-KLĒ-ĭk) acid (DNA) - Nucleotide that stores the genetic information of the organism.

Depolarization (dē-pōl-ăr-ĭ-ZĀ-shŭn) - Change in the membrane potential across the cell membrane with the inside of the cell becoming less negative or less polarized.

Dermatome (DĔR-mă-tōm) - Area of the body that is supplied by a spinal nerve.

Dermis - Thick layer of dense connective tissue that lies under the epidermis of the skin.

Detrusor (dē-TROO-sĕr) muscle - Smooth muscle located in the urinary bladder.

Dialysis (dī-ĂL-ĭsĭs) - A passive transport process that allows small particles to diffuse through a semipermeable membrane.

Diaphragm (DĪ-ă-frăm) - Dome-shaped skeletal muscle that separates the thoracic and abdominal cavities; it is the chief muscle of inspiration (inhalation).

Diaphysis (dī-ĂF-ĭ-sĭs) - Shaft of a long bone.

Diastole (dī-ĂS-tō-lē) - Relaxation phase of the cardiac cycle.

Diastolic (dī-ə-STŎL-ĭk) blood pressure - Blood pressure in the large arteries when the heart is resting (diastole); the bottom number of a blood pressure reading.

Differentiation (dĭf-ĕr-ĔN-shē-ā-shŭn) - Process whereby a cell becomes specialized.

Diffusion - Passive transport process that causes movement of a substance from an area of high concentration to an area of low concentration.

Digestion - Process of breaking down food into absorbable particles.

Disease - Failure of the body to function normally.

Diuresis (dī-ŭr-RĒ-sĭs) - Increased excretion of urine.

Dominant gene - Gene whose trait is expressed.

Dorsal cavity - Body cavity that is located toward the back part of the body; divided into the cranial cavity and the spinal cavity.

Dorsal root - Sensory nerve of a spinal nerve as it attaches to the spinal cord.

Duodenum (dŭ-ō-DĒ-nŭm) - First part of the small intestine.

Eccrine (ĔK-krĭn) gland - Type of sweat gland that secretes a watery substance; plays an important role in the regulation of body temperature.

Edema (ĕ-DĒ-mă) - Abnormal collection of fluid, usually causing swelling.

Efferent (ĔF-ĕr-ĕnt) - Movement away from a central point, such as a motor neuron that carries information away from the central nervous system.

Efferent neuron (ĔF-ĕr-ĕnt) - A motor neuron; brings information from the CNS to the periphery.

Electrocardiogram (ECG) (ĕ-LĔK-trō-KĂR-dē-ō-grăm) - Graphic recording of the electrical events that occur during the cardiac cycle.

Electrolyte (ĕ-LĔK-trŏ-līt) - Compound that dissociates into ions when dissolved in water.

Electrolyte (ĕ-LĔK-trŏ-līt) balance - Having normal amounts of electrolytes in each fluid compartment.

Element - Substance composed of only one kind of atom.

Embryo (ĔM-brē-ō) - The developing human between the gestational ages of 2 and 8 weeks.

Emulsification (ī-mŭl-sə-fī-KĀ-shən) - The physical breakdown of a large fat globule into many smaller fat globules.

Endocardium (ĕn-dō-KĂR-dē-ŭm) - Inner lining of the heart wall.

Endocrine (ĔN-dŏ-krĭn) gland - Ductless gland that secretes hormones, usually into the blood.

Endocytosis (ĔN-dō-cī-TŌ-sĭs) - Uptake of material through the cell membrane by forming a vesicle; includes pinocytosis and phagocytosis.

Endometrium (ĕn-dō-MĒ-trē-ŭm) - Inner mucous membrane lining of the uterus.

Endoplasmic reticulum (ER) (ĕn-dō-PLĂs-mĭk rĕ-TĬK-ū-lŭm) - Intracellular membrane system that is concerned with the synthesis and transportation of protein; called the rough ER if ribosomes are attached; called the smooth ER if there are no ribosomes.

Energy - Ability to perform work.

Enzyme - Organic catalyst; it speeds up the rate of a chemical reaction.

Eosinophil (ē-ō-SĬN-ō-fĭl) - Type of granular leukocyte; stains red.

Epicardium (ĕp-ĭ-KĂR-dē-ŭm) - Outer layer of the heart; forms part of the pericardium.

Epidermis (ĕp-ĭ-DĔR-mĭs) - Outer epithelial layer of the skin.

Epididymis (ĕp-ĭ-DĬD-ĭ-mĭs) - Coiled tube that carries sperm from the testis to the vas deferens.

Epiglottis (ĕp-ĭ-GLŎT-ĭs) - Cartilage that guards the opening into the larynx; directs food and water into the esophagus.

Epiphysis (ĕ-PĬF-ĭ-sĭs) - End of a long bone.

Epithelial (ĕp-ĭ-THĒL-ē-ăl) tissue - One of the four types of tissues; found on the surface of the body (skin) and lining the body cavities; it also forms glands.

Equilibrium - Balance.

Erythrocyte (ĕ-RĬTH-rō-sīt) - Red blood cell.

Erythropoietin (ĕ-rĭth-rō-PŌ-ĕ-tĭn) - Hormone secreted by the kidneys that stimulates the bone marrow to produce red blood cells.

Esophagus (ĕ-SŎF-ă-gŭs) - The tubelike structure that connects the pharynx to the stomach; the food tube.

Estrogen (ĔS-trō-jĕn) - Female sex hormone secreted by the developing ovarian follicle.

Eustachian (ū-STĀ-shŭn) tube - Tube that connects the pharynx with the middle ear; also called the auditory tube.

Evaporation - Loss of heat as water changes from the liquid to the vapor or gas state.

Exchange vessel - See *Capillaries*.

Exhalation - Process of moving air out of the lungs; the breathing-out phase of ventilation; also called expiration.

Exocrine (ĕx-ŏ-krĭn) gland - Type of gland that secretes its products into ducts that open onto a surface.

Exocytosis (ĕx-ō-cī-TŌ-sĭs) - Elimination of material from a cell through the formation of vesicles.

Extension - Increase in the angle of a joint.

Extracellular fluid - Fluid that is located outside of the cell, such as the plasma and interstitial fluid.

Facilitated diffusion - Process by which a substance moves with the assistance of a carrier molecule from an area of high concentration to an area of low concentration.

Fallopian (fă-LŌ-pē-ăn) tube - Passageway through which the egg or zygote moves from the ovary to the uterus; also called the oviduct or uterine tube.

Fascia (FĂSH-ē-ă) - Fibrous connective tissue membrane that covers individual skeletal muscles or certain organs.

Fertilization - Union of an ovum and a sperm to form a zygote; also called conception.

Fetus - Name given to the developing human at the end of the embryonic period; from the end of the 8th week of pregnancy to birth.

Fibrin (FĪ-brĭn) - Protein strands formed by the action of thrombin on fibrinogen; the clot.

Filtration - Process by which water and dissolved substances move through a membrane in response to pressure.

Flexion - Decrease in the angle of a joint; a bending movement.

Fontanel (fŏn-tă-NĔL) - Membranous gap between the cranial bones of an infant's skull.

Frontal lobe - Anterior portion of the cerebrum that controls voluntary skeletal activity and plays an important role in emotions, critical thinking, and ethical decision making.

Frontal plane - Vertical plane that divides the body into front (anterior) and back (posterior parts); the coronal plane.

Fungus - Plantlike organisms such as mushrooms; cause mycotic infections.

Gene - Part of the chromosome that codes for a specific trait; the biologic unit of heredity.

Glomerular (glō-MĔR-ū-lăr) filtration - The filtration (pushing) of water and dissolved solute across the glomerular membrane. The rate of glomerular filtration is called the glomerular filtration rate (GFR).

Glomerulus (glō-MĔR-ū-lŭs) - Tuft of capillaries located within the Bowman's capsule of the nephron unit of the kidney.

Glottis (GLŎT-ĭs) - Opening between the vocal cords; an air passage for the respiratory tract.

Gluconeogenesis (glōō-kə-nē-ə-JĔN-ĭ-sĭs) - Biochemical process that makes glucose from nonglucose substances, especially protein.

Glucose - A monosaccharide, or simple sugar, that serves as the principal fuel for the cells of the body.

Glycogen (GLĪ-kō-jĕn) - Polysaccharide that is the storage form of glucose; also called animal starch.

Glycolysis (glī-kŏl-Ĭ-sĭs) - Anaerobic catabolism of glucose into lactic acid.

Golgi (GŌL-jē) apparatus - Membranous organelle that is concerned with the final trimming and packaging of protein for exocytosis.

Gonad (GŌ-năd) - Organ that produces gametes (ova or sperm); term for ovaries and testes.

Gonadotropin (gō-nă-dō-TRŌ-pĭn) - Hormone "aimed at" the gonads; includes follicle-stimulating hormone (FSH), luteinizing hormone (LH), and human chorionic gonadotropin (hCG).

Graafian (GRÄ-fē-ən) follicle - Mature ovarian follicle.

Gray matter - Part of the central nervous system that is composed of cell bodies and unmyelinated fibers.

Haversian (hă-VĔR-shăn) system - Structural unit of compact bone; bone is layered in concentric circles around an osteonic canal; an osteon.

Helminth (HĔL-mĭnth) - Parasitic worm.

Hematocrit (hē-MĂT-Ăō-krĭt) - Laboratory test that expresses the percentage of red blood cells present in a volume of blood.

Hematopoiesis (hē-măt-ō-poi-Ē-sĭs) - Production of blood cells.

Hemoglobin (HĒ-mō-GLŌ-bĭn) - Iron-containing protein in the red blood cell that has the ability to take up and release oxygen; also transports carbon dioxide.

Hemolysis (hē-MOL-ĭ-sĭs) - Break down of erythrocytes.

Hemostasis (hē-mō-STĀ-sĭs) - The stopping of blood loss.

Homeostasis (hō-mē-ō-STĀ-sĭs) - Ability of the body to maintain a constant internal environment.

Hormone - Substance secreted by an endocrine gland into the blood.

Human chorionic gonadotropin (kŏr-rē-ŎN-ĭk gō-nă-dō-TRŌ-pĭn) - Hormone secreted by the trophoblastic cells; maintains the corpus luteum until the placenta can take over its glandular function.

Hydrogen bond - Weak intermolecular bond formed between hydrogen and a negatively charged atom such as oxygen or nitrogen.

Hyperkalemia (hī-pĕr-kă-LĒ-mē-ă) - Abnormally high blood potassium level.

Hypertension - Blood pressure that is higher than normal.

Hypertonic (hī-pĕr-TŎN-ĭk) - Having a solute concentration greater than a reference solution.

Hypertrophy (hī-PĔR-trŏ-fē) - Increase in the size of a body part, usually referring to a muscle.

Hyperventilation (hī-pĕr-vĕn-tĭ-LĀ-shŭn) - Abnormally rapid, deep breathing.

Hypokalemia (hī-pō-kă-LĒ-mē-ă) - A lower than normal amount of potassium in the blood.

Hypophysis (hī-PŎF-ĭ-sĭs) - Pituitary gland.

Hypotension - Blood pressure that is lower than normal.

Hypothalamus (hī-pō-THĂL-ă-mŭs) - Part of the diencephalon (below the thalamus) that regulates the pituitary gland, the autonomic nervous system, water balance, appetite, temperature, and the emotions.

Hypotonic (hī-pō-TŎN-ĭk) - Having a solute concentration less than a reference solution.

Hypoventilation (hī-pō-vĕn-tĭ-LĀ-shŭn) - Abnormally slow and/or shallow respiratory rate.

Ileum (ĬL-ē-ŭm) - Distal end of the small intestine.

Immunity - Ability to resist and overcome injury by pathogens or antigenic substances.

Immunoglobulin (ĭm-ū-nō-GLŎB-ū-lĭn) - Antibodies produced by plasma cells in response to antigenic stimulation.

Infection - Disease caused by a pathogen.

Inflammation - Body's response to infection or injury; characterized by redness, heat, swelling, and pain.

Inhalation - Process of moving air into the lungs; the breathing-in phase of ventilation. Also called inspiration.

Inotropic (ĭn-ō-TRŌ-pĭk) effect - A change in the strength or force of myocardial contraction that does not involve stretching the myocardial fibers.

Insertion - The more movable attachment point of a muscle to a bone.

Intake - Amount of fluid taken into the body.

Integumentary (ĭn-tĕg-ū-MĔN-tăr-ē) system - Organ system that consists of the skin and the accessory organs.

Intercellular - Between the cells.

Interferons (ĭn-tĕr-FĒR-ŏnz) - Substances produced by a virus-infected cell; the substance protects other cells from viral infection.

Interneuron - An association neuron; links the sensory and motor neurons in the central nervous system.

Interstitial (ĭn-tĕr-STĬSH-ăl) fluid - Fluid located between the cells; tissue fluid.

Intracellular fluid - Fluid located within cells.

Intrapleural (ĭn-tră-PLOOR-ăl) pressure - The pressure within the intrapleural space; must be negative in order for the lungs to be expanded.

Ion (Ī-On) - An electrically charged atom or group of atoms; either cations or anions.

Ionic (ī-ŎN-ĭk) bond - Bond formed by the exchange of electrons between atoms.

Ischemia (ĭ-SKĒ-mē-ə) - Insufficient blood flow to a tissue, sometimes resulting in tissue damage and death.

Isotonic (ī-sō-TŎN-ĭk) - Having the same concentration as the reference solution.

Isotope (Ī-sŏ-tōp) - Element that has the same number of protons and electrons but a different number of neutrons.

Jaundice (JĂWN-dĭs) - Yellow coloring of the skin and "whites" of the eyes caused by an increase in bilirubin in the blood.

Jejunum (jĕ-JOO-nŭm) - Second or middle part of the small intestine.

Joint - Union of two or more bones; an articulation.

Karyotype (KĂR-ē-ō-tīp) - Arrangement of the chromosomes by pairs in a fixed order.

Keratin (KĔR-ă-tĭn) - A protein found in the skin, hair, and nails; it hardens the cells and makes them water-resistent.

Ketone bodies - Products of faulty fatty acid catabolism; includes acetone, acetoacetic acid, and beta hydroxybutyric acid.

Kidney - Organ of the urinary system that produces urine.

Kussmaul (KOOS-mŭl) respirations - Increase in the rate and depth of respirations in order to correct a metabolic acidosis.

Lacrimal (LĂK-rĭ-măl) gland - Gland that secretes tears.

Lacteal (LĂK-tē-ăl) - Lymph vessel in a villus of the small intestine.

Larynx (LĂR-ĭnks) - Structure that contains the vocal cords; voice box.

Leukocyte (LOO-kō-sīt) - White blood cell; it functions primarily to defend the body against infection.

Ligament - Strong band of connective tissue that joins bone to bone.

Limbic system (LĬM-bĭk) - The emotional brain.

Lipase - Enzyme that digests fats into fatty acids and glycerol.

Lipid - Organic molecule that includes fats, oils, and steroids.

Loop of Henle (HĔN-lē) - A hairpin looped tubular structure of the nephron unit that receives urine from the proximal tubule and delivers it to the distal tubule.

Lymph (lĭmf) - Fluid that has the same composition as tissue fluid and is carried by the lymph vessels.

Lymph node - Mass of lymphoid tissue located along the course of a lymphatic vessel.

Lymphatic duct - Large tube or vessel that carries lymph, such as the thoracic duct; same as lymphatic vessel.

Lymphatic vessels - The tubes through which lymph flows.

Lymphocyte (LĬM-fō-sīt) - Agranular leukocyte. There are T and B lymphocytes.

Lysosome (LĪ-sō-sōmz) - Organelle that contains powerful enzymes; engages in phagocytosis and does the "intracellular housecleaning."

Macrophage (MĂK-rō-fāj) - Enlarged monocyte that eats foreign material; a "big eater."

Mammary (MĂM-ŏr-ē) gland - Gland of the female breast that secretes milk.

Matter - Anything that occupies space; may occur as solid, liquid, or gas.

Mechanoreceptor (mĕ-KĂN-ō-rĕ-SĔP-tŏr) - Receptor that is stimulated by bending, pressing, or pushing.

Mediastinum (mē-dē-ă-STĪ-nŭm) - Space between the lungs that contains the heart, trachea, thymus gland, esophagus, and large blood vessels.

Medulla oblongata (mĕ-DŪL-ă ŏb-lŏn-GĂ-tă) - Part of the brain stem that controls vital functions such as respiratory and cardiovascular function.

Meiosis (mī-Ō-sĭs) - Type of cell division used by the sex cells to reduce the number of chromosomes in each from 46 to 23.

Melanin (MĔL-ă-nĭn) - Pigment that is responsible for the color of the skin and hair.

Melanocyte (MĔL-ă-nō-sīt) - Melanin-producing cell.

Meninges (mĕ-NĬN-jēz) - Membranes that cover the brain and spinal cord and include the dura mater, arachnoid mater, and pia mater.

Menopause - Normal developmental stage in women that marks the end of the ovarian and uterine cycles.

Menses (MĔN-sēz) - Menstruation; the monthly discharge of blood from the uterus.

Metabolic acidosis - A condition in which blood pH decreases below 7.35; the cause is nonrespiratory.

Metabolic alkalosis - A condition in which blood pH increases above 7.45; the cause is nonrespiratory.

Metabolism - All the chemical reactions that occur within the cells; consists of anabolism and catabolism.

Micturition (mĭk-chə-RĬSH-ən) - Urination.

Milk let-down reflex - An oxytocin-mediated reflex that results in the release of milk from the breast in response to suckling.

Mineral - Inorganic substance such as sodium or potassium.

Mitochondria (mī-tō-KŎN-drē-ă) - Organelles that produce most of the ATP; the "powerplants" of the cell.

Mitosis (mī-TŌ-sĭs) - Type of cell division that produces two identical daughter cells, each containing 46 chromosomes.

Mitral (MĪ-trăl) valve - See *Bicuspid valve*.

Mixed nerve - Nerve that contains both sensory and motor fibers.

Mixture - Combination of two or more substances that can be separated by ordinary physical means.

Molecule - Chemical combination of two or more atoms.

Monocyte (MŎN-ō-sīt) - Agranular phagocytic leukocyte that can become a macrophage.

Monosaccharide (mŏn-ō-SĂK-ă-rīd) - A simple sugar consisting of hexoses (glucose, fructose, galactose) or pentoses (ribose, deoxyribose).

Morphology - Structure of the body.

Motor nerve - Collection of motor neurons that carries information away from the central nervous system.

Mucous membrane - Type of membrane that lines the cavities and tubes that open to the exterior of the body.

Muscarinic (mŭs-kə-RĬN-ĭk) receptor - Cholinergic receptor that is activated by acetylcholine; located primarily on the target organs of the parasympathetic nerves.

Muscle tissue - Type of tissue that contains the contractile proteins, actin and myosin; three types of muscle are smooth, skeletal, and cardiac.

Myelin (MĪ-ĕ-lĭn) - White, fatty material that covers some nerve fibers.

Myocardium - Heart muscle.

Myometrium (mī-ō-MĒ-trē-ŭm) - Muscle layer of the uterus that contracts and causes the delivery of the infant.

Myosin (MĪ-Ō-sĭn) - Muscle protein that interacts with actin to cause muscle contraction; also called the thick filament.

Naturally acquired immunity - Immunity that is acquired through natural means, such as getting a disease or receiving antibodies from your mother.

Negative feedback - A mechanism that is activated by an imbalance; activation of the mechanism then corrects the imbalance.

Nephron unit - Structural and functional unit of the kidney that makes urine.

Nerve - Bundle of nerve fibers and blood vessels.

Nerve impulse - Action potential that occurs in neurons.

Nerve tract - Group of neurons that share a common function within the central nervous system; may be ascending (sensory) or descending (motor).

Nervous tissue - A type of tissue that includes neurons and neuroglia.

Neuroglia (nū-rō-GLĒ-ă) - Nerve cells that support, protect, and nourish the neurons.

Neurohypophysis (nū-rō-hī-PŎF-ĭ-sĭs) - The posterior pituitary gland; secretes oxytocin and antidiuretic hormone.

Neuromuscular junction - Junction or space that occurs between a motor neuron and a muscle fiber.

Neuron - Nerve cell that conducts the action potential (nerve impulse).

Neurotransmitters (nū-rō-trăns-MĬ-tĕrs) - Chemical made within the axon terminal that is responsible for transmission of the signal across the synapse or junction.

Neutrophil (NŪ-trō-fĭl) - Granular, motile, and highly phagocytic leukocyte.

Nicotinic receptor - A type of cholinergic receptor that is activated by acetylcholine; located in the autonomic ganglia and within the neuromuscular junction.

Nociceptor (nō-sĭ-SĔP-tŏr) - Pain receptor.

Norepinephrine - A neurotransmitter secreted by the adrenergic fibers of the sympathetic nervous system; activates adrenergic receptors.

Normal flora - A population of microorganisms that normally inhabit an area such as the skin, intestines, or vagina.

Nosocomial (nō-sō-KŌ-mē-ăl) infection - Hospital-acquired infection.

Nucleus (*pl.* nuclei) - Large organelle separated from the cytoplasm by a nuclear membrane; stores the DNA in chromosomes and acts as the control center of the cell.

Occipital (ŏk-SĬP-ĭ-tăl) lobe - Cerebral lobe located in the back of the head; concerned primarily with vision.

Olfactory (ŏl-FĂK-tĕr-ē) receptor - Chemoreceptor associated with the sense of smell.

Oliguria (ŏl-ĭ-GŪ-rē-ă) - Scanty urine formation.

Oncotic pressure - The part of the osmotic pressure of the blood that is due to the plasma proteins.

Optic chiasm (KĪ-azm) - Site for the crossing of the medial fibers of the optic nerve to the opposite side of the brain; located in front of the pituitary gland.

Organ - Group of tissues that performs a specialized function, such as the lungs.

Organelle (ŏr-gă-NĔL) - Part of the cell that performs a specialized function, such as the energy-producing mitochondrion.

Organic compound - Carbon-containing substance.

Organ of Corti (KŎR-tē) - Hearing receptors (mechanoreceptors) located in the inner ear.

Organ system - Group of organs that perform a particular function, such as the organs of digestion.

Origin - Part of the muscle that is attached to the more immovable structure.

Osmosis (ŏz-MŌ-sĭs) - Movement of water across a membrane from an area where there is more water to an area where there is less water.

Osseous (ŎS-ē-ŭs) tissue - Bone tissue.

Ossicles (ŎS-ĭ-k'lz) - Tiny bones found in the middle ear.

Osteoblast - Bone-building cell.

Osteoclast - Cell that causes the breakdown of bone.

Output - Amount of fluid that is eliminated from the body.

Ovarian follicle - Ovarian structure that releases an egg at maturation; graafian follicle.

Ovulation - Discharge of the mature ovum from the graafian follicle.

Oxyhemoglobin (ŏks-ē-HĒ-mō-glō-bĭn) - Hemoglobin that contains oxygen.

Pain receptor - Nociceptor; free nerve endings that sense pain.

Pancreas (PĂN-krē-ăs) - Organ that has both endocrine and exocrine functions. The islets of Langerhans secrete the hormones insulin and glucagon. The exocrine glands secrete the most important of the digestive enzymes.

Parasite - An organism that requires another living organism for its growth and survival.

Parasympathetic (păr-ă-sĭm-pă-THĔT-ĭk) nervous system - Division of the autonomic nervous system that is concerned with "feeding and breeding."

Parathyroid (păr-ă-THĪ-royd) gland - Gland that secretes parathyroid hormone (PTH) and helps regulate calcium balance.

Parietal (pă-RĪ-ĕ-tăl) - Pertaining to the wall of a cavity, as in the parietal pleura that lines the wall of the thoracic cavity.

Parietal (pă-RĪ-ĕ-tăl) lobe - Lobe of the cerebrum that is concerned primarily with somatosensory function.

Partial pressure - Pressure exerted by one gas in a gas mixture.

Passive immunity - Short-acting immunity achieved when the person is given antibodies made by another animal.

Passive transport - Transport process that requires no additional energy in the form of ATP.

Pathogen - Disease-causing organism.

Pectoral girdle - Portion of the skeleton that supports and attaches to the upper extremities.

Pelvic girdle - Portion of the skeleton to which the lower extremities are attached.

Peptide bond - Bond formed between two amino acids.

Pericardium (pĕr-ĭ-KĂR-dē-ŭm) - Slinglike serous membrane that partially encloses the heart; supports the weight of the heart.

Perineum (pĕ-rĭ-NĒ-ŭm) - Pelvic floor; extends from the anus to the vulva in the female and from the anus to the scrotum in the male.

Periosteum (pĕr-ē-ŎS-tē-ŭm) - Fibrous connective tissue that covers the surface of a long bone.

Peripheral nervous system - Nerves and ganglia that lie outside the central nervous system.

Peristalsis (pĕr-ĭ-STĂL-sĭs) - Rhythmic contraction of smooth muscle that propels a substance forward; peristalsis in the digestive tract moves food from the esophagus toward the anus.

Peritoneum (pĕ-rĭ-tō-NĒ-ŭm) - Serous membrane located in the abdominal cavity; there is a parietal peritoneum and a visceral peritoneum.

pH - A measure of the hydrogen ion concentration.

Phagocytosis (fă-gō-sī-TŌ-sĭs) - Eating of pathogens or cellular debris.

Pharynx (FĂR-ĭnks) - The throat.

Photoreceptor - Receptor stimulated by light; include the rods and cones of the retina.

Physiology (fĭz-ē ŎL-ĕ-jē) - Study of the functioning of the body.

Pineal (pĭ-NĒ-ăl) gland - Small gland located in the brain; secretes melatonin and is involved in regulating biorhythms.

Placenta (plă-SĔN-tă) - A gland and site of exchange of nutrients, oxygen, and waste between mom and baby-to-be.

Plasma - The yellow liquid portion of blood.

Platelet (PLĀT-lĕt) - A fragment of a megakaryocyte that functions in hemostasis; also called a thrombocyte.

Preload - The degree of ventricular myocardial stretch; end diastolic volume.

Pleura (PLOOR-ă) - Serous membrane located in the thoracic cavity; there is a visceral pleura and a parietal pleura.

Plexus - Network of nerves such as the cervical plexus.

Polysaccharide (pŏl-ē-SĂK-ă-rīd) - Carbohydrate made of more than two simple sugars, such as glycogen.

Precordium (prē-cor-DĒ-əm) - Area of the anterior chest that overlies the heart.

Preganglionic fiber - A neuron that transmits action potentials from the central nervous system to a ganglion.

Postganglionic fiber - A neuron that transmits action potentials from a ganglion to a distal target organ.

Prime mover - The muscle that is most responsible for a particular movement.

Progesterone (prō-JĔS-tĕ-rōn) - Hormone secreted by the corpus luteum of the ovary; it stimulates the growth of the endometrium and helps maintain the pregnancy.

Projection - Process by which the brain causes a sensation to be felt at the point of stimulation.

Proprioception (prō-prē-ō-SĔP-shŭn) - Sensation of movement and position of the body.

Prostaglandins (prŏs-tă-GLĂN-dĭnz) - Group of compounds that are made from fatty acids in cell membranes; they exert powerful hormonelike effects.

Prostate gland - Gland that surrounds the upper portion of the urethra in the male and contributes to the formation of semen.

Protease (PRŌ-tē-ās) - Enzyme that digests protein.

Protein - Large, nitrogen-containing molecule that is composed of many amino acids.

Protozoa (prō-tō-ZŌ-ă) - Single-cell, animal-like microbe, classified as amebas, ciliates, flagellates, and sporozoa.

Pulmonary circulation - Path of blood through vessels that takes unoxygenated blood from the right ventricle to the lungs and oxygenated blood from the lungs to the left atrium.

Pulmonary edema - Abnormal collection of fluid in the lungs causing difficulty in oxygenation of hemoglobin.

Pulse - Vibration of the arteries caused by rhythmic expansion and recoil of the large arteries following contraction of the ventricles.

Purkinje (PŬR-kĭn-jē) fibers - Fast-conducting fibers located in the ventricular walls; conduct the electrical impulses from the bundle of His to the ventricular myocardium.

Pyramidal (pĭ-RĂM-ĭ-dăl) tract - Major motor tract that descends from the precentral gyrus of the frontal lobe to the spinal cord; also called the corticospinal tract.

Radiation - Loss of heat as it leaves a warm object, such as the body, to the surrounding cooler air.

Receptor - Sensory structure that responds to specific stimuli such as light, chemicals, or touch.

Recessive gene - Gene whose trait is not expressed.

Recruitment - Enlistment of additional muscle fibers to increase the force of muscle contraction.

Red blood cell - Blood cell that contains mostly hemoglobin; an erythrocyte.

Referred pain - Pain that feels that it originates in an area other than the part being stimulated.

Reflex - Automatic response (nervous or chemical) to a stimulus.

Reflex arc - A nerve pathway that includes a receptor, sensory neuron, interneuron, motor neuron, and effector organ.

Refraction - Bending of light waves so that they can focus on the retina.

Refractory period - Period during which nervous tissue cannot respond to a second stimulus.

Renal tubule - Tubular part of the nephron unit that helps make and transport urine; consists of Bowman's capsule, proximal convoluted tubule, loop of Henle, distal convoluted tubule, and collecting duct.

Renin (RĒ-nĭn) - Enzyme secreted by the kidneys that causes the activation of angiotensinogen.

Repolarization (rē-pō-lăr-ĭ-ZĀ-shŭn) - Return of the membrane potential to its resting state after the nerve impulse.

Resistance vessel - Blood vessel that can change its diameter and therefore determine resistance to the flow of blood; the functional name for the arterioles.

Respiratory acidosis - Increased H^+ concentration (decreased pH) caused by hypoventilation.

Respiratory alkalosis - Decreased H^+ concentration (increased pH) caused by hyperventilation.

Reticular formation - Complex network of nerve fibers that arises within the brain stem and projects into the lower cerebrum; causes arousal of the cerebrum so that the person does not slip into a coma.

Reticulocyte (rĕ-TĬK-ū-lō-sīt) - Immature red blood cell.

Retina (RĔT-ĭ-nă) - Nervous inner layer of the eye; contains the photoreceptors, the rods, and cones.

Rh factor - Type of antigen on the surface of the red blood cell.

Ribonucleic (rī-bō-nū-KLĒ-ĭK) acid (RNA) - Nucleotide that copies or transcribes the genetic code from DNA; also involved in translation.

Ribosomes (RĪ-bō-sōmz) - Organelles that are concerned with the synthesis of protein; ribosomes either are bound to endoplasmic reticulum or are free in the cytoplasm.

Rickettsia (rĭ-KĔT-sē-ă) - Type of small bacteria that must reproduce in a living organism.

Sagittal (SĂJ-ĭ-tl) plane - Vertical plane that divides the organ or body into right and left parts. A midsagittal plane divides the body into right and left halves.

Sarcomere (SĂR-kō-mĭr) - Contractile unit of a muscle extending from Z line to Z line; contains the contractile proteins, actin, and myosin.

Sarcoplasmic reticulum (săr-kō-PLĂZ-mĭK rĕ-TĬK-ū-lŭm) - Calcium-storing endoplasmic reticulum located in muscle.

Sclera (SKLĔ-ră) - Outer layer of the eyeball.

Scrotum - Pouch of skin that encloses the testes.

Sebaceous (sĕ-BĀ-shŭs) gland - Exocrine gland located in the skin that secretes sebum.

Sebum (SĒ-bŭm) - Oily secretion of a sebaceous gland.

Second messenger - Chemical that is activated in response to hormone stimulation, such as cAMP.

Semen - Sperm-containing secretion of the male.

Semilunar valve - Valve shaped like a half-moon located between the ventricles and their attached vessels; pulmonic valve and aortic valve.

Sensory nerves - Collection of sensory neurons that carry information toward the central nervous system.

Serous membrane - Membrane that covers an organ or lines cavities that do not open to the outside; includes the pleurae.

Serum - Blood plasma minus the clotting factors.

Sex-linked trait - Any trait that is carried on a sex chromosome (X or Y chromosome).

Sinus - Cavity such as the paranasal sinuses in the head.

Sinusoid (SĪ-nŭ-soyd) - Large, highly permeable capillary that permits free movement of proteins between the tissue fluid and the blood.

Skeletal muscle - Striated, voluntary muscle that lies over parts of the skeleton; causes movement of the skeleton.

Skin turgor (TŬR-gŏr) - Turgor is a condition of normal tension within a cell. Skin turgor refers to the degree of elasticity of the skin.

Smooth muscle - Nonstriated, involuntary muscle found in tubes and organs.

Solute - A substance that is dissolved in another substance (solvent).

Solution - Mixture in which the particles that are mixed together remain evenly distributed.

Solvent - Substance in which the solute is dissolved or mixed.

Somatic nervous system - Part of the peripheral nervous system that stimulates the skeletal muscles.

Specific gravity - Weight of urine compared with the weight of an equal volume of water.

Spermatogenesis (spĕr-mă-tō-JĔN-ĕ-sĭs) - Formation of sperm.

Sphincter (SFINGK-tĕr) - Circular muscle that opens and closes a tube, such as the anal sphincter.

Spinal cavity - Elongated cavity that contains the spinal cord; the vertebral cavity.

Spinal cord - Part of the central nervous system located in the vertebral canal.

Spinal nerves - Nerve that arises from the spinal cord.

Splanchnic (SPLĂNGK-nĭk) circulation - Blood supply of the abdominal organs of digestion.

Spleen (splēn) - Lymphoid organ located in the left upper quadrant of the abdominal cavity.

Spores - An encasement that allows the organism to withstand harsh environmental conditions.

Squamous (SKWĀ-mŭs) epithelium - Flattened, scalelike epithelial cells; simple or stratified.

Starling's law of the heart - Refers to the relationship between myocardial stretch and the strength of myocardial contraction.

Steroid - Lipid-soluble hormone such as estrogen, testosterone, and cortisol.

Stomach - A digestive organ located between the esophagus and the duodenum.

Stratum corneum (STRĀ-tŭm KŎR-nē-ŭm) - Outermost layer of the epidermis.

Stratum germinativum (STRĀ-tŭm jĕr-mĭ-NĀ-tĭv-ŭm) - Innermost layer of the epidermis where cell division takes place.

Stroke volume - Amount of blood that the ventricle pumps in one beat.

Subcutaneous (sŭb-kū-TĀ-nē-ŭs) layer - Tissue beneath the dermis that contains fat cells.

Sudoriferous (sū-dŏ-RĬF-ĕr-ŭs) gland - Sweat gland.

Surfactant (sŭr-FĂK-tănt) - Chemical substance that reduces surface tension thereby preventing the collapse of alveoli.

Suspension - Mixture in which the large particles gradually settle to the bottom unless continuously shaken or agitated.

Suture (SOO-chŭr) - Type of immovable joint found between the bones of the skull.

Sympathetic nervous system - A division of the autonomic nervous system that causes the "fight or flight" response.

Synapse (SĬN-ăps) - The interaction between two nerves where chemical transmission of the electrical signal occurs.

Synergist (SĬN-ĕr-jĭst) - A muscle that assists or works with another muscle.

Synovial joint (sĭ-NŌ-vē-ăl joint) - Freely movable joint.

Systemic circulation - Part of the circulatory system that serves all parts of the body except the blood vessels that supply the gas-exchanging portions of the lungs.

Systole (SĬS-tō-lē) - Contraction of the myocardium.

Systolic blood pressure - The blood pressure in the large arteries during cardiac contraction (systole); the upper part of a blood pressure reading.

Target tissue - Tissue at which a hormone is aimed.

T cell - Type of lymphocyte that engages in cell-mediated immunity; a T lymphocyte.

Temporal (TĔM-pŏr-ăl) lobe - Lobe of the cerebrum that is responsible for hearing, smelling, speech, and memory.

Tendon - Strong band of connective tissue that anchors muscle to bone.

Teratogen (TĔR-ă-tō-jĕn) - Means "monster-producing"; anything that causes developmental abnormalities in the embryo or fetus, such as the rubella virus, alcohol, or radiation.

Testes (TĔS-tēz) (*s.* testis) - Male gonads that produce sperm and testosterone.

Testosterone (tĕs-TŎS-tĕ-rōn) - Most important androgen (male hormone).

Tetanus - Sustained muscle contraction; also a disease caused by the *Clostridium tetani* pathogen.

Thermoreceptor (THĔR-mō-rĕ-SĔP-tor) - Receptor that detects changes in temperature.

Thermoregulation - Homeostatic regulation of body temperature by adjustments in the heat-producing and heat-losing mechanisms.

Thoracic (thō-RĂS-ĭk) cavity - Upper part of the ventral cavity that is superior to the diaphragm; it is filled largely by the lungs and heart.

Thoracic (thō-RĂS-ĭk) duct - Large lymphatic vessel that receives lymph and empties it into the left subclavian vein.

Thrombocyte (THRŎM-bō-sīt) - See *Platelet.*

Thoracolumbar outflow - Sympathetic nerve activity; "fight or flight."

Thymus gland - Lymphoid organ that plays an important role in immunity.

Thyroid gland - Gland that secretes T_3, T_4 (thyroxine), and calcitonin.

Tidal volume - Amount of air that is inhaled and exhaled during one ventilatory cycle.

Tissue - Group of cells that perform a similar function.

Tonsil - Patches of lymphoid tissue embedded in the throat region.

Tonus (TŌN-ŭs) - The continuous contraction of a muscle.

Toxoid - Inactivated toxin that retains its antigenic properties.

Trachea (TRĀ-kē-ă) - Large airway located between the larynx and the bronchus; windpipe.

Transcellular fluid - Extracellular fluid that includes cerebrospinal fluid, aqueous and vitreous humor, synovial fluid of the joints, serous fluid within body cavities, and exocrine gland secretions (e.g., gastric juice).

Transverse plane - Plane that divides the body into a top (superior) and bottom (inferior) part.

Tricuspid (trī-KŬS-pĭd) valve - Atrioventricular valve found between the right atrium and the right ventricle.

Tubular reabsorption - Movement of water and dissolved substances from the tubules into the peritubular capillaries.

Tubular secretion - Movement of substances from the peritubular capillaries into the tubules.

Turgor - See *Skin turgor.*

Umbilical (ŭm-BĬL-ĭ-kăl) cord - Long structure that connects the fetus to the placenta; contains the umbilical arteries and umbilical vein.

Urea (ū-RĒ-ă) - Nitrogenous waste product formed by the liver and excreted by the kidneys.

Ureter (ū-RĒ-tĕr) - Tube that conducts urine from the kidney to the urinary bladder.

Urethra (ū-RĒ-thră) - Tube that conducts urine from the bladder to the exterior of the body.

Uterus - Hollow reproductive organ in which the fetus grows; the womb.

Vaccine - Antigens that have been altered so as to produce active immunity without causing the disease.

Vascular resistance - The amount of opposition that the blood vessels offer to the flow of blood; most resistance is caused by the arterioles (resistance vessels).

Vas deferens (văs DĔF-ĕr-ĕnz) - Tube that carries sperm from the epididymis to the ejaculatory duct; the ductus deferens.

Vasoconstriction (văz-ō-kŏn-STRĬK-shŭn) - Narrowing of blood vessels; usually refers to arterioles.

Vasodilation (văz-ō-dī-LĀ-shŭn) - Widening of blood vessels; usually refers to arterioles.

Vector - A carrier of pathogens from host to host; mechanical or animal.

Vein - Blood vessel that takes blood toward the heart.

Vena cava (VĒnă KĀ-vă) - Large vein that takes unoxygenated blood to the right atrium; superior and inferior vena cava.

Ventilation - Moving air into and out of the lungs. Two phases: inhalation (breathing in) and exhalation (breathing out).

Ventral cavity - Cavity that is located toward the front part of the body; divided by the diaphragm into the upper thoracic cavity and the lower abdominopelvic cavity.

Ventral root - Attachment of a motor branch of a spinal nerve to the spinal cord.

Ventricle (VĔN-trĭ-k'l) - Cavity in an organ, such as the ventricles in the heart and brain.

Venule (VĔN-ūl) - Tiny vein.

Vernix caseosa (VĔR-nĭks kă-sē-Ō-să) - Cheeselike substance covering the skin of the fetus; secreted by the sebaceous glands.

Vestibule (VĔS-tĭ-būl) - Part of the inner ear that is concerned with equilibrium.

Villi (*s.* villus) - Fingerlike projections such as the villi that line the intestine; function in absorption.

Virus - Pieces of either DNA or RNA surrounded by a protein shell; viruses are parasitic in that they require other living cells for reproduction.

Viscera (VĬS-ĕr-ă) - Internal organs of the body.

Vital capacity - The greatest amount of air that can be exhaled following maximal inhalation.

Vitamin - Organic substance that is necessary for normal metabolism.

White blood cell - See *Leukocyte*.

White matter - Myelinated fibers, mostly axons, that are located in the central nervous system.

Zoonosis (zō-ō-NŌ-sĭs) - A disease that occurs primarily in the wild but can be transmitted from animals to humans.

Zygote (ZĪ-gōt) - Fertilized ovum.

From Chabner D: *The language of medicine,* ed 6, Philadelphia, 2001, WB Saunders.

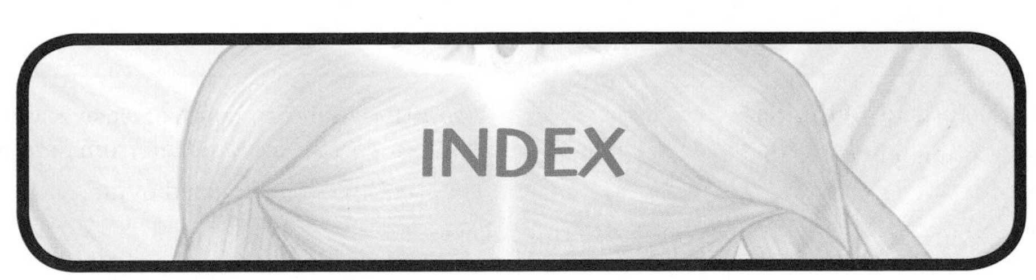

INDEX

Page numbers followed by *b* indicate boxes; *f*, figures; *t*, tables.

C

D

E

I

M

N

O

P

Q

R

T

U

V